The GALE ENCYCLOPEDIA of ALTERNATIVE MEDICINE

SECOND EDITION

The GALE
ENCYCLOPEDIA of
ALTERNATIVE
MEDICINE

SECOND EDITION

VOLUME

4

S-Z
ORGANIZATIONS
GLOSSARY
GENERAL INDEX

JACQUELINE L. LONGE, PROJECT EDITOR

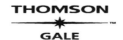

THOMSON
GALE

Detroit • New York • San Francisco • San Diego • New Haven, Conn. • Waterville, Maine • London • Munich

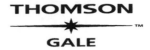

The Gale Encyclopedia of Alternative Medicine, Second Edition

Project Editor
Jacqueline L. Longe

Editorial
Deirdre S. Blanchfield, Laurie Fundukian, Erin Watts

Editorial Support Services
Andrea Lopeman

Rights Acquisition Management
Margaret Abendroth, Ann Taylor

Imaging
Randy Bassett, Lezlie Light, Dan W. Newell, Robyn V. Young

Product Design
Michelle DiMercurio, Tracey Rowens

Composition and Electronic Prepress
Evi Seoud, Mary Beth Trimper

Manufacturing
Wendy Blurton, Dorothy Maki

Indexing
Synapse Corp. of Colorado

LIBRARY OF CONGRESS CATALOGING-IN-PUBLICATION DATA

The Gale encyclopedia of alternative medicine / Jacqueline L. Longe, project editor.-- 2nd ed.
     p. ; cm.
   Includes bibliographical references and index.
   ISBN 0-7876-7424-9 (set hardcover : alk. paper) -- ISBN 0-7876-7425-7 (v. 1 : alk. paper) -- ISBN 0-7876-7426-5 (v. 2 : alk. paper) -- ISBN 0-7876-7427-3 (v. 3 : alk. paper) -- ISBN 0-7876-7428-1 (v. 4 : alk. paper)
   1. Alternative medicine--Encyclopedias.
   [DNLM: 1. Complementary Therapies--Encyclopedias--English. 2. Internal Medicine--Encyclopedias--English. WB 13 G1507 2005] I. Title: Encyclopedia of alternative medicine. II. Longe, Jacqueline L.
   R733.G34 2005
   615.5'03--dc22
                                                         2004022502

This title is also available as an e-book
ISBN 7876-9396-0 (set)
Contact your Gale sales representative for ordering information

ISBN 0-7876-7424-9(set)
0-7876-7425-7 (Vol. 1)
0-7876-7426-5 (Vol. 2)
0-7876-7427-3 (Vol. 3)
0-7876-7428-1 (Vol. 4)

Printed in the United States of America
10 9 8 7 6 5 4 3 2

CONTENTS

LIST OF ENTRIES

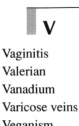

PLEASE READ – IMPORTANT INFORMATION

The Gale Encyclopedia of Alternative Medicine is a medical reference product designed to inform and educate readers about a wide variety of complementary therapies and herbal remedies and treatments for prevalent conditions and diseases. Thomson Gale believes the product to be comprehensive, but not necessarily definitive. It is intended to supplement, not replace, consultation with a physician or other healthcare practitioner. While Thomson Gale has made substantial efforts to provide information that is accurate, comprehensive, and up-to-date, Thomson Gale makes no representations or warranties of any kind, including without limitation, warranties of merchantability or fitness for a particular purpose, nor does it guarantee the accuracy, comprehensiveness, or timeliness of the information contained in this product. Readers should be aware that the universe of complementary medical knowledge is constantly growing and changing, and that differences of medical opinion exist among authorities. They are also advised to seek professional diagnosis and treatment for any medical condition, and to discuss information obtained from this book with their healthcare provider.

ABOUT THE ENCYCLOPEDIA

The Gale Encyclopedia of Alternative Medicine (GEAM) is a one-stop source for alternative medical information that covers complementary therapies, herbs and remedies, and common medical diseases and conditions. It avoids medical jargon, making it easier for the layperson to use. The Gale Encyclopedia of Alternative Medicine presents authoritative, balanced information and is more comprehensive than single-volume family medical guides.

Scope

Over 800 full-length articles are included in The Gale Encyclopedia of Alternative Medicine. Many prominent figures are highlighted as sidebar biographies that accompany the therapy entries. Articles follow a standardized format that provides information at a glance. Rubrics include:

Therapies

- Origins
- Benefits
- Description
- Preparations
- Precautions
- Side effects
- Research & general acceptance
- Resources
- Key terms

Herbs/remedies

- General use
- Preparations
- Precautions
- Side effects
- Interactions
- Resources
- Key terms

Diseases/conditions

- Definition
- Description
- Causes & symptoms
- Diagnosis
- Treatment
- Allopathic treatment
- Expected results
- Prevention
- Resources
- Key terms

Inclusion criteria

A preliminary list of therapies, herbs, remedies, diseases, and conditions was compiled from a wide variety of sources, including professional medical guides and textbooks, as well as consumer guides and encyclopedias. The advisory board, made up of three medical and alternative healthcare experts, evaluated the topics and made suggestions for inclusion. Final selection of topics to include was made by the medical advisors in conjunction with Thomson Gale editors.

About the Contributors

The essays were compiled by experienced medical writers, including alternative healthcare practitioners and educators, pharmacists, nurses, and other complementary healthcare professionals. GEAM medical advisors reviewed over 95% of the completed essays to insure that they are appropriate, up-to-date, and medically accurate.

How to Use this Book

The Gale Encyclopedia of Alternative Medicine has been designed with ready reference in mind:

- Straight **alphabetical arrangement** allows users to locate information quickly.

- Bold faced terms function as *print hyperlinks* that point the reader to related entries in the encyclopedia.

- A list of **key terms** is provided where appropriate to define unfamiliar words or concepts used within the context of the essay. Additional terms may be found in the **glossary**.

- **Cross-references** placed throughout the encyclopedia direct readers to where information on subjects without their own entries can be found. Synonyms are also cross-referenced.

- A **Resources section** directs users to sources of further complementary medical information.

- An appendix of alternative medical organizations is arranged by type of therapy and includes valuable **contact information**.

- A comprehensive **general index** allows users to easily target detailed aspects of any topic, including Latin names.

Graphics

The Gale Encyclopedia of Alternative Medicine is enhanced with over 450 images, including photos, tables, and customized line drawings. Each volume contains a color insert of 64 important herbs, remedies, and supplements.

ADVISORY BOARD

An advisory board made up of prominent individuals from complementary medical communities provided invaluable assistance in the formulation of this encyclopedia. They defined the scope of coverage and reviewed individual entries for accuracy and accessibility. We would therefore like to express our appreciation to them:

Mirka Knaster, PhD
author, editor, consultant in Eastern and Western body-mind disciplines and spiritual traditions
Oakland, CA

Lisa Meserole, MS, ND
President, Botanical Medicine Academy
One Sky Medicine Clinic
Seattle, WA

Katherine E. Nelson, ND
Naturopathic Physician
Naples, FL

Jamison Starbuck, JD, ND
Naturopathic Family Physician
Former president, American Association of Naturopathic Physicians
Member, Homeopathic Academy of Naturopathic Physicians
Missoula, MT

CONTRIBUTORS

Margaret Alic, PhD
Medical Writer
Eastsound, WA

Greg Annussek
Medical Writer
American Society of Journalists and Authors
New York, NY

Barbara Boughton
Health and Medical Writer
El Cerrito, CA

Ruth Ann Prag Carter
Freelance Writer
Farmington Hills, MI

Linda Chrisman
Massage Therapist and Educator
Medical Writer
Oakland, CA

Gloria Cooksey, CNE
Medical Writer
Sacramento, CA

Amy Cooper, MA, MSI
Medical Writer
Vermillion, SD

Sharon Crawford
Writer, Editor, Researcher
American Medical Writers Association
Periodical Writers Association of Canada and the Editors'
    Association of Canada
Toronto, ONT Canada

Sandra Bain Cushman
Massage Therapist
Alexander Technique Practitioner and Educator
Charlottesville, VA

Tish Davidson, MA
Medical Writer
Fremont, CA

Lori DeMilto, MJ
Medical Writer
Sicklerville, NJ

Doug Dupler, MA
Medical Writer
Boulder, CO

Paula Ford-Martin, PhD
Medical Writer
Warwick, RI

Rebecca J. Frey, PhD
Medical Writer
New Haven, CT

Lisa Frick
Medical Writer
Columbia, MO

Kathleen Goss
Medical Writer
Darwin, CA

Elliot Greene, MA
former president, American Massage Therapy Association
Massage Therapist
Silver Spring, MD

Peter Gregutt
Medical Writer
Asheville, NC

Clare Hanrahan
Medical Writer
Asheville, NC

David Helwig
Medical Writer
London, ONT Canada

Beth A. Kapes
Medical Writer, Editor
Bay Village, OH

Katherine Kim
Medical Writer
Oakland, CA

Erika Lenz
Medical Writer
Lafayette, CO

Lorraine Lica, PhD
Medical Writer
San Diego, CA

Contributors

Whitney Lowe, LMT
Orthopedic Massage Education & Research Institute
Massage Therapy Educator
Bend, OR

Mary McNulty
Freelance Writer
St.Charles, IL

Katherine E. Nelson, ND
Naturopathic physician
Naples, FL

Teresa Odle
Medical Writer
Ute Park, NM

Jodi Ohlsen Read
Medical Writer
Carver, MN

Carole Osborne-Sheets
Massage Therapist and Educator
Medical Writer
Poway, CA

Lee Ann Paradise
Freelance Writer
Lubbock, TX

Patience Paradox
Medical Writer
Bainbridge Island, WA

Belinda Rowland, PhD
Medical Writer
Voorheesville, NY

Joan M. Schonbeck, RN
Medical Writer
Marlborough, MA

Gabriele Schubert, MS
Medical Writer
San Diego, CA

Kim Sharp, M Ln
Medical Writer
Houston, TX

Kathy Shepard Stolley, PhD
Medical Writer
Virginia Beach, VA

Judith Sims, MS
Science Writer
Logan, UT

Patricia Skinner
Medical Writer
Amman, Jordan

Genevieve Slomski, PhD
Medical Writer
New Britain, CT

Jane E. Spear
Medical Writer
Canton, OH

Liz Swain
Medical Writer
San Diego, CA

Judith Turner, DVM
Medical Writer
Sandy, UT

Samuel Uretsky, PharmD
Medical Writer
Wantagh, NY

Ken R. Wells
Science Writer
Laguna Hills, CA

Angela Woodward
Science Writer
Madison, WI

Kathleen Wright, RN
Medical Writer
Delmar, DE

Jennifer L. Wurges
Medical Writer
Rochester Hills, MI

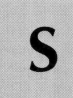

S

Sacro-occipital technique *see* **Craniosacral therapy**

SAD *see* **Seasonal affective disorder**

Safflower flower

Description

Safflower is an annual herb whose botanical name is *Carthamus tinctorius*. It is a member of the Asteraceae family. It has long, spiny leaves and yellow or reddish flowers on a stiff, upright stem. The seeds produce an edible oil. Safflower grows to a height of about 3 ft (1 m) in poor, dry soils in full sun. The origins of this plant are not clear, although some herbalists suggest the basin of the Euphrates River. Today safflower grows wild in Iran, northwest India, and North Africa. It has also spread to the Far East and North America. Safflower is cultivated extensively both as a herb and as a food crop.

Other names for safflower include false **saffron**, dyer's saffron, American saffron, bastard saffron, Mexican saffron, and zaffer. Despite these names, safflower is in no way related to true saffron, although it is sometimes used to adulterate that spice because true saffron is very expensive and safflower is relatively cheap. In Chinese medicine, safflower flower is called *hong hua*; in India it is known as *koosumbha*.

General use

Safflower flower has been used in **traditional Chinese medicine** for thousands of years. It is used to treat menstrual disorders. Safflower flower is an emmenagogue, meaning that it is given to bring on **menstruation**. Safflower is also used to treat menstrual **pain**, to firm up the uterus after **childbirth**, to ease stiffness and pain in the joints, and sometimes also to treat trauma to the abdomen. According to traditional Chinese usage,

safflower flower is a blood regulator; that is, it invigorates and harmonizes the blood and dissolves **blood clots**. Safflower is said to have a warm nature and a pungent taste. Chinese practitioners use safflower oil in *tui na* massage.

Safflower flowers are also used to treat such childhood problems as **measles**, fevers, and skin **rashes**. Applied externally, safflower flower is used to cleanse **wounds** . Interestingly, on the other side of the world, North Americans used safflower flower in the nineteenth century in much the same way as the Chinese—to bring on menstruation and to treat **measles**. They also used it to induce sweating.

Safflower seeds can be pressed to produce an edible oil. The unpurified form of this oil is used as a laxative or purgative to cleanse the bowels. Processed safflower oil does not have laxative properties. The processed oil is used extensively in cooking and for making margarine and salad dressings. The oil is also used in paints and varnishes, and is burned for lighting where electricity is unavailable.

Safflower has other nonmedicinal uses. Its flowers produce a dye that in times past was used for dyeing silk yellow or red. Today, chemical dyes have largely replaced safflower dye. The flowers were also dried and ground together with finely powdered talc to produce cosmetic rouge.

Modern scientific research shows that safflower oil lowers serum **cholesterol** levels, making it useful in preventing **heart disease**. The claim has also been made that safflower flowers prevent coronary artery disease because they are a digestive bitter and assist in the digestion of oils. Infusions of safflower flowers are used to lower the accumulation of lactic acid in the muscles during athletic competition. In addition, a compound has been isolated from safflower that stimulates the immune system in mice. Additional studies are ongoing to confirm this effect.

More recently, safflower has been identified as the source of several flavonoids with strong antioxidative ac-

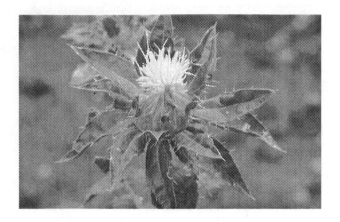

Safflower plant. (© PlantaPhile, Germany. Reproduced by permission.)

tivity. Flavonoids are water-soluble plant pigments that help to lower inflammation as well as counteract the damaging effects of oxidation on body tissues. Quercetin, which is one of the flavonoids found in safflower, is a well-known antioxidant.

As of 2002, several groups of Asian researchers are studying the effectiveness of traditional herbal medicines containing safflower extract in treating bone disease. Although these studies are still in their early stages, preliminary findings indicate that safflower extract inhibits bone resorption and thus may be useful in treating diseases involving bone loss.

Many other medicinal claims have been made for safflower that are less well documented by modern scientists. These include claims that it reduces pain; has antibacterial action; reduces **fever**; reduces enlarged breasts; and can be used to purge the body of parasitic **worms**.

Preparations

Harvesting safflower flowers requires some care. The flowers are picked just as they begin to wilt and can be used fresh or dried. If they are to be dried, they must be kept away from sunlight during the drying process or they will lose their distinctive reddish-yellow color. Dried flowers are not normally kept more than one year.

Safflower flowers can be used alone or in formulas. They can be prepared as dried powder, tinctures, or decoctions. Used alone, a common daily dosage is 3 g of decoction or 1 g of powder. A standard infusion of safflower flowers uses 4–8 oz of dried flowers. A common Chinese formula that uses safflower flower is pseudoginseng and dragon blood formula. This formula is used to treat traumatic injuries such as sprains or **fractures** that are accompanied by pain and swelling. The role of the safflower flower in this formula is to move congealed blood and reduce pain.

KEY TERMS

Antioxidant—An enzyme or other organic substance that is able to counteract the damaging effects of oxidation in living tissue.

Decoction—An extract of a plant's flavor or essence made by boiling or simmering parts of the plant in water.

Emmenagogue—A substance or medication that brings on a woman's menstrual period. Safflower flowers have been used as an emmenagogue.

Flavonoid—Any of a group of water-soluble plant pigments that are thought to have antioxidative, anti-inflammatory, and antiviral properties.

Quercetin—An important flavonoid found in safflower that has strong anti-inflammatory and antioxidative activity.

Resorption—The breakdown or dissolving of bone tissue by biochemical processes in the body.

Precautions

Because safflower flower brings on menstruation, it should not be used by pregnant women. Large doses can cause spontaneous abortion. In addition, because safflower may prolong blood clotting time, it should not be given to patients with peptic ulcers or hemorrhagic illnesses.

Side effects

The unprocessed oil of safflower seed can cause severe **diarrhea**.

Interactions

Safflower flower is often used in conjunction with other Chinese herbs with no reported interactions. As of 2002, there are no reported interactions of safflower extract or oil with standard pharmaceuticals. Its use in dissolving clots, however, suggests that it should not be taken with allopathic medications given to thin the blood.

Resources

BOOKS

Chevallier, Andrew. *Encyclopedia of Medicinal Plants.* London, UK: Dorling Kindersley Publishers, 1996.

Molony, David. *Complete Guide to Chinese Herbal Medicine.* New York: Berkeley Books, 1998.

Reid, Daniel. *Chinese Herbal Medicine.* Boston, MA: Shambhala, 1996.

PERIODICALS

Hong, H. T., H. J. Kim, T. K. Lee, et al. "Inhibitory Effect of a Korean Traditional Medicine, Honghwain-Jahage (Water

Extracts of *Carthamus tinctorius L.* seed and Hominis Placenta) on Interleukin-1-Mediated Bone Resorption." *Journal of Ethnopharmacology* 79 (February 2002): 143-148.

Lee, J. Y., E. J. Chang, H. J. Kim, et al. "Antioxidative Flavonoids from Leaves of *Carthamus tinctorius.*" *Archives of Pharmacal Research* 25 (June 2002): 313-319.

Yuk, T. H., J. H. Kang, S. R. Lee, et al. "Inhibitory Effect of *Carthamus tinctorius L.* Seed Extracts on Bone Resorption Mediated by Tyrosine Kinase, COX-2 (Cyclooxygenase) and PG (Prostaglandin) E2." *American Journal of Chinese Medicine* 30 (2002): 95-108.

ORGANIZATIONS

American Association of Oriental Medicine (AAOM). 909 22nd Street, Sacramento, CA 95816, (916) 451-6950 <http://www.aaom.org>.

Centre for International Ethnomedicinal Education and Research (CIEER). <www.cieer.org>.

OTHER

Herbal Dave. http://www.herbaldave.com.

Tish Davidson
Rebecca J. Frey, PhD

Saffron

Description

Saffron is a herbal preparation harvested from the stigma of the *Crocus sativus* flower. It is dark orange and threadlike in appearance, with a spicy flavor and pungent odor. The plant is grown in India, Spain, France, Italy, the Middle East, and the eastern Mediterranean region.

General use

In addition to its culinary uses, saffron is prescribed as a herbal remedy to stimulate the digestive system, ease **colic** and stomach discomfort, and minimize **gas**. It is also used as an emmenagogue, to stimulate and promote menstrual flow in women.

Preliminary studies have shown that saffron may also be a useful tool in fighting **cancer**. According to a 1999 study, use of the herb slowed tumor growth and extended lifespan in female rats. A 2002 study done at Indiana University indicates that saffron may not only be effective in treating certain types of cancer, but significantly less likely to cause birth defects if given to pregnant women than all-trans-retinoic acid (ATRA), the compound most often given to treat these cancers. Saffron may thus be a preferable alternative

to treating ATRA-sensitive cancers in women of child-bearing age.

Additional human studies have indicated that saffron has powerful antioxidant properties; that is, it helps to protect living tissues from free radicals and other harmful effects of oxidation.

Two chemical components of saffron extract, crocetin and crocin, reportedly improved memory and learning skills in learning-impaired rats in a Japanese study published in early 2000. These properties indicate that saffron extract may be a useful treatment for neurodegenerative disorders and related memory impairment.

Preparations

Saffron is harvested by drying the orange stigma of the *Crocus sativus* flower over fire. Over 200,000 crocus stigmas must be harvested to produce one pound of saffron. This volume makes the herb extremely expensive, and it is often cut with other substances of a similar color (e.g., marigold) to keep the price down.

Because saffron is frequently used as a spice to flavor a variety of dishes, particularly in Mediterranean recipes, it can often be purchased by mail order and at gourmet food stores as well as at health food stores. The herb is usually sold in either powdered form or in its original threadlike stigma form. Saffron can cost as much to $10.00 per gram.

For medicinal purposes, saffron can be taken by mouth in powder, tincture, or liquid form. To make a liquid saffron decoction, mix 6–10 stigmas or strands of saffron in one cup of cold water, bring the mixture to a boil, and then let it simmer. The saffron is then strained out of the decoction, which can be drunk either hot or cold. An average recommended dose of saffron decoction is 1/2–1 cup daily.

Saffron should be stored in an airtight container in a cool location away from bright light to maintain its potency. The herb can be frozen. Properly stored saffron can be used for up to two years. A good measure of the herb's freshness and potency is its odor. If the saffron does not have a noticeable pungent smell, it is probably past its peak.

Precautions

Because saffron can stimulate uterine contractions, pregnant women should never take the herb for medicinal purposes.

Saffron should always be obtained from a reputable source that observes stringent quality control procedures and industry-accepted good manufacturing practices. Be-

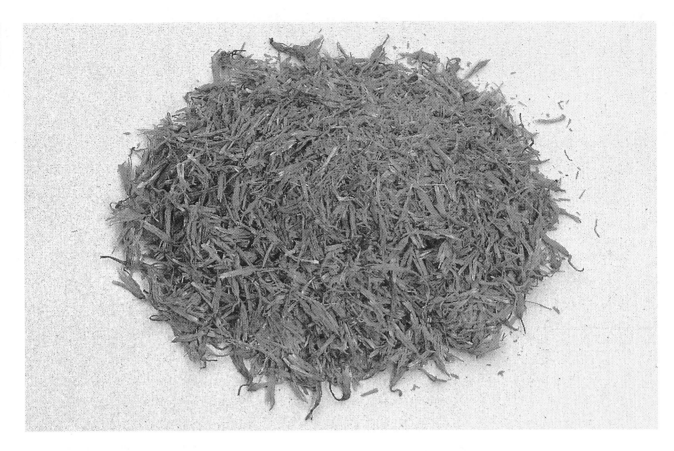

Saffron. *(© PlantaPhile, Germany. Reproduced by permission.)*

cause of its high cost, saffron is often found in adulterated form, so package labeling should be checked carefully for the type and quality of additional ingredients.

Botanical supplements are regulated by the FDA; however, they are currently not required to undergo any approval process before reaching the consumer market, and are classified as nutritional supplements rather than drugs. Legislation known as the Dietary Supplement Health and Education Act (DSHEA) was passed in 1994 in an effort to standardize the manufacture, labeling, composition, and safety of botanicals and supplements. In January 2000, the FDA's Center for Food Safety and Applied Nutrition (CFSAN) announced a ten-year plan for establishing and implementing these regulations by the year 2010.

Side effects

Although there are no known side effects or health hazards associated with recommended dosages of saffron preparations in healthy individuals, people with chronic medical conditions should consult with their healthcare professional before taking the herb. In addition, pregnant women should never take saffron, as the herb stimulates uterine contractions and may cause miscarriage.

Saffron can cause severe illness, kidney damage, central nervous system paralysis, and possible death at dosages of 12 g and higher. The symptoms of saffron poisoning include:

- vomiting
- uterine bleeding
- intestinal cramping
- bloody diarrhea
- skin hemorrhaging
- dizziness
- stupor
- paralysis

If any of these symptoms occur, the user discontinue the use of saffron immediately and seek emergency medical assistance.

Interactions

As of 2002, there are no reported negative interactions between saffron and other medications and herbs, although certain drugs with the same therapeutic properties as saffron may enhance the effect of the herb.

KEY TERMS

Antioxidants—Enzymes that bind with free radicals to neutralize their harmful effects.

Crocetin—A reddish-yellow plant pigment found in saffron that is being studied for its anticancer effectiveness.

Decoction—A herbal extract produced by mixing a herb with cold water, bringing the mixture to a boil, and letting it simmer to evaporate the excess water. Decoctions are usually chosen over infusion when the botanical or herb in question is a root, seed, or berry.

Emmenagogue—A medication or substance given to bring on a woman's menstrual period.

Free radicals—Reactive molecules created during cell metabolism that can cause tissue and cell damage like that which occurs in aging and with such disease processes as cancer.

Stigma—The thread-like filament found in the center of a flower where pollen collects.

Tincture—A liquid extract of a herb prepared by steeping the herb in an alcohol and water mixture.

Resources

BOOKS

Hoffman, David. *The Complete Illustrated Herbal.* New York: Barnes & Noble Books, 1999.

Medical Economics Corporation. *The PDR for Herbal Medicines.* Montvale, NJ: Medical Economics Corporation, 1998.

PERIODICALS

Martin, G., E. Goh, and A. W. Neff. "Evaluation of the Developmental Toxicity of Crocetin on *Xenopus.*" *Food and Chemical Toxicology* 40 (July 2002): 959-964.

ORGANIZATIONS

Office of Dietary Supplements. National Institutes of Health. Building 31, Room 1B25. 31 Center Drive, MSC 2086. Bethesda, MD 20892-2086. (301) 435-2920. Fax: (301) 480-1845. http://odp.od.nih.gov/ods/

United States Food and Drug Administration (FDA), Center for Food Safety and Applied Nutrition. 5100 Paint Branch Parkway, College Park, MD 20740. (888) SAFEFOOD. <www.cfsan.fda.gov>.

Paula Ford-Martin
Rebecca J. Frey, PhD

Sage

Description

Sage (*Salvia officinalis*) is native to the Mediterranean and naturalized throughout Europe and North America. Known as garden sage, meadow sage, and true sage, this pungent herb is a member of the Lamiaceae, or mint, family. The genus name is taken from the Latin *salvare* meaning "to save." The specific name *officinalis* indicates that sage was included on official lists of medicinal herbs. There are numerous species of sage, including clary sage (*S. sclarea*) named because of its traditional use as an eyewash. Native Americans used the roots and leaves of lyre-leafed sage (*S. lyrata L.*), also known as cancerweed, as a salve for sores and in a tea to treat colds and coughs. Another species, known as divine sage (*S. divinorum*), a native of Oaxaca, Mexico, has been used for centuries by local shamans to achieve altered states of consciousness in healing rituals. There are many more garden varieties, including red or purple sage (*S. officinalis purpurascens*), which is valued particularly for its medicinal purposes.

Sage thrives in full sun and well-drained soils, growing wild in some areas. It is a hardy evergreen shrub with a deep taproot and an erect root stalk that produces woody, square, slightly downy, branching stems that may reach a height of 4 ft (1.2 m). This familiar garden perennial has long, light-green leaf stalks that bear simple opposite lance- or oval-shaped leaves. The strong and pliable leaves are veined, with a velvet-like somewhat crinkled texture and may grow to 2 in (5.1 cm) long in some varieties. Leaf margins resemble a fine embroidery finish with rounded minutely toothed edges. They are a gray-green on the top and lighter on the underside. The entire plant is strongly aromatic, with a familiar pungency. Fresh leaves are bitter to the taste. Sage blossoms in the middle of summer with small white, blue, or purple flowers.

General use

Sage is a celebrated herb long valued for its many uses in medicine, magic, and meal preparation. Poets, shamans, herbalists, cooks, emperors, and common folk have touted its virtues for thousands of years. The Romans revered the herb as a sacred plant, and the Egyptians used it to treat the plague. Nicholas Culpeper, the seventeenth-century herbalist and astrologer, believed sage was under the dominion of Jupiter. Folk belief placed the herb under the influence of Venus, and sage was traditionally used to aid conception. One folk tradition encouraged eating a bit of sage each day during the month of May to assure immortality. Although it failed to live up to this promise, sage was traditionally planted on graves.

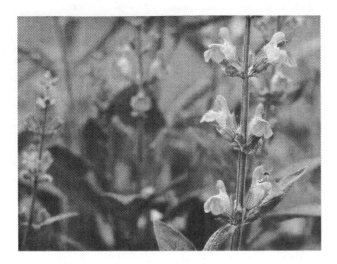

Sage plant in Michigan. *(Photograph by Robert J. Huffman/Field Mark Publications. Reproduced by permission.)*

Sage's main constituents include volatile oil, diterpene **bitters**, thujone, camphor, tannins, triterpenoids, resin, flavonoids, estrogenic substances, phenolic acids, including rosmarinic and caffeic acids, and saponins. It acts as a carminative, antiperspirant, antispasmodic, astringent, antiseptic, and antibiotic. More recently, sage has been discovered to have antiallergic effects.

Sage has been used as a general tonic. It is the preferred beverage tea in many cultures, particularly in China, where the root of the species *S. miltiorrhiza*, known as *dan shen*, is used for its soothing and healing qualities. Sage has antioxidant properties that have recently been used by the food industry to improve the stability of oils that must be kept in storage for long periods of time.

Sage is also high in **calcium**. It provides **potassium**, **magnesium**, and **zinc** as well as vitamins C and B-complex. Sage is calming to the central nervous system and may reduce **anxiety**. It can soothe spasms in smooth and skeletal muscles. Sage is a bitter digestive stimulant and acts to relieve digestive problems. The herb also contains estrogenic substances that help to regulate **menstruation**.

Taken cold, the tea is astringent and diuretic, and will help to reduce night sweats in menopausal women and reduce milk flow in breast-feeding mothers. Taken hot, a sage infusion acts as an expectorant and is good for common colds and flu. A strong infusion of sage used as a hair rinse may darken hair color and help reduce **hair loss**. The antibacterial properties in sage make it a useful mouthwash for gingivitis and an antiseptic **sore throat** gargle. Sage is still listed in the *United States Pharmacopoeia* as a treatment for bleeding gums and sore throats. A tea made from the leaves may be used as an antiseptic wash for **wounds** and sores. Crushed leaves may be applied to relieve insect bites. The powdered herb, added to toothpaste and powders, helps to whiten teeth.

Some research indicates that sage may boost insulin action and be helpful to treat non-insulin dependent diabetes. The herb may reduce blood sugar levels and promote bile flow. Among its many virtues, sage is said to improve memory and bring prosperity to the household. Dried sage, burned as a smudge, is used in Native American rituals as a purifying and cleansing herb believed to promote healing, wisdom, protection, and longevity.

Preparations

The leaf is the medicinal part of the herb. Both fresh and dried leaves may be used for medicinal or culinary purposes. The leaves are harvested when the herb begins to flower in the summer of its second year. The leaves are removed from the woody branches and spread in a single layer on a tray or screen in a warm, airy, and shady place. Exposure to direct sunlight during the drying process will result in a significant loss of the volatile oil. Dried leaves are stored in a dark, airtight container.

To make an infusion, 1 pint of nonchlorinated water that has just reached the boiling point is poured over 2–3 tsp of dried or fresh sage leaves in a glass container. The mixture is covered and steeped for 10–15 minutes. This liquid can be drunk warm or cold, up to 3 cups daily, or used as a gargle or hair rinse.

Tinctures of sage are available commercially. A standard dose is 16–40 drops, taken up to three times daily.

To make a sage compress, a clean cotton cloth is soaked in an infusion of sage leaves and then applied to wounds or sores to aid healing.

Precautions

Sage preparations in medicinal doses should not be used during **pregnancy**, although use of small amounts of sage for culinary purposes is safe. Breast-feeding women should avoid sage unless they are using the herb to reduce the flow of breast milk when weaning. People with **epilepsy** should not use sage due to the thujone content in the herb. Thujone may trigger convulsions in these people, and the essential oil contains as much as 25% thujone. The **essential oils** may accumulate in the system, so long-term use of essential oils (more than two weeks at a time) should be avoided. Those allergic to sage or other plants in the mint family should avoid this herb.

KEY TERMS

Antioxidant—Any one of a group of substances that destroy cell-damaging free radicals in the body.

Carminative—A Preparation that prevents the formation of intestinal gas or allows it to be expelled.

Thujone—A natural chemical compound found in sage as well as in wormwood and certain other spices. Thujone in large quantities can cause hallucinations and convulsions.

Tonic—A preparation or medicine that invigorates, strengthens, or restores tone to body tissues.

Side effects

There are no adverse side effects when sage is taken in designated therapeutic doses. However, sage may interfere with absorption of **iron** and other minerals

Interactions

As of 2002, no interactions have been reported between sage and standard prescription medications.

Resources

BOOKS

The Herbal Healer, Prevention Health Library. Emmaus, PA: Rodale Press, Inc., 1998.

McIntyre, Anne. *The Medicinal Garden.* New York: Henry Holt and Company, 1997.

PDR for Herbal Medicines. Montvale, NJ: Medical Economics Company, 1998.

Prevention's 200 Herbal Remedies, 3rd edition. Emmaus, PA: Rodale Press, Inc., 1997.

Reid, Daniel. *Chinese Herbal Medicine.* Boston, MA: Shambhala, 1996.

PERIODICALS

Miura, K., H. Kikuzaki, and N. Nakatani. "Antioxidant Activity of Chemical Components from Sage (*Salvia officinalis L.*) and thyme (*Thymus vulgaris L.*) Measured by the Oil Stability Index Method." *Journal of Agricultural and Food Chemistry* 50 (March 27, 2002): 1845-1851.

Shi, T. Y., and H. M. Kim. "Inhibition of Immediate-Type Allergic Reactions by the Aqueous Extract of *Salvia plebeia*." *Immunopharmacology and Immunotoxicology* 24 (May 2002): 303-314.

Zainuddin, A., J. Pokorny, and R. Venskutonis. "Antioxidant Activity of Sweetgrass (*Hierochloe odorata Wahlnb.*) Extract in Lard and Rapeseed Oil Emulsions." *Nahrung* 46 (February 2002): 15-17.

ORGANIZATIONS

United States Pharmacopoeia (USP). 12601 Twinbrook Parkway, Rockville, MD 20852. (800) 822-8772. <www. usp.org>.

OTHER

"1001 Herbs for a Healthy Life." <www.herb.com>.

Clare Hanrahan
Rebecca J. Frey, PhD

Saliva sample testing

Definition

Saliva sample testing is a technique used to collect samples of a person's saliva, or spit, to check for or monitor certain drugs, hormones (chemical messengers from one cell or group of cells to another), antibodies (substances in the body's blood or fluids that act against such foreign substances as bacteria), and other molecules present in the body. With a saliva sample, diagnostic data for such diseases or conditions as human immunodeficiency virus (HIV), hypogonadism (reduced or absent secretion of hormones from the sex glands, the gonads), **measles**, **hepatitis** (a liver disease caused by the hepatitis A virus), certain cancers, low fertility, **menopause** and others are available without having to draw a person's blood. Saliva can reveal use of alcohol and many drugs. With simple use-at-home kits, women can self-determine when they are ovulating, which is especially useful when trying to conceive a child. Researchers also have found they can detect **stress** in a person through saliva samples.

Origins

In ancient times, saliva served as "judge and jury" when a person was accused of a wrong-doing. The suspect was given a mouthful of dry rice; and if his **anxiety** reduced saliva flow to the point that he could not swallow the rice, he was considered guilty as charged. To this day, a **dry mouth** signals nervousness. Spittoons were common in history until it was discovered that saliva carries germs.

Scientists began to realize that along with germs, saliva carries clues about our bodies. Saliva contains important enzymes (organic substances that accelerate chemical changes) that help digest food, and this natural body fluid serves as an antimicrobial, fighting viruses and diseases that enter our bodies. Additional properties in saliva help fight off bacteria.

In the twentieth century, researchers learned that saliva reveals to the presence of diseases and conditions that once were monitored only by measuring blood, urine, or other fluids. For example, a Spanish gynecologist named Biel Cassals, M.D., noticed in 1969 that saliva would "fern," or crystallize during hormonal changes, almost identically to the changes observable in cervical mucus. These changes in cervical mucus have helped predict when a woman is about to ovulate. Further studies of salivary ferning through the 1990s showed that saliva also could also help predict ovulation (when an egg is released from an ovary in response to a hormonal signal) with a high degree of accuracy. By the twentieth-first century, at-home kits using saliva to help women trying to conceive children were introduced and marketed.

Since the 1980s, some nutritional practitioners have used saliva samples to measure certain imbalances and disease processes in order to determine a person's need for a nutritional plan and dietary supplements. In addition to hormones related to ovulation, some physicians and other practitioners have measured other hormone levels in saliva, including testosterone, cortisol, and **melatonin**. Melatonin levels are much higher at night than in the daytime. Sometimes supplements are suggested for people who have trouble sleeping.

By 2004, more and more uses for saliva sample testing were in experimental stages or being approved by the U.S. Food and Drug Administration (FDA). In fact, saliva research has led to many important discoveries. Saliva holds a complete imprint of a person's DNA, or genetic makeup. In effect, saliva once again serves as judge and jury, since a crime laboratory can determine who committed a crime, based on the saliva left after licking an envelope seal, for example. Saliva tests are increasingly being used to test people for the presence of drugs and alcohol and may one day be used to test them immediately after being pulled over or at police checkpoints.

Benefits

Such laboratory tests as saliva sample tests are used to help a person detect a disease or other condition. Saliva sample testing is particularly beneficial because it is less invasive or noninvasive. Noninvasive means the skin does not have to be broken or an organ or cavity of that the body entered. As a result, test results may be more accurate in that less stress on the system during the production of the specimen means less interference with the factors being tested. In some cases, a swab is put in the mouth to collect the saliva or sufficient quantities of saliva, are gathered by spitting for several minutes into a collecting tube, but studies have shown that many patients prefer this collection method to being pricked in the arm or finger with a needle. Health care workers say saliva samples are much easier to obtain, especially from children.

Saliva sample tests offer other benefits as well, depending on the specific test and its use. The saliva test for HIV provides results in about 20 minutes while the person waits at the testing facility. In the past, people having HIV tests had to wait for days or weeks to learn results and often did not return. Another major benefit of oral HIV tests is that they can reduce transmission of HIV to healthcare workers, who once had to worry about accidentally pricking themselves with the needle they had used to test an HIV-infected patient. Those who test for HIV with saliva kits will not have to worry about handling blood. No cases of HIV transmission through saliva have been documented. The HIV sample test's noninvasive nature and rapid results may even lead to increased screening, especially among young people. The ease and rapid results could make the test valuable in Africa and other countries with widespread need for testing.

Finding less invasive methods to test for a number of diseases is a benefit for many people. Research has been done on a saliva test to detect a person's immune response to the anthrax vaccine, in the event of a bioterror attack, which would help emergency workers rapidly determine who has been immunized and who has not without having to gain access to their medical records.

At-home kits that use saliva instead of urine to help determine ovulation have made it more convenient for women trying to conceive children to track their hormonal cycles, eliminating a lot of guesswork. Instead of simply predicting ovulation, the new saliva-based tests more precisely indicate the timing of ovulation. They also allow women to save results from previous months and compare cycles to determine patterns. The tests are reportedly accurate up to 98% for timing of ovulation.

Saliva sampling is also a more accurate way of measuring a woman's hormone levels, pre-, peri-, and post-menopause, for fertility studies and hormone replacement therapy. The reproductive hormones of estrogen and progesterone weave a complex pattern throughout the length of a woman's cycle. For women who are still menstroating, a blood test for hormone levels reveals only a single snapshot of this very complex pattern, whereas the saliva sampling, done throughout the cycle, reveals the relationships and balance of the hormones. For women who are no longer menstruating, saliva sampling is able to quantify and qualify the amounts and rates of hormone level changes, and may reveal that a woman's symptoms, for example, are a result of low progesterone rather than low estrogen. Saliva sampling may be used as a very effective diagnostic tool in helping a woman balance her hormone levels, thereby guiding the **aging** process to a more fluid, and graceful adjustment over time.

Description

In most cases, the saliva sample test works by using a plastic stick with a pad on the end to swab or rub against the patient's gums to gather saliva. Other tests work by simply inserting a foam pad on a stick into the person's mouth, having the person pucker his or her lips, and moving the pad slightly around for a period of time until enough saliva fluid has been gathered. Still others rely on asking the patient to spit directly into a collecting container.

The collected saliva then is exposed to a reagent, a chemical substance that is known to react a certain way, to indicate a positive result or measures ranges. For instance, the pad from an HIV saliva collection is put in a vial of reagent solution. Within 20 minutes, certain colored lines may appear, indicating a positive result. Other samples may be collected at home, mailed to a laboratory, and may take longer to be analyzed and reported back.

Women who test at home for ovulation will place a drop of saliva onto the device, let it dry and look through a dial that magnifies and lights up the sample for about 45 seconds.

Preparation

Preparation may depend on the use of the test. It is best to follow any instructions given by laboratory personnel or on a home test kit package. For some saliva tests, it is recommended that the person have nothing in his or her mouth for at least five minutes before sample collection. Certain foods may need to be avoided for a period of time prior to testing. These foods are indicated in the instructions. One such set of instructions advises the avoidance of eating, drinking and brushing the teeth for a minimum of 60 minutes prior to collection. If sublingual (under the tongue) hormone drops are being used, a person will need to wait until after collecting the saliva before taking the drops. Saliva sampling may not be accurate or useful if a person has gingivitis, or **gum disease**.

Precautions

If a person has a condition such as **Sjögren's syndrome**, which causes dry mouth and poor saliva production, he or she may not be a candidate for saliva sample testing. Certain medications also can cause a dry mouth.

When using at-home ovulation saliva test kits, women must remember not to use them to help prevent **pregnancy**. The kits are not designed for that purpose. **Smoking**, eating, drinking, and brushing the teeth can affect test results, as can the way in which the person puts saliva on the slide. Further, any home test kit is not intended or recommended to take the place of periodic visits to a physician or other health professional.

Some medical professionals involved in HIV prevention have expressed concerns about saliva sampling for HIV, including an unintended effect of making the general population wrongly believe that HIV can be spread through saliva. Others have been concerned that the ease of saliva testing could lead to abuses, with authorities testing without first obtaining the person's consent.

Caution should be used when having saliva sample tests for nutritional measurements. It is best to check with a registered alternative medicine practitioner or licensed physician before paying for at-home saliva tests for this purpose. Some saliva sample tests will be completed at medical offices or sent to laboratory facilities. Those done at home should be completed with kits approved by the FDA or by a professional healthcare provider.

Side effects

There are no known side effects to saliva sample testing.

Research & general acceptance

In March 2004, the FDA approved saliva sample testing for HIV. Home-based test kits have been approved by the FDA for use in determining ovulation. Many other tests were under constant experimentation or in the approval process throughout the early twenty-first century. Manufacturers must go through an exhaustive process of clinical trials and application with the FDA before marketing these types of products to the public.

Training & certification

The Clinical Laboratory Improvement Amendments (CLIA) passed by Congress in 1988 and finalized in 1992, regulate clinical laboratories in the United States, including education and training of laboratory personnel. Generally, test samples are processed by medical laboratory technicians (MLTs) or clinical laboratory technicians (CLTs). They usually have an associate degree and have completed an accredited program for technicians. The technicians are supervised by other laboratory professionals with more advanced scientific training. Technologists with special training reviewing results under microscopes or preparing tissue samples to diagnose disease also will handle a sample, depending on the type of test involved. A laboratory director oversees the operation. He or she usually is a physician (an M.D. or, as allowed in some states, an N.D.) or scientist holding a doctorate (Ph.D.) with training in interpreting disease via cell samples. Often, the physician is a board-certified pathologist.

Resources

PERIODICALS

Berger, Abi. "Saliva Test Could Diagnose Cancers." *British Medical Journal* (March 25, 2000): 825.

KEY TERMS

Cervical—Having to do with the lower part of the uterus (womb), which reaches into the vagina and leads to the outside of the body.

Cortisol—A hormone related to performance and stress levels, detectable in saliva.

Melatonin—A hormone, detectable in saliva, sometimes called "the chemical equivalent of night" that is involved in regulating sleeping and waking cycles or the complex rhythms related to light and dark, the seasons of the year, and fertility.

N.D. or Doctor of Naturopathic Medicine—In some states, Naturopathic doctors, medically trained in diagnostics and natural and alternative therapies, are licensed as Naturopathic physicians. In other states, they may be licensed or registered as Naturopathic doctors. They are distinct from other naturopathic doctors, who may be correspondence school trained in traditional alternatives, by being medically trained graduates of accredited programs in naturopathic medicine, and board certified by a state's Department of Health. Information on finding a naturopathic physician may be found at www.naturopathic.org.

Ovulation—When an ovum, or egg, is released from a woman's ovary. Ovulation is determined by certain hormonal activity, which reveals itself in patterns seen in a woman's cervical mucous. For example, the ferning pattern at the time of greatest fertility, a pattern which facilitates sperm conductance for fertilization of the egg.

Pathologist—A physician specializing in the study of disease, particularly as is involves cellular changes in the body and laboratory tests and methods.

"FDA Approves Oral HIV Rapid Saliva Test 99 Percent Accuracy Results in 20 Minutes." *British Medical News Today* (March 27, 2004).

"Oral HIV Testing Can Increase Belief in Disease Transmission Through Saliva." *Biotech Week* (September 10, 2003): 229.

"Saliva-Based Rapid Test Kit Hits Market." *Medical Devices & Surgical Technology Week* (September 23, 2001).

Young, Karen. "FDA Clears New Saliva-Based Test for Determining Ovulation." *Diagnostics & Imaging Week* (August 14, 2003): 3–4.

ORGANIZATIONS

U.S. Food and Drug Administration Office of In Vitro Diagnostic Device Evaluation and Safety. HFZ-440 2098 Gaither Road, Rockville, MD 20850. (301) 594-3084. <http://www.fda.gov/cdrh/oivd>.

OTHER

Barrett, Stephen, M.D. *Dubious Urine/Saliva Testing.* [cited June 14, 2004]. <http://www.canoe.ca/HealthAlternativeColumns/001220.html>.

Consumer Information. Home-use Tests. U.S. Food and Drug Administration. 2004. <http://www.fda.gov/cdrh/oivd.>.

History of Method Development. Website. Craig Medical Distribution Inc. 1997. <http://www.craigmedical.com/ovulation_abstract.htm>.

Home-use Tests. Ovulation (Saliva Test). U.S. Food and Drug Administration. 2004. <http://www.fda.gov/cdrh/oivd>.

Latest Defense Against Bioterrorism: Saliva. Montana State University. 2003. <http:// techlink.msu.montana.edu/articles/saliva.html.>.

New Saliva Test Offers Fast, Simple Means of Measuring Stress. Northwestern University. 1997. <http://www.northwestern.edu/univ-relations/media>.

Saliva. National Institute of Dental and Carniofacial Research, National Institutes of Health. <http://www.nidcr.nih.gov/spectrum/nidcr2/2textsec5.htm>.

The Saliva Story—Part 1. Website. Aeron Life Cycles Clinical Laboratory. <http://www. areon.com/volume_2_number_1.htm>.

The Young Prefer Rapid Saliva HIV Test. David Douglas, HIV and AIDS News Stories. August 3, 2001. <http://www.hivandhepatitis.com>.

Teresa G. Odle

Sargassum seaweed

Description

Sargassum seaweed is a type of seaweed found along the coasts of Japan and China. Two species, *Sargassum fusiforme* and *Sargassum pallidum*, are both referred to as sargassum seaweed or gulfweed in English and *hai zao* in Chinese.

Sargassum seaweed is a brown algae with leafy segments supported at the surface of the ocean by air bladders. Many species of sargassum are found worldwide. In fact, the Sargasso Sea, an area of the Caribbean near the West Indies, is named for its large floating masses of sargassum seaweed. However, sargassum used in healing is usually of Asian origin.

General use

Sargassum seaweed, or *Hai zao*, has been used in **traditional Chinese medicine** (TCM) since at least the eighth century A. D. In TCM it is characterized as having a cold nature and a salty, bitter taste.

The primary use of sargassum seaweed is to treat goiters. A goiter is a nodule in the neck caused by enlargement of the thyroid gland. The thyroid needs **iodine** to produce a critical hormone, thyroxin, that regulates body metabolism. When not enough iodine is consumed in the diet, the thyroid gland enlarges. The primary natural sources of dietary iodine are sea salt, fish, and vegetables that live in the ocean. In the days before mechanical refrigeration, it was often difficult for people living far from the ocean to get enough iodine in their **diets**. Today, widespread refrigeration or freezing of fish and rapid transportation to inland markets has made iodine deficiency and goiters rare in the developed world. In addition, commercial salt manufacturers often produce a version of their product, called iodized salt, that is available in supermarkets and has iodine artificially added. However, iodine deficiency is still a worldwide problem and a major cause of mental and learning disabilities.

Using sargassum seaweed as a source of iodine to treat goiters is a scientifically sound practice. In TCM, sargassum seaweed is also used to treat such other thyroid disorders as Hashimoto's disease. In addition it is prescribed as a diuretic to increase the production of urine and reduce **edema**. It is also used to treat **pain** from hernia and swollen testes. Sargassum seaweed is found in many common Chinese formulas. In combination with silkworm, prunella, and scrophularia, it is used to treat scrofuloderma. When sargassum seaweed is combined with water chestnut, it is used to treat silicosis, a lung disease.

Sometimes modern herbalists use sargassum seaweed to promote weight loss because it encourages the body to discharge water through the urine. This can be risky because of the role iodine plays in setting the metabolic rate of the body. In China and Japan, fresh sargassum seaweed is sometimes stir-fried and eaten as a vegetable.

Reliable scientific evidence shows that sargassum seaweed provides enough dietary iodine to make it useful as a treatment for goiter. There is little scientific evidence that sargassum seaweed is useful in treating such other thyroid problems as Hashimoto's disease. Research shows that sargassum seaweed also has mild diuretic and anti-fungal properties. Studies done in Japan (1998) and Hong Kong (2000) using different but related species of sargassum seaweed showed that sargassum seaweed contained **antioxidants** that helped protect the livers of rats when they were subjected to chemical damage in laboratory experiments. In general, antioxidants are thought to slow **aging** and protect the body from damage caused by free radicals.

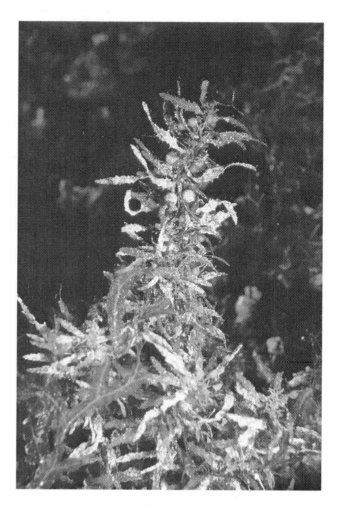

Sargassum seaweed. *(© Lawson Wood/Corbis. Reproduced by permission.)*

Preparations

Sargassum seaweed is collected from the ocean throughout the year and dried at cool temperatures away from direct sunlight for future use. This plant is a component of several Chinese formulas, including *haizao yuhu tang*, used to treat goiter and *neixiao lei li wan*, used to treat scrufuloderma. Dosage varies depending on the condition being treated.

Precautions

Because thyroid problems are serious, people with enlarged thyroid or nodules in their neck should seek professional help from a physician and not try to treat these problems solely with alternative remedies. Sargassum seaweed should be used with caution for weight loss because of the interactions of this product and the thyroid gland.

Side effects

No side effects have been reported when using sargassum seaweed in recommended dosages.

KEY TERMS

Diuretic—A diuretic is any substance that increases the production of urine.

Edema—Water retention in the body that often causes swelling of the hands and feet is called edema.

Hashimoto's disease—Disease in which the body makes antibodies to destroy the thyroid. Tendency toward this disease is thought to be inherited.

Scrofuloderma—Abscesses on the skin that are a symptom of the lung disease tuberculosis.

Silicosis—A serious lung disease caused by prolonged inhaling of dust from stone or sand that contains silicon dioxide. It is also called grinder's disease.

Interactions

Some traditional Chinese herbalists claim that **licorice** and sargassum seaweed should not be used together; however, no scientific research supports this claim. No interactions between sargassum seaweed and Western pharmaceuticals have bveen reported as of 2004; however, anyone taking medication for thyroid disorders should discuss the use of this remedy with their healthcare provider before using it.

Resources

BOOKS

Chevallier, Andrew. *Encyclopedia of Medicinal Plants.* London: Dorling Kindersley, 1996.

PERIODICALS

"In Case You Haven't Heard." *Mental Health Weekly* (July 1, 2002): 8.

ORGANIZATIONS

American Association of Oriental Medicine (AAOM) 433 909 22nd St. Sacramento, CA 95816. (916) 451-6950 <http://www.aaom.org>.

OTHER

"Sargassum Seaweed." *OnHealth.* http://onhealth.com/alternative/.

Tish Davidson
Teresa G. Odle

Sassafras

Description

Sassafras is a small tree, *Sassafras albidum*, belonging to the laurel family native to eastern North America.

Sassafras grows in woodlands in rich sandy well-drained soil from Maine to Florida, reaching a height of about 75 ft (25 m). The tree has also been imported to Europe, probably by the Spaniards who discovered it in Florida.

All parts of the sassafras tree are aromatic with a pleasant odor and a slightly sweet but astringent taste. The root and root bark were formerly used medicinally. The root is thick and woody. When alive, it is whitish but rapidly turns cinnamon-brown on exposure to air. Other names for sassafras are ague tree, cinnamon wood, saxifrax, saxafrax, and saloop. There are other plants that have the word sassafras in their name that are completely unrelated to *Sassafras albidum*. These include black sassafras (*Oliveri cortex*); swamp sassafras (*Magnolia glauca*); Australian sassafras (*Antherosperma moschatum*); sassafras goesianum (*Massoja aromatica,*); and California sassafras (*Umbellularia californica*).

General use

Sassafras should not be taken internally or used for healing except for topical applications. In the 1960s scientists determined that the volatile oil derived from sassafras root contains safrole as its chief component. Safrole is a known carcinogen in animal studies. Safrole in concentrations of 80–90%, similar to its concentration in the volatile oil, produced tumors in the livers of laboratory animals. In 1960 the United States Food and Drug Administration (FDA) banned sassafras volatile oil as a food and flavoring additive. In 1976 it prohibited the interstate shipment of sassafras bark for making tea. A safrole-free sassafras extract is now available; however, there are questions about its potentially cancer-causing properties.

Prior to the discovery that sassafras contains a carcinogen, it had a long and widespread history of use as a folk medicine. Native Americans used sassafras to cure many different conditions, but especially as a spring blood tonic. Before long, Native Americans introduced the European settlers to sassafras. It became a sought-after herb in Europe. Sassafras root bark was imported from the United States, and sassafras trees were also planted in Europe. Sassafras tea, sold under the name saloop, was a popular beverage in London.

Before sassafras was discovered to be a carcinogen, it was used as a diuretic as well as to treat urinary tract disorders and kidney problems. It was also used as an ineffective treatment for **syphilis**. Other herbal practitioners used sassafras to treat rheumatism and arthritis. It was given to women to ease painful **menstruation** and help their recovery from **childbirth**. Other conditions treated with sassafras include high blood pressure, colds, flu, and **bronchitis**. The volatile oil was used in dentistry in combination with cloves and other herbs to relieve

toothache. By far the most common use of sassafras, however, was to flavor root beer.

Externally, sassafras washes were used to soothe the eyes. The volatile oil was used as a liniment and to treat **bruises** and swellings. The volatile oil was also used to control head and body lice. The risks in applying sassafras oil externally are still unclear.

Despite the fact that sassafras contains a proven carcinogen, it is still used today in many parts of the Appalachian Mountains, where the root is locally gathered. In 1994, there was evidence that teas containing sassafras were still being sold in some health food stores. Even the health community has not fully grasped the harmful effects of sassafras. A 1993 article in *Midwifery Today and Childbirth Education* recommended sassafras as a cure for breast inflammation after childbirth. Many reputable studies, however, indicate that there is a definite health hazard in using even small amounts of sassafras either as oil or tea.

Preparations

Sassafras should not be used. In times past, before its potentially harmful effects were recognized, it was available as a volatile oil, as bark that could be brewed into tea, and as a component of tonic formulas and tonic teas. Since use of sassafras is not recommended, there is no recommended dosage.

Precautions

Sassafras should not be used.

Side effects

It has been reported that as little as one teaspoon of pure sassafras oil can kill an adult, and only a few drops can kill a toddler. The signs of sassafras poisoning include **nausea**, **vomiting**, confusion, and paralysis. The potentially hazardous dose of safrole has been determined to be 0.66 mg/kg of a person's body weight. This amount is less than the dose often found in sassafras tea.

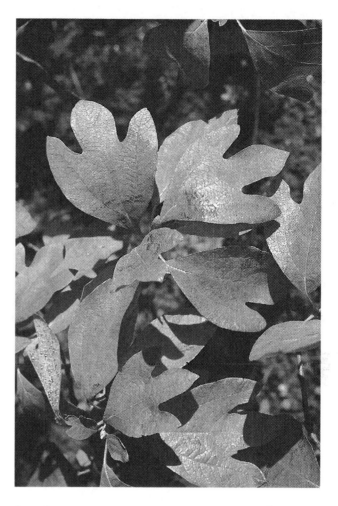

Sassafras. *(© PlantaPhile, Germany. Reproduced by permission.)*

Interactions

Sassafras should not be used. Since it is toxic, drug interactions have not been investigated.

Resources

BOOKS

Lawless, Julia. *The Illustrated Encyclopedia of Essential Oils.* Rockport, MA: Element, 1995.

PDR for Herbal Medicines. Montvale, New Jersey: Medical Economics Company, 1998.

Peirce, Andrea. *The American Pharmaceutical Association Practical Guide to Natural Medicines.* New York: William Morrow and Company, 1999.

OTHER

Plants for the Future: Sassafras albidum. http://www.metal-ab.unc.edu.

Tish Davidson

Saw palmetto

Description

Saw palmetto is an extract derived from the deep purple berries of the saw palmetto fan palm (*Serenoa repens*), a plant indigenous to the coastal regions of the southern United States and southern California. There is an estimated one million acres of wild saw palmetto palms in Florida, where the bulk of commercial saw palmetto is grown.

General use

Saw palmetto is used by natural health practitioners to treat a variety of ailments in men and women, such as testicular inflammation, urinary tract inflammation, coughs, and respiratory congestion. It is also used to strengthen the thyroid gland, balance the metabolism, stimulate appetite, and aid digestion. Most of the evidence supporting these uses is anecdotal and has not been proven by controlled clinical trials. However, there is much scientific documentation outlining the effectiveness of the herb in treating irritable bladder and urinary problems in men with benign prostate hyperplasia (BPH), an enlargement of the prostatic gland. BPH produces a swelling of the prostate gland that obstructs the urethra. This causes painful urination, reduced urine flow, difficulty starting or stopping the flow, dribbling after urination, and more frequent nighttime urination. Saw palmetto does not reduce **prostate enlargement**. Instead, it is thought to work in a variety of ways. First, it inhibits the conversion of testosterone into dihydrotestosterone (DHT). BPH is thought to be caused by an increase in the ratio of testosterone to DHT. Secondly, saw palmetto is believed to interfere with the production of estrogen and progesterone, hormones associated with DHT production.

In addition to causing **pain** and embarrassment, BPH can lead to serious kidney problems if undiagnosed and left untreated. It is a common problem in men over the age of 40. Estimates are that 50-60% of all men will develop BPH in their lifetimes. The Agency for Health Care Policy and Research estimates there are six million men between the ages of 50-79 who have BPH serious enough to require some type of therapy. Yet only half of them seek treatment from physicians. Health practitioners in both the allopathic and natural medicine communities recommend annual prostate for men over the age of 50, and an annual blood test that measures prostate-specific antigen (PSA), a marker for prostate **cancer**.

Recently, a number of clinical trials have confirmed the effectiveness of saw palmetto in treating BPH. Many of these trials have shown saw palmetto works better than the most commonly used prescription drug, finasteride, sold unter the trade name Proscar. Saw palmetto is effective in nearly 90% of patients after six weeks of use, while Proscar is effective in less than 50% of patients. In addition, Proscar may take up to six months to achieve its full effect. Since Proscar blocks the production of testosterone, it can cause **impotence** and breast enlargement. Also, saw palmetto is significantly less expensive than Proscar. A one-month supply of saw palmetto costs $12-25, while a one_month supply of Proscar costs $65-75. Other prescription drugs used to treat BPH are Cardura (doxazosin), Hytrin (terazosin), and Flomax (tamsulosin hydrochloride). Originally prescribed to treat **hypertension**, Cardura and Hytrin can cause a drop in blood pressure, causing lightheadedness and fainting. Presently, saw palmetto is being evaluated by the U.S. Food and Drug Administration (FDA) for treatment of BPH. If approved, it would become the first herbal product to be licensed by the agency as a treatment for a specific condition. Saw palmetto is listed in the *Physicians Desk Reference for Herbal Medicine* (1998 edition) as a treatment for prostate complaints and irritable bladder.

Since the 1960s, extensive clinical studies of saw palmetto have been done in Europe. A review of 24 European trials appeared in the November 1998 issue of the *Journal of the American Medical Association*. The trials involved nearly 3,000 men, some taking saw palmetto, others taking Proscar, and a third group taking a placebo. The men taking saw palmetto had a 28% improvement in urinary tract symptoms, a 24% improvement in peak urine flow, and 43% improvement in overall urine flow. The results were nearly comparable to the results from the group taking Proscar and superior to the results from men taking the placebo. As of 2002, however, many American physicians still regard the effectiveness of saw palmetto as requiring further proof.

Uses in women

There is very little documentation or scientific research regarding saw palmetto use in women. However, several studies in the 1990s show that the BPH drug Proscar can be effective in stopping unwanted facial and body hair growth, and in treating thinning hair in women. It works by blocking the action of an enzyme called 5-alpha reductase. Anecdotal reports suggest that saw palmetto may be as effective as Proscar in treating unwanted hair growth and thinning hair, and in preventing some types of **acne**. It has also been used to treat urinary tract inflammation and help relieve the symptoms of **menstruation**. There are claims that it can be used to enlarge breasts, but these claims have not been scientifically tested.

History

Saw palmetto berries have been used in American folk medicine for several hundred years as an aphrodisiac and for treating prostate problems. Native Americans

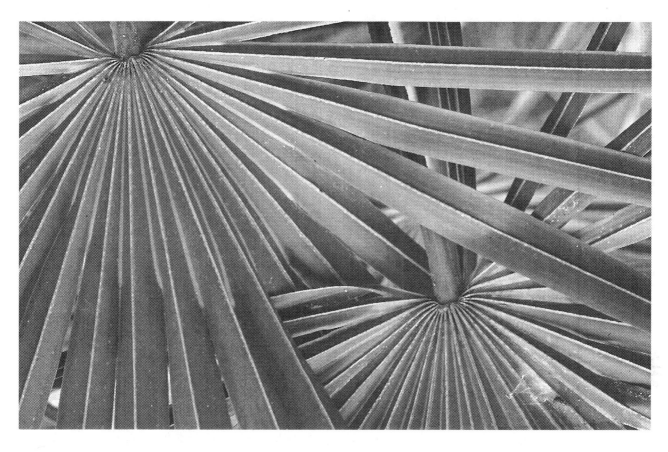

Saw palmetto leaves. *(Photo Researchers, Inc. Reproduced by permission.)*

in the southeast United States have used saw palmetto since the 1700s to treat male urinary problems. In the 1800s, the medical botanist John Lloyd noted that animals that ate saw palmetto appeared healthier and fatter than other livestock. Early American settlers noticed the same effects and used the juice from saw palmetto berries to gain weight, to improve general disposition, as a sedative, and to promote reproductive health.

In the United States, the medicinal uses of saw palmetto were first documented in 1879 by Dr. J.B. Read, a physician in Savannah, Georgia, who published a paper on the medicinal benefits of the herb in the April 1879 issue of the *American Journal of Pharmacy*. He found the herb useful in treating a wide range of conditions. "By its peculiar soothing power on the mucous membrane it induces sleep, relieves the most troublesome coughs, promotes expectoration, improves digestion, and increases fat, flesh and strength. Its sedative and diuretic properties are remarkable," Read wrote. "Considering the great and diversified power of the saw palmetto as a therapeutic agent, it seems strange that it should have so long escaped the notice of the medical profession."

A pungent tea made from saw palmetto berries was commonly used in the early 1900s to treat prostate enlarge-

ment and urinary tract **infections**. It was also used in men to increase sperm production and sex drive, although these uses are discounted today. One of the first published medical recommendations that saw palmetto was effective in treating prostate problems appeared in the 1926 edition of the *United States Dispensatory*. In the late 1920s, the use of medicinal plants, including saw palmetto, began to decline in the United States, while at the same time, it was on the rise in Europe.

Preparations

People taking saw palmetto should use only standardized extracts that contain 85–95% fatty acids and sterols. Dosages vary depending on the type of saw palmetto used. A typical dose is 320 mg per day of standardized extract, or 1–2 g per day of whole berries that have been dried and ground. It may take up to four weeks of use before beneficial effects are seen. In late 1999, the web-based independent consumer organization ConsumerLab.com tested 27 leading brands of saw palmetto for fatty acid and sterol content. Ten of the brands contained less than the minimum recommended level of 85% fatty acids and sterols. The 17 brands that passed the test are listed on the organization's web site at http://www.consumerlab.com/results/sawpalmetto.html.

Precautions

There are no special precautions associated with taking saw palmetto, even in high doses. BPH can become a serious problem, however, if left untreated. Men who are experiencing symptoms should be examined by a physician, since the symptoms of BPH are similar to those of **prostate cancer**. Men over the age of 50 should have a yearly prostate examination. Saw palmetto should be used only under a doctor's supervision by people with prostate cancer, **breast cancer**, or any sex hormone related diseases. Although the effects of saw palmetto on a fetus is unknown, pregnant women are advised not to take saw palmetto. Saw palmetto can alter hormonal activity that could have an adverse effect on the fetus. Women taking birth control pills or estrogen replacement products should consult a physician before taking saw palmetto. Persons taking testosterone or other anabolic steroids should not take saw palmetto without first consulting their doctor.

Physicians who accept saw palmetto as an effective remedy for prostate problems nevertheless point out that it is not completely free of side effects. In rare cases, allergic reactions to saw palmetto have been reported. Symptoms include difficulty breathing, constricting of the throat, **hives**, and swelling of the lips, tongue, or face. Persons experiencing any of these symptoms should stop taking saw palmetto and seek immediate medical attention.

Side effects

Other reported minor side effects are rare. They include cramps, **nausea**, **diarrhea**, and **headache**.

Interactions

Saw palmetto may interfere with such hormone-related drugs as testosterone and estrogen replacements, including Premarin, Cenestin, Vivelle, Fempatch, and Climara. It may also interact with birth control pills, such as Triphasil, Ovral, Lo-Ovral, Nordette, Alesse, Demulen, and Ortho-Novum. Anyone on these types of medications should consult with their doctor before taking saw palmetto. There are no known restrictions on food, beverages, or physical activity while taking saw palmetto.

Several herbs and minerals have been used in conjunction with saw palmetto in treating BPH. A 1996 European study showed positive results in treating patients with a daily dose of 320 mg of saw palmetto extract and 240 mg of **nettle** root extract. Many alternative health practitioners also recommend saw palmetto be used in combination with the herb pygeum africanung, pumpkin seeds, **zinc**, **flaxseed** oil, certain **amino acids**, antioxi-

---

KEY TERMS

Anabolic steroids—A group of mostly synthetic hormones sometimes taken by athletes to temporarily increase muscle size.

Aphrodisiac—Any substance that excites sexual desire.

Estrogen—A hormone that stimulates development of female secondary sex characteristics.

Hyperplasia—Enlargement of a part of the body, such as the prostate gland, due to an abnormal increase in the number of its cells.

Placebo—An inert or innocuous substance used in controlled experiments testing the efficacy of another substance.

Progesterone—A steroid hormone that is a biological precursor to corticoid (another steroid hormone) and androgen (a male sex hormone).

Testosterone—A male hormone produced in the testes or made synthetically that is responsible for male secondary sex characteristics.

Urethra—The canal that carries urine from the bladder to the outside of the body.

---

dants, and **diets** high in protein and soy products. Some factors that can impair the effectiveness of saw palmetto include beer, cigarette smoke, and some chemical pesticides used on fruit and vegetables. Some physicians recommend using saw palmetto in addition to a prescription medicine, such as Proscar, Hytrin, or Cardura.

Resources

BOOKS

Fleming, Thomas, editor. *PDR for Herbal Medicine*. Montvale, NJ: Medical Economics Co., 1998.

Foster, Steven W. *101 Medicinal Herbs*. Loveland, CO: Interweave Press, 1998.

Foster, Steven W. *Guide to Herbal Dosages*. Loveland, CO: Interweave Press, 2000.

Sahelian, Ray. *Saw Palmetto, Nature's Prostate Healer*. New York: Kensington Publishing Corp., 1998.

Winston, David. *Saw Palmetto for Men & Women: Herbal Healing for the Prostate, Urinary Tract, Immune System, and More*. North Adams, MA: Storey Books, 1999.

PERIODICALS

PERIODICALS

D'Epiro, Nancy Walsh. "Saw Palmetto and the Prostate." *Patient Care* (April 15, 1999): 29.

Ernst, E. "The Risk-Benefit Profile of Commonly Used Herbal Therapies: Ginkgo, St. John's Wort, Ginseng, Echinacea,

Saw Palmetto, and Kava." *Annals of Internal Medicine* 136 (January 1, 2002): 42-53.

Lowe, F. C., and E. Fagelman. "Phytotherapy in the Treatment of Benign Prostatic Hyperplasia." *Current Opinion in Urology* 12 (January 2002): 15-18.

Overmyer, Mac. "Saw Palmetto Shown to Shrink Prostatic Epithelium." *Urology Times* (June 1999): 1, 42.

Wilt, Timothy J., et al. "Saw Palmetto for Benign Prostatic Hyperplasia." *Nutritional Research Newsletter* (March 1999): 1.

Ken R. Wells
Rebecca J. Frey, PhD

Scabies

Definition

Scabies, also known as *sarcoptic acariasis,* is a contagious, parasitic skin infection caused by a tiny mite (*sarcoptes scabiei*).

Description

Scabies is caused by a tiny, 0.3 mm-long, parasitic insect called a mite. When a human comes into contact with the female mite, the mite burrows under the skin, laying eggs along the lines of its burrow. These eggs hatch, and the resulting offspring rise to the surface of the skin; mate; and repeat the cycle either within the skin of the original host; or within the skin of its next victim, causing red lesions.

The intense **itching**, or pruritus, that is almost always caused by scabies is due to a reaction within the skin to the feces of the mite. The first time someone is infected with scabies, he or she may not notice any itching for four to six weeks. With subsequent **infections**, the itchiness will begin within hours of picking up the first mite.

Causes & symptoms

Scabies is most common among people who live in overcrowded conditions, and whose ability to practice good hygiene is limited. Scabies can be passed between people by close skin contact. Although the mites can only live away from human skin for about three days, sharing clothing or bedclothes can pass scabies among family members or close contacts. In May 2002, the Centers for Disease Control (CDC) included scabies in its updated guidelines for the treatment of sexually transmitted diseases.

Scabies mites have penetrated under the skin of this person's hand. *(Custom Medical Stock Photo. Reproduced by permission.)*

Mite burrows within the skin are seen as winding, slightly raised gray lines along a person's skin. The female mite may be found at one end of the burrow, as a tiny pearl-like bump underneath the skin. Because of the intense itching, burrows may be obscured by scratch marks left by the patient. The most common locations for burrows include the sides of the fingers, between the fingers, the top of the wrists, around the elbows and armpits, around the nipples of the breasts in women, in the genitalia of men, around the waist (beltline), and on the lower part of the buttocks. Babies may have burrows on the soles of their feet, palms of their hands, and faces. The itching from scabies becomes worse after a hot shower and at night. Scratching, however, seems to serve some purpose in scabies, as the mites are apparently often inadvertently removed. Most infestations with scabies are caused by no more than 15 mites altogether.

Infestation with huge numbers of mites (on the order of thousands to millions) occurs when an individual does not scratch, or when an individual has a weakened immune system. These patients include those who live in institutions; are mentally retarded, or physically infirm; have other diseases which affect the amount of sensation they have in their skin (leprosy or syringomyelia); have **leukemia** or diabetes; are taking medications that lower their immune response (**cancer** chemotherapy, drugs given after organ transplantation); or have other diseases which lower their immune response (such as acquired immunodeficiency syndrome or **AIDS**). This form of scabies, with its major infestation, is referred to as crusted scabies or Norwegian scabies. Infected patients have thickened crusty areas all over their bodies, including over the scalp. Their skin appears scaly, and their fingernails may be thickened and horny.

Diagnosis

Diagnosis can be made simply by observing the characteristic burrows of the mites causing scabies. A sterilized needle can be used to explore the pearly bump at the end of a burrow, remove its contents, and place it on a slide to be examined. The mite itself may then be identified under a microscope.

Occasionally, a type of mite carried on dogs (*Sarcoptes scabiei var. canis*) may infect humans. These mites cannot survive for very long on humans, however, so the infection is less severe.

Treatment

A paste made from two herbs, **neem** (*Azadirachta indica*) and **turmeric** (*Curcuma longa,*) applied to the affected area daily for 15 days has been found to be effective in treating scabies.

Allopathic treatment

Several types of lotions (usually containing 5% permethrin) can be applied to the body and left on for 12–24 hours. One topical application is usually sufficient, although the scabicide may be reapplied after a week if mites remain. Preparations containing lindane are no longer recommended for treating scabies as of 2003 because of the potential for damage to the nervous system. Itching can be lessened by the use of calamine lotion or antihistamine medications.

In addition to topical medications, the doctor may prescribe oral ivermectin. Ivermectin is a drug that was originally developed for veterinary practice as a broad-spectrum antiparasite agent. Studies done in humans, however, have found that ivermectin is as safe and effective as topical medications for treating scabies. A study published in 2003 reported that ivermectin is safe for people in high-risk categories, including those with compromised immune systems.

Expected results

The prognosis for complete recovery from a scabies infestation is excellent. In patients with weak immune systems, the biggest danger is that the areas of skin involved with scabies will become secondarily infected with bacteria.

KEY TERMS

. . . .

Mite—An insect parasite belonging to the order Acarina. The organism that causes scabies is a mite.

Pruritus—An unpleasant itching sensation. Scabies is characterized by intense pruritus.

Topical—A type of medication applied to the skin or body surface.

Prevention

Good hygiene is essential in the prevention of scabies. When a member of a household is diagnosed with scabies, all that person's recently worn clothing and bedding should be washed in very hot water. Extensive cleaning of the household, however, is not necessary because the mite does not live long away from the human body.

Resources

BOOKS

Darmstadt, Gary L., and Al Lane. "Arthropod Bites and Infestations." In *Nelson Textbook of Pediatrics,* edited by Richard Behrman. Philadelphia: W.B. Saunders Co., 1996.

Maguire, James H. "Ectoparasite Infestations and Arthropod Bites and Stings." In *Harrison's Principles of Internal Medicine,* edited by Anthony S. Fauci, et al. New York: McGraw–Hill, 1998.

"Scabies (The Itch)." Section 10, Chapter 114 in *The Merck Manual of Diagnosis and Therapy,* edited by Mark H. Beers, MD, and Robert Berkow, MD. Whitehouse Station, NJ: Merck Research Laboratories, 2002.

Stoffman, Phyllis. *The Family Guide to Preventing and Treating 100 Infectious Diseases.* New York: John Wiley and Sons, Inc., 1995.

PERIODICALS

Burroughs, R. F., and D. M. Elston. "What's Eating You? Canine Scabies." *Cutis* 72 (August 2003): 107–109.

Burstein, G. R., and K. A. Workowski. "Sexually Transmitted Diseases Treatment Guidelines." *Current Opinion in Pediatrics* 15 (August 2003): 391–397.

Fawcett, R. S. "Ivermectin Use in Scabies." *American Family Physician* 68 (September 15, 2003): 1089–1092.

Santoro, A. F., M. A. Rezac, and J. B. Lee. "Current Trend in Ivermectin Usage for Scabies." *Journal of Drugs in Dermatology* 2 (August 2003): 397–401.

ORGANIZATIONS

American Academy of Dermatology (AAD). 930 East Woodfield Road, Schaumburg, IL 60173. (847) 330-0230. <http://www.aad.org>.

Kathleen D. Wright
Rebecca J. Frey, PhD

Scallion

Description

A variety of onion, the scallion (*Allii fistulosi*) is a pointy-leafed perennial that can reach about 20 inches in height. The herb has been a popular remedy in Asian folk medicine for thousands of years, having been first described about 2,000 years ago in the Chinese herbal classic *Shen Nong Ben Cao Jing*. The plant, which flourishes in warm climates, is native to Asia but has been found growing in many parts of the world.

While the scallion's fresh bulb is the part that is most often used as a drug, the entire plant is believed to have medicinal properties. Scallion, which belongs to the Liliaceae family, is sometimes called green onion, spring onion, Welsh onion, or Japanese bunching onion. The scallion bulb is called *Cong Bai* in Chinese and the root of the scallion is called *Cong Xu*.

General use

While not approved by the Food and Drug Administration (FDA) or widely used by Western herbalists, scallion is believed by Eastern herbalists to possess a number of important properties. Often used to treat the **common cold**, it is also believed to fight fungal and bacterial **infections** and to cause or increase perspiration. The herb may also act as a metabolic stimulant.

Because scallion has not been studied extensively in people, its effectiveness is based mainly on the results of animal and laboratory studies as well as its ancient reputation as a folk remedy. In a 1999 investigation, scallion was shown to block the growth of several types of fungi. In a 1998 study, scallion extract was shown to inhibit the activity of *Aspergillus niger* and *Aspergillus flavus*. In a 1985 Chinese study of scallion's antibacterial properties, the herb was shown to be effective against microorganisms such as *Pseudomonas aeruginosa* and *Micrococcus luteus* .

Exactly how scallion works is unknown. Its therapeutic effects (as well as its pungent flavor) are often attributed to the herb's volatile oils, which include sulfurous compounds such as allicin, dipropyl disulfide, and allyl sulfide. Allicin may be of particular importance. This agent, also found in **garlic** (*Allium sativum*), has been shown to fight bacteria and fungi, help prevent **atherosclerosis**, lower **cholesterol** levels, and act as an antioxidant. Other constituents of scallion include starch, sugars, cellulose, fatty acids, pectin, and vitamins A and C.

In the philosophy of Chinese folk medicine in which diseases are often believed to result from disruptions in the flow of bodily energy, scallion is considered warm and acrid. The whitish bulb of the scallion, called *Cong Bai* by Chinese herbalists, is mainly used to treat the common cold. Often combined with other herbs, it may be used to shorten the duration of a cold or alleviate symptoms such as runny nose, **fever** and **chills**, nasal congestion, and **headache**. It is also recommended for **diarrhea**, stomachache, abdominal bloating, **earache**, mastitis (breast inflammation), pinworms, **kidney stones**, carbuncles, urinary difficulties, and sores or abscesses. In a more general sense, the bulb is believed to improve digestion, remove impurities from the body, and restore vital functions.

While the bulb of the scallion is usually favored, other parts of the plant have been used to treat a long list of maladies. The roots, called *Cong Xu* in Chinese herbalism, are sometimes recommended for cold-related headaches, throat sores, and frostbite. The leaves are employed to treat cold symptoms, carbuncles, **stroke**, and traumatic injuries. Scallion seeds are reputed to enhance vision and improve kidney function. They may also be used to treat **dizziness** as well as **impotence** due to kidney problems, among other health complaints. Juice derived from the bulb (or from the whole plant) is thought to detoxify the body and thin the blood. It may also be used for **nosebleeds**, headaches, carbuncles, hematuria (the presence of blood in the urine), internal parasites, and traumatic injuries.

Some of the more intriguing research related to scallion has been conducted in China and Japan. One Japanese investigation focused on scallion and the common cold. In the study, which involved 107 people suffering from colds, equal amounts (15 g) of scallion bulb and **ginger** were combined with a few grams of salt. The mixture was applied externally to a number of areas on the body, including the back, chest, palms, and soles of the feet. All of the study participants treated with the scallion mixture recovered in a day or two. One application of scallion was usually sufficient to achieve results, though a few people in the study required two treatments. In several instances, the mixture reduced **fever** completely within half an hour.

An enema prepared by combining scallion, ginger juice, and **pinellia** root may be helpful in treating acute mastitis (breast inflammation), according to one study.

Preparations

The optimum dosage of scallion has not been established with any certainty. When scallion bulb is used internally, the dosage is typically 9–15 g a day. A preparation can be made by boiling scallion in water or wine. Mashed bulbs can also be applied externally to an affected area of skin.

When other parts of scallion (such as the leaves, roots, and seeds) are used internally, daily dosage is 3–15 g. Like the bulbs, scallion's leaves and roots may be applied externally.

Tablets containing scallion in combinations are also available.

Scallion may be included in the diet. The herb is a favorite ingredient in Chinese cooking, where it is used in raw and cooked form.

Because scallion has been recommended for a variety of purposes and can be used internally and externally, consumers are advised to consult a doctor experienced in the use of alternative remedies or Chinese medicine to determine proper dosage.

Precautions

Scallion is not known to be harmful when taken in recommended dosages. It is important to note that the long-term effects of taking the herb (in any amount) have not been investigated. Due to lack of sufficient medical study, scallion should be used with caution in children, women who are pregnant or breast-feeding, and people with liver or kidney disease.

The volatile oils present in the herb may cause skin irritation or **eczema** in susceptible people. Because scallion can increase sweating, people who are perspiring heavily should avoid this herb.

Side effects

When taken in recommended dosages, scallion is not associated with any bothersome or significant side effects.

Interactions

Scallion should not be combined with honey, according to some practitioners of Chinese folk medicine. When used internally, scallion has been mixed with ginger, white pepper, and pig's feet without apparent harm. When used externally, scallion has been safely combined with a variety of other herbs, including ginger and powdered **fennel** seed.

Resources

BOOKS

Editors of Time-Life Books. *The Drug and Natural Medicine Advisor.* Alexandria, Va.: Time-Life Books, 1997.

PERIODICALS

Abramovitz, D., et al. "Allicin-Induced Decrease in Formation of Fatty Streaks (Atherosclerosis) in Mice Fed a Choles-

terol-Rich Diet." *Coronary Artery Disease* 10, no. 7 (1999): 515–9.

Chen, H. C., M. D. Chang, and T. J. Chang. "Antibacterial Properties of Some Spice Plants Before and After Heat Treatment." *Chung-Hua Min Kuo Wei Sheng Wu Chi Mien I Hsueh Tsa Chih* 18, no. 3 (1985): 190–5.

Eilat, S., et al. "Alteration of Lipid Profile in Hyperlipidemic Rabbits by Allicin, an Active Constituent of Garlic." *Coronary Artery Disease* 6, no. 12 (1995): 985–90.

Prasad, K., et al. "Antioxidant Activity of Allicin, an Active Principle in Garlic." *Mol Cell Biochemistry* 148, no. 2 (1995): 183–9.

Yin, M. C., and W. S. Cheng. "Inhibition of *Aspergillus Niger* and *Aspergillus Flavus* by Some Herbs and Spices." *Journal of Food Protection* 61, no. 1 (1998): 123–5.

Yin, M. C., and S. M. Tsao. "Inhibitory Effect of Seven Allium Plants upon Three Aspergillus Species." *International Journal of Food Microbiology* 49, no. 1-2 (1999): 49–56.

ORGANIZATIONS

American Botanical Council. P. O. Box 144345, Austin, TX 78714-4345. http://www.herbalgram.org.

OTHER

Internet Grateful Med: Medline. http://igm.nlm.nih.gov.

Greg Annussek

Scarlet fever

Definition

Scarlet fever is an infection caused by a streptococcus bacterium. It can be transmitted through the air or by physical contact and primarily affects children between four and eight years of age. In temperate climates, scarlet fever is most common during the late fall, winter, and early spring.

Scarlet fever is characterized by a **sore throat**, a fever of 103–104°F (39.4–40°C), and a sandpaper-like rash on reddened skin. If scarlet fever is untreated, such serious complications can develop; as **rheumatic fever** (a **heart disease**) or kidney inflammation (glomerulonephritis).

Description

Scarlet fever, or scarlatina, gets its name from the characteristic flush of the patient's skin, especially on the cheeks. Fever and sluggishness accompany a sore throat and raised rash that progressively covers much of the body. Symptoms usually begin within two to five days after a person is exposed. The fever usually subsides within a few days, and recovery is complete by two weeks. After the fever is gone, the skin on the face and body forms flakes, with the skin on the palms of the hands and soles of the feet peeling more dramatically.

Scarlet fever is highly contagious when the patient is in the early stages and is not being treated with antibiotics. It is spread by **sneezing**, coughing, or direct contact with an infected person. Early in the twentieth century, severe scarlet fever epidemics were common. As of the early 2000s, the disease is rare, partially because of the availability of antibiotics. However, antibiotics are not the entire reason, since the decline began before their widespread use. One theory is that the strain of bacteria that causes scarlet fever has become weaker over time.

Causes & symptoms

Scarlet fever is caused by Group A streptococcal bacteria (*Streptococcus pyogenes*). In addition to causing scarlet fever, Group A streptococci bacteria cause many different illnesses, such as **strep throat**, wound or skin **infections**, **pneumonia**, serious **kidney infections**, and **toxic shock syndrome**. The strain of streptococcus that causes scarlet fever is slightly different from the strain that causes most strep throats. The scarlet fever strain produces an erythrogenic toxin, which is what causes the skin to turn red.

The main symptoms and signs of scarlet fever are fever, sluggishness, sore throat, and a bumpy rash that blanches (turns white) when it's pressed. The rash appears first on the upper chest and spreads to the neck, abdomen, legs, arms, and in folds of skin such as under the arm or in the groin. The skin around the mouth tends to be pale while the cheeks are flushed. In children, the disease causes a "strawberry tongue," in which inflamed bumps on the tongue rise above a bright red coating. Strawberry tongue is rarely seen in adults. Finally, dark red lines (called Pastia's lines) may appear in the creases of skin folds.

Diagnosis

A medical practitioner must diagnose and treat scarlet fever. The doctor notes the symptoms and eliminates

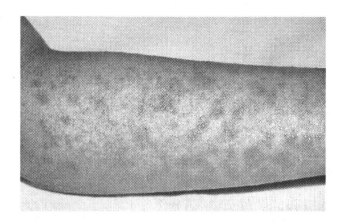

The scarlet fever rash on this person's arm was caused by a streptococcal infection. *(Custom Medical Stock Photo. Reproduced by permission.)*

the possibility of other diseases. **Measles** is a viral infection that is also associated with a fever and rash. However, scarlet fever can be distinguished from measles by the quality of the rash, the presence of a sore throat in scarlet fever, and the absence of the severe eye inflammation and runny nose that usually accompany measles.

Because scarlet fever may begin with a sore throat, the doctor will first determine if the problem is bacterial or viral in nature by checking for specific symptoms. For example, inflammation of the lymph nodes in the neck is typical in strep infections but not viral infections. On the other hand, **cough**, **laryngitis**, and stuffy nose tend to be associated with viral infections rather than strep infections.

Laboratory tests are necessary to make a definitive diagnosis of a strep infection and to distinguish a strep throat from a viral sore throat. One test that can be performed is a blood cell count. Bacterial infections are associated with an elevated white blood cell count. In viral infections, the white blood cell count is generally below normal. A throat culture can distinguish between a strep infection and a viral infection. A throat swab from the infected person is brushed over a nutrient gel containing red blood cells (a sheep blood agar plate) and incubated overnight. If streptococcal bacteria are present in the sample, they will break down the red blood cells and leave a clear zone in the gel surrounding the bacteria.

The doctor will also distinguish between a strep throat and scarlet fever. In a strep infection, the throat is sore and appears beefy and red. White spots appear on the tonsils. Lymph nodes under the jaw line may swell and become tender. These symptoms may or may not be present with scarlet fever. The main feature that distinguishes scarlet fever from a strep throat is the presence of the sandpapery red rash.

Treatment

Because of the nature of the infection and the danger of serious complications, scarlet fever cannot be treated solely with alternative therapies. A course of antibiotics and treatment by a physician is imperative. However, alternative therapies may be used to relieve the symptoms of fever and sore throat.

Fever

For fever, especially in children, there are some alternative treatments. Naturopathy recommends sponging with tepid water if the fever rises over 102°F (38.9°C). Rest and plenty of water are advised.

Homeopathy treats the specific type of fever, so it will be necessary to consult with a homeopath to determine the correct remedy for the patient. Some common homeopathic remedies for fever are:

- Aconite 6c at the onset of fever that is accompanied by thirst, **chills**, dry burning skin, and restlessness.
- Belladonna 6c for high fever with dry burning skin, red face, dilated pupils, and swollen glands.
- *Arsenicum album* 6c for patients who are restless and agitated, alternately hot and cold, thirsty, and patients whose fever is worse after midnight.
- Byronia 6c for the patient who is shivery and sweating, very thirsty at long intervals, and having headaches and **pain**.
- *Ferrum phosphoricum* (**iron** phosphate) 6c for a mild fever of slow onset accompanied by frequent bouts of sweating, shivering, and headaches.

Western herbalism may be used to treat fever, but treatment requires a qualified medical herbalist. The herbalist may recommend a bath with tepid infusions of limeflower, elderflower, **yarrow**, or German **chamomile**. Herbs such as **catnip**, **hyssop**, **lemon balm**, and vervain can lower the temperature and increase perspiration. German chamomile, **lavender**, and limeflower promote **relaxation**, and **echinacea** and **garlic** fight infection.

Chinese herbs in combinations can treat specific patterns of fever. They can also be used to balance the energies, specifically the yin (cool and moist) energies after the illness subsides.

Sore throat

Some recommended treatments for sore throat are:

- Aromatherapy, in which the patient gargles with water and very small amounts of geranium or tea tree **essential oils**. A massage using diluted **eucalyptus** oil may also be helpful.

- Naturopathy may suggest **fasting** to eliminate toxins and the use of garlic to fight infection. Naturopaths will also recommend fruit juices high in **vitamin C**, especially citrus fruit juices, to soothe irritation.

- Hydrotherapy, in which water is utilized to restore health, uses humidifiers to prevent the irritation of a sore throat by dry air. A practitioner may also recommend using a cold abdominal pack and throat compress to stimulate both circulation and the immune system.

- Western herbalists will recommend gargling with an infusion of antiseptic herbs such as **calendula** or **sage**, and may use echinacea to fight infection.

Allopathic treatment

Although the symptoms of scarlet fever often clear within a few days, the patient should receive antibiotic treatment to reduce the severity of symptoms, prevent complications, and avoid spreading the infection to others. Antibiotics may be taken either orally or by injection. After a patient has been on antibiotics for 24 hours, he or she is no longer contagious. The rash itself is not contagious. Antibiotic treatment will shorten the course of the illness in small children but may not do so in adolescents or adults. Nevertheless, a full course of treatment with antibiotics is important for preventing complications.

Since penicillin injections are painful, oral penicillin may be preferable. If the patient is unable to tolerate penicillin, alternative antibiotics such as erythromycin or clindamycin may be substituted. The patient must take the entire course of medication—usually 10 days—for the therapy to be effective and to ensure that the bacteria have been killed. Because symptoms subside quickly, there is a temptation to stop therapy prematurely. However, not completing the medication increases the risk of developing rheumatic fever and kidney inflammation. If the patient is considered too unreliable to take all of the pills or is unable to take oral medication, daily injections of procaine penicillin can be given in the hip or thigh muscle.

After the contagious period has passed, the patient does not need to be isolated. Bed rest is not necessary. Aspirin or Tylenol (acetaminophen) may be given for fever or pain relief.

Expected results

If the patient is treated promptly with antibiotics, full recovery can be expected. Patients who have had scarlet fever develop immunity to the disease and cannot be infected again. However, about 10% of children don't respond to an initial antibiotic treatment, so it may be necessary for a second throat culture and the use of a different antibiotic.

KEY TERMS

Clindamycin—An antibiotic that can be used instead of penicillin.

Erythrogenic toxin—A toxin or agent produced by the scarlet fever-causing bacteria that causes the skin to turn red.

Erythromycin—An antibiotic that can be used instead of penicillin.

Glomerulonephritis—A serious inflammation of the kidneys that can be caused by streptococcal bacteria; a potential complication of untreated scarlet fever.

Pastia's lines—Red lines in the folds of the skin, especially in the armpit and groin, that are characteristic of scarlet fever.

Penicillin—An antibiotic that is used to treat bacterial infections.

Procaine penicillin—An injectable form of penicillin that contains an anesthetic to reduce the pain of the injection.

Rheumatic fever—A heart disease that is a complication of a strep infection.

Sheep blood agar plate—A petri dish filled with a nutrient gel containing red blood cells that is used to detect the presence of streptococcal bacteria in a throat culture. Streptococcal bacteria will break down the red blood cells, leaving a clear spot around the bacterial colony.

Strawberry tongue—A sign of scarlet fever in which the tongue appears to have a red coating with large raised bumps.

Prevention

Although scarlet fever is only contagious before treatment with antibiotics is begun, it is wise to avoid exposure to children at any stage of the disease. Doing so will help prevent the spread of scarlet fever.

Resources

BOOKS

Berkow, Robert M.D., ed. *The Merck Manual of Diagnosis and Therapy.* 16th ed. Rahway, NJ: Merck, 1992.

Driscoll, John. "Scarlet Fever." In *The Columbia University College of Physicians and Surgeons Complete Home Medical Guide.* 3rd rev. ed. New York: Crown Publishers, 1995.

Woodham, Anne, and David Peters, M.D. *Encyclopedia of Healing Therapies.* New York: DK Pub., 1997.

Wyngaarden, James B., Lloyd H. Smith, and J. Claude Bennett, eds. *Cecil Textbook of Medicine.* 19th ed. New York: W.B. Saunders Company, 1992.

PERIODICALS

Gregory, Tanya. "Scarlet Fever and Its Relatives." *Patient Care* (June 15, 1998): 109.

Schmitt, B. D. "Scarlet Fever" *Clinical Reference Systems* (July 1, 1999): 1293.

Amy Cooper

Schisandra

Description

Schisandra (*Schisandra chinensis*) is an aromatic woody vine that is native to northern and northeastern China. It is predominately cultivated in the Chinese provinces of Jilin, Hebei, Heilongjiang, and Lianoning. Schisandra is also found in Russia and Korea.

The schisandra plant reaches a height of up to 25 ft (7.5 m) and has pink flowers. Schisandra fruit is fully ripened in the fall and appears as numerous spikes of tiny, bright red berries. The berries have sweet, sour, hot, salty and bitter tastes—hence the Chinese name for schisandra, "Wu Wei Zi" (five-flavored herb). Other names for schisandra include schizandra, five-taste fruit, and herb of five tastes.

Constituents and bioactivities

Schisandra fruit contains a wide variety of compounds with biological activities. Constituents of schisandra include:

- acids
- lignans (deoxyschizandrin, gomisins, pregomisin, schizandrin, and others)
- phytosterols (beta-sitosterol and stigmasterol)
- vitamins C and E
- volatile oils

Schisandra fruit contains at least 30 different lignans. Lignans, which are sometimes described as phytoestrogens (plant-derived compounds with estrogen-like activity), are known to have liver-protective (anti-hepatotoxic) action and to regenerate damaged liver tissue. In addition, lignans interfere with a compound called platelet activating factor, which promotes inflammation. The results of a study in rats showed that a lignan-enriched extract of *Schisandra chinensis* protected against liver damage from either aflatoxin (a toxin produced by a mold) or cadmium chloride (a toxic chemical). The liver-protective function is partly due to schisandra's antioxidant activity. However, treating the rats with **vitamin E**, an antioxidant, did not protect them from liver damage. This finding indicates that schisandra's liver-protective activity is not due to its vitamin E content. Schisandra increases liver function, which helps the body's metabolism become more efficient.

Research has shown that schisandra has adaptogenic properties, which means that it helps the body to fight disease and adapt to stresses from physical, mental, chemical, and environmental sources. Schisandra also has tonic (restoring tone to tissues), expectorant (promoting the clearing of lung mucus), and cough-suppressant (reducing coughing) activities. It stimulates the nervous system by increasing the speed of nervous responses, leading to quicker and stronger reflexes. Schisandra has been shown to stimulate breathing, lower blood pressure, act as a vasodilator (causing blood vessels to dilate), improve blood circulation, improve heart function, strengthen uterine contractions, improve vision, normalize blood sugar levels, and assist in food digestion and absorption of nutrients. It can activate all major body systems.

General use

Schisandra is a Chinese tonic herb used in **traditional Chinese medicine** as a lung astringent and kidney tonic. Historically, it was used to treat mental illness, night sweats, coughs, thirst, **insomnia**, chronic dysentery (**diarrhea** containing blood and mucus), premature ejaculation, and physical exhaustion. The Chinese consider it an energy tonic that can be used to restore lost vitality. Schisandra can improve overall health and increase energy levels.

Schisandra is an overall tonic that is used to treat the following conditions:

- Fluid imbalance. Because of its kidney tonic effect, schisandra is useful in treating thirst, night sweats, excessive sweating, **urinary incontinence**, and the frequent urge to urinate.

- Circulatory disorders. Schisandra may be used to treat poor circulation and poor heart function.

- Intestinal disease. Schisandra has been used to treat diarrhea and dysentery.

- **Fatigue**. Schisandra may help to reduce fatigue, improve endurance, improve work performance, and build strength. It is recommended for persons who need high levels of energy, such as athletes.

- Liver disease. Schisandra is used to treat **hepatitis** and poor liver function. In one clinical study, schisandra successfully treated 76% of the patients with hepatitis.

It has been shown to improve both virally and chemically induced hepatitis. More recently, schisandra has been found to protect the liver against the side effects of anti-Alzheimer's medications.

- Mental and emotional illness. Schisandra has been shown to improve mental clarity, concentration, and coordination. It reduces forgetfulness, irritability, and nervous exhaustion. Schisandra is used to treat **stress** and may be part of a useful treatment for depression.

- Respiratory disease and disorder. Schisandra is used to treat **allergies**. It treats respiratory symptoms such as shortness of breath, chronic **cough**, and wheezing.

- Sensory organ failure. Schisandra has been used to help improve failing sight and hearing. It enhances the sensation of touch.

- Sexual disorder. Schisandra tones the sexual organs of both men and women. It increases the production of sexual fluids, improves male sexual stamina, and treats premature ejaculation and low sex drive.

- Skin rash. Schisandra has been used to treat skin conditions, including **hives** and eczema.

- Sleep disorder. Because of its adaptogenic properties, schisandra can relieve insomnia and dream-disrupted sleep.

- Other. Schisandra counteracts respiratory paralysis caused by morphine overdose, and strengthens uterine contractions to promote healthy labor and childbirth.

Schisandra is one of nine herbs combined in a Chinese dietary supplement called Equiguard, which is given to support the functioning of the kidneys and prostate gland in men. A recent study indicates that Equiguard may be helpful in treating **prostate cancer** because it appears to prevent the **cancer** cells from forming new colonies.

Preparations

Only the fruit of schisandra is used for medicinal purposes. Schisandra berries are harvested when fully ripe and allowed to dry in the sun. Schisandra's dried fruit is used, and the herb is prepared in the form of powder, tincture (an alcoholic extract), and wine. It is also found, usually in combination with other herbs, in capsules, tea, and decoctions (a water extract). Schisandra may be found in Chinese herb shops or health food stores. Recommended doses of schisandra are 1.5–15 g of dried fruit daily, 2–4 ml of tincture three times daily, 1.5–6 g of powder daily, one to three cups of tea once daily, or 1.5 g in capsule form daily.

The decoction is prepared by boiling 5 g of crushed berries in 100 ml of water. This decoction is divided into three doses, which are taken over a 24-hour period. The tea is prepared by steeping 1–6 g of dried schisandra berries in one to three cups of boiling water.

For use as a general tonic in China, patients are advised to chew dried schisandra berries daily for 100 days. Skin conditions are usually treated with a medicinal wine formulation.

It may take several weeks for the energy-increasing effects of schisandra to be felt.

Precautions

Schisandra should not be used during **pregnancy** or in patients who are having trouble urinating.

Side effects

Schisandra is safe for long-term use; it has relatively few side effects. It has, however, been reported to cause upset stomach, **heartburn**, decreased appetite, and skin rash.

Interactions

Schisandra interacts with acetaminophen in a positive way. In a laboratory study, gomisin A, a lignan found in schisandra, offered some degree of liver protection to rats given doses of acetaminophen high enough to cause liver damage.

Schisandra has been reported to increase the effects of antidiabetic medications and anesthetics; it should therefore be discontinued before major surgery. Schisandra should not be taken together with terfenadine (seldane) because it appears to increase the risk of cardiac arrhythmia as a side effect of this medication.

Schisandra is often used in Chinese herbal formulas as a harmonizing agent because it complements and coordinates well with other herbs. Schisandra is often found in combination with **Korean ginseng** (*Panax ginseng*).

Resources

BOOK

Chevallier, Andrew. "Schisandra." In *The Encyclopedia of Medicinal Plants*. New York: DK Publishing, 1996.

PERIODICALS

Hsieh, T. C., X. Lu, J. Guo et al. "Effects of Herbal Preparation Equiguard on Hormone-Responsive and Hormone-Refractory Prostate Carcinoma Cells: Mechanistic Studies." *International Journal of Oncology* 20 (April 2002): 681-689.

Ip, Siu Po, et al. "Effect of a Lignan-Enriched Extract of *Schisandra Chinensis* on Aflatoxin B1 and Cadmium Chloride-Induced Hepatotoxicity in Rats." *Pharmacology & Toxicology* 78 (1996): 413–416.

KEY TERMS

Adaptogen—A medicine that increases the body's ability to fight disease and any stress it encounters including those from chemical, environmental, mental, and physical sources.

Lignans—Chemicals found in plants that have estrogen-like, liver-protective, and anti-inflammatory activities.

Phytosterols—Plant-based oils that appear to have a cholesterol-lowering effect.

Tonic—A preparation or medicine that invigorates, strengthens, or restores tone to tissues. Schisandra is considered to be an overall tonic that is good for any organ or system of the body.

Volatile oil—The fragrant oil that can be obtained from a plant by distillation. The word "volatile" means that the oil evaporates in the open air.

Pan, S. Y., Y. F. Han, P. R. Carlier, et al. "Schisandrin B Protects Against Tacrine- and Bis(7)-Tacrine-Induced Hepatotoxicity and Enhances Cognitive Function in Mice." *Planta Medica* 68 (March 2002): 217-220.

Schar, Douglas. "5 Cutting-Edge Superherbs." *Prevention* 51 (December 1999): 110+.

ORGANIZATIONS

American College of Acupuncture and Oriental Medicine. 9100 Park West Drive, Houston, TX 77063. (800) 729-4456. <www.acaom.edu>.

American College of Traditional Chinese Medicine. 455 Arkansas Street, San Francisco, CA 94107. (415) 282-7600. <www.actcm.edu>.

OTHER

"Schisandra." *Healthnotes Online.* http://www.puritan.com/healthnotes/Herb/Schisandra.htm.

"Schizandra." *Planet Botanic.* http://www.planetbotanic.com/schizand.htm.

Belinda Rowland
Rebecca J. Frey, PhD

Schizophrenia

Definition

Schizophrenia is a psychotic disorder (or group of disorders) marked by severely impaired thinking, emotions, and behaviors. The term schizophrenia comes from two Greek words that mean "split mind." It was coined around 1908 by a Swiss doctor named Eugen Bleuler to describe the splitting apart of mental functions that he regarded as the central characteristic of schizophrenia. (Note that the splitting apart of mental functions in schizophrenia differs from the split personality of people with multiple personality disorder.) Schizophrenic patients are typically unable to filter sensory stimuli and may have enhanced perceptions of sounds, colors, and other features of their environment. Most schizophrenics, if untreated, gradually withdraw from interactions with other people, and lose their ability to take care of personal needs and grooming.

Although schizophrenia was described by doctors as far back as Hippocrates (500 B.C.), it is difficult to classify. Many writers prefer the plural terms schizophrenias or schizophrenic disorders to the singular schizophrenia because of the lack of agreement in classification, as well as the possibility that different subtypes may eventually be shown to have different causes.

Description

The schizophrenic disorders are a major social tragedy because of the large number of persons affected and the severity of their impairment. It is estimated that people who suffer from schizophrenia fill 50% of the hospital beds in psychiatric units and 25% of all hospital beds. A number of studies indicate that about 1% of the world's population is affected by schizophrenia, without regard to race, social class, level of education, or cultural influences. (However, outcome may vary from culture to culture, depending on the familial support of the patient.) Most patients are diagnosed in their late teens or early 20s, but the symptoms of schizophrenia can emerge at any point in the life cycle. The male/female ratio in adults is about 1.2:1. Males typically have their first acute episode in their late teens or early 20s, while females are usually well into their 20s when diagnosed.

Schizophrenia is rarely diagnosed in preadolescent children, although patients as young as five or six have been reported. Childhood schizophrenia is at the upper end of the spectrum of severity and shows a greater gender disparity. It affects one or two children in every 10,000; the male/female ratio is 2:1.

The course of schizophrenia in adults can be divided into three phases or stages. In the acute phase, the patient has an overt loss of contact with reality (psychotic episode) that requires intervention and treatment. In the second or stabilization phase, the initial psychotic symptoms have been brought under control but the patient is at risk for relapse if treatment is interrupted. In the third or maintenance phase, the patient is relatively stable and can be kept indefinitely on antipsychotic medications. Even in the maintenance phase, however, relapses are not unusual and patients do not always return to full functioning.

Recently, some psychiatrists have begun to use a classification of schizophrenia based on two main types. People with Type I, or positive schizophrenia, have a rapid (acute) onset of symptoms and tend to respond well to drugs. They also tend to suffer more from the positive symptoms, such as delusions and hallucinations. People with Type II, or negative schizophrenia, are usually described as poorly adjusted before their schizophrenia slowly overtakes them. They have predominantly negative symptoms, such as withdrawal from others and a slowing of mental and physical reactions (psychomotor retardation).

The fourth revised (2000) edition of the *Diagnostic and Statistical Manual of Mental Disorders* (*DSM-IV*) specifies five subtypes of schizophrenia:

Paranoid

The key feature of this subtype of schizophrenia is the combination of false beliefs (delusions) and hearing voices (auditory hallucinations), with more nearly normal emotions and cognitive functioning. (Cognitive functions include reasoning, judgment, and memory.) The delusions of paranoid schizophrenics usually involve thoughts of being persecuted or harmed by others or exaggerated opinions of their own importance, but may also reflect feelings of jealousy or excessive religiosity. The delusions are typically organized into a coherent framework. Paranoid schizophrenics function at a higher level than other subtypes, but are at risk for suicidal or violent behavior under the influence of their delusions.

Disorganized

Disorganized schizophrenia (formerly called hebephrenic schizophrenia) is marked by disorganized speech, thinking, and behavior on the patient's part, coupled with flat or inappropriate emotional responses to a situation (affect). The patient may act silly or withdraw socially to an extreme extent. Most patients in this category have weak personality structures prior to their initial acute psychotic episode.

Catatonic

Catatonic schizophrenia is characterized by disturbances of movement that may include rigidity, stupor, agitation, bizarre posturing, and repetitive imitations of the movements or speech of other people. These patients are at risk for malnutrition, exhaustion, or self-injury. This subtype is presently uncommon in Europe and the United States. Catatonia as a symptom is most commonly associated with mood disorders.

Undifferentiated

Patients in this category have the characteristic positive and negative symptoms of schizophrenia but do not meet the specific criteria for the paranoid, disorganized, or catatonic subtypes.

Residual

This category is used for patients who have had at least one acute schizophrenic episode but do not presently have such strong positive psychotic symptoms as delusions and hallucinations. They may have negative symptoms, such as withdrawal from others, or mild forms of positive symptoms, which indicate that the disorder has not completely resolved.

Causes & symptoms

One of the reasons for the ongoing difficulty in classifying schizophrenic disorders is incomplete understanding of their causes. It is thought that these disorders are the end result of a combination of genetic, neurobiological, and environmental causes. A leading neurobiological hypothesis looks at the connection between the disease and excessive levels of dopamine, a chemical that transmits signals in the brain (neurotransmitter). The genetic factor in schizophrenia has been underscored by recent findings that first-degree biological relatives of schizophrenics are 10 times as likely to develop the disorder as are members of the general population.

Prior to recent findings of abnormalities in the brain structure of schizophrenic patients, several generations of psychiatrists advanced a number of psychoanalytic and sociological theories about the origins of schizophrenia. These theories ranged from hypotheses about the patient's problems with **anxiety** or aggression to theories about **stress** reactions or interactions with disturbed parents. Psychosocial factors are now thought to influence the expression or severity of schizophrenia, rather than cause it directly.

Another hypothesis suggests that schizophrenia may be caused by a virus that attacks the hippocampus, a part of the brain that processes sense perceptions. Damage to the hippocampus would account for schizophrenic patients' vulnerability to sensory overload. As of mid-1998, researchers were preparing to test antiviral medications on schizophrenics.

In 2002, scientists at the University of Southern California (UCLA) used a special technique to determine that people with schizophrenia have significantly less gray matter in certain regions of the brain than others, even than their identical twins. This discovery shows that gray matter reductions are partly due to genetics and partly due to environmental factors. It also helps show the difficulty schizophrenic patients face in focusing and organizing information in their brains. The scientists hope that their work will eventually lead to targeting of exactly how and where gray matter loss occurs so that maybe researchers can develop methods to stop the process and prevent or reduce loss of brain function in those areas.

Patients with a possible diagnosis of schizophrenia are evaluated on the basis of a set or constellation of symptoms; there is no single symptom that is unique to schizophrenia. In 1959, the German psychiatrist Kurt Schneider proposed a list of so-called first-rank symptoms, which he regarded as diagnostic of the disorder:

• delusions

• somatic hallucinations

• hearing voices commenting on behavior

• thought insertion or withdrawal

Somatic hallucinations refer to sensations or perceptions concerning body organs that have no known medical cause or reason, such as the notion that one's brain is radioactive. Thought insertion and/or withdrawal refer to delusions that an outside force (for example, the FBI, the CIA, Martians, etc.) has the power to put thoughts into one's mind or remove them.

POSITIVE SYMPTOMS. The positive symptoms of schizophrenia are those that represent an excessive or distorted version of normal functions. Positive symptoms include Schneider's first-rank symptoms as well as disorganized thought processes (reflected mainly in speech) and disorganized or catatonic behavior. Disorganized thought processes are marked by such characteristics as looseness of associations, in which the patient rambles from topic to topic in a disconnected way; tangentiality, which means that the patient gives unrelated answers to questions; and word salad, in which the patient's speech is so incoherent that it makes no grammatical or linguistic sense. Disorganized behavior means that the patient has difficulty with any type of purposeful or goal-oriented behavior, including personal self-care or preparing meals. Other forms of disorganized behavior may include dressing in odd or inappropriate ways, sexual self-stimulation in public, or agitated shouting or cursing.

NEGATIVE SYMPTOMS. The *DSM-IV* definition of schizophrenia includes three so-called negative symptoms. They are called negative because they represent the lack or absence of behaviors. The negative symptoms that are considered diagnostic of schizophrenia are a lack of emotional response (affective flattening), poverty of speech, and absence of volition or will. In general, the negative symptoms are more difficult for doctors to evaluate than the positive symptoms.

Diagnosis

A doctor must make a diagnosis of schizophrenia on the basis of a standardized list of outwardly observable symptoms, not on the basis of internal psychological processes. There are no specific laboratory tests that can be used to diagnose schizophrenia. Researchers have, however, discovered that patients with schizophrenia have certain abnormalities in the structure and functioning of the brain compared to normal test subjects. These discoveries have been made with the help of such imaging techniques as computed tomography (CT) scans, magnetic resonance imaging (MRI), and positron emission tomography (PET) scans.

When a psychiatrist assesses a patient for schizophrenia, he or she will begin by excluding physical conditions that can cause abnormal thinking and some other behaviors associated with schizophrenia. These conditions include organic brain disorders (including traumatic injuries of the brain), temporal lobe **epilepsy**, Wilson's disease, Huntington's chorea, and encephalitis. The doctor will also need to rule out substance abuse disorders, especially amphetamine use.

After ruling out organic disorders, the doctor will consider other psychiatric conditions that may include psychotic symptoms or symptoms resembling psychosis. These disorders include mood disorders with psychotic features; delusional disorder; dissociative disorder not otherwise specified (DDNOS) or multiple personality disorder; schizotypal, schizoid, or paranoid personality disorders; and atypical reactive disorders. In the past, many individuals were incorrectly diagnosed as schizophrenic. Some patients who were diagnosed prior to the changes in categorization introduced by *DSM-IV* should have their diagnoses and treatment reevaluated. In children, the doctor must distinguish between psychotic symptoms and a vivid fantasy life, and also identify learning problems or disorders. After other conditions have been ruled out, the patient must meet a set of criteria specified by *DSM-IV*:

- Characteristic symptoms. The patient must have two (or more) of the following symptoms during a one-month period: delusions; hallucinations; disorganized speech; disorganized or catatonic behavior; negative symptoms.

- Decline in social, interpersonal, or occupational functioning, including self-care.

- Duration. The disturbed behavior must last for at least six months.

- Diagnostic exclusions. Mood disorders, substance abuse disorders, medical conditions, and developmental disorders have been ruled out.

Treatment

The treatment of schizophrenia depends in part on the patient's stage or phase. Patients in the acute phase are hospitalized in most cases, to prevent harm to the patient or others and to begin treatment with antipsychotic medications. A patient having a first psychotic episode should be given a CT or MRI scan to rule out structural brain disease.

Psychotic patients require conventional antipsychotic medications. Once a patient is stabilized and nonpsychotic, other alternative treatments may be used. A 2002 study reported that patients who received **ginkgo biloba** extract showed enhanced effectiveness and reduced toxicity of haloperidol. This raised the possibility that ginkgo might be useful as an adjunct to antipsychotic drugs. **Essential fatty acids** (**fish oil**, flax oil, etc.), multivitamins with a high vitamin B potency, and ginseng may help to balance the mind and decrease or improve the side effects of antipsychotic medication, but should not be taken without consultation with a doctor. Grounding and stress-reducing therapies such as breathwork and **movement therapy** (**yoga, t'ai chi**, and **qigong**) are also beneficial. However, long-term compliance with a medication regime is critical to controlling the disorder.

Allopathic treatment

The primary form of treatment for schizophrenia is antipsychotic medication. Antipsychotic drugs help to control almost all the positive symptoms of the disorder. They have minimal effects on disorganized behavior and negative symptoms. Between 60–70% of schizophrenics will respond to antipsychotics. In the acute phase of the illness, patients are usually given medications by mouth or by intramuscular injection.

One of the most difficult challenges in treating schizophrenia patients with medications is helping them stay on medication. After the patient has been stabilized, an antipsychotic drug may be given in a long-acting form called a depot dose. Depot medications last for two to four weeks; they have the advantage of protecting the patient against the consequences of forgetting or skipping daily doses. In addition, some patients who do not respond to oral neuroleptics have better results with depot form. In 2002, scientists at the University of Pennsylvania Medical School designed an implantable device that can deliver medication to patients over a five-month period. While still in clinical trials, the device showed promise in allowing for measured, consistent doses of antipsychotic drugs to schizophrenic patients. The device can be implanted in a simple 15-minute procedure under local anesthesia. Most people with schizophrenia are kept indefinitely on antipsychotic medications during the maintenance phase of their disorder to minimize the possibility of relapse.

The most frequently used antipsychotics fall into two classes: the older dopamine receptor antagonists, or DAs, and the newer serotonin dopamine antagonists, or SDAs. (Antagonists block the action of some other substance; for example, dopamine antagonists counteract the action of dopamine.) The exact mechanisms of action of these medications are not known, but it is thought that they lower the patient's sensitivity to sensory stimuli and so indirectly improve the patient's ability to interact with others.

The dopamine antagonists include the older antipsychotic (also called neuroleptic) drugs, such as haloperidol (Haldol), chlorpromazine (Thorazine), and fluphenazine (Prolixin). These drugs have two major drawbacks: it is often difficult to find the best dosage level for the individual patient, and a dosage level high enough to control psychotic symptoms frequently produces extrapyramidal side effects, or EPSs. EPSs include parkinsonism, in which the patient cannot walk normally and usually develops a tremor; dystonia, or painful muscle spasms of the head, tongue, or neck; and akathisia, or restlessness. A type of long-term EPS is called tardive dyskinesia, which features slow rhythmic automatic movements. Schizophrenics with **AIDS** are especially vulnerable to developing EPS.

The serotonin dopamine antagonists, also called atypical antipsychotics, are newer medications that include clozapine (Clozaril), risperidone (Risperdal), and olanzapine (Zyprexa). The SDAs have a better effect on the negative symptoms of schizophrenia than do the older drugs and are less likely to produce EPS than the older compounds. These drugs are significantly more expensive in the short term, although the SDAs may reduce long-term costs by reducing the need for hospitalization.

Most schizophrenics can benefit from **psychotherapy** once their acute symptoms have been brought under control by antipsychotic medication. Psychoanalytic approaches are not recommended. Behavior therapy, however, is often helpful in assisting patients to acquire skills for daily living and social interaction. It can be combined with occupational therapy to prepare the patient for eventual employment.

Family therapy is often recommended for the families of schizophrenic patients, to relieve the feelings of guilt that they often have as well as to help them understand the patient's disorder. The family's attitude and be-haviors toward the patient are key factors in minimizing relapses (for example, by reducing stress in the patient's life), and family therapy can often strengthen the family's ability to cope with the stresses caused by the schizophrenic's illness. Family therapy focused on communication skills and problem-solving strategies is particularly helpful. In addition to formal treatment, many families benefit from support groups and similar mutual help organizations for relatives of schizophrenics.

Expected results

Patients with early onset of schizophrenia are more often male, have a lower level of functioning prior to onset, a higher rate of brain abnormalities, more noticeable negative symptoms, and worse outcomes. Patients with later onset are more likely to be female, with fewer brain abnormalities and thought impairment, and more hopeful prognoses.

The average course and outcome for schizophrenics are less favorable than those for most other mental disorders, although as many as 30% of patients diagnosed with schizophrenia recover completely and the majority experience some improvement. Schizophrenics with a high number of stressful changes in their lives, or who have frequent contacts with critical or emotionally involved family members, are more likely to relapse. Overall, the most important component of long-term care of schizophrenic patients is complying with their regimen of antipsychotic medications.

Resources

BOOKS

Clark, R. Barkley. "Psychosocial Aspects of Pediatrics & Psychiatric Disorders." *Current Pediatric Diagnosis & Treatment.* Edited by William W. Hay Jr., et al. Stamford, CT: Appleton & Lange, 1997.

Day, Max, and Elvin V. Semrad. "Schizophrenia: Comprehensive Psychotherapy." *The Encyclopedia of Psychiatry, Psychology, and Psychoanalysis.* Edited by Benjamin B. Wolman. New York: Henry Holt and Company, 1996.

Eisendrath, Stuart J. "Psychiatric Disorders." *Current Medical Diagnosis & Treatment 1998.* Edited by Lawrence M. Tierney Jr., et al. Stamford, CT: Appleton & Lange, 1997.

Marder, Stephen R. "Schizophrenia." *Conn's Current Therapy.* Edited by Robert E. Rakel. Philadelphia: W. B. Saunders Company, 1998.

"Schizophrenia and Other Psychotic Disorders." *Diagnostic and Statistical Manual of Mental Disorders.* 4th ed. rev Washington, DC: The American Psychiatric Association, 2000.

Schultz, Clarence G. "Schizophrenia: Psychoanalytic Views." *The Encyclopedia of Psychiatry, Psychology, and Psychoanalysis.* Edited by Benjamin B. Wolman. New York: Henry Holt and Company, 1996.

KEY TERMS

Affective flattening—A loss or lack of emotional expressiveness. It is sometimes called blunted or restricted affect.

Akathisia—Agitated or restless movement, usually affecting the legs and accompanied by a sense of discomfort. It is a common side effect of neuroleptic medications.

Dopamine receptor antagonists (DAs)—The older class of antipsychotic medications, also called neuroleptics. These primarily block the site on nerve cells that normally receives the brain chemical dopamine.

Dystonia—Painful involuntary muscle cramps or spasms. Dystonia is one of the extrapyramidal side effects associated with antipsychotic medications.

Extrapyramidal symptoms (EPSs)—A group of side effects associated with antipsychotic medications. EPSs include parkinsonism, akathisia, dystonia, and tardive dyskinesia.

Huntington's chorea—A hereditary disease that typically appears in midlife, marked by gradual loss of brain function and voluntary movement. Some of its symptoms resemble those of schizophrenia.

Neuroleptic—Another name for the older type of antipsychotic medications given to schizophrenic patients.

Parkinsonism—A set of symptoms originally associated with Parkinson's disease that can occur as side effects of neuroleptic medications. The symptoms include trembling of the fingers or hands, a shuffling gait, and tight or rigid muscles.

Serotonin dopamine antagonists (SDAs)—The newer second-generation antipsychotic drugs, also called atypical antipsychotics. SDAs include clozapine (Clozaril), risperidone (Risperdal), and olanzapine (Zyprexa).

Wilson's disease—A rare hereditary disease marked by high levels of copper deposits in the brain and liver. It can cause psychiatric symptoms resembling those of schizophrenia.

PERIODICALS

"Brain Defects Identified by UCLA Scientists." *Pain & Central Nervous System Week* (April 1, 2002):3.

Gaby, Alan R. "Ginkgo for Schizophrenia (Literature Review & Commentary)." *Townsend Letter for Doctors and Patients*. (June 2002):31.

"Implant May Stabilize Treatment." *Pain & Central Nervous System Week*, (June 17, 2002):2.

Winerip, Michael. "Schizophrenia's Most Zealous Foe." *The New York Times Magazine*. (February 22, 1998): 26-29.

Paula Ford-Martin
Teresa G. Odle

Sciatica

Definition

Sciatica refers to **pain** or discomfort associated with the sciatic nerve. This nerve runs from the lower part of the spinal cord down the back and side of the leg to the foot. Injury to or pressure on the sciatic nerve can cause the characteristic pain of sciatica: a sharp or burning pain or even numbness that radiates from the lower back or hip, possibly following the path of the sciatic nerve to the foot.

Description

The sciatic nerve is the largest and longest nerve in the body. About the thickness of a person's thumb, it spans from the lower back to the foot. The nerve originates in the lower part of the spinal cord, the so-called lumbar region. As the sciatic nerve branches off from the spinal cord, it passes between the bony vertebrae (the component bones of the spine) and runs through the pelvic girdle, or hip bones, and the buttock area. The nerve passes through the hip joint and continues down the back and side of the leg to the foot.

Sciatica is a fairly common disorder, approximately 40% of the population experiences it at some point in their lives. However, only about 1% have coexisting sensory or motor deficits. Sciatic pain has several root causes and treatment may hinge upon the underlying problem.

Of the identifiable causes of sciatic pain, lumbosacral radiculopathy and back strain are the most frequently suspected. The term lumbosacral refers to the lower part of the spine, and radiculopathy describes a problem with the spinal nerve roots that pass between the vertebrae and give rise to the sciatic nerve. This area between the vertebrae is cushioned with a disk of shock-absorbing tissue. If this disk shifts or is damaged through injury or disease, the spinal nerve root may be compressed by the shifted tissue or the vertebrae.

This compression of the nerve roots sends a pain signal to the brain. Although the actual injury is to the nerve roots, the pain may be perceived as coming from any point along the sciatic nerve.

The sciatic nerve can be compressed in other ways. Back strain may cause muscle spasms in the lower back, placing pressure on the sciatic nerve. In rare cases, infection, **cancer**, bone inflammation, or other diseases may cause the pressure. More likely, but often overlooked, is the piriformis syndrome. As the sciatic nerve passes through the hip joint, it shares the space with several muscles. One of these muscles, the piriformis muscle, is closely associated with the sciatic nerve. In some people, the nerve actually runs through the muscle. If this muscle is injured or has a spasm, it places pressure on the sciatic nerve—in effect, compressing it.

In many sciatica cases, the specific cause is never identified. About half of affected individuals recover from an episode within a month. Some cases can linger a few weeks longer and may require aggressive treatment. In other cases, the pain may return or potentially become chronic.

Causes & symptoms

Persons with sciatica may experience some lower back pain, but the most common symptom is pain that radiates through one buttock and down the back of the adjoining leg. The most identified cause of the pain is compression or pressure on the sciatic nerve. The extent of the pain varies among individuals. Some people describe pain that centers in the area of the hip, and others perceive discomfort all the way to the foot. The quality of the pain also varies; it may be described as tingling, burning, prickly, aching, or stabbing.

Onset of sciatica can be sudden, but it can also develop gradually. The pain may be intermittent or continuous. Certain activities, such as bending, coughing, **sneezing**, or sitting, may make the pain worse.

Chronic pain may arise from more than just compression on the nerve. According to some pain researchers, physical damage to a nerve is only half of the equation. A recent theory proposes that some nerve injuries result in a release of neurotransmitters and immune system chemicals that enhance and sustain a pain message. Even after the injury has healed or the damage has been repaired, the pain continues. Control of this abnormal type of pain is difficult.

Diagnosis

Before treating sciatic pain, as much information as possible must be collected. The individual is asked to recount the location and nature of the pain, how long it has continued, and any accidents or unusual activities prior to its onset. This information provides clues that may

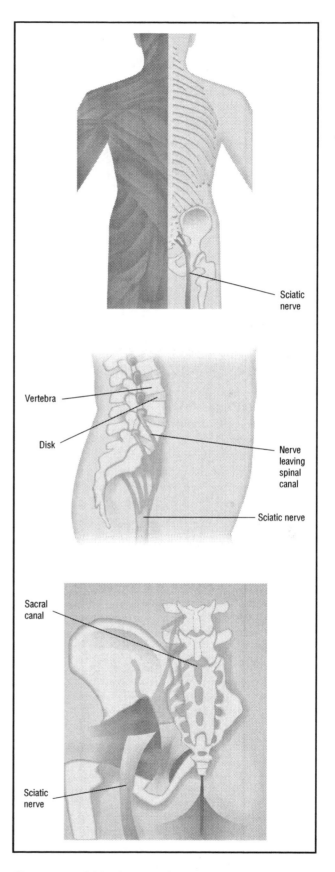

(Illustration by GGS Information Services, Inc. The Gale Group.)

point to back strain or injury to a specific location. Back pain from disk disease, piriformis syndrome, and back strain must be differentiated from more serious conditions such as cancer or infection. Lumbar stenosis, an overgrowth of the covering layers of the vertebrae that narrows the spinal canal, must also be considered. The possibility that a difference in leg lengths is causing the pain should be evaluated; the problem can be easily be treated with a foot orthotic or built-up shoe.

Often, a straight-leg-raising test is done, in which the person lies face upward and the healthcare provider raises the affected leg to various heights. This test pinpoints the location of the pain and may reveal whether it is caused by a disk problem. Other tests, such as having the individual rotate the hip joint, assess the condition of the hip muscles. Any pain caused by these movements may provide information about involvement of the piriformis muscle, and piriformis weakness is tested with additional leg-strength maneuvers.

Further tests may be done depending on the results of the physical examination and initial pain treatment. Such tests might include magnetic resonance imaging (MRI) and computed tomography (CT) scans. Other tests examine the conduction of electricity through nerve tissues, and include studies of the electrical activity generated as muscles contract (electromyography), nerve conduction velocity, and evoked potential testing. A more invasive test involves injecting a contrast substance into the space between the vertebrae and making x-ray images of the spinal cord (myelography), but this procedure is usually done only if surgery is being considered as an option. All of these tests can reveal problems with the vertebrae, the disk, or the nerve itself.

Treatment

Massage is a recommended form of therapy, especially if the sciatic pain arises from muscle spasm. Symptoms may also be relieved by icing the painful area as soon as the pain occurs. Ice should be left on the area for 30–60 minutes several times a day. After two or three days, a hot water bottle or heating pad can replace the ice. **Chiropractic** or **osteopathy** may offer possible solutions for relieving pressure on the sciatic nerve and alleviating the accompanying pain. **Biofeedback** may also be useful as a pain control method. Bodywork, such as the **Alexander technique**, can assist an individual in improving posture and preventing further episodes of sciatic pain.

Acupuncture is another alternative approach that appears to offer relief to many persons with sciatica, as indicated by several clinical trials in the United States and Europe. The World Health Organization (WHO) lists sciatica as one of 40 conditions for which acupuncture is recognized as an appropriate complementary treatment.

Practitioners of **Ayurvedic medicine** regard sciatica as a disorder resulting from an imbalance in vata, one of three doshas or energies in the human body. The traditional Ayurvedic treatment for vata disorders is vasti, or administration of an oil-based enema to cleanse the colon. An Ayurvedic herbal preparation that is used to treat sciatica is made from the leaves of *Nyctanthes arbor tristis*, which is also known as Parijat or "sad tree." A recent study of an alcohol-based extract of this plant indicates that it is effective as a tranquilizer and local anesthetic, which supports its traditional Ayurvedic use.

Western herbalists typically treat sciatica with **valerian** root to relax the muscle spasms that often accompany sciatica, and with **white willow** bark for pain relief.

Homeopathic remedies for sciatica include *Ruta graveolens*, *Colocynth* (for sciatic pain that is worse in cold or damp weather), or *Magnesium phosphoric* (for lightning-like pains that are soothed by heat and made worse by coughing).

Allopathic treatment

Initial treatment for sciatica focuses on pain relief. For acute or very painful flare-ups, bed rest is advised for up to a week in conjunction with medication for the pain. Pain medication includes acetaminophen, nonsteroidal anti-inflammatory drugs (NSAIDs), such as aspirin, or muscle relaxants. If the pain is unremitting, opioids may be prescribed for short-term use, or a local anesthetic will be injected directly into the lower back. Massage and heat application may be suggested as adjuncts.

If the pain is chronic, different pain relief medications are used to avoid long-term dosing of NSAIDs, muscle relaxants, and opioids. Antidepressant drugs, which have been shown to be effective in treating pain, may be prescribed alongside short-term use of muscle relaxants or NSAIDs. Local anesthetic injections or epidural steroids are used in selected cases.

As the pain allows, physical therapy is introduced into the treatment regime. Stretching exercises that focus on the lower back, buttock, and hamstring muscles are suggested. The exercises also include finding comfortable, pain-reducing positions. Corsets and braces may be useful in some cases, but evidence for their general effectiveness is lacking. However, they may be helpful to prevent exacerbations related to certain activities.

With less pain and the success of early therapy, the individual is encouraged to follow a long-term program to maintain a healthy back and prevent re-injury. A physical therapist may suggest exercises and regular activity, such as water **exercise** or walking. Patients are instructed in proper body mechanics to minimize symptoms during light lifting or other activities.

If the pain is chronic and conservative treatment fails, surgery to repair a **herniated disk** or to cut out part or all of the piriformis muscle may be suggested, particularly if there is evidence of nerve or nerve-root damage.

A new minimally invasive surgical treatment for sciatica was introduced in 2002. It is known as microscopically assisted percutaneous nucleotomy, or MAPN. MAPN allows the surgeon to repair a herniated disk with less damage to surrounding tissues; it shortens the patient's recovery time and relieves the pain of sciatica as effectively as more invasive surgical procedures.

Expected results

Most cases of sciatica are treatable with pain medication and physical therapy. After four to six weeks of treatment, an individual should be able to resume normal activities.

Prevention

Some sources of sciatica are not preventable, such as disk degeneration, back strain due to **pregnancy**, or accidental falls. Other sources of back strain, such as poor posture, overexertion, being overweight, or wearing high heels, can be corrected or avoided. Cigarette **smoking** may also predispose people to pain, and should be discontinued with the onset of pain.

General suggestions for avoiding sciatica or preventing a repeat episode include sleeping on a firm mattress; using chairs with firm back support; and sitting with both feet flat on the floor. Habitually crossing the legs while sitting can place excess pressure on the sciatic nerve. Sitting for long periods of time can also place pressure on the sciatic nerves, so it is recommended to take short breaks and move around during the work day, during long trips, or in other situations that require sitting for extended periods of time. If lifting is required, the back should be kept straight and the legs should provide the lift. Regular exercise, such as swimming and walking, can strengthen back muscles and improve posture. Exercise can also help maintain a healthy weight and lessen the likelihood of back strain.

Resources

BOOKS

Maigne, Robert. "Sciatica." In *Diagnosis and Treatment of Pain of Vertebral Origin: A Manual Medicine Approach.* Baltimore: Williams & Wilkins, 1996.

Pelletier, Kenneth R., MD. *The Best Alternative Medicine*, Part II, "CAM Therapies for Specific Conditions: Sciatica." New York: Simon & Schuster, 2002.

KEY TERMS

Bodywork—Any healing technique involving hands-on massage or manipulation of the body. Types of bodywork that involve movement reeducation or movement patterning are also categorized as movement therapy.

Disk—Dense tissue between the vertebrae that acts as a shock absorber and prevents damage to nerves and blood vessels along the spine.

Electromyography—A medical test in which a nerve's ability to conduct an impulse is measured.

Lumbosacral—Referring to the lower part of the backbone or spine.

Myelography—A medical test in which a special dye is injected into a nerve to make it visible on an x ray.

Piriformis—A muscle in the pelvic girdle, or hip bones, that is closely associated with the sciatic nerve.

Radiculopathy—A condition in which the spinal nerve root of a nerve has been injured or damaged.

Spasm—Involuntary contraction of a muscle.

Vertebrae—The component bones of the spine.

Rydevik, Björn, Mitsuo Hasue, and Peter Wehling. *Etiology of Sciatic Pain and Mechanisms of Nerve Root Compression,* vol. 1: The Lumbar Spine, 2d ed., edited by Sam W. Wiesel, et al. Philadelphia: W.B. Saunders Company, 1996.

PERIODICALS

Chiodo, A., and A. J. Haig. "Lumbosacral Radiculopathies: Conservative Approaches to Management." *Physical Medicine and Rehabilitation Clinics of North America* 13 (August 2002): 609-621.

Douglas, Sara. "Sciatic Pain and Piriformis Syndrome." *The Nurse Practitioner* 22 (May 1997): 166.

Greiner-Perth, R., H. Bohm, and H. El Saghir. "Microscopically Assisted Percutaneous Nucleotomy, An Alternative Minimally Invasive Procedure for the Operative Treatment of Lumbar Disc Herniation: Preliminary Results." *Neurosurgical Review* 25 (August 2002): 225-227.

Parziale, John R., Thomas H. Hudgins, and Loren M. Fishman. "The Piriformis Syndrome." *The American Journal of Orthopedics* (December 1996): 819.

Saxena, R. S., B. Gupta, and S. Lata. "Tranquilizing, Antihistaminic and Purgative Activity of *Nyctanthes arbor tristis* Leaf Extract." *Journal of Ethnopharmacology* 81 (August 2002): 321-325.

Wheeler, Anthony H. "Diagnosis and Management of Low Back Pain and Sciatica." *American Family Physician* (October 1995): 1333.

ORGANIZATIONS

American Academy of Medical Acupuncture (AAMA). 4929 Wilshire Blvd., Suite 428, Los Angeles, CA 90010. (323) 937-5514. <www.medicalacupuncture.org>.

American Academy of Orthopaedic Surgeons (AAOS). 6300 North River Road, Rosemont, IL 60018. (847) 823-7186 or (800) 346-AAOS. <www.aaos.org>.

American Physical Therapy Association (APTA). 1111 North Fairfax Street, Alexandria, VA 22314. (703)684-APTA or (800) 999-2782. <www.apta.org>.

National Center for Homeopathy. 801 North Fairfax Street, Alexandria, VA 22314. (703) 548-7790. <www.homeopathic.org>.

National Institute of Ayurvedic Medicine. 584 Milltown Road, Brewster, NY 10509. (845) 278-8700. <www.niam.com>.

Kathleen Wright
Rebecca J. Frey, PhD

Scoliosis

Definition

Scoliosis is defined as an abnormal side-to-side or front-to-back curvature of the spine.

Description

When viewed from the rear, the spine usually appears perfectly straight. Scoliosis is a lateral (side-to-side) curve in the spine, usually combined with a rotation of the vertebrae. The lateral curvature of scoliosis should not be confused with the normal set of front-to-back spinal curves visible from the side. While a small degree of lateral curvature does not cause any medical problems, larger curves can cause postural imbalance and lead to muscle **fatigue** and **pain**. More severe scoliosis can interfere with breathing and lead to arthritis of the spine (spondylosis).

Approximately 10% of all adolescents have some degree of scoliosis, though fewer than 1% have curves that require medical attention beyond monitoring. Scoliosis is found in both boys and girls, but a girl's spinal curve is much more likely to progress than a boy's. Girls require scoliosis treatment about five times as often. The reason for these differences is not known.

Causes & symptoms

Four out of five cases of scoliosis are *idiopathic*, meaning that the cause is unknown. Idiopathic scoliosis tends to run in families; genetic screening has identified several different patterns of genetic transmission as of late 2001. In some families, idiopathic scoliosis is transmitted in an autosomal dominant pattern, while in others the mode of inheritance is X-linked. Children with idiopathic scoliosis appear to be otherwise entirely healthy, and have not had any bone or joint disease early in life. Scoliosis is not caused by poor posture, diet, or carrying a heavy book-bag exclusively on one shoulder.

Idiopathic scoliosis is further classified according to age of onset:

- Infantile. Curvature appears before age three. This type is quite rare in the United States, but is more common in Europe.

- Juvenile. Curvature appears between ages three and 10. This type may be equivalent to the adolescent type, except for the age of onset.

- Adolescent. Curvature appears between ages of 10 and 13, near the beginning of puberty. This is the most common type of idiopathic scoliosis.

- Adult. Curvature begins after physical maturation is completed.

Causes are known for three other types of scoliosis:

- Congenital scoliosis is due to congenital birth defects in the spine, often associated with other organ defects.

- Neuromuscular scoliosis is due to loss of control of the nerves or muscles that support the spine. The most common causes of this type of scoliosis are **cerebral palsy** and muscular dystrophy.

- Degenerative scoliosis may be caused by degeneration of the discs that separate the vertebrae or arthritis in the joints that link them.

Scoliosis causes a noticeable asymmetry in the torso when viewed from the front or back. The first sign of scoliosis is often seen when a child is wearing a bathing suit or underwear. A child may appear to be standing with one shoulder higher than the other, or to have a tilt in the waistline. One shoulder blade may appear more prominent than the other due to rotation. In girls, one breast may appear higher than the other, or larger if rotation pushes that side forward.

Curve progression is greatest near the adolescent growth spurt. Scoliosis that begins early is more likely to progress significantly than scoliosis that begins later in puberty.

More than 30 states have screening programs in schools for adolescent scoliosis, usually conducted by trained school nurses or physical education teachers.

Diagnosis

Diagnosis for scoliosis is typically continued by an orthopedist. A complete medical history is taken, including questions abouta a family history of scoliosis. The physical examination includes determination of pubertal development in adolescents, a neurological examination (which may reveal a neuromuscular cause), and measurements of trunk asymmetry. Examination of the trunk is done while the patient is standing, bending over, and lying down. The forward bending test is sometimes referred to as the Adams test. It involves both visual inspection and use of a simple mechanical device called a scoliometer.

If a curve is detected, one or more x rays will usually be taken to define the curve or curves more precisely. An x ray is used to document spinal maturity, any pelvic tilt or hip asymmetry, and the location, extent, and degree of curvature. The curve is defined in terms of its beginning and ending points, its direction, and by an angle measure known as the Cobb angle. The Cobb angle is found by projecting lines parallel to the vertebrae tops at the extremes of the curve, projecting perpendiculars from these lines, and measuring the angle of intersection. To properly track the progress of scoliosis, it is important to project from the same points of the spine each time.

Occasionally, magnetic resonance imaging (MRI) is used, primarily to look more closely at the condition of the spinal cord and nerve roots extending from it if neurological problems are suspected.

Treatment

Although important for general health and strength, **exercise** has not been shown to prevent or slow the progression of scoliosis. It may help to relieve pain from scoliosis by helping to maintain range of motion. Good **nutrition** is also important for general health, but no specific dietary regimen has been shown to control scoliosis development. In particular, dietary **calcium** levels do not influence scoliosis progression.

Chiropractic treatment may relieve pain but cannot halt scoliosis development, and should not be a substitute for conventional treatment of progressive scoliosis. **Acupuncture** and **acupressure** may also help reduce pain and discomfort, but they cannot halt scoliosis development either.

Other movement therapies (**yoga, t'ai chi, qigong,** and dance) improve flexibility and are useful when used with such movement education therapies as **Feldenkrais,** the **Rosen method,** the **Alexander technique,** and **Pilates.**

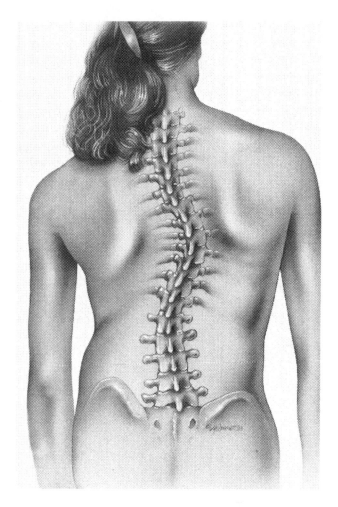

Illustration of spinal curvature occurring with scoliosis. *(J. Mc-Dermott. Custom Medical Stock Photo. Reproduced by permission.)*

Allopathic treatment

Treatment decisions for scoliosis are based on the degree of curvature, the likelihood of significant progression, and the presence of pain, if any.

Curves less than 20° are not usually treated, except by regular follow-up for children who are still growing. Watchful waiting is usually all that is required in adolescents with curves of 20–30°, or adults with curves up to 40° or slightly more, as long as there is no pain.

For children or adolescents whose curves progress to 30°, and who have a year or more of growth left, bracing may be required. Bracing cannot correct curvature but may be effective in halting or slowing progression. Bracing is rarely used in adults, except where pain is significant and surgery is not an option, as in some elderly patients.

Two general styles of braces are used for daytime wear. The Milwaukee brace consists of metal uprights attached to pads at the hips, rib cage, and neck. The under-arm brace uses rigid plastic to encircle the lower rib cage, abdomen, and hips. Both of these brace types hold the spine in a vertical position. Because it can be worn out of sight beneath clothing, the underarm brace is better tolerated and often leads to better compliance. A third style, the Charleston bending brace, is used at night to bend the spine in the opposite direction. Braces are often prescribed to be worn for 22–23 hours per day, though some clinicians allow or encourage removal of the brace for exercise.

Bracing may be appropriate for scoliosis due to some types of neuromuscular disease, including spinal muscular atrophy, before growth is finished. Duchenne muscular dystrophy is not treated by bracing, since surgery is likely to be required and later surgery is complicated by loss of respiratory capacity.

Surgery for idiopathic scoliosis is usually recommended if:

• The curve has progressed despite bracing.

• The curve is greater than 40–50° before growth has stopped in an adolescent.

• The curve is greater than 50° and continues to increase in an adult.

• There is significant pain.

Orthopedic surgery for neuromuscular scoliosis is often done earlier. The goals of surgery are to correct the deformity as much as possible, to prevent further deformity, and to eliminate pain as much as possible. Surgery can usually correct 40–50% of the curve, sometimes as much as 80%. Surgery cannot always completely remove pain.

The surgical procedure for scoliosis is called spinal fusion, because the goal is to straighten the spine as much as possible, and then to fuse the vertebrae together to prevent further curvature. To achieve fusion, the involved vertebra are first exposed, and then scraped to promote regrowth. Bone chips are usually used to splint together the vertebrae to increase the likelihood of fusion. To maintain the proper spinal posture before fusion occurs, metal rods are inserted alongside the spine and attached to the vertebrae by hooks, screws, or wires. Fusion of the spine makes it rigid and resistant to further curvature. The metal rods are no longer needed once fusion is complete but are rarely removed unless their presence leads to complications.

Spinal fusion leaves the involved portion of the spine permanently stiff and inflexible. While this stiffness leads to some loss of normal motion, most functional activities are not strongly affected, unless the very lowest portion of the spine (the lumbar region) is fused.

KEY TERMS

Adams test—A screening test in which a child being examined for scoliosis is asked to bend forward with the feet together and the knees straight.

Cobb angle—A measure of the curvature of scoliosis, determined by measurements made on x rays.

Scoliometer—A tool for measuring trunk asymmetry; it includes a bubble level and angle measure.

Spondylosis—Arthritis of the spine.

Normal mobility, exercise, and even contact sports are usually all possible after spinal fusion. Full recovery takes approximately six months.

Expected results

The prognosis for a person with scoliosis depends on many factors, including the age at which scoliosis begins and the treatment received. More importantly, mostly unknown individual factors affect the likelihood of progression and the severity of the curve. Most cases of mild adolescent idiopathic scoliosis need no treatment and do not progress. Untreated severe scoliosis often leads to spondylosis and may impair breathing.

Prevention

There is no known way to prevent the development of scoliosis. Progression of scoliosis may be prevented through bracing or surgery.

Resources

BOOKS

Neuwirth, Michael, and Kevin Osborn. *The Scoliosis Handbook.* New York: Henry Holt & Co., 1996.

PERIODICALS

Justice, C.M., N. H. Miller, B. Marosy, et al. "Genetic Heterogeneity Comprising Both X-Linked and Autosomal Dominant Forms of Inheritance in Families with Familial Idiopathic Scoliosis." *American Journal of Human Genetics* 69 (October 2001): 384.

Splete, Heidi. "Catch Curves Like Scoliosis in Time for Bracing (Watch Your Patients' Backs)." *Pediatric News* 35 (November 2001): 42–43.

ORGANIZATIONS

National Scoliosis Foundation. 5 Cabot Place Stoughton, MA 02072. (800) 673-6922. NSF@scoliosis.org. <http://www.scoliosis.org>.

The Scoliosis Association. PO Box 811705 Boca Raton, FL 33481-1705. (407) 368-8518. normlipin@aol.com. <http://www.scoliosis-assoc.org>.

Scoliosis Research Society. 611 East Wells Street Milwaukee, WI 53202. (414) 289-9107. Tjackson@execinc.com. <http://www.srs.org>.

Paula Ford-Martin
Rebecca J. Frey, PhD

Scratches *see* **Cuts and scratches**

Scullcap *see* **Skullcap**

Seasickness *see* **Motion sickness**

Seasonal affective disorder

Definition

Seasonal affective disorder (SAD) is a form of depression most often associated with lack of daylight in extreme northern and southern latitudes from the late fall to the early spring.

Description

Although researchers are not certain what causes seasonal affective disorder, they suspect that it has something to do with the hormone **melatonin**. Melatonin is thought to play an active role in regulating the "internal body clock," which dictates when humans feel like going to bed at night and getting up in the morning. Although seasonal affective disorder is most common when light is low, it may occur in the spring, which is often called reverse or spring-onset SAD. Recent research also indicates that SAD has a genetic factor; about 29% of cases in the United States run in families.

Causes & symptoms

The body produces more melatonin at night than during the day, and scientists believe it helps people feel sleepy at nighttime. There is also more melatonin in the body during winter, when the days are shorter. Some researchers believe that excessive melatonin release during winter in people with SAD may account for their feelings of drowsiness or depression. One variation on this idea is that people's internal clocks may become out of sync during winter with the light-dark cycle, leading to a long-term disruption in melatonin release. Another possible cause of SAD is that people may not adjust their habits to the season, or sleep more hours when it is darker, as would be natural.

Seasonal affective disorder, while not an official category of mental illness listed by the American Psychi-

SYMPTOMS OF SEASONAL AFFECTIVE DISORDER (SAD)
Increased sleep
Depression
Lethargy
Weight gain
Carbohydrate cravings
Decreased sex drive
Avoidance of social interaction
Difficulty performing daily tasks
Crying fits
Suicidal thoughts

atric Association, is estimated to affect 6% of the American population. Another 25 million Americans may have a mild form of SAD, sometimes called the "winter blues" or "winter blahs." The risk of SAD increases the further from the equator a person lives; one early study of SAD found a 1.4% incidence of the disorder among people living in Florida, compared with 9.7% among residents of New Hampshire. Other factors that influence the incidence and severity of SAD are sex and age. Women are more likely than men to develop SAD, but men with the disorder are more severely depressed than most women who have it. SAD appears to decrease in severity with age; the elderly have milder SAD symptoms than adolescents.

Comparative studies indicate that the incidence of SAD in the United States and Canada is about twice as high as in European countries at the same latitudes north of the Equator. These findings suggest that cultural factors are also involved in the disorder.

The symptoms of SAD are similar to those of other forms of depression. People with SAD may feel sad, irritable, or tired, and may find themselves sleeping too much. They may also lose interest in normal or pleasurable activities (including sex), become withdrawn, crave carbohydrates, and gain weight.

Diagnosis

Doctors usually diagnose seasonal affective disorder based on the patient's description of symptoms, including the time of year they occur. There is also a diagnostic questionnaire called the Seasonal Pattern Assessment Questionnaire, or SPAQ, used in all Canadian university hospitals and widely used in the United States to assess SAD patients.

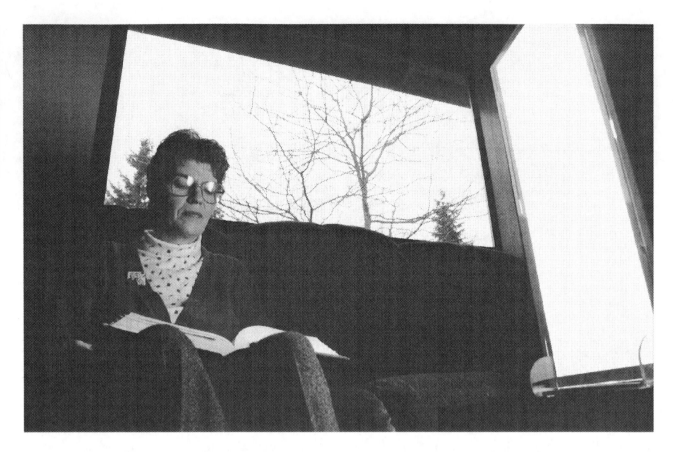

This woman is treating her seasonal affective disorder with exposure to a full-spectrum light box. *(A/P Wide World Photos. Reproduced by permission.)*

Treatment

The first-line treatment for seasonal affective disorder is **light therapy** (also known as phototherapy). The most commonly used phototherapy equipment is a portable lighting device known as a light box. The box may be mounted upright to a wall or slanted downward toward a table. The patient sits in front of the box for a pre-prescribed period of time (anywhere from 15 minutes to several hours). Some patients with SAD undergo light therapy sessions two or three times daily, others only once. The time of day and the number of times treatment is administered depend on the physical needs and lifestyle of the patient. Light therapy treatment for SAD typically begins in the fall as the days begin to shorten, and continues throughout the winter and possibly the early spring.

The light from a slanted light box is designed to fall on the table supporting the box, so patients may look down to read or do other sedentary activities during therapy. Patients using an upright light box must face the light source (although they need not look directly into the light). The light sources in these light boxes typically range from 2,500 to 10,000 lux (in contrast, average indoor lighting is 300 to 500 lux; a sunny summer day is about 100,000 lux).

A recent British study suggests that dawn simulation, a form of light therapy in which the patient is exposed to white light of gradually increasing brightness (peaking at 250 lux after 90 min) may be even more effective in treating SAD than exposure to bright light. Dawn simulation is started around 4:30 or 5 o'clock in the morning while the patient is still asleep.

Patients with eye problems should see an ophthalmologist regularly both before and during light therapy. Because some UV rays are emitted by the light boxes used in phototherapy, patients taking photosensitizing medications and those who have sun-sensitive skin should consult with a health care professional before beginning treatment. Patients with medical conditions that make them sensitive to UV rays should also see a doctor before starting phototherapy.

Light therapy appears to be safe for most people. However, it can cause side effects of eyestrain, headaches, **insomnia, fatigue, sunburn,** and dry eyes and nose in some patients. Most of these effects can be managed by adjusting the timing and duration of light therapy sessions. A strong sun block and eye and nose drops can alleviate the others.

Recently, researchers have begun testing whether people who do not completely respond to light therapy can benefit from tiny doses of the hormone melatonin to reset the body's internal clock. Early results look promising, but the potential benefits must be confirmed in larger studies before this type of treatment becomes widely accepted.

Allopathic treatment

Like other types of mood disorders, seasonal affective disorder may also respond to medication and **psychotherapy**. Common drugs prescribed for mood disorders are:

• Selective serotonin reuptake inhibitors (SSRIs), such as fluoxetine (Prozac), paroxetine (Paxil), and sertraline (Zoloft)

• Monoamine oxidase inhibitors (MAO inhibitors), such as phenelzine sulfate (Nardil) and tranylcypromine sulfate (Parnate)

• Lithium salts, such as lithium carbonate (Eskalith), often used in people with bipolar mood disorders, are often useful with SAD patients who also suffer from **bipolar disorder** (excessive mood swings; formerly known as manic depression)

A number of psychotherapy approaches are useful as well. Interpersonal psychotherapy helps patients recognize how their mood disorder and their interpersonal relationships interact. Cognitive-behavioral therapy explores how the patient's view of the world may be affecting mood and outlook.

A new treatment for SAD that is still in the experimental phase as of 2001 is the use of high-density negative air ionization.

Expected results

Most patients with seasonal affective disorder respond to light therapy, dawn simulation, and/or antidepressant drugs. Others respond to sleeping more hours in a dark room. Some researchers estimate that as much as 9.5 hours of sleep are important in winter months and that getting more sleep will increase the person's levels of natural melatonin.

Resources

BOOKS

Lam, Raymond, ed. *Seasonal Affective Disorder and Beyond: Light Treatment for SAD and Non-SAD Conditions.* Washington, DC: American Psychiatric Press, 1998.

KEY TERMS

Cognitive behavioral therapy—Psychotherapy aimed at helping people change their attitudes, perceptions, and patterns of thinking.

Dawn simulation—A form of light therapy in which the patient is exposed while asleep to gradually brightening white light over a period of an hour and a half.

Lux—The International System unit for measuring illumination, equal to one lumen per square meter.

Melatonin—A naturally occurring hormone involved in regulating the body's "internal clock."

Serotonin—A chemical messenger in the brain thought to play a role in regulating mood.

Partonen, Timo, and Andres Magnusson, eds. *Seasonal Affective Disorder: Practice and Research.* Oxford, UK: Oxford University Press, 2001.

Peters, Celeste A. *Don't Be SAD: Your Guide to Conquering Seasonal Affective Disorder.* Calgary, Alberta: Good Health Books, 1994.

Rosenthal, Norman. *Winter Blues: Seasonal Affective Disorder—What It Is and How to Overcome It.* New York: Guilford Press, 1998.

PERIODICALS

Anderson, Janis L., and Gabrielle I. Warner. "Seasonal Depression." *Harvard Health Letter* (February 1996): 7-8.

Eagles, John M. "SAD—Help arrives with the dawn?" *Lancet* 358 (December 22, 2001): 2100.

Singer, Ethan A. "Seasonal Affective Disorder: Autumn Onset, Winter Gloom." *Clinician Reviews* 11 (November 2001): 49-54.

"Winter Depression: Seeing the Light." *The University of California Berkeley Wellness Letter* (November 1996): 4.

ORGANIZATIONS

National Depressive and Manic Depressive Association. 730 N. Franklin Street, Ste. 501, Chicago, IL 60610. (312) 642-0049.

National Institute of Mental Health. Mental Health Public Inquiries, 5600 Fishers Lane, Room 15C-05, Rockville, MD 20857. (301) 443-4513. (888) 826-9438. <http://www.nimh.nih.gov>.

Society for Light Treatment and Biological Rhythms. 824 Howard Ave., New Haven, CT 06519. Fax (203) 764-4324. <http://www.sltbr.org. sltbr@yale.edu>.

Paula Ford-Martin
Rebecca J. Frey, PhD

Seaweed *see* **Kelp**

Seaweed, sargassum *see* **Sargassum seaweed**

Seborrhea *see* **Cradle cap**

Seizure disorder *see* **Epilepsy**

Selenium

Description

Selenium is a nonmetallic element with an atomic number of 34 and an atomic weight of 78.96. Its chemical symbol is Se. Selenium is most commonly found in nature in its inorganic form, **sodium** selenite. An organic form of selenium, selenomethionine, is found in foods.

General use

The role of selenium in human **nutrition** and other therapeutic applications has provoked intense controversy over the past two decades. In contrast to such major minerals as **magnesium** and **calcium**, neither selenium's benefits nor its toxic aspects are yet fully understood. Until very recently, selenium was considered a toxic element that was not necessary to human health. In 1989, selenium was reclassified as an essential micronutrient in a balanced human diet when the National Research Council established the first recommended daily allowance (RDA) for it. It is considered a minor mineral, or a *trace element*, as distinct from a *major mineral* such as calcium or **phosphorus**, or an *electrolyte* such as sodium or chloride. There is less than 1 mg of selenium in the average human body. The selenium is concentrated in the liver, kidneys, and pancreas. In males, selenium is also found in the testes and seminal vesicles. Selenium currently has a variety of applications, ranging from standard external preparations for skin problems to experimental and theoretical applications in nutrition and internal medicine.

Alternative medicine

Naturopaths use selenium supplements to treat **asthma**, **acne**, **tendinitis**, **infertility** problems in men, and postmenopausal disorders in women. Selenium is also considered an important component in naturopathic life extension (longevity) **diets**, because of its role in tissue repair and maintaining the youthful elasticity of skin.

Dermatology

Selenium has been used since the 1960s in **dandruff** shampoos and topical medications for such skin disorders as folliculitis ("hot tub" syndrome) and tinea versicolor, a mild infection of the skin caused by the yeast-like fungus *Pityrosporum orbiculare*. When selenium is compounded with **sulfur** to form a sulfide, it has antibiotic and antifungal properties. Selenium sulfide is absorbed by the outermost layer of skin cells, the epithelium. Inside the cells, the compound splits into selenium and sulfide ions. The selenium ions counteract the enzymes that are responsible for producing new epithelial cells, thus lowering the turnover of surface skin cells. As a result, **itching** and flaking of the skin associated with dandruff and tinea versicolor is reduced.

Nutrition

Prior to 1989, there were no established RDA values for selenium. In 1989, the National Research Council of the National Academy of Sciences defined the RDAs for selenium as follows: Males aged 15–18 years, 50 g; 19–24 years, 70 g; 25–50 years, 70 g; 51 years and older, 70 g. Females: aged 15–18 years, 50 g; 19–24 years, 55 g; 25–50 years, 55 g; 51 years and older, 55 g; pregnant, 65 g; lactating, 75 g. The generally higher levels for males are related to the importance of selenium in producing vigorous sperm.

The amount of selenium in the diet is influenced by its level in the soil. Most selenium is absorbed from food products, whether plants grown in the soil or animals that have eaten the plants. Much of the selenium in foods is lost during processing. About 60% of dietary selenium is absorbed as food passes through the intestines. Selenium leaves the body in the urine and feces; males also lose some selenium through ejaculation of sperm. Selenium levels in soil vary widely, not only in different countries but also across different regions. For example, in the United States the western states have higher levels of selenium in the soil than the eastern states. South Dakota has the highest rates of soil selenium in the United States, while Ohio has the lowest.

Foods that are high in selenium contain the element in an organic form, selenomethionine. This form of selenium is considerably less toxic than inorganic sodium selenite or elemental selenium. Good sources of selenium include brewer's yeast, **wheat germ**, wheat bran, **kelp** (seaweed), shellfish, Brazil nuts, barley, and oats. Onions, **garlic**, mushrooms, broccoli, and Swiss chard may contain high amounts of selenium if they are grown in selenium-rich soil. Selenium is also present in drinking water in some parts of the world and can be added to drinking water as a health measure. Nursing mothers should note that human milk is much richer in selenium than cow's milk.

There is no widely recognized deficiency syndrome for selenium, unlike the syndromes associated with calcium or magnesium (hypocalcemia and hypomagnesemia, respectively). However, many researchers who

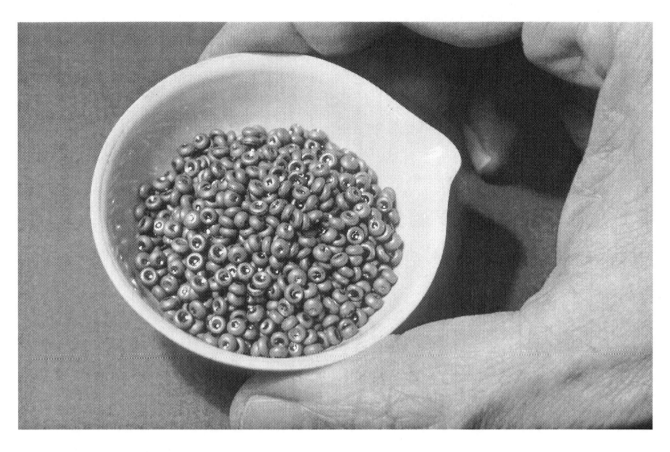

Sample of selenium. *(Rich Treptow, National Audubon Society Collection/Photo Researchers, Inc. Reproduced by permission.)*

have investigated Keshan disease, a form of **heart disease** in children, believe that it is caused by selenium deficiency. The disease can be prevented but not cured with supplemental selenium; it responds to treatment with 50 g per day. The symptoms of Keshan disease, which is named for the region of China where it was discovered, include enlargement of the heart and congestive heart failure. The soil in the Keshan region is low in selenium. The researchers observed that the local Chinese treat Keshan disease with **astragalus** (*Astragalus membranaceus*), a plant that absorbs selenium from the soil.

Selenium toxicity is still a matter of controversy. It is a known fact that humans can tolerate higher levels of selenium in its organic form (selenomethionine) than in its inorganic forms. Humans can show symptoms of selenium toxicity after doses as low as 1 mg of sodium selenite. On the other hand, some researchers speculate that the organic forms of selenium may accumulate in the body and interfere with the functioning of sulfur molecules in the body, or that they may cause genetic mutations. These long-term questions await further research. In addition, researchers disagree about how much selenium will produce symptoms of toxicity. It has been suggested that toxicity can result from a daily intake of 2 mg in people

who already have body stores of 2.5 mg of selenium or higher. Another measurement suggests that selenium toxicity may occur wherever the food or water regularly contains more than 5 or 10 parts per million of selenium. Patients with symptoms of selenium toxicity usually have blood plasma levels of 100 g/dl or higher, which is about four times the upper limit of normal levels.

The symptoms of selenium toxicity are not always clearly defined. People living in areas of selenium-rich soil sometimes develop heart, eye, or muscular problems. Eating foods containing high amounts of selenium over a long period of time increases the risk of tooth decay. It is thought that the selenium may compete with the fluoride in teeth, thus weakening their structure. Other symptoms associated with high levels of selenium include a metallic taste in the mouth, garlic-like breath odor, **dizziness**, **nausea**, skin inflammation, **fatigue**, and the loss of hair or nails. The symptoms of acute selenium poisoning include **fever**, kidney and liver damage, and eventual death.

Internal medicine

Selenium is most widely recognized as a substance that speeds up the metabolism of fatty acids and works together with **vitamin E** (tocopherol) as an antioxidant. **Antioxidants** are organic substances that are able to counteract the damage done to human tissue by oxidation (the breakdown of fatty acids). Selenium's antioxidant properties have been studied with respect to several diseases and disorders. In addition to its antioxidant properties, selenium also appears to work as an anti-inflammatory agent in certain disorders.

CARDIOVASCULAR DISEASES. Low levels of selenium have been associated with high risk of heart attacks and strokes. It is thought that the antioxidant properties of selenium can help prevent **atherosclerosis** (narrowing and hardening of the arteries) by decreasing the formation of fatty deposits in the arteries. It does so by soothing the inflamed arterial walls and binding the free radicals that damage the tissues lining the arteries. Other studies indicate that selenium reduces the symptoms of **angina** pectoris.

CATARACTS. **Cataracts** in the eye contain only one-sixth as much selenium as normal lens tissue. The healthy lens requires adequate levels of three antioxidant enzymes: superoxide dismutase, catalase, and **glutathione** peroxidase. Glutathione peroxidase in the human eye is dependent on selenium, which suggests that a selenium deficiency speeds up the progression of cataracts.

CANCER. Low dietary levels of selenium have been associated with an increased incidence of **cancer**. Cancers of the respiratory system and the gastrointestinal tract seem to be especially sensitive to the level of selenium in the body. In a recent study, patients with histories of **skin cancer** were given 200 g of selenium per day. Results indicated that the patients had a reduced incidence of rectal, prostate, and lung cancers as well as a lower rate of mortality from all cancers. In addition, cervical dysplasias (abnormal growths of tissue) in women are associated with low levels of selenium in the patient's diet. In animal studies, as little as 1–4 parts per million of selenium added to the water or food supply is associated with a decreased incidence of cancer. It is not yet known, however, exactly how selenium protects against cancer. Some researchers believe that it may prevent mutations or decrease the rate of cell division, particularly on the outer surfaces of the body. A recent study of the effects of a selenium compound on mammary tissue indicates that selenium may inhibit the growth of tumors in deeper layers of tissue, not just cancers arising from the epithelium.

As of 2002, selenium is being studied as a possible chemopreventive for **prostate cancer**. The researchers hope to learn more about the mechanisms by which selenium slows the progress of an established cancer as well as discover a preventive strategy that makes use of selenium.

PERIODONTAL DISEASE. Selenium appears to speed up the healing of fragile gum tissue as well as opposing the actions of free radicals, which are extremely damaging to gum tissue.

RHEUMATOID ARTHRITIS. Selenium may be useful for treating several autoimmune diseases, especially lupus and **rheumatoid arthritis** (RA). It has been discovered that patients suffering from RA have low selenium levels. Selenium is necessary for production of the enzyme glutathione peroxidase, which reduces the production of inflammatory substances in the body (prostaglandins and leukotrienes) as well as opposing free radicals. Although supplemental selenium by itself has not been shown to cause improvement in RA, selenium taken together with vitamin E appears to have measurable positive results.

OSTEOARTHRITIS. Recent research in Germany indicates that selenium is beneficial in the prevention and treatment of **osteoarthritis** (OA), particularly OA resulting from physical wear and tear or structural problems in the patient's joints. Selenium supplements are even more effective when given together with vitamins in treating OA.

Preparations

Selenium is available in topical preparations and as a dietary supplement.

External preparations

Selenium sulfide for the treatment of dandruff is available as over-the-counter (OTC) scalp preparations or shampoo containing 1% or 2.5% solutions of the drug. A topical 2.5% solution of selenium sulfide is available for the treatment of tinea versicolor. Common trade names include Exsel™, Selsun™, and Selsun Blue™.

Dietary supplements

Selenium is widely available in vitamin/mineral dietary supplements and in nutritional antioxidant formulas. Although the average diet supplies enough selenium, some naturopaths recommend daily supplements of 100–200 g for adults and 30–150 g for children. Sexually active males are advised to take higher doses. Some naturopaths recommend taking selenium together with vitamin E on the grounds that their combined effect is greater than the sum of their individual effects. There are at present no definitive studies on the positive effects on health of selenium taken as a dietary supplement.

Precautions

Topical preparations

Persons using selenium compounds to control dandruff or tinea versicolor should be careful to avoid applying the product to damaged or broken skin. In addition to irritating skin, selenium can enter the body through broken skin. This process is known as percutaneous absorption and can cause selenium toxicity if the preparation is used for a long period of time. Patients should wash their hands carefully after applying the selenium product to affected areas. Doing so will minimize absorption through small breaks in the skin of the hands.

Nutritional supplements

It is difficult to assess the effectiveness of dietary supplements containing selenium because there is little agreement on standards for interpreting selenium levels in human blood. Depending on their intake, healthy adults may have blood plasma levels of selenium in the range of 8–25 g/dl. In addition, most of the selenium in the body is not carried in the blood but is stored in tissue. Analysis of hair has not been useful in measuring selenium. In the absence of a useful test, people who wish to take supplemental selenium should first find out whether they live in an area that already has high levels of selenium in the drinking water and soil. Most people will probably not need more selenium than is in standard vitamin/mineral supplements. In addition, the body seems to utilize selenium more efficiently when it is taken together with vitamin E.

Side effects

The side effects of contact with compounds containing selenium sulfide include stinging of the skin; irritation of the lining of the eyes; hair discoloration or loss; and oily scalp. Both topical products and megadoses of selenium taken by mouth can cause selenium toxicity. The symptoms of selenium toxicity include nausea, **vomiting**, tiredness, abdominal **pain**, a garlicky breath odor, and the loss of hair and fingernails. These symptoms usually last 10–12 days after the selenium preparation is discontinued.

Interactions

Topical preparations containing selenium may interact with the metals in costume jewelry. Patients should remove all their jewelry before applying the shampoo or lotion.

With regard to dietary supplements, there is some evidence that **vitamin C** inactivates selenium within the digestive tract. Persons who are concerned about their selenium intake may prefer to take supplemental selenium in the absence of vitamin C.

Resources

BOOKS

Baron, Robert B., M.D. "Nutrition." In *Current Medical Diagnosis and Treatment*, edited by Lawrence M. Tierney, M.D., et al. 39th ed. New York: McGraw-Hill, 2000.

KEY TERMS

Antioxidant—A substance that works to counteract the damage done to human tissue by the breakdown of fatty acids. Dietary antioxidants include beta-carotene and vitamins C and E as well as selenium.

Epithelium—The layer of tissue that covers body surfaces or lines the inner surfaces of body cavities and hollow organs.

Free radical—A highly reactive molecule that binds to and destroys compounds in tissue cells. Most free radicals in the human body are produced in the body, while others come from the environment and foods.

Glutathione peroxidase—An enzyme that functions as an antioxidant, in the activation of other enzymes, and in the transport of minerals and amino acids. Human glutathione is dependent on selenium.

Keshan disease—A form of heart disease in children, first discovered in the Keshan region of China. It may represent a selenium deficiency syndrome.

Percutaneous absorption—The process by which certain strong medications, such as selenium compounds, can enter the body through the skin.

Trace element—An element that is required in only minute quantities for the maintenance of good health. Trace elements are also called micronutrients.

Beers, Mark H., M.D., and Robert Berkow, M.D., eds. *The Merck Manual of Diagnosis and Therapy*. Whitehouse Station, NJ: Merck Research Laboratories, 2002.

Berger, Timothy G., M.D. "Skin, Hair, and Nails." In *Current Medical Diagnosis and Treatment*, edited by Lawrence M. Tierney, M.D., et al. 39th ed. New York: McGraw-Hill, 2000.

Burton Goldberg Group, comp. *Alternative Medicine: The Definitive Guide*. Fife, WA: Future Medicine Publishing, 1995.

Murray, Michael, N.D., and Joseph Pizzorno, N.D. *Encyclopedia of Natural Medicine*. Rocklin, CA: Prima Publishing, 1991.

PERIODICALS

Dong, Y., C. Ip, and H. Ganther. "Evidence of a Field Effect Associated with Mammary Cancer Chemoprevention by Methylseleninic Acid." *Anticancer Research* 22 (1A)(January-February 2002): 27-32.

Kurz, B., B. Jost, and M. Schunke. "Dietary Vitamins and Selenium Diminish the Development of Mechanically Induced Osteoarthritis and Increase the Expression of Antioxidative Enzymes in the Knee Joint of STR/1N Mice." *Osteoarthritis and Cartilage* 10 (February 2002): 119-126.

Nelson, M. A., M. Reid, A. J. Duffield-Lillico, and J. R. Marshall. "Prostate Cancer and Selenium." *Urology Clinics of North America* 29 (February 2002): 67-70.

Tan, J., W. Zhu, W. Wang, et al. "Selenium in Soil and Endemic Diseases in China." *The Science of the Total Environment* 4 (February 2002): 227-235.

Ujiie, S., and H. Kikuchi. "The Relation Between Serum Selenium Value and Cancer in Miyagi, Japan: 5-Year Follow-Up Study." *Tohoku Journal of Experimental Medicine* 196 (March 2002): 99-109.

Rebecca J. Frey, PhD

Senior nutrition

Definition

Senior **nutrition** is concerned with the special dietary requirements of the elderly. In his book, *Earl Mindell's Vitamin Bible for the 21st Century,* Earl Mindell, Ph.D, R.Ph (Registered Pharmacist), Master Herbalist, and best-selling author of books about maintaining health through nutrition for the last 20 years, states, "Aging is caused by the degeneration of cells. Our bodies are made up of millions of these cells, each with a life of somewhere around two years or less. But before a cell dies, it reproduces itself. Why then, you might wonder, shouldn't we look the same now as we did ten years ago? The reason for this is that with each successive reproduction, the cell goes through some alteration—basically deterioration. So as our cells change, deteriorate, we grow old. The good news is that deteriorating cells can be rejuvenated if provided with substances that directly nourish them . .

Origins

After age 50, adults experience significant reduction in metabolism (chemical action in living cells that provide energy for life's activities and assimilation of new restorative material, or the rate at which the body burns energy) and changes in physiology (body and organ functions during life) that significantly affect their nutritional needs. These changes often call for decreased-calorie **diets**, but there are many complications that can affect a senior's balance of food intake and energy needs.

Aging causes a decrease in lean tissue mass and an increase in body fat. These changes are significant because an older person utilizes dietary protein less efficiently and may need more than the recommended amount of high-quality protein to maintain lean tissue mass. Complications may also arise because of age-related digestive problems, oral/dental problems, and eating/nutrient problems related to medication. Other complicating factors for the elderly include loneliness, **depression**, economic concerns, and lack of cooking skills and nutritional knowledge (such as eating too many processed/refined foods devoid of nutritional value). These factors often result in seniors under-consuming the proper foods to meet their energy and nutrient requirements and can lead to weakness, chronic **fatigue**, and a weakened immune system.

Benefits

Nutritional studies have clearly demonstrated that sound dietary habits adopted by seniors can promote longevity and reverse some of the effects of aging; reduce the risks and severity of illness and disease; increase overall levels of wellness and vitality; and improve quality of life.

The three leading causes of death among adults are **heart disease**, strokes, and **cancer**. Diabetes, **atherosclerosis**, and liver disease are also in the top ten causes of human mortality. All of these diseases have been correlated with dietary habits and alcohol intake, and research has shown that these and many other diseases can be reversed or eliminated through dietary and lifestyle changes. Seniors, who face the most risk from these diseases, can therefore greatly benefit from healthy nutritional practices, especially if they are initiated early in life.

Description

Nearly 90% of Americans above age 65 have one or more degenerative disorders (diseases that develop over time), including heart disease, cancer, arthritis, diabetes, and **osteoporosis**. Once considered diseases of old age, these conditions are now also being seen as lifestyle-related diseases, which means that changes in habits, including diet, can significantly reduce their risks. For instance, Dr. **Dean Ornish**, a California cardiologist, demonstrated that heart disease could be reversed by a low-fat vegetarian diet combined with **exercise** and **stress** reduction techniques such as **meditation** and **yoga**. Furthermore, it has been strongly demonstrated that improper diet is directly correlated with disease and premature aging. **Obesity**, for example, shortens life expectancy and increases the risk of diabetes, **hypertension**, and heart disease. For seniors, it is never too late to adopt informed nutritional practices to improve health and chances for longer, healthier life.

Longevity studies (in which researchers attempt to determine the behaviors that contribute to long life in human populations) have shown that moderation is a key component to a life-extending diet. In the longest-living people, stability of overall body weight—where people remain consistently at no more than 5% under their ideal weight or no more than 10–20% overweight—implying moderation of diet, has been found to be very important. Moderation of alcohol intake, meaning no more than two drinks per day, is also important, as is the consistency of eating breakfast every day. As people age, their metabolism slows, making it easier to gain weight and harder to lose weight after it is put on. This factor underscores the importance for seniors to adopt diets that reduce large fluctuations in weight.

In the marketplace of dietary knowledge, the numerous fads and claims can be extremely confusing for the conscientious eater. For instance, there are diets that restrict fats and favor carbohydrates, such as the **Ornish diet** as mentioned above. Then there are diets that restrict carbohydrates and recommend higher amounts of fats and proteins to be consumed, like the **Atkins diet** that has been very popular in the mainstream of the early 2000s. The confusion can be compounded by the fact that different people and different age groups, including seniors, have different dietary requirements and tastes.

Within the alternative health care model, there are many diets that have been shown to improve health. These include **vegetarianism**, **veganism**, the Ornish diet, macrobiotics, the **Mediterranean diet**, juicing, the raw food diet, and others. Seniors may not have the time or energy to experiment with various diets until finding a satisfactory one, nor is it advisable that seniors enforce strict guidelines that might take the pleasure and freedom out of eating and preparing food. Nutrition is made easier within the alternative health care model because there are simple principles that can be applied to make any senior's diet more nutritionally sound.

Another healthy diet model for seniors contains a wide variety of fresh fruits and vegetables, whole grains, and legumes (peas, lentils and beans, including soybeans and soy products), and is moderate in the consumption of animal products including meat, eggs, and dairy products. In this diet, the majority of daily calories, or energy, comes from fruits, vegetables, whole grains, legumes, and nuts and seeds—all plant sources. This plant-based diet is naturally high in fiber, which is important for seniors because fiber assists in the digestive process, which is slower and more sensitive in the elderly. Eating fiber also lowers blood **cholesterol** levels. A sound senior diet also contains adequate protein, derived primarily from vegetable and low-fat animal sources; avoids the intake of saturated fat, which raises cholesterol levels in the blood; and emphasizes the careful intake of healthy fats.

In the alternative health care model, there are general principles that make dietary choices easy and uncomplicated, which in itself is important for the elderly. First, food should be as fresh and in as close to its natural state as available. Fresh and natural food contains the highest amount of life energy, sometimes known as *chi* or *prana,* which can be lost when food is overly processed, overcooked, or stale. Furthermore, fresh food, such as fresh fruits and vegetables, contains no harmful food additives and no added ingredients such as sugar and fat, both of which should be consumed only in moderate amounts by seniors. Fresh and natural foods are also more nutrient-dense than processed foods, which means that they contain more vitamins and minerals for the same amount of calories. This is particularly important for seniors, who should strive to maximize the intake of nutrients while maintaining consistent body weight and not consuming more calories than are needed. Foods that contain empty calories—that is, calories without other nutrients, such as foods that are high in sugar or junk foods— should be reduced to very minimal levels in the diet.

More and more health-conscious people have turned to the alternative of juicing fresh vegetables and fruits as a healthy supplement to daily meals because they provide concentrated essential nutrients, vitamins and minerals that the body does not have to first chew and digest. This process requires the purchase of a juicer, the price of which runs from $100 to $500.

Another principle within the alternative health model is a holistic view of the world. Humans are connected to the whole living system of the earth. Food choices that are healthiest for the individual would also be better for the earth; and likewise, keeping the earth's living system healthy improves the health of the human population. It has been estimated that worldwide, 33% of all disease is related to environmental degradation. Thus, organically grown foods are the healthiest choice for consumers. The production of those foods is safest for them and the environment because they contain no toxic chemicals. Healthy fresh organic food choices would also eliminate unnecessary packaging and artificial ingredients. Healthy choices also emphasize locally grown foods, which reduce the loss of nutrients due to transportation and refrigeration. Finally, eating seasonal fruits and vegetables keeps the diet aligned with the natural rhythm of the seasons.

Food can be broken down into the categories of carbohydrates, fats, and proteins. Nutritional science attempts to determine the optimal quantities of each in the diet. Some diets are very rigorous about the measurement of overall calories and exactly how many carbohydrates, fats, and proteins should be included, but general dietary guidelines should suffice for most seniors.

Carbohydrates are a basic energy source found in foods and can provide up to 70% of daily calories in a senior's diet. The simplest carbohydrates are sugars, such as those found in fruits, honey, table sugar, and corn syrup, while complex carbohydrates are found in whole grains and legumes and other plant and animal sources. Small amounts of sugar are not unhealthy, although sugar is no substitute for nutrient-rich foods. A piece of fresh fruit, for instance, would be a far better choice for a sweet tooth than a soft drink. As Dr. Earl Mindell indicates, "The big problem with sugar is that we eat way too much of it and often don't even know it." He implicates sugar in tooth decay and obesity, which can lead to heart disease, diabetes, hypertension, **gallstones**, back problems, and arthritis. He also points out that its presence in foods tempts one to eat more; and that if calories are reduced without reducing sugar intake, more nutrients than pounds will be lost. Complex carbohydrates are a healthier source of energy and fiber, and whole grains, pastas, breads, beans, cereals, fruits, and vegetables are recommended to supply them in the diet.

Seniors should pay close attention to the amount and type of fat in the diet. The Ornish diet, shown to reverse the effects of heart disease, recommends no more than 10% of all calories coming from fat, and cautions against any saturated fats, or those fats that are present mainly in meat and dairy products as well as in tropical oils like palm and coconut oils, and some nuts and seeds. Some seniors may not need to be this stringent about fats in the diet, but just getting fat content down to 20–30% of total calories will reduce the risks of disease and improve overall health. Generally saturated fats, for seniors, should be greatly reduced and avoided as much as possible. The best fats to consume are generally from such plant sources as olive oil and canola oil, which are the healthiest choices for cooking oils; and occasional use of avocados, nuts, seeds, and nut butters. Clarified butter (ghee) is a substitute for butter, which contains high amounts of saturated fat and should be avoided.

Seniors should also take care to get plenty of **essential fatty acids** (EFAs) in the diet, particularly omega-3 EFA and omega-6 EFA, important nutrients for the elderly and essential fats for the body. Omega-3 EFA is found in cold-water fish like salmon and mackerel as well as in walnuts, **wheat germ**, and **flaxseed**. EFAs can also be obtained in such nutritional supplements as **evening primrose oil**, wheat germ oil, **borage oil**, flaxseed oil, and hemp seed oil.

Finally, seniors should take care to avoid the consumption of trans-fatty acids (TFAs). These are artificial fats that are created during industrial cooking processes, and have been widely implicated in heart disease and atherosclerosis. These unhealthy oils are found in margarine, vegetable shortening, and partially hydrogenated oils, which are present in many processed foods. Deep-fried foods should also be avoided, which contribute these unhealthy fats to the diet. By paying close attention to ingredients and then avoiding partially hydrogenated oils, seniors can avoid many unhealthy foods.

Proteins are the basic building blocks used by the body. Americans in general consume more protein than is required, and the excess consumption of red meat, dairy products, and eggs, all high in saturated fats, contributes to the prevalence of many degenerative diseases. Seniors should be careful to not eat too much protein, particularly from meat, dairy, and egg sources. Excess protein in the diet can stress the digestive system, liver, and kidneys, and also contribute to the development of osteoporosis, or weakness of the bones due to **calcium** loss—a condition afflicting many seniors, particularly women. Two to four ounces (57–113 g) of protein per day is sufficient for most seniors, which would be a piece of lean meat the size of a deck of cards, or a several servings of soy or beans. Healthy sources of protein include legumes, tofu, nuts and seeds, low-fat dairy products, fish, egg whites, and lean meats. Soy products are an excellent addition to the senior diet, providing high-quality and low-fat protein while containing several age-protective nutrients.

Other dietary habits can help seniors optimize nutrition. Sound diets contain a variety of wholesome foods. At least five servings per day of fruits and vegetables are recommended. Variety is important to provide a full range of vitamins and minerals, and helps seniors avoid eating too much of any food that may not be the healthiest. Furthermore, seniors should strive to eat less rather than more at mealtime, and to stop eating while still slightly hungry. Overeating inhibits digestion and causes weight gain, which healthy seniors avoid doing. Regular exercise also contributes to sound nutrition by improving metabolism and digestion and thus the absorption of nutrients by the body. Food choices should not inhibit seniors' autonomy and freedom but enhance them. Food preparation should emphasize taste and the pleasure of eating. Seniors should also drink plenty of fresh clean water as part of their diet. Spring water or filtered water is best, and up to eight glasses per day is recommended. Drinking plenty of water prevents dehydration (which can lead to low blood pressure, heat **stroke**, **nausea**, dryness of mouth, **vomiting**, and **constipation**); improves digestion; and helps the body flush out impurities. **Green tea** is a healthy substitute for coffee, as it contains an antioxidant shown to have anti-aging effects as well as less **caffeine**.

Caffeine is really a drug with many unhealthy side effects. Although it acts quickly on the central nervous system, resulting in almost immediate increased mental clarity and energy, caffeine accumulates in the fat tissues of the body and can lead to nervousness, exhaustion of the adrenal gland, the loss of important vitamins and minerals from the body, and increased acidity in the gastrointestinal tract, caffeine can also dangerously increase heart and blood pressure rates when consumed with decongestants or bronchodilators. It is considered by some doctors to be implicated in hypertensive heart disease. Medical schools and journals have linked excessive caffeine consumption to benign breast disease, prostate problems, cancer of the bladder and lower urinary tract, and **heart attack**.

Nutritional and Herbal Supplementation

Seniors can inform and avail themselves of the many nutritional and herbal supplements available for specific health problems by consulting alternative physicians—M.D.s, osteopaths, naturopaths, homeopaths, chiropractors—and herbalists for recommendations. They can also consult many books on vitamins, minerals, and nutritional/herbal supplements, and find a great deal of information on this subject on the Internet.

Senior nutrition includes two additional ways in which the elderly can fulfill their nutritional requirements. Although there is ample evidence that a varied and plant-based diet consisting of fresh fruits, vegetables, whole grains, legumes, and moderate amounts of animal products prolongs life expectancy and improves overall health, informed use of nutritional supplements can add extra protection and support for the mature body, and herbal supplements can be safely used to support the treatment of age-related illnesses and as general health tonics.

It should again be noted that there is general acceptance that the best way for seniors to get plenty of nutrients is through a varied diet, because supplements cannot make up for a diet that is not nutritionally balanced in the first place; that nutrients from food sources are more efficiently utilized by the body; that seniors should try to add natural foods to their diets that are high in nutrients known or recommended to help in the treatment of certain disease or degenerative conditions; and that nutritional supplements can then be properly used to supply any extra support or protection that seniors may need.

Generally if a senior is eating a balanced, healthy diet over 1,200 calories a day, vitamin-mineral supplement may be unnecessary. However, some physicians think that much of today's food is grown in soil depleted of nutrients and a high-quality, broad-spectrum multivitamin and mineral supplement, taken once per day, is fre-

quently recommended to seniors to supplement their diets by providing a range of nutrients. It should contain the B vitamins B_6, B_{12}, and **folic acid**, which may help prevent heart disease, and the minerals **zinc** and **copper**, which aid the immune system. Some nutritionists advise that seniors should take a multi vitamin/mineral supplement that provides no more than 100% of the recommended daily allowance (RDA), and caution against taking one nutrient by itself because nutrients interact with each other and single-dose nutrient interaction can be harmful, even toxic, and may actually cause a deficiency of another nutrient.

In addition to a multivitamin, many health professionals, however, advise seniors to add **antioxidants** to their supplementation routine. These include **vitamin A** (or **beta carotene**), **vitamin C**, **vitamin E**, and the mineral **selenium**. Antioxidants may have several positive effects on the body, such as slowing the aging process, reducing the risks of cancer and heart disease, and reducing the risks of illness and infection by supporting the immune system.

Coenzyme Q_{10} is another antioxidant that is gaining use by the elderly, as it may retard aging, improve the health of the heart and reduce the effects of heart disease, help lower blood pressure, aid in treatment of periodontal disease, help lower blood pressure, and aid in the prevention of toxicity from drugs used to treat many diseases associated with aging.

Essential fatty acids, particularly omega-3, are also recommended for seniors, as, according to **Andrew Weil**, M.D., author of *Spontaneous Healing*," they appear to reduce inflammatory changes in the body, protect against abnormal blood clotting, and, possibly, protect against cancer and degenerative changes in cells and tissues."

Calcium supplementation is recommended for the elderly, particularly for women, to strengthen bones and prevent bone loss. Also, the senior stomach may secrete less hydrochloric acid—the enzyme involved in food digestion, which may reduce the amount of calcium that is absorbed. Calcium supplements that are balanced with **magnesium** have a less constipating effect on the bowels and are better absorbed.

Another nutrient concern is sufficient intake of **iron**. Many sources of iron need to be eaten to get enough. While the best source or iron is meat, people can also get iron from whole grains, cooked dry beans, and some fruits and vegetables. Vitamin C aids absorption of iron, so such vitamin C foods as citrus fruits, greens, and tomatoes should be included in the same meal with iron.

The supplement **glucosamine** sulfate, together with **chondroitin** and MSN, may be useful for seniors with joint problems and **pain**.

KEY TERMS

Arthritis—An inflammatory condition affecting joints.

Atherosclerosis—Disease characterized by hardening and narrowing of the arteries, leading to strokes and heart disease.

Cancer—A disease caused by uncontrolled abnormal cell growth.

Carbohydrates—Digestible sugars and starches in food that are the major sources of energy.

Chi—Basic life energy in traditional Chinese medicine, contained in food, air, and water.

Diabetes—Lack of the hormone insulin leading to uncontrolled carbohydrate metabolism.

Fats—Long chains of fatty acids that are stored in animal tissue.

Macrobiotics—A diet emphasizing grains, certain vegetables, legumes, and fish.

Osteoporosis—A reduction in the amount of bone mass leading to fractures after minimal trauma.

Prana—Basic life energy, found in food, air, and water, as defined in the East Indian Ayurveda and yoga philosophies.

Proteins—Organic compounds of amino acids in vegetable and animal matter.

Saturated fat.—A fatty acid that is totally hydrogenated (chemically bound) and holds the greatest risk for development of atherosclerosis.

Stroke—A blood clot or blood vessel bursting and interrupting blood flow to the brain, which may cause coma, paralysis, speech problems, dementia.

Vegan—A vegetarian who omits all animal and dairy products from the diet.

Vegetarianism—The theory or practice of living only on vegetables and fruits.

traditional East Indian system, **ashwaganda** and **gotu kola** are herbs prescribed for their rejuvenating effects on the elderly, and **triphala** is used to improve digestion and as a mild laxative. Seniors can inform themselves of the many herbs available for specific problems, and also consult alternative physicians and herbalists for recommendations on herbal supplements.

Resources

BOOKS

Chopra, Deepak, M.D., and David Simon, M.D. *Grow Younger, Live Longer.* New York: Harmony Books, 2001.

Kordich, Jay. *The Juiceman's Power of Juicing.* New York: Warner Books, 1993.

Mindell, Earl, Ph.D, R.Ph. *Vitamin Bible for the 21st Century.* New York: Warner Books, 1999.

Null, Gary, Ph.D. *Gary Null's Ultimate Anti-Aging Program.* New York: Kensington Books, 1999.

Walford, Roy, M.D. and Lisa Walford. *The Anti-Aging Plan.* New York: Four Walls Eight Windows, 1994.

Weil, Andrew, M.D. *Eating Well for Optimum Health.* New York: Alfred A. Knopf, 2000.

Weil, Andrew, M.D. *Spontaneous Healing.* New York: Ballantine Books, 1995.

PERIODICALS

Natural Health. <http://www.naturalhealthmag.com.>.

Vegetarian Times. <http://www.vegetariantimes.com.>.

ORGANIZATIONS

Center for Science in the Public Interest. 1875 Connecticut Avenue NW, Suite 300. Washington, D.C. 20009. (202) 332-9110. <http://www.cspinet.org.>.

OTHER

U.S.D.A. Food and Nutrition Information Center. <http://www.nal.usda.gov/fnic>.

Vegetarian Resource Group. <http://www.vrg.org.>.

Douglas Dupler
Ruth Ann Carter

Such natural sources of fiber as **psyllium** seed husks may be used by those seniors who need added fiber in their diet.

There are many herbs that support vitality and health in old age. In Chinese medicine, ginseng has been the fabled elixir of youth, and **astragalus** and ginkgo are also recommended to the elderly. Ginkgo has been shown to enhance memory and brain function. **Grape seed extract** and **pine bark extract** (pycnogenol) are herbal derivatives that have powerful antioxidant, and thus anti-aging, effects in the body. In the Ayurvedic or

Senna

Description

Senna, *Cassia angustifolia*, is known by the name Egyptian senna. A member of the Leguminaceae family, senna is a shrub-like plant whose leaves and pods have been used for centuries in the East and West as a purgative. This property of senna was first described in the ninth century A.D. by Arabian physicians in the service of the caliph of Baghdad. Senna's reputation as a powerful laxative has grown through the ages. Senna can be found as an ingredient in many over-the-counter laxative products in the United States. Senna is also considered an important herb in **traditional Chinese medicine,** Indian Ayurvedic, and unani medicine. The two species used most often for medicinal purposes are Alexandrian senna and Tinnevelly senna. The Alexandrian variety is obtained mainly from Egypt and the Sudan. Tinnevelly senna is primarily cultivated in India.

Senna contains naturally occurring chemicals called anthraquinone glycosides. They are strong laxatives that soften stools and increase the contractions of intestinal muscle, thereby stimulating bowel movements. "Like **aloe, buckthorn,** and cascara sagrada, senna contains anthraquinone glycosides, chemicals that stimulate the colon," reports James A. Duke, Ph.D. Senna usually starts to work in three to nine hours. Anthraquinone laxatives, such as senna, are believed to alleviate **constipation** by increasing the amount of water and electrolytes in the intestine. They also work by stimulating contractions of the colon muscles, which help to accelerate the passage of stool. Senna is considered among the strongest of the anthraquinone laxatives. Its effectiveness as a purgative has been supported by centuries of anecdotal reports as well as modern human and animal studies.

General use

Senna is widely accepted as a stool softener and a short-term treatment for **constipation.** Senna leaf is approved by the World Health Organization (WHO) for short-term use in occasional constipation. Senna is also approved in the United States and in European countries as an ingredient in over-the-counter and prescription laxative preparations. The herb is approved by the German government for any condition in which alleviating constipation or softening stools is desirable. Senna may be recommended for people with **hemorrhoids,** anal fissures, or those undergoing surgery involving the abdomen, anus, or rectum. Senna may also be used to clear the bowel in order to improve the visibility of abdominal organs during an ultrasound procedure.

Clinical studies in the United States and abroad involving various age groups suggest that senna is effective in managing constipation associated with a number of causes including surgery, **childbirth,** and use of narcotic **pain** relievers. A study in the medical journal *Diseases of the Colon and Rectum* showed that senna was able to prevent or treat postoperative constipation after proctologic surgery. The *South African Medical Journal* shows that treatment with senna was successful in 93%-96% of women suffering from postpartum constipation. By comparison, only 51%-59% of women in the placebo group experienced relief. Senna is considered to be one of the more effective agents for relieving constipation

caused by such narcotic pain relievers as morphine. In another study published in the *Journal of Pain and Symptom Management*, researchers recommended the use of senna in terminal **cancer** patients with opiate-induced constipation, citing the effectiveness of the herb and its relatively low cost. A study published in the medical journal *Pharmacology* suggests that a combination of senna and bulk laxatives can alleviate chronic constipation in geriatric patients.

Preparations

The recommended dosage of senna, which is generally taken at bedtime, ranges from 0.6-2.0 g a day. Tablets, syrups, oral solutions, and other medications that list senna as an ingredient usually contain standardized amounts of the herb and its active agents. People who choose to prepare senna using unprocessed leaves or pods may have difficulty determining exact dosages. No matter which form or preparation of senna is chosen, using the lowest effective dosage helps to avoid side effects.

Consumers who wish to brew a medicinal tea from unprocessed senna should use 1-2 tsp of the dried leaves of the herb per cup of boiling water and let it steep for about 10 minutes. Senna is generally considered to have an unpleasant taste, so adding sugar or honey to the mixture may help to make it more palatable. **Anise, ginger, chamomile,** coriander, **fennel,** and **peppermint** can also be added to the tea to improve its taste and to reduce **gas** and cramping. Up to one cup of senna tea a day is recommended to alleviate constipation. It should not be taken for longer than one or two weeks.

Precautions

Senna and other stimulant laxatives should not be used for longer than two to four weeks without medical supervision. Using senna longer than recommended can result in lazy bowel syndrome and permanent damage to the intestinal lining. Chronic use or misuse can also cause electrolyte and fluid imbalances, which can have adverse effects on the heart. To prevent or treat constipation, most doctors recommend making dietary changes or trying milder bulk-forming laxatives such as **psyllium** before using senna or other anthraquinone purgatives. Dietary approaches involve eating a **high-fiber diet,** drinking six to eight glasses of water a day, and getting plenty of regular **exercise**.

Unless otherwise indicated by a doctor, senna should not be used by anyone with an intestinal obstruction, stomach inflammation, or intestinal inflammatory diseases such as **Crohn's disease,** colitis, **irritable bowel syndrome,** or **appendicitis.** Senna should also be avoided by those with undiagnosed abdominal pain.

Senna should not be used by children younger than age 12. Senna should not be used by pregnant or breast-feeding women. It may significantly reduce drug absorption and lessen the efficiency of any over-the-counter or prescription medication. Children and seniors, who may be more susceptible to senna's effects, should start with smaller dosages of the herb.

Side effects

Such stimulant laxatives as senna tend to have more side effects than other purgatives, so it is important to take the lowest effective dosage. The side effects of senna include stomach cramps, **diarrhea**, and gas, which can be severe if the herb is used longer than recommended or in large amounts. The effects of senna can be immediate, sometimes too fast or intense. These problems may be avoided by reducing the dosage and adding other herbs. More serious effects include fainting, dehydration, and such electrolyte disorders as low blood **potassium**, albuminuria, and hematuria. **Potassium** deficiency can lead to muscle weakness and disorders of heart function. Potassium levels may drop even further if senna is combined with cardiac glycoside medications, diuretics, or corticosteroids. People using diet pills or teas should be sure that if senna is an ingredient they use the products short-term (a month or less).

Interactions

Because of its potential effect on potassium levels, senna should not be combined with antiarrhythmic drugs, thiazide diuretics, corticoadrenal steroids, or **licorice** root without the supervision of a doctor.

Resources

BOOKS

Duke, James A., Michael Castleman, and Alice Feinstein. *The Green Pharmacy*. Emmaus, PA: Rodale Press, 1997.

Foster, Steven and Varro E. Tyler. *Tyler's Honest Herbal: A Sensible Guide to the Use of Herbs and Related Remedies*. Binghamton, NY: Haworth, 1998.

Goldberg, Burton. *Alternative Medicine: The Definitive Guide*. Fife, WA: Future Medicine Publishing, 1993.

PERIODICALS

Agra, Y. Sacristan and M.A. Gonzalez. "Efficiency of Senna versus Lactulose in Terminal Cancer Patients Treated with Opioids." *Journal of Pain and Symptom Management* (1998) 15(1): 1-7.

Corman, M.L. "Management of Postoperative Constipation in Anorectal Surgery." *Diseases of the Colon and Rectum* (1979) 22(3): 149-51.

"Go for Natural Laxative Relief, but Best if not from Senna or Cascara." *Environmental Nutrition* (May 2002): 7.

KEY TERMS

Albuminuria—The presence of high levels of the protein albumin in the urine.

Electrolytes—Substances in the blood, such as sodium and potassium, that help to regulate fluid balance in the body.

Hematuria—The presence of blood in the urine.

Lazy bowel syndrome—An inability to have a bowel movement without the aid of chemical laxatives.

Licorice root—An herb believed to be helpful in treating ulcers, respiratory problems, and a variety of other conditions.

Purgative—A substance that encourages bowel movements.

Stimulant laxatives—Powerful laxatives that increase the frequency of bowel movements by stimulating muscle contractions that accelerate the passage of stool.

Shelton, M.G. "Standardized Senna in the Management of Constipation in the Puerperium: A Clinical Trial." *South African Medical Journal* (1980) 57(3): 78-80.

ORGANIZATIONS

American Botanical Council. P.O. Box 144345, Austin, TX 78714-4345. (512) 926-4900. http://www.herbalgram.org.

Herb Research Foundation. 1007 Pearl Street, Suite 200, Boulder, CO 80302. (303) 449-2265. Info@herbs.org. http://www.herbs.org.

OTHER

Prevention Magazine. http://www.prevention.com.

Greg Annussek
Teresa G. Odle

Sensory deprivation

Definition

Sensory deprivation, or Restricted Environmental Stimulation Therapy (REST), is a technique by which sensory input (sound, light, smell, etc.) is minimized. This practice encourages an extremely deep level of **relaxation**. REST is typically conducted in a float tank, in which the person is suspended in a solution of warm water and

Epsom salt without sound or light. This relaxation technique produces significant physical and mental benefits.

Origins

In the 1950s, sensory deprivation experiments were conducted to determine the effects of restricted environmental stimulation on mental and physical functions. For 24 hours a day, students were confined to a bed in cramped cubicles with their vision and hearing blocked by various means, such as opaque goggles and U-shaped pillows around their heads. The students' physical and psychological functions quickly deteriorated under these harsh conditions.

In 1954, Dr. John Lilly, a neurophysiologist at the National Institute of Mental Health in Bethesda, Maryland, developed the Floatation Restricted Environmental Stimulation Technique. By suspending a person in water, external stimuli (such as light and sound) were reduced almost completely, but without the harsh conditions of similar experiments.

Dr. Lilly refined his technique between 1960 and 1970, allowing subjects to float freely in an Epsom salt and water solution contained within a dark soundproof chamber. The solution was warmed to skin temperature so that the person would not react to cold or heat.

From his experiments, Lilly determined that such external stimuli as gravity, light, sound, and touch accounted for 90% of the central nervous system's workload. Although extended sensory deprivation could be harmful, extended sensory overload could also have detrimental effects on a person's mental and physical well-being. By reducing excess stimuli appropriately, he could actually lower **stress** levels. Drs. Peter Suedfeld and Roderick Borrie of the University of British Columbia began experimenting on the therapeutic benefits of this technique in the late 1970s. However, they renamed the technique Restricted Environmental Stimulation Therapy (REST) or, more appropriately, Floatation REST.

Since that time, several studies have been conducted on the benefits of Floatation REST, as well as other forms of REST. The consistently positive findings of these studies have led to the incorporation of Floatation REST into physical and mental health care programs, as well as fitness training and professional sports medicine. Currently, floatation centers can be found in major cities in Asia, Australia, Europe, and North America. Individuals can also purchase float tanks for their homes.

Benefits

Floatation REST has many physical and mental benefits because it provides an unparalleled level of relaxation. With the elimination of external stimuli, the central nervous system's workload is reduced by as much as 90%. This reduction draws a person's energy inward and promotes relaxation (the parasympathetic response). The parasympathetic response is the mechanism by which the body naturally regenerates itself and maintains chemical and metabolic balance. Old **wounds** and injuries are allowed to heal faster. Increased T-cell production strengthens the immune system. This deep level of relaxation also benefits the cardiovascular system. Known as the vasodilatory effect, the body's circulation is increased while the blood pressure and heart rate are reduced. Furthermore, the elimination of gravity on the body allows muscles and joints to release tension and heal more rapidly. For this reason, people suffering from musculoskeletal and rheumatic conditions greatly benefit from Floatation REST, as can women throughout the length of their **pregnancy**.

As the brain relaxes into a *theta* state, endorphins are released into the bloodstream, reducing **pain** and **fatigue**. The increased endorphin levels also promote a general sense of well-being and happiness and therefore increase vitality and further reduce levels of stress and tension. The blood levels of stress hormones such as adrenaline and cortisol are reduced by various body messages, receptor site activity, and organ processes. Combined, these positive effects help reduce the risks of high blood pressure and cardiovascular disease. Stress-related health problems as **migraine headache**, **hypertension**, and **insomnia** are similarly reduced.

The brain, freed of external stimuli, begins working more efficiently. This change provides the floater with an accelerated ability to learn, process information, and use his or her creative mind. This increased level of mental performance and concentration can be carried over into daily life. Equally important, Floatation REST can help with eliminating compulsive behaviors such as **alcoholism** and **smoking**. People with psychological and emotional problems as **anxiety** and **depression** can also benefit from this therapy.

An added benefit to Floatation REST stems from the Epsom salts used to provide buoyancy. According to the Archangel Vitamin, Health, and Nutrition Center's *Health Newsletter*, Epsom salt "draws toxins from the body, sedates the nervous system, reduces swelling, relaxes muscles, and is a natural emollient (and exfoliative)." Also, because the solution does not leach salt from the skin, the floater's skin will not wrinkle during the treatment.

Description

Modern float tanks are large enough in size and shape to allow a full-sized adult to easily enter, exit, and lie comfortably. The bottom of the light-proof and sound-insulated chamber is filled with a shallow 10–12-in (24.4–31 cm) pool of 30% **magnesium** sulfate (Epsom salt) solution. The density of this solution provides the floater with complete buoyancy and weightlessness. Indeed, the solution's density makes it impossible for the user to sink.

A float session begins when the tank's door is closed. Light is completely eliminated and sound is reduced to near zero through the combination of the tank's insulation and submersion of the floater's ears. Earplugs can further block outside noises. The air and water within the tank are maintained at a constant skin temperature. This neutral temperature prevents the physical and mental distractions caused by cold and heat. The silky nature of the solution further reduces the separation between the floater's skin and its surroundings, so that the body seems to gradually disappear. The combined elements of the tank, therefore, virtually eliminate all external stimulation for the floater.

Without environmental stimuli to process, the central nervous system's level of activity drops dramatically, sending the floater into a state of deep relaxation. The body undergoes positive physiological changes that work toward achieving homeostasis—the state of physical equilibrium. Muscular tension is released and proper blood flow is enhanced. Additionally, the body begins to balance any neurochemical imbalances caused by tension and stress. There is increased production of endorphins and T-cells, which provide pain relief and increased immunity, respectively. In essence, relieved of outward stimuli, the floater's central nervous system can concentrate most of its energies inward for the restoration of physical and mental health.

During a float session, the brain also enters the *theta* state, usually accessible only in the brief moments before falling asleep. This level of consciousness provides access to the right hemisphere of brain, which is associated with concentration, creativity, and learning. The brain can more easily retain information while in the *theta* state.

A typical float session lasts an hour, although longer sessions are available. After the floater rinses off the salt solution in a shower, most float centers provide a rest area to recuperate and reflect on the float session. This downtime with other floaters and staff enhances the relaxation process. In total, the entire session lasts one-and-one-half to two hours. Repeated weekly sessions are suggested to achieve the full benefits of Floatation REST.

Preparations

Persons interested in Flotation REST should consult with the local floatation center before the session. Most centers provide items such as towels, shampoo, soap, and hairdryers for their clients. Bathing suits are not required, and most people float without wearing one. It is recommended that a session be scheduled in advance to avoid a long wait.

Precautions

People suffering from high blood pressure, **heart disease**, or kidney conditions should consult a physician or family doctor before undergoing Floatation REST. Those who have claustrophobia, certain psychological disorders, or discomfort in the dark may find the treatment unpleasant.

Side effects

Prolonged exposure to the Epsom salt solution may cause **diarrhea** and dry skin. Otherwise, Floatation REST has no known negative side effects.

Research & general acceptance

Unfortunately, sensory deprivation remains stigmatized by the general public. Many people continue to associate it negatively with the experiments conducted in the 1950s and 1960s. Science fiction movies such as *Altered States* have done little to improve the therapy's public image. For this reason, the term floatation REST is more accurately and commonly used. Floatation centers have begun appearing in cities throughout the world, and are growing in popularity. Studies confirming the positive physical and mental benefits of Floatation REST further enhance their popularity.

Floatation REST has been researched and studied for decades. The positive findings have impressed even those who were once strongly opposed to it. Journalist Michael Hutchinson tried to debunk the therapy but ended up writing what some call the "definitive" book on Floatation REST. Hutchinson says in *The Book of Floating* that "there's no doubt that floatation therapy works—as a therapeutic, educational, and entertainment tool, it has powerful effects on a number of levels, including the physical, emotional, intellectual, and spiritual."

Research scientists and physicians confirm the benefits of floatation REST. In their study for *Health Psychology*, Jacobs and colleagues found that the results indicated that, "Floatation REST can be an effective means of teaching normal subjects to lower systolic and diastolic pressure and heighten their perception of relaxation."

In their literature review, *Floatation REST in Applied Psychophysiology*, Drs. Thomas Fine and Roderick Borrie concluded that floatation REST can have positive psychophysiological effects and clinical applications as well as uses in pain management, performance enhancement, and the treatment of chronic illness and depression. Further studies support these findings.

Training & certification

There is no training or certification required for those undergoing floatation REST. The floater does not even need to know how to swim.

All floatation centers must adhere to strict health and safety regulations. Ultraviolet lights, chemicals, and filtration help assure that water hygiene within the tanks is maintained at all times. Tanks can be easily opened from within so that a floater cannot be locked inside.

Resources

BOOKS

Barabasz, Arreed, and Marianne Barabasz, eds. *Clinical and Experimental Restricted Environmental Stimulation.* New York: Springer-Verlag, 1993.

Hutchison, Michael. *The Book of Floating: Exploring the Private Sea.* New York: William Morrow, 1985.

Lilly, John. *The Deep Self: Profound Relaxation and the Tank Isolation Technique.* New York: Simon & Schuster, 1977.

Suedfeld, Peter. *Restricted Environmental Stimulation.* Hoboken, NJ: Wiley, 1980.

PERIODICALS

Borrie, Roderick. "The Use of Restricted Environmental Stimulation Therapy in Treating Addictive Behaviors." *International Journal of Addiction* (1990–1991): 995–1015.

Fine, Thomas, and John Turner. "Rest-assisted Relaxation and Chronic Pain." *Health and Clinical Psychology* (1985): 511–18.

Jacobs G., R. Heilbronner, and J. Stanley. "The Effects of Short Term Flotation REST on Relaxation: A Controlled Study." *Health Psychology* (March 1984): 99–112.

Kjellgren, A., U. Sundequist, T. Norlander, and T. Archer. "Effects of Floatation-REST on Muscle Tension Pain." *Pain Research and Management* (Winter 2001): 181–9.

Turner, John, and Thomas Fine. "Restricting Environmental Stimulation Influences Levels and Variability of Plasma Cortisol." *Journal of Applied Psychology* (October 1991): 2010–13.

Wallbaum, A.B., R. Rzewnicki, H. Steele, and P. Suedfeld. "Progressive Muscle Relaxation and Restricted Environmental Stimulation Therapy for Chronic Tension Headache: A Pilot Study." *International Journal of Psychosomatics* (1991): 33–9.

OTHER

Fine, Thomas, and Roderick Borrie. *Floatation REST in Applied Psychophysiology.* [cited June 14, 2004]. <http://www.drborrie.com/rest2.html>.

"Float Tank Australia." *Introduction to Floating.* [cited June 14, 2004]. <http://www.floattank.com/what.html>.

KEY TERMS

Adrenaline—Also known as the "emergency hormone," adrenaline is produced by the body during times of stress. Excess adrenaline levels can increase blood pressure and heart rate, leading to heart disease.

Cortisol—Also known as the "stress hormone," cortisol is produced by the body during stress. Excess levels of cortisol can lead to a variety of health-related issues.

Endorphin—A natural substance released by the body to relieve fatigue and pain and bring on a sense of well-being.

Homeostasis—The state in which the body reaches its optimal level of internal balance and stability.

Parasympathetic response—A state of deep relaxation and the mechanism by which the body naturally regenerates itself and maintains chemical and metabolic balance.

Floatation.com. [cited May 30, 2004]. <http://www.floatation.com/index.html>.

London Floatation Tank Centre. [cited June 14, 2004]. <http://www.londonfloatcentre.com>.

Think Tank International. *About Floatation.* [cited June 14, 2004]. <http://www.thinktank.com.sg/float.htm>.

Tudor, Silke. "Going into the Tank." [cited June]. <http://www.sfweekly.com/issues/2000-03-01/nightcrawler.html>,

Lee Ann Paradise

Sensory integration disorder

Definition

Sensory integration disorder or dysfunction (SID) is a neurological disorder that results from the brain's inability to integrate certain information received from the body's five basic sensory systems. These sensory systems are responsible for detecting sights, sounds, smell, tastes, temperatures, **pain**, and the position and movements of the body. The brain then forms a combined picture of this information in order for the body to make sense of its surroundings and react to them appropriately. The ongoing relationship between behavior and brain functioning is called sensory integration (SI), a theory that was first pioneered by A. Jean Ayres, Ph.D., OTR, in the 1960s.

Description

Sensory experiences include touch, movement, body awareness, sight, sound, smell, taste and the pull of gravity. Distinguishing among these is the process of sensory integration (SI). While the process of SI occurs automatically and without effort for most, for some the process is inefficient. Extensive effort and attention are required in these individuals for SI to occur, without a guarantee of its being accomplished. When this happens, goals are not easily completed, resulting in sensory integration disorder (SID).

The normal process of SI begins before birth and continues throughout life, with the majority of SI development occurring before the early teenage years. The increased refinement and effectiveness of SI coincides with the **aging** process, as it determines how well motor and speech skills and emotional stability develop. Ayres' initial work on the SI theory instigated ongoing research that looks at the crucial foundation that SI provides for complex learning and behavior throughout life.

Causes & symptoms

The presence of a sensory integration disorder is typically detected in young children. While most children develop SI during the course of ordinary childhood activities, which helps establish such things as the ability for motor planning and adapting to incoming sensations, others SI ability does not develop as efficiently. When their process is disordered, a variety of problems in learning, development, or behavior become obvious.

Those who have sensory integration dysfunction may be unable to respond to certain sensory information by planning and organizing what needs to be done in an appropriate and automatic manner. This failure may trigger a primitive survival mechanism called "fright, flight, and fight," or withdrawal response, which originates from the "primitive" part of the brain, the limbic system. This response often appears extreme and inappropriate to the particular situation.

The neurological disorganization resulting in SID occurs in three different ways: the brain does not receive messages due to a disconnection in the neuron cells; sensory messages are received inconsistently; or sensory messages are received consistently, but do not connect properly with other sensory messages. When the brain poorly processes sensory messages, inefficient motor, language, or emotional output is the result.

According to Sensory Integration International (SII), a non-profit corporation concerned with the impact of sensory integrative problems on people's lives, the following are some signs of sensory integration disorder (SID):

- oversensitivity to touch, movement, sights, or sounds
- underreactivity to touch, movement, sights, or sounds

- a tendency to be easily distracted
- social and/or emotional problems
- activity level that is unusually high or unusually low
- physical clumsiness or apparent carelessness
- impulsivity or lack of self-control
- difficulty in making transitions from one situation to another
- inability to unwind or calm self
- poor self-concept
- delays in speech, language, or motor skills
- academic under achievement

While research indicates that sensory integrative problems are found in up to 70% of children who are considered learning-disabled by schools, the problems of sensory integration are not confined to children with learning disabilities. SID is found in people of all age groups, as well as intellectual levels and socioeconomic groups. Factors that contribute to SID include: premature birth; **autism** and other developmental disorders; learning disabilities; delinquency and substance abuse due to learning disabilities; stress-related disorders; and brain injury. Two of the biggest contributing conditions are autism and **attention-deficit hyperactivity disorder** (ADHD).

Diagnosis

In order to determine the presence of SID, an evaluation may be conducted by a qualified occupational or physical therapist. An evaluation normally consists of both standardized testing and structured observations of responses to sensory stimulation, posture, balance, coordination, and eye movements. These test results and assessment data, along with information from other professionals and parents, are carefully analyzed by the therapist, who then makes recommendations about appropriate treatment.

Treatment

Sensory integration disorder (SID) is treatable with occupational therapy, but some alternative methods are emerging to complement the conventional methods used for SID.

Therapeutic body brushing is often used on children (not infants) who overreact to tactile stimulation. A specific nonscratching surgical brush is used to make firm brisk movements over most of the body, especially the arms, legs, hands, back, and soles of the feet. A technique of deep joint compression follows the brushing. Usually begun by an occupational therapist, the technique is taught to parents, who must carry out the procedure for three to five minutes six to eight times a day. The time needed for brushing is reduced as the child begins to respond more normally to touch. In order for this therapy to be effective, the correct brush and technique must be used.

A report in 1998 indicates that the use of cerebral electrical stimulation (CES) is helpful to children with such conditions such as moderate to severe autistic spectrum disorders, learning disabilities, and sensory integration dysfunction. CES is a modification of Transcutaneous Electrical Nerve Stimulation (TENS) technology that has been used to treat adults with various **pain** problems, including arthritis and **carpal tunnel syndrome**. TENS therapy uses a low voltage electric current applied to the body through the skin with the goal of replacing painful impressions with a massage-like sensation. A much lower current is used for CES than that used for traditional TENS, and the electrodes are placed on the scalp or ears. Occupational therapists who have studied the use of CES suggest that CES for children with SID can result in improved brain activity. The device is worn by children at home for 10 minutes at a time twice per day.

Music therapy helps promote active listening. Hypnosis and **biofeedback** are sometimes used, along with **psychotherapy**, to help those with SID, particularly older patients.

Allopathic treatment

Occupational therapists play a key role in the conventional treatment of SID. By providing sensory integration therapy, occupational therapists are able to supply the vital sensory input and experiences that children with SID need to grow and learn. Also referred to as a "sensory diet," this type of therapy involves a planned and scheduled activity program implemented by an occupational therapist, with each "diet" being designed and developed to meet the needs of the child's nervous system. A sensory diet stimulates the "near" senses (tactile, vestibular, and proprioceptive) with a combination of alerting, organizing, and calming techniques.

Motor skills training methods that normally consist of adaptive physical education, movement education, and gymnastics are often used by occupational and physical therapists. While these are important skills to work on, the sensory integrative approach is vital to treating SID.

The sensory integrative approach is guided by one important aspect—the child's motivation in selection of the activities. By becoming actively involved, and explore activities that provide sensory experiences most beneficial to them, children become more mature and efficient at organizing sensory information.

Expected results

By combining alternative and conventional treatments and providing these therapies at an early age,

---

KEY TERMS

Axon—A process of a neuron that conducts impulses away from the cell body. Axons are usually long and straight.

Cortical—Regarding the cortex, or the outer layer of the brain, as distinguished from the inner portion.

Neurotransmission—When a neurotransmitter, or chemical agent released by a particular brain cell, travels across the synapse to act on the target cell to either inhibit or excite it.

Proprioceptive—Pertaining to proprioception, or the awareness of posture, movement, and changes in equilibrium and the knowledge of position, weight, and resistance of objects as they relate to the body.

Tactile—The perception of touch.

Vestibular—Pertaining to the vestibule; regarding the vestibular nerve of the ear which is linked to the ability to hear sounds.

---

sensory integration disorder may be managed successfully. The ultimate goal of both types of treatment is for the individual to be better able to interact with his or her environment in a more successful and adaptive way.

Resources

PERIODICALS

"Body Brushing Therapy for Tactile Defensiveness." *Latitudes* (April 30, 1997).

"Brain Stimulation for Autism?" *Latitudes* (October 31, 1998).

"Sensory Integration Therapy." *Latitudes* (December 31, 1994).

Morgan, Nancy. "Strategies for Colic." *Birth Gazette* (September 30, 1996).

ORGANIZATIONS

Sensory Integration International/The Ayres Clinic, 1514 Cabrillo Avenue, Torrance, CA 90501-2817. http://www.sensoryint.com.

OTHER

"Sensory Integration Dysfunction." http://home.ptd.net/blnelson/SIDEWEBPAGE2.htm.

Sensory Integration Network. http://www.sinetwork.org.

Southpaw Enterprises, Inc. http://www.southpawenterprises.com.

Beth Kapes

Sepia

Description

Sepia (*Sepia officinalis*) is the homeopathic name for "cuttlefish" or squid remedy. The remedy is made from the contents of the "ink bag" of the cuttlefish.

General use

Sepia's primary role in the world of alternative medicine is as one of the homeopathic remedies. In fact, it is classed as one of the 20 polychrests, which are those homeopathic remedies having the widest range of application, and which are also recommended for inclusion in the set of basic remedies that should be kept on hand in every household.

Homeopathy is a method of treatment devised by **Samuel Hahnemann** that works on the principle of treating "like with like," *(similia similibus curentur)*. Hahnemann devised a system of more than 100 remedies formulated to be administered in minute doses; effective, yet safe and without side effects. He discovered the principle of minute doses by gradually reducing medicines until he arrived at an effective dose with no side effects.

Hahnemann also discovered the method of "potentizing" his remedies by sucussing (similar to shaking) them vigorously. Until now, no one has been able to discover exactly why potentizing works. Even in his lifetime, Hahnemann's new methods were proven to be effective and safe.

According to homeopathy, the chief centers of action of the sepia remedy are those of the mind, mental processes and reproductive organs, upon which it is considered to act deeply over extended periods of time and to which it is more appropriate as a long-term remedy rather than a "quick fix."

Sepia is considered one of the chief remedies for the treatment of female ailments. It is particularly indicated for the following type of person: Irritable, tall thin girls who have pale sallow skin. These girls may often be ill, in fact never really well, and tired most of the time. They may often be at odds with others because of their attitudes. They feel better after **exercise** and improve with company, and when sociably occupied forget their ailments. These girls often suffer from heavy prolonged periods with intense cramping and general discomfort. Backache and **constipation** may also be experienced.

The ink of the cuttlefish was previously known as Indian ink, and was widely used by artists in the past because of its dark reddish brown pigment.

Uses for sepia

• women's problems related to **menstruation**

• costipation, particularly as a result of **pregnancy** or menstruation

• dandruff, particularly when associated with "pigmented patches"

• delayed menstruation, particularly if yeast **infections** are a problem

• problems associated with **menopause**, especially menstrual flooding and feeling that the womb will "drop out"

• amenorrhea when accompanied by **depression** and general aches and pains

• menorrhagia when accompanied by dragging **pain** in the lower abdomen, backache, depression, and irritability

• miscarriage when accompanied by dragging pains and irritability

• nonmalignant swellings and tumors of the uterus (such as fibroids), again, when accompanied by the dragging pains and emotional make-up outlined above

• bedwetting in children when it occurs soon after falling asleep, and involuntary passing of urine on **sneezing** or coughing

• irritability, especially when connected with menstruation

• morning sickness, especially when cravings are worse in the morning and there is a craving for vinegar or pickles

• thrush or candidiasis

• young mothers who are having difficulty developing maternal feelings

• babies who dislike being held

• depression accompanied by irritability and an exaggerated sense of responsibility

• infertility, particularly when associated with loss of libido, exhaustion, and apathy

Preparations

Homeopathic remedies come in several strengths, or potencies. Common examples include 6x, 12c, and 30c. For minor ailments, the 6x potency may be taken twice daily for seven to ten days. For acute conditions, either the 6x remedy may be taken every two to four hours for three to five days, or the 30 remedy may be taken once every four hours three times only.

For extremely serious conditions, such as severe pain or accidents, **burns** or hemorrhage, the patient can take either the 6x remedy once every fifteen minutes for six to eight doses or until the condition improves, or the

KEY TERMS

Amenorrhea—Absence of menstual periods.

Candidiasis—An infection caused by a fungus of the genus Candida, most commonly affectine the skin or mucus.

Fibroids—Fibrous non-cancerous growths on the uterus or surrounding tissue.

Ink bag—The part of a cuttlefish that contains their dye, also known as sepia.

Menorrhagia—Heavy and painful periods.

Potentize—To trigger the effectiveness of a substance.

30c potency once every 15 to 30 minutes for four to six doses or until the condition improves.

Precautions

Homeopathic remedies work best if the correct remedy is picked. The best person to do this is an experienced homeopathic physician. Some naturopathic physicians are among the finest homeopathic practitioners.

Homeopathic remedies should be dissolved under the tongue. Handling of the remedies should be kept to a minimum as they react to handling and may be spoiled. They should also be kept away from heat and light, and should not be swallowed with a drink. After taking a homeopathic dose, patients should not eat, drink, smoke, or clean their teeth for about fifteen minutes if possible.

Side effects

Homeopathic remedies are not known to produce side effects, as they have no effect except when matched with particular symptoms. Individual aggravations may occur.

Interactions

Homeopathic remedies can be taken in conjunction with allopathic medicine. Sepia should not be taken at the same time as **bryonia** or **lachesis**, as they may react adversely to each other. Coffee, peppermints, and some **essential oils** may counteract the effects of homeopathic remedies. Dental treatment may also affect the action of remedies.

Resources

BOOKS

Smith, Trevor. *Homeopathic Medicine, A Doctor's Guide to Remedies for Common Ailments*. UK: Thorsons Publishers, 1982.

Treacher, Sylvia. *Practical Homeopathy, A Beginner's Guide to Natural Remedies*. Bath: Parragon Books, 2000.

OTHER

American Association of Naturopathic Physicians. http://www.naturopathic.org.

Holistic-online.http://www.holisticonline.com.

Patricia Skinner

Septicemia *see* **Blood poisoning**

Sesame oil

Description

Sesame oil is derived from a plant species called *Sesamum indicum*, which is a herbaceous annual belonging to the Pedaliaceae family that reaches about 6 ft (1.8 m) in height. Sesame has been used for millennia in Chinese and Indian systems of medicine. Though often recommended as a laxative, the herb was used as early as the 4th century A.D. as a Chinese folk remedy for toothaches and **gum disease**. In modern times, sesame has been embraced by Western herbalists for a variety of therapeutic purposes. The oil is also used in cooking and as an ingredient in margarine and salad dressings as well as in certain cosmetics and skin softening products. Native to Asia and Africa, sesame is primarily cultivated in India, China, Africa, and Latin America. Only the seeds and oil of the sesame plant are used for medicinal purposes.

Sesame oil, which is also referred to as benne, gingili, or teel oil, is made from the black seeds of *Sesamum indicum*. The large round seeds are extracted by shaking the dried plant upside down after making an incision in the seed pods. The oil and seeds are believed by herbalists to have several important properties, including anticancer, antibacterial, and anti-inflammatory effects. Some of these claims have been supported by cell culture and human studies. Sesame may also have some power as an analgesic. In *The Green Pharmacy*, the prominent herbalist James Duke states that sesame contains at least seven pain-relieving compounds and is a rich source of **antioxidants** and other therapeutic agents. Some authorities believe that sesame also has weak estrogen-like effects.

Sesame oil is high in polyunsaturated fat. When used in moderation, this type of fat can benefit the heart by helping the body to eliminate newly made **cholesterol**, according to the American Heart Association.

General use

Nutrition and digestion

While not approved by the Food and Drug Administration (FDA) as a medication, sesame oil is reputed to have a number of therapeutic uses. Its centuries-old reputation as a laxative persists to this day. It is also used to treat blurred vision, **dizziness**, headaches, and to generally fortify the constitution during recuperation from severe or prolonged illness. When used in place of saturated fats, sesame oil may help to lower cholesterol levels and prevent **atherosclerosis**. The oil is taken internally for all the purposes mentioned above.

Menopausal symptoms

Due to its estrogen-like effects, sesame oil is sometimes recommended to alleviate the vaginal dryness associated with change of life. During **menopause**, women often experience this problem due to a decline in levels of female hormone. The vaginal lining becomes drier, thinner, and less elastic, which may lead to **pain** or irritation during intercourse. Some women insert cotton pads treated with sesame oil to increase lubrication and relieve symptoms associated with vaginal dryness.

Cancer

Research suggests that sesame oil may have potential as a **cancer** fighter. One cell culture study, published in the journal *Prostaglandins, Leukotrienes, and Essential Fatty Acids* in 1992, found that sesame oil blocked the growth of malignant melanoma in human cells. The researchers speculated that the **linoleic acid** (an essential fatty acid) in sesame oil may be responsible for its anticancer properties. Another test tube study, published in *Anticancer Research* in 1991, investigated the effects of sesame oil on human colon **cancer** cells. The results suggest that the oil may inhibit the development of the disease.

Traditional Asian medicine

Sesame oil plays a prominent role in Indian **Ayurvedic medicine**. It is sometimes rubbed into the skin during abhyanga, a form of Indian massage that focuses on over 100 points on the body (called marma points). Abhyanga is believed to improve energy flow and help free the body of impurities. Some practitioners of **Ayurvedic medicine** recommend sesame oil as an antibacterial mouthwash. In one small study involving 25 subjects in general good health, sesame oil was shown to reduce the growth of oral bacteria. These results suggest that the oil may help to prevent tooth and gum disease. According to tradition, sesame oil may also be applied externally to the abdomen to relieve cramps and stomach pain associated with **premenstrual syndrome** (PMS).

Sesame oil also has a reputation as a sedative in Indian and **Tibetan medicine**. It can be used to relieve **anxiety** and **insomnia** by applying a few drops directly into the nostrils. Its calming effects are supposedly carried to the brain by way of blood vessels in the nose.

Preparations

The optimum daily dosage of sesame oil has not been established with any certainty. People generally take 1 tsp of the oil at bedtime to relieve **constipation**.

Vaginal dryness associated with **menopause** may be relieved by following this procedure: Soak a quilted cotton cosmetic pad in sesame oil and then wring out the excess oil. A freshly treated cotton square may be inserted into the vagina overnight and removed each morning for seven days. After the first week, this treatment is typically used once a week (or as often as needed) as a form of maintenance therapy.

To relieve **anxiety** or insomnia, place one drop of pure raw sesame oil into each nostril.

Because sesame oil has been recommended for so many different purposes, and can be used internally and externally, consumers are advised to consult a doctor experienced in the use of alternative remedies or Chinese/Ayurvedic medicine to determine the proper dosage.

Precautions

Sesame oil is not known to be harmful when taken in recommended dosages, though it is important to remember that the long-term effects of taking sesame-derived remedies (in any amount) have not been investigated. Due to lack of sufficient medical study, sesame oil should be used with caution in children, women who are pregnant or breast-feeding, and people with liver or kidney disease.

Because of its laxative effects, sesame oil should not be used by people who have **diarrhea**.

Sesame oil is best kept refrigerated to protect it from oxidation. It should also be protected from light and heat. While the oil may be added to cooked food, it should not be employed during the cooking process because high temperatures can compromise its therapeutic effects. In other words, do not use it during frying, boiling, or baking. Sesame oil may be used in a low-temperature sauté without losing much of its medicinal value, according to some authorities.

No more than 10% of a person's total caloric intake should be derived from polyunsaturated fats such as those found in sesame oil, according to the American Heart Association.

KEY TERMS

Analgesic—Any substance that functions as a pain reliever.

Antioxidant—An agent that helps to protect cells from damage caused by free radicals, the destructive fragments of oxygen produced as a byproduct during normal metabolic processes.

Linoleic acid—An essential fatty acid that is found in sesame oil.

Melanoma—A common form of skin cancer originating in the cells that provide the skin with coloring.

While some body builders inject themselves with sesame oil to enhance muscles, this practice is not recommended and may be potentially dangerous. According to a report published in the *Journal of the American Academy of Dermatology* in 2000, injecting sesame or other plant-derived oils may lead to the development of cysts. Scarring, skin thickening, and scleroderma or other connective tissue diseases may also occur as a result of such injections.

Side effects

When taken in recommended dosages, sesame oil is not associated with any bothersome or significant side effects.

Interactions

Sesame oil is not known to interact adversely with any drug or dietary supplement. Sesame seeds have been combined with **biota** seeds, **dong quai**, and white mulberry leaf without apparent harm.

Resources

BOOKS

Collinge, William. *The American Holistic Health Association Complete Guide to Alternative Medicine.* New York: Warner Books, 1996.

ORGANIZATIONS

American Botanical Council. PO Box 144345. Austin, TX 78714-4345.

OTHER

Medline.http://igm.nlm.nih.gov.

Greg Annussek

Sexual dysfunction

Definition

Sexual dysfunction is broadly defined as the inability to fully enjoy sexual intercourse. Specifically, sexual dysfunction is a group of disorders that interfere with a full sexual responsiveness. These disorders make it difficult for a person to enjoy or to have sexual intercourse. While sexual dysfunction rarely threatens physical health, it can take a heavy psychological toll, bringing on **depression**, **anxiety**, and debilitating feelings of inadequacy.

Description

Sexual dysfunction takes different forms in men and women. A dysfunction can be lifelong and always present, or it can be temporary and sporadic. It can be situational or generalized. In either gender, symptoms of a sexual problem include the lack or loss of sexual desire, anxiety during intercourse, **pain** during intercourse, or the inability to achieve orgasm. In addition, a man may have a sexual problem if he:

• Ejaculates before he or his partner desires.

• Does not ejaculate, or experiences delayed ejaculation.

• Is unable to have or maintain an erection sufficient for pleasurable intercourse.

Also, a woman may have a sexual problem if she:

• Feels vaginal or other muscles contract involuntarily before or during sex.

• Has inadequate vaginal lubrication.

The most common sexual dysfunctions in men include:

• Erectile dysfunction: an impairment of a man's ability to have or maintain an erection that is firm enough for coitus or intercourse.

• Premature ejaculation, or rapid ejaculation, with minimal sexual stimulation before, on, or shortly after penetration and before the person wishes it.

• Ejaculatory incompetence: the inability to ejaculate within the vagina despite a firm erection and relatively high levels of sexual arousal.

• Retarded ejaculation: a condition in which the bladder neck does not close off properly during orgasm so that the semen spurts backward into the bladder.

Female sexual dysfunctions include:

• Sexual arousal disorder: the general arousal aspect of sexual response is inhibited. A woman with this disorder does not lubricate, her vagina does not swell, and the muscle that surrounds the outer third of the vagina does not tighten—a series of changes that normally prepare the body for orgasm ("the orgasmic platform"). Also, in this disorder, the woman typically does not feel erotic sensations.

• Orgasmic disorder: the orgasmic component of the female sexual response is impaired. The woman may be sexually aroused but never reach orgasm.

• Vaginismus: a condition in which the muscles around the outer third of the vagina have involuntary spasms in response to attempts at vaginal penetration.

• Painful intercourse also known as dyspareunia.

Causes & symptoms

Many factors of both physical and psychological origin can affect sexual response and performance. Injuries, such ailments as **infections**, and drugs of abuse are among the physical influences. Certain prescription medications, such as drugs to regulate blood **cholesterol** levels, may also affect sexual functioning. In addition, there is increasing evidence that chemicals and other environmental pollutants depress sexual function. As for psychological factors, sexual dysfunction may have roots in traumatic events such as rape or incest, guilt feelings, a poor self-image, depression, chronic **fatigue**, certain religious beliefs, or marital problems. Dysfunction is often associated with anxiety. If a man operates under the misconception that all sexual activity must lead to intercourse and to orgasm by his partner, he may consider the act a failure if his expectations are not met.

In Chinese medicine, sexual dysfunction is considered an imbalance of yin and yang. Yin and yang are the two dependent and constantly interacting forces of energy in the world, according to ancient Chinese thought. Yin energy is receptive, dark, feminine, and cool. It is associated with the heavy, the cold, and the moist. Yang energy is masculine, active, bright, and warm. It is associated with the dry, the light, and the hot. People with sexual dysfunction who have yin deficiency are too dry and tired, causing premature ejaculation or dry and spastic conditions. Symptoms of a yang deficiency may include erectile dysfunction as well as lack of sexual appetite or excitement. There are other imbalances that can cause sexual dysfunction.

Other types of alternative medicine, such as herbalism, regard sexual dysfunction as stemming from the same causes as those recognized by Western medicine. In such alternative approaches as **homeopathy**, sexual dysfunction is seen as an energy deficiency in the sexual organs or the glands that regulate these organs.

Diagnosis

In deciding whether sexual dysfunction is present, it is necessary to remember that each person has a different level of sexual interest. While some people may be interested in sex at almost any time, others have low or seemingly nonexistent levels of sexual interest. A sexual condition is classified as sexual dysfunction only when it is a source of personal or interpersonal distress instead of a voluntary choice.

The first step in diagnosing a sexual dysfunction is usually discussing the problem with a doctor or an alternative practitioner, who will need to ask further questions so he or she can differentiate among the types of sexual dysfunction. The physician may also perform a physical exam of the genitals, and may order further medical tests, including measurement of hormone levels in the blood.

An expert in Chinese medicine will take the pulses at the wrist to assess the patient's overall health. According to Chinese thought, there are 12 pulses at the wrist, six on each wrist. The practitioner will ask questions that relate to yin and yang energy, such as whether the patient's hands and feet are cold or warm most of the time. An alternative practitioner is also likely to query the patient about his diet and any issues in his life that may be contributing to **stress**.

In allopathic medicine, men may be referred to a urologist, a specialist in diseases of the urinary and genital organs, and women may be referred to a gynecologist.

Treatment

A variety of alternative therapies can be useful in the treatment of sexual dysfunction. Counseling or **psychotherapy** is highly recommended to address any emotional or mental components of the disorder. Nutritional supplementation, as well as Western, Chinese, or ayurvedic **botanical medicine**, can help resolve biochemical causes of sexual dysfunction.

Beneficial supplements and herbs include gingko biloba, which improves circulation to the genitals and has been shown to be effective in a number of studies. If the cause is a psychological, emotional, or energy disorder, such adrenal tonics as **licorice**, **epimedium**, eucommia, and **cuscuta** can restore the patient's mood and increase sexual interest. These herbs increase the ability to adapt to physical and mental stress because they increase the power of the adrenal system, which secretes the brain chemical epinephrine. If the patient's reproductive organs are not producing enough of the hormones that regulate sex drive and function, vitex is also a good solution. When a patient lacks sexual drive, such tonics as deer antler can increase interest in sex.

One drug derived from herbal sources that is used in mainstream medicine to treat **impotence** in men is yohimbine, an alkaloid derived from the bark of the **yohimbe** or rauwolfia tree. Yohimbine is used to treat inadequate circulation in the arms and legs and to dilate the pupil of the eye as well as to treat impotence. It is available as a prescription medication under such brand names as Yocon and Yohimex. Yohimbine does not work for all men affected by impotence, but appears to have fewer side effects than sildenafil (Viagra).

Homeopathic treatment can be helpful by focusing on the energetic aspects of the disorder. A Chinese medicine practitioner might address sexual dysfunction by using **acupuncture**, in which hair-thin needles are used to stimulate the body's energy (or qi). According to ancient Chinese theory, the body has 12 meridians that correspond to various organs, their functions, and the patient's emotions. Acupuncture needles might be applied at points on these meridians that regulate the kidney, which forms the foundation for the reproductive system in **traditional Chinese medicine**, or to other meridians that have roles in sexual function.

Yoga and **meditation** provide needed mental and physical **relaxation** for conditions such as vaginismus. A yoga teacher may advise forward bends to calm the patient and yoga twists to help the body produce hormones that increase sexual drive and a feeling of well-being.

Relaxation therapy eases and relieves anxiety about dysfunction. Massage is extremely effective at reducing stress, especially if performed by the partner.

A massage therapist or aromatherapist can also provide sandalwood or jasmine oils to boost sexual drive. An aromatherapist usually prescribes singular scents or a mixture created with the person's preferences and his or her symptoms in mind.

Allopathic treatment

Allopathic treatments break down into two main categories: behavioral psychotherapy and physical treatment. Sex therapy, ideally provided by a member of the American Association of Sexual Educators, Counselors, and Therapists (AASECT), emphasizes correction of sexual misinformation, the importance of improved partner communication and honesty, anxiety reduction, sensual experience and pleasure, and interpersonal tolerance and acceptance. Sex therapists believe that many sexual disorders are rooted in learned patterns and values. These disorders or symptoms are termed psychogenic. An underlying assumption of sex therapy is that relatively short-term outpatient therapy can alleviate learned patterns, restrict symptoms, and allow a greater satisfaction with sexual experiences.

In some cases, a specific technique may be used during intercourse to correct a dysfunction. One of the most common is the "squeeze technique" to prevent premature ejaculation. When a man feels that an orgasm is imminent, he withdraws from his partner. Then, the man or his partner gently squeezes the head of the penis to halt the orgasm. After 20-30 seconds, the couple may resume intercourse. The couple may repeat this technique several times before the man proceeds to ejaculation.

In cases in which significant sexual dysfunction is linked to a broader emotional problem such as depression or substance abuse, intensive psychotherapy and/or medications may be appropriate. People who are taking such medications as fluoxetine (Prozac), paroxetine (Paxil), or reboxetine (Edronax) for depression, however, should be advised that sexual dysfunction in adults of either sex is a fairly common side effect of these medications.

In many cases, doctors prescribe medications to treat an underlying physical cause of sexual dysfunction. Possible medical treatments include:

• Clomipramine and fluoxetine for premature ejaculation.

• Papaverine and prostaglandin for erectile difficulties.

• Hormone replacement therapy or androgen therapy for female dysfunctions.

• Sildenafil (Viagra), a drug approved in 1998 as a treatment for impotence. As of 2002, however, sildenafil has been shown to have potentially serious side effects, including headaches, **nausea**, sudden changes in blood pressure, and eye disorders.

Expected results

There is no single cure for sexual dysfunction, but almost all of the individual conditions can be controlled. Most people who have a sexual dysfunction fare well once they get into a treatment program. Most alternative therapies, however, take at least several weeks to take effect. If the patient doesn't see improvement in that time, he or she should consider trying another practitioner.

Prevention

It often helps to continue such treatments, such as acupuncture and massage after the initial problem is resolved. Doing so keeps sexual energy high and the genital organs and sex glands healthy. By continuing to use alternative therapies, the patient can help maintain sexual interest even when normal sexual doldrums occur. Continuing to take alternative medicines or treatment also ensures the problem won't return.

Resources

BOOKS

American Psychiatric Association. *Diagnostic and Statistical Manual of Mental Disorders,* 4th ed., text revision. Washington, D.C.: American Psychiatric Association, 2000.

Masters, William H., Virginia E. Johnson, and Robert C. Kolodny. *Human Sexuality.* New York: HarperCollins, 1992.

Molony, David. *The American Association of Oriental Medicine's Complete Guide to Herbal Medicine.* New York: Berkley Books, 1998.

PERIODICALS

Guay, A. T., R. F. Spark, J. Jacobson, et al. "Yohimbine Treatment of Organic Erectile Dysfunction in a Dose-Escalation Trial." *International Journal of Impotence Research* 14 (February 2002): 25-31.

Haberfellner, E. M. "Sexual Dysfunction Caused by Reboxetine." *Pharmacopsychiatry* 35 (March 2002): 77-78.

Hensley, P. L., and H. G. Nurnberg. "SSRI Sexual Dysfunction: A Female Perspective." *Journal of Sex and Marital Therapy* 28 (2002, Suppl. 1): 143-153.

Pomerantz, H. D., K. H. Smith, W. M. Hart, Jr., and R. A. Egan. "Sildenafil-Associated Nonarteritic Anterior Ischemic Optic Neuropathy." *Ophthalmology* 109 (March 2002): 584-587.

Traish, A. M., N. Kim, K. Min, et al. "Androgens in Female Genital Sexual Arousal Function: A Biochemical Perspective." *Journal of Sex and Marital Therapy* 28 (2002, Suppl. 1): 233-244.

Wagstaff, A. J., S. M. Cheer, A. J. Matheson, et al. "Spotlight on Paroxetine in Psychiatric Disorders in Adults." *CNS Drugs* 16 (2002): 425-434.

ORGANIZATIONS

American Academy of Clinical Sexologists. 1929 18th Street NW, Suite 1166, Washington, DC 20009. (202) 462-2122.

American Association for Marriage and Family Therapy. 1100 17th Street NW, 10th Floor, Washington, DC 20036-4601. (202) 452-0109.

American Association of Oriental Medicine. 909 22nd St. Sacramento, CA 95816. (916) 451-6950. <http://www.aaom.org>.

American Association of Sex Educators, Counselors & Therapists. P.O. Box 238, Mt. Vernon, IA 52314. <http://www.aasect.org>.

Yoga Research and Education Center. P.O. Box 1386, Lower Lake, CA 95457. (707) 928-9898. <http://www.yrec.com.>.

Barbara Boughton
Rebecca J. Frey, PhD

Sexually transmitted diseases *see*
Chlamydia; Genital herpes; Genital warts; Gonorrhea; Syphilis

Shamanism

Definition

A complex pattern of diverse rites and beliefs, shamanism is a tribal religion in societies without a literary tradition. Healing is one function of the shaman and the most important along with prophecy. The shaman uses mystical powers to journey to other worlds or realities and communicate with spirits in order to bring about a balance between the physical and spiritual worlds.

Origins

Shamanism is the oldest form of human healing. It is a type of religious medicine that originated over 25,000 years ago in the Paleolithic hunting cultures of Siberia and Central Asia. The English word shaman is derived from the Siberian Tungus word "saman," which is defined as a technique of ecstasy. The shaman is considered a great master of trance and ecstasy. He or she is the dominating figure in certain indigenous populations.

Most early cultures' healing practices stem from a shamanic tradition. For instance, when visiting the sick, Egyptian magicians often brought a papyrus roll filled with incantations and amulets in order to drive out demons.

The shaman is often the religious leader or priest of the tribe. He is believed to have magical powers that can heal the sick. The shaman is called upon to mediate between the people of the community and the spirit world to cure disease, exorcize evil spirits, and to promote success in hunting and food production and to keep the tribal community in balance. Traditional shamanic rituals included singing, dancing, chanting, drumming, storytelling, and healing. The shaman is a specialist in human souls. He is able to see them and know their form and destiny. The shaman controls the spirits. Rather than being possessed by them, he communicates with the dead, demons, and nature spirits.

The shaman's work is based on the belief that the soul can forsake the body even while a person is alive and can stray into other cosmic realms where it falls prey to demons and sorcerers. The shaman diagnoses the problem, then goes in search of the wandering soul and makes it return to the body.

Shamanism is still practiced all over the world, although each culture's shamanic tradition has evolved in different ways. **Native American medicine** men perform soul flights and vision quests to heal. North American Inuit shamans undertake undersea spirit journeys to ensure a plentiful supply of game. Tibetan shamans use a drum to help them in spirit flight and soul retrieval. Central and South American shamans often use hallucinogenic plants to invoke their shamanic journeys. Australian aborigine shamans believe that crystals can be inserted into the body for power. Some cultures have female as well as male shamans.

Benefits

Shamanism is based on the belief that the condition of the soul must be addressed in order for healing to occur. Relief of **pain**, **anxiety**, and **stress**, as well as spiritual and emotional healing, are common benefits of a shamanic healing.

Description

Shamans believe that there are realities that exist beyond the dimension that we experience on Earth. They believe that all creation is alive—rocks, plants, animals, trees, fish—and work regularly with these forces of nature.

The role of the shaman is to mediate between different realities to treat disease and create harmony between the physical and spiritual dimensions. Shamanism is a combination of "magic" and medicine. A shaman is a warrior who uses his power to combat disease, demons, and practitioners of black magic. They also perform rights to assure success in hunting and fishing, to protect the tribe's lands, and increase and develop the family. Although shamans have traditionally been male, there are many female shamans in contemporary Asia and Africa.

Shamans can see and exorcize spirits, perceive when a person's soul has fled from the body, and return souls to their rightful owners. They specialize in soul healing, heal-

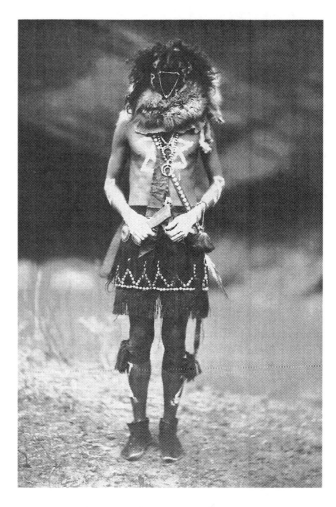

A Navajo medicine man in 1904. *(Photograph by Edward S. Curtis. The Library of Congress.)*

ing physical sickness, and delivering a deceased person's soul to the underworld of death. They also communicate with ancestral spirits, gods, and demons through ceremony, sacred dance, vision quests, by visiting places of power, and through dreams and out-of-body experiences.

The basis of a shaman's work stems from his or her mastery of the ecstasy technique, in which he or she enters an altered state of consciousness known as the trance state. During this state, the shaman's soul leaves his or her body to travel to nonphysical realities, in order to communicate with spirits and gain information for healing.

The state of ecstasy is brought about in several ways, depending upon the shaman's culture. Native American shamans use drumming, dancing, and chanting to enter the trance state. Some Central and South American shamans use peyote or other hallucinogenic plants to enter a state of altered consciousness.

During their spiritual journey, shamans may travel to heavens and hells, higher levels of existence, parallel physical worlds, or other regions of the world. The shaman is protected during his travels by spirit helpers and such animal guides as bears, wolves, stags, hares, and birds.

According to Central and North American shamanism, disease is caused when the soul strays or is stolen from the body. To restore health a shaman goes in search of the spirit, captures it, and persuades it to return. Illness may also be caused when the body becomes possessed by evil spirits, or by a magical object such as a pebble or insect that has been telepathically implanted in the body by sorcerers of black magic. The shaman removes the item by sucking it out of the patient's body.

Shamans often wear ritual costumes such as feathers, masks, or animal skins. They may also use ritual objects, charms, and herbs.

Training & certification

Becoming a shaman is not an ordinary task that occurs overnight. Shamans go through strenuous training before they begin to practice as a shaman. They are usually chosen or "called" by the spirits. This call to become a shaman may involve a series of tests to prove intent and worth.

A personal crisis, severe trauma, near-death experience, lightning strike, or life-threatening illness may serve as the calling to become a shaman. Initiation may also occur though dreams or visions as the spirits are made known to the chosen one. This connection between a call to become a shaman and physical or emotional trauma is one reason why some historians and psychiatrists regard shamanism as evidence of mental illness. They see resemblances between the dreams, visions, and other unusual experiences reported by shamans and the delusions and hallucinations associated with **schizophrenia** and other psychotic disorders.

In many cultures, the shamanic tradition is passed from father to son, from mother to daughter, or to those outside the shaman's family who have answered the call. The teaching involves training by master shamans in the ecstatic trance; a thorough understanding of traditional shamanic techniques; the names and functions of spirits; and the mythology and genealogy of the clan. While in the apprentice stage, the shaman-to-be learns about the soul: the forces that can threaten it and where it may flee or be captured by evil spirits.

A shaman's initiation typically involves a visionary death or dismemberment of the body during the trance journey. By knowing death and returning from it, the shaman attains the secret of life and the power to heal. The shaman-in-training must also undergo an initiation

in which he faces and resolves his fears. After the initiation, the shaman is trained by a more experienced shaman until he has reached a level of mastery.

In modern times, shamanic knowledge is being shared with the general population. One does not have to belong to a native tribe to become a shaman. Carlos Casteneda, one of the most well-known writers of shamanism, studied under a Native American Yaqui shaman. Dr. Michael Harner, an anthropologist, is one of the world's leading authorities on shamanism and has even started a nonprofit educational organization, The Foundation for Shamanic Studies. Modern shamanism is often practiced in groups and lodges and through workshops and classes. Shamanic training may be obtained through similar schools or psychological or spiritual teachers.

Several schools of shamanism are located in the United States:

• Dance of the Deer Foundation, Center for Shamanic Studies, P.O. Box 699, Soquel, CA 95073. (831)475-9560. www.shamanism.com.

• The Foundation for Shamanic Studies, P.O. Box 1939, Mill Valley, CA 94942. (415) 380-8282.

Resources

BOOKS

Goldberg, Dr. Bruce. *Soul Healing.* Minneapolis, MN: Llewellyn Publications, 1997.

Harner, Michael. *The Way of the Shaman.* San Francisco, CA: Harper, 1990.

Mindell, Arnold. *The Shaman's Body.* San Francisco, CA: Harper, 1993.

Moorey, Teresa. *Shamanism: A Beginner's Guide.* London, UK: Hodder and Stoughton, 1997.

PERIODICALS

Polimeni, J., and J. P. Reiss. "How Shamanism and Group Selection May Reveal the Origins of Schizophrenia." *Medical Hypotheses* 58 (March 2002): 244-248.

Jennifer Wurges
Rebecca J. Frey, PhD

Sheep sorrel

Description

Sheep sorrel (*Rumex acetosella*) is a tall herb that is found in grasslands, prairies, meadows, fields, pastures, and roadsides of Europe, Asia, and North America. This perennial plant from the buckwheat (Polygonaceae) family was originally from Eurasia, but is now naturalized throughout Canada and the United States. Sheep sorrel is also known as field sorrel, red top sorrel, sour grass, common sorrel, and dog-eared sorrel. The plant is related to other highly acidic members of the *Rumex* genus, including French or garden sorrel (*Rumex acetosa*).

Sheep sorrel is considered a common weed in the United States. Its slim reddish stems grow to a height of 4-24 in (10-60 cm). Narrow arrow-shaped leaves that have a pungent lemon scent grow to 1-4 in (2-10 cm) long. The slender roots grow to a depth of 5 feet (1.5 m). Near the upper part of the stem are small yellow or red flowers that bloom in the spring and summer, generally from April to September. The male plant has yellow flowers while the female plant has red flowers.

Sheep sorrel has antioxidant, diuretic, detoxifying, laxative, astringent, and diaphoretic properties. The herb is a rich source of vitamins and minerals. Vitamins B-complex, C, D, E, K, and P are included in sheep sorrel. It contains **sodium, calcium, sulfur, iron, magnesium,** chlorine, silicon, **copper, iodine, manganese, zinc,** and **beta carotene.** The silicon in sheep sorrel may help the nervous system. Other constituents of sheep sorrel are malic, oxalic, tannic, and tartaric acids; chlorophyll; rutins; polysaccharides; protein; and **carotenoids.**

The oxalic acid in sheep sorrel is the substance that gives the leaves a sour lemony taste. Large intakes of sheep sorrel can be poisonous due to the oxalic acid content. Livestock that have eaten excessive quantities of sheep sorrel have been poisoned. It has also been reported that large consumption of sheep sorrel causes **dermatitis** in some animals. Too much oxalic acid can prevent the body from using important nutrients, especially calcium. When the plant is cooked, the oxalic acid content is reduced.

Origins

French sorrel has been used as a food for hundreds of years. Native Americans ate the leaves, stems, seeds, and roots, and seasoned their meats and bread with the herb. The Irish used French sorrel as an ingredient in soup, and the French added the leaves to salads. In colonial times, sugar and vinegar were added to French sorrel leaves to create a sauce that was eaten over cold meat. A dark green, brown, or dark gray dye was made from the roots. Medicinally, sheep sorrel was used as a folk remedy to treat **cancer.**

General use

Today, French sorrel is still used as a food. The leaves are used as a thickener in soups, ground into a powder and made into noodles, or added to salads.

Sheep sorrel is gaining popularity as an anticancer agent and for its ability to break down and reduce tumors. A poultice made from sheep sorrel is reported to have a drawing effect on tumors or cysts. Sheep sorrel's rutins and polysaccharides act to prevent tumors and other cancerous growths. The beta carotene contained in sheep sorrel acts as an antioxidant, increasing the production of white blood cells and T-cells (cancer-killing cells). The chlorophyll in sheep sorrel acts to purify the liver, promote regeneration of tissue, decrease swelling of the pancreas, strengthen cell walls, cleanse the blood, and may increase resistance to x rays. The oxalic acid also has antitumor and anticancer properties.

Sheep sorrel is an ingredient in **essiac tea,** an herbal preparation that was adopted from an Ojibwa recipe and is used to treat a variety of cancers. The tea also contains rhubarb, **burdock root,** and **slippery elm.** Sheep sorrel has also been used to treat the side effects of chemotherapy.

Herbalists recommend sheep sorrel for treating mouth and throat ulcers, digestive disorders, **hemorrhoids,** loss of appetite, fevers, scurvy, and **infections.** The juice extracted from the fresh plant is used to treat urinary and kidney disease. Sheep sorrel can be applied externally as a topical wash for skin problems such as herpes, **eczema,** and itchy **rashes** including poison ivy and **hives.**

Preparations

All parts of sheep sorrel (leaves, flowers, roots, and stems) are used medicinally. The leaves and stems should be harvested in the spring or summer before the flowers form. The roots are harvested in the fall.

Small quantities of the leaves of sheep sorrel may be eaten in salads or boiled as a green vegetable. Sheep sorrel is also available in tincture, capsule, or tea form.

For the tincture, 30-120 drops may be diluted in a glass of water and drunk daily.

The leaves are brewed as a tea to treat **fever**, inflammation, and scurvy. A tea made from the roots is used for **diarrhea** and excessive menstrual bleeding. To create an infusion, the leaves and stems are steeped in hot water for five minutes, or the roots are steeped 10 minutes, and 2-3 cups can be drunk daily.

Precautions

Due to the high oxalic acid content, large doses of sheep sorrel can be toxic. Oxalic acid can cause **kidney stones**, irritate the kidneys, or worsen an existing kidney disorder. For these reasons, those with kidney problems or who are prone to kidney ailments should not use sheep sorrel.

When using the leaves as a food, one should eat small quantities, or cook them to reduce the oxalic content.

People with arthritis, rheumatism, **endometriosis**, **gout**, or kidney stones should use caution when taking sheep sorrel since it may aggravate their condition.

Sheep sorrel should not be used by children, infants, or pregnant or breast-feeding women.

Side effects

High doses of sheep sorrel may cause **nausea**, a tingling sensation of the tongue, or a severe **headache**.

Interactions

There are no known interactions between sheep sorrel and standard prescription medications as of 2004.

Resources

BOOKS

Duke, James A. *The Green Pharmacy*. Emmaus, PA: Rodale Press, 1997.

Jennifer Wurges

Shiatsu

Definition

Shiatsu is a manipulative therapy developed in Japan and incorporating techniques of *anma* (Japanese traditional massage), **acupressure**, stretching, and Western massage. Shiatsu involves applying pressure to special points or areas on the body in order to maintain physical and mental well being, treat disease, or alleviate discomfort. This therapy is considered holistic because it attempts to treat the whole person instead of a specific medical complaint. All types of **acupressure** generally focus on the same pressure points and so-called energy pathways, but may differ in terms of massage technique. Shiatsu, which can be translated as finger pressure, has been described as needle-free **acupuncture**.

Origins

Shiatsu is an offshoot of anma that developed during the period after the Meiji Restoration in 1868. Traditional massage (anma) used during the age of the shoguns was being criticized, and practitioners of *koho anma* (ancient way) displeased with it introduced new practices and new names for their therapies.

During the twentieth century, shiatsu distinguished itself from anma through the merging of Western knowledge of anatomy, koho anma, *ampuku* (abdominal massage), acupressure, *Do-In* (breathing practices), and Buddhism. Based on the work of Tamai Tempaku, shiatsu established itself in Japan and worldwide. The Shiatsu Therapists Association was found in 1925 and clinics and schools followed. Students of Tempaku began teaching their own brand of shiatsu, creating branch disciplines. By 1955, the Japanese Ministry of Health and Welfare acknowledged shiatsu as a beneficial treatment and licensing was established for its practitioners.

Benefits

Shiatsu has a strong reputation for reducing **stress** and relieving **nausea** and **vomiting**. Shiatsu is also believed to improve circulation and boost the immune sys-

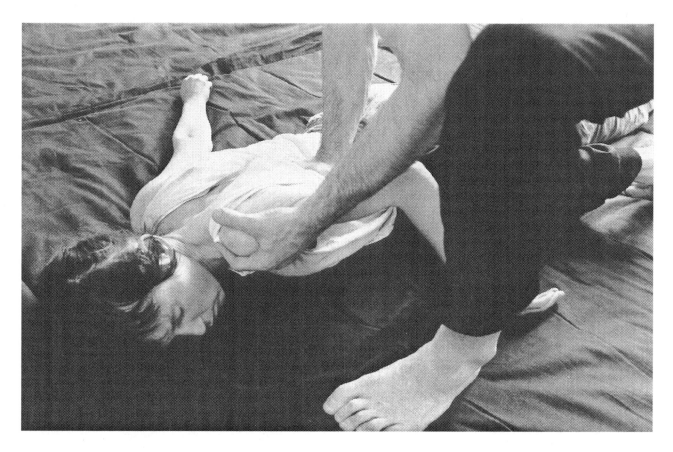

A woman receiving shiatsu massage on her shoulder. *(Photo Researchers, Inc. Reproduced by permission.)*

tem. Some people use it to treat **diarrhea**, **indigestion**, **constipation**, and other disorders of the gastrointestinal tract; menstrual and menopausal problems; chronic **pain**; migraine; arthritis; **toothache**; **anxiety**; and **depression**. Shiatsu can be used to relieve muscular pain or tension, especially neck and back pain. It also appears to have sedative effects and may alleviate **insomnia**. In a broader sense, shiatsu is believed to enhance physical vitality and emotional well-being.

Description

Shiatsu and other forms of Japanese acupressure are based on the concept of *ki*, the Japanese term for the all-pervading energy that flows through everything in the universe. (This notion is borrowed from the Chinese, who refer to the omnipresent energy as *qi* or *chi*.) Ki tends to flow through the body along special energy pathways called meridians, each of which is associated with a vital organ. In Asian systems of traditional medicine, diseases are often believed to occur due to disruptions in the flow of this energy through the body. These disruptions may stem from emotional factors, the climate, or a host of other causes including **stress**, the presence of impurities in the body, and physical trauma.

The aim of shiatsu is to restore the proper flow of bodily energy by massaging the surface of the skin along the meridian lines. Pressure may also be applied to any of the 600 or so acupoints. Acupoints, which are supposedly located just under the skin along the meridians, are tiny energy structures that affect the flow of ki through the body. When ki either stagnates and becomes deflected or accumulates in excess along one of these channels, stimulation of the acupoints, which are sensitive to pressure, can unblock and regulate the ki flow through toning or sedating treatment.

Western medicine hasn't proven the existence of meridians and acupoints. However, in one study, two French medical doctors conducted an experiment at the Necher Hospital in Paris to test the validity of theory that energy is being transported along acupuncture meridians. They injected and traced radioactive isotopes with gamma-camera imaging. The meridians may actually correspond to nerve transmission lines. In this view, shiatsu and other forms of healing massage may trigger the emission of naturally occurring chemicals called neurotransmitters. Release of these chemical messengers may be responsible for some of the therapeutic effects associated with shiatsu, such as pain relief.

Preparations

People usually receive shiatsu therapy while lying on a floor mat or massage table or sitting up. The massage is performed through the clothing—preferably a thin garment made from natural fibers—and disrobing is not required. Pressure is often applied using the thumbs, though various other parts of the body may be employed, including fingertips, palms, knuckles, elbows, and knees—some therapists even use their feet. Shiatsu typically consists of sustained pressure (lasting up to 10 seconds at a time), squeezing, and stretching exercises. It may also involve gentle holding as well as rocking motions. A treatment session lasts anywhere from 30 to 90 minutes.

Before shiatsu treatment begins, the therapist usually performs a general health assessment. This involves taking a family medical history and discussing the physical and emotional health of the person seeking therapy. Typically, the practitioner also conducts a diagnostic examination by palpating the abdomen or back for any energy imbalances present in other parts of the body.

Precautions

While shiatsu is generally considered safe, there are a few precautions to consider. Because it may increase blood flow, this type of therapy is not recommended in people with bleeding problems, **heart disease** , or **cancer. Massage therapy** should always be used with caution in those with **osteoporosis**, fresh **wounds** or scar tissue, bone **fractures**, or inflammation.

Applying pressure to areas of the head is not recommended in people with **epilepsy** or high blood pressure, according to some practitioners of shiatsu.

Shiatsu is not considered effective in the treatment of **fever, burns**, and infectious diseases.

Shiatsu should not be performed right after a meal.

Side effects

When performed properly, shiatsu is not associated with any significant side effects. Some people may experience mild discomfort, which usually disappears during the course of the treatment session.

Research & general acceptance

Like many forms of massage, shiatsu is widely believed to have a relaxing effect on the body. There is also a significant amount of research suggesting that acupressure techniques can relieve nausea and **vomiting** associated with a variety of causes, including **pregnancy** and anesthetics and other drugs. In one study, published in the *Journal of Nurse-Midwifery* in 1989, acupressure was shown to significantly reduce the effects of nausea in 12 of 16 women suffering from **morning sickness**. Five days of this therapy also appeared to reduce anxiety and improve mood. Another investigation, published in the *British Journal of Anaesthesia* in 1999, studied the effects of acupressure on nausea resulting from the use of anesthetics. Pressure applied to an acupoint on the inside of the wrist appeared to alleviate nausea in patients who received anesthetics during the course of laparoscopic surgery.

Shiatsu may also produce sedative and analgesic effects. The sedative powers of acupressure were investigated in a study published in the *Journals of Gerontology* in 1999, which involved over 80 elderly people who suffered from sleeping difficulties. Compared to the people in the control groups, the 28 participants who received acupressure were able to sleep better. They slept for longer periods of time and were less likely to wake up during the night. The researchers concluded that acupressure may improve the quality of sleep in older adults. The use of acupressure in postoperative pain was investigated in a study published in the *Clinical Journal of Pain* in 1996. In this study, which involved 40 knee surgery patients, one group received acupressure (15 acupoints were stimulated) while the control group received sham acupressure. Within an hour of treatment, members of the acupressure group reported less pain than those in the control group. The pain-relieving effects associated with acupressure lasted for 24 hours.

Shiatsu may benefit **stroke** victims. The results of at least one study (which did not include a control group) suggest that shiatsu may be useful during stroke rehabilitation when combined with other treatments.

Training & certification

A qualified shiatsu therapist must have completed courses in this form of therapy and should be nationally certified or licensed by the state (most are certified by the American Oriental Bodywork Therapy Association). Asking a medical doctor for a recommendation is a good place to start. It can also be helpful to consult friends and family members who have tried shiatsu. There are several massage-related organizations that offer information on locating a qualified therapist. These include the National Certification Board for Therapeutic Massage and Bodywork, the American **Massage Therapy** Association, the International School of Shiatsu, and the American Oriental Bodywork Therapy Association.

Resources

BOOKS

Cook, Allan R. *Alternative Medicine Sourcebook*. Detroit: Omnigraphics, 1999.

KEY TERMS

....

Acupressure—An ancient form of Asian healing massage that involves applying pressure to special points or areas on the body in order to maintain good health, cure disease, and restore vitality.

Analgesic—Pain reliever.

Osteoporosis—A disease of the bones due to deficiency of bone matrix, occurring most frequently in postmenopausal women.

Palpate—Feel.

PERIODICALS

Chen, M.L., L.C. Lin, S.C. Wu, et al. "The effectiveness of acupressure in improving the quality of sleep of institutionalized residents." *J Gerontol A Biol Sci Med Sci* (1999): M389-94.

Felhendler, D. and B. Lisander. "Pressure on acupoints decreases postoperative pain." *Clin J Pain* (1996): 326-329.

Harmon, D., J. Gardiner, R. Harrison, et al. "Acupressure and the prevention of nausea and vomiting after laparoscopy." *Br J Anaesth* (1999): 387-390.

Hogg, P.K. "The effects of acupressure on the psychological and physiological rehabilitation of the stroke patient." *Dissertation Abstracts Int* (1986): 841.

Hyde, E. "Acupressure therapy for morning sickness. A controlled clinical trial." *J Nurse Midwifery* (1989): 171-178.

ORGANIZATIONS

Acupressure Institute. 1533 Shattuck Avenue, Berkeley, CA 94709.

American Massage Therapy Association. 820 Davis Street, Suite 100, Evanston, IL.

American Oriental Bodywork Therapy Association. 50 Maple Place, Manhassett, NY 11030.

International School of Shiatsu. 10 South Clinton Street, Doylestown, PA 18901.

National Certification Board for Therapeutic Massage and Bodywork. 8201 Greensboro Drive, Suite 300, McLean, VA 22102.

OTHER

International School of Shiatsu. http://www.shiatsubo.com.

Medline. http://igm.nlm.nih.gov.

Greg Annussek

Shiitake mushroom

Description

Shiitake mushroom (*Lentinus edodes*) is a fungus native to Japan, China, and Korea. Although these mushrooms are cultivated worldwide as of 2004, Japan is still the largest producer of shiitake mushrooms, producing 80% of the total supply. Used in Asian cuisine for over 2,000 years, cultivation of shiitake began almost 700 years ago in Japan. The Japanese consider the shiitake not only a flavorful food but also "the elixir of life." During the Ming Dynasty (1368–1644), the shiitake was reserved only for the emperor and his family and it became known as the emperor's food. The word shiitake comes from *shii* (a type of chestnut tree) and *take* (mushroom). Shiitake is an excellent source for **amino acids**; vegetable proteins; **iron**; **thiamine** (vitamin B_1); **riboflavin** (vitamin B_2); **niacin**; and vitamins B_6, B_{12}, and D_2. Shiitake is known as *hsaing ku* (fragrant mushroom) in China.

General use

Traditionally, shiitake was used medicinally for a number of conditions.

- colds and influenza
- headaches
- sexual dysfunction
- constipation
- measles
- hemorrhoids
- diabetes
- gout

Presently, shiitake has been shown to boost the immune system, act as an antiviral and antibacterial agent, and possibly shrink tumors. Since shiitake has been part of the Asian diet, particularly in Japanese cuisine, for hundreds of years, its health benefits have been documented. Most of the formal studies conducted have been in Japan; however Western interest in the mushroom as a possible treatment for **cancer** and HIV infection has encouraged researchers in the United States and elsewhere to begin formalized studies of its medicinal properties. A 1998 study done in San Francisco of lentinan, a glucan (complex sugar) found in shiitake, found that patients with HIV infection who were given lentinan together with a standard drug for **AIDS** maintained higher CD4 cell counts for longer periods of time than those who were given the standard drug alone.

The possible health benefits of lentinan have also led to agricultural experiments intended to raise the level of the compound in commercially grown shiitake. Researchers found that mushrooms grown on logs had higher levels of lentinan than mushrooms grown on other types of organic material.

Shiitake contains over 50 different enzymes, including pepsin and trypsin that help digestion, and asparagi-

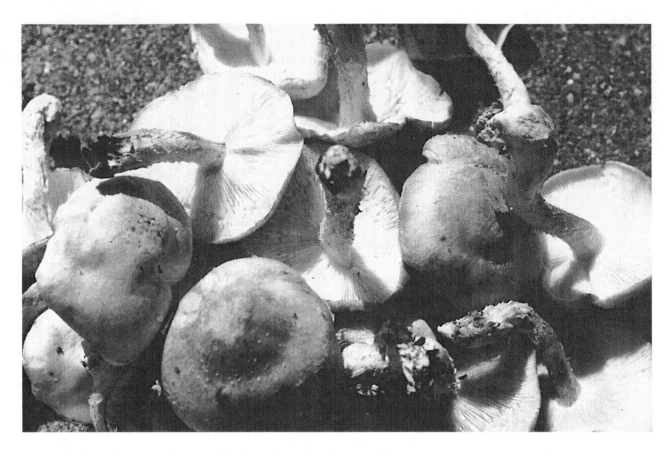

Fresh shiitake mushrooms. *(Photo by Kelly Quinn. Reproduced by permission.)*

nase, which that has been used to treat childhood **leukemia**. The mushroom also contains chitin, eritadenine, and lentinacin, all of which have been shown to lower serum **cholesterol**. Further studies completed in 2002 have confirmed the beneficial effects of shiitake in lowering serum cholesterol levels.

Perhaps shiitake's most beneficial ingredient is an activated hexose-containing compound (also known as 1,3-beta glucan). Japanese studies of this compound have supported evidence that it has anticancer properties in humans as well as in animals. The compound is already produced by a private company as a nutritional supplement and is available in Europe, Japan, and the United States. It is also regularly used in hospitals in Asia and Japan in conjunction with allopathic treatments of several kinds of cancer. According to a Hokkaido University School of Medicine study of cancer patients taking the supplement on a daily basis, the compound may slow tumor growth and decrease the side effects caused by allopathic cancer treatments. The University of California Davis School of Medicine is conducting the first human trial outside of Japan to determine the antitumor effects that the activated hexose-containing compound may have on cancer patients. The focus of the study will be on patients with

prostrate cancer because the characteristic symptom of the cancer—elevated PSA levels in the blood—are easily detected and monitored for change.

Activated hexose-containing compound is isolated from partially grown mushroom spores that have undergone a treatment that releases the compound. It is not abundant in the mushrooms that are readily available in grocery stores, but the overall health benefits from shiitake mushrooms have been corroborated by research.

Preparations

Shiitake production in the United States has risen markedly since 1980. Since shiitake is now being marketed as a nutraceutical, or food that is thought to provide health benefits above and beyond its nutritional value, its production is expected to rise even further.

Shiitake mushrooms can be prepared and eaten in the same way the more common white mushrooms are, by grilling, sautéing, and stir-frying. Dried shiitake mushrooms are used in soups, stews, and sauces. Eat one to two fresh mushrooms or 1–2 tsp of dried shiitake daily.

Shiitake supplements are also available in gel-cap form, as well as powders, extracts, and tea at health food stores. Shiitake is also an ingredient in compound formulas to boost the immune system. The newest product of this type is a mixture of dried shiitake, reishi, and **maitake** mushrooms that have been grown on a base of therapeutic herbs. Consumers who use these products should follow the recommended daily dosage on the label.

Injections of shiitake should be prescribed and monitored by a healthcare provider.

Precautions

Shiitake is nontoxic and safe to ingest.

Side effects

Large daily doses over a prolonged period of time can cause **diarrhea** in some users.

Interactions

Shiitake has been reported to interact supportively with didanosine (Videx), a drug given to treat HIV infection. Because shiitake can lower blood pressure, it should not be taken together with drugs given to control blood pressure (antihypertensives). For the same reason, it should be discontinued before any operation requiring general anesthesia.

Resources

BOOKS

Atkins, Robert C. M.D. *Dr. Atkins' Vita-Nutrient Solution.* New York: Simon & Schuster, 1998.

Carper, Jean. *Food—Your Miracle Medicine: How Food Can Prevent And Cure Over 100 Symptoms and Problems.* New York: HarperCollins, 1993.

Duke, James A. *The Green Pharmacy.* Emmaus, PA: Rodale Press, 1997.

Harrar, Sari, and Sara Altshul O'Donnell. *The Woman's Book of Healing Herbs.* Emmaus, PA: Rodale Press, 1999.

Mindell, Earl. *Earl Mindell's Herb Bible.* New York: Simon & Schuster, 1992.

PERIODICALS

Brauer, D., T. Kimmons, and M. Phillips. "Effects of Management on the Yield and High-Molecular-Weight Polysaccharide Content of Shiitake (*Lentinula edodes*) Mushrooms." *Journal of Agricultural and Food Chemistry* 50 (September 11, 2002): 5333-5337.

Fuchs, Nan Kathryn. "A Brand New Super Nutrient!" *Women's Health Letter* 8 (August 2002): 1-3.

Gordon, M., B. Bihari, E. Goosby, et al. "A Placebo-Controlled Trial of the Immune Modulator, Lentinan, in HIV-Positive Patients: A Phase I/II Trial." *Journal of Medicine* 29 (5-6): 305-330.

Shimada, Y., T. Morita, and K. Sugiyama. "Effects of *Lentinus edodes* on Fatty Acid and Molecular Species Profiles of

Phosphatidylcholine in Rats Fed Different Levels of Corn Oil." *Bioscience, Biotechnology, and Biochemistry* 66 (August 2002): 1759-1763.

ORGANIZATIONS

American Association of Oriental Medicine. 909 22nd Street, Sacramento, CA 95816, (916) 451-6950 <http://www.aaom.org>.

United States Department of Agriculture (USDA), Agricultural Research Service (ARS). 5601 Sunnyside Avenue, Beltsville, MD 20705. (301) 504-1651. <www.ars.usda.gov>.

Jacqueline L. Longe
Rebecca J. Frey, PhD

Shingles

Definition

Shingles, also called herpes zoster, gets its name from both the Latin and French words for belt or girdle and refers to girdle-like skin eruptions that may occur on the trunk of the body. The virus that causes **chickenpox**, the *Varicella zoster* virus (VSV), can become dormant in nerve cells after an episode of chickenpox and later re-emerge as shingles.

Initially, red patches of rash develop into **blisters**. Because the virus travels along the nerve to the skin, it can damage the nerve and cause it to become inflamed. This condition can be very painful. If the **pain** persists long after the rash disappears, it is known as post-herpetic **neuralgia** (PHN).

Description

Any individual who has had chickenpox can develop shingles. Between 600,000 and one million Ameri-

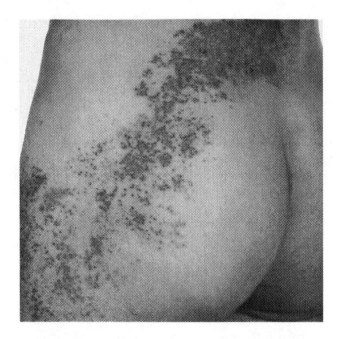

Shingles, or herpes zoster, on patient's buttocks and thigh.
(Custom Medical Stock Photo. Reproduced by permission.)

cans are diagnosed with shingles each year. Overall, approximately 20% of those who have had chickenpox as children develop shingles at some time in their lives. People of all ages—even children—can be affected, but the incidence increases with age. Newborns, bone marrow and other transplant recipients, and individuals with immune systems weakened by disease or drugs are also at increased risk. However, most individuals who develop shingles do not have any underlying malignancy or other immunosuppressive condition.

Causes & symptoms

Shingles erupts along the course of the affected nerve, producing lesions anywhere on the body. The condition may cause severe nerve pain. The most common areas to be affected are the face and trunk, which correspond to the areas where the chickenpox rash is most concentrated. There is usually a line of eruptions running from the spine along the path of the affected nerve on one side of the body.

The disease is caused by a reactivation of the chickenpox virus that has lain dormant in certain nerves following an episode of chickenpox. Exactly how or why this reactivation occurs is not clear. In 2002 clinicians pointed out that one of the causes of increasing cases of shingles was actually the success of chicken pox vaccinations. It is believed that the reactivation is triggered when the immune system becomes weakened as a result of age, **stress**, **fatigue**, certain medications, chemotherapy, or diseases such as **cancer** or HIV. Furthermore, in persons with HIV, shingles can be an early sign that the immune system has deteriorated.

Early signs of shingles are often vague and can easily be mistaken for other illnesses. The condition may begin with **fever** and malaise (a vague feeling of weakness or discomfort). Within two to four days, severe pain, **itching**, and numbness/tingling (paresthesias) or extreme sensitivity to touch (hyperesthesia) can develop, usually on the trunk and occasionally on the arms and legs.

Pain may be continuous or intermittent, usually lasting one to three weeks. It may occur at the time of the eruption, but can precede the eruption by days, occasionally making the diagnosis difficult.

Signs and symptoms may include the following:

• itching, tingling, or severe burning pain

• red patches that develop into blisters

• dense clusters of small blisters that ooze and crust

• swollen lymph nodes

Diagnosis

Diagnosis usually is not possible until the skin lesions develop. Once they develop, however, the pattern and location of the blisters and the type of cell damage displayed are characteristic of the disease. This feature allows an accurate diagnosis based primarily upon the physical examination. Although tests are rarely necessary, they may include the following:

• Viral culture of skin lesion.

• Microscopic examination using a Tzanck preparation. This involves staining a smear obtained from a blister. Cells infected with the herpes virus appear very large and contain many dark cell centers or nuclei.

• Complete blood count (CBC) may show an elevated white blood cell count (WBC), a nonspecific sign of infection.

Treatment

A person with shingles should immediately see a doctor or health practitioner. Although the condition generally clears up within three to five weeks, treatment can ease the painful symptoms. Alternative medicine remedies and therapies will not cure shingles, but they will provide pain relief, reduce inflammation, and speed recovery.

Herbal remedies

Many herbs can be used to treat shingles. Some remedies involve brewing tea and then consuming and/or applying it to the affected area. Herbs used to treat shingles include:

• Red pepper, also known as capsicum or **cayenne**, is so effective that it's an ingredient in commercial ointments approved by the U.S. Food and Drug Administration. Commercial preparations include Zostrix and Capzasin-P. Red pepper is hot, so the ointment should be applied only to healed blisters. Red pepper is useful for treating painful PHN.

- Topical applications of **lemon balm**, **licorice**, or **peppermint** may reduce pain and blistering. These herbs may be brewed as teas and then consumed and applied to the skin.

- Herbal antivirals, such as **echinacea**, can be effective in fighting infection and boosting the immune system.

- Calendula ointment or lotion works to counter the virus.

- Sedative herbs such as **passionflower** can be brewed for a tea. Such herbs can help with treatment of postherpetic neuralgia.

- Vervain helps relieve pain and inflammation. St. John's wort, **lavender**, **chamomile**, and marjoram also help relieve inflammation.

Homeopathic remedies

A person with shingles should consult a homeopath for specific remedies and dosages. Homeopathic remedies include *Ranunculus,* which is effective for shingles on the trunk. It is also taken for itching. A homeopath may recommend *Rhus toxicodendron* for blisters and *Arsenicum album* or *Hypericum* for pain.

Traditional Chinese medicine

Practitioners of **traditional Chinese medicine** (TCM) recommend **acupressure** and **acupuncture** to alleviate pain. Acupuncture can help with post-herpetic neuralgia. In addition, a TCM practitioner may recommend herbal remedies such as Chinese gentian root, which is used to treat the liver. In addition, Chinese **skullcap** root is combined with water and used as a folk remedy for treating shingles in China. Also, certain herbal combinations can treat specific symptoms and contributing causes. For example, *Long Dan Xie Gan Tang* can quell the accumulation of damp toxic heat in the liver. For damp infected painful eruptions on the torso, *Huang Qin Gao* can be applied to the surrounding area.

Diet and nutrition

To boost the immune system, supplement the diet with vitamin B during the first one or two days. Until health returns, continue to supplement with **vitamin B complex**, high levels of **vitamin C** with **bioflavonoids**, and **calcium**.

Food seasoned with red pepper (capsicum) may provide relief, as may foods containing the amino acid **ly-sine**. High-lysine foods include soybeans, black bean sprouts, lentils, **parsley**, and peas.

Home remedies

Cool wet compresses may help reduce pain while blisters or crusting is present. Patients may be made more comfortable with the application of a cloth dipped in one-quarter cup (60 ml) of white vinegar mixed in two quarts (1.9 l) of lukewarm water. Compresses should be used twice daily for 10 minutes. When blisters dry up, the compresses may be discontinued.

Soothing treatments such as colloidal oatmeal baths, starch baths or lotions, and calamine lotion may help to relieve itching and discomfort.

When the crusts and scabs are separating, the skin may become dry, tight, and cracked. If that happens, a small amount of plain petroleum jelly can be applied to the area three or four times daily.

Ayurvedic medicine

Ayurveda is an Indian healing science that is more than 5,000 years old. Treatment is based on maintaining a balance between the body and the world. Treatment for shingles may include applying a **turmeric** paste to the skin.

Relaxation techniques

Relaxation techniques can be used to treat symptoms of shingles. Techniques such as **hypnotherapy** and **yoga** can help a person relax.

Flower remedies

Flower remedies are liquid concentrates made by soaking flowers in spring water. Also known as flower essences, 38 remedies were developed by the homeopathic physician Edward Bach during the 1930s. A 39th combination formula, known as **Rescue Remedy** is taken to relieve stress. The remedy is taken by placing several drops under the tongue four times daily. Alternately, the drops may be added to a glass of water. The patient drinks the mixture throughout the day.

Reflexology

Reflexology is the manipulation of the foot to bring the body into balance. Reflex points on the foot correspond to parts of the body. These points can be treated by a reflexologist or at home by following instructions on a reflex chart.

Allopathic treatment

The antiviral drugs acyclovir, valacyclovir, and famciclovir can be used to treat shingles. These drugs may shorten the course of the illness. More rapid healing of the blisters results when drug therapy is started within 72 hours of the onset of the rash. In fact, the earlier the drugs are administered the better, because early cases can sometimes be halted. If taken later, these drugs are less effective but may still lessen the pain. Antiviral drug treatment does not seem to reduce the incidence of post-herpetic neuralgia (PHN), but recent studies suggest famciclovir may cut the duration of PHN in half.

Side effects of typical oral doses of these antiviral drugs are minor, with **headache** and **nausea** reported by 8–20% of patients. Severely immuno compromised individuals, such as those diagnosed with **AIDS**, may require intravenous administration of antiviral drugs. Corticosteroids such as prednisone may be used to reduce inflammation but they interfere with the functioning of the immune system. Corticosteroids in combination with antiviral therapy are also used to reduce severe pain and to treat severe **infections**, such as those affecting the eyes.

After the blisters heal, some people continue to experience PHN for months or even years. This pain can be excruciating. Consequently, the doctor may prescribe tranquilizers, sedatives, or antidepressants to be taken at night. Attempts to treat PHN with famciclovir have shown some promising results. When all else fails, severe pain may require a permanent nerve block.

Expected results

Shingles usually clears up within three to five weeks and rarely recurs. There have been reports that shingles cleared up several days after licorice ointment was applied to the skin or when the homeopathic remedy *Ranunculus* was taken.

If the nerves that cause movement are affected, temporary or permanent nerve paralysis and/or **tremors** may occur. Elderly or debilitated patients may have a prolonged and difficult course and recovery. For them, the eruption is typically more extensive and inflammatory, occasionally resulting in blisters that bleed, areas in which the skin actually dies, secondary bacterial infection, or extensive and permanent scarring.

Similarly, patients with compromised immune systems usually have more severe courses that are often prolonged for weeks to months. They develop shingles frequently and the infection can spread to the skin, lungs, liver, gastrointestinal tract, brain, or other vital organs.

Cases of chronic shingles have been reported in AIDS patients, especially when they have a decreased number of one particular kind of immune cell called CD4 lymphocytes. Depletion of CD4 lymphocytes is associated with more severe, chronic, and recurrent varicella zoster virus infections. Lesions are typical at the onset but may turn into ulcers that do not heal. Herpes zoster can lead to potentially serious complications.

Many individuals continue to experience persistent pain long after the blisters heal. This post-herpetic neuralgia can be severe and debilitating. The incidence of post-herpetic neuralgia increases with age, and episodes in older individuals tend to be of longer duration. Most patients under 30 years of age experience no persistent pain. By age 40, the risk of prolonged pain lasting longer than one month increases to 33%. By age 70, the risk increases to 74%. The pain can adversely affect quality of life, but it usually diminishes over time.

Other complications include secondary bacterial infections.

Prevention

Strengthening the immune system by making lifestyle changes is thought to help prevent the development of shingles. These changes include eating a well-balanced diet rich in essential vitamins and minerals, getting enough sleep, exercising regularly, and reducing stress.

In 2002, reports from a large, five-year study showed that researchers might be nearing a workable vaccine for shingles. The vaccine is 10 times stronger than the chickenpox vaccine and similar in nature. Study results were planned for release in mid-2004.

Resources

BOOKS

Cummings, Stephen, and Dana Ullman. *Everybody's Guide to Homeopathic Medicines.* New York: Putnam, 1997.

Duke, James A. *The Green Pharmacy.* Emmaus, PA.: Rodale Press, 1997.

Gottlieb, Bill. *New Choices in Natural Healing.* Emmaus, PA.: Rodale Press, 1995.

Keville, Kathi. *Herbs for Health and Healing.* Emmaus, PA.: Rodale Press, 1996.

L'Orange, Darlena. *Herbal Healing Secrets of the Orient.* Paramus, NJ: Prentice Hall, 1998.

Squier, Thomas Broken Bear, with Lauren David Peden. *Herbal Folk Medicine.* New York: Henry Holt, 1997.

Ullman, Dana. *The Consumer's Guide to Homeopathy.* New York: Putnam, 1995.

PERIODICALS

Landers, Susan J. "Rash of Pain: With an Increasingly Large Patient Population at Risk for Shingles, Researchers Focus on Uncovering New Ways to Prevent and Treat this Viral Response." *American Medical News* (April 1, 2002):32.

MacKenzie, Deborah. "The Hidden Catch: Although Chickenpox is Nasty, Vaccination Might Not be the Answer." *New Scientist* (May 4, 2002):7.

ORGANIZATIONS

American Academy of Dermatology. 930 N. Meacham Road, P.O. Box 4014, Schaumberg, IL 60168-4014. (708) 330-0230. http://www.aad.org/zoster.html.

American Botanical Council. P.O. Box 201660, Austin TX, 78720. (512) 331-8868. http://www.herbalgram.org.

Herb Research Foundation. 1007 Pearl St., Suite 200, Boulder, CO 80302. (303) 449-2265. http://www.herbs.org.

OTHER

MotherNature.com Health Encyclopedia. http://www.mother-nature.com/ency.

Liz Swain
Teresa G. Odle

Shin splints

Definition

Shin splints can be defined as an inflammation of the tissues in the lower leg causing **pain** with **exercise** . The disorder is also referred to as medial tibial **stress** syndrome.

Description

Shin splints are an inflammation of the tendons, muscles, and periosteum most commonly seen in those who walk, jog, or run on hard, uneven surfaces. The resulting pain may indicate either anterior shin splints, with radiation down the front and lateral leg, or posterior shin splints, extending down the back and inner leg and ankle. Depending on the body tissues involved, shin splints may indicate myositis (an inflammation of the muscle), **tendinitis** (inflammation of the tendons), or periostitis (an inflammation of the tissue covering the bone).

Causes & symptoms

The inflammation of shin splints is caused by an imbalance of the calf and shin muscles used to mobilize the forefoot with **exercise**. The associated pain in the lower leg usually worsens with exercise.

Diagnosis

The identification of shin splints is often made by the affected individual's observation of the symptoms. X rays of the lower extremity may be requested to prevent a misdiagnosis when **stress fractures** are suspected.

Treatment

Exercise should not be resumed until it can be performed without pain. Switching from high-impact work-

---

outs to swimming or cycling will allow for healing to the inflamed areas. A gentle massage with lubricating oil will provide comfort and decrease swelling. An ice massage may also facilitate healing, using a circular movement over the affected area three to four times daily for 10-15 minutes. Some find heat more comforting and beneficial, applied via a heating pad or lamp, a hot shower, or whirlpool.

A well-balanced, high-protein diet, dietary **antioxidants**, and **essential fatty acids** may also promote healing. As the patient's activity level may be lower than usual during the initial healing phase of shin splints, adequate fluid and fiber intake is vital to promote normal bowel function.

After at least a two-week rest period, a gradual resumption of exercise is recommended. Icing the legs for 5-10 minutes before stretching and after cool-down is recommended. Crisscross taping of the anterior leg maybe be helpful for the individual with anterior shin splints, as well as raising the heel portion of the shoe approximately one-eighth of an inch. The individual with posterior shin splints should remember to hold the body erect rather than leaning forward while running, and to avoid landing directly on the toes. An extra pair of socks for warmth while running is also recommended.

KEY TERMS

Myositis—Inflammation of the muscle.

Periosteum—Tissue covering the bone.

Periostitis—Inflammation of the tissue covering the bone.

Tendinitis—Inflammation of the tendon.

Tibia—One of the long bones of the lower leg.

Allopathic treatment

For minor discomfort associated with shin splints, over-the-counter anti-inflammatory medications such as ibuprofen or aspirin may provide relief. If these are found to be ineffective for pain relief, prescription-strength, nonsteriodal, anti-inflammatory drugs (NDAIDs) may be ordered by the physician. Physical therapy sessions and ice and/or heat application may also be helpful.

Expected results

A complete resolution of the pain associated with shin splints requires an adequate period of rest followed by a slow rehabilitation or gradual resumption of activity ranging from two weeks to two months. Resuming activities too soon may result in a prolonged healing time and recurrence of symptoms. The change in gait and posture associated with shin splint pain may result in inflammatory or arthritic changes in the local joints, i.e. the ankle, knee, hip, or back.

Prevention

Those who exercise by running or doing high-impact aerobics should be sure to wear well-fitting shoes that offer adequate lateral and arch support with cushioning for the ball and heel of the foot. Footwear should be reevaluated for adequacy of support and cushioning about every six months. Warming up before and cooling down after the activity is vital, and the shins should also be kept warm during exercise. Jogging on soft surfaces such as dirt or grass is preferred over hard or uneven surfaces.

Resources

BOOKS

Gottlieb, Bill. *New Choices in Natural Healing.* Emmaus, Pennsylvania: Rodale press, Inc., 1995.

Mercier, Lonnie. *Practical Orthopedics.* St. Louis, Missouri: Mosby-Year Book, Inc., 1995.

OTHER

Thriveonline.http://www.thriveonline.com/health/Library/sports.

Kathleen Wright

Shintaido

Definition

Shintaido is a noncombative form of **martial arts** designed to improve physical and mental health.

Origins

Although shintaido has its roots in the ancient and traditional Japanese martial arts, including elements of sword fencing, karate, and aikido. Hiroyuki Aoki, an actor, artist, and shotokai karate master, developed shintaido in Yokohama, Japan, in 1965. He formed *rakutenkai* or "meeting of people," a group that brought together several dozen people, including martial arts instructors, artists, musicians, and actors, to create a new art form and health **exercise**. Translated from Japanese, shintaido means "new body way."

Benefits

Like many other martial arts, shintaido promotes a healthy mind and spirit as much as a healthy body. The benefits of practicing shintaido include:

- Enhancing physical health through a series of body movements, including warm-ups, vigorous exercises, fundamental movements, traditional movements, and exercises with a partner.
- Eliminating **stress** and amplifying natural energies of the body and mind.
- Developing *ki*, a Japanese word meaning internal spirit or vital energy.
- Opening the mind and fostering a cheerful attitude.
- Improving the ability to interact with other people.
- Fostering love, peace, and magnanimity.
- Increasing concentration.
- Strengthening individuality and enhancing creativity.

Description

The body movements in shintaido are influenced by traditional and contemporary aspects of Japanese culture, including dance, music, Noh theatre, and abstract art. It involves a series of movements ranging from slow and meditative to rapid and energetic. One shintaido movement, *bojutsu*, involves using a six-foot staff, while another, *kenjutsu*, uses a wooden sword.

Most formal shintaido classes offered by schools sanctioned through the International Shintaido Federation or Shintaido of America are taught by an instructor and teaching assistant. The classes consist of wrap-ups, vigorous exercises, fundamental movements, partner practice, and traditional movements called *kata*.

Preparations

No preparations are required to begin shintaido. It can be practiced by anyone who desires, including children and the elderly.

Precautions

There are no precautions associated with learning shintaido.

Side effects

No serious adverse side effects have been reported from shintaido. In rare cases, beginning students of the art may experience slight muscle or joint soreness if practice is overdone.

Research & general acceptance

Shintaido, like other martial arts, is almost universally accepted in Japan as beneficial for physical exercise, stress reduction, and as a tool for bringing mental clarity. It is generally accepted in Western cultures, including medical science, as a legitimate and effective exercise for the mind and body. However, few if any controlled scientific studies on measurable benefits of shintaido have been conducted in the United States.

Training & certification

Most shintaido classes are taught by trained and certified instructors. There are four levels of teachers: instructor, senior instructor, general instructor, and master instructor. Most qualified teachers in the United States are examined and certified by Shintaido of America or the International Shintaido Federation. During an examination, all levels of instructors are judged on technical expertise and leadership qualities. There are also specified years of practice required for each level and apprenticeship with a more advanced instructor.

Resources

BOOKS

Aoki, Hiroyuki. *Shintaido: An Art of Movement and Life Expression.* Cambridge, MA: Shintaido of America, 1982.

Aoki, Hiroyuki. *Total Stick Fighting: Shintaido Bojutsu.* Tokyo: Kodansha International, 2000.

PERIODICALS

"A Way to Stop the Spear." *The Economist* (May 15, 1993): 114.

KEY TERMS

....

Aikido—A Japanese martial art developed during the early twentieth century by Morihei Ueshiba. Literally translated, aikido means "the way of harmony with universal energy" or "the way of a loving spirit."

Karate—A native Okinawan fighting style brought to Japan in the early twentieth century.

Noh theatre—A Japanese theatrical form developed in the fourteenth century, featuring masks, extravagant costumes, bare stages, and restrained movements.

ORGANIZATIONS

Shintaido of America. P.O. Box 38-1672, Cambridge, MA 02238. http://www.shintaido.org.

Ken R. Wells

Sick building syndrome

Definition

Sick building syndrome (SBS) is a term used to describe certain health effects people experience that may be related to poor air in buildings. The problems can be localized, for instance experienced by workers in only one section of an office or factory; or they may be widespread and experienced throughout an entire building. SBS has been reported in various settings such as hospitals, schools, industrial and art business, and care homes, or any building or home with off gassing carpets, paints, and fumes, as well as buildings with ventilation problems and concentration of vapors, gases, solvents, or other airborne agents toxic to the skin, lungs or nervous system. In fact, sick building syndrome is a condition related to poor ventilation in some of America's schools.

Description

People who have SBS generally experience symptoms related to the eyes, nose, throat, and skin. They also may complain of overall symptoms such as feeling very tired. When caused by SBS, these symptoms have no other known cause or explanation. Other similar symptoms are related to SBS and may be confused with the syndrome. For instance, "building-related illness" (BRI) is the term used for a diagnosed illness attributed to contaminants that can be identified in a building. Often, the contaminants come from the ventilation system. Legionnaire's disease is a well-known example of BRI. **Multiple chemical sensitivity** (MCS) is another closely related condition; however, it is not caused by SBS. People with MCS have high sensitivity or allergy to many chemicals and other substances in the environment. They may experience symptoms in many organs and systems of their bodies from low levels of exposure to chemicals.

Like MCS, SBS is largely a modern phenomenon, first recognized by the World Health Organization (WHO) as a medical condition in 1982. When building designers sought to save energy during the 1970s oil embargo, they began creating virtually airtight buildings. However, the new energy-efficient structures reduced ventilation, even to the point of reducing health and comfort for occupants. SBS has resulted in lost productivity among affected workers and increased costs for those who own and operate the buildings with poor air quality and other problems. An entire industry has developed around producing air filters and other products, as well as engineering and design consulting.

Causes & symptoms

People who complain of SBS report symptoms of acute discomfort such as eye, nose, and throat irritation, a dry **cough**, and **dizziness** or **nausea**. Many also report dry, itchy skin. Some will have difficulty concentrating of experience sensitivity to odors, **fatigue**, and headaches. While many of these symptoms are common to other conditions, their relation to time spent in a specific building suggests the possibility of SBS.

The specific causes of SBS are unknown, but several factors may contribute to the condition. The most notable factor is poor indoor air quality. If air is not properly ventilated, it may become too dry or too humid. Also, chemicals or biological contaminants (molds, pollen, viruses, etc.) may collect in the air. The World Health Organization (WHO) estimates that up to 30% of office buildings worldwide have significant indoor air quality problems. A 1995 study found that about one-half of schools in the United States had poor ventilation and sources of pollution inside the buildings.

More than 700,000 chemicals are in common use today. Chemical contaminants can enter indoor air from the outside or from the inside. For example, vehicle exhaust can enter a building through windows or through poorly located air intake vents. However, most chemical contaminants come from indoor sources. Commonly used materials for construction and cleaning emit byproducts that can cause acute health effects in people when concentrated at high levels. Even low or moderate levels of these contaminants can cause health effects in some people with certain sensitivities. Called volatile organic compounds (VOCs), the contaminants come from carpet glues, copy machines, manufactured wood products, cleaning agents, pesticides, and tobacco smoke. Formaldehyde is one of the most common VOCs.

Radon, a radioactive gas that forms when radium breaks down in certain rock formations, can be found in homes in several states. It enters the home through foundation cracks. Radon is colorless and odorless and can go undetected, building up to dangerous levels that can lead to **lung cancer**.

Biological contaminants can enter a building's ventilation system. They are formed in standing water from humidifiers, drain pans, or ducts. They also may form where water has collected on wet ceiling tiles, carpet, or insulation. Some biological contaminants are pollen, bacteria, viruses, and molds.

Dust also has been found to contribute to SBS. Dust irritates the mucous membranes. A study showed that improved methods of office cleaning reduced symptoms for at least two months after cleaning.

Diagnosis

Diagnosing SBS differs from diagnosing many other medical conditions. First, the diagnosis is made by patient history, physical and clinical finding. Rarely do laboratory or imaging tests confirm abnormalities. Second, the diagnosis involves a thorough review of the building and its occupants as much as an individual's symptoms. Finally, the medical community has debated for many years about whether or not SBS is a "real medical condition." Because many of the symptoms are self–reported and can't easily be measured, and since some reported cases of sick buildings have shown no signs of chemicals or other problems, some professionals dispute whether the syndrome exists. In addition, there are people who are more sensitive to low levels of VOCs who may experience symptoms even though other people in the building experience no symptoms.

For these reasons, SBS often remains undiagnosed or misdiagnosed. Schools may blame such other diseases as winter flu outbreaks or perhaps assign a child's symptoms to a condition such as attention deficit hyperactivity disorder. When a patient goes to a physician with symptoms typical of SBS — **headache**, fatigue, dizziness, nausea, runny or stuffy nose, a dry cough, dry and itchy skin, itchy or watery eyes, and difficulty concentrating — a complete history is critical. If no other medical condition can explain these symptoms, the physician needs to ask questions that might lead to a diagnosis of SBS. The trigger will come in questions involving time. For instance, if a child's symptoms worsen when he or she enters the school building, SBS is likely to blame. If an office worker didn't start having these symptoms until changing jobs or office locations, the office building could be the culprit.

To diagnose a "sick building," trained occupational health or industrial experts will perform a "walkthrough" to survey building occupants for common SBS symptoms and to check the building for signs of problems. If a number of occupants have these symptoms and there are problems in the building such as overcrowding, poor cleaning, poor ventilation, or water damage, the surveyor may recommend work that done to improve the building's indoor air quality.

Treatment

No specific treatment has proven effective at eliminating SBS. Many experts agree that the best treatment for SBS is prevention — removing the contaminants or other identified sources that are causing SBS. Individuals with SBS may be encouraged to avoid the building that is making them sick. However, this is not always possible and can lead to isolation or job loss.

A person with suspected SBS may ask that a building be inspected for possible contaminants. A course of **detoxification** under the guidance of a qualified practitioner can be helpful. This includes stimulating lung, liver, kidney and skin expulsion and release of toxic compounds, some of which are stored in fat tissues. If the affected individual cannot leave the building or if the source is not removed, treating the symptoms of SBS may help ease some discomfort. In this case, it is wise to see an environmental medicine specialist and other providers who can help with detoxification and symptom relief (**acupuncture**, massage, etc.) However, these therapies should be coordinated by a physician, since treating multiple symptoms with multiple remedies may possibly create additional interactions. And even herbal remedies may interact with the various chemical substances that are producing the sensitivities; they should be started in small doses and recommended only by trained practitioners.

Some patients with MCS will test for **allergies** to determine the sources of their sensitivities; similar testing might prove helpful for SBS patients who do not know the exact source of their symptoms. Efforts to relieve **stress** also may help deal with or lessen SBS symptoms. **Aromatherapy**, **yoga**, **biofeedback**, and massage may be helpful.

Allopathic treatment

Again, tests have shown that among those with chemical sensitivities, avoiding chemicals has proven to be the most effective treatment. If the environmental problem is not corrected, the individual must decide how to best avoid the SBS source. Clinicians will aim their treatment at easing patients' symptoms while trying to help them avoid or adapt to triggers. Like many conditions that are difficult to pinpoint, physicians must listen respectfully to patients and should not prematurely label symptoms as psychological. Once SBS is suspected, the building that is likely the source of trouble should be evaluated and improvements made as needed.

Expected results

Avoiding the source of SBS or making necessary environmental improvements to the building should improve most symptoms of SBS in a short time. No permanent complications of SBS have been reported as of 2004.

Prevention

Preventing SBS begins with the proper design and maintenance of buildings. In particular, attention should be paid to the heating, ventilation, and air conditioning (HVAC) systems. WHO has set guidelines for proper management of building ventilation systems that include avoiding introduction of biological contaminants as well as conducting regular inspection and maintenance. In late 2003, a medical journal reported that use of ultraviolet light irradiation in cooling coils and drip pans could kill the germs that cause SBS. In addition, designing buildings to minimize introduction of contaminants or inspecting older buildings for possible VOCs and correcting potential problems can prevent SBS in building occupants. Education and communication are essential for effective air quality management in any building.

Resources

PERIODICALS

Anderson, Ashley. "Ultraviolet Light Reduces Sick Building Syndrome." *Supply House Times* (January 2004): 28–29.

Burge, P. S. "Sick Building Syndrome." *Occupational and Environmental Medicine* (February 2004): 185–191.

Henckel, Leslie. "IAQ FYI: Proactive Management Can Help to Clear Buildings of Indoor Air Quality Problems." *Journal of Property Management* (July-August 2003): 48–52.

Sadovsky, Richard. "Assessing Patients with Medically Unknown Symptoms." *American Family Physician* (June 1, 2000): 3455.

Yurkovsky, Savely. "Multiple Chemical Sensitivity. From Treatments to Cure." *Townsend Letter for Doctors and Patients* (January 2001): 58.

ORGANIZATIONS

American Academy of Environmental Medicine. East Kellogg, Suite 625, Wichita, KS 67207. (316) 684-5500. <http://www.aaem.com>.

American Industrial Hygiene Association. 2700 Prosperity Avenue, Suite 250, Fairfax, VA 22031. (703) 849-8888. <http://www.aiha.org>.

Environmental Health Center. 1025 Connecticut Avenue, NW, Suite 1200, Washington, DC 20036. (202) 293-2270. <http://www.nsc.org>.

National Institute for Occupational Safety and Health, US Department of Health and Human Services. 4676 Columbia Parkway (Mail Drop R2), Cincinnati, OH 45226. <http://www.cdc.gov/niosh/homepage.html>.

OTHER

"Sick School Syndrome." KidsHealth for Parents and Nemours Foundation. 2004. [cited June 5, 2004]. <http://www.kidshealth.org>.

"Top Ten Tips for a Healthy Home." American Lung Association. 2004. [cited June 5, 2004]. <http://www.lungusa.org/>.

Teresa G. Odle

Sickle cell anemia

Definition

Sickle cell anemia, which is also known as meniscocytosis or sicklemia, is an inherited blood disorder that arises from a gene mutation. As a result, affected hemoglobin molecules have a tendency to stick to one another, forming abnormal strands of hemoglobin within the red blood cells. The cells that contain these strands become stiff and elongated—sickle-shaped.

Because sickle cell anemia is characterized by the rapid loss of red blood cells as they enter the circulation, it is classified as a hemolytic anemia, "hemolytic" referring to the destruction of the cell membrane of red blood cells, resulting in the release of hemoglobin.

Description

Sickle-shaped cells die much more rapidly than normal red blood cells and the body cannot create replacements fast enough. Anemia develops due to the chronic shortage of red blood cells. Further complications arise because sickle cells do not fit well through small blood vessels, and can become trapped. The trapped sickle cells form blockages that prevent oxygenated blood from reaching associated tissues and organs. The damaged tissues and organs cause considerable **pain** and can lead to serious complications, including **stroke** and an impaired immune system. Sickle cell anemia primarily affects people with African, Mediterranean, Middle Eastern, and Indian ancestry. In the United States, one in 12 African Americans are carriers. An additional 72,000 Americans have sickle cell anemia, meaning they have inherited the trait from both parents. Among African Americans, approximately one in every 500 babies is diagnosed with sickle cell anemia. Hispanic Americans are also heavily affected; sickle cell anemia occurs in one of every 1,000-1,400 births. Worldwide, it has been estimated that 250,000 children are born each year with sickle cell anemia.

Hemoglobin structure

Normal hemoglobin is composed of a heme molecule and two pairs of proteins called globins. Humans have the genes to create six different types of globins—alpha, beta, gamma, delta, epsilon, and zeta—but do not use all of them at once. The type of genes expressed depends upon the stage of development: embryonic, fetal, or adult. Virtually all of the hemoglobin produced in humans from ages 2-3 months and onward contains a pair of alpha-globin and beta-globin molecules.

Sickle cell hemoglobin

A change, or mutation, in a gene can alter the formation or function of its product. In the case of sickle cell hemoglobin, the gene that carries the blueprint for beta-globin has a tiny alteration that makes it different from the normal gene. This mutation affects a single nucleic acid along the entire DNA strand that makes up the beta-globin gene. (Nucleic acids are the chemicals that make up deoxyribonucleic acid [DNA].) Specifically, the nucleic acid adenine is replaced by a different nucleic acid called thymine.

Because of this seemingly slight mutation, called a point mutation, the finished beta-globin molecule has a single amino acid substitution: valine occupies the spot normally taken by glutamic acid. (**Amino acids** are the building blocks of all proteins.) This substitution is incorporated into the beta-globin molecule—and eventually returning in a hemoglobin molecule—that does not function normally.

Normal hemoglobin, referred to as hemoglobin A, transports oxygen from the lungs to tissues throughout the body. In the smallest blood vessels, the hemoglobin exchanges the oxygen for carbon dioxide, which it carries back to the lungs for removal from the body. The defective hemoglobin, designated hemoglobin S, can also transport oxygen. However, once the oxygen is released, hemoglobin S molecules have an abnormal tendency to clump together. Aggregated hemoglobin molecules form strands within red blood cells, which then lose their usual shape and flexibility.

The rate at which hemoglobin S aggregation and cell sickling occurs depends on many factors, such as the blood flow rate and the concentration of hemoglobin in the blood cells. If the blood flows at a normal rate, hemoglobin S is reoxygenated in the lungs before it has a chance to aggregate. The concentration of hemoglobin within red blood cells is influenced by an individual's hydration level—that is, the amount of water contained in the cells. If a person becomes dehydrated, hemoglobin becomes more concentrated in the red blood cells. In this situation, hemoglobin S has a greater tendency to clump together and induce sickle cell formation.

Sickle cell anemia

Genes are inherited in pairs, one copy from each parent. Therefore, each person has two copies of the gene that makes beta-globin. As long as a person inherits one normal beta-globin gene, the body can produce sufficient quantities of normal beta-globin. A person who inherits a copy of each of the normal and abnormal beta-globin genes is referred to as a carrier of the sickle cell trait. Generally, carriers do not have symptoms, but their red blood cells contain some hemoglobin S.

A child who inherits the sickle cell trait from both parents—a 25% possibility if both parents are carriers—will develop sickle cell anemia. These cells have a decreased life span in comparison to normal red blood cells. Normal red blood cells survive for approximately 120 days in the bloodstream; sickle cells last only 10-12 days. As a result, the bloodstream is chronically short of red blood cells and the affected individual develops anemia.

The sickle cells can create other complications. Due to their shape, they do not fit well through small blood vessels. As an aggravating factor, the outside surfaces of sickle cells may have altered chemical properties that in-

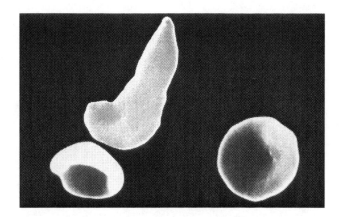

A scanning electron micrograph (SEM) of red blood cells taken from a person with sickle cell anemia. The blood cells at the bottom are normal; the diseased, sickle-shaped cell appears at the top. *(Photograph by Dr. Gopal Murti, Photo Researchers, Inc. Reproduced by permission.)*

crease the cell's "stickiness." These sticky sickle cells are more likely to adhere to the inside surfaces of small blood vessels as well as to other blood cells. As a result of the sickle cells' shape and stickiness, blockages occasionally form in small blood vessels. Such blockages prevent oxygenated blood from reaching areas where it is needed, causing extreme pain as well as organ and tissue damage.

The severity of the symptoms cannot be predicted based solely on the person's genetic inheritance. Some individuals with sickle cell anemia develop health- or life-threatening problems in infancy but others may have only mild symptoms throughout their lives. For example, genetic factors, such as the continued production of fetal hemoglobin after birth can modify the course of the disease. Fetal hemoglobin contains gamma-globin in place of beta-globin; if enough of it is produced, the potential interactions between hemoglobin S molecules are reduced.

Affected populations

Worldwide, millions of people carry the sickle cell trait. Individuals whose ancestors lived in sub-Saharan Africa, the Middle East, India, or the Mediterranean region are the most likely to have the trait. The areas of the world associated with the sickle cell trait are also strongly affected by **malaria**, a disease caused by blood-borne parasites transmitted through mosquito bites. According to a widely accepted theory, the genetic mutation associated with the sickle cell trait occurred thousands of years ago. Coincidentally, this mutation increased the likelihood that carriers would survive malaria outbreaks. Survivors then passed the mutation on to their offspring, and the trait became established throughout areas where malaria was common.

Causes & symptoms

Symptoms typically appear during the first year or two of life. However, some individuals do not develop symptoms until adulthood and may not be aware that they have the genetic inheritance for sickle cell anemia.

Anemia

Sickle cells have a high turnover rate, and there is an ongoing deficit of red blood cells in the bloodstream. Common symptoms of anemia include **fatigue**, paleness, and shortness of breath. A particularly severe form of anemia—aplastic anemia—occurs following infection with parvovirus. Though temporary, parvovirus infection causes extensive destruction of the bone marrow, bringing production of new red blood cells to a halt. Bone marrow production resumes after 7–10 days, but given the short lives of sickle cells, even a brief shutdown in red blood cell production can cause a major decline in hemoglobin concentrations. This event is called "aplastic crisis."

Painful crises

Painful crises, also known as vasoocclusive crises, are a primary symptom of sickle cell anemia in children and adults. The pain may be caused by small blood vessel blockages that prevent oxygen from reaching tissues. An alternate explanation, particularly with regard to bone pain, is that blood is shunted away from the bone marrow but through some mechanism other than blockage by sickle cells.

These crises are unpredictable and can affect any area of the body, although the chest, abdomen, and bones are frequently affected sites. There is some evidence that cold temperatures or infection can trigger a painful crisis, but most crises occur for unknown reasons. The frequency and duration of the pain can vary tremendously. Crises may be separated by more than a year or possibly only by weeks, and they can last from hours to weeks.

The hand-foot syndrome is a particular type of painful crisis, and is often the first sign of sickle cell anemia in an infant. Common symptoms include pain and swelling in the hands and feet, possibly accompanied by a **fever**. Hand-foot syndrome typically occurs only during the first four years of life, with the greatest incidence at one year.

Enlarged spleen and infections

Sickle cells can impede blood flow through the spleen and cause organ damage. In infants and young children, the spleen is usually enlarged. After repeated incidence of blood vessel blockage, the spleen usually atrophies by late childhood. Damage to the spleen can have a negative impact on the immune system, leaving individuals with sickle cell anemia more vulnerable to **infections**. Infants and young children are particularly prone to life-threatening infections.

Anemia can also impair the immune system, because stem cells—the precursors of all blood cells—are earmarked for red blood cell production rather than white blood cell production. White blood cells form the cornerstone of the immune system within the bloodstream.

Delayed growth

The energy demands of the bone marrow for red blood cell production compete with the demands of a growing body. Children with sickle cell anemia have delayed growth and reach puberty at a later age than normal. By early adulthood, they catch up on growth and attain normal height, but their weight typically remains below average.

Stroke

Blockage of blood vessels in the brain can have particularly harsh consequences and can be fatal. When areas of the brain are deprived of oxygen, control of the associated functions may be lost. Sometimes this loss is permanent. Common stroke symptoms include weakness or numbness that affects one side of the body, sudden loss of vision, confusion, loss of speech or the ability to understand spoken words, and **dizziness**. Children between the ages of 1 and 15 have a 30% risk of suffering a stroke. Approximately two-thirds of the children who have a stroke will have at least one more; those who survive typically suffer severe learning disabilities. As of 2003, researchers are investigating various techniques for helping children with **memory loss** related to strokes caused by sickle cell disease.

Acute chest syndrome

Acute chest syndrome can occur at any age, and is caused by sickle cells blocking the small blood vessels of the lungs. This blockage is complicated by accompanying problems such as infection and pooling of blood in the lungs. Affected persons experience fever, **cough**, chest pain, and shortness of breath. Recurrent attacks can lead to permanent lung damage.

Other problems

Males with sickle cell anemia may experience a condition called priapism, characterized by a persistent and painful erection of the penis. Due to blood vessel blockage by sickle cells, blood is trapped in the tissue of the penis. Damage to this tissue can result in permanent **impotence** in adults.

Both genders may experience kidney damage. The environment of the kidney is particularly conducive to sickle cell formation; even otherwise asymptomatic carriers may experience some level of kidney damage. Kidney damage is indicated by blood in the urine, incontinence, and enlarged kidneys.

Jaundice and an enlarged liver are also commonly associated with sickle cell anemia. Jaundice, indicated by a yellow tone in the skin and eyes, may occur if bilirubin levels increase. Bilirubin is the final product of hemoglobin degradation, and is typically removed from the bloodstream by the liver. Bilirubin levels often increase with high levels of red blood cell destruction, but jaundice can also be a sign of a poorly functioning liver.

Some individuals with sickle cell anemia may experience vision problems. The blood vessels that feed into the retina—the tissue at the back of the eyeball—may be blocked by sickle cells. New blood vessels can form around the blockages, but these vessels are typically weak or otherwise defective. Bleeding, scarring, and **retinal detachment** may eventually lead to blindness.

Diagnosis

Sickle cell anemia is suspected based on an individual's ethnic or racial background, and on the symptoms of anemia. A blood count reveals the presence of anemia, and a sickle cell test reveals the presence of the sickle cell trait.

To confirm a diagnosis of the sickle cell trait or sickle cell anemia, another laboratory test called gel electrophoresis is performed. This test uses an electric field applied across a slab of gel-like material to separate protein molecules based on their size, shape, or electrical charge. Although hemoglobin S (sickle) and hemoglobin A (normal) differ by only one amino acid, they can be clearly separated using gel electrophoresis. If both types of hemoglobin are identified, the individual is a carrier of the sickle cell trait; if only hemoglobin S is present, the person most likely has sickle cell anemia.

The gel electrophoresis test is also used as a screening method for identifying the sickle cell trait in newborns. More than 40 states screen newborns in order to identify carriers and individuals who have inherited the trait from both parents.

Treatment

In general, treatment of sickle cell anemia relies on conventional medicine. However, alternative therapies may be useful in pain control.

Massage

The daily pain caused by sickle cell disease has been shown to be managed by massage. A pilot study whose results were published in 1999 indicated that those who received massage reported less perception of pain than those who were part of a **relaxation** control group during the research. Massage is recommended as a complementary treatment in the management of the chronic disease.

Pain diaries

A 2001 study revealed that diaries kept by children and adolescents could help the patients and their families better manage sickle cell pain from home. If children (who are old enough to read and write) can record pain episodes, they have better recall and provide improved documentation for physicians and parents so they can relate pain episodes to possible causes.

Acupuncture

Acupuncture may relieve some of the pain caused by sickle cell disease. For longer-lasting results, acupuncturists indicate that the treatment works with the body's subtle energies by manipulating the "chi" to remove blockages and allow the body to heal itself. Acupuncture uses extremely thin needles that are inserted into various areas of the body, with placement depending on the patient's condition. Each treatment usually takes 20-45 minutes.

Diet

While the pain of sickle cell disease ranges from acute to chronic, simple alterations to the diet are one way to help those who endure the illness. Foods like horseradish, cassava, yams, corn, bamboo shoots, sweet potatoes, and lima beans contain cyanogenic glucosides, or natural plant compounds that are recommended additions to the diet. These natural plant compounds interact with bacteria in the large intestine and aid the body in producing a type of hemoglobin that can effectively carry oxygen through blood cells—possibly leading to less pain.

Allopathic treatment

Early identification of sickle cell anemia can prevent many problems. The highest death rates occur during the first year of life due to infection, aplastic anemia, and acute chest syndrome. If anticipated, steps can be taken to avert these crises. With regard to long-term treatment, prevention of complications remains a main goal. Sickle cell anemia cannot be cured—other than through a risky bone marrow transplant—but treatments are available for symptoms.

Pain management

Pain is one of the primary symptoms of sickle cell anemia, and controlling it is an important concern. The methods necessary for pain control are based on individual factors. Some people can gain adequate pain control through over-the-counter oral painkillers (analgesics), local application of heat, and rest. Others need stronger methods, which can include administration of narcotics.

Blood transfusions

Blood transfusions are usually not given on a regular basis but are used to treat painful crises, severe anemia, and other emergencies. In some cases, such as treating spleen enlargement or preventing stroke from recurring, blood transfusions are given as a preventative measure. Regular blood transfusions have the potential to decrease formation of hemoglobin S and reduce associated symptoms.

Drugs

Infants are typically started on a course of penicillin that extends from infancy to age six. This treatment is meant to ward off potentially fatal infections. Infections at any age are treated aggressively with antibiotics. Vaccines for common infections, such as pneumococcal **pneumonia**, are administered when possible.

Emphasis is being placed on developing drugs that treat sickle cell anemia directly. The most promising of these drugs in the late 1990s is hydroxyurea, a drug that was originally designed for anticancer treatment. Hydroxyurea has been shown to reduce the frequency of painful crises and acute chest syndrome in adults, and to lessen the need for blood transfusions. Hydroxyurea seems to work by inducing a higher production of fetal hemoglobin. The major side effects of the drug include decreased production of platelets, red blood cells, and certain white blood cells. The effects of long-term hydroxyurea treatment are unknown; however, a nine-year follow-up study of 299 adults with frequent painful crises reported in 2003 that taking hydroxyurea was associated with a 40% reduction in mortality.

Bone marrow transplantation

Bone marrow transplantation has been shown to cure sickle cell anemia in severely affected children. Indications for a bone marrow transplant are stroke, recurrent acute chest syndrome, and chronic unrelieved pain. Bone marrow transplants tend to be the most successful in children; adults have a higher rate of transplant rejection and other complications.

Gene research

Replacing the gene that produces the defective hemoglobin in sickle cell disease patients with one that makes normal hemoglobin may be a possible treatment due to recent research. According to a 1998 report in *Science*, researchers studied the blood cells from people who carry the sickle cell gene. By using an enzyme called a ribosome, the study was able to alter sickle cells into normal cells. The ribosome cut out the mutated instructions in the cells' genetic pattern and replaced them with the correct instructions. Researchers hope that this gene therapy will allow the cells to make normal hemoglobin— leading to the ultimate treatment for those with sickle cell disease.

In late 2001 genetic scientists reported that they had designed a gene that might lead to a future treatment of sickle cell anemia. Although the gene had not tested in humans, early results showed that the injected gene protected cells from sickling. As of 2003, experiments in gene therapy for sickle cell disease have been carried out in mice, using lentiviral vectors to transfer the corrective gene into the mouse's stem cells. This technique, however, has not yet been attempted in human subjects as of late 2003.

Expected results

Several factors aside from genetic inheritance determine the prognosis for affected individuals. Therefore, predicting the course of the disorder based solely on genes is not possible. In general, given proper medical care, persons with sickle cell anemia are in fairly good health most of the time. The life expectancy for these individuals has steadily increased over the last 30 years, and many are now surviving past the age of 50. In the United States, the average life expectancy for men with sickle cell anemia is 42 years; for women, it is 48 years. The most common causes of death are infections, lung disease, the blocking of a blood vessel supplying a vital organ, and kidney failure. Pregnant women with sickle cell disease are particularly vulnerable to infection, most often pneumonia or urinary tract infections.

Prevention

The sickle cell trait is a genetically linked, inherited condition. Inheritance cannot be prevented but may be predicted. Screening is recommended for individuals in high-risk populations; in the United States, African Americans, and Hispanic Americans have the highest risk of being carriers.

Screening at birth offers the opportunity for early intervention; more than 40 states include sickle cell screening as part of the usual battery of blood tests done for newborns. Pregnant women and couples planning to have children may also wish to be screened to determine their carrier status. Carriers have a 50% chance of passing the trait to their offspring. Children born to two carriers have a 25% chance of inheriting the trait from both

KEY TERMS

Amino acid—A type of molecule used as a building block for protein construction.

Anemia—A condition in which the level of hemoglobin falls below normal values due to a shortage of mature red blood cells. Common symptoms include paleness, fatigue, and shortness of breath.

Bilirubin—A yellow pigment that is the end result of hemoglobin degradation. Bilirubin is cleared from the blood by the action of liver enzymes and excreted from the body.

Bone marrow—A spongy tissue located in the hollow centers of certain bones, such as the skull and hip bones. Bone marrow is the site of blood cell generation.

Bone marrow transplantation—A medical procedure in which normal bone marrow is transferred from a healthy donor to an ailing recipient. An illness that prevents production of normal blood cells—such as sickle cell anemia—may be treated with a bone marrow transplant.

Gel electrophoresis—A laboratory test that separates molecules based on their size, shape, or electrical charge.

Globin—One of the component protein molecules found in hemoglobin. Normal adult hemoglobin has a pair each of alpha-globin and beta-globin molecules.

Heme—The iron-containing molecule in hemoglobin that serves as the site for oxygen binding.

Hemoglobin—The red pigment found within red blood cells that enables them to transport oxygen throughout the body. Hemoglobin is a large molecule composed of five component molecules, a heme molecule and two pairs of globin molecules.

Hemoglobin A—Normal adult hemoglobin which contains a heme molecule, two alpha-globin molecules, and two beta-globin molecules.

Hemoglobin S—Hemoglobin that is produced in association with the sickle cell trait; the beta-globin molecules of hemoglobin S are defective.

Hemolytic—Referring to the destruction of the cell membranes of red blood cells, resulting in the release of hemoglobin from the damaged cell.

Jaundice—A condition characterized by higher-than-normal levels of bilirubin in the bloodstream and an accompanying yellowing of the skin and eyes.

Meniscocytosis—Another word for sickle cell disease.

Mutation—A change in a gene's DNA. Whether a mutation is harmful is determined by the effect on the product for which the gene codes.

Nucleic acid—A type of chemical that is used as a component for building DNA. The nucleic acids found in DNA are adenine, thymine, guanine, and cytosine.

Red blood cell—Hemoglobin-containing blood cells that transport oxygen from the lungs to tissues. In the tissues, the red blood cells exchange their oxygen for carbon dioxide, which is brought back to the lungs to be exhaled.

---

parents and having sickle cell anemia. Carriers may consider genetic counseling to assess any risks to their offspring. The sickle cell trait can also be identified through prenatal testing, specifically through use of amniotic fluid testing or chorionic villus sampling.

By maintaining a good diet, staying well hydrated with plenty of fluids, exercising regularly, and getting enough sleep those with sickle cell disease may help their bodies remain strong and ward off fatigue and dehydration.

Resources

BOOKS

"Anemias Caused by Excessive Hemolysis: Sickle Cell Diseases." Section 11, Chapter 127 in *The Merck Manual of Diagnosis and Therapy*, edited by Mark H. Beers, MD, and Robert Berkow, MD. Whitehouse Station, NJ: Merck Research Laboratories, 2002.

Beutler, Ernest. *The Sickle Cell Diseases and Related Disorders*. Williams Hematology, edited by Ernest Beutler, et al. 5th ed. New York: McGraw-Hill,1995.

Bloom, Miriam. *Understanding Sickle Cell Disease*. Jackson, MS: University Press of Mississippi, 1995.

The Editors of Time-Life Books. *Sickle Cell Anemia*. The Medical Advisor: The Complete Guide to Alternative & Conventional Treatments, Richmond, VA: Time-Life Inc., 1996.

Embury, Stephen H., et al., eds. *Sickle Cell Disease: Basic Principles and Clinical Practice*. New York: Raven Press, 1994.

"Pregnancy Complicated by Disease: Hemoglobinopathies." Section 18, Chapter 251 in *The Merck Manual of Diagno-*

sis and Therapy, edited by Mark H. Beers, MD, and Robert Berkow, MD. Whitehouse Station, NJ: Merck Research Laboratories, 2002.

PERIODICALS

Davies, S. C., and A. Gilmore. "The Role of Hydroxyurea in the Management of Sickle Cell Disease." *Blood Reviews* 17 (June 2003): 99–109.

Egbert Maikler, Virginia, et al. "Children's and Adolescents' Use of Diaries for Sickle Cell Pain." *Journal of the Society of Pediatric Nurses* 6. no. 4 (October – December 2001): 161 – 169.

Harris, Leslie. "Living Well with Sickle Cell." *Essence* (September 1999): 58.

Nienhuis, A. W., H. Hanawa, N. Sawai, et al. "Development of Gene Therapy for Hemoglobin Disorders." *Annals of the New York Academy of Science* 996 (May 2003): 101–111.

Seppa, N. "Gene Therapy for Sickle-cell Disease?." *Science News* 160, no. 24 (December 15, 2001): 372.

"Sickle Cell Pain Relieved by Massage." *Massage Magazine* (June 30, 1999): 52.

Steinberg, M. H., F. Barton, O. Castro, et al. "Effect of Hydroxyurea on Mortality and Morbidity in Adult Sickle Cell Anemia: Risks and Benefits up to 9 Years of Treatment." *Journal of the American Medical Association* 289 (April 2, 2003): 1645–1651.

Winrow, N., and E. R. Melhem. "Sickle Cell Disease and Stroke in a Pediatric Population. Evidence-Based Diagnostic Evaluation." *Neuroimaging Clinics of North America* 13 (May 2003): 185–196.

Yerys, B. E., D. A. White, C. F. Salorio, et al. "Memory Strategy Training in Children with Cerebral Infarcts Related to Sickle Cell Disease." *Journal of Pediatric Hematology and Oncology* 25 (June 2003): 495–498.

ORGANIZATIONS

Mayo Foundation for Medical Education and Research. <http://www.mayohealth.org>.

Sickle Cell Disease Association of America. 200 Corporate Point, Suite 495, Culver City, CA 90230-7633. (310) 216-6363. (800) 421-8453. <http://sicklecelldisease.org/>.

Sickle Cell Disease Program, Division of Blood Diseases and Resources. National Heart, Lung, and Blood Institute. II Rockledge Centre, 6701 Rockledge Dr. MSC 7950, Bethesda, MD 20892-7950. (301) 435-0055.

Beth Kapes
Teresa Norris
Rebecca J. Frey, PhD

Silica

Description

Silica, sometimes called *Silicea terra* or abbreviated as sil., is a homeopathic remedy. Silica is a mineral and is prepared from silicon dioxide found in flint, quartz, sandstone, and many other common rocks.

General use

Homeopathic medicine operates on the principle that "like heals like." This principle means that a disease can be cured by treating it with products that produce the same symptoms as the disease. These products follow another homeopathic law, the Law of Infinitesimals. In opposition to traditional medicine, the Law of Infinitesimals states that the *lower* a dose of curative, the more effective it is. To achieve a very low dose, the curative is diluted many, many times until only a tiny amount remains in a huge amount of the diluting liquid.

In homeopathic terms, remedies are "proved" by experimentation and reports made by famous homeopathic practitioners. Silica was proved as a remedy by the German founder of **homeopathy**, Dr. Samuel Hahnemann (1775–1843).

In homeopathy, silica is often used to treat symptoms of chronic diseases where there is general weakness and a lack of either physical or emotional strength. The rocks silica comes from are hard and compact. Silica is used to strengthen many parts of the body and impart to them silica's hard, dense, strong characteristics.

Silica is used to treat conditions associated with frequent and recurrent illnesses that occur because of a weakened immune system. These include frequent colds, flu, and chronic ear **infections** (especially those with a thick, yellow discharge or fluid in the middle ear).

Silica is also useful in expelling material from the body. It is used to remove splinters, bits of embedded glass, and other foreign irritants. It also aids in the elimination of stools from the rectum.

Certain skin and bone complaints can also be treated with silica. These include **fractures** that are slow to heal, rough or peeling lips, **acne**, weak nails, and ingrown toenails. Other ailments for which silica is considered an appropriate homeopathic remedy are migraines that begin in the back of the head and extend to the eyes, heavy sweating around the head and neck, **mumps**, dental abscesses, vaginal cysts, mastitis in breast-feeding women, and general low stamina.

One diagnostic tool in homeopathy is to observe when symptoms improve or worsen as a clue to which remedy to use.

Symptoms benefiting from silica worsen:

- in cold damp weather
- in the morning
- after getting feet wet

- at the time of the new moon
- if sweating is suppressed
- from washing or swimming
- from lying on the left side

    Symptoms improve:
- in hot, humid weather
- with warmth
- with wrapping the head

Homeopathy also ascribes certain personality types to certain remedies. The silica personality is said to be chronically exhausted and lacking in stamina. These people are happy to sit and take no action. The silica personality type feels cold intensely. These people are often intellectually bright but lack confidence. They obsess about small details to the point of exhaustion because they fear failure and being hurt. They tend to be shy and have good manners but are also willful to the point of resenting any outside interference.

Preparations

For homeopathic remedies, the remedy material is finely ground and then prepared by extensive dilutions. In the early days of homeopathy, silica was prepared from powered rock. Today, most silica is manufactured chemically.

There are two homeopathic dilution scales: the decimal (x) scale with a dilution of 1:10 and the centesimal (c) scale with a dilution of 1:100. Once the mixture is diluted, shaken, strained, then rediluted many times to reach the desired degree of potency, the final mixture is added to lactose (a type of sugar) tablets or pellets. These are then stored away from light. *Silica* is available commercially in tablets in many different strengths. Dosage depends on the symptoms being treated.

Homeopathic and orthodox medical practitioners agree that by the time the initial remedy solution is diluted to strengths used in homeopathic healing, it is likely that very few molecules of the original remedy remain. Homeopaths, however, believe that these remedies continue to work through an effect called "potentization" that has not yet been explained by mainstream scientists.

Precautions

Homeopaths recommend that anyone with implants or artificial body components avoid silica because of its tendency to cause foreign materials to be expelled from the body.

Side effects

When taken in the recommended dilute form, no side effects have been reported.

Interactions

Studies on interactions between silica and conventional pharmaceuticals have not been found.

Resources

BOOKS
Hammond, Christopher. *The Complete Family Guide to Homeopathy.* London: Penguin Studio, 1995.
Lockie, Andrew, and Nicola Geddes. *The Complete Guide to Homeopathy.* London: Dorling Kindersley, 1995.

ORGANIZATIONS
Foundation for Homeopathic Education and Research. 21 Kittredge St., Berkeley, CA 94704. (510) 649-8930.
International Foundation for Homeopathy. P. O. Box 7, Edmonds, WA 98020. (206) 776-4147.
National Center for Homeopathy. 801 N. Fairfax St., Suite 306, Alexandria, VA 22314. (703) 548-7790.

Tish Davidson

Silymarin *see* **Milk thistle**

Sinus infection

Definition

Sinusitis, or sinus infection, refers to an inflammation of the sinuses, the air spaces within the bones of the face, due to an infection within these spaces.

Description

The sinuses are paired air pockets located within the bones of the face. They are:

- The frontal sinuses. Located above the eyes, in the center region of each eyebrow.
- The maxillary sinuses. Located within the cheekbones, just to either side of the nose.
- The ethmoid sinuses. Located between the eyes, just behind the bridge of the nose.
- The sphenoid sinuses. Located just behind the ethmoid sinuses, and behind the eyes.

The sinuses are connected with the nose. They are lined with the same kind of skin found elsewhere within

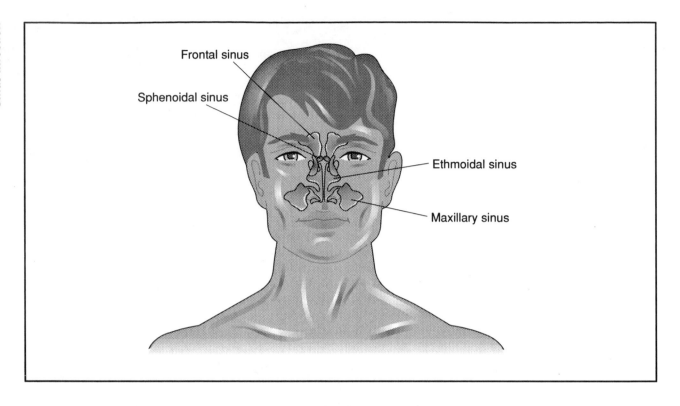

Frontal sinus

Sphenoidal sinus

Ethmoidal sinus

Maxillary sinus

Sinusitis is inflammation of the sinuses caused by a bacterial infection. Sometimes diagnosis may be problematic because the symptoms often mimic those of the common cold. Sinusitis is usually treated with antibiotics. *(Illustration by Electronic Illustrators Group. Gale Group.)*

the respiratory tract. This skin has tiny little hairs projecting from it called cilia. The cilia beat constantly to help move the mucus produced in the sinuses into the respiratory tract. The ciliary action sweeps mucus along the respiratory tract and helps to clear the tract of debris or any organisms which may be present. When the lining of the sinuses swells,, the swelling interferes with the normal flow of mucus. Trapped mucus can then fill the sinuses, causing an uncomfortable sensation of pressure and providing an excellent environment for the growth of infection-causing bacteria.

Causes & symptoms

Although swelling from **allergies** can mimic the symptoms of pressure, **pain**, and congestion, allergies can set the stage for a bacterial infection. Bacteria have usually been considered the most common cause of sinus infection; however, recent research has suggested that fungi are the most common cause. *Streptococcus pneumoniae* causes about 33% of all cases, while *Haemophilus influenzae* causes about 25% of all cases. Twenty percent of sinus **infections** in children may be caused by *Moraxella catarrhalis.* In people with weakened immune systems (including patients with diabetes; acquired immunodeficiency syndrome or **AIDS**; and patients who are taking medications that lower their immune

resistance, such as **cancer** and transplant patients), sinus infections may be caused by fungi such as *Aspergillus, Candida,* or *Mucorales.* Additionally, those repeatedly on antibiotics may be predisposed to sinus infections.

Acute sinus infections usually follow some type of upper respiratory tract infection or cold. Instead of ending, the cold seems to linger, with constant or even worsening congestion. Drainage from the nose often changes from a clear color to a thicker yellowish-green discharge. There may be **fever. Headache** and pain over the affected sinuses may occur, as well as a feeling of pressure that may worsen when the patient bends over. There may be pain in the jaw or teeth. Some children, get upset stomachs from the infected drainage going down the back of their throats and into their stomachs. Other patients develop a **cough.** In recent years, however, physicians have cautioned patients not to assume that the presence of colored mucus or pain automatically means a bacterial infection. It may be of viral origin, and patients can avoid overusing antibiotics with proper diagnosis.

Diagnosis

Medical practitioners have differing levels of trust in certain basic examinations commonly conducted in the office. For example, tapping over the sinuses may cause pain in patients with sinus infection, but it may not. A procedure called sinus transillumination may, or may not, also be helpful. Using a flashlight pressed up against the skin of the cheek, the practitioner will look in the patient's open mouth. When the sinuses are full of air (under normal conditions), the light will project through the sinus and will be visible on the roof of the mouth as a lit-up reddened area. When the sinuses are full of mucus, the light will be blocked. While this simple test can be helpful, it is certainly not a completely reliable way to diagnose or rule out the diagnosis of a sinus infection.

X-ray pictures and CT scans of the sinuses are helpful for both acute and chronic sinus infections. Those experiencing chronic sinus infections may need a procedure with a scope to see if any kind of anatomic obstruction is causing their illness. For example, the septum (the cartilage that separates the two nasal cavities) may be slightly displaced. This condition is called a deviated septum. It can result in chronic obstruction, setting the person up for the recurrent development of infection.

Treatment

A 2001 telephone survey in northern California revealed that use of alternative treatments for rhinosinusitis and **asthma** is common in the population, with 52% reporting use of alternative treatment in the past 12 months to treat breathing or nasal symptoms. Of these, most used herbal treatments, primarily ephedra-containing products.

Chronic sinus inflammation often is associated with food allergies. An elimination/challenge diet is recommended to identify and eliminate allergenic foods. Irrigating the sinuses with a salt water solution is often recommended for sinusitis and allergies, in order to clear the nasal passages of mucus. Another solution for nasal lavage, or washing, utilizes powdered **goldenseal** (*Hydrastis canadensis*) added to the salt water solution. Other herbal treatments taken internally include a mixture made of **eyebright** (*Euphrasia officinalis*), goldenseal, **yarrow** (*Achillea millefolium*), horseradish, and **ephedra** (*Ephedra sinica*); or, when infection is present, a mixture made of **echinacea** (*Echinacea*), wild indigo, and poke root (*Phytolacca decandra-americana*).

Homeopathic practitioners find a number of remedies useful for treating sinusitis. Among those they recommend are: *Arsenicum album, Kalium bichromium,* **Nux vomica,** Mercurius iodatus, and **silica**. Andrographics paniculata, commonly known as Kalmegh, is a herbal remedy from India that is recommended for fighting winter infections and sinus infection. It is usually combines with Echinacea.

Acupuncture has been used to treat sinus inflammation, as have a variety of dietary supplements, including vitamins A, C, and E, and the mineral **zinc**. Contrast **hydrotherapy** (hot and cold compresses, alternating 3 minutes hot, 30 seconds cold, repeated 3 times always ending with cold) applied directly over the sinuses can relieve pressure and enhance healing. A direct inhalation of an essential oil solution using a combination of two cups of water and two drops of a mixture of **thyme**, **rosemary**, or **lavender essential oils** can help open the sinuses and kill bacteria that cause infection.

Allopathic treatment

Antibiotic medications are often used to treat an acute sinus infection, once it has been diagnosed as a bacterial infection. Suitable antibiotics include sulfa drugs, amoxicillin, and a variety of cephalosporins. These medications are usually given for about two weeks but may be given for even longer periods of time. A 2001 study found that the type of antibiotic used for mild to moderate sinus infection did not seem to matter. In other words, any of about 16 antibiotics stopped the infection, so cost could help physicians determine the best therapy. Also, the study suggests that physicians might sometimes delay giving antibiotics to patients with milder symptoms and prescribe them only when moderately severe symptoms last seven days or more or severe symptoms occur.

Decongestants, or the short-term use of decongestant nose sprays, can be useful. Acetaminophen and ibuprofen can decrease the associated pain and headache. Also, running a humidifier can prevent mucus within the nasal passages from uncomfortably drying out, and can help soothe an accompanying **sore throat** or cough.

Chronic sinus infections are often treated initially with antibiotics. Steroid nasal sprays may be used to decrease swelling in the nasal passages. If an anatomic reason is found for chronic infections, it may require corrective surgery. If a surgical procedure is necessary, samples are usually taken at the same time to allow identification of any organisms present which may be causing infection.

Fungal sinus infection may require surgery to clean out the sinuses. Then, a relatively long course of a very strong antifungal medication called amphotericin B is given intravenously through a needle in the vein. This type of infection also can be treated with **botanical medicine**.

Expected results

Prognosis for sinus infections is usually excellent, although some individuals may find that they are particularly prone to contracting such infections after a cold. Fungal sinus infection, however, has a relatively high death rate.

Prevention

Prevention involves maintaining usual standards of good hygiene to cut down on the number of colds an individual catches. Avoiding exposure to cigarette smoke, identifying and treating allergies, and avoiding deep dives into swimming pools or other aquatic areas may help prevent sinus infections. Prevention may include avoiding dairy products and/or wheat products. During the winter, it is a good idea to use a humidifier, as dry nasal passages may develop breaks in the tissues, allowing bacteria to enter. When allergies are diagnosed, a number of nasal sprays are available to try to prevent inflammation within the nasal passageways, thus allowing the normal flow of mucus. A 2003 report from Sweden recommended regular humming. It appears that when people hum, they exhale about 15 times more air and thus expel potentially harmful microbes from nasal passages.

Resources

BOOKS

Durand, Marlene, et al. *Infections of the Upper Respiratory Tract.* Harrison's Principles of Internal Medicine, 14th ed., edited by Anthony S. Fauci, et al. New York: McGraw-Hill, 1998.

Ray, C. George. "Eye, Ear, and Sinus Infections." In *Sherris Medical Microbiology: An Introduction to Infectious Diseases,* edited by Kenneth J. Ryan. Norwalk, CT: Appleton and Lange, 1994.

Stoffman, Phyllis. *The Family Guide to Preventing and Treating 100 Infectious Diseases.* New York: John Wiley and Sons, 1995.

PERIODICALS

Blanc, Paul D., et al. "Alternative Therapies Among Adults with a Reported Diagnosis of Asthma or Rhinosinusitis: Data from a Population-Based Survey." *Chest* (November 2001): 1461.

Bone, Kerry. "Andrographis for Colds and Sinus Infection." *Townsend Letter for Doctors and Patients* (January 2003):36–44.

Kaliner, Michael A. "The Signs of Sinusitis." *Discover* 19 (March 1998): S16+.

O'Brien, Katherine L., et al. "Acute Sinusitis: Principles of Judicious Use of Antimicrobial Agents." *Pediatrics* 101 (January 1998): 174+.

Piccirillo, Jay F., et al. "Impact of First-Line vs. Second-Line Antibiotics for the Treatment of Acute Uncomplicated Sinusitis." *JAMA, The Journal of the American Medical Association* (October 17, 2001): 1849.

"Save Your Schnozz: Hum a Few Bars." *Bicycling* (November 2002):24.

"Sinus Infection Detection." *Harvard Health Letter* (December 2003):

William, J.W., et al. "Clinical Evaluation for Sinusitis: Making the Diagnosis by History and Physical Examination." *Annals of Internal Medicine* 117 (1992): 705+.

ORGANIZATION

American Academy of Otolaryngology-Head and Neck Surgery, Inc. 1 Prince Street, Alexandria, VA 22314–3357. (703) 836–4444.

Kathleen D. Wright
Teresa G. Odle

Sinusitis *see* **Sinus infection**

Sjögren's syndrome

Definition

Sjögren's syndrome is an autoimmune disorder in which the mouth and eyes become extremely dry. Sjögren's syndrome is often associated with other autoimmune disorders.

Description

Like other autoimmune disorders, Sjögren's syndrome occurs when the body's immune system mistakenly considers parts of the body as foreign invaders. People with this disease have abnormal proteins in their blood, suggesting that their immune system is reacting against their own tissue. While the immune cells should attack and kill invaders like bacteria, viruses, and fungi, these cells should not attack the body itself. In autoimmune disorders, however, cells called antibodies see tissues of the body as foreign, and help to start a chain of events that results in damage and destruction of those tissues.

There are three types of Sjögren's syndrome. Primary Sjögren's syndrome occurs by itself with no other associated disorders. Secondary Sjögren's syndrome occurs along with other autoimmune disorders, like **systemic lupus erythematosus, rheumatoid arthritis**, scleroderma, vasculitis, or polymyositis. When the disorder is limited to involvement of the eyes, with no other organ or tissue involvement evident, it is called sicca complex.

Women are about 10 times more likely to suffer from Sjögren's syndrome than are men. It affects all age groups, although most patients are diagnosed when they are between 45 and 55 years old. Sjögren's syndrome is commonly associated with other autoimmune disorders. In fact, 30% of patients with certain autoimmune disorders will also have Sjögren's syndrome.

Causes & symptoms

The cause of Sjögren's syndrome has not been clearly defined, but several causes are suspected. For instance, genetic factors play a role, in that the syndrome sometimes runs in families. In fact, autoimmune diseases in general tend to occur in families with certain genetic characteristics. In late 2001, researchers announced discovery of the genetic markers that predict increased risk of many autoimmune disorders like rheumatoid arthritis, **multiple sclerosis,** and lupus.

Other potential causes include hormonal factors (since there are more women than men with the disease) and viral factors. The viral theory suggests that the immune system is activated in response to a viral invader, but then fails to turn itself off. Some other immune malfunction then causes the overly active immune system to begin attacking the body's own tissues. Sjögren's syndrome is thought to be the end result of several factors including genetic, immunologic, hormonal, and possibly infectious.

The main problem in Sjögren's syndrome is dryness. The salivary glands and secretory glands (mucous/liquid) are often attacked and slowly destroyed, leaving the mouth extremely dry and sticky-feeling. Swallowing and talking become difficult. Normally, the saliva washes the teeth clean. Saliva cannot perform this function in Sjögren's syndrome, so the teeth develop many cavities and decay quickly. The parotid glands produce the majority of the mouth's saliva. These glands are located over the jaw bones, behind the area of the cheeks and in front of the ears, and may become significantly enlarged in Sjögren's syndrome.

The eyes also become extremely dry as the tear glands (called lacrimal glands) are slowly destroyed. Eye symptoms include **itching**, burning, redness, increased sensitivity to light, and thick secretions gathering at the eye corners closest to the nose. The cornea may have small irritated pits in its surface (ulcerations).

Destruction of secretary glands in other areas of the body may cause a variety of symptoms. In the nose, dryness may result in **nosebleeds**. In the rest of the respiratory tract, the rates of **ear infection**, hoarseness, **bronchitis**, and **pneumonia** may increase. Vaginal dryness can be quite uncomfortable. Rarely, the pancreas may slow production of enzymes critical for digestion. The kidney may malfunction. About 33% of all patients with Sjögren's syndrome have other symptoms unrelated to gland destruction. These symptoms include **fatigue**, decreased energy, fevers, muscle aches and pains, and joint **pain**.

Patients who also have other autoimmune diseases will suffer from the symptoms specific to those conditions. A rare but serious complication of Sjögren's syndrome is inflammation of the blood vessels (vasculitis), which can damage tissues supplied by these blood vessels.

Diagnosis

Diagnosis of Sjögren's syndrome is based on the patient having at least three consecutive months of bothersome eye and/or mouth dryness. A variety of tests can then be done to determine the quantity of tears produced, the quantity of saliva produced, and the presence or absence of antibodies that could be involved in the destruction of glands.

Treatment

There is no cure for Sjögren's syndrome. Instead, treatment usually attempts to reduce the discomfort and complications associated with dryness of the eyes and mouth (and other areas). Artificial tears are available, and may need to be used up to every 30 minutes. By using these types of products, the patient is more comfortable and avoids the complications associated with eyes that are overly dry. **Dry mouth** is treated by sipping fluids slowly but constantly throughout the day. Sugarless chewing gum can also be helpful. An artificial saliva is available for use as a mouthwash. Careful dental hygiene is important in order to avoid tooth decay, and it is wise for patients to decrease sugar intake.

Allopathic treatment

Vaginal dryness can be treated with certain gel preparations. Steroid or immunosuppressive medications may be required when other symptoms of autoimmune disorders complicate Sjögren's syndrome. However, these medications should be avoided when possible because they may thin the cornea and make it even more susceptible to injury.

Expected results

The prognosis for patients with primary Sjögren's syndrome is particularly good. Although the condition is quite annoying, serious complications rarely occur. The prognosis for patients with secondary Sjögren's syndrome varies, since it depends on the prognosis for the accompanying autoimmune disorder.

Prevention

Since the cause of Sjögren's syndrome is unknown, there are no known ways to prevent this syndrome.

Resources

BOOKS

Aaseng, Nathan. *Autoimmune Diseases.* New York: F. Watts, 1995.

Koopman, D. *Arthritis and Allied Conditions.* New York: Williams and Wilkins, 1997.

Moutsopoulos, Haralampos M. "Sjögren's Syndrome." In *Harrison's Principles of Internal Medicine,* edited by Anthony S. Fauci, et al. New York: McGraw-Hill, 1998.

Talal, N., et al. *Sjögren's syndrome: Clinical and Immunological Aspects.* Berlin: Springer, 1987.

PERIODICALS

Moran, M. "Autoimmune Diseases Could Share Common Genetic Etiology." *American Medical News.* 44, no. 38: (October 8, 2001):38.

Moutsopoulos, H. M., and P. G. Vlachoyiannopoulos. "What Would I Do If I Had Sjögren's syndrome?" *Rheumatology Review* 2 (1993): 17+.

Moutsopoulos, H. M., and P. Youinou. "New Developments in Sjögren's syndrome." *Current Opinion in Rheumatology* 3 (1991): 815+.

ORGANIZATIONS

National Institute of Arthritis & Skin Diseases. Building 31, Room 4C05, Bethesda, MD 20892-2350. (301) 496-8188. http://nih.gov/niams.

National Organization for Rare Disorders (NORD). 55 Kenosia Avenue, Danbury, CT 06813 (203) 744-0100 (toll-free # is the same).

National Sjögren's Syndrome Association. 5815 N. Black Canyon Highway, #103, Phoenix, AZ 85015-2200. (602) 443-9844.

Kim Sharp
Teresa Norris

Skin cancer

Definition

Skin cancer is a malignant growth of the external surface or epithelial layer of the skin.

Description

Skin cancer is the growth of abnormal cells capable of invading and destroying other associated skin cells. Skin cancer is often subdivided into either melanoma or non-melanoma. Melanoma is a dark-pigmented, usually malignant, tumor arising from a skin cell capable of making the pigment melanin (a melanocyte). Melanoma can spread throughout the body via the bloodstream or lymphatic system. Non-melanoma skin cancer most often originates from the external skin surface as a squamous cell carcinoma or a basal cell carcinoma.

The cells of a cancerous growth originate from a single cell that reproduces uncontrollably, resulting in the formation of a tumor. Exposure to sunlight is documented as the main cause of almost 800,000 cases of skin cancer diagnosed each year in the United States. The incidence increases for those living where direct sunshine is plentiful, such as in regions near the equator.

Basal cell carcinoma affects the skin's basal layer and has the potential to grow progressively larger in size, although it rarely spreads to distant areas (metastasizes). Basal cell carcinoma accounts for 80% of skin cancers (excluding melanoma), whereas squamous cell cancer makes up about 20%. Squamous cell carcinoma is a malignant growth of the external surface of the skin. Squamous cell cancers metastasize at a rate of 2–6%, with up to 10% of lesions affecting the ear and lip.

Causes & symptoms

Cumulative sun exposure is considered a significant risk factor for non-melanoma skin cancer. High incidence has been noted in individuals with freckles, light hair, and light complexion; in individuals with darker skin, the palms, soles, mucous membranes, and other areas of light pigmentation are the most common sites for melanomas.

Pre-existing moles can change into melanomas, and should be observed for any particular change in appearance, specifically the classic *ABCD* appearance, in which asymmetrical borders, colors, and diameter are observed. Lesions typically are circular with irregular or *asymmetrical borders*. Melanomas typically have a combination of *colors*, including tan, brown, black, or gray; there may also be a dull pink or rose pigmentation within a small area of the lesion. The *diameter* of a malignant melanoma is typically greater than that of a pencil eraser.

There is evidence suggesting that early intense sun exposure causing blistering **sunburn** in childhood may also play an important role in the cause of non-melanoma skin cancer. Basal cell carcinoma most frequently affects the skin of the face, with the next most

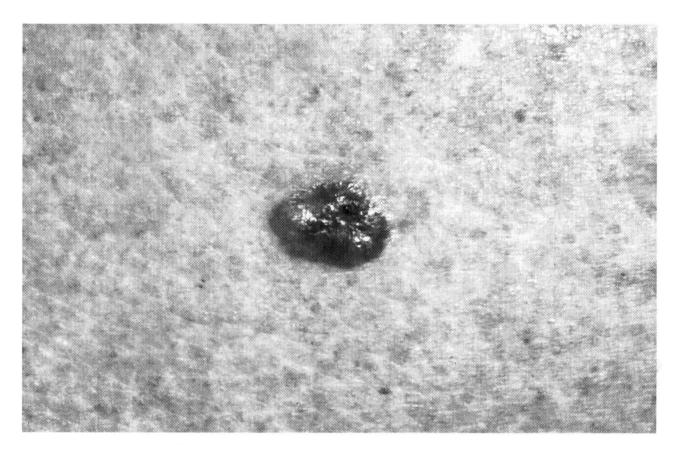

Basal cell type of skin cancer. Basal cell cancers grow more slowly than melanomas. *(Custom Medical Stock Photo. Reproduced by permission.)*

common sites being the ears, the backs of the hands, the shoulders, and the arms. It is prevalent in both sexes, and most commonly occurs in people over the age of 40.

Basal cell carcinoma usually appears as a small skin lesion that persists for at least three weeks. This form of non-melanoma cancer looks flat and waxy, with the edges of the lesion translucent and rounded. The edges also contain small fresh blood vessels. An ulcer found in the center gives the lesion a dimpled appearance. Basal cell carcinoma lesions vary from 4–6 mm in size, but can slowly grow larger if left untreated.

Squamous cell carcinoma also involves skin exposed to the sun, such as the face, ears, hands, or arms. This form of non-melanoma cancer also is most common among people over the age of 40. Squamous cell carcinoma presents itself as a small, scaling, raised bump on the skin with a crusting ulcer in the center, but without **itching**.

Basal cell and squamous cell carcinomas can grow more easily when people have a suppressed immune system because they are taking immunosuppressive drugs or are exposed to radiation. Some people must take immunosuppressive drugs to prevent the rejection of a trans-

planted organ or because they have a disease in which the immune system attacks the body's own tissues, referred to as autoimmune illnesses; others may need radiation therapy to treat another form of cancer. Because of the increased risk of skin cancer, all people taking these immunosuppressive drugs or receiving radiation treatments should undergo complete skin examination at regular intervals. If proper treatment is delayed and the tumor continues to grow, the tumor cells can spread, or metastasize, to other muscles, bones, nerves, and possibly to the brain.

About 1–2% of all skin cancers develop within burn scars; squamous cell carcinomas account for about 95% of these cancers, with 3% being basal cell carcinomas and the remainder malignant melanomas.

Diagnosis

To diagnose skin cancer, doctors must carefully examine the lesion and ask the patient how long it has been there, whether it itches or bleeds, and other questions about the patient's medical history. If skin cancer cannot be ruled out, a biopsy is performed, in which a sample of the tissue is removed and examined under a microscope. A definitive diagnosis of melanoma, squamous, or basal cell cancer can only be made with microscopic examination of the tumor cells. Once skin cancer has been diagnosed, the stage of the disease's development is determined. The information from the biopsy and staging allows the physician and patient to plan for treatment and possible surgical intervention.

Treatment

Alternative medicine aims to prevent rather than treat skin cancer. Vitamins have been shown to prevent sunburn and possibly skin cancer. Some dermatologists have suggested that taking antioxidant vitamins E and C by mouth may help prevent sunburn. In one particular study, men and women took these vitamins for eight days prior to being exposed to ultraviolet light. The researchers found that those who consumed vitamins required about 20% more ultraviolet light to induce sunburn than did people who did not take vitamins. This is the first study that indicates the oral use of vitamins E and C increases resistance to sunburn. These **antioxidants** are thought to reduce the risk of skin cancer and are thought to provide protection from the sun even if taken in lower doses. Other antioxidant nutrients, including **beta carotene**, **selenium**, **zinc**, and the bioflavonoid quercetin, may also help prevent skin cancer, as may such antioxidant herbs as **bilberry** (*Vaccinium myrtillus*), **hawthorn** (*Crataegus laevigata*), **turmeric** (*Curcuma longa*), and ginkgo (*Ginkgo biloba*).

A team of researchers at Duke University reported in 2003 that topical application of a combination of 15% **vitamin C** and 1% **vitamin E** over a four-day period offered significant protection against sunburn. The researchers suggest that this combination may protect skin against **aging** caused by sunlight as well.

Another antioxidant that appears to counter the effects of severe sun exposure is superoxide dismutase, or SOD. SOD must be given in injectable form, however, because it is destroyed in the digestive tract.

As of 2003, researchers are also looking at botanical compounds that could be added to skin care products applied externally to lower the risk of skin cancer. Several botanical compounds have been tested on animals and found to be effective in preventing skin cancer, but further research needs to be done in human subjects.

Allopathic treatment

A wide surgical removal of the melanoma and surrounding tissue is usually necessary. Surgery may also include removal of affected lymph nodes, usually followed by skin grafting, which is a process in which a piece of skin that is taken from a donor area replaces the skin removed.

Since the early 1990s, some melanomas have been treated with chemotherapy (usually carmustine or lomustine); other biological therapies are also being used as of 2003.

A variety of treatment options are available for those diagnosed with non-melanoma skin cancer. Some carcinomas can be removed by cryosurgery, the process of freezing with liquid nitrogen. Uncomplicated and previously untreated basal cell carcinoma of the torso and arms is often treated with curettage and electrodesiccation, which is the scraping of the lesion and the destruction of any remaining malignant cells with an electrical current. Moh's surgery, or removal of a lesion layer by layer down to normal margins, is an effective treatment for both basal and squamous cell carcinoma. Radiation therapy is best reserved for older, debilitated patients, or those whose tumors are considered inoperable. Laser therapy is sometimes useful in specific cases; however, this form of treatment is not widely used to treat skin cancer.

Expected results

Both squamous and basal cell carcinoma are curable with appropriate treatment. Early detection remains critical for a positive prognosis.

Prevention

Avoiding exposure to the sun reduces the incidence of non-melanoma skin cancer. Sunscreen with a sun-protective factor (SPF) of 15 or higher is helpful in prevention, along with a hat and clothing to shield the skin from sun damage. Individuals who are physically active while exposed to sunlight should consider using waterproof sunscreen, or reapply it. There are many different brands of sunscreen for those with certain skin **allergies**. People should examine their skin monthly for unusual lesions, especially if previous skin cancers have been experienced.

Advances in photographic technique have now made it easier to track the development of moles with the help of whole-body photographs. A growing number of hospitals are offering these photographs as part of outpatient mole-monitoring services.

Resources

BOOKS

Chandrasoma, Parakrama, and Clive R. Taylor. *Concise Pathology*. East Norwalk, CT: Appleton and Lange, 1991.

Copstead, Lee-Ellen C. "Alterations in the Integument." In *Perspectives on Pathophysiology*. Philadelphia: W.B. Saunders, 1994.

"Dermatologic Disorders: Malignant Tumors." Section 10, Chapter 126 in *The Merck Manual of Diagnosis and Therapy*, edited by Mark H. Beers, MD, and Robert Berkow,

MD. Whitehouse Station, NJ: Merck Research Laboratories, 2002.

"Dermatologic Disorders: Reactions to Sunlight." Section 10, Chapter 119 in *The Merck Manual of Diagnosis and Therapy*, edited by Mark H. Beers, MD, and Robert Berkow, MD. Whitehouse Station, NJ: Merck Research Laboratories, 2002.

Pelletier, Kenneth R., MD. *The Best Alternative Medicine*, Part I: Food for Thought. New York: Simon & Schuster, 2002.

PERIODICALS

Bray, C. "The Development of an Improved Method of Photography for Mole-Monitoring at the University Hospital of North Durham." *Journal of Audiovisual Media in Medicine* 26 (June 2003): 60–66.

Brown, C. K., and J. M. Kirkwood. "Medical Management of Melanoma." *Surgical Clinics of North America* 83 (April 2003): 283–322.

F'guyer, S., F. Afaq, and H. Mukhtar. "Photochemoprevention of Skin Cancer by Botanical Agents." *Photodermatology, Photoimmunology and Photomedicine* 19 (April 2003): 56–72.

Jellouli-Elloumi, A., L. Kochbati, S. Dhraief, et al. "Cancers Arising from Burn Scars: 62 Cases." [in French] *Annales de dermatologie et de venereologie* 130 (April 2003): 413–416.

Lin, J. Y., M. A. Selim, C. R. Shea, et al. "UV Photoprotection by Combination Topical Antioxidants Vitamin C and Vitamin E." *Journal of the American Academy of Dermatology* 48 (June 2003): 866-874.

ORGANIZATIONS

American Academy of Dermatology. 930 N. Meacham Road, Schaumburg, IL 60173. (847) 330–0230 or (888) 462–DERM (227–3376).

American Cancer Society. 1599 Clifton Road NE, Atlanta, GA 30329. (800) ACS-2345.

Centers for Disease Control and Prevention (CDC) Cancer Prevention and Control Program. 4770 Buford Highway, NE, MS K64, Atlanta, GA 30341. (888) 842-6355. <http://www.cdc.gov/cancer/comments.htm>.

National Cancer Institute (NCI). NCI Public Inquiries Office, Suite 3036A, 6116 Executive Boulevard, MSC8332, Bethesda, MD 20892-8322. (800) 4-CANCER or (800) 332-8615 (TTY). <http://www.nci.nih.gov>.

Kathleen Wright
Rebecca J. Frey, PhD

Skullcap

Description

Skullcap is a name that refers to any of the dozens of species (*Scutellaria*) of the mint family Lamiaceae. The plant's name refers to the helmet-shaped calyx on the outer whorl of the plant's tiny flowers. The flowers range in color from blue to pink. In herbal medicine, the name skullcap refers to *Scutellaria lateriflora*, a perennial herb native to North America and cultivated in Europe. The leaves, flowers, and stems are used as herbal remedies. Skullcap is also known as scullcap, American skullcap, Western skullcap, European skullcap, blue skullcap, greater skullcap, hoodwort or hoodwart, blue pimpernel, Quaker bonnet, helmet flower, hooded willow herb, side-flowering skullcap, mad-dog weed, and mad weed.

Chinese skullcap (*Scutellaria baicalensis*) is a related species. The species *Scutellaria baicalensis Georgi* is native to eastern Asia, and the skinless yellow root of this plant is used in **traditional Chinese medicine** (TCM). Its Chinese name is *huang qin*. Chinese skullcap is sometimes called baikal, baical skullcap root, scute, and scutellaria. Another species used in Chinese medicine is *Scutellaria barbata* , whose Chinese name is *ban zhi lian*.

General use

Skullcap was once called mad-dog weed because of its use during the eighteenth century to treat **rabies**. In addition, Native Americans used skullcap as a sedative, tranquilizer, and a digestive aid. Other cultures have used it as a sedative and to lower fevers.

In contemporary practice, both common skullcap and Chinese skullcap are used as remedies for **anxiety**, nervous tension, premenstrual syndrome (PMS), **insomnia, stress** headaches, muscle spasms, seizures, and **epilepsy**. In addition, each herb is used for a variety of other conditions, and even in these conditions they are used differently.

Skullcap

Skullcap (*Scutellaria lateriflora*) is currently known best as a herbal sedative. By reducing tension, skullcap may contribute to lower blood pressure. Skullcap is also used as a remedy for exhaustion, convulsions, menstrual cramps, and as a treatment for withdrawal from alcohol and tobacco. The herb may be taken as a bitter tonic to boost digestion. Skullcap is also sometimes used as a remedy for **hiccups**, hangovers, and **asthma**.

Chinese skullcap

In traditional Chinese medicine, baical skullcap (*Scutellaria baicalensis*) is prescribed for irritability, dysentery, **diarrhea**, **infections** accompanied by **fever**, **hay fever**, urinary tract infections, **gout**, **jaundice**, potential miscarriages, nosebleed, abdominal **pain**, and redness in the eyes or face. The herb is used for **hepatitis** and has been said to improve liver function. The root of baical skullcap is also given in formulas together with other herbs for vaginal bleeding, blood in the stool, and coughing or **vomiting** blood. Chinese skullcap is frequently among the ingredients in herbal compounds used for disorders involving high **cholesterol** and triglycerides levels, high blood pressure, allergic diseases, and inflammatory skin conditions.

As of the late 1990s, research in countries including China indicated that Chinese skullcap showed "promise" in treating **allergies**, **cancer**, and as an aspirin-like anti-inflammatory remedy. Research at that time also indicated that the herb might be used in the future to prevent strokes and **heart disease** . A team of researchers in Hong Kong reported in 2002 that baicalein, a flavonoid derived from skullcap, appears to have chemoprotective effects against cancer.

Another recent discovery is that a group of flavones in skullcap appear to protect nerve cells against the damage caused by oxidation. This finding may have potential applications in treating **Alzheimer's disease**.

Preparations

Skullcap (*scutellaria lateriflora*) and Chinese skullcap (*scutellaria baicalensis*) are both taken internally. Skullcap is generally sold commercially as a liquid extract, as a tea, in dried form, and in capsules. The leaves and flowers are used as remedies for such conditions as insomnia. In the United States, "blue skullcap" refers to scutellaria that is frequently harvested without determining the species, according to *Tyler's Honest Herbal* . Tyler, a respected pharmacognosist, wrote that "pink

scullcap" is an adulterant with pink flowers. It costs the manufacturer less than blue skullcap.

Chinese skullcap root is sold usually in bulk or capsule form, the capsules usually containing other herbs. Both Chinese skullcap and common skullcap have a bitter taste, and there are customary dosages for both herbs.

Skullcap dosages

Skullcap tea can be purchased commercially or brewed at home for conditions including anxiety, tension, and PMS. Skullcap preparations include:

• A tea prepared by pouring 1 cup (250 ml) of boiling water over 1–2 tsp. (5–10 g) of dried leaves. The mixture is covered and steeped for 10–15 minutes. From two to three cups of tea may be consumed daily.

• A liquid tincture that can be taken three times daily. The tincture, 1/2–1 tsp (2–4 ml) of solution, is added to an 8 oz (250 ml) glass of warm water. Skullcap tincture can be purchased over the counter, or made at home by mixing the herb with water or alcohol in a ratio of 1:5 or 1:10.

• To ease insomnia, skullcap leaves can be placed inside a dream pillow. Also known as a sleep pillow, it can be made by sewing together two 8-in (20.3-cm) pieces of fabric. The dream pillow is placed under the bed pillow.

Chinese skullcap dosages

Chinese skullcap tea is prepared by adding 1–3 tsp (5–15 g) of the powdered root to 1 cup (250 ml) of boiling water. The mixture is covered and steeped for 10–20 minutes. From three to four cups may be consumed daily.

Baikal skullcap is also available in capsule form. Three capsules of the standard dosage may be taken for treatment of liver ailments and chronic inflammatory conditions.

The root of Chinese skullcap is usually decocted, but it may be fried dry and consumed for conditions such as **diarrhea** and urinary tract infections. The root can be cooked in wine to treat upper respiratory infections and redness in the face and eyes. A practitioner of traditional Chinese medicine can provide information about specific dosages.

Skullcap combinations

Skullcap may be combined with other herbs such as oats or **St. John's wort**. It works well in combination with such sedative herbs as **valerian**, **passionflower** , and **black cohosh**. Skullcap is included among the herbal ingredients in a tincture that people take to quit **smoking**. Other herbs in this tincture include **mullein**, St. John's wort, and **licorice**.

Precautions

Before beginning herbal treatment, people should consult a physician, practitioner of TCM, or herbalist. This precaution is especially important when taking skullcap or Chinese skullcap because there is disagreement among health care professionals about whether these herbs are safe to use. Advocates of both remedies state that research conducted in China and Russia proves that skullcap is safe and effective. Although the United States Food and Drug Administration does not subject herbal preparations (which are regarded as dietary supplements) to the same types of regulatory procedures as prescription drugs, it does monitor reports of adverse interactions to herbal products. Between 1996, when the FDA's MedWatch program began, and January 2003, there have been no reports or alerts for American consumers regarding products containing skullcap. There have, however, been reports of liver toxicity from products containing skullcap in the Netherlands and Norway in the early 1990s. Until more is known, some experts advise that skullcap should be avoided on the grounds that it can cause liver damage.

That is also the position of **Hepatitis** Foundation International, which rates skullcap as toxic to the liver. That position that had not changed by May of 2000. It is also possible, however, that skullcap may have been mistakenly identified as dangerous. Tyler was among the herbal experts who pointed out that germander, a herb that causes liver damage, was found in the skullcap products taken by people who experienced liver damage. In addition, some supporters of skullcap maintain that prejudice against the herb stems from its previous use as a rabies treatment.

Skullcap is safe for adults when taken in proper dosages.

Skullcap advocates state that the herb can be used safely for relieving conditions such as PMS. Some experts, however, recommend medical supervision when taking skullcap for medicinal purposes. That precaution is particularly important for pregnant women and those who are lactating. Skullcap may cause drowsiness, so the person taking it should not drive or operate heavy equipment.

Chinese skullcap should not be taken when a person has diarrhea or a deficiency of heat in the lungs.

Side effects

Possible side effects include diarrhea, an upset stomach, and drowsiness. If the first two conditions occur, the person should reduce the dosage of skullcap or stop taking it. In addition, large amounts of the tincture may cause giddiness, twitching, confusion, erratic pulse, and seizures.

Interactions

In traditional Chinese medicine, Chinese skullcap is said to offset the effects of some Chinese remedies. For this reason, it is important that persons using Chinese skullcap consult a traditional practitioner, as Chinese skullcap is usually given in combinations of herbs that are specific to each symptom.

With regard to standard prescription medications, people who are taking antihistamines, barbiturates, benzodiazepines, or sedative medications should not use skullcap because it will intensify their effects on the central nervous system, particularly drowsiness.

People who are taking skullcap should discontinue its use two weeks before any surgical procedure requiring general anesthesia, as skullcap interacts with anesthetics to lower blood pressure. For the same reason, skullcap should not be used by persons who are taking drugs to control high blood pressure (antihypertensives).

Skullcap also interferes with the body's absorption of **iron** and other minerals; persons who are taking mineral supplements should therefore use skullcap with caution.

Resources

BOOKS

Duke, James A. *The Green Pharmacy.* Emmaus, PA: Rodale Press, Inc., 1997.

Keville, Kathi. *Herbs for Health and Healing.* Emmaus, PA: Rodale Press, Inc., 1996

L'Orange, Darlena. *Herbal Healing Secrets of the Orient.* Paramus, NJ: Prentice Hall, 1998.

PDR for Herbal Medicines. Montvale, NJ: Medical Economics Company, 1998.

Reid, Daniel. *Chinese Herbal Medicine.* Boston: Shambhala, 1996.

Squier, Thomas Broken Bear, with Lauren David Peden. *Herbal Folk Medicine.* New York: Henry Holt and Company, 1997.

Tyler, Varro and Steven Foster. *Tyler's Honest Herbal.* Binghamton, NY: The Haworth Herbal Press, 1999.

PERIODICALS

Chan, H. Y., Z. Y. Chen, D. S. Tsang, and L. K. Leung. "Baicalein Inhibits DMBA-DNA Adduct Formation by Modulating CYP1A1 and CYP1B1 Activities." *Biomedicine and Pharmacotherapy* 56 (August 2002): 269-275.

Choi, J., C. C. Conrad, C. A. Malakowsky, et al. "Flavones from *Scutellaria baicalensis Georgi* Attenuate Apoptosis and Protein Oxidation in Neuronal Cell Lines." *Biochimica et Biophysica Acta* 1571 (July 3, 2002): 201-210.

Xie, L. H., X. Wang, P. Basnet, et al. "Evaluation of Variation of Acteoside and Three Major Flavonoids in Wild and

KEY TERMS

Adulterant—A substance that makes something impure or inferior.

Baicalein—A compound found in skullcap that appears to be a cancer chemopreventive.

Barbiturate—Any of an older group of sedatives derived from barbituric acid. Barbiturates were frequently prescribed in the 1950s and 1960s as sleeping pills.

Benzodiazepine—Any of a group of minor tranquilizers given to relieve anxiety; they produce sedation and muscle relaxation.

Decoction—A method for releasing the herbal essence of bark or roots by boiling or simmering them in a non-aluminum pan.

Flavone—A colorless crystalline compound found in skullcap and other plants that is the parent substance of a group of yellow plant pigments.

Germander—A plant, *Teucrium chamaedrys*, that belongs to the mint family and may have been used to adulterate skullcap products reported to cause liver damage.

Infusion—A method for releasing the herbal essence of herbal leaves and flowers by pouring boiling water over the plant matter and allowing it to steep.

Pharmacognosist—A person involved in pharmacognosy, the science concerned with the medical products of plants in their natural state.

Sedative—A preparation or medication given to calm or soothe.

Tincture—A method of preserving herbs in a solution of alcohol or water.

Cultivated *Scutellaria baicalensis* Roots by Micellar Electrokinetic Chromatography." *Chemical and Pharmaceutical Bulletin (Tokyo)* 50 (July 2002): 896-899.

ORGANIZATIONS

American Botanical Council. P.O. Box 201660. Austin TX, 78720.(512) 331-8868.

Herb Research Foundation. 1007 Pearl St., Suite 200. Boulder, CO 80302. (303) 449-2265. <www.herbs.org>.

Liz Swain
Rebecca J. Frey, PhD

Sleep disorders *see* **Insomnia; Narcolepsy**

Sleep apnea

Definition

Sleep apnea is a condition in which breathing stops for more than ten seconds during sleep. Sleep apnea is a major, though often unrecognized, cause of daytime sleepiness. It can have serious negative effects on a person's quality of life, and is thought to be considerably underdiagnosed in the United States.

Description

A sleeping person normally breathes continuously and without interruption throughout the night. A person with sleep apnea, however, has frequent episodes (up to 400-500 per night) in which he or she stops breathing. This interruption of breathing is called "apnea." Breathing usually stops for about 30 seconds; then the person usually startles awake with a loud snort and begins to breathe again, gradually falling back to sleep.

There are two forms of sleep apnea. In *obstructive sleep apnea* (OSA), breathing stops because tissue in the throat closes off the airway. In *central sleep apnea*, (CSA), the brain centers responsible for breathing fail to send messages to the breathing muscles. OSA is much more common than CSA. It is thought that about 1–10% of adults are affected by OSA; only about one tenth of that number have CSA. OSA can affect people of any age and of either sex, but it is most common in middle-aged, somewhat overweight men, especially those who use alcohol.

Causes & symptoms

Obstructive sleep apnea

Obstructive sleep apnea occurs when part of the airway is closed off (usually at the back of the throat) while a person is trying to inhale during sleep. People whose airways are slightly narrower than average are more likely to be affected by OSA. Obesity, especially obesity in the neck, can increase the risk of developing OSA, because the fat tissue tends to narrow the airway. In some people, the airway is blocked by enlarged tonsils, an enlarged tongue, jaw deformities, or growths in the neck that compress the airway. Blocked nasal passages may also play a part in some people's apnea.

When a person begins to inhale, expansion of the lungs lowers the air pressure inside the airway. If the muscles that keep the airway open are not working hard enough, the airway narrows and may collapse, shutting off the supply of air to the lungs. OSA occurs during sleep because the neck muscles that keep the airway

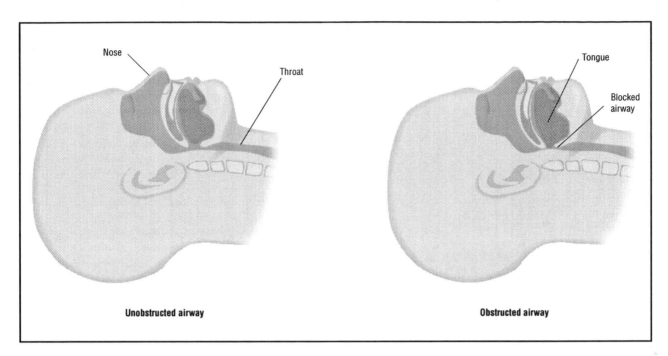

Nose

Throat

Tongue

Blocked airway

Unobstructed airway

Obstructed airway

Sleep apnea is caused when the airway of the sleeping person becomes obstructed. (Illustration by GGS Information Services, Inc. The Gale Group.)

open are not as active then. Congestion in the nose can make collapse more likely, since the extra effort needed to inhale will lower the pressure in the airway even more. Drinking alcohol or taking tranquilizers in the evening worsens this situation, because these substances cause the neck muscles to relax. These drugs also lower the "respiratory drive" in the nervous system, reducing breathing rate and strength.

People with OSA almost always snore heavily, because the same narrowing of the airway that causes **snoring** can also cause OSA. Snoring may actually help cause OSA as well, because the vibration of the throat tissues can cause them to swell. However, most people who snore do not go on to develop OSA.

Other risk factors for developing OSA include male sex; **pregnancy**; a family history of the disorder; and **smoking**. With regard to gender, it has been found that male sex hormones sometimes cause changes in the size or structure of the upper airway. The weight gain that accompanies pregnancy can affect a woman's breathing patterns during sleep, particularly during the third trimester. With regard to family history, OSA is known to run in families even though no gene or genes associated with the disorder have been identified as of 2002. Smoking increases the risk of developing OSA because it causes inflammation, swelling, and narrowing of the upper airway.

Some patients being treated for head and neck **cancer** develop OSA as a result of physical changes in the muscles and other tissues of the neck and throat. Doctors

recommend prompt treatment of the OSA to improve the patient's quality of life.

Central sleep apnea

In central sleep apnea, the airway remains open, but the nerve signals controlling the respiratory muscles are not regulated properly. This loss of regulation can cause wide fluctuations in the level of carbon dioxide (CO_2) in the blood. Normal activity in the body produces CO_2, which is brought by the blood to the lungs for exhalation. When the blood level of CO_2 rises, brain centers respond by increasing the rate of respiration, clearing the CO_2. As blood levels fall again, respiration slows down. Normally, this interaction of CO_2 and breathing rate maintains the CO_2 level within very narrow limits. CSA can occur when the regulation system becomes insensitive to CO_2 levels, allowing wide fluctuations in both CO_2 levels and breathing rates. High CO_2 levels cause very rapid breathing (hyperventilation), which then lowers CO_2 so much that breathing becomes very slow or even stops. CSA occurs during sleep because when a person is awake, breathing is usually stimulated by other signals, including conscious awareness of breathing rate.

A combination of the two forms is also possible, and is called "mixed sleep apnea." Mixed sleep apnea episodes usually begin with a reduced central respiratory drive, followed by obstruction.

OSA and CSA cause similar symptoms. The most common symptoms are:

- daytime sleepiness

- morning headaches

- a feeling that sleep is not restful

- disorientation upon waking

- memory loss and difficulty paying attention

- poor judgment

- personality changes

Sleepiness is caused not only by the frequent interruption of sleep, but by the inability to enter long periods of deep sleep, during which the body performs numerous restorative functions. OSA is one of the leading causes of daytime sleepiness, and is a major risk factor for motor vehicle accidents. Headaches and disorientation are caused by low oxygen levels during sleep, from the lack of regular breathing.

Other symptoms of sleep apnea may include **sexual dysfunction**, loss of concentration, **memory loss**, intellectual impairment, and behavioral changes including **anxiety** and **depression**.

Sleep apnea is also associated with night sweats and nocturia, or increased frequency of urination at night. **Bedwetting** in children is also linked to sleep apnea.

Sleep apnea can also cause serious changes in the cardiovascular system. Daytime **hypertension** (high blood pressure) is common. An increase in the number of red blood cells (polycythemia) is possible, as is an enlarged left ventricle of the heart (cor pulmonale), and left ventricular failure. In some people, sleep apnea causes life-threatening changes in the rhythm of the heart, including heartbeat slowing (bradycardia), racing (tachycardia), and other types of arrhythmias. Sudden death may occur from such arrhythmias. Patients with the Pickwickian syndrome (named after a Charles Dickens character) are obese and sleepy, with right heart failure, pulmonary hypertension, and chronic daytime low blood oxygen (hypoxemia) and increased blood CO_2 (hypercapnia).

Diagnosis

Excessive daytime sleepiness is the complaint that usually brings a person to see the doctor. A careful medical history will include questions about alcohol, tobacco, or tranquilizer use; family history; snoring (often reported by the person's partner); and morning headaches or disorientation. A physical examination will include examination of the mouth, nose and throat to look for narrowing or obstruction, or unusual size or shape of the tonsils or adenoids. Blood pressure is also measured. Measuring heart rate or blood levels of oxygen and CO_2 during the daytime will not usually be done, since these are abnormal only at night in most patients.

In some cases the person's dentist may suggest the diagnosis of OSA on the basis of a dental checkup or evaluation of the patient for oral surgery.

Confirmation of the diagnosis usually requires making measurements while the person sleeps. These tests are called a polysomnography study, and are conducted during an overnight stay in a specialized sleep laboratory. Important parts of the polysomnography study include measurements of:

- heart rate

- airflow at the mouth and nose

- respiratory effort

- sleep stage (light sleep, deep sleep, dream sleep, etc.)

- oxygen level in the blood, using a noninvasive probe (ear oximetry)

Simplified studies done overnight at home are also possible, and may be appropriate for people whose profile strongly suggests the presence of obstructive sleep apnea; that is, middle-aged, somewhat overweight men, who snore and have high blood pressure. The home-based study usually includes ear oximetry and cardiac measurements. If these measurements support the diagnosis of OSA, initial treatment is usually suggested without polysomnography. Home-based measurements are not used to rule out OSA, however, and if the measurements do not support the OSA diagnosis, polysomnography may be needed to define the problem further.

Treatment

Treatment of obstructive sleep apnea begins with reducing the use of alcohol or tranquilizers in the evening, if these have been contributing to the problem. Quitting smoking is recommended for a number of health concerns in addition to OSA. Weight loss is also effective, but if the weight returns, as it often does, so does the apnea. Changing sleeping position may be effective. Snoring and sleep apnea are both most common when a person sleeps on his back. Turning to sleep on the side may be enough to clear up the symptoms. Raising the head of the bed may also help.

There are few reports of OSA being treated by alternative and complementary approaches. In 2002, however, some Japanese researchers reported on the case of a 44-year-old male who was successfully treated for OSA by taking a Kampo extract, or traditional Japanese herbal formulation.

Allopathic treatment

Opening of the nasal passages can provide some relief for sleep apnea sufferers. There are a variety of nasal devices such as clips, tapes, or holders which may help, though discomfort may limit their use. Nasal decongestants may be useful, but should not be taken for sleep apnea without the consent of the treating physician. Supplemental nighttime oxygen can be useful for some people with either central and obstructive sleep apnea. Tricyclic antidepressant drugs such as protriptyline (Vivactil) may help by increasing the muscle tone of the upper airway muscles, but their side effects may severely limit their usefulness.

For moderate to severe sleep apnea, the most successful treatment is nighttime use of a ventilator, called a CPAP machine. CPAP (continuous positive airway pressure) blows air into the airway continuously, preventing its collapse. CPAP requires the use of a nasal mask. The appropriate pressure setting for the CPAP machine is determined by polysomnography in the sleep lab. Its effects are dramatic; daytime sleepiness usually disappears within one to two days after treatment begins. CPAP is used to treat both obstructive and central sleep apnea.

CPAP is tolerated well by about two-thirds of patients who try it. Bilevel positive airway pressure (BiPAP), is an alternative form of ventilation. With BiPAP, the ventilator reduces the air pressure when the person exhales. This form of treatment is more comfortable for some.

Another approach to treating OSA involves the use of oral appliances intended to improve breathing either by holding the tongue in place or by pushing the lower jaw forward during sleep to increase the air volume in the upper airway. The first type of oral appliance is known as a tongue retaining device or TRD. The second type is variously called an oral protrusive device (OPD) or mandibular advancement splint (MAS), because it holds the mandible, or lower jaw, forward during sleep. These oral devices appear to work best for patients with mild-to-moderate OSA, and in some cases can postpone or prevent the need for surgery. Their rate of patient compliance is about 50%; most patients who stop using oral appliances do so because their teeth are in poor condition. TRDs and OPDs can be fitted by dentists; however, most dentists work together with the patient's physician following a polysomnogram rather than prescribing the device by themselves.

Surgery can be used to correct obstructions in the airway. The most common surgery is called UPPP, for uvulopalatopharyngoplasty. This surgery removes tissue from the rear of the mouth and top of the throat. The tissues removed include parts of the uvula (the flap of tissue that hangs down at the back of the mouth), the soft palate, and the pharynx. Tonsils and adenoids are usually removed as well. This operation significantly improves sleep apnea in slightly more than half of all cases. More recently, oral surgeons have been performing region-spe-

cific surgery for OSA, which grew out of the recognition that obstructions may exist in more than one level of the patient's upper airway. Region-specific surgery has a cure rate of over 90%, though it may involve more than one surgical operation.

A modified tracheotomy may also be performed to treat OSA. This procedure involves the surgical placement of a tiny breathing tube that fits in a 2 mm incision in the throat.

Reconstructive surgery is possible for those whose OSA is due to constriction of the airway by lower jaw deformities. Genioplasty, which is a procedure that plastic surgeons usually perform to reshape a patient's chin to improve his or her appearance, is now being done to reshape the upper airway in patients with OSA.

Expected results

Appropriate treatment enables most people with sleep apnea to be treated successfully, although it may take some time to determine the most effective and least intrusive treatment. In many cases consultation and cooperation between the person's physician and dentist help in finding the best treatment option. Polysomnography testing is usually required after beginning a treatment to determine how effective it has been.

Prevention

For people who snore frequently, weight control, smoking cessation, avoidance of evening alcohol or tranquilizers, and adjustment of sleeping position may help reduce the risk of developing obstructive sleep apnea.

Resources

BOOKS

"Disorders of the Oral Region." Section 9, Chapter 105 in *The Merck Manual of Diagnosis and Therapy*, edited by Mark H. Beers, MD, and Robert Berkow, MD. Whitehouse Station, NJ: Merck Research Laboratories, 1999.

Pascualay, Ralph, and Sally Warren Soest. *Snoring and Sleep Apnea,* 2nd ed. New York, NY: Demos Vermande, 1996.

"Sleep Disorders." Section 14, Chapter 173 in *The Merck Manual of Diagnosis and Therapy*, edited by Mark H. Beers, MD, and Robert Berkow, MD. Whitehouse Station, NJ: Merck Research Laboratories, 1999.

PERIODICALS

Chasens, E. R., and M. G. Umlauf. "Nocturia: A Problem That Disrupts Sleep and Predicts Obstructive Sleep Apnea" *Geriatric Nursing* 24 (March-April 2003): 76–81, 105.

Chung, S. A., S. Jairam, M. R. Hussain, and C. M. Shapiro. "How, What, and Why of Sleep Apnea. Perspectives for Primary Care Physicians." *Canadian Family Physician* 48 (June 2002): 1073–1080.

Edwards, N., P. G. Middleton, D. M. Blyton, and C. E. Sullivan. "Sleep Disordered Breathing and Pregnancy." *Thorax* 57 (June 2002): 555–558.

Hisanaga, A., T. Itoh, Y. Hasegawa, et al. "A Case of Sleep Choking Syndrome Improved by the Kampo Extract of Hange-Koboku-To." *Psychiatry and Clinical Neuroscience* 56 (June 2002): 325–327.

Kapur, V., K. P. Strohl, S. Redline, et al. "Underdiagnosis of Sleep Apnea Syndrome in U.S. Communities." *Sleep and Breathing* 6 (June 2002): 49–54.

Koliha, C. A. "Obstructive Sleep Apnea in Head and Neck Cancer Patients Post Treatment .. Something to Consider?" *ORL—Head and Neck Nursing* 21 (Winter 2003): 10–14.

Neill, A., R. Whyman, S. Bannan, et al. "Mandibular Advancement Splint Improves Indices of Obstructive Sleep Apnoea and Snoring but Side Effects Are Common." *New Zealand Medical Journal* 115 (June 21, 2002): 289–292.

Rose, E., R. Staats, J. Schulte-Monting, et al. "Long-Term Compliance with an Oral Protrusive Appliance in Patients with Obstructive Sleep Apnoea." [in German] *Deutsche medizinische Wochenschrift* 127 (June 7, 2002): 1245–1249.

Shiomi, T., A. T. Arita, R. Sasanabe, et al. "Falling Asleep While Driving and Automobile Accidents Among Patients with Obstructive Sleep Apnea-Hypopnea Syndrome." *Psychiatry and Clinical Neuroscience* 56 (June 2002): 333–334.

Stanton, D. C. "Genioplasty." *Facial Plastic Surgery* 19 (February 2003): 75–86.

Umlauf, M. G., and E. R. Chasens. "Bedwetting—Not Always What It Seems: A Sign of Sleep-Disordered Breathing in Children." *Journal for Specialists in Pediatric Nursing* 8 (January-March 2003): 22–30.

Veale, D., G. Poussin, F. Benes, et al. "Identification of Quality of Life Concerns of Patients with Obstructive Sleep Apnoea at the Time of Initiation of Continuous Positive Airway Pressure: A Discourse Analysis." *Quality of Life Research* 11 (June 2002): 389–399.

Viera, A. J., M. M. Bond, and S. J. Yates. "Diagnosing Night Sweats." *American Family Physician* 67 (March 1, 2003): 1019–1024.

ORGANIZATIONS

American Academy of Otolaryngology, Head and Neck Surgery, Inc. One Prince Street, Alexandria, VA 22314-3357. (703) 836-4444. <http://www.entnet.org>.

American Dental Association. 211 East Chicago Avenue, Chicago, IL 60611. (312) 440-2500. <www.ada.org>.

American Sleep Apnea Association. 1424 K Street NW, Suite 302, Washington, DC 20005. (202) 293-3650. Fax: (202) 293-3656. <www.sleepapnea.org>.

Canadian Coordinating Office for Health Technology Assessment. <www.ccohta.ca/pubs/english/sleep/treatmnt>.

National Sleep Foundation. 1522 K Street, NW, Suite 500, Washington, DC 20005. <www.sleepfoundation.org>.

OTHER

American Sleep Apnea Association (ASAA). *Considering Surgery for Snoring?* <http://www.sleepapnea.org/snoring. html>.

National Heart, Lung, and Blood Institute (NHLBI). *Facts About Sleep Apnea* . NIH Publication No. 95-3798. <http://www.nhlbi.nih.gov/health/public/sleep/sleepapn.htm>.

Paula Ford-Martin
Rebecca J. Frey, PhD

KEY TERMS

Continuous positive airway pressure (CPAP)—A ventilation system that blows a gentle stream of air into the nose to keep the airway open.

Genioplasty—An operation performed to reshape the chin. Genioplasties are often done to treat OSA because the procedure changes the structure of the patient's upper airway.

Mandible—The medical term for the lower jaw. One type of oral appliance used to treat OSA pushes the mandible forward in order to ease breathing during sleep.

Nocturia—Excessive need to urinate at night. Nocturia is a symptom of OSA and often increases the patient's daytime sleepiness.

Polysomnography—A group of tests administered to analyze heart, blood, and breathing patterns during sleep.

Tracheotomy—A surgical procedure in which a small hole is cut into the trachea, or windpipe, below the level of the vocal cords.

Uvulopalatopharyngoplasty (UPPP)—An operation to remove excess tissue at the back of the throat to prevent it from closing off the airway during sleep.

Sleep disorders

Definition

Sleep disorders are a group of syndromes characterized by disturbances in the amount, quality, or timing of sleep, or in behaviors or physiological conditions associated with sleep.

Description

Although sleep is a basic behavior in all animals, its functions in maintaining health are not completely understood. In the past 30 years, however, researchers have learned about the cyclical patterns of different types of sleep and their relationships to breathing, heart rate, brain waves, and other physical functions.

There are five stages of human sleep. Four stages are characterized by non-rapid eye movement (NREM) sleep, with unique brain wave patterns and physical changes. Dreaming occurs in the fifth stage during rapid eye movement (REM) sleep.

• Stage 1 NREM sleep. This stage occurs while a person is falling asleep and represents about 5% of a normal adult's sleep time.

• Stage 2 NREM sleep. This stage marks the beginning of "true" sleep. About 50% of sleep time is stage 2 REM sleep.

• Stages 3 and 4 NREM sleep. Also called delta or slow wave sleep, these are the deepest levels of human sleep and represent 10–20% of sleep time. They usually occur during the first 30–50% of the sleeping period.

• REM sleep. REM sleep accounts for 20–25% of total sleep time. It usually begins about 90 minutes after the person falls asleep, an important measure called REM latency. REM sleep alternates with NREM sleep about every hour and a half throughout the night. REM periods increase in length over the course of the night.

The average length of nighttime sleep varies among people. Most adults sleep between seven and nine hours a night.

Sleep disorders are classified according to their causes. Primary sleep disorders are distinguished as those that are not caused by other mental disorders, prescription medications, substance abuse, or medical conditions. The two major categories of primary sleep disorders are the dyssomnias and the parasomnias.

Dyssomnias

Dyssomnias are primary sleep disorders in which the patient suffers from changes in the amount, restfulness, and timing of sleep. The most important dyssomnia is primary insomnia, which is defined as difficulty in falling asleep or remaining asleep that lasts for at least one month. It is estimated that 35% of adults in the United States experience insomnia during any given year. Primary insomnia usually begins during young adulthood or middle age.

Hypersomnia is a condition marked by excessive sleepiness during normal waking hours. The patient has either lengthy episodes of daytime sleep or episodes of daytime sleep on a daily basis even though he or she is sleeping normally at night. The number of people with primary hypersomnia is unknown, although 5–10% of patients in sleep disorder clinics have the disorder. Pri-

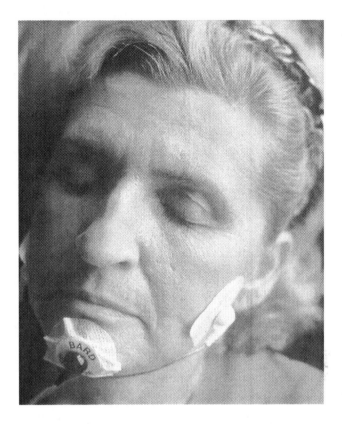

This woman with insomnia is receiving biofeedback to learn self-relaxation techniques. *(Peter Berndt, Custom Medical Stock Photo. Reproduced by permission.)*

mary hypersomnia usually affects young adults between the ages of 15 and 30.

Nocturnal myoclonus and restless legs syndrome (RLS) can cause either insomnia or hypersomnia in adults. Patients with nocturnal myoclonus, sometimes called periodic limb movement disorder (PLMD), awaken because of cramps or twitches in the calves and feel sleepy the next day. RLS patients have a crawly or aching feeling in their calves that can be relieved by moving or rubbing the legs. RLS often prevents the patient from falling asleep until the early hours of the morning.

Narcolepsy is a dyssomnia characterized by recurrent "sleep attacks" (abrupt loss of consciousness) lasting 10–20 minutes. The patient feels refreshed by the sleep, but typically feels sleepy again several hours later. Narcolepsy has three major symptoms in addition to sleep attacks: cataplexy (sudden loss of muscle tone and stability), hallucinations, and sleep paralysis. About 40% of patients with narcolepsy have or have had another mental disorder. Although narcolepsy is considered an adult disorder, it has been reported in children as young as three years old. Almost 18% of patients with narcolepsy are 10 years old or younger. It is estimated that 0.02–0.16% of the general population suffers from narcolepsy.

Breathing-related sleep disorders are syndromes in which the patient's sleep is interrupted by problems with his or her breathing. There are three types of breathing-related sleep disorders:

- Obstructive **sleep apnea** syndrome is the most common form, marked by episodes of blockage in the upper airway during sleep. It is found primarily in obese people. Patients with this disorder typically alternate between periods of **snoring** or gasping (when their airway is partly open) and periods of silence (when their airway is blocked). Very loud snoring is characteristic of this disorder.

- Central sleep apnea syndrome is primarily found in elderly patients with heart or neurological conditions that affect their ability to breathe properly.

- Central alveolar hyperventilation syndrome is found most often in extremely obese people. The patient's airway is not blocked, but his or her blood oxygen level is too low.

- Mixed-type sleep apnea syndrome combines symptoms of both obstructive and central sleep apnea.

Circadian rhythm sleep disorders are dyssomnias resulting from a discrepancy between the person's daily sleep/wake patterns and the demands of social activities, shift work, or travel. There are three circadian rhythm sleep disorders: delayed sleep phase (going to bed and arising later than most people); **jet lag** (traveling to a new time zone); and shift work.

Parasomnias

Parasomnias are primary sleep disorders in which the patient's behavior is affected by specific sleep stages or transitions between sleeping and waking.

Nightmare disorder is a parasomnia in which the patient is repeatedly awakened by frightening dreams. Approximately 10–50% of children between three and five years old have nightmares. They occur during REM sleep, usually in the second half of the night.

Sleep terror disorder is a parasomnia in which the patient awakens screaming or crying. Unlike nightmares, sleep terrors typically occur in stage 3 or stage 4 NREM sleep during the first third of the night. The patient may be confused or disoriented for several minutes and may not remember the episode the next morning. Sleep terror disorder is most common in children 4–12 years old. It affects about 3% of children and fewer than 1% of adults.

Sleepwalking disorder (somnambulism) occurs when the patient is capable of complex movements during sleep, including walking. Sleepwalking occurs during stage 3 and stage 4 NREM sleep during the first part of the night. In addition to walking around, patients with sleepwalking disorder have been reported to eat, use the bathroom, unlock doors, or talk to others. It is estimated that 10–30% of children have at least one episode of sleepwalking. However, only 1–5% meet the criteria for sleepwalking disorder. The disorder is most common in children 8–12 years old.

Sleep disorders related to other conditions

Substances, living situations, and physical or mental disorders that can cause sleep disorders include:

- Mental disorders, especially **depression** or one of the **anxiety** disorders, can cause sleep disturbances. Psychiatric disorders are the most common cause of chronic insomnia.

- Medical conditions like **Parkinson's disease**, Huntington's disease, viral encephalitis, brain disease, and thyroid disease may cause sleep disorders.

- Such substances as drugs, alcohol, and **caffeine** frequently produce disturbances in sleep patterns.

- Emotional **stress** and hormone imbalances can also cause sleep problems.

- Job-related stress is a common factor in sleep disorders. Police officers, firefighters, and other emergency workers have a higher-than-average rate of sleep disorders.

- Sleeping arrangements can be a factor. People who must share a bedroom with someone who snores heavily sometimes develop sleep disorders. In addition, research has shown that co-sleeping (small children sleeping in the same bed as their parents) is stressful for the children and contributes to sleep disorders.

- Such prescription medications as antihistamines, corticosteroids, **asthma** medicines, and drugs that affect the central nervous system can affect sleep patterns.

Causes & symptoms

The causes of sleep disorders have already been discussed with respect to the *Diagnostic and Statistical Manual of Mental Disorders (DSM-IV)* classification of these disorders.

The most important symptoms of sleep disorders are insomnia and sleepiness during waking hours. Insomnia is the more common of the two symptoms and encompasses the inability to fall asleep at bedtime, repeated awakening during the night, and/or inability to go back to sleep once awakened.

Sleep disorders can have a number of negative health consequences in addition to general feelings of tiredness. Studies have shown that people with sleep disorders are at increased risk of having serious motor vehicle accidents and fatal workplace accidents.

Diagnosis

Diagnosis of sleep disorders usually requires a psychological history as well as a medical history. With the exception of sleep apnea syndromes, physical examinations are not usually revealing. The doctor may also talk to other family members in order to obtain information about the patient's symptoms. Psychological tests or inventories are used because insomnia is frequently associated with mood or affective disorders.

Patients may be asked to keep a sleep diary for one to two weeks to evaluate the sleep disturbance. Medications taken, the length of time spent in bed, and the quality of sleep are recorded.

If breathing-related sleep disorders, myoclonus, or narcolepsy are suspected, the patient may be tested in a sleep laboratory or at home with portable instruments. Polysomnography records physiological functions that can be used to help diagnose sleep disorders as well as conduct research into sleep.

Treatment

General recommendations

General recommendations for getting more restful sleep include:

- Waiting until one feels sleepy before going to bed.

- Not using the bedroom for work, reading, or watching television.

- Arising at the same time every morning.

- Avoiding **smoking** and drinking caffeinated liquids.

- Limiting fluids after dinner and avoiding alcohol.

- Avoiding high-sugar or high-calorie snacks at bedtime.

- Avoiding highly stimulating activities before bed, such as watching a frightening movie, playing competitive computer games, etc.

- Avoiding tossing and turning in bed. Instead, the patient should get up and listen to relaxing music or read.

Herbal remedies

Herbal remedies that are helpful in relieving insomnia include:

- catnip (*Nepeta cataria*): poor sleep

- **chamomile** (*Matricaria recutita*): anxiety

- chrysanthemum (*Chrysanthemum morifolium*): insomnia

- hops (*Humulus lupulus*): overactive mind

- lime blossom (*Tilia cordata*): anxiety

- linden (*Tilia* species): anxiety

- oats (*Avena sativa*): poor sleep and nervous exhaustion

- passionflower (*Passiflora incarnata*): anxiety and muscle cramps

- skullcap (*Scutellaria lateriflora*): nervous tension

- squawvine (*Mitchella repens*): insomnia

- St. John's wort (*Hypericum perforatum*): depression

- valerian (*Valeriana officinalis*): anxiety

- vervain (*Verbena officinalis*): nervous tension, sleep apnea

According to *Prevention* magazine, insomnia is the sixth most common condition treated with herbal formulas in the United States; it accounts for 18% of all use of herbal preparations. Some herbs used for insomnia are safer than others. Persons who are using alternative remedies, whether to treat insomnia or other conditions, *should always tell their doctor what they are taking, how much, and how often.* This warning is important because some herbal preparations that are safe in themselves can interact with prescription medications.

Dietary supplements and modifications

Some naturopaths recommend Vitamins B_6, B_{12}, and D for the relief of insomnia. **Calcium** and **magnesium** are natural sedatives, which helps to explain the traditional folk recommendation of drinking a glass of warm milk at bedtime. Tryptophan may relieve insomnia; as turkey is high in tryptophan, a turkey sandwich as a bedtime snack may be helpful. **Melatonin** is widely used to induce sleep although adequate studies of its effectiveness are lacking.

Other treatments

A wide variety of other alternative treatments that may be helpful in treating sleep disorders include:

- Acupressure. The pressure points on both heels, the base of the skull, between the eyebrows, and on the inside of the wrists can be used to relieve insomnia.

- Acupuncture. The specific treatment for insomnia depends upon the cause.

- Aromatherapy. The use of **essential oils** of bergamot, **lavender**, basil, chamomile, neroli, marjoram, or rose promotes **relaxation**.

- Ayurvedic medicine. Ayurvedic remedies for insomnia include scalp and soles massage with sesame, brahmi, or jatamamsi oils, a warm bath, or a **nutmeg** ghee paste applied to the forehead and around the eyes. Nightmares are treated with scalp and soles massage with brahmi or bhringaraj oils, tranquility tea (jatamamsi, brahmi, ginkgo, and **licorice** root), and **yoga**. Sleep apnea is treated by changing sleep positions, humidifying the air, and nasya (nose drops) with warm brahmi ghee.

- Biofeedback. This technique can promote relaxation.

- Chinese medicine. Practitioners of **traditional Chinese medicine** usually treat insomnia as a symptom of excess yang energy. Either magnetite or "dragon bones" are recommended for insomnia associated with hysteria or fear.

- Chiropractic. Spinal manipulation can reduce stress upon the nervous system, thus allowing relaxation.

- Colored **light therapy**. Treatment with true green light can balance the nervous system and may relieve insomnia.

- Homeopathy. Homeopathic remedies are chosen according to the specific causes of insomnia. They may include: *Nux vomica* (alcohol or substance-related sleeplessness), *Ignatia* (emotional upset), *Arsenicum* (anxiety), *Passiflora* (mental stress, aches, and pains), and *Lycopodium* (talking and laughing during sleep).

- Light/dark therapy involves making the bedroom very dark at night and exposing the patient to early morning sunlight (or a light box).

- Low-energy emission therapy (LEET) is a clinically proven treatment for chronic insomnia. LEET treatment involves delivering electromagnetic fields through a mouthpiece.

- Massage. Therapeutic massage can relieve the muscular tension associated with chronic insomnia.

- **Meditation**. Regular meditation practice can counteract emotional stress.

- **Reflexology**. The use of the reflexology points for the diaphragm, pancreas, ovary/testicle, pituitary, parathyroid, thyroid, and adrenal gland helps to relieve insomnia.

- Visualization may help to promote relaxation.

- Yoga can promote relaxation by releasing muscular tension.

Allopathic treatment

Treatment for a sleep disorder depends on its cause. In some cases, rearrangement of the bedroom or changes in sleeping arrangements may be all that is needed. Sedative or hypnotic medications are generally recommended only for insomnia related to a temporary stress because of the potential for addiction or overdose. Trazodone, a sedating antidepressant, is often used for chronic insomnia that does not respond to other treatments. Hypnotic agents include lorazepam, temazepam, and zolpidem.

Bright-light therapy, which was originally introduced as a treatment for **seasonal affective disorder**, is being tried as a treatment for insomnia in elderly adults. Although the results are not conclusive as of 2002, this form of treatment does appear to benefit many patients. In addition, it does not involve medications, which are more likely to produce side effects in the elderly than in younger patients.

Narcolepsy is treated with such stimulants as dextroamphetamine sulfate or methylphenidate. Nocturnal myoclonus has been successfully treated with clonazepam.

Children with sleep terror disorder or sleepwalking are usually treated with benzodiazepines. Children with nightmare disorder may benefit from limits on violent or frightening television programs or movies.

Psychotherapy is recommended for patients with sleep disorders associated with other mental disorders.

Patients with sleep apnea or hypopnea are encouraged to stop smoking, avoid alcohol or drugs of abuse, and lose weight to improve the stability of the upper airway. In children and adolescents, removal of the tonsils and adenoids is a fairly common and successful treatment for sleep apnea. Most sleep apnea patients are treated with continuous positive airway pressure (CPAP). Sometimes an oral prosthesis is used for mild sleep apnea.

Expected results

The prognosis depends on the specific disorder. Natural remedies often require several weeks to have noticeable effects. Children usually outgrow sleep disorders. Narcolepsy, however, is a lifelong disorder.

Resources

BOOKS

Becker, Philip M. "Sleep Disorders." In *Current Diagnosis 9,* edited by Rex B. Conn, et al. Philadelphia: W. B. Saunders, 1997.

DeGeronimo, Theresa Foy. *Insomnia: 50 Essential Things To Do.* New York: Penguin Group, 1997.

Eisendrath, Stuart J. "Psychiatric Disorders: Sleep Disorders." In *Current Medical Diagnosis & Treatment 1998,* edited by Lawrence M. Tierney, Jr., et al. Stamford, CT: Appleton & Lange, 1997.

Goldson, Edward. "Behavioral Disorders and Developmental Variations: Sleep Disorders." In *Current Pediatric Diagnosis & Treatment,* edited by William W. Hay, Jr., et al. Stamford, CT: Appleton & Lange, 1997.

Pelletier, Kenneth R., MD. *The Best Alternative Medicine*, Part II, "CAM Therapies for Specific Conditions: Insomnia." New York: Simon & Schuster, 2002.

KEY TERMS

Apnea—The temporary absence of breathing.

Cataplexy—Sudden loss of muscle tone, often causing a person to fall.

Circadian rhythm—Any body rhythm that recurs in 24-hour cycles such as the sleep-wake cycle.

Dyssomnia—A primary sleep disorder in which the patient suffers from changes in the quantity, quality, or timing of sleep.

Hypersomnia—An abnormal increase of 25% or more in time spent sleeping.

Hypopnea—Shallow or excessively slow breathing usually caused by partial closure of the upper airway during sleep.

Narcolepsy—A lifelong sleep disorder marked by four symptoms: sudden brief sleep attacks, cataplexy, temporary paralysis, and hallucinations.

Nocturnal myoclonus—A disorder in which the patient is awakened repeatedly during the night by cramps or twitches in the calf muscles. Also called periodic limb movement disorder (PLMD).

Parasomnia—A primary sleep disorder in which the person's physiology or behaviors are affected by sleep, the sleep stage, or the transition from sleeping to waking.

Polysomnography—Laboratory measurement of a patient's basic physiological processes during sleep.

Restless legs syndrome (RLS)—A disorder in which the patient experiences crawling, aching, or other disagreeable sensations in the calves that can be relieved by movement.

Sleep latency—The amount of time that it takes a person to fall asleep.

Reichenberg-Ullman, Judyth, and Robert Ullman. *Homeopathic Self-Care: The Quick and Easy Guide for the Whole Family.* Rocklin, CA: Prima Publishing, 1997.

Sanders, Mark H. "Sleep Apnea and Hypopnea." In *Conn's Current Therapy.* Edited by Robert E. Rakel. Philadelphia: W.B. Saunders, 1998.

"Sleep Disorders." In *Diagnostic and Statistical Manual of Mental Disorders.* 4th ed., text revision. Washington, DC: American Psychiatric Association, 2000.

Vasant, Lad. *The Complete Book of Ayurvedic Home Remedies.* New York: Harmony Books, 1998.

Wiedman, John. *Desperately Seeking Snoozin': The Insomnia Cure from Awake to Zzzz.* Memphis, TN: Towering Pines Press, 1997.

PERIODICALS

Akerstedt, T., P. Fredlund, M. Gillberg, and B. Jansson. "A Prospective Study of Fatal Occupational Accidents— Relationship to Sleeping Difficulties and Occupational Factors." *Journal of Sleep Research* 11 (March 2002): 69-71.

Hunsley, M., and E. B. Thoman. "The Sleep of Co-Sleeping Infants When They Are Not Co-Sleeping: Evidence That Co-Sleeping Is Stressful." *Developmental Psychobiology* 40 (January 2002): 14-22.

Lushington, K., and L. Lack. "Non-Pharmacological Treatments of Insomnia." *Israeli Journal of Psychiatry and Related Sciences* 39 (2002): 36-49.

Montgomery, P., and J. Dennis. "Bright Light Therapy for Sleep Problems in Adults Aged 60+ (Cochrane Review)." *Cochrane Database Systems Review* 2002: CD003403.

Neylan, T. C., T. J. Metzler, S. R. Best, et al. "Critical Incident Exposure and Sleep Quality in Police Officers." *Psychosomatic Medicine* 64 (March-April 2002): 345-352.

Powell, N. B., K. B. Schechtman, R. W. Riley, et al. "Sleepy Driving: Accidents and Injury." *Otolaryngology, Head and Neck Surgery* 126 (March 2002): 217-227.

ORGANIZATIONS

American Sleep Disorders Association. 1610 14th Street NW, Suite 300. Rochester, MN 55901. (507) 287-6006.

National Sleep Foundation. 1367 Connecticut Avenue NW, Suite 200. Washington, DC 20036. (202) 785-2300.

Belinda Rowland
Rebecca J. Frey, PhD

Slippery elm

Description

Slippery elm (*Ulmus rubra*), known variously as Indian elm, sweet elm, red elm, and moose elm, is a deciduous tree native to North America, particularly the eastern and central United States and eastern Canada. Slippery elm is smaller in stature than other members of the Ulmaceae, or elm, family. There are about twenty species of elm. The slippery elm can grow 50-60 ft (15-18 m) in height with a trunk measuring one to four feet in diameter. Its exterior bark is dark brown, rough, and fissured. The mucilaginous inner bark is white with a distinctive scent. The tree flowers in early spring before it comes into leaf. Flowers bloom in dense and inconspicuous clusters at the tips of the branches that spread out into an open crown. The stigmas of the blossoms are bright red. The downy leaf buds are rust colored with orange tips. The alternate leaves are dark-green, hairy, and abrasive on top, and a lighter green, hairy, and less abrasive on the underside. Leaves are 4-7 in (10-18 cm) long and oblong to ovate with irregularly toothed margins.

The seeds are contained in flat round paper-thin fruits and grow in clusters.

The slippery elm is a rare or threatened species in some parts of the United States, particularly in the northeastern U.S. where Dutch elm disease has devastated the elm forests. Its usual habitat is along stream banks and in woods. Harvesting the medicinally valuable and nutritious inner rind involves stripping the tree of large segments of the outer bark. This often results in the death of the tree, further diminishing its presence in the wild forests. Planting additional trees to replace those harvested is vital to the preservation of this beneficial native American tree. The National Center for the Preservation of Medicinal Herbs lists slippery elm as one of the "at-risk botanicals."

Native American herbalists included the mucilaginous inner bark in their medicine bags, and found numerous other uses for the pliable slippery elm bark, including using the fiber for making canoes and baskets. Native American herbalists shared their herbal knowledge with the early colonists, who came to rely on the slippery elm as one of their most valued home remedies. Midwives used slippery elm as a birth aid because its lubricant properties eased labor. Early settlers called the inner bark of the tree "slippery-elm food." The boiled bark was an important survival food for both the Native Americans and the colonists during times of famine. George Washington and his troops are believed to have subsisted for several days on gruel made from slippery elm bark during the cold winter at Valley Forge, Pennsylvania. A poultice made from the inner bark was a field dressing for gunshot **wounds** during the Revolutionary War.

General use

The dried inner bark of the slippery elm, known as the bast, is a calcium-rich, nutritive substance containing **bioflavonoids**, a high amount of mucilage, starch, a small quantity of tannins, and **vitamin E**. Slippery elm in various preparations acts as a demulcent, emollient, expectorant, diuretic, and is a soothing and nutritive tonic benefiting the adrenal glands, the respiratory system, and the gastrointestinal tract. The inner bark, taken as an infusion or syrup, has been used to treat **sore throat**, **laryngitis**, **bronchitis**, and stomach or duodenal ulcers. Slippery elm is a healing remedy once widely used to treat consumption, known now as **tuberculosis**, and typhoid **fever**. The mucilaginous substance in the inner bark is soothing to irritated tissues in the lungs, intestines, colon and urinary tract, and may be helpful in the treatment of **Crohn's disease**, an inflammation of the walls of the small intestines and colon. Slippery elm helps to draw out toxins from the body and assists the body in expelling mucus. It is beneficial externally in poultice form. When the inner bark is mixed with water, the soothing and emollient substance can be applied to the skin as a healing salve for numerous skin problems. It can be used for **diaper rash**, bed sores, **abscess**, **burns**, scalds, **infections**, and **boils**.

Slippery elm may be combined with such other soothing herbs, such as **echinacea**, **goldenseal**, and **comfrey**, in a salve preparation to soothe and bring healing to inflamed and infected skin. A gruel or paste of slippery elm mixed with water is useful as a nutritive food for invalids who may be unable to keep down regular food. When an infusion of ginseng is used in place of the water, the tonic effect of this herbal food will be enhanced. Slippery elm was listed in the *U.S. Pharmacopoeia* and the *National Formulary* from 1820 until 1960. The Food and Drug Administration has listed slippery elm as a safe and effective remedy for soothing throat and respiratory inflammations and as a digestive aid.

More recently, slippery elm has been studied as a possible antioxidant. **Antioxidants** are compounds that counteract **aging** and other destructive effects of oxidation in living tissue. One group of Korean researchers found that slippery elm extract inactivates peroxynitrite, an oxidizing compound that causes cell death. British researchers have also studied the antioxidant effects of slippery elm, which they think explains its effectiveness as a treatment for irritable bowel disease (IBD).

Preparations

Maude Grieve recommended in her 1931 book, *A Modern Herbal*, that only 10-year-old bark should be harvested. She listed numerous recipes for medicinal preparations using slippery elm bark in combination with other healing herbs for specific applications for many illnesses. The most common commercially available slippery elm products on the market today are in the form of throat lozenges and teas.

Powdered bark: Euell Gibbons, an American herbalist, suggested a way to prepare slippery elm for storage or use. Separate the inner rind from the outer bark and place the strips on an oven shelf at a very low temperature. Leave the door slightly ajar. When the inner rind is brittle, cut into small pieces across the grain and put it through a food processor, one cupful at a time. Coarser material is useful in preparing a poultice. The finer powder is used for decoctions, syrup, or slippery elm "gruel."

Slippery elm "gruel": Slowly add fresh, cold water, a little at a time, to the finely powdered bark. Stir until the mixture reaches the consistency of a thick porridge. Sweeten with honey and add cinnamon and **ginger** to taste. Refrigerate unused portions. Milk may also be used in place of water.

Infusion: Bring one pint of fresh unchlorinated water just to the point of a boil. Pour over one ounce of

KEY TERMS

Antioxidant—An enzyme or other organic substance that is able to counteract the damaging effects of oxidation in living tissue.

Mucilaginous—Having a moist, soft, and sticky quality. The inner rind of slippery elm bark is an example of a mucilaginous plant product.

Poultice—A soft moist mass of cloth, often stuffed with herbs, applied warm as a treatment for wounds or injuries.

the powdered slippery elm bark. Steep until the mixture is cool. Add lemon and honey to taste. Drink freely throughout the day.

Precautions

Use care when purchasing slippery elm products. Avoid those that are wildcrafted (harvested in the wild) to minimize depletion of this endangered American native tree.

Side effects

No known side effects have been reported.

Interactions

As of 2002, slippery elm has not been reported to interact with any prescription medications. it is best to take slippery elm several hours before or after other herbs or medications because of possible interference with speed of absorption.

Resources

BOOKS

Duke, James A. *The Green Pharmacy.* Emmaus, PA: Rodale Press, 1997.

Elias, Jason, and Shelagh Ryan Masline. *The A to Z Guide to Healing Herbal Remedies.* New York: Dell Books, 1995.

Medical Economics Company. *PDR for Herbal Medicines,* 1st ed. Montvale, NJ: Medical Economics Company, 1998.

Tierra, Lesley. *The Herbs of Life, Health & Healing Using Western & Chinese Techniques.* Santa Cruz, CA: The Crossing Press, 1997.

Tyler, Varro E., ed. *Prevention's 200 Herbal Remedies.* Emmaus, PA: Rodale Press, Inc., 1997.

PERIODICALS

Choi, H. R., J. Choi, Y. N. Han, et al. "Peroxynitrite Scavenging Activity of Herb Extracts." *Phytotherapy Research* 16 (June 2002): 364-367.

Langmead, L., C. Dawson, C. Hawkins, et al. "Antioxidant Effects of Herbal Therapies Used by Patients with Inflammatory Bowel Disease: An In Vitro Study." *Alimentary Pharmacological Therapy* 16 (February 2002): 197-205.

ORGANIZATIONS

American Herbalists Guild. 1931 Gaddis Road, Canton, GA 30115. (770) 751-6021. <www.americanherbalistsguild.com>.

OTHER

Grieve, Mrs. M. "Elm, Slippery." *A Modern Herbal.* http://botanical.com/botanical/mgmh/e/elmsli09.html.

"Slippery Elm." http://www.mothernature.com/ency/Herb/Slippery_Elm.asp.

Clare Hanrahan
Rebecca J. Frey, PhD

Smoking

Definition

Smoking is the inhalation of the smoke of burning tobacco encased in cigarettes, pipes, and cigars. Casual smoking is the act of smoking only occasionally, usually in a social situation or to relieve **stress**. A smoking habit is a physical addiction to tobacco products. Many health experts now regard habitual smoking as a psychological addiction, too, and one with serious health consequences.

Description

The U.S. Food and Drug Administration (FDA) has asserted that cigarettes and smokeless tobacco should be considered nicotine delivery devices. Nicotine, the active ingredient in tobacco, is inhaled into the lungs, where most of it stays. The rest passes into the bloodstream, reaching the brain in about ten seconds and dispersing throughout the body in about 20 seconds.

Depending on the circumstances and the amount consumed, nicotine can act as either a stimulant or tranquilizer. This can explain why some people report that smoking gives them energy and stimulates their mental activity, while others note that smoking relieves **anxiety** and relaxes them. The initial "kick" results in part from the drug's stimulation of the adrenal glands and resulting release of epinephrine into the blood. Epinephrine causes several physiological changes—it temporarily narrows the arteries, raises the blood pressure, raises the levels of fat in the blood, and increases the heart rate and flow of blood from the heart. Some researchers think epinephrine contributes to smokers' increased risk of high blood pressure.

THERAPIES FOR TREATING SYMPTOMS OF SMOKING CESSATION		
Treatment	*Description*	*Symptom treated*
Lobelia	Used as a nicotine substitute, it can bolster the nervous system	Withdrawal and craving
Wild oats or kava kava	Relaxant	Withdrawal
Licorice	Can be chewed to help withdrawal	Oral fixation
Hawthorn, gingko biloba, and bilberry	All contain bioflavonoids that can help repair free radical damage	Damage to lungs and cardiovascular system
Acupuncture	Stimulation of points in ears and feet helps cessation	Addiction and withdrawal
Vitamin C	Antioxidant that helps fight infection	Boosts immune system
Vitamin B_{12}	Helps protect body from disease	Smoking-induced cancers
Omega-3 fatty acids	Helps protect body from disease	Smoking-related illness, such as emphysema, and depression

Nicotine by itself increases the risk of **heart disease**. However, when a person smokes, he or she is ingesting a lot more than nicotine. Smoke from a cigarette, pipe, or cigar is made up of many additional toxic chemicals, including tar and carbon monoxide. Tar is a sticky substance that forms into deposits in the lungs, causing lung **cancer** and respiratory distress. Carbon monoxide limits the amount of oxygen that the red blood cells can convey throughout the body. Also, it may damage the inner walls of the arteries, which allows fat to build up in them.

Besides tar, nicotine, and carbon monoxide, tobacco smoke contains 4,000 different chemicals. More than 200 of these chemicals are known be toxic. Nonsmokers who are exposed to tobacco smoke also take in these toxic chemicals. They inhale the smoke exhaled by the smoker as well as the more toxic *sidestream* smoke—the smoke from the end of the burning cigarette, cigar, or pipe.

Here's why sidestream smoke is more toxic than exhaled smoke: When a person smokes, the smoke he or she inhales and then breathes out leaves harmful deposits inside the body. But because lungs partially cleanse the smoke, exhaled smoke contains fewer poisonous chemicals. That's why exposure to tobacco smoke is dangerous even for a nonsmoker.

Causes & symptoms

No one starts smoking to become addicted to nicotine. It isn't known how much nicotine may be consumed before the body becomes addicted. However, once smoking becomes a habit, the smoker faces a lifetime of health risks associated with an addiction that has been shown to be stronger than alcohol addiction and at least as strong as narcotics addiction.

About 70% of smokers in the United States would like to quit; in any given year, however, only about 3.6% of the country's 47 million smokers quit successfully.

Although specific genes have not yet been identified as of 2003, researchers think that genetic factors contribute substantially to developing a smoking habit. Several twin studies have led to estimates of 46–84% heritability for smoking. It is thought that some genetic variations affect the speed of nicotine metabolism in the body and the activity level of nicotinic receptors in the brain.

Smoking risks

Smoking is recognized as the leading preventable cause of death, causing or contributing to the deaths of approximately 430,700 Americans each year. Anyone with a smoking habit has an increased chance of lung, cervical, and other types of cancer; respiratory diseases such as emphysema, **asthma**, and chronic **bronchitis**; and cardiovascular disease, such as **heart attack**, high blood pressure, **stroke**, and **atherosclerosis** (narrowing and hardening of the arteries). The risk of stroke is especially high in women who take birth control pills.

Smoking can damage fertility, making it harder to conceive, and it can interfere with the growth of the fetus during **pregnancy**. It accounts for an estimated 14% of premature births and 10% of infant deaths. There is some evidence that smoking may cause **impotence** in some men.

Because smoking affects so many of the body's systems, smokers often have vitamin deficiencies and suffer oxidative damage caused by free radicals. Free radicals are molecules that steal electrons from other molecules, turning the other molecules into free radicals and destabilizing the molecules in the body's cells.

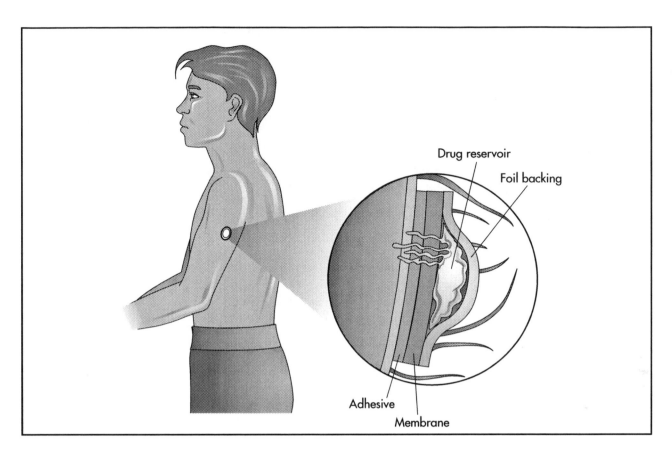

The nicotine patch is a type of transepidermal patch designed to deliver nicotine, the addictive substance contained in cigarettes, directly through the skin and into the blood stream. The patch contains a drug reservoir sandwiched between a nonpermeable back layer and a permeable adhesive layer that attaches to the skin. The drug leaches slowly out of the reservoir, releasing small amounts of the drug at a constant rate for up to 16 hours. *(Illustration by Electronic Illustrators Group. The Gale Group.)*

Smoking is recognized as one of several factors that might be related to a higher risk of hip **fractures** in older adults.

Studies reveal that the more a person smokes, the more likely he is to sustain illnesses such as cancer, chronic bronchitis, and emphysema. But even smokers who indulge in the habit only occasionally are more prone to these diseases.

Some brands of cigarettes are advertised as "low tar," but no cigarette is truly safe. If a smoker switches to a low-tar cigarette, he is likely to inhale longer and more deeply to get the chemicals his body craves. A smoker has to quit the habit entirely in order to improve his health and decrease the chance of disease.

Though some people believe chewing tobacco is safer, it also carries health risks. People who chew tobacco have an increased risk of heart disease and mouth and throat cancer. Pipe and cigar smokers have increased health risks as well, even though these smokers generally do not inhale as deeply as cigarette smokers do. These groups haven't been studied as extensively as cigarette

smokers, but there is evidence that they may be at a slightly lower risk of cardiovascular problems but a higher risk of cancer and various types of circulatory conditions.

Recent research reveals that passive smokers, or those who unavoidably breathe in secondhand tobacco smoke, have an increased chance of many health problems such as **lung cancer**, ischemic heart disease, and asthma; and in children, sudden infant death syndrome. A Swedish study published in 2001 found that people who were exposed to environmental tobacco smoke (ETS) as children were both more likely to develop asthma as adults, and to become smokers themselves. In the fall of 2001 the Environmental Protection Agency (EPA) partnered with the American Academy of Allergy, Asthma, and Immunology (AAAAI) to educate parents about the risks to their children of secondhand smoke, and to persuade parents to sign a Smoke Free Home Pledge. The AAAAI reported that many parents cut down on or gave up smoking when they recognized the damage that smoking was causing to their children's lungs. A study of secondhand smoke in the workplace done by the European Union found that it can affect workers as severely as smoke in the home can affect children. The study noted that workers exposed to secondhand smoke from their colleagues had significantly higher rates of asthma and upper respiratory **infections** than those who were employed in smoke-free workplaces.

Smokers' symptoms

Smokers are likely to exhibit a variety of symptoms that reveal the damage caused by smoking. A nagging morning **cough** may be one sign of a tobacco habit. Other symptoms include shortness of breath, **wheezing**, and frequent occurrences of respiratory illness, such as bronchitis. Smoking also increases **fatigue** and decreases the smoker's sense of smell and taste. Smokers are more likely to develop poor circulation, with cold hands and feet and premature wrinkles.

Sometimes the illnesses that result from smoking come on silently with little warning. For instance, coronary artery disease may exhibit few or no symptoms. At other times, there will be warning signs, such as bloody discharge from a woman's vagina, a sign of cancer of the cervix. Another warning sign is a hacking cough, worse than the usual smoker's cough, that brings up phlegm or blood—a sign of lung cancer.

Withdrawal symptoms

A smoker who tries to quit may expect one or more of these withdrawal symptoms: **nausea, constipation** or **diarrhea**, drowsiness, loss of concentration, **insomnia**, **headache**, nausea, and irritability.

Diagnosis

It's not easy to quit smoking. That's why it may be wise for a smoker to turn to his physician for help. For the greatest success in quitting and to help with the withdrawal symptoms, the smoker should talk over a treatment plan with his doctor or alternative practitioner. He should have a general physical examination to gauge his general health and uncover any deficiencies. He should also have a thorough evaluation for some of the serious diseases that smoking can cause.

Treatment

There are a wide range of alternative treatments that can help a smoker quit the habit, including **hypnotherapy**, herbs, acupuncture, and **meditation**. For example, a controlled trial demonstrated that self-massage can help smokers crave less intensely, smoke fewer cigarettes, and in some cases give them up completely.

Hypnotherapy

Hypnotherapy helps the smoker achieve a trance-like state, during which the deepest levels of the mind are accessed. A session with a hypnotherapist may begin with a discussion of whether the smoker really wants to and truly has the motivation to stop smoking. The therapist will explain how hypnosis can reduce the stress-related symptoms that sometimes come with kicking the habit.

Often the therapist will discuss the dangers of smoking with the patient and begin to "reframe" the patient's thinking about smoking. Many smokers are convinced they can't quit, and the therapist can help persuade them that they can change this behavior. These suggestions are then repeated while the smoker is under hypnosis. The therapist may also suggest while the smoker is under hypnosis that his feelings of worry, anxiety, and irritability will decrease.

In a review of 17 studies of the effectiveness of hypnotherapy, the percentage of people treated by hypnosis who still were not smoking after six months ranged from 4% to 8%. In programs that included several hours of treatment, intense interpersonal interaction, individualized suggestions, and follow-up treatment, success rates were above 50%.

Aromatherapy

One study demonstrated that inhaling the vapor from black pepper extract can reduce symptoms associated with smoking withdrawal. Other **essential oils** can be used for relieving the anxiety a smoker often experiences while quitting.

Herbs

A variety of herbs can help smokers reduce their cravings for nicotine, calm their irritability, and even reverse the oxidative cellular damage done by smoking. Lobelia, sometimes called Indian tobacco, has historically been used as a substitute for tobacco. It contains a substance called lobeline, which decreases the craving for nicotine by bolstering the nervous system and calming the smoker. In high doses, lobelia can cause **vomiting**, but the average dose—about 10 drops per day— should pose no problems.

Herbs that can help relax a smoker during withdrawal include wild oats and **kava kava**.

To reduce the oral fixation supplied by a nicotine habit, a smoker can chew on licorice root—the plant, not the candy. Licorice is good for the liver, which is a major player in the body's **detoxification** process. Licorice also acts as a tonic for the adrenal system, which helps reduce stress. And there's an added benefit: If a smoker tries to light up after chewing on licorice root, the cigarette tastes like burned cardboard.

Other botanicals that can help repair free-radical damage to the lungs and cardiovascular system are those high in flavonoids, such as hawthorn, gingko biloba, and **bilberry**, as well as **antioxidants** such as **vitamin A, vitamin C, zinc**, and **selenium**.

Acupuncture

This ancient Chinese method of healing is used commonly to help beat addictions, including smoking. The acupuncturist will use hair-thin needles to stimulate the body's *qi*, or healthy energy. Acupuncture is a sophisticated treatment system based on revitalizing qi, which supposedly flows through the body in defined pathways called meridians. During an addiction like smoking, qi isn't flowing smoothly or gets stuck, the theory goes.

Points in the ear and feet are stimulated to help the smoker overcome his addiction. Often the acupuncturist will recommend keeping the needles in for five to seven days to calm the smoker and keep him balanced.

Vitamins

Smoking seriously depletes vitamin C in the body and leaves it more susceptible to infections. Vitamin C can prevent or reduce free-radical damage by acting as an antioxidant in the lungs. Smokers need additional C, in higher dosage than nonsmokers. Fish in the diet supplies **Omega-3 fatty acids**, which are associated with a reduced risk of chronic obstructive pulmonary disease (emphysema or chronic bronchitis) in smokers. Omega-3 fats also provide cardiovascular benefits as well as an anti-depressive effect. Vitamin therapy doesn't reduce craving but it can help beat some of the damage created by smoking. **Vitamin B$_{12}$** and **folic acid** may help protect against smoking-induced cancer.

Allopathic treatment

Research shows that most smokers who want to quit benefit from the support of other people. It helps to quit with a friend or to join a group such as those organized by the American Cancer Society. These groups provide support and teach behavior modification methods that can help the smoker quit. The smoker's physician can often refer him to such groups.

Other alternatives to help with the withdrawal symptoms of kicking the habit include nicotine replacement therapy (NRT) in the form of gum, patches, nasal sprays, and oral inhalers. These are available by prescription or over the counter. A physician can provide advice on how to use them. They slowly release a small amount of nicotine into the bloodstream, satisfying the smoker's physical craving. Over time, the amount of gum the smoker chews is decreased and the amount of time between applying the patches is increased. This tapering helps wean the smoker from nicotine slowly, eventually beating his addiction to the drug. But there's one important caution: If the smoker lights up while taking a nicotine replacement, a nicotine overdose may cause serious health problems.

The prescription drug Zyban (bupropion hydrochloride) has shown some success in helping smokers quit. This drug contains no nicotine, and was originally developed as an antidepressant. It isn't known exactly how bupropion works to suppress the desire for nicotine. A five-year study of bupropion reported in 2003 that the drug has a very good record for safety and effectiveness in treating tobacco dependence. Its most common side effect is insomnia, which can also result from nicotine withdrawal.

Researchers are investigating two new types of drugs as possible treatments for tobacco dependence as of 2003. The first is an alkaloid known as 18-methoxycoronaridine (18-MC), which selectively blocks the nicotinic receptors in brain tissue. Another approach involves developing drugs that inhibit the activity of cytochrome P450 2A6 (CYP2A6), which controls the metabolism of nicotine.

Expected results

Research on smoking shows that most smokers desire to quit. But smoking is so addictive that fewer than 20% of the people who try ever successfully kick the habit. Still, many people attempt to quit smoking over and over again, despite the difficulties—the cravings and withdrawal symptoms, such as irritability and restlessness.

For those who do quit, the rewards of better health are well worth the effort. The good news is that once a smoker quits the health effects are immediate and dramatic. After the first day, oxygen and carbon monoxide levels in the blood return to normal. At two days, nerve endings begin to grow back and the senses of taste and smell revive. Within two weeks to three months, circulation and breathing improve. After one year of not smoking, the risk of heart disease is reduced by 50%. After 15 years of abstinence, the risks of health problems from smoking virtually vanish. A smoker who quits for good often feels a lot better too, with less fatigue and fewer respiratory illnesses.

Prevention

How do you give up your cigarettes for good and never go back to them again?

KEY TERMS

Antioxidant—Any substance that reduces the damage caused by oxidation, such as the harm caused by free radicals.

Chronic bronchitis—A smoking-related respiratory illness in which the membranes that line the bronchi, or the lung's air passages, narrow over time. Symptoms include a morning cough that brings up phlegm, breathlessness, and wheezing.

Cytochrome—A substance that contains iron and acts as a hydrogen carrier for the eventual release of energy in aerobic respiration.

Emphysema—An incurable, smoking-related disease, in which the air sacs at the end of the lung's bronchi become weak and inefficient. People with emphysema often first notice shortness of breath, repeated wheezing and coughing that brings up phlegm.

Epinephrine—A nervous system hormone stimulated by the nicotine in tobacco. It increases heart rate and may raise smokers' blood pressure.

Flavonoid—A food chemical that helps to limit oxidative damage to the body's cells and protects against heart disease and cancer.

Free radical—An unstable molecule that causes oxidative damage by stealing electrons from surrounding molecules, thereby disrupting activity in the body's cells.

Nicotine—The addictive ingredient of tobacco, it acts on the nervous system and is both stimulating and calming.

Nicotine replacement therapy (NRT)—A method of weaning a smoker away from both nicotine and the oral fixation that accompanies a smoking habit by giving the smoker smaller and smaller doses of nicotine in the form of a patch or gum.

Passive smoking—A term that refers to a person's having to breathe in smoke from someone else's cigarette or pipe. Other terms for passive smoking are exposure to secondhand smoke or exposure to environmental tobacco smoke (ETS).

Sidestream smoke—The smoke that is emitted from the burning end of a cigarette or cigar, or that comes from the end of a pipe. Along with exhaled smoke, it is a constituent of second-hand smoke.

Here are a few tips from the experts:

- Have a plan and set a definite quit date.

- Get rid of all the cigarettes and ashtrays at home or in your desk at work.

- Don't allow others to smoke in your house.

- Tell your friends and neighbors that you're quitting. Doing so helps make quitting a matter of pride.

- Chew sugarless gum or eat sugar-free hard candy to redirect the oral fixation that comes with smoking. This will prevent weight gain, too.

- Eat as much as you want, but only low-calorie foods and drinks. Drink plenty of water. This may help with the feelings of tension and restlessness that quitting can bring. After eight weeks, you'll lose your craving for tobacco, so it's safe then to return to your usual eating habits.

- Stay away from social situations that prompt you to smoke. Dine in the nonsmoking section of restaurants.

- Spend the money you save by not smoking on an occasional treat for yourself.

Resources

BOOKS

"Acupuncture." In *The American Medical Association Encyclopedia of Medicine,* edited by Charles B. Clayman. New York: Random House, 1989.

Molony, David, and Ming Ming Pan. *The American Association of Oriental Medicine's Complete Guide to Herbal Medicine.* New York: Berkley Books, 1998.

"Tobacco Addiction." Section 21, Chapter 290 in *The Merck Manual of Diagnosis and Therapy*, edited by Mark H. Beers, MD, and Robert Berkow, MD. Whitehouse Station, NJ: Merck Research Laboratories, 2002.

Tyler, Varro E. *The Honest Herbal: a Sensible Guide to the Use of Herbs and Related Remedies.* New York: Haworth Press, 1993.

PERIODICALS

"AAAAI, EPA Mount Effort to Raise Awareness to Dangers of Secondhand Smoke." *Immunotherapy Weekly* (November 30, 2001): 30.

Batra, V., A. A. Patkar, W. H. Berrettini, et al. "The Genetic Determinants of Smoking." *Chest* 123 (May 2003): 1338–1340.

Ferry, L., and J. A. Johnston. "Efficacy and Safety of Bupropion SR for Smoking Cessation: Data from Clinical Trials and Five Years of Postmarketing Experience." *International al Journal of Clinical Practice* 57 (April 2003): 224–230.

Janson, Christer, Susan Chinn, Deborah Jarvis, et al. "Effect of Passive Smoking on Respiratory Symptoms, Bronchial Responsiveness, Lung Function, and Total Serum IgE in the European Community Respiratory Health Survey: A Cross-Sectional Study." *Lancet* 358 (December 22, 2001): 2103.

Lerman, C., and W. Berrettini. "Elucidating the Role of Genetic Factors in Smoking Behavior and Nicotine Dependence." *American Journal of Medical Genetics* 118-B (April 1, 2003): 48–54.

Maisonneuve, I. M., and S. D. Glick. "Anti-Addictive Actions of an Iboga Alkaloid Congener: A Novel Mechanism for a Novel Treatment." *Pharmacology, Biochemistry, and Behavior* 75 (June 2003): 607–618.

Richmomd, R., and N. Zwar. "Review of Bupropion for Smoking Cessation." *Drug and Alcohol Review* 22 (June 2003): 203–220.

Sellers, E. M., R. F. Tyndale, and L. C. Fernandes. "Decreasing Smoking Behaviour and Risk through CYP2A6 Inhibition." *Drug Discovery Today* 8 (June 1, 2003): 487–493.

"Study Shows Link Between Asthma and Childhood Exposure to Smoking." *Immunotherapy Weekly* (October 10, 2001): np.

Yochum, L., L. H. Kushi, and A. R. Folsom. "Dietary Flavonoid Intake and Risk of Cardiovascular Disease in Postmenopausal Women." *American Journal of Epidemiology* 149, no. 10 (May 1999): 943–9.

ORGANIZATIONS

American Association of Oriental Medicine. 909 22nd Street, Sacramento, CA 95816, (916) 451-6950 <http://www.aaom.org>.

American Cancer Society. Contact the local organization or call (800) 227-2345. <http://www.cancer.org>.

American Lung Association. 1740 Broadway, New York, NY 10019. (800) 586-4872 or (212) 315-8700. <http://www.lungusa.org>.

Herb Research Foundation. 1007 Pearl St., Suite 200, Boulder CO 80302. (303) 449-2265. <http://www.herbs.org>.

National Heart, Lung, and Blood Institute (NHLBI). Building 31, Room 5A52, 31 Center Drive, MSC 2486, Bethesda, MD 20892. (301) 592-8573. <http://www.nhlbi.nih.gov>.

Smoking, Tobacco, and Health Information Line; Centers for Disease Control and Prevention. Mailstop K-50, 4770 Buford Highway NE, Atlanta, GA 30341-3724. (800) 232-1311. <http://www.cdc.gov/tobacco>.

OTHER

Virtual Office of the Surgeon General: Tobacco Cessation Guideline. <http://www.surgeongeneral.gov/tobacco>.

Barbara Boughton
Rebecca J. Frey, PhD

SMT *see* **Spinal manipulative therapy**

Sneezing

Definition

Sneezing, also known as sternutation, is the response of the mucous membrane of the nose to an irritant or foreign body that causes allergy in a hypersensitive person.

Description

A sneeze is an involuntary explosive burst of air from the nose and mouth that removes offending material from the nasal passages.

Causes & symptoms

Sneezing can occur from a number of causes, or may itself be a symptom of an underlying condition, most likely an allergy or **common cold**. Sneezing may simply be triggered by a small foreign object or substance in the nose, including particles of pepper, smoke, irritating chemical fumes, or gases. It may also be a symptom of a common cold, upper respiratory tract infection, hay **fever**, or other **allergies** to pollen, dust, dust mites, mold, dander, grass, or other substances. Additional potential causes of sneezing include withdrawal from opiate drugs, inhaling corticosteroids, whooping **cough**, or anaphylaxis. Many people sneeze when they step outdoors into bright sunlight. Others report sneezing whenever they tweeze their eyebrows.

In a January 2000 paper in the journal *Neurology*, Dr. Mark Hersch of Australia's New South Wales University reported that some **stroke** patients find themselves temporarily unable to sneeze, leading to speculation that a "sneeze center" may exist in the medulla of the brainstem.

Diagnosis

An attempt to determine the cause of sneezing is likely to include an examination of the upper respiratory tract. A doctor might perform skin tests to uncover any allergies, or antibody tests. In some cases, x rays are also useful.

Treatment

Herbs and supplements

Echinacea, Yin Chiao Chieh Tu Pien (a Chinese over-the-counter formulation), **zinc**, and **vitamin C** are all potentially useful against sneezing and other cold symptoms. Stinging **nettle** (*Urtica dioica*) and **red clover** (*Trifolium pratense*) may be used for allergies.

Homeopathy and acupuncture

Either of these disciplines may offer individualized relief. A local practitioner should be consulted. Homeo-

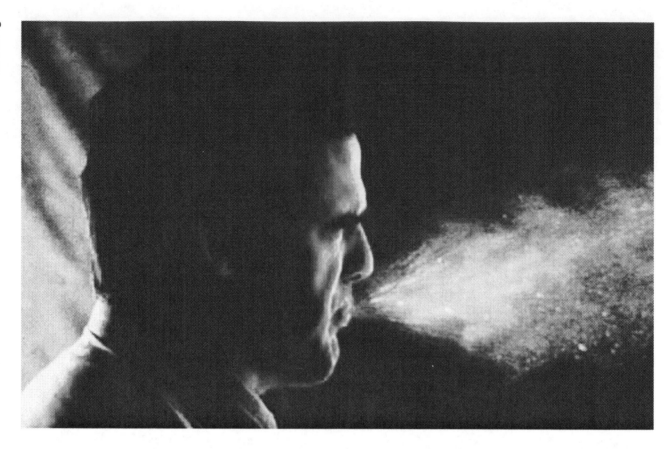

A man sneezing. *(Linda Steinmark. Custom Medical Stock Photo, Inc. Reproduced by permission.)*

pathic remedies may include *Allium cepa, Sabadilla, Nux vomica, Euphrasia, Natrum muriaticum*, and others.

Acupressure

Acupressure points that may be effective against sneezing include Large Intestine 4 (between the thumb and the index finger), Governing Vessel 26 (on the upper lip), and Triple Warmer 5 (on the forearm).

Relaxation

Some **hay fever** sufferers report benefits from hot baths, massage, and other **relaxation** therapies.

Allopathic treatment

This most commonly consists of over-the-counter antihistamines. Although these drugs often result in drowsiness, newer versions including Allegra and Claritin do not cause that problem.

Other treatment options may include an allergen-free diet, or a series of allergy shots, injecting increased amounts of an allergen to desensitize the body.

Expected results

Most commonly, sneezing is a mild and temporary problem. In those cases in which medical intervention is needed, the results are usually favorable, although allergy patients sometimes develop **asthma**.

Prevention

With allergies, the best way to prevent sneezing is to avoid exposure to allergens, the substances that provoke allergic attacks. Depending on the substance, this can be done by timely replacement of furnace filters, removing animals from the house, or even getting out of town during particularly sensitive seasons.

Handwashing and careful hygiene are good ways to avoid common colds and other **infections**.

Resources

ORGANIZATIONS

National Institute of Allergies and Infectious Diseases. 9000 Rockville Pike, Building 31, Room 7A-03, Bethesda, MD, 20205. (800) 644-6627. http://www.niaid.nih.gov/.

David Helwig

Snoring

Definition

Snoring is a sound generated during sleep by vibration of loose tissue in the upper airway.

Description

Snoring is one symptom of a group of disorders known as sleep-disordered breathing. It occurs when the soft palate, uvula, tongue, tonsils, and/or muscles in the back of the throat rub against each other and generate a vibrating sound during sleep. Twenty percent of all adults are chronic snorers, and 45% of normal adults snore occasionally. As people grow older, their chance of snoring increases. Approximately half of all individuals over 60 snore regularly.

In some cases, snoring is a symptom of a more serious disorder called obstructive **sleep apnea** (OSA). OSA occurs when part of the airway is closed off (usually at the back of the throat) while a person is trying to inhale during sleep, and breathing stops for more than 10 seconds before resuming again. These breathless episodes can occur as many as several hundred times a night.

People with OSA almost always snore heavily because the same narrowing of the airway that causes snoring can also cause OSA. Snoring may actually contribute to OSA as well, because the vibration of the throat tissues that occurs in snoring can cause the tissue to swell.

Snoring is associated with physical problems as well as social **stress**. People who do not suffer from OSA may be diagnosed with socially unacceptable snoring (SUS), which refers to snoring that is loud enough to prevent the sleeper's bed partner or roommate from sleeping. SUS is a factor in the breakup of some marriages and other long-term relationships. Moreover, a study published in 2002 indicates that people who snore are at increased risk of developing type 2 diabetes. Snoring appears to be a risk factor that is independent of body weight or a family history of diabetes.

Causes & symptoms

There are several major causes of snoring, including:

- Excessively relaxed throat muscles. Alcohol, drugs, and sedatives can cause the throat muscles to become lax, and/or the tongue to pull back into the airway.
- Large uvula. The piece of tissue that hangs from the back of the throat is called the uvula. Individuals with a large or longer than average uvula can suffer from snoring when the uvula vibrates in the airway.

- Large tonsils and/or adenoids. The tonsils (tissue at the back of either side of the throat) can also vibrate if they are larger than normal, as can the adenoids.
- Excessive weight. Overweight people are more likely to snore. Their snoring is frequently caused by the extra throat and neck tissue they are carrying around.
- Nasal congestion. Colds and **allergies** can plug the nose, creating a vacuum in the throat that results in snoring as airflow increases.
- Cysts and tumors. Cysts and/or tumors of the throat can trigger snoring.
- Structural problems of the nose. A deviated septum or other nasal problems can also cause snoring.

Diagnosis

A patient interview, and possibly an interview with the patient's spouse or anyone else in the household who has witnessed the snoring, is usually enough for a diagnosis of snoring. A medical history that includes questions about alcohol or tranquilizer use; past ear, nose, and throat problems; and the pattern and degree of snoring will be completed, and a physical examination will be performed to determine the cause of the problem. This will typically include examination of the throat to look for narrowing, obstruction, or malformations.

In some cases the patient may be referred to a dentist or orthodontist for evaluation of the jaw structure and dentition.

In addition, the patient may be examined by sleep endoscopy. In this procedure, the patient is given a medication (midazolam) to induce sleep. His or her throat and nasal passages are then examined with a flexible laryngoscope. In many cases, sleep endoscopy reveals obstructions that are not apparent during a standard physical examination of the throat. Many patients are found to have obstructions at more than one level in their breathing passages.

If the snoring is suspected to be a symptom of a more serious disorder such as obstructive sleep apnea, the patient will require further testing. This testing is called a polysomnography study, and is conducted during an overnight stay in a specialized sleep laboratory. The polysomnography study includes measurements of heart rate, airflow at the mouth and nose, respiratory effort, sleep stage (light sleep, deep sleep, dream sleep, etc.), and oxygen level in the blood.

Treatment

There are a number of remedies for snoring, but few are proven clinically effective. Popular treatments include:

- Mechanical devices. Many splints, braces, and other devices are available to reposition the nose, jaw, and/or mouth in order to clear the airways. Other devices are designed to wake an individual when snoring occurs. Patients should consult a dentist or orthodontist about these devices, as most require custom fitting. In addition, persons with certain types of **gum disease** or dental problems should not be fitted with oral appliances to stop snoring.

- Nasal strips. Nasal strips that attach like an adhesive bandage to the bridge of the nose are available at most drugstores, and can help stop snoring in some individuals by opening the nasal passages.

- Continuous positive airway pressure (CPAP). Some chronic snorers find relief by sleeping with a nasal mask that provides air pressure to the throat.

- Decongestants. Snoring caused by nasal congestion may be successfully treated with decongestants. Some effective herbal remedies that clear the nasal passages include golden rod (*Solidago virgauria*) and golden seal (*Hydrastis canadensis*). Steam inhalation of **essential oils** of **eucalyptus** blue gum (*Eucalyptus globulus*) or **peppermint** (*Mentha x piperata*) can also relieve congestion.

- Weight loss. Snoring thought to be caused by excessive weight may be curtailed by a sensible weight loss and **exercise** program.

- Sleep position. Snoring usually worsens when an individual sleeps on his or her back, so sleeping on one's side may alleviate the problem. Those who have difficulty staying in a side sleeping position may find sleeping with pillows behind them helps them maintain the position longer. Other devices include a new vest designed to prevent the sleeper from lying on his or her back.

- Bed adjustments. For some people, raising the head of the bed solves their snoring problem. A slight incline can prevent the tongue from retracting into the back of the throat. Bricks, wooden blocks, or specially designed wedges can be used to elevate the head of the bed approximately 4–6 in.

Alternative treatments that have been reported to be effective for patients whose snoring is caused by colds or allergies include **acupuncture**, **homeopathy**, and **aromatherapy** treatments. Aromatherapy treatments for snoring typically make use of marjoram oil, which is thought to be particularly effective in clearing the nasal passages.

Allopathic treatment

Several surgical procedures are available for treating chronic snoring. These include:

- Uvulopalatopharyngoplasty (UPPP), a surgical procedure that involves removing excess throat tissues (e.g., tonsils, parts of the soft palate) to expand the airway. The success rate of UPPP is about 53% after five years. The success of the surgery is related to the patient's body mass before the operation.

- Laser-assisted uvulopalatoplasty (LAUP) uses a surgical laser to remove part of the uvula and palate. Its chief drawback is a period of discomfort that lasts for about a week following surgery.

- Palatal stiffening is a minimally invasive surgical technique in which a laser or cauterizer is used to produce scar tissue in the soft palate in order to stop the vibrations that produce snoring.

- Radiofrequency ablation is another technique that uses scarring to shrink the uvula and/or soft palate. A needle electrode is used to shrink and scar the mouth and throat tissues. Like other surgical treatments for snoring, radiofrequency ablation has a relapse rate over the long term. One of its advantages, however, is that it is less painful than other surgical treatments.

Prevention

Adults with a history of snoring may be able to prevent snoring episodes with the following measures:

- Avoid alcohol and sedatives before bedtime.

- Remove allergens from the bedroom.

- Use a decongestant before bed.

- Sleep on the side of the body, not the back.

Resources

BOOKS

"Disorders of the Oral Region." Section 9, Chapter 105 in *The Merck Manual of Diagnosis and Therapy*, edited by Mark H. Beers, MD, and Robert Berkow, MD. Whitehouse Station, NJ: Merck Research Laboratories, 1999.

Pascualy, Ralph A. and Sally Warren Soest. *Snoring and Sleep Apnea: Personal and Family Guide to Diagnosis and Treatment*. New York: Demos Medical Publishing, 1996.

Pelletier, Kenneth R., MD. *The Best Alternative Medicine*, Part I, Chapter 5, "Acupuncture," and Chapter 8, "Homeopathy." New York: Simon & Schuster, 2002.

Price, Shirley. *Practical Aromatherapy*, 3rd ed. London, UK: Thorsons, 1994.

"Sleep Disorders." Section 14, Chapter 173 in *The Merck Manual of Diagnosis and Therapy*, edited by Mark H. Beers, MD, and Robert Berkow, MD. Whitehouse Station, NJ: Merck Research Laboratories, 1999.

PERIODICALS

Al-Delaimy, W. K., J. E. Manson, W. C. Willett, et al. "Snoring as a Risk Factor for Type II Diabetes Mellitus: A Prospective Study." *American Journal of Epidemiology* 155 (March 1, 2002): 394-395.

Ayappa, I., and D. M. Rapoport. "The Upper Airway in Sleep: Physiology of the Pharynx." *Sleep Medicine Reviews* 7 (February 2003): 3–7.

Blumen, M. B., S. Dahan, I. Wagner, et al. "Radiofrequency Versus LAUP for the Treatment of Snoring." *Otolaryngology and Head and Neck Surgery* 126 (January 2002): 67-73.

Ellis, S. G., N. W. Craik, R. F. Deans, and C. D. Hanning. "Dental Appliances for Snoring and Obstructive Sleep Apnoea: Construction Aspects for General Dental Practitioners." *Dental Update* 30 (January-February 2003): 16–22, 24–26.

Hassid, S., A. H. Afrapoli, C. Decaesteker, and G. Choufani. "UPPP for Snoring: Long-Term Results and Patient Satisfaction." *Acta Otorhinolaryngologica Belgica* 56 (2002): 157-162.

Hessel, N. S., and N. de Vries. "Diagnostic Work-Up of Socially Unacceptable Snoring. II. Sleep Endoscopy." *European Archives of Otorhinolaryngology* 259 (March 2002): 158-161.

Maurer, J. T., B. A. Stuck, G. Hein, et al. "Treatment of Obstructive Sleep Apnea with a New Vest Preventing the Supine Position." [in German] *Deutsche medizinische Wochenschrift* 128 (January 17, 2003): 71–75.

Nakano, H., T. Ikeda, M. Hayashi, et al. "Effects of Body Position on Snoring in Apneic and Nonapneic Snorers." *Sleep* 26 (March 15, 2003): 169–172.

Remacle, M., E. Jouzdani, G. Lawson, and J. Jamart. "Laser-Assisted Surgery Addressing Snoring Long-Term Outcome Comparing CO_2 Laser vs. CO_2 Laser Combined with Diode Laser." *Acta Otorhinolaryngologica Belgica* 56 (2002): 177-182.

Stevenson, J. E. "Diagnosis of Sleep Apnea." *Wisconsin Medical Journal* 102 (2003): 25–27, 46.

Trotter, M. I., A. R. D'Souza, and D. W. Morgan. "Medium-Term Outcome of Palatal Surgery for Snoring Using the Somnus Unit." *Journal of Laryngology and Otology* 116 (February 2002): 116-118.

ORGANIZATIONS

American Academy of Otolaryngology, Head and Neck Surgery, Inc. One Prince Street, Alexandria, VA 22314-3357. (703) 836-4444. <http://www.entnet.org>.

American Academy of Sleep Medicine (AASM). One Westbrook Corporate Center, Suite 920, Westchester, IL 60154. (708) 492-0930. <http://www.aasmnet.org>.

American Dental Association. 211 East Chicago Avenue, Chicago, IL 60611. (312) 440-2500. <http://www.ada.org>.

American Sleep Apnea Association. *Wake-Up Call: The Wellness Letter for Snoring and Apnea.* 1424 K Street NW, Suite 302, Washington, DC 20005. (202) 293-3650. http://www.sleepapnea.org.

National Sleep Foundation. 1522 K Street, NW, Suite 500, Washington, DC 20005. http://www.sleepfoundation.org.

KEY TERMS

. . . .

Ablation—The removal of abnormal tissue growths by surgery.

Cauterize—To seal tissue or blood vessels using a heat or electrical source.

Continuous positive airway pressure (CPAP)—A ventilation device that blows a gentle stream of air into the nose during sleep to keep the airway open.

Deviated septum—A hole or perforation in the septum, the wall that divides the two nasal cavities.

Endoscope—A slender optical instrument that allows a doctor to examine the inside of the throat or other hollow organ. Sleep endoscopy is a technique that allows the doctor to detect previously unsuspected obstructions in the patient's nose and throat.

Obstructive sleep apnea (OSA)—A potentially life-threatening condition characterized by episodes of breathing cessation during sleep alternating with snoring or disordered breathing. The low levels of oxygen in the blood of patients with OSA may eventually cause heart problems or stroke.

Polysomnography—A technique for diagnosing sleep disorders with the use of a machine that records the pulse, breathing rate and other variables while the patient sleeps.

Soft palate—The structure at the roof of the mouth that separates the mouth and the pharynx

---

OTHER

American Sleep Apnea Association (ASAA). *Considering Surgery for Snoring?* <http://www.sleepapnea.org/snoring.html>.

National Heart, Lung, and Blood Institute (NHLBI). *Facts About Sleep Apnea*. NIH Publication No. 95-3798. <http://www.nhlbi.nih.gov/health/public/sleep/sleepapn.htm>.

Paula Ford-Martin
Rebecca J. Frey, PhD

Sodium

Description

Known to most people in the form of table salt, sodium is one of the minerals that the body needs in relatively large quantities. Humankind's taste for sodium reaches far back into the distant past. Much like today, sodium was popular in antiquity as a food preservative and an ingredient in snacks. In some ancient societies, sodium was even used as a form of currency.

In modern times, most Americans and other Westerners consume far too much of the mineral, and it is easy to see why. One obvious culprit is table salt, which has a high sodium content. The mineral is also found in many of America's favorite foods (or the chemicals used to preserve those foods). Sodium can be found in potato chips and a variety of other snacks, processed foods, meat, fish, butter and margarine, soft drinks, dairy products, canned vegetables, and bread, just to name a few sources. A single slice of pizza can supply the body with all the sodium it needs for one day (about 500 mg), while a teaspoon of table salt contains four times that amount.

A certain intake of sodium is considered essential to life. The mineral is a vital component of all bodily fluids, including blood and sweat. Often working in combination with other minerals such as **potassium**, sodium helps to manage the distribution and pH balance of these fluids inside the body and plays an important role in blood pressure regulation. Sodium is referred to as an electrolyte because it possesses a mild electrical charge when dissolved in bodily fluids. Due to this charge, sufficient amounts of the mineral are necessary for the normal functioning of nerve transmissions and muscle contractions. Sodium also helps the body to retain water and prevent dehydration, and may have some activity as an antibacterial.

The important benefits associated with sodium become apparent in cases of sodium deficiency, which is relatively uncommon. Sodium deficiency is most likely to occur in cases of starvation, **diarrhea**, intense sweating, or other conditions that cause rapid loss of water from the body. People who suffer from low sodium levels may experience a wide range of bothersome or serious health problems, including digestive disorders, muscle twitching or weakness, **memory loss**, **fatigue**, and lack of concentration or appetite. Arthritis may also develop. These problems usually occur when fluids that belong in the bloodstream take a wrong turn and enter cells.

General use

Most Americans consume anywhere from 3,000 mg to 20,000 mg of sodium a day. These amounts are much more than the body needs to function at an optimal level. Many **nutrition** experts are concerned about the rise in sodium intake in the general population in the last twenty years. Much of this increase is due to the popularity of fast foods and salty snacks, including the sale of high-sodium snack foods in school cafeterias or vending machines.

While sodium deficiencies are rare, supplements may be required in people with certain medical conditions such as Addison's disease, adrenal gland tumors, kidney disease, or low blood pressure. More sodium may also be needed by those who experience severe dehydration or by people who take diuretic drugs.

Though taking extra amounts of sodium is not known to improve health or cure disease, the mineral may have some therapeutic value when used externally. A number of medical studies in people suggest that soaking in water from the Dead Sea may be beneficial in the treatment of various diseases such as **rheumatoid arthritis**, psoriatic arthritis, and **osteoarthritis** of the knees. Located in Israel, the Dead Sea is many times saltier than ocean water and rich in other minerals such as **magnesium**, potassium, and **calcium**. In one small study, published in 1995 by researchers from the Soroka Medical Center in Israel, nine people with rheumatoid arthritis showed significant improvement in their condition after bathing in the Dead Sea for 12 days. The control group in the study, whose members did not bathe in the Dead Sea, failed to improve. The beneficial effects of the Dead Sea soaks lasted for up to three months after they had stopped bathing in the famous body of water. Despite intriguing findings such as these, no one knows for certain if sodium plays a major role in the therapeutic powers associated with the Dead Sea soaks.

Sodium has a reputation as a germ killer. Some people use a sodium solution as an antibacterial mouthwash to combat microorganisms that cause **sore throat** or inflamed gums. Plain saltwater soaks have also been recommended as a remedy for sweaty feet. Salt is believed to have a drying effect by soaking up excess perspiration. In ages past, saltwater soaks were used to relieve sore or aching muscles.

Preparations

In the late 1990s the National Academy of Sciences established the recommended daily allowance (RDA) of sodium as between 1,100 and 3,300 milligrams.

To prepare a sodium mouthwash, mix 1 tsp of table salt with a glass of warm water. The solution should be swished around in the mouth for about a minute or so. Then spit the mixture out. Try not to swallow the solution, as it contains about 2,000 mg of sodium.

Sodium is available in tablet form, but supplements should only be taken under the supervision of a doctor. As mentioned earlier, most people already get far too much sodium in their **diets**.

A trip to the Dead Sea is not necessary in order to enjoy its potential benefits. Dead Sea bath salts are also available.

Precautions

People who wish to take sodium supplements or increase their sodium intake should talk to a doctor first if they have high blood pressure (or a family history of the disease), congestive heart failure (or other forms of heart or blood vessel disease), hepatic **cirrhosis**, **edema**, **epilepsy**, kidney disease, or bleeding problems.

Studies investigating the role of sodium in the development of high blood pressure have produced mixed results. However, sodium is widely believed to contribute to the development of the disease in susceptible people. For this reason, most doctors and major health organizations around the world recommend a diet low in sodium. Eating a low-sodium diet may actually help to lower blood pressure, especially when that diet includes sufficient amounts of potassium.

A 20-year-long follow-up study to the National Health and Nutrition Examination Survey that was conducted between 1971–1975 reported in 2002 that high levels of sodium in the diet are an independent risk factor for congestive heart failure (CHF) in overweight adults. The authors of the study suggested that lowering the rate of sodium intake may play an important role in lowering the risk of CHF in overweight populations as well as individuals.

Another good reason for limiting one's intake of sodium is the link between high levels of dietary sodium and an increased risk of stomach **cancer**. This risk is increased if a person's diet is also low in fresh fruits and vegetables.

Apart from an increase in blood pressure, high levels of sodium may cause confusion, **anxiety**, edema, **nausea**, **vomiting**, restlessness, weakness, and loss of potassium and calcium.

People who are concerned about consuming too much sodium should try to keep their sodium intake below 2500 mg per day. This is the level recommended by the US Department of Health and Human Services and the US Department of Agriculture in their 2000 Dietary Guidelines for Americans. Ways to reduce sodium intake include the following:

- Reading the Nutrition Facts labels on processed food items. The amount of sodium in a specific processed food, such as cake mix or canned soup, can vary widely from brand to brand.

- Retraining the taste buds. A taste for salt is acquired. A gradual decrease in the use of salt to season foods gives the taste buds time to adjust.

- Using other spices and herbs to season food.

- Cooking from scratch rather than using processed foods.

- Substituting fresh fruits and vegetables for salty snack foods.

- Tasting food at the table before adding salt. Many people salt their food automatically before eating it, which often adds unnecessary sodium to the daily intake.

- Choosing foods that are labeled "low sodium" or "sodium free."

- Watching the sodium content of over-the-counter medications, and asking a pharmacist for information about the sodium content of prescription drugs.

Restricting sodium intake is not usually recommended for women who are pregnant or breast-feeding.

Side effects

Dietary sodium is not associated with any bothersome or significant short-term side effects. In some people, however, salt tablets may cause upset stomach or affect kidney function.

Interactions

Sodium may promote the loss of calcium and potassium from the body. In addition, sodium in the diet should be restricted for such medications as antihypertensives (drugs to control blood pressure) and anticoagulants (blood thinners) to be fully effective.

Resources

BOOKS

Pelletier, Kenneth R., MD. *The Best Alternative Medicine*, Part I: Food for Thought. New York: Simon & Schuster, 2002.

Sifton, David W. *PDR Family Guide to Natural Medicines and Healing Therapies*. New York: Three Rivers Press, 1999.

PERIODICALS

Becker, Elizabeth, and Marian Burros. "Eat Your Vegetables? Only at a Few Schools." *New York Times*, January 13, 2003.

He, J., L. G. Ogden, L. A. Bazzano, et al. "Dietary Sodium Intake and Incidence of Congestive Heart Failure in Overweight US Men and Women: First National Health and Nutrition Examination Survey Epidemiologic Follow-up Study." *Archives of Internal Medicine* 162 (July 22, 2002): 1619-1624.

Ngoan, L. T., T. Mizoue, Y. Fujino, et al. "Dietary Factors and Stomach Cancer Mortality." *British Journal of Cancer* 87 (July 1, 2002): 37-42.

Nielsen, S. J., A. M. Siega-Riz, and B. M. Popkin. "Trends in Food Locations and Sources Among Adolescents and Young Adults." *Preventive Medicine* 35 (August 2002): 107-113.

KEY TERMS

Calcium—A mineral necessary for strong bones and the proper functioning of organs and muscles.

Diuretic—An agent that increases the production of urine.

Edema—Abnormal swelling of tissue due to fluid buildup. Edema, which typically occurs in the legs, liver, and lungs, is often a complication of heart or kidney problems.

Electrolytes—Substances in the blood, such as sodium and potassium, that help to regulate fluid balance in the body.

Sukenik, S."Balneotherapy for Rheumatic Diseases at the Dead Sea Area." *Israeli Journal of Medicine and Science.* (1996): S16–9.

Sukenik, S., D. Flusser, and S. Codish et al."Balneotherapy at the Dead Sea Area for Knee Osteoarthritis." *Israeli Journal of Medicine and Science.* (1999):83–5.

ORGANIZATIONS

American Heart Association. 7272 Greenville Avenue, Dallas, TX 75231. http://www.americanheart.org/.

National Academy of Sciences. 500 Fifth Street, NW, Washington, DC 20001. <www4.nationalacademies.org/nas>.

Greg Annussek
Rebecca J. Frey, PhD

Somatics

Definition

Somatics, from *soma*, a Greek word for living body, is a **movement therapy** that employs mind-body training to manage muscular **pain** and spasticity, improve balance and posture, and increase ease of motion. It presents an alternative to treatment by **osteopathy**, physical therapy, chiropractics, and/or **massage therapy**.

Origins

Somatic therapy was developed by Thomas Hanna in 1976. Hanna was a follower of **Moshe Feldenkrais**, a twentieth-century physicist whose self-named method is based on the philosophy that all movement, thought, speech, and feelings are a reflection of one's self-image. The **Feldenkrais method** is practiced in group sessions called Awareness Through Movement and in individual sessions called Functional Integration. Hanna, a former philosophy professor by training, became a Functional Integrationist. He also subscribed to the teachings of Hans Selye, a medical researcher who taught that physiological diseases have their origins in psychological causes, especially the presence of **stress**.

In creating what he called Hanna Somatic Education, Hanna hypothesized that the body's sensory-motor system responds to the stresses and traumas of daily life with specific muscular reflexes that become involuntary and habitual contractions. These contractions cause stiffness and soreness. Eventually, the individual suffers from sensory-motor amnesia (SMA), a loss of meaning of how muscles feel and how to control them.

Benefits

Practitioners believe that by re-educating the muscular system, somatic therapy can cure or relieve a variety of complaints including but not limited to adhesive capsulitis, arthritis, back pain, balance problems, dislocation of joints, displaced patella, **dizziness**, foot pain, frequent urination, hamstring pulls, headaches, joint pain, **obesity**, sacroiliac pain, **sciatica**, **scoliosis**, shoulder tightness and pain, spinal stenosis, **temporomandibular joint syndrome** (TMJ), thoracic outlet syndrome, uneven leg length, and whiplash injuries. Somatic education is also taught to combat the decreased ease of motion associated with **aging**.

Description

Hanna named three reflexes that lead to SMA. The red light reflex (startle response) is a withdrawal response in the abdominal muscles in which the body curves in on itself in response to distress. The green light reflex (Landau arousal response) involves the back muscles and the action response in which the body is constantly thrusting forward in response to daily responsibilities. The trauma reflex occurs when the body suffers an injury.

Hanna theorized that because these reflexes are learned, they can be unlearned. To that end, he developed a series of exercises. During somatic education sessions, the individual is taught to release the chronic tension-holding patterns.

Somatic exercises are slow-motion movements performed in prone or sitting positions. During the various movements, the individual is instructed to be aware of the way his or her muscles feel at each step. Deep breathing techniques are also used at various stages.

The goal of the therapy is to teach the individual the ability to control muscle problems. Relief should occur within two to eight sessions. The effects are cumulative, increasing as flexibility and ease of movement improve. As the body gives up restricted physical patterns, it also tends to release rigid psychological habits.

After the education sessions, the individual is encouraged to continue the exercises on his or her own. Sessions can range from as little as 15 minutes per day to as long as three to four hours.

Sessions can cost between $50 and $175 each, depending on the practitioner's level of experience. Insurance coverage varies with the carrier but is more likely if a physician prescribes somatic therapy.

Gradual movement and awareness of the body are emphasized throughout Hanna Somatic Education.

• Always move slowly, gently, and without forcing the movement.

• Always focus your attention on the internal sensations of the movement.

Preparations

The exercises should be performed in a comfortable and quiet setting. Clothing should be loose and allow for easy movement. A floor mat or other comfortable surface is recommended.

Precautions

Before embarking on any type of therapy to relieve pain, the patient should consult a physician. Severe pain in any part of the body could indicate serious disease or injury.

Side effects

There are no known adverse side effects to somatic therapy.

Research & general acceptance

The bulk of the research into the effects of somatic therapy has been conducted within the discipline itself. Not surprisingly, these studies show positive results across the board. Somatic education is a slow-growing field; there are currently less than 100 certified practitioners worldwide.

However, the scientific medical profession has conducted studies on the effects of various types of **exercise** on chronic musculoskeletal pain. Although results are inconclusive, findings show that pain is minimized somewhat during the period in which the exercise is undertak-

---

KEY TERMS

Adhesive capsulitis—Adhesions and inflammation in the shoulder capsule that restrict movement.

Kinesiology—The study of the principles of mechanics and anatomy in relation to human movement.

Sacroiliac—The joint at which the upper hip bone joins the backbone to the pelvis.

Sciatica—Pain along one of the two sciatic nerves that run from the pelvic area down the backs of the thighs to the feet.

Scoliosis—A lateral (sideways) curvature of the spine.

Spinal stenosis—Pain and tension in the spine due to abnormal constriction.

Thoracic outlet syndrome—Spasticity of the muscles of the upper back, neck, and/or shoulders.

TMJ syndrome—Tightness and pain in the jaw and neck muscles

---

en. In addition, preliminary research points to a possible link between muscles, memory, and emotion.

Training & certification

The Novato Institute for Somatic Research and Training, which Hanna founded in 1976 conducts a three-year training program that covers studies in anatomy, functional and structural kinesiology, physical evaluation, neurophysiology, and practical methods. Applicants must pass three annual examination in order to be certified. Admittance to the program is usually limited to individuals with training in related fields, particularly physicians, chiropractors, physical therapists, and certified massage therapists.

Resources

BOOKS

Credit, Larry P., Sharon G. Hartunian, and Margaret J. Nowak. *The Feldenkrais Method in Your Guide to Complementary Medicine.* Garden City, New Jersey: Avery Publishing Group, 1998.

Hanna, Thomas. *Somatics.* Reading, Massachusetts: Addison-Wesley, 1988.

ORGANIZATIONS

Novato Institute for Research & Training. 1516 W. Grant Avenue, Suite 212, Novato, California 94945. 415-897-0336. http://www.somatics.com/.

Mary McNulty

Sore throat

Definition

Sore throat, also called pharyngitis, is a painful inflammation of the back of the throat. It is a symptom of many conditions, but most often is associated with colds or **influenza**. Sore throat may be caused by either viral or bacterial **infections** or by environmental conditions. Most sore throats heal without complications, but they should not be ignored because some develop into serious illnesses.

Description

Almost everyone gets a sore throat at one time or another, although children in child care or grade school have them more often than adolescents and adults. Sore throats are most common during the winter months when upper respiratory infections (colds) and influenza are more frequent.

Sore throats can be either acute or chronic. Acute sore throats are the more common. They may appear suddenly and last approximately three to about seven days. A chronic sore throat that is still present after three weeks may be a symptom of an unresolved underlying condition or disease, such as a **sinus infection** or **mononucleosis**.

Causes & symptoms

Sore throats have many different causes, and may or may not be accompanied by cold symptoms, **fever**, or swollen lymph glands. Proper treatment depends on identifying the cause.

Viral sore throat

Viruses cause 90–95% of all sore throats. Cold and flu viruses are the main culprits. These viruses cause an inflammation in the throat and occasionally the tonsils (**tonsillitis**). Cold symptoms usually accompany a viral sore throat. These can include a runny nose, **cough**, congestion, hoarseness, **conjunctivitis**, fever, and swollen lymph nodes in the neck. The level of throat **pain** varies from uncomfortable to excruciating, when it is painful for the patient to eat, breathe, swallow, or speak.

Another group of viruses that cause sore throat are the adenoviruses. These may also cause infections of the lungs and ears. In addition to a sore throat, symptoms that accompany an adenovirus infection may include cough, runny nose, white bumps on the tonsils and throat, mild **diarrhea**, **vomiting**, and a rash. The sore throat lasts about one week.

A third type of virus that can cause severe sore throat is the coxsackie virus. It can cause a disease called herpangina. Although anyone can get herpangina, it is most common in children up to age 10 and is more prevalent in the summer or early autumn. Herpangina is sometimes called summer sore throat.

Three to six days after being exposed to the virus, an infected person develops a sudden sore throat that is usually accompanied by a fever usually between 102–104°F (38.9–40°C). Tiny grayish-white **blisters** form on the throat and in the mouth. These fester and become small ulcers. Throat pain is often severe, interfering with swallowing. Children may easily become dehydrated if they are reluctant to eat or drink because of the pain. In addition, people with herpangina may vomit, have abdominal pain, and generally feel ill and miserable.

Another common cause of a viral sore throat is mononucleosis. Mononucleosis occurs when the Epstein-Barr virus infects one specific type of lymphocyte. The infection may spread to the lymphatic system, respiratory system, liver, spleen, and throat. Symptoms appear 30–50 days after exposure.

Mononucleosis, sometimes called the kissing disease, is extremely common in young adults. It is estimated that by the age of 35–40, 80–95% of Americans will have had mononucleosis. Often, symptoms are mild, especially in young children, and are diagnosed as a cold. Since symptoms are more severe in adolescents and adults, more cases are diagnosed as mononucleosis in this age group. One of the main symptoms of mononucleosis is a severe sore throat.

Although a runny nose and cough are much more likely to accompany a sore throat caused by a virus than one caused by a bacteria, there is no absolute way to tell what is causing the sore throat without a laboratory test. Viral sore throats are contagious and are passed directly from person to person by coughing and **sneezing**.

Bacterial sore throat

From 5–10% of sore throats are caused by bacteria. The most common bacterial sore throat results from an infection by group A *Streptococcus*. This type of infection is commonly called **strep throat**, or GABHS pharyngitis. The acronym stands for "Group A beta-hemolytic streptococci." Anyone can get strep throat, but it is most common in school age children. Since three is a low risk of strep throat invading and damaging heart valves (**rheumatic fever**), it is important to see a doctor who may prescribe antibiotics to eliminate the risk.

Pharyngeal **gonorrhea**, a sexually transmitted bacterial disease, causes a severe sore throat. Gonorrhea in the throat is transmitted by having oral sex with an infected person.

Noninfectious sore throat

Not all sore throats are caused by infection. Postnasal drip from **allergies** and airborne irritants can cause sore throat. It can be caused by **hay fever** and other allergies that irritate the sinuses. Environmental and other conditions, such as heavy **smoking** or breathing secondhand smoke, breathing polluted air or chemical fumes, or swallowing substances that burn or scratch the throat can also cause pharyngitis. Dry air, like that in airplanes or from forced hot air furnaces, can make the throat sore. People who breathe through their mouths at night because of nasal congestion often get sore throats that improve as the day progresses. Sore throat caused by environmental conditions is not contagious.

Diagnosis

It is easy for people to tell if they have a sore throat, but difficult to diagnose its cause without seeing a doctor and having laboratory tests. Most sore throats are minor and heal without any complications. A small number of bacterial sore throats develop into serious diseases. It is advisable to see a doctor if a sore throat lasts more than a few days or is accompanied by fever, **nausea**, or abdominal pain.

Diagnosis of a sore throat by a doctor begins with a physical examination of the throat and chest. The doctor will also look for signs of other illness, such as a sinus infection or **bronchitis**. Since both bacterial and viral sore throats are contagious and pass easily from person to person, the doctor will seek information about whether the patient has been around other people with flu, sore throat, colds, or strep throat. If it appears that the patient may have strep throat, the doctor will do laboratory tests.

One test that doctors are using more often in diagnosing a sore throat is the rapid antigen test. While a throat culture may require 2 days for the laboratory to identify the causative organism, a rapid antigen test gives results in a few hours.

If mononucleosis is suspected, the doctor may do a Monospot test to look for antibodies indicating the presence of the Epstein-Barr virus. The test in inexpensive, takes only a few minutes, and can be done in a physician's office. An inexpensive blood test can also determine the presence of antibodies to the mononucleosis virus.

Treatment

Effective treatment varies depending on the cause of the sore throat. As frustrating as it may be to the patient,

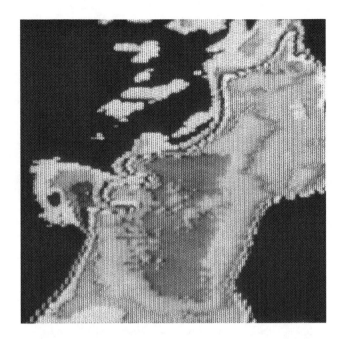

A thermographic image showing a sore throat. *(Photograph by Howard Sochurek, The Stock Market. Reproduced by permission.)*

viral sore throat is best left to run its course without drug treatment. Antibiotics have no effect on a viral sore throat. They do not shorten the length of the illness, nor do they lessen the symptoms.

Treatment uses antiviral plants and herbs and vitamins to boost immunity and speed recovery.

• Aromatherapists recommend inhaling the fragrances of **essential oils** of **lavender** (Lavandula officinalis), **thyme** (*Thymus vulgaris*), **eucalyptus** (*Eycalyptus globulus*), **sage** (*Salvia officinalis*), and sandalwood.

• Ayurvedic practitioners suggest gargling with a mixture of water, salt, and **turmeric** (*Curcuma longa*) powder or astringents such as alum, sumac, sage, and **bayberry** (*Myrica* spp.).

• Herbalists recommend taking **osha** root (*Ligusticum porteri*)internally for infection, or drinking **ginger** (*Zingiber officinale*) or **slippery elm** (*Ulmus fulva*) tea for pain.

• Homeopaths may treat sore throats with superdilute solutions of *Lachesis, Belladonna,* or *Phytolacca,* yellow jasmine (*Gelsemium*), or mercury *(Mercurius).*

• Nutritional recommendations include **zinc** lozenges every two hours along with **vitamin C** with **bioflavonoids, vitamin A**, and beta-carotene supplements.

In the case of chronic sore throat, it is necessary to treat the underlying disease to heal the sore throat. If a sore throat is caused by environmental factors, the aggravating stimulus should be eliminated from the sufferer's environment. In the case of chronic sore throat in a child, the doctor may recommend a tonsillectomy (surgical removal of the tonsils).

Home care for sore throat

Regardless of the cause of a sore throat, there are some home care steps that people can take to ease their discomfort. These include:

- Gargling with warm double strength tea or warm salt water made by adding one teaspoon of salt to 8 oz of water.

- Drinking plenty of fluids, but avoiding acid juices like orange juice, which can irritate the throat. Sucking on popsicles is a good way to get fluids into children.

- Eating soft, nutritious foods like noodle soup and avoiding spicy foods.

- Refraining from smoking.

- Resting until the fever is gone, then resuming strenuous activities gradually.

- A room humidifier may make sore throat sufferers more comfortable.

- Antiseptic lozenges and sprays may aggravate the sore throat rather than improve it.

Allopathic treatment

Sore throat caused by a streptococci or another bacteria must be treated with antibiotics. Penicillin is the preferred medication. Oral penicillin must be taken for 10 days. Patients need to take the entire amount of antibiotic prescribed, even after symptoms of the sore throat improve. Stopping the antibiotic early can lead to a return of the sore throat. Sometimes a single injection of long-acting penicillin G is given instead of 10 days of oral treatment. These medications generally cost under $15.

Because mononucleosis is caused by a virus, there is no specific drug treatment available. Rest, a healthy diet, plenty of fluids, limiting heavy **exercise** and competitive sports, and treatment of aches with acetaminophen (Datril, Tylenol, Panadol) or ibuprofen (Advil, Nuprin, Motrin, Medipren) are the prescribed treatments. Nearly 90% of mononucleosis infections are mild. The infected person does not normally get the disease again.

Aspirin should not be given to children because of its association with increased risk for Reye's Syndrome, a serious disease.

Expected results

Sore throat caused by a viral infection generally clears up on its own within one week with no complica-

KEY TERMS

Antigen—A foreign protein to which the body reacts by making antibodies

Conjunctivitis—An inflammation of the membrane surrounding the eye. Conjunctivitis is sometimes called "pinkeye."

Lymphocyte—A type of white blood cell. Lymphocytes play an important role in fighting disease.

Pharynx—The part of the throat that lies between the mouth and the larynx or voice box.

Toxin—A poison. In the case of scarlet fever, the toxin is secreted as a byproduct of the growth of the streptococcus bacteria and causes a rash.

tions. The exception is mononucleosis. Ninety percent of cases of mononucleosis clear up without medical intervention or complications, so long as dehydration does not occur. In young children the symptoms may last only a week, but in adolescents the symptoms last longer. Adults over age 30 have the most severe and long lasting symptoms. Adults may take up to six months to recover. In all age groups **fatigue** and weakness may continue for up to six weeks after other symptoms disappear.

In rare cases of mononucleosis, breathing may be obstructed because of swollen tonsils, adenoids, and lymph glands. If this happens, the patient should immediately seek emergency medical care.

Patients with bacterial sore throat begin feeling better about 24 hours after starting antibiotics. Untreated strep throat has the potential to cause **scarlet fever**, kidney damage, or rheumatic fever. Scarlet fever causes a rash, and can cause high fever and convulsions. Rheumatic fever causes inflammation of the heart and damage to the heart valves. Taking antibiotics within the first week of a strep infection will prevent these complications. People with strep throat remain contagious until after they have been taking antibiotics for 24 hours.

Prevention

There is no way to prevent a sore throat; however, the risk of getting one or passing one on to another person can be minimized by:

- Washing hands with warm water and soap frequently.

- Maintaining a balanced life with adequate sleep, **nutrition**, and personal fulfillment.

- Avoiding close contact with someone who has a sore throat.

• Not sharing food and eating utensils with anyone.

• Not smoking.

• Optimizing the functioning of the immune system by exercising and eating such immune-boosting foods as carrots, yams, shiitake mushrooms, etc.

• Avoiding sources of air pollution.

Resources

BOOK

Berkow, Robert. *The Merck Manual of Diagnosis and Therapy* Rahway, NJ: Merck Research Laboratories, 1992.

PERIODICALS

Larkin, Marilynn. "A Single, Rapid Test Suffices for Pharyngitis Diagnosis in High-Risk Patients." *Lancet* 358 (December 8, 2001): 1969.

National Institute of Allergy and Infectious Diseases. *Infectious Mononucleosis Fact Sheet* http://www.niaid.nih.gov/factsheets/infmono.htm (September 1997).

Kathleen Wright
Rebecca J. Frey, PhD

Soul revival *see* **Shamanism**

Sound therapy

Definition

Sound therapy refers to a range of therapies in which sound is used to treat physical and mental conditions. One of these therapies is **music therapy**, which can involve a person listening to music for conditions such as **stress** and muscle tension.

Music is one component of this therapy. Others use sound wave vibrations to treat physical and mental conditions. In general, this therapy is based on the theory that all of life vibrates, including people's bodies. When a person's healthy resonant frequency is out of balance, physical and emotional health is affected.

Treatment by sound waves is believed to restore that healthy balance to the body. Healing is done by transmitting beneficial sound to the affected area. The healing sound may be produced by a voice or an instrument such as electronic equipment, chanting bowls, or tuning forks.

Origins

Indigenous societies around the world have traditionally used sound in healing ceremonies, including drumming, hand-clapping, singing, dancing, and pulsat-

ing. The broad spectrum of sound therapy includes chanting, an activity long connected to healing and religion, and sounds of nature. Different sounds have elicited a variety of emotional responses and altered mental and physical states in people. One recent brain-imaging study found that spine-tingling music "lights up" the same parts of the brain that are stimulated by food, sex, and certain types of drugs.

For example, the chimes of a church bell pealed for such happy occasions as weddings and harvest festivals, and tolled slowly to announce a death. The connection between sound and healing was chronicled in 1896 when American physicians discovered that certain types of music improved thought processes and spurred blood flow. More advances in sound therapy came after World War II. Music therapy began in the 1940s, when it was used as part of rehabilitation treatment for soldiers.

During the 1950s and 1960s, sound wave therapy developed in Europe. The British osteopath Sir Peter Guy Manners developed a machine that treated patients with healing vibrations. The machine is placed on the area to be treated and a frequency is set to match the cells of a healthy body. Advocates believe that the treatment makes the body's cells vibrate at a healthy resonance.

By the 1990s, Manners had developed a computerized system with about 800 frequencies used to treat a range of conditions. Similar therapies are also known by names such as bioresonance and vibrational therapy. This therapy is used to treat such conditions as **cancer**.

After Manners developed his therapy, two ear specialists in France developed therapies that focus on listening. Dr. Alfred Tomatis' method and Dr. Guy Berard's **auditory integration training** involve the patient listening to sounds through headphones. Currently, the Tomatis method is used to treat conditions ranging from learning disabilities to **anxiety** in both children and adults.

From the 1960s on, interest in alternative medicine and New Age healing has led to a wide variety of sound healing therapies. These range from the ancient practice of chanting and the use of singing bowls to vibroacoustic furniture. A person sits or lies on a chair or bed and music is directed into the body. Benefits are said to include lowered blood pressure.

Benefits

Sound therapy focuses on balancing energy to treat a condition. Advocates maintain that sound therapy is effective in treating such conditions as stress, anxiety, high blood pressure, **depression**, and **autism**. Chanting and overtone chanting are used in therapy with Alzheimer's patients. This form of sound therapy is said to help with memory function. Some researchers think that music

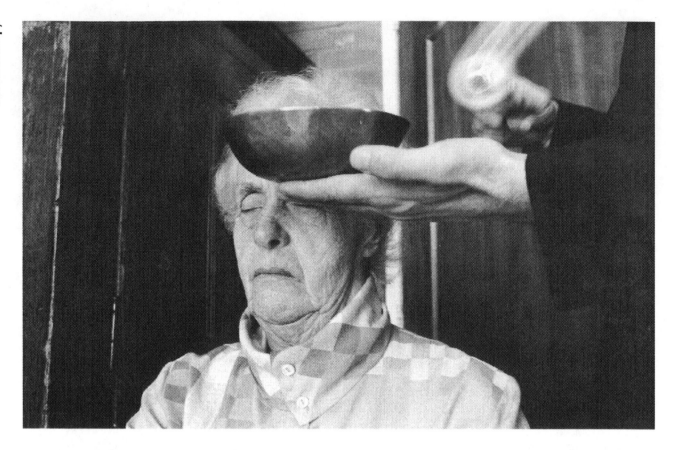

A practitioner of Tibetan sound therapy with patient. In this therapy, metal bowls are struck to produce specific sounds that are said to resonate in the body. *(Photo Researchers, Inc. Reproduced by permission.)*

memories may outlast some other types of memories because music involves many parts of the brain.

A newer form of sound therapy that is used with Alzheimer's patients is called multisensory or Snoezelen therapy. The name "Snoezelen" comes from two Dutch words that mean "to sniff" and "to doze." It was originally developed to treat disabled children by stimulating all the senses. Snoezelen therapy takes place in specially constructed rooms in which patients can, for example, produce music simply by walking in front of a sound beam. The sound beam, which looks like a microphone, "translates" the patient's movements into music. Other Snoezelen devices include fiber-optic cables that glow when patients wrap them around their bodies, and a chair that vibrates as it plays music through internal speakers. In this way, even deaf patients can "feel" the music as it plays. Snoezelen therapy has been found to reduce **pain** in Alzheimer's patients without the need for extra medication.

Physical conditions treated by sound therapy include pain during labor, muscle and joint pain like arthritis, back pain, sports injuries, soft tissue damage, and cancer.

The Tomatis method is used for conditions including **dyslexia**, attention deficit hyperactivity disorder (ADHD), Down syndrome, **chronic fatigue syndrome**, autism, depression, and behavioral problems. The method, also known as listening therapy, is used to help older people with coordination and motor problems. Furthermore, performers take the therapy to refine their skills.

Description

The spectrum of sound therapy is so broad that a person has many choices about the type of treatment and its cost. Some therapies can be done at home; others require a practitioner or therapist to perform the therapy or to provide initial instruction. As of 2002, most health plans did not cover the cost of any form of sound therapy, including music therapy. However, some sound therapies may be part of integrative treatment for a condition.

Chanting and toning

Chanting and toning are among the complementary therapies offered through the integrative medicine program at Memorial Sloan-Kettering Cancer Center in New York City. The program, which opened in April 1999, is one example of how the traditional medical community is incorporating alternative therapies into treatment.

People learn to reach a meditative state by producing a "pure" sound such as a drawn-out vowel. The chanting is said to produce a state of well-being in mind and body. The cost of therapy will vary since a person could take a class or workshop or opt for longer therapy. Treatment could involve weekly hour-long sessions over a period of several months.

Toning refers to using the voice to let out pain or stress. Sound healers point out that people do this naturally when they cry out or sigh. In toning therapy, a healer will help the patient learn healing sounds. Overtoning involves the therapist using his or her voice to assess a client's condition from the feet to the head. The therapist then treats the person by projecting healing sounds or "overtones."

Sounding, also known as toning, strives to improve vocal and listening abilities for emotional release and better communication. It was developed by Don Campbell, who established the Institute for Music, Health, and Education in Boulder, Colorado, in 1988. The discipline is being used in hospitals, schools, and educational centers to release stress. Toning or sounding is the way to massage the body from the inside out.

The Tomatis method

The Tomatis method involves the client using special headphones with bone and air conduction to listen to electronically recorded music frequencies. These are believed to open the brain to greater frequencies of sound. As of 2002, there were more than 250 Tomatis centers located around the world.

Furthermore, the Mozart Center in northern California began offering home treatment in the late 1990s. Treatment for the three-phase program cost $3,210 in mid-2000. Therapy lasted about three months and started with initial testing and instruction about how to use equipment.

The client used the equipment for two hours per day for 15 days. A diary was kept during that time, and a practitioner made weekly check-up calls. A month after therapy started, the practitioner returned to the home and reinstalled the equipment. The two-hour daily therapy continued for 10 days, along with the diary entries. The third phase of therapy continued six weeks later with 10 days of therapy and diary-keeping.

Vibrational therapy

Sound therapies like cymatics have been compared to **acupressure**. An instrument is placed on a point of the body and beneficial sound is directed at that point. The sound directed through the skin is believed to establish healthy resonance in unhealthy tissue.

Other forms of sound therapy

The spectrum of sound therapy includes such other treatments as:

- Audiotapes with special frequencies or music are designed for conditions ranging from **AIDS** to weight problems. Costs will vary. Some recordings are said to target both the emotional and physical aspects of these conditions.

- Tuning forks are used to give the person resonance. This is said to help the person relax and give balance. Costs vary.

- Hemi-sync therapy involves listening to synthesized sounds to balance both hemispheres of the brain. This is said to produce an altered state of consciousness.

- Adaptation of age-old instruments such as the Tibetan singing bowls. Sound from these bowls can be used in conjunction with chanting or **meditation**. Tibetan monks used bronze bowls.

Preparations

Pre-treatment preparation varies with the type of therapy to be undertaken. Some therapies such as the Tomatis method require an assessment and then treatment is administered. Other therapies can be taught by therapists and done at home. Some therapies require little or no training. Equipment such as audiotapes and chanting bowls can be purchased and used with minimal instruction.

Furthermore, organizations like the Sound Healers Association can provide information about training in other types of sound therapy. In addition, some companies sell equipment such as bioresonance machines.

Precautions

Although treatments like the Tomatis method and cymatics require training in those therapies, there are no certification programs for practitioners of other therapies.

While there is no danger from such therapies as chanting, other forms of sound therapy should not be undertaken until a doctor or health practitioner is consulted. People with pacemakers should not do cymatics.

Side effects

Sound therapy has produced no known side effects or complications.

Research & general acceptance

Sound therapy is so diverse that the amount of research and general acceptance in the United States is varied. Music therapy has been accepted within the traditional medical community. Other therapies such as chanting and toning have been integrated into traditional treatment of cancer. Furthermore, some studies indicated that auditory integration training and the Tomatis method could be used for behavioral problems.

Much of the medical community remains dubious about the healing effects of treating patients' unhealthy cells with sound waves. Although a clinic or center may provide testimonials from cured patients, there has been no scientific research to prove this.

While the traditional medical community remains skeptical about some aspects of sound therapy, treatment has been undertaken by people around the world. Therapies are available in areas including North America, Europe, and Japan.

Training & certification

Unlike music therapy, in which the therapist must have a degree and pass a national board certification examination, there are no licensing and training requirements for sound therapists. However, some disciplines may require training in their therapies. The directors of Tomatis Centers are certified specialists in fields including music, speech therapy, and psychology. Furthermore, the Sound Healers Association provides training and sells a national directory of sound healers and such other sound therapy items as books and tapes.

Resources

BOOKS

Albright, Peter. *The Complete Book of Complementary Therapies.* Allentown, PA: People's Medical Society, 1997.

Editors of Time-Life Books. *The Alternative Advisor.* Alexandria, VA: Time-Life Books, 1997.

Gottlieb, Bill. *New Choices in Natural Healing.* Emmaus, PA: Rodale Press, Inc., 1995.

Nash, Barbara. *From Acupuncture to Zen: An Encyclopedia of Natural Therapies.* Alameda, CA: Hunter House, 1996.

Ortiz, John M. *The Tao of Music, Sound Psychology: Using Music to Change Your Life.* Samuel Weiser Inc., 1997.

PERIODICALS

"Brain Health—Music and the Mind." *Harvard Health Letter* 27 (December 2001): np.

Green, Chris. "Light, Sound Prescribed for Pain Relief." *Capper's* 123 (October 16, 2001): 12.

ORGANIZATIONS

Memorial Sloan-Kettering Cancer Center. 1275 York Ave. 68th St., New York, NY 10021. (212) 639-2000. <http://www.mskcc.org>.

Mozart Center (Tomatis method). P.O. Box 76, Jenner, CA 95450. (707) 632-6976. <http://www.mozartcenter.com>.

Sound Healers Association. P.O. Box 2240, Boulder CO, 80306. (303) 443-8181. <http://www.healingsounds.com/sha/sha-about.asp>.

Telesound LTD. 31 Hall Green, Malvern, Worcestershire, UK, WR14 3QY. (0)1684 572506. E-mail: sales@telesound.co.uk. <http://www.telesound.co.uk>.

The Tomatis Method. <http://www.tomatis.com>.

Liz Swain

South Beach diet

Definition

The South Beach diet is a three-phase, carbohydrate-restrictive diet. It emphasizes foods that are low on the glycemic index (GI) and low in saturated fat, such as lean meats, vegetables, cheeses, nuts, and eggs. Unlike other carbohydrate-restrictive **diets**, such as the Atkins and Zone diets, the South Beach diet promotes "good" carbohydrates, such as whole grains and fruit.

Origins

The creator of the South Beach diet, Dr. Arthur Agatston, is considered a leading cardiologist and is the director of the Mount Sinai Cardiac Prevention Center in Miami Beach. Originally, he had intended to design an eating plan to improve the **cholesterol** and insulin levels of his patients. However, Dr. Agatston soon discovered that his patients also lost weight on his plan. After further research, he approached Marie Almon, R.D., chief clinical dietician at the hospital, to help develop the eating plan into an effective diet. The results became the South Beach diet. Having sold more than a million copies since its publication in April 2003, *The South Beach Diet* book has remained on the *New York Times* bestseller list for over a year.

Benefits

The primary benefit of the South Beach diet is considered by many to be its initial rapid and significant weight loss—8–13 lb(4–6 kg) in the first two weeks. After the first two weeks, weight loss continues at a slower rate, averaging 1–2 lb (0.4–1 kg) weekly. In addition to weight loss, the diet reduces cholesterol and insulin levels, thus reducing the risks of diabetes and **heart disease**. It is claimed that the diet is easy to follow because it is designed to eliminate cravings and has more flexible food options after the first two weeks.

Description

In his book, *The South Beach Diet*, Dr. Agatston states that "this diet is not low-carb. Nor is it low-fat."

Instead, the diet focuses on eating the "good" carbohydrates (fruits, vegetables, and whole grains) and "good" fats (olive oil and nuts) rather than eliminating them from the diet entirely.

Dr. Agatston based the core of his dietary plan around the glycemic index –the increase in blood sugar levels by foods containing carbohydrates during a set amount of time.

After consumption, food is metabolized into sugars and promotes the release of the hormone insulin. When the blood contains excess sugar, insulin removes it from the blood stream by storing it in cells, including fat cells. High-glycemic carbohydrates (greater than 70 GI) are metabolized rapidly, which causes elevated insulin production. High levels of insulin result in more blood sugar being stored as fat, thus causing weight gain. This pattern induces craving for more carbohydrates, thus leading to the consumption of more high-GI foods. Low to moderate-GI foods, however, raise insulin levels more slowly and sugars are metabolized more effectively, thus reducing the amount of blood sugar stored as fat. Cravings for more food is reduced. In addition, by eating these low-GI foods, the risk of **insulin resistance** that can lead to **atherosclerosis** and diabetes is reduced. As such, Dr. Agatston designed the South Beach diet to promote foods low on the GI and eliminate the body's craving for high-GI foods.

The South Beach diet consists of three phases. Phase one is the strictest part of the diet and lasts for two weeks. The purpose of Phase one is to banish the dieter's cravings for high-GI foods such as bread, rice, potatoes, pasta, and sugar. Alcohol, fruits, cereal, and such vegetables as carrots and corn are also restricted during Phase one. Instead, protein-rich foods are emphasized, such as lean meat, fish, eggs, cheese, nuts, and vegetables. Coffee and tea are also allowed. Three regular-sized meals are eaten each day, supplemented by mid-morning and mid-afternoon snacks as well as dessert. During this period, the body chemistry will change dramatically until cravings for high-GI foods are eliminated and insulin resistance is improved/lowered. In addition, rapid weight loss is typically experienced.

Phase two reintroduces several of the restricted foods and encourages eating from all the dietary food groups, the expected result being that the body will neither crave high-GI foods nor store food as excess fat to the same degree. Such high-fiber carbohydrates as whole-wheat pasta and bread and most fruits are now permitted. Moderation remains the key to success for this phase and low-GI foods are strongly encouraged. Phase two continues until the dieter reaches his or her ideal weight, ideally averaging a loss of one to two pounds per week.

Phase three, the ultimate goal, focuses solely on weight maintenance. Having reached the ideal weight, the dieter now makes the changed eating habits a lifestyle from this point forward. Basic dietary techniques are still maintained. Only the high-GI foods and "bad" fats from the previous two phases continue to be restricted. Altered body chemistry will promote long-term cardiovascular health and reduce the risk of diabetes. Should weight gain occur, Phase one of South Beach diet is reintroduced until the weight goal is achieved.

Preparations

There are no initial preparations required for the South Beach diet. However, as with most diets, it is wise to consult with a physician beforehand. Blood testing for insulin, glucose, and cholesterol levels is suggested. It is strongly recommended that dieters taking medications for medical conditions such as heart disease consult a physician before going on the South Beach diet. Similarly, diabetics on insulin or other medications are advised to have a doctor monitor their blood sugar regularly and determine if they are at risk of kidney impairment while on the diet. It is also recommended that a registered dietitian be consulted to determine the dietary needs of certain medical conditions, such as **pregnancy**.

Precautions

The South Beach diet is not recommended for people suffering from or at risk of kidney problems. The diet's high protein content can place increased strain on the kidneys, possibly causing long-term damage as well as **kidney stones** and bone loss. Additionally, the possibility of ketosis-induced dehydration during Phase one can increase the risk of further kidney impairment. Dehydration occurs when the body experiences water loss with accompanying loss of important blood salts like **potassium** and **sodium**. Ketosis occurs when carbohydrates are not available and the body burns an excessive amount of fat, during which some ketones, or fat fragments, are excreted. The restrictive nature of Phase one may also induce mineral and vitamin deficiencies. Remaining in Phase one of the diet for longer than two weeks greatly increases the risk of losing bone and muscle mass. Dieters should remain in Phase one for no longer than three or four weeks.

Some **nutrition** professionals contend that the South Beach diet menus provided in the book lack important nutritional information and detailed portion sizes as well as specific substitutes for foods the dieter cannot or will not eat. They claim that these aspects, combined with the restrictive nature of the diet, can make sticking with the South Beach diet on a long-term basis difficult for some people. Also, they assert that the diet does not emphasize an **exercise** regimen and that exercise is vitally important to avoid the loss of muscle and bone mass, especially during Phase one of the diet.

Side effects

Despite Dr. Agatston's claims to the contrary, the South Beach diet is both a low carbohydrate and a low fat diet. For this reason, one main concern regarding the diet is the risk of ketosis, especially during Phase one. Ketosis can cause such symptoms as dehydration, **dizziness**, heart palpitations, **fatigue**, lightheadedness, and irritability. **Hypoglycemia**, low blood sugar, headaches, and excessive fluid loss are also commonly associated with this diet. Cramping and tired muscles can be incited by salt depletion. Kidney functions can be impaired, possibly leading to serious health issues. Kidney function can be further impaired by the diet's high protein requirements. These side effects typically lessen or fade at the beginning of Phase two, when a more balanced diet is undertaken.

Research & general acceptance

Unlike the majority of low-carbohydrate diets, the medical community generally accepts the South Beach diet. The South Beach diet contains all the major food groups, promotes ingestion of "good" fats for maintaining heart health, and is flexible enough to accommodate most dietary needs.

However, many clinicians and dietitians agree that the rapid initial weight loss results mostly from water loss. Much of this weight can return once the dieter rehydrates.

Another important criticism by medical and nutritional professionals is the lack of evidence to support Dr. Agatston's claims connecting the consumption of low-GI foods and weight loss. They assert that as of the early 2000s, there is no scientific proof that eating low-GI foods will have any more weight loss effect than eating a normal, calorie-reduced diet that includes carbohydrates; that Dr. Agatston also fails to take into account the interaction of different foods when eaten together, which can dramatically alter glucose metabolism; and that this failure means that utilizing the Glycemic Index as a gauge for what foods to eat is not only confusing but also slightly misleading.

Resources

BOOKS

Agatston, Arthur. *The South Beach Diet: The Delicious, Doctor–designed, Foolproof Plan for Fast and Healthy Weight Loss.* New York:Rodale Press, 2003.

PERIODICALS

Abel, Lee. "Somewhere on South Beach." *The Journal of the Arkansas Medical Journal.* (February, 2004): 255–256.
Center for Science in the Public Interest. "Weighing the Diet Books (Cover Story)." *Nutrition Action Healthletter.* (January/February, 2004):3–8.

KEY TERMS

. . . .

Atherosclerosis—The process in which deposits of fatty substances, such as cholesterol, build up in the inner lining of an artery.

Carbohydrates—Neutral compounds of carbon, hydrogen, and oxygen found in sugar, starches, and cellulose.

Glycemic index (GI)—A numeric scale for measuring the level and speed of blood glucose increase that carbohydrate-containing food creates upon consumption.

Insulin—The hormone responsible for converting, in the blood, incoming nutrients into cells.

Insulin resistance—A metabolic state in which the body's cells fail to respond properly to insulin, thus allowing high blood glucose levels to remain in the blood stream longer. This can produce hyperglycemia, diabetes, and other complications including high-blood pressure and elevated fat levels in the blood.

Ketosis—An abnormal increase in ketones (fat fragments) in the body, usually found in people with uncontrolled diabetes mellitus. Ketosis can cause serious side effects, including bad breath, dehydration, and kidney stones.

Goodnough, Abby. "New Doctor, New Diet, but Still No Cookies." *New York Times.* (October 7, 2003): F1.
Harvard Medical School. "Sizing up South Beach." *Harvard Health Letter.* (November, 2003): 5.
Schnirring, Lisa. "The South Beach Diet." *Physician & Sports Medicine.* (January, 2004): 9–10.

OTHER

Keefe, Sarah. "The Lowdown on the South Beach Diet." Askmen.com [cited May 22, 2004] <http://www.askmen.com/sports/foodcourt_100/102_eating_well.html>.
"The South Beach Diet." DietSurf.com. <http://www.dietsurf.com/diet/south_beach_diet.htm>.
"The South Beach Diet." South Beach Diet Online. <http://www.southbeachdiet.com>.
"WebMD Interview with Arthur Agatston, MD." WebMD. <http://my.webmd.com/content/article/71/81355.htm>.

Lee Ann Paradise

Soy protein

Description

Soy protein is derived from the soya bean (*Glycine max*), which has been cultivated in Asia for centuries but has only recently begun to attain wide acceptance in the United States. In the natural product industry, soy has been a staple for years. Recently, soy protein has been recognized as a dietary ingredient that has tremendous potential benefit.

General use

Soy protein is used in many forms for its health benefits, but these claims have only recently been substantiated. Over the course of 20 years, more than 40 studies were conducted to gather human clinical data, which proved that soy helps to reduce the risk of **heart disease**, the number one killer in the United States. In October 1999, the United States Food and Drug Administration (FDA) allowed soy product manufacturers to claim that eating soy as a part of a low fat, low **cholesterol** diet may reduce the risk of coronary (**heart**) disease. The FDA recommendations are for 0.9 oz (25 g) of soy protein per day.

The benefits of soy primarily come from its isoflavone content. Isoflavones are a type of antioxidant that combats cell damage. Genistein and daidzein, the isoflavones present in soy protein, possess antioxidant properties that protect LDL cholesterol from oxidation and are linked to the reduction of cholesterol levels in the blood. Studies have shown that soy protein reduced total cholesterol by 9.3% and lowered LDL (or "bad") cholesterol by almost 13%. Soy also raised HDL (or "good") cholesterol in the blood by over 2%. This result is due to the structure of the amino acid in soy protein. Soy protein differs from meat protein, and changes the way the liver creates and metabolizes cholesterol. Since high cholesterol levels are a major risk factor for the development of heart disease, the benefit of soy in reducing that health problem could be significant for a large segment of the population.

Soy also contains phytoestrogens (plant hormones) that mimic the female hormone estrogen. This fact encourages promoters to tout the benefits of soy for relief of the symptoms of **menopause**. Studies show that eating 20 grams of soy daily for six weeks will help reduce **hot flashes** and other symptoms. Supporters also claim that soy may lower the risk of **osteoporosis, Alzheimer's disease, cancer**, and kidney disease. Unlike the claim for lowering cholesterol, none of these have been conclusively proven, nor has soy received FDA approval for these uses. Because of the potential estrogenic effects of soy proteins, the British Dietetic Association has recommended that soy based infant formulas be used with extreme caution. They warn: "Dietitians should discourage the use of soya protein in children with atopy or cow's milk allergy in the first six months of life to avoid sensitization to soya protein and exposure to phytoestrogens while organ systems remain at their most vulnerable. This would include soy infant formula and soya products such as desserts, etc." Note that this warning is limited to soy protein and does not apply to other soybean products such as soy *lecithin*, which has been used as a cholesterol-lowering agent. The United States FDA and the German Commission E have placed no limits on the use of this soy product and consider it safe even for nursing mothers.

Preparations

Soy is available in a number of forms and is found in many foods:

- Tofu is soy bean curd. It can be used as a meat substitute in many dishes.

- Soy milk is a beverage that can replace cow's milk.

- Soy burgers are specially processed meat substitutes that use a base of soy protein. They may also contain vegetables, cheese, and spices to enhance flavor, but the primary base is usually soy. Some of these products may have a high salt content.

- Soy protein powders are used by mixing them into foods and beverages.

It is important for consumers to realize that the FDA has approved the cholesterol-lowering claim only for products containing "soy protein." Products that are labeled "soy" in general, or isoflavone tablets, cannot make this claim. There is not enough evidence to support claims that soy isoflavones alone lower blood lipid levels or reduce the risk of heart disease. Research has indicated that isoflavones must be present along with soy protein for the cholesterol-lowering effect to take place. In addition, soy products must adhere to strict guidelines in order to make the claim that they are beneficial to a person's health. One serving of a product must contain at least 6.25 grams of soy protein, no more than 20 mg of cholesterol, less than 1 gram of saturated fat, no more than 3 grams of total fat, and no more than 480 milligrams of **sodium**.

Precautions

Some soy products may not meet the standards for the FDA's approval because they are too low in soy protein or too high in saturated fat.

Some researchers warn that adding isoflavones to the diet of postmenopausal women may put them at risk for **breast cancer**. Researchers distinguish between soy protein and isoflavones, and warn that taking isoflavone supplements could result in overdose. A maximum safe level of isoflavones has not been established. In one study, 64 postmenopausal women who took soy protein supplements for one year showed a reduction in breast tenderness and *fibrocystic disease*.

KEY TERMS

. . . .

Atopy—An allergy that is related to a genetic predisposition.

Fibrocystic disease—A common condition in middle aged women, characterized by the growth of one or more cysts in the breasts. Cysts are small inclusions filled with fluid. These are harmless, but may cause pain and tenderness.

Protein—A complex molecule that contains carbon, hydrogen, oxygen, nitrogen, and usually sulfur, which forms an amino acid chain. Proteins are essential for tissue growth and repair.

Soybean—The seed of the plant *Glycine max*.

Side effects

There is no concrete evidence of negative effects from incorporating additional food-based sources of soy protein into the diet. Soy **allergies**, however, are fairly common.

Resources

BOOKS

Blumenthal, M., A. Goldberg, and J. Brinchmann. *Herbal Medicine*. Austin, TX: Amer. Botanical Council, 2000.

PERIODICALS

The British Dietetic Association. "Paediatric group position statement on the use of soya protein for infants." *Journal of Family Health Care* (2003): 93.

Burros, Marian. "Doubts Cloud Rosy News on Soy." *New York Times* (January 26, 2000): F1.

"Soy: The Superfood." *Psychology Today* (March/April 2000): 48.

Stein, Karen. "FDA Approves Health Claim Labeling for Foods Containing Soy Protein." *Journal of the American Dietetic Association* (March 2000): 292.

Zreik, Marwan. "The Great Soy Protein Awakening." *Total Health* (January/February 2000): 52-4.

OTHER

"Say Soy Long to High Cholesterol." *MotherNature.com Health Journal Newsletter*. <http:\\www.mothernature.com>. (October 27, 1999).

Amy Cooper
Samuel Uretsky, Pharm.D.

Spastic colitis *see* **Irritable bowel syndrome**

Spearmint

Description

Spearmint, *Mentha spicata* (sometimes referred to as *M. viridis* and *M. crispa*), is a Mediterranean native known from ancient times as an herb of hospitality. In the symbolism of plants, spearmint conveys wisdom. Common names for this aromatic herb include garden mint, lamb's mint, Our Lady's mint, spire mint, and **sage** of Bethlehem. The Romans brought mints to Britain, and English colonists brought spearmint and other mints to their settlements in North America.

Spearmint is one of at least thirty species in the extensive Lamiaceae, or mint, family. Only the members of the *Mentha* genus, however, are considered "true mints." Mints interbreed quite easily. There are hundreds of hybrids and varieties in this sprawling genus of aromatic herbs, and many have naturalized throughout North America.

A mint used in Chinese medicine is *M. arvensis*, commonly known as field mint or wild mint. The name in China for this highly variable species is *bo he*. This lilac-blossomed herb is used as a cooling remedy in the treatment of **influenza**, **sore throat**, inflammations of the eyes, and head colds. *M. arvensis* is widely prescribed by Chinese herbalists as a carminative (medication given to expel **gas** from the digestive tract) and stomachic (medication given to improve digestive functions). It is also effective in relieving some types of **headache**. In general, field mint is said to be helpful in stimulating movement of the *qi* or life energy that may become stagnated in the liver.

Some herbalists categorize *M. arvensis* and *M. canadensis* as wild mint, a native American species. The species *M. arvensis* var. *piperescens* is known as Japanese mint. It is widely cultivated as a primary commercial source of menthol.

Mints are hardy perennials which spread by underground runners. They may become troublesome weeds in the garden if not tended and controlled. Mints thrive in semi-shade and rich, moist soil. All mints have a square stem with simple leaves growing in opposite pairs. Spearmint leaves are about two inches long, bright green, oblong or lance-shaped, veined and somewhat wrinkled with unevenly toothed margins. The upper leaves are sessile, and the lower leaves have a short stalk. The herb is unbranched and grows in thick clumps in moist areas along roadsides, near streams, and in low meadows and pastures where it may reach a height of two to three feet. The flowers form in a cluster in the leaf axils at the tip of the purple or green stem, tapering nearly to a point. One or more flowering stems flank the central spike. Blossoms are a pale to deep violet color and bloom in July and August. The small tubular flowers each have two long and two short stamens. The brown seeds are tiny and round.

Spearmint contains volatile oil, the flavonoid thymonin, caffeic acid derivatives, rosmaric acid, carvone, and limonene. Spearmint's distinctive, pungent aroma is attributed to the primary constituent of the volatile oil, the chemical carvone.

According to the United States Department of Agriculture (USDA), spearmint is regarded as an invasive weed only in Tennessee and other parts of the South. In the northern Plains states and parts of the Midwest, however, spearmint is raised as a cash crop; it is presently on the list of the 50 top cash crops in the United States. Researchers in Montana are studying spearmint, hoping to discover why it resists a plant disease known as verticillium wilt when **peppermint** is not resistant.

History

Like most medicinal herbs, the mints have found a place in ancient myth and legend. The generic name *Mentha* is derived from the story of the goddess Persephone, who was jealous of Pluto's love for the nymph Minthe, and transformed her rival into a common garden plant. The god Pluto, unable to retrieve the lovely Minthe, assured that her fragrance would waft on the garden breezes, releasing more of the pleasant aroma each time it was trod upon.

In the first century A.D., the naturalist Pliny suggested that students wrap a braid of mint around their heads to bring delight to the soul, thus benefiting the mind and enhancing their scholarship. Aristotle forbade mints to be used by soldiers prior to battle because he believed that the qualities of this herb might diminish their willingness to fight. The smell of "Spere Mynte," according to the herbalist John Gerard writing in 1568, "rejoiceth the heart of man." Mints were commonly used as strewing herbs, both for their fragrance and because they repel mice. Sprigs of fresh mint were also put in grain storage sacks to repel rodents. The steam vapor of infused mint was used to freshen the air in a sickroom. Mints were also used to scent bath water and to "strengthen the nerves and sinews," according to the herbalist Parkinson. Mints were used to whiten the teeth and in a wash to ease irritation of chapped hands. In the Middle Ages, when the bites of mad dogs must have been a common complaint, mints, particularly spearmint and peppermint, were among the many herbs recommended to treat the **wounds** . The mints were mixed with salt and applied directly to the bite. Mints were mentioned in the Bible as herbs the Pharisees used for tithing. Mints were a highly

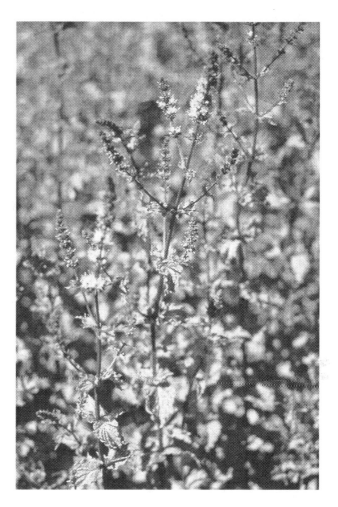

Spearmint (*Mentha spicata*). *(Photo by Henriette Kress. Reproduced by permission.)*

valued medium of exchange in ancient times. Refreshing mint teas were a popular drink during the time of the American Revolution because they were not taxed by the English; in fact, spearmint was an important cash crop in Connecticut at the time of the Revolution. The aromatic tea also enjoyed popularity during the Civil War, when imported black teas were less available.

General use

The various mint species have many common chemical properties and beneficial actions. The fresh or dried leaves and the volatile oil, extracted by steam distillation, are the medicinally useful parts. Spearmint is slightly less medicinally potent than peppermint (*M. piperita*), a popular and well-known hybrid of spearmint and water mint *(M. aquatica)*. Spearmint is used similarly to peppermint in medicinal preparations. These mints are particularly beneficial in relieving digestive disorders, **colic**, and flatulence due to their carminative and antispasmodic actions, and may be helpful in the treatment of **irritable bowel syn-**

drome. Spearmint may also relieve **motion sickness, hiccups,** and **nausea.** The milder spearmint is a safe remedy when prepared as an infusion for children. Spearmint is diuretic and has been used to treat cases of suppressed or painful urination. It is high in vitamins A and C, and has been employed both to prevent and cure scurvy, to improve eyesight and reduce **night blindness,** and to bring a sparkle to dull eyes and a gloss to the hair. A vinegar decoction of spearmint applied as a hair rinse has been used to treat head sores. Spearmint is commonly used in culinary preparations to season meat, fish, and vegetable dishes. Mints are also used to flavor candy, toothpaste, antacid medicines, chewing gum, shaving cream, liqueurs, and even cigarettes. Spearmint is the preferred herb used to prepare the traditional drink of the American South, the mint julep.

Recent research indicates that spearmint may have useful antibacterial properties in addition to its traditional uses as a digestive aid. A group of Japanese researchers reported in 2001 that essential oil of spearmint showed significant bactericidal activity against such disease agents as *Staphylococcus aureus*, *Escherichia coli*, and *Helicobacter pylori*.

Spearmint is also being studied for its effectiveness in counteracting the damaging effects of oxidation in human and animal tissue. It has already been shown in animal studies to offer some protection against the growth of certain types of tumors.

Preparations

Spearmint should be harvested on a dry day, after the dew has evaporated and before the sun robs the plant of its volatile oil. The plant should just be coming into bloom. Stalks are cut a few inches from the ground, and any insect-damaged or brown leaves should be trimmed from the stem. The stalks should be tied in bundles and hung to dry in a warm, airy room out of direct sunlight. After the herb is crisply dry, the leaves are removed from the stems. The discarded stems may be added to a compost pile. The dried leaf is stored in clearly labeled, tightly sealed dark-glass containers.

Infusion: Place 6 tbsp of fresh mint leaves in a warmed glass container. Bring 2.5 cups of fresh, nonchlorinated water to the boiling point, and add it to the herbs. Cover and infuse the tea for about five minutes. Strain and sweeten to taste. Mints may also be infused with warm milk for easing abdominal **pain.** The prepared tea will store for about two days in the refrigerator in a sealed container. Drink three cups a day. Spearmint combines well with white **horehound** (*Marrubium vulgare*) in infusions for feverish children. The infusion of spearmint may also be used as a gargle to soothe the throat and freshen the breath.

Tincture: Combine four ounces of finely-cut fresh or powdered dry herb with one pint of brandy, gin, or vodka, in a glass container. The alcohol should be enough to cover the plant parts. Place the mixture away from light for about two weeks, shaking several times each day. Strain and store in a tightly capped, dark glass bottle. A standard dose is 10 to 30 drops of the tincture three times a day.

Essential oil: The essential oil is obtained by steam distillation of the fresh, flowering tops of the mint. A few drops on a sugar cube are a safe dosage several times a day. A few drops of oil added to water and applied externally will relieve **itching, burns,** insect bites, **scabies,** and other skin irritations. The essential oil may also be diluted with almond or sunflower oil for massage.

Precautions

Spearmint is a mild herb and generally considered safe. Some herbalists counsel against administering mint tea to young children, infants, and pregnant women. People with **hiatal hernia** or having an acute gallstone attack should not use spearmint.

Side effects

When spearmint is taken internally at normal dose levels, there are no side effects. The plant has, however, been reported to cause an allergic skin rash in some susceptible people.

Interactions

Preparations containing spearmint are believed to interfere with the beneficial action of homeopathic remedies when taken in close proximity. On the other hand, homeopaths in the United States disagree as of 2002 as to whether spearmint can antidote a remedy. Many maintain that if the remedy has been properly selected by the practitioner, there will be no interference from mint-flavored products.

Resources

BOOKS

Duke, James A. *The Green Pharmacy.* Emmaus, PA: Rodale Press, 1997.

PDR for Herbal Medicines, 1st ed. Montvale, NJ: Medical Economics Company, 1998.

Pelletier, Kenneth R., MD. *The Best Alternative Medicine*, Part I: Homeopathy. New York: Simon & Schuster, 2002.

Reid, Daniel. *Chinese Herbal Medicine*. Boston, MA: Shambhala, 1996.

Tyler, Varro E., ed. *Prevention's 200 Herbal Remedies*. Emmaus, PA: Rodale Press, Inc., 1997.

KEY TERMS

Carminative—Any medication or preparation given to expel gas from the digestive tract.

Carvone—The chemical compound that gives spearmint its characteristic flavor. Carvone is a pale yellow or colorless liquid when extracted from the plant.

Decoction—A herbal extract obtained by boiling parts of the plant in water or alcohol.

Stomachic—A medication or herbal preparation given to improve the functioning of the digestive system.

Volatile oil—The essential oil of a plant, usually extracted by steam distillation. The oil is called "volatile" because it evaporates at room temperature.

PERIODICALS

Bonamonte, D., L. Mundo, M. Daddabbo, and C. Foti. "Allergic Contact Dermatitis from *Mentha spicata* (Spearmint)." *Contact Dermatitis* 45 (November 2001): 298.

Imai, H., K. Osawa, H. Yasuda, et al. "Inhibition by the Essential Oils of Peppermint and Spearmint of the Growth of Pathogenic Bacteria." *Microbios* 106 (2001) (Supplement 1): 31-39.

Saleem, M., A. Alam, and S. Sultana. "Attenuation of Benzoyl Peroxide-Mediated Cutaneous Oxidative Stress and Hyperproliferative Response by the Prophylactic Treatment of Mice with Spearmint (*Mentha spicata*)." *Food Chemistry and Toxicology* 38 (October 2000): 939-948.

ORGANIZATIONS

Institute of Traditional Medicine. 2017 SE Hawthorne Blvd., Portland, OR 97214. (503) 233-4907. <www.itmonline.org>.

National Center for Homeopathy. 801 N. Fairfax St., Suite 306, Alexandria, VA 22314. (703) 548-7790.

United States Department of Agriculture. Washington, DC 20250. <www.usda.gov>.

OTHER

"*Mentha arvensis Linn.*" <www.modern-natural.com/mentha_arvensis.htm>.

Taylor, Suzi. "Young Scientists Wage War on Wilt." *Montana State University News*, May 24, 2002. <www.montana.edu>.

Clare Hanrahan
Rebecca J. Frey, PhD

Spinal manipulative therapy

Definition

Spinal manipulative therapies are those that are used on the human skeleton, particularly the spinal area, to relieve muscular or skeletal **pain**, relieve tension, improve the mobility of joints and, in the case of the oriental therapies, to "unblock energy channels." The idea behind spinal manipulation is that when the vertebrae are subluxated (misaligned), the resulting pressure on nerves can have negative effects on organ system function and general health, in addition to impeding proper joint motion.

Origins

Forms of manipulative therapy have been used for thousand of years in Asia. The nineteenth century, however, saw the introduction of many new forms of manipulative therapy in the West. The best known and most widely used of these approaches are **osteopathy** and **chiropractic**. Most areas and societies have some tradition of manipulation or massage and osseous adjustments.

Benefits

Osteopathy and chiropractic in particular have been used to relieve spinal pain and immobility. Both of these therapies can be used in cases of a "slipped disk," and are also used after accidents or surgery to restore mobility. Osteopathy and chiropractic can treat problems of the bones, muscles, joints, or ligaments. They have been used in the treatment of headaches of nervous origin, and even **osteoarthritis**. Athletes and dancers commonly seek osteopathic or chiropractic treatment for sports or occupational injuries to restore function.

Description

A common practice among the spinal manipulative therapies is that the therapist will generally work on patients while they are lying on a special treatment couch adjusted to the height of the practitioner. The therapies vary from light touching to fairly vigorous manipulation.

The cost of treatment across the various disciplines varies a great deal according to the practitioner's level of qualification, the area of competence, and other factors.

Osteopathy

Osteopathy was founded by an American doctor, **Andrew Taylor Still**. He applied his engineering study and detailed knowledge of human anatomy to the treatment of the human body. He deduced that since misalignment of the skeleton could cause illness, manipulation could theoretically restore good health. The manipulative techniques that Still recommended are commonly referred to as Osteopathic Manipulative Treatment (OMT). OMT is a form of noninvasive, "hands-on" care used for prevention, diagnosis, and treatment to reduce pain and restore motion, as well as help the body heal itself. OMT may be used to facilitate the movement of body fluids and normal tissue functioning, and release painful joints or dysfunctional areas. These therapies take different forms depending on patient needs. In addition to OMT, Dr. Still emphasized the importance that a nutritious diet and overall physical fitness play in maintaining good health. Osteopathy is now widely accepted by the allopathic medical profession, to the extent that they often refer patients to an osteopath. In fact, as of 2002, osteopaths were the fastest growing segment of the total population of physicians and surgeons in the United States.

Chiropractic

Chiropractic was developed by a "magnetic healer," Daniel David Palmer, who founded the Palmer School of Chiropractic. This therapy aims to treat pain and other disorders caused by misalignment of the skeleton with manipulation. Upon consultation with a chiropractor, the patient will be asked for a detailed medical history. The chiropractor may take a set of x rays to obtain a more accurate picture of the condition of the patient's spine. The consultant will decide what form the treatment should take, and treatment will begin on a subsequent visit.

Conditions that may benefit from manipulative treatment:

- whiplash injuries
- immobility of the spine due to arthritis
- strain injuries
- immobility due to previous injuries
- muscular problems
- sciatica
- poor posture
- tinnitus
- neuralgia
- partial paralysis due to stroke
- cerebral palsy

Preparations

Generally, no special preparation is required prior to treatment with the various kinds of spinal manipulative therapy, but some practitioners insist on x rays before treatment.

Precautions

The licensing credentials of spinal manipulation practitioners should always be checked. They should also be given any information regarding the health of the patient that may be relevant to treatment.

Side effects

In the presence of serious spinal problems, damage could result if the practitioner is not properly qualified. A registered practitioner should always be consulted, and should be made aware of all relevant patient information.

Research & general acceptance

Osteopathy and chiropractic are now well accepted as options for the treatment of back pain and many types of sports injuries. The field of sports medicine has found particular benefit in osteopathic practitioners because of their emphasis on the musculoskeletal system, manipulation, diet, **exercise**, and fitness. Many professional sports team physicians, Olympic physicians, and personal sports medicine physicians are doctors of osteopathy (DOs).

Training & certification

Osteopathy

Fully qualified osteopaths undergo four years of post-collegiate training in a college of osteopathy. They must pass state licensing examinations, and are entitled to use MRO (Member of the Register of Osteopaths) after their name. A DO is one of only two types of qualified physician in the United States, the other being an MD (allopathic physician). DOs are qualified to practice surgery, prescribe medications, and offer the same health care services that their allopathic counterparts are. The chief difference between the two groups of physicians is that MDs are more likely to enter specialized branches of medicine, while most DOs enter primary care practice.

Many aspects of traditional osteopathic philosophy, such as advice about diet and **smoking**, have entered mainstream medicine to the point that the lines between DOs and MDs are blurring. In addition, the dedication of osteopaths to **holistic medicine** and primary care has been a great benefit to rural areas of the United States that are often understaffed by mainstream practitioners.

Chiropractic

Chiropractors are required to take two years of college with a relevant biological curriculum, and four years of resident study that must include supervised clinical experience. A further two years of practical or clinical studies is required, which must include diagnosis and disease treatment.

The Council on Chiropractic Education (CCE) and its Commission on Accreditation is an autonomous national organization recognized by the United States De-

KEY TERMS

Neuralgia—Severe nerve pain.

Osteopathic manipulative treatment (OMT)—A collective term that refers to the variety of hands-on manipulative techniques practiced by osteopaths to diagnose and prevent disorders as well as to treat them.

Sciatica—Pain along the course of the sciatic nerve, running from pelvis down the back of leg to the foot caused by a compression or irritation of the fifth lumbar spinal root.

Tinnitus—Ringing or other noises in the ears, sometimes caused by skeletal misalignment.

partment of Education as the authority on the quality of training offered by colleges of chiropractic.

Resources

BOOKS

Shealy, Norman C. *Alternative Medicine, An Illustrated Encyclopedia of Natural Healing.* Boston, MA: Element Books, 1996.

PERIODICALS

"Osteopathic Manipulative Treatment May Benefit Patients." *Health & Medicine Week* (October 8, 2001).

Shepard, Scott. "Health Philosophies on Common Ground." *Cincinnati Business Courier* 18 (November 9, 2001): 38.

ORGANIZATIONS

American Association of Colleges of Osteopathic Medicine. 5550 Friendship Blvd., Suite 310, Chevy Chase, MD 20815-7231. (301) 968-4100. <http://www.aacom.org>.

The American Chiropractic Association. 1701 Clarendon Blvd, Arlington, VA 22209. (800) 986-4636. Memberinfo@amerchiro.org. <http://www.amerchiro.org>.

American College of Chiropractic Consultants (ACCC). 28 E. Jackson Bldg., 10th Fl., Suite 1020 Chicago, IL 60604. <http://www.accc-chiro.com>.

American Osteopathic Association. 142 East Ontario Street, Chicago, IL 60611 (800) 621-1773. msc@aoa-net.org. <http://www.aoa-net.org>.

American Osteopathic Board of Neuromusculoskeletal Medicine. 3500 DePauw Boulevard, Suite 1080, Indianapolis, IN 46268-1136.

The General Council and Register of Osteopaths. 56 London Street, Reading, Berkshire RG1 4SQ, United Kingdom.

Patricia Skinner
Rebecca J. Frey, PhD

Spirulina

Description

Spirulina is a genus of blue-green algae used as a nutritional supplement. Blue-green algae, which are microscopic fresh-water organisms, are also known as cyanobacteria. Their color is derived from the green pigment of chlorophyll, and the blue from a protein called phycocyanin. The species most commonly recommended for use as a nutritional supplement are *Spirulina maxima* and *Spirulina platensis*. These occur naturally in warm, alkaline, salty, brackish lakes, but are also commonly grown by aquaculture and harvested for commercial use. Spirulina contains many nutrients, including B vitamins, beta-carotene, gamma-linolenic acid, **iron, calcium, magnesium, manganese, potassium, selenium, zinc, bioflavonoids**, and protein.

Spirulina is about 65% protein by composition. These proteins are complete, in that they contain all essential **amino acids**, plus some nonessential ones. In that regard, it is similar to animal protein, but does not contain saturated fats, or residues of hormones or antibiotics that are in some meats. Since spirulina is normally taken in small amounts, the quantity of dietary protein supplied for the average reasonably well-nourished person would not be significant. However, it is a good source of trace minerals, some vitamins, bioflavonoids, and other phytochemicals. It also has high digestibility and bioavailability of nutrients.

General use

Spirulina has been used as a source of protein and nutrients, particularly beta-carotene, by the World Health Organization (WHO) to feed malnourished Indian children. The program resulted in a decrease of a type of blindness that results from inadequate dietary **vitamin A**. The dose used in this year-long study was 1 gram per day.

There is a high **vitamin B$_{12}$** content in spirulina. For this reason, it has often been recommended as a supplemental source of the vitamin for vegans and other strict vegetarians, who are unlikely to have adequate dietary vitamin B$_{12}$. Unfortunately, spirulina is not an effective source of the usable vitamin. Much of the vitamin B$_{12}$ is in the form of analogs that are unusable for humans, and may even block the active forms of vitamin B$_{12}$ consumed from other sources.

Gamma linolenic acid (GLA) is present in significant amounts in a small percent of spirulina species. This essential fatty acid can be used in the body to form products that are anti-inflammatory and antiproliferative. It is potentially useful for individuals with **rheumatoid arthritis** and diabetic neuropathy. It may also play a role in lowering plasma triglycerides and increasing HDL **cholesterol**.

Spirulina is a good source of available iron and zinc. A study done in rats found that those consuming spirulina had equivalent or better absorption than those given a ferrous sulfate iron supplement. A small human study of iron-deficient women had good response to iron supplementation with spirulina, although the amounts used were large (4 grams after each meal). Similarly, a study of zinc deficient children found that those taking spirulina had a superior response to those taking zinc sulfate, and had fewer side effects.

In addition to serving as a source of nutrients itself, spirulina has been used in the manufacture of fermented dairy products to guarantee the survival of the bacteria used to ferment the milk.

A stronger immune system is one claim made by boosters of spirulina. A number of animal studies appear to support stimulation of both antibody and cellular types of immunity. Immune function was markedly improved in children living in the areas surrounding Chernobyl. The measurements were made after 45 days, with each child consuming 5 grams of spirulina per day.

The growth of beneficial intestinal bacteria, including *Lactobacillus*, appears to be stimulated by the consumption of spirulina, based on a study of rats who consumed it as 5% of their **diets**. The absorption of vitamin B$_1$ was also improved.

Cholesterol, serum lipids, and low-density lipoprotein (LDL) cholesterol may be lowered by a small but significant percentage by the consumption of spirulina. One study group of men with high cholesterol took 4.2 grams per day of spirulina, and experienced a 4.5% decrease in cholesterol after one month.

Spirulina is also thought to be helpful in the treatment of oral leukoplakia, a precancerous condition that is manifested as white patches in the mouth. It improves experimentally induced oral carcinoma (**cancer** in the mouth) as supported by studies done in animals.

The evidence for the ability of spirulina to promote weight loss is not very strong. Results have been mixed, and the phenylalanine content does not appear to be an appetite suppressant as is sometimes claimed. Whether other components of the algae are beneficial for weight loss is uncertain and unproven.

Spirulina has been recommended to alleviate the symptoms of **attention-deficit hyperactivity disorder** (ADHD), although evidence for this indication is lacking.

Spirulina has the highest concentration of evercetin found in a natural source. Evercetin is a potent antioxidant and anti-inflammatory compound that can be used

to alleviate the symptoms of sinusitis and **asthma**. Phycocyanin, the protein that gives spirulina its blue color, has also been shown to relieve inflammation associated with arthritis and various **allergies**.

One recommended dose is 3–5 grams per day, but the amount used may depend on the product, the individual using it, and the indication for which it is being taken.

Preparations

Spirulina supplements are available in powder, flake, capsule, and tablet form. These supplements are generally expensive and have a strong flavor that many people find unpleasant.

Precautions

Because spirulina is sensitive to pollutants in sea water, it can be used as a biosensor to measure the toxicity of a given body of water. Unfortunately, this sensitivity means that spirulina grown in water contaminated with heavy metals can concentrate these toxic substances. Mercury levels are of particular concern. Infectious organisms may also be present and contaminate harvested algae, so reputable sources of spirulina should be used.

Phenylketonurics should avoid spirulina due to the potential content of phenylalanine.

A number of varieties of blue-green algae, including *Aphanizomenon flos-quae* and *Anabaena*, have been found to sometimes produce toxins that may affect the nervous system or the liver.

Side effects

The potential side effects of spirulina are primarily gastrointestinal, and include **diarrhea**, **nausea**, and **vomiting**. Allergic reactions occur rarely, but can cause **insomnia** and **anxiety**.

Interactions

No interactions of spirulina with foods, conventional medications, or herbs have been documented as of 2002.

Resources

BOOKS

Bratman, Steven, and David Kroll. *Natural Health Bible*. Rocklin, CA: Prima Publishing, 1999.

Griffith, H. Winter. *Vitamins, Herbs, Minerals & supplements: the complete guide*. New York: Fisher Books, 1998.

Jellin, Jeff, Forrest Batz, and Kathy Hitchens. *Pharmacist's Letter/Prescriber's Letter Natural Medicines Comprehensive Database*. California: Therapeutic Research Faculty, 1999.

KEY TERMS

Algae (sing., alga)—Any of numerous groups of one-celled organisms containing chlorophyll. Spirulina is a blue-green alga.

Neuropathy—Condition of weakness affecting the nervous system.

Phenylalanine—An essential amino acid that cannot be consumed by people with a metabolic disease known as phenylketonuria (PKU).

Phycocyanin—A protein found in spirulina that gives the alga its blue color. Phycocyanin has anti-inflammatory effects.

Phytochemicals—Nutritional substances contained in plants.

PERIODICALS

Remirez, D., R. Gonzalez, N. Merino, et al. "Inhibitory Effects of Spirulina in Zymosan-Induced Arthritis in Mice." *Mediators of Inflammation* 11 (April 2002): 75-79.

Remirez, D., N. Ledon, and R. Gonzalez. "Role of Histamine in the Inhibitory Effects of Phycocyanin in Experimental Models of Allergic Inflammatory Response." *Mediators of Inflammation* 11 (April 2002): 81-85.

Tonnina, D., et al. "Integral Toxicity Test of Sea Waters by an Algal Biosensor." *Annali di Chimica (Rome)* 92 (April 2002): 477-484.

Varga, L., J. Szigeti, R. Kovacs, et al. "Influence of a *Spirulina platensis* Biomass on the Microflora of Fermented ABT Milks During Storage (R1)." *Journal of Dairy Science* 85 (May 2002): 1031-1038.

OTHER

EarthNet. *EarthNet Scientific Health Library.* http://www.spirulina.com/SPLAbstracts1.html (2000).

Earthrise. *Spirulina Library Abstracts and Summaries.* http://www.earthrise.com/ERLibAbstracts2.html (2000).

Mayo Clinic. *Mayo Clinic: Blue-green algae.* http://www.mayohealth.org/mayo/askdiet/htm/new/qd970618.htm (1997).

Judith Turner
Rebecca J. Frey, PhD

Sports massage

Definition

Sports massage is a form of bodywork geared toward participants in athletics. It is used to help prevent injuries, to prepare the body for athletic activity and maintain it in optimal condition, and to help athletes recover from workouts and injuries. Sports massage has three basic forms: pre-event massage, post-event massage, and maintenance massage.

Origins

Sports massage has antecedents in earlier periods of history. The ancient Greeks and Romans combined massage and **exercise** in their athletic training. Various Asian cultures also developed forms of massage for dancers and for students of **martial arts**. As a formal practice, however, sports massage began in the Soviet Union and Communist bloc countries in the 1960s. Soviet teams were the first to have a massage therapist travel with them and work on their athletes on a regular and ongoing basis. Through sports and cultural exchanges, the concept of sports massage moved to Europe and the United States in the 1970s. Over time the benefits of sports massage became accepted, and sports massage became a part of the training regimen, first of professional athletes, then of college and amateur athletes. Today sports massage is recognized as a specialty by the American **Massage Therapy** Association.

Benefits

Sports massage is a generic term for three different types of **massage** associated with athletic performance. Each type of massage has its own benefits and uses different techniques.

Pre-event sports massage is done to help prevent serious athletic injury. It helps to warm up the muscles, stretching them and making them flexible for optimal athletic performance. A pre-event massage stimulates the flow of blood and nutrients to the muscles, reduces muscle tension, loosens the muscles, and produces a feeling of psychological readiness.

Whenever athletes exercise heavily, their muscles suffer microtraumas. Small amounts of swelling occur in the muscle because of tiny tears. Post-event sports massage helps reduce the swelling caused by microtraumas; loosens tired, stiff muscles; helps maintain flexibility; promotes blood flow to the muscle to remove lactic acid and waste build-up; and reduces cramping. In addition, post-event massage helps speed the athlete's recovery time and alleviates pulls, strains, and soreness.

Maintenance sports massage is done at least once a week as a regular part of athletic training programs, although professional athletes who have their own massage therapists may have maintenance massage daily. Maintenance massage increases the flow of blood and nutrients to the muscles. It also keeps the tissues loose so that different layers of muscle slide easily over each other. Maintenance sports massage also helps reduce the development of scar tissue while increasing flexibility and range of motion.

The goal of all sports massage is to maximize athletic performance. Athletes in different sports will concentrate the massage on different parts of the body.

Conditions that generally respond well to massage as a complementary therapy include:

• muscle **pain** and stiffness

• muscle strain

• edema (swelling)

• muscle soreness

• muscle sprains

• muscle tension

• sore spots

• repetitive strain injuries

• tendinitis

Massage can help these conditions, but it should never be used to replace skilled medical care.

Description

Each type of sports massage uses different massage techniques. Effleurage is a light stroking that can be performed with the palms or the thumbs. The pressure and speed is varied depending on the muscle and the desired result. Effleurage increases blood flow to the muscle. Petrissage is a form of two-handed kneading in which both hands pick up the muscle and compress it. This technique loosens tight bunches of muscles. Percussive strokes are blows or strikes on the muscle, often performed with the little fingers. They are used to tone the muscles. **Cupping** involves percussing or striking the muscles with cupped hands. It stimulates the skin and causes muscle contractions that help tone the muscles. There are variations on all these strokes, such as deep cross-fiber friction to separate muscle fibers and break down scar tissue, and jostling to relieve muscle tension. A good sports massage therapist will combine techniques to achieve the maximum desired result. Sports massage sessions generally last 30-60 minutes.

Pre-event massage is given shortly before an athlete competes. It consists mainly of brisk effleurage to stimulate and warm the muscles and petrissage to help muscles move fluidly and to reduce muscle tension. Effleurage is generally a relaxing **stroke**, but when done briskly it is stimulating. As the massage progresses, the pressure increases as the massage therapist uses percussive strokes and cupping to stimulate the muscles to contract and flex. The part of the body being massaged varies from sport to sport, although leg and back muscles are common targets for this type of massage.

Post-event massage is usually given 1–2 hours after the competition is over in order to give dilated blood vessels a chance to return to their normal condition. Post-event massage is light and gentle in order not to damage already stressed muscles. The goal is to speed up removal of toxic waste products and reduce swelling. Very light effleurage will decrease swelling while light petrissage will help clear away toxins and relieve tense, stiff muscles. Post-event massage can be self-administered on some parts of the body, such as the legs.

Maintenance massage is performed at least once a week while the athlete is in training. It is frequently administered to the back and legs. Deep effleurage and petrissage are used to relax and tone knotted muscles.

Preparations

No special preparations are needed to participate in a sports massage. Athletes should wait 1–2 hours after competing before having a post-event massage.

Precautions

Massage may be an appropriate technique for helping certain sports injuries, especially muscle injuries, to heal. When treating an injury, however, it is best to seek advice from a qualified sports therapist or a specialist in sports medicine before performing any massage. Certain ligament and joint injuries that need immobilization and expert attention may be aggravated by massage.

People who suffer from the following conditions or disorders should consult a physician before participating in a sports massage: acute infectious disease; aneurysm; heavy bruising; **cancer**; hernia; high blood pressure; inflammation due to tissue damage; **osteoporosis**; **phlebitis**; **varicose veins**; and certain skin conditions. Individuals who are intoxicated are not good candidates for sports massage.

Side effects

Sports massage is safe and effective. When given correctly, there are no undesirable side effects.

Research & general acceptance

Sports massage has become an established and accepted practice. Various studies done in both the United States and Europe have shown that when properly used, massage will produce greater blood flow to the muscles and better athletic performance. The practice of sports massage is not considered controversial.

Training & certification

Accredited sports massage therapists must first complete a course in general massage from a school accredited by the American Massage Therapy Association/Commission on Massage Training Accreditation/Approval (AMTA/COMTAA) or their State Board of Education. They must then complete an additional training program approved by the AMTA National Sports Massage Certification Program. Many sports massage practitioners also complete the National Certification Examination for Therapeutic Massage and Bodywork.

Resources

BOOKS

Cassar, Mario-Paul. *Massage Made Easy.* Allentown, PA: People's Medical Society, 1995.

Johnson, Joan. *The Healing Art of Sports Massage.* Emmaus, PA: Rodale Press, 1995.

ORGANIZATIONS

American Massage Therapy Association. 820 Davis Street, Suite 100. Evanston, IL 60201. (847) 864-0123.

National Certification Board for Therapeutic Massage and Bodywork. 8201 Greensboro Drive, Suite 300. McLean, VA 22102. (703) 610-9015.

Tish Davidson

Sprains & strains

Definition

Sprain refers to damage or tearing of ligaments or a joint capsule. Strain refers to damage or tearing of a muscle.

Description

When excessive force is applied to a joint, the ligaments that hold the bones together may be torn or damaged. This results in a sprain, and its seriousness depends on how badly the ligaments are torn. Any ligament can be sprained, but the most frequently injured ligaments are at the ankle, knee, and finger joints.

Strains are tears in the muscle. Sometimes called pulled muscles, they usually occur because a muscle lacks the flexibility, strength, or endurance to perform a certain activity. The majority of strains occur where the muscle meets the tendon, although they may occur in the middle of the muscle belly as well.

Children under age eight are less likely to have sprains than are older people. Children's ligaments are tighter, and their bones are more apt to break before a ligament tears. People who are active in sports suffer more strains and sprains than less active people. Repeated sprains in the same joint make the joint less stable and more prone to future sprains. Muscle strains are also more likely to occur in muscles that have been previously injured.

Causes & symptoms

There are three grades of sprains. Grade I sprains are mild injuries in which there is a stretching or mild tearing of the ligament, yet no joint function is lost. However, there may be tenderness and slight swelling.

Grade II sprains are caused by a partial tear in the ligament. These sprains are characterized by obvious swelling, localized tenderness, **pain**, joint laxity, difficulty bearing weight if the injury is to a lower extremity, and reduced function of the joint.

Grade III, or third degree, sprains are caused by complete tearing of the ligament. There is severe pain, loss of joint function, widespread swelling, and the inability to bear weight if in the lower extremity. While a Grade III sprain may be very painful when it occurs, it is sometimes not painful after the injury because the ligament fibers have been completely torn and nothing is pulling on them. If this is true, the injury will be accompanied by a significant loss in joint stability.

Strains, like sprains, are also graded in three different categories. Grade I strains are considered mild. They are categorized by some localized swelling with no significant disruption of the muscle tendon unit. Stretching or contraction of the muscle may be painful.

Grade II strains indicate some disruption of the muscle tendon unit. They will often show a loss of strength and limitation in active motion, but the muscle has not been completely disrupted.

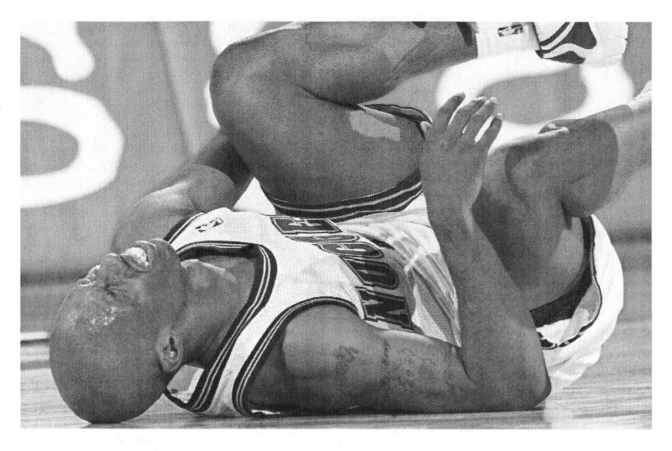

Chauncy Billups, a guard for the Denver Nuggets, grimaces after spraining his ankle during a game. *(AP/Wide World Photos. Reproduced by permission.)*

Grade III, or third degree, strains indicate a complete rupture in the muscle tendon unit. This injury is likely to be very painful and often the individual will report hearing a loud pop or snap when the injury occurred. The site of injury is often quite visible and there will be a significant defect in the muscle that can be felt with the fingers. A Grade III muscle strain will often have very serious bruising with it as well.

Diagnosis

Grade I sprains and strains are usually self-diagnosed. Grade II and III sprains are often seen by a physician, who may x ray the area to differentiate between a sprain and other serious joint injuries. Since muscles don't show up on x ray, Grade II and III muscle strains are usually diagnosed by physical examination.

Treatment

While the primary problem with sprains and strains is a torn or damaged ligament or muscle fiber, additional complications may develop as a result of swelling and immobilization of the injured area. In order to prevent these complications from worsening, alternative practitioners endorse RICE: Rest, Ice for 48 hours, Compression (wrapping in an elastic bandage), and Elevation of the sprain or strain above the level of the heart.

Nutritional therapists recommend **vitamin C** and **bioflavonoids** to supplement a diet high in whole grains, fresh fruits, and vegetables. Anti-inflammatories, such as **bromelain** (a proteolytic enzyme from pineapples) and **turmeric** (*Curcuma longa*), may also be helpful. The homeopathic remedy *Arnica* (*Arnica montana*) may be used initially for a few days, followed by *Rhus tox* (*Rhus toxicodendron*) for joint-related injuries or *Ruta rutagraveolens* for muscle-related injuries. **Arnica** gel or ointment, such as *Traumeel*, or a homeopathic combination of arnica and other remedies, has also been found effective with certain joint sprains.

Traditional Chinese medicine has been effectively used to treat soft tissue injuries like sprains and strains. **Acupuncture** is used to treat pain and speed the healing process in the damaged tissues by moving blocked energy from the area. The radiant heat of **moxibustion** may also be used to speed up the healing response in the damaged tissues.

Specialized forms of massage and soft tissue manipulation may be used by a variety of practitioners. Massage has significant effects in enhancing local circulation, promoting earlier mobility, and speeding the healing response in the damaged tissue. It will most often be used in combination with other approaches, including stretching and range of motion exercises.

Allopathic treatment

Grade I sprains and strains can be treated at home. Basic first aid for sprains consists of RICE (Rest, Ice, Compression, and Elevation). Such over-the-counter pain medication such as acetaminophen (Tylenol) or ibuprofen (Motrin) can be taken for pain.

People with grade II sprains or strains may often be referred to physical therapy. Crutches or splints may be used during the healing process to help maintain stability. Surgery may be required for Grade III sprains or strains as a greater amount of damage will often prevent adequate healing without surgery.

Expected results

Moderate sprains and strains heal within two to four weeks, but it can take months to recover from severe injuries. Until recently, tearing the ligaments of the knee meant the end of an athlete's career. Improved surgical and rehabilitative techniques now offer the possibility of complete recovery. However, once a ligament has been sprained, it may not be as strong as it was before. A muscle that has been strained is also more susceptible to reinjury.

Prevention

Sprains and strains can be prevented by warming up before exercising, using proper form when performing activities and conditioning, being careful not to **exercise** past the point of **fatigue**, and taping or bracing certain joints to protect them from injury.

Resources

BOOKS

Benjamin, Ben. *Listen to Your Pain.* New York: Penguin, 1984.

Burton Goldberg Group. "Sprains." In *Alternative Medicine: The Definitive Guide,* edited by James Strohecker. Puyallup, WA: Future Medicine Publishing, 1994.

Corrigan, Brian, and G.D. Maitland. *Musculoskeletal & Sports Injuries.* Oxford: Butterworth–Heinemann, 1994.

Pelletier, Kenneth R. *The Best Alternative Medicine.* New York: Simon & Schuster, 2000.

"Sprains and strains." In *The Medical Advisor: The Complete Guide to Alternative and Conventional Treatments.* Alexandria, VA: Time–Life Books, 1996.

KEY TERMS

Ligament—Tough, fibrous connective tissue that holds bones together at joints.

Moxibustion—A treatment in which crushed leaves of the plant *Vulgaris* are formed into a cigar-like form that is lit and held directly over the skin of the area being treated.

PERIODICALS

Wexler, Randall K. "The Injured Ankle." *American Family Physician* 57 (February 1, 1998): 474.

Whitney Lowe

Sprue *see* **Celiac disease**

Squaw root *see* **Black cohosh**

Squawvine

Description

Squawvine (*Mitchella repens*) is a plant that is native to North America. It is an evergreen herb belonging to the madder or Rubiaceae family. It grows in the forests and woodlands of the eastern United States and Canada. Squawvine is usually found at the base of trees and stumps. Although squawvine grows year round, herbalists recommend collecting the herb when the plant flowers during the months of April through June.

Squawvine's name refers to its use by Native American women as a remedy for a range of conditions. Squawvine is also referred to as "partridge berry" because some people consider the other name to be insulting to Native American women. Squawvine is also known as squaw vine, squaw berry, checkerberry, deerberry, winter clover, twinberry, and hive vine.

General use

Squawvine's name stems from its use by Native American women for conditions related to childbearing. The plant was used to ease menstrual cramps, strengthen the uterus for **childbirth**, and prevent miscarriage. During the final 2 to 4 weeks of a Native American woman's **pregnancy**, she drank tea made from squawvine leaves so that childbirth was less painful. The herb was said to regulate contractions so that the baby was delivered safely, easily, and quickly. After the baby was born, the Native American mother who nursed her child would put a squawvine solution on her nipples to relieve the soreness.

In folk medicine, squawvine continued to be a remedy for women's disorders. In addition to conditions related to childbirth, the herb was used to treat postpartum **depression**, irregular **menstruation**, and bleeding. In addition to treating internal ailments, a squawvine wash was said to provide relief to sore eyes. Squawvine is still used in folk medicine to treat conditions including **anxiety**, **hemorrhoids**, **insomnia**, muscle spasms, **edema**, and inflammation.

Current uses of squawvine

Squawvine is used in alternative medicine to tone the uterine lining and prepare a woman's body for childbirth. The herb is taken for painful menstruation and to tone the prostate. It is also said to help promote fertility and to increase the flow of mother's milk.

Furthermore, squawvine is recognized by practitioners of alternative medicine for its effectiveness as a diuretic. It is used to treat such urinary conditions as suppression of urine. Squawvine is also a remedy for **diarrhea**, shrinking tissues, muscle spasms, and nerves.

Squawvine is still used as an eye wash. It is also used as a skin wash and to treat colitis.

Preparations

Squawvine is available in various forms. Commercial preparations include tinctures, extracts and powdered herb.

Squawvine tea, which is also known as an infusion, is made by pouring 1 cup (240 ml) of boiling water over 1 tsp (1.5 g) of the dried herb. The mixture is steeped for 10 to 15 minutes and then strained. Squawvine tea may be taken up to three times a day. Women seeking relief for difficult or painful menstruation can combine squawvine with **cramp bark** and pasque flower.

Squawvine tincture can be used in an infusion. The dosage is 1–2mL in 1 cup (240 ml) of boiling water. The tincture dosage can be taken three times a day.

Use in pregnancy and lactation

Pregnant women should not take squawvine during the first two trimesters of **pregnancy**. Some herbalists, however, recommend taking the herb during the eighth and ninth month to make labor easier. During those months, squawvine can be taken once or twice daily. It can be combined with **raspberry** leaves in this remedy to prepare for childbirth.

Nursing mothers with sore nipples can try a nineteenth-century folk remedy. A squawvine ointment is prepared by first making a decoction. A non-aluminum pan is used to boil 2 oz. (2 ml) of the powdered herb and 1 pint (470 ml) of water. The mixture is simmered for 10 minutes. It is then strained and the juice is squeezed out. The liquid is measured and an equal amount of cream is added to it. This mixture is boiled until it reaches a soft, ointment-like consistency. It is cooled and can be applied to the nipples after the baby has finished nursing.

Precautions

Some herbal remedies have been studied in Europe, but no information was available about the safety of squawvine as of June 2000. Squawvine is believed to be safe when taken in recommended dosages for a short time. There should be no problems when this remedy is used by people beyond childhood and those who are above age 45. Some of the assessment that squawvine is a safe remedy, however, is based on the fact that no problems had been reported when squawvine was used by people including pregnant women and nursing mothers.

Squawvine is an herbal remedy and not regulated by the U.S. Food and Drug Administration (FDA). The regulation process involves research into whether the remedy is safe to use. In addition, the effectiveness of squawvine for its traditional uses in childbirth and during lactation has not been clinically tested.

People should consult a doctor or health care practitioner before taking squawvine. The patient should inform the doctor about other medications or herbs that he or she takes. Once treatment with squawvine begins, people should see their doctors if their conditions haven't improved within two weeks.

Opinion is divided about whether squawvine is safe for women to use. On one side are those who caution that squawvine should be avoided by women who are currently pregnant or are planning to conceive within the short term. Herbalists advise that it should not be taken during the first two trimesters of pregnancy. Furthermore, squawvine and other herbal remedies should not be given to children under the age of two.

Side effects

There are no known side effects from using squawvine. Little research has been done, however, on its safety.

Interactions

No interactions have been reported between squawvine and other herbs or medications. Before using

KEY TERMS

Decoction—A herbal extract produced by mixing a herb with cold water, bringing the mixture to a boil, and letting it simmer to evaporate the excess water.

Tincture—A liquid extract of a herb prepared by steeping the herb in an alcohol and water mixture.

this herb as a remedy, however, a person should first consult with a doctor or health practitioner to discuss potential interactions.

Resources

BOOKS

Duke, James A. *The Green Pharmacy.* Emmaus, PA: Rodale Press, Inc., 1997.

Keville, Kathi. *Herbs for Health and Healing.* Emmaus, PA: Rodale Press, Inc., 1996.

Ritchason, Jack. *The Little Herb Encyclopedia.* Pleasant Grove, UT: Woodland Health Books, 1995.

Squier, Thomas Broken Bear, with Lauren David Peden. *Herbal Folk Medicine.* New York: Henry Holt and Company, 1997.

ORGANIZATIONS

American Botanical Council. P.O. Box 201660. Austin TX, 78720. (512) 331-8868.

Herb Research Foundation. 1007 Pearl St., Suite 200. Boulder, CO 80302. (303) 449-2265. http://www.herbs.org.

Liz Swain

St. John's wort

Description

Hypericum perforatum is the most medicinally important species of the Hypericum genus, commonly known as St. John's wort or Klamath weed. There are as many as 400 species in the genus, which belongs to the Clusiaceae family. Native to Europe, St. John's wort is found throughout the world. It thrives in sunny fields, open woods, and gravelly roadsides. Early colonists brought this plant to North America, and it has become naturalized in the eastern United States and California, as well as in Australia, New Zealand, eastern Asia, and South America. As of 2004, St. John's wort is one of the most commonly used herbs in the United States, especially among women.

The entire plant, particularly its round black seeds, exudes a slight turpentine-like odor. The woody-branched root spreads from the base with runners that produce numerous stalks. The simple dark green leaves are veined and grow in opposite, oblong, or oval pairs on round branching stalks that reach as high as 3 ft (91.4 cm). Tiny holes, visible when the leaf is held to the light, are actually transparent oil glands containing a chemical known as hypericin. These characteristic holes inspired the species name, Perforatum, which is the Latin word for "perforated." The bright yellow star-shaped flowers, often clustered in groups of three, have five petals. Black dots along the margins of the blossom contain more hypericin. The flowers bloom in branching flat-topped clusters atop the stalks, around the time of the summer solstice. St. John's wort, sometimes called devil's flight or grace of God, was believed to contain magical properties that ward off evil spirits. Its generic name, Hypericum, is derived from a Greek word meaning "over an apparition." The herb was traditionally gathered on midsummer's eve, June 23. This date was later celebrated in the Christian Church as the eve of the feast day of St. John the Baptist. This folk custom gave the plant its popular name. The Anglo-Saxon word "wort" means "medicinal herb."

General use

St. John's wort has been known for its medicinal properties as far back as Roman times. On the battlefield, it was a valued remedy that promoted healing from trauma and inflammation. The herb is regarded as a vulnerary, and can speed the healing of **wounds**, **bruises**, ulcers, and **burns**. It is also popularly used as a nervine for its calming effect, easing tension and **anxiety**, relieving mild **depression**, and soothing women's mood swings during **menopause**. The bittersweet herb is licensed in Germany for use in mild depression, anxiety, and sleeplessness. It is said to be helpful in nerve injury and trauma, and was used in the past to speed healing after brain surgery. Its antispasmodic properties have been thought to ease uterine cramping and menstrual difficulties. St. John's wort may also be used as an expectorant.

The hypericin in St. John's wort possesses antiviral properties that are said to be effective against certain cancers. An infusion of the plant taken as a tea has been helpful in treating **bedwetting** in children. The oil has been used internally to treat **colic**, intestinal **worms**, and abdominal **pain**. The plant's medicinal parts are its fresh leaves and flowers. This herbal remedy has been extensively tested in West Germany, and is dispensed throughout Germany as a popular medicine called *Johanniskraut*. Commercially prepared extracts are commonly standardized to contain 0.3% hypericin.

Clinical studies

In contrast to early European reports made in the 1980s, more recent clinical studies tend to undermine the

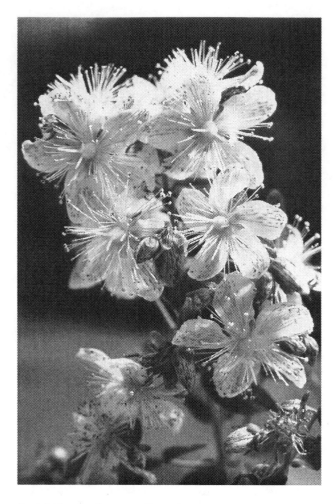

St. John's wort flowers. *(Photo Researchers, Inc. Reproduced by permission.)*

claims made for St. John's wort as a possible treatment for HIV infection and depression. As of 2002, health care professionals and regulatory agencies in Europe were advised to warn **AIDS** patients that St. John's wort decreases the effectiveness of drugs known as HIV protease inhibitors. In addition, the National Center for Complementary and Alternative Medicine (NCCAM) in the United States released the results of a large-scale multi-site study in April 2002, which reported that St. John's wort is no more effective than a placebo for treating major depression of moderate severity. The study was also published in the *Journal of the American Medical Association*. Additional studies being conducted in several countries are researching the interactions between St. John's wort and various types of prescription medications.

Preparations

An oil extract can be purchased commercially or prepared by combining fresh St. John's wort flowers and leaves in a glass jar with sunflower or olive oil. The con-

tainer should be sealed with an airtight lid, and placed on a sunny windowsill for four to six weeks. It should be shaken daily. When the oil absorbs the red pigment, the mixture is strained through muslin or cheesecloth, and stored in a dark container. The medicinal oil maintains its potency for two years or more. The oil of St. John's wort has been known in folk culture as "Oil of Jesus." This oil forms a rub used for painful joints, **varicose veins**, muscle strain, arthritis, and rheumatism. Placed in a compress, it can help to heal wounds and inflammation, and relieve the pain of deep bruising.

An infusion is made by pouring one pint of boiling water over 1 oz (28 g) of dried herb, or 2 oz (57 g) of fresh, minced flower and leaf. It is steeped in a glass or enamel pot for five to 10 minutes, then strained and covered. The tea should be consumed while it is warm. A general dose is one cup, up to three times daily.

To prepare a capsule, the leaves and flowers are dried, and ground with a mortar and pestle into a fine powder. The mixture is then placed in gelatin capsules. The potency of the herb varies with the soil, climate, and harvesting conditions of the plant. A standardized extract of 0.3% hypericin extract, commercially prepared from a reputable source, is more likely to yield reliable results. Standard dosage is up to three 300 mg capsules of 0.3% standardized extract daily.

A tincture is prepared by combining one part fresh herb to three parts alcohol (50% alcohol/water solution) in a glass container. The mixture is placed in a dark place, and shaken daily for two weeks. Then it is strained through muslin or cheesecloth, and stored in a dark bottle. The tincture should maintain potency for two years. Standard dosage, unless otherwise prescribed, is 0.24–1 tsp added to 8 oz (227 g) of water, up to three times daily.

A salve can be made by warming 2 oz (57 g) of prepared oil extract in a double boiler. Once warmed, 1 oz (28 g) of grated beeswax is added and mixed until melted. The mixture is poured into a glass jar and allowed to cool. The salve can be stored for up to one year. The remedy keeps best if refrigerated after preparation. The salve is useful in treating burns, wounds, and soothing painful muscles. It is also a good skin softener. St. John's wort salve may be prepared in combination with **calendula** extract (*Calendula officinalis*) for application on bruises.

Precautions

There are a number of important precautions to observe in using St. John's wort. Pregnant or lactating women should not use the herb at all. Persons taking prescription antidepressants of any kind should not use St. John's wort at the same time, as the herb may precipitate a health crisis known as serotonin syndrome. Serotonin syndrome is potentially life-threatening, and is characterized by changes in level of consciousness, behavior, and neuromotor functioning as a result of increased levels of the neurotransmitter serotonin in the central nervous system. Drug interactions are the most common cause of serotonin syndrome. Several cases of serotonin syndrome have been reported in patients who were taking St. John's wort by itself or in combination with SSRIs, fenfluramine (Pondimin), or nefazodone (Serzone). Persons using the herb should discontinue it a minimum of two weeks prior to any surgery requiring general anesthesia, as it interacts with a number of intravenous and inhaled anesthetics.

It is also important for persons using St. John's wort to purchase the herb from a reputable source, as the quality of herbal products sold in the United States and Canada varies widely. One study of 10 popular herb samples, including St. John's wort, reported in 2003 that each herb had "a large range in label ingredients and recommended daily dose (RDD) across available products." The researchers recommended that physicians and consumers pay very close attention to labels on over-the-counter (OTC) herbal products.

In addition to the herb's potential risks to humans, it can be toxic to livestock. Toxic effects in cattle include reports of **edema** of the ears, eyelids, and the face due to photosensitization after the animal eats the herb. Exposure to sunlight activates the hypericin in the plant. Adverse effects have been reported in horses, sheep, and swine, including a staggering gait and blistering or peeling of the skin. Smaller animals, such as rabbits, suffer severe side effects from accidental ingestion of St. John's wort. The Veterinary **Botanical Medicine** Association (VBMA), which was founded in 2002 as an offshoot of the American Veterinary Medical Association (AVMA), offers a page on its website for reporting adverse effects of St. John's wort or any other herb in cats, dogs, or other animals.

Side effects

When used either internally or externally, the herb may cause photodermatitis in humans with fair or sensitive skin, following exposure to sunlight or other sources of ultraviolet light. There have also been some case reports of side effects in breast-feeding women taking hypericum extract. Changes in the nutritional quality and flavor of the milk, as well as reduction or cessation of lactation, have been reported. In addition, St. John's wort has been known to cause headaches, stiff neck, **nausea** or **vomiting**, and high blood pressure in susceptible individuals.

Interactions

St. John's wort has a number of problematic interactions with many drugs. It has been reported to interact with amphetamines, **asthma** inhalants, decongestants, diet pills, narcotics, tryptophan and tyrosine (**amino acids**), as well as antidepressant medications and certain foods. It has also been reported to interfere with the effectiveness of birth control pills as well as with indinavir (Crixivan) and other AIDS medications. Moreover, anesthesiologists have reported that the herb increases bleeding time in patients under general anesthesia. Patients should always consult a mainstream health practitioner before using St. John's wort, and should discontinue taking it at least two weeks prior to major surgery.

Resources

BOOKS

Blumenthal, Mark. *The Complete German Commission E Monographs, Therapeutic Guide to Herbal Medicines.* American Botanical Council, Boston: Integrative Medicine Communications, 1998.

Bown, Deni. *The Herb Society of America, Encyclopedia of Herbs & Their Uses.* New York: DK Publishing, Inc., 1995.

Foster, Steven, and James A. Duke. *A Field Guide to Medicinal Plants.* New York: Peterson Field Guides, Houghton Mifflin Company, 1990.

Hoffmann, David. *The New Holistic Herbal.* Massachusetts: Element Books, 1992.

McIntyre, Anne. *The Medicinal Garden.* New York: Henry Holt and Company Inc., 1997.

PERIODICALS

Deshmukh, R., and K. Franco. "Talking to Patients About St. John's Wort." *Cleveland Clinic Journal of Medicine* 70 (November 2003): 990.

Finfgeld, D. L. "Serotonin Syndrome and the Use of SSRIs." *Journal of Psychosocial Nursing and Mental Health Services* 42 (February 2004): 16–20.

Garrard, J., S. Harms, L. E. Eberly, and A. Matiak. "Variations in Product Choices of Frequently Purchased Herbs: Caveat Emptor." *Archives of Internal Medicine* 163 (October 27, 2003): 2290–95.

Henderson, L., Q. Y. Yue, C. Bergquist, et al. "St. John's Wort (*Hypericum perforatum*): Drug Interactions and Clinical Outcomes." *British Journal of Clinical Pharmacology* 54 (October 2002): 349–56.

Hodges, P. J., and P. C. Kam. "The Peri-Operative Implications of Herbal Medicines." *Anaesthesia* 57 (September 2002): 889–99.

Hypericum Depression Trial Study Group. "Effect of *Hypericum perforatum* (St. John's Wort) in Major Depressive Disorder: A Randomized, Controlled Trial." *Journal of the American Medical Association (JAMA)* 287 (April 10, 2002): 1807–14.

Pfrunder, A., M. Schiesser, S. Gerber, et al. "Interaction of St. John's Wort with Low-Dose Oral Contraceptive Therapy: A Randomized Controlled Trial." *British Journal of Clinical Pharmacology* 56 (December 2003): 683–90.

Steinbach, Harvey, M.D. "Serotonin Syndrome: How to Avoid, Identify, and Treat Dangerous Drug Interactions." *Current*

KEY TERMS

Antispasmodic—A drug or medication given to relieve mild intestinal cramping or muscle spasms.

Expectorant—A medication or preparation that encourages the discharge of mucus from the respiratory system.

Nervine—A medication or preparation given to calm the nervous system.

Neurotransmitter—Any of several compounds produced in the body that relay nerve impulses from one nerve cell to another. St. John's wort has been reported to affect the balance of neurotransmitters in the brain.

Serotonin syndrome—A potentially life-threatening reaction to increased levels of the neurotransmitter serotonin in the central nervous system, most often as a result of drug interactions. St. John's wort has been implicated in several cases of serotonin syndrome.

Vulnerary—A medication or preparation used to heal wounds, bruises, sprains, and ulcers.

Psychiatry Online 2 (May 2003). <http://www.currentpsy-chiatry.com/2003_05/0503_serotonin.asp>.

Yu, S. M., R. M. Ghandour, and Z. J. Huang. "Herbal Supplement Use Among US Women, 2000." *Journal of the American Medical Women's Association* 59 (Winter 2004): 17–24.

ORGANIZATIONS

American Botanical Council. P.O. Box 201660, Austin, TX 78720-1660.

Food and Drug Administration (FDA). 5600 Fishers Lane, Rockville, MD 20857. (888) 463-6332. <http://www.fda.gov>.

Herb Research Foundation. 1007 Pearl St., Suite 200, Boulder, CO 80302. (303) 449-2265. <http://www.herbs.org>.

National Center for Complementary and Alternative Medicine (NCCAM) Clearinghouse. P. O. Box 7923, Gaithersburg, MD 20898-7923. (888) 644-6226. Fax: (866) 464-3615. <http://nccam.nih.gov>.

Veterinary Botanical Medicine Association (VBMA). c/o Susan G. Wynn, DVM, 334 Knollwood lane, Woodstock, GA 30188. E-mail: s.wynn@vbma.org. <http://www.vbma.org>.

OTHER

National Center for Complementary and Alternative Medicine (NCCAM) Fact Sheet. *St. John's Wort and the Treatment of Depression* . Bethesda, MD: NCCAM, 2002. <http://nccam.nih.gov/health/stjohnswort/>.

National Center for Complementary and Alternative Medicine (NCCAM) press release, 9 April 2002. "Study Shows St. John's Wort Ineffective for Major Depression of Moderate Severity." <http://nccam.nih.gov/news/2002/stjohnswort/pressrelease.htm>.

Clare Hanrahan
Rebecca J. Frey, PhD

Staphylococcal infections

Definition

Staphylococcal (staph) **infections** are communicable infections caused by staph organisms and often characterized by the formation of abscesses. They are the leading cause of primary infections originating in hospitals (nosocomial infections) in the United States.

Description

Classified since the early twentieth century as among the deadliest of all disease-causing organisms, staph exists on the skin or inside the nostrils of 20–30% of healthy people. These bacteria are sometimes found in breast tissue, the mouth, and the genital, urinary, and upper respiratory tracts.

Although staph bacteria are usually harmless, when injury or a break in the skin enables the organisms to invade the body and overcome the body's natural defenses, consequences can range from minor discomfort to death. Infection is most apt to occur in:

• Newborns (especially those born prematurely).

• Women who are breast-feeding.

• Persons whose immune systems have been weakened by radiation treatments, chemotherapy, HIV, or medication.

• Intravenous drug users.

• Those with surgical incisions, skin disorders, and serious illness like **cancer**, diabetes, and lung disease.

• The elderly, particularly those who are confined to nursing homes.

Types of infections

Staph skin infections often produce pus-filled pockets (abscesses) located just beneath the surface of the skin or deep within the body. Risk of infection is greatest among the very young and the very old.

A localized staph infection is confined to a ring of dead and dying white blood cells and bacteria. The skin above it feels warm to the touch. Most of these abscesses eventually burst, and pus leaking onto the skin can cause new infections.

A small fraction of localized staph infections enter the bloodstream and spread through the body. In children, these systemic (affecting the whole body) or disseminated infections frequently affect the ends of the long bones of the arms or legs, causing a bone infection called osteomyelitis. When adults develop invasive staph infections, bacteria are most apt to cause abscesses of the brain, heart, kidneys, liver, lungs, or spleen.

TOXIC SHOCK. Toxic shock syndrome is a life-threatening infection characterized by severe **headache**, **sore throat**, **fever** as high as 105°F (40.6°C), and a sun-burn-like rash that spreads from the face to the rest of the body. Symptoms appear suddenly; they also include de-hydration and watery **diarrhea**.

Inadequate blood flow to peripheral parts of the body (shock) and loss of consciousness occur within the first 48 hours. Between the third and seventh day of illness, skin peels from the palms of the hands, soles of the feet, and other parts of the body. Kidney, liver, and muscle damage often occur.

SCALDED SKIN SYNDROME. Rare in adults and most common in newborns and other children under the age of five, scalded skin syndrome originates with a localized skin infection. A mild fever and/or an increase in the number of infection-fighting white blood cells may occur.

A bright red rash spreads from the face to other parts of the body and eventually forms scales. Large, soft **blisters** develop at the site of infection and elsewhere. When they burst, they expose inflamed skin that looks as if it had been burned.

MISCELLANEOUS INFECTIONS. *Staphylococcus aureus* can also cause:

- arthritis

- bacteria in the bloodstream (bacteremia)

- pockets of infection and pus under the skin (carbuncles)

- tissue inflammation that spreads below the skin, causing **pain** and swelling (cellulitis)

- inflammation of the valves and walls of the heart(endocarditis)

- inflammation of tissue that enclosed and protects the spinal cord and brain (meningitis)

- inflammation of bone and bone marrow (osteomyelitis).

- pneumonia

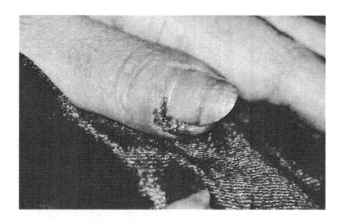

A close-up of woman's finger and nail cuticle infected with *Staphyloccus aureus.* (Custom Medical Stock Photo. Reproduced by permission.)

Types of staph infections

STAPHYLOCOCCUS AUREUS. Named for the golden color of the bacterium when grown under laboratory conditions, *S. aureus* is a hardy organism that can survive in extreme temperatures or other inhospitable circumstances. About 70–90% of the population carry this strain of staph in the nostrils at some time. Although present on the skin of only 5–20% of healthy people, as many as 40% carry it elsewhere, such as in the throat, vagina, or rectum, for varying periods of time, from hours to years, without developing symptoms or becoming ill.

S. aureus flourishes in hospitals, where it infects healthcare personnel and patients who have had surgery; who have acute **dermatitis**, insulin-dependent diabetes, or dialysis-dependent kidney disease; or who receive frequent allergy-desensitization injections. Staph bacteria can also contaminate bedclothes, catheters, and other objects. In many cases, staph contamination in hospitals is made worse by overprescribing and misuse of antibiotics. The result is the emergence of strains of *S. aureus* that are resistant to antibiotics.

S. aureus causes a variety of infections. **Boils** and inflammation of the skin surrounding a hair shaft (folliculitis) are the most common. Toxic shock syndrome (TSS) and scalded skin syndrome (SSS) are among the most serious. *S. aureus* is also emerging as a leading cause of infective endocarditis and of a higher mortality rate from this disorder.

Together with *S. pyogenes*, *S. aureus* is known to be a major producer of superantigens, which are bacterial exotoxins that trigger abnormal and excessive activation of T-cells. T cells are produced in the thymus gland and regulate the human immune system's response to infection. Superantigens are being studied intensively for their roles in causing disease. Staphylococci are responsible for at least 19 different superantigens.

S. EPIDERMIDIS. Capable of clinging to tubing (as in that used for intravenous feeding, etc.), prosthetic devices, and other non-living surfaces, *S. epidermidis* is the organism that most often contaminates devices that provide direct access to the bloodstream.

The primary cause of bacteremia in hospital patients, this strain of staph is most likely to infect cancer patients, whose immune systems have been compromised, and high-risk newborns receiving intravenous supplements.

S. epidermidis also accounts for two of every five cases of prosthetic valve endocarditis. Prosthetic valve endocarditis is an infection that develops as a complication of the implantation of an artificial valve in the heart. Although contamination usually occurs during surgery, symptoms of infection may not become evident until a year after the operation. More than half of the patients who develop prosthetic valve endocarditis die.

STAPHYLOCOCCUS SAPROPHYTICUS. Existing within and around the tube-like structure that carries urine from the bladder (urethra) of about 5% of healthy males and females, *S. saprophyticus* is the second most common cause of unobstructed urinary tract infections (UTIs) in sexually active young women. This strain of staph is responsible for 10-20% of infections affecting healthy outpatients.

Causes & symptoms

Staph bacteria can spread through the air, but infection is almost always the result of direct contact with open sores or body fluids contaminated by these organisms.

Warning signs

Common symptoms of staph infection include:

- Pain or swelling around a cut or an area of skin that has been scraped.
- Boils or other skin abscesses.
- Blistering, peeling, or scaling of the skin. This symptom is most common in infants and young children.
- Enlarged lymph nodes in the neck, armpits, or groin.

A family physician should be notified whenever:

- A boil or carbuncle appears on any part of the face or spine. Staph infections affecting these areas can spread to the brain or spinal cord.
- A boil becomes very sore. Usually a sign that infection has spread, this condition may be accompanied by fever, **chills**, and red streaks radiating from the site of the original infection.

- Boils that develop repeatedly. This type of recurrent infection could be a symptom of diabetes.

Diagnosis

Blood tests that show unusually high concentrations of white blood cells can suggest staph infection, but diagnosis is based on laboratory analysis of material removed from pus-filled sores, and on analysis of normally uninfected body fluids, such as blood and urine. Also, x rays can enable doctors to locate internal abscesses and estimate the severity of infection. Needle biopsy (removing tissue with a needle, then examining it under a microscope) may be used to assess bone involvement.

Treatment

Superficial staph infections can generally be cured by keeping the area clean and antiseptic and applying warm moist compresses to the affected area for 20 to 30 minutes three or four times a day.

Among the therapies believed to be helpful for the person with a staph infection are **yoga** (to stimulate the immune system and promote **relaxation**), **acupuncture** (to draw heat away from the infection), and herbal remedies. Herbs that may help the body overcome, or withstand, staph infection include:

- **Garlic** (*Allium sativum*). This herb is believed to have antibacterial properties. Herbalists recommend consuming three garlic cloves or three garlic oil capsules a day, starting when symptoms of infection first appear.

- Cleavers (*Galium aparine*). This anti-inflammatory herb is believed to support the lymphatic system. It may be taken internally to help heal staph abscesses and reduce swelling of the lymph nodes. A cleavers compress can also be applied directly to a skin infection.

- **Goldenseal** (*Hydrastis canadensis*). Another herb believed to fight infection and reduce inflammation, goldenseal may be taken internally when symptoms of infection first appear. Skin infections can be treated by making a paste of water and powdered goldenseal root and applying it directly to the affected area. The preparation should be covered with a clean bandage and left in place overnight.

- Echinacea (*Echinacea* spp.). Taken internally, this herb is believed to have antibiotic properties and is also thought to strengthen the immune system.

- Thyme (*Thymus vulgaris*), **lavender** (*Lavandula officinalis*), or bergamot (*Citrus bergamot*) oils. These oils are believed to have antibacterial properties and may help to prevent the scarring that may result from skin infections. A few drops of these oils are added to water and a compress soaked in the water is then applied to the affected area.

• Tea tree oil (*Melaleuca* spp., or ylang ylang). Another infection-fighting herb, this oil can be applied directly to a boil or other skin infection.

Allopathic treatment

Severe or recurrent staphylocoecal infections may require a seven- to 10-day course of treatment with penicillin or other oral antibiotics. The location of the infection and the identity of the causal bacterium determines which of several effective medications should be prescribed. In recent years, doctors have turned to such newer medications as vancomycin or the fluoroquinolones to treat staph infections because strains of *S. aureus* have emerged that are resistant to penicillin and the older antibiotics.

In case of a more serious infection, antibiotics may be administered intravenously for as long as six weeks. Intravenous antibiotics are also used to treat staph infections around the eyes or on other parts of the face.

Surgery may be required to drain or remove abscesses that form on internal organs, or on shunts or other devices implanted inside the body.

Expected results

Most healthy people who develop staph infections recover fully within a short time. Others develop repeated infections. Some become seriously ill, requiring long-term therapy or emergency care. A small percentage die.

Prevention

Healthcare providers and patients should always wash their hands thoroughly with warm water and soap after treating a staph infection or touching an open wound or the pus it produces. Pus that oozes onto the skin from the site of an infection should be removed immediately. This affected area should then be cleansed with antiseptic or with antibacterial soap.

To prevent infection from spreading from one part of the body to another, it is important to shower rather than bathe during the healing process. Because staph infection is easily transmitted from one member of a household to others, towels, washcloths, and bed linens used by someone with a staph infection should not be used by anyone else. They should be changed daily until symptoms disappear, and laundered separately in hot water with bleach.

Children should frequently be reminded not to share:

• brushes, combs, or hair accessories

• caps

• clothing

• sleeping bags

• sports equipment

• other personal items

A diet rich in green, yellow, and orange vegetables can bolster natural immunity. A doctor or nutritionist may recommend vitamins or mineral supplements to compensate for specific dietary deficiencies. Drinking eight to 10 glasses of water a day can help flush disease-causing organisms from the body.

Because some strains of staph bacteria are known to contaminate artificial limbs, prosthetic devices implanted within the body, and tubes used to administer medication or drain fluids from the body, catheters and other devices should be removed on a regular basis if possible and examined for microscopic signs of staph. Symptoms may not become evident until many months after contamination has occurred, so this practice should be followed even with patients who show no sign of infection.

A vaccine against *S. aureus* was developed in the late 1990s for use with patients with low resistance to infection. A trial of the vaccine in hemodialysis patients indicates that it offers partial protection against bacteremia for about 40 weeks.

Resources

BOOKS

Bennett, J. Claude, and Fred Plum, eds. *Cecil Textbook of Medicine.* Philadelphia, PA: W. B. Saunders Company, 1996.

Civetta, Joseph M., et al, eds. *Critical Care.* Philadelphia, PA: Lippincott-Raven Publishers, 1997.

Fauci, Anthony, et al, eds. *Harrison's Principles of Internal Medicine.* New York, NY: McGraw-Hill, Inc., 1998.

PERIODICALS

Al-Ghamdi, S., M. Gedebou, and N. E. Bilal. "Nosocomial Infections and Misuse of Antibiotics in a Provincial Community Hospital, Saudi Arabia." *Journal of Hospital Infection* 50 (February 2002): 115-121.

Amir, L. "Breastfeeding and *Staphylococcus aureus*: Three Case Reports." *Breastfeeding Review* 10 (March 2002): 15-18.

Bradley, S. F. "*Staphylococcus aureus* Infections and Antibiotic Resistance in Older Adults." *Clinical Infectious Diseases* 34 (January 15, 2002): 211-216.

Cabell, C. H., J. G. Jollis, G. E. Peterson, et al. "Changing Patient Characteristics and the Effect on Mortality in Endocarditis." *Archives of Internal Medicine* 162 (January 14, 2002): 90-94.

KEY TERMS

Abscess—A localized accumulation of pus in a body tissue.

Bacteremia—The presence of bacteria in the bloodstream.

Endocarditis—Inflammation of the lining of the heart, and/or the heart valves, caused by infection.

Fluoroquinolones—A group of newer antibiotics that are used to treat penicillin-resistant staphylococcal infections.

Nosocomial—Contracted in a hospital. Staph infections are the most common type of nosocomial infections.

Superantigen—A type of bacterial toxin that triggers abnormal activation of T-cells, which regulate the body's response to infected or malignant cells. *S. aureus* is responsible for the production of a number of different superantigens.

Llewelyn, M., and J. Cohen. "Superantigens: Microbial Agents That Corrupt Immunity." *Lancet Infectious Diseases* 2 (March 2002): 156-162.

Shinefeld, H., S. Black, A. Fattom et al. "Use of a *Staphylococcus aureus* Conjugate Vaccine in Patients Receiving Hemodialysis." *New England Journal of Medicine* 346 (February 14, 2002): 491-496.

Paula Ford-Martin
Rebecca J. Frey, PhD

Sties

Definition

Also known as an external hordeolum, a stye is an infection or small **abscess** formation within the hair follicle glands on the free edge of the eyelid. These sebaceous glands are also known as Zeis's or Moll's glands.

Description

A stye may develop on or under the eyelid with an eyelash within a yellow point. The area becomes red, warm, swollen, and painful. It may also cause blepharitis, an inflammation of the eyelid.

Causes & symptoms

A stye is caused by staphylococcal or other bacterial infection of the sebaceous gland. This infection may be only on the eyelid, or may also be present elsewhere in the body. The presence of a stye may be a sign of the need for glasses, or indicate declining overall health status.

In addition to localized redness, **pain** and swelling, the affected eye may be sensitive to bright light. The individual with a stye may complain of a gritty sensation in the affected eye, and notice that the eye has increased tearing. Once the abscess drains, localized pain and other symptoms quickly resolve.

Diagnosis

Individuals can usually identify a stye from its accompanying symptoms. A laboratory culture of the drainage from the stye may be done to determine the causative organism, allowing identification of the appropriate topical antibiotic drop, ointment or cream, if necessary, to prevent bacterial infection of the rest of the eye.

Treatment

Application of a warm-water compress for 15–20 minutes several times daily will help bring the stye to a point. Most sties drain spontaneously, or with gentle removal of the affected eyelash. The affected individual should avoid hand-to-eye contact, and wash hands frequently, drying thoroughly with clean towels.

A somewhat unusual local treatment that was recommended by a pediatric ophthalmologist for sties that will not drain after several days of warm-water compresses is the application of a hot potato. The hot potato holds heat longer than a washcloth.

Because a stye may also be the result of overall poor health, intake of a well-balanced diet and other measures to strengthen the immune system are helpful in healing and preventing recurrences. Foods rich in **beta carotene**, along with **vitamin C** and A are beneficial in early stages of bacterial infection; herbal remedies include **garlic, echinacea, goldenseal, calendula**, and **tea tree oil**. Focus on a healthy lifestyle will also include getting enough rest, exercising regularly, and limiting negative **stress. Yoga, meditation**, and **guided imagery** may be helpful for stress reduction and **relaxation**. Eye irritation from **smoking** or other chemical or environmental factors should be avoided.

Allopathic treatment

Self-care is often adequate in resolving a stye; however, surgical incision and drainage of the abscess may occasionally be necessary. While oral or injectable antibiotics are not usually needed, antibiotic drops, ointments or creams may be prescribed to hasten healing and prevent spread of the infection. A physician should

1926

KEY TERMS

Blepharitis—An inflammation of the eyelid.

Hordeolum—The medical term for stye; an infection or small abscess formation in the hair follicle glands of the eyelids.

Sebaceous glands—The oil- or grease-producing glands of the body.

also be consulted for any notable change in vision or pain in the eye.

Expected results

A stye usually resolves completely within five to seven days after it has drained. Even with treatment, recurrence is not uncommon, especially in children. Patients with seborrheic blepharitis (nonulcerated inflammation of the eyelid) are also more likely to develop recurrent sties.

Prevention

Measures to improve overall health and strengthen the immune status will help prevent complications and recurrence. Crowded or unsanitary living conditions will predispose individuals to illnesses that can lower resistance to **infections**. Frequent exposure to dust and other chemical/environmental factors will irritate the eyes and can increase the risk of stye formation.

Resources

BOOKS

Dillard, James, and Terra Ziporyn. *Alternative Medicine for Dummies.* Foster City, CA: IDG Books Worldwide, Inc., 1998.

PERIODICALS

Giusti, Robert. "Don't Pass This Hot Potato." *Contemporary Pediatrics* 18 (November 2001): 116.

Skorin Jr., Leonid. "Eyelid Swelling: What's the Underlying Cause?" *Consultant* 41 (October 2001): 1624–1630.

OTHER

Thrive Online. <http://www.thriveonline.com/health/Library>.

Kathleen Wright
Rebecca J. Frey, PhD

Stiff neck *see* **Neck pain**
Stinging nettle *see* **Nettle**

Stomachaches

Definition

Stomachache is **pain** or discomfort in the stomach that is a symptom of many different gastrointestinal diseases or conditions.

Description

Stomachache, also called dyspepsia, is a symptom of an underlying disease or condition of the gastrointestinal system. Stomachache is defined as pain or discomfort in the upper abdomen. Discomfort refers to any negative feeling including fullness, bloating, or early satiety (quenched thirst or appetite).

Dyspepsia accounts for 2–5% of all visits to a physician. Unfortunately, no cause is found for 30–60% of patients with dyspepsia. When no cause is found, the disorder is termed nonulcer dyspepsia. Several factors may lead to nonulcer dyspepsia. Delayed emptying of the stomach contents and stomach and intestinal rhythmic movement (motility) disorders can lead to dyspepsia. Some persons have lower sensory thresholds for stomach distension and more readily experience stomachache. Abnormal release of stomach acids may also be associated with dyspepsia.

Studies performed around the world have determined that between 7–41% of the population suffer from dyspepsia. This wide variation is most likely due to differences in study methods, not differences in the prevalence of dyspepsia.

Causes & symptoms

The occasional stomachache is usually caused by overeating, stomach **gas**, eating foods that do not agree with a person's digestive system, drinking too much alcohol, **food poisoning**, or gastrointestinal infection. **Obesity** places extra pressure on the stomach that can cause pain. **Smoking** increases stomach acid production and relaxes the valve between the stomach and the esophagus, both of which can cause stomach pain.

Because there are many causes of dyspepsia, physicians try to fit each case into one of five categories based upon the set of symptoms. Nonulcer dyspepsia refers to long-term or recurrent pain in the upper abdomen that has no identified structural cause. Ulcer-like dyspepsia refers to abdominal pain with three or more of the following symptoms: well-localized pain, pain relieved by eating, pain relieved by antacids, pain occurring when hungry, pain that disrupts sleep, or pain that comes and goes for at least two week intervals. Dysmotility-like dyspepsia refers to upper abdominal discomfort, not pain, with three or more of the following: early satiety, **nausea**, fullness after eating, recurrent retching or **vomiting**, bloating, or abdominal discomfort worsened by food. Reflux-like dyspepsia is stomach pain accompanied by **heartburn**. Nonspecific dyspepsia refers to patients whose symptoms do not fit into the other categories.

Specific causes of stomachaches include:

- Biliary tract disease, disorders of the gallbladder, bile, and bile ducts. Biliary pain is a severe persistent pain in the upper middle or upper right region of the abdomen.

- Drug-induced dyspepsia, which may be caused by digitalis, theophylline, antibiotics, and **iron** or **potassium** supplements.

- Dysmotility disorders, gastrointestinal motility that is either too fast or too slow, and may lead to abdominal pain.

- Gastric **cancer**, although a rare cause of stomachache, needs to be considered in the differential diagnosis because of the seriousness of the disease.

- Gastroesophageal reflux causes a burning pain or discomfort that travels up to the throat. This common disorder affects up to 50% of adults.

- Irritable bowel syndrome, a chronic disease characterized by abdominal pain and changes in bowel functioning (**diarrhea** and/or constipation).

- Pancreatic disease, including **pancreatitis** (inflammation of the pancreas) and pancreatic cancer, can cause severe persistent pain that may travel to the back.

- Peptic ulcer refers to any ulcer (a defect or hole) of the upper digestive tract.

- Such psychiatric disorders as **depression**, **panic disorder**, and eating disorders can lead to stomach pains.

- Other disorders. Stomachaches may be caused by **diabetes mellitus**, **hypothyroidism**, hypercalcemia, ischemic **heart disease**, intestinal **angina**, certain cancers, **Crohn's disease**, **tuberculosis**, and **syphilis**. In addition, abdominal muscle strain, myositis, and nerve entrapment can cause abdominal pain which could be confused with dyspepsia.

Stomachache itself is a discomfort or pain in the upper abdomen. The patient may experience other symptoms as well, depending upon the cause of the stomachache. Stomachache must be experienced for three months to be considered chronic (long-term). Persons who experience recurrent vomiting, weight loss, dysphagia (swallowing difficulty), or bleeding should seek prompt medical attention.

Diagnosis

Stomachache may be diagnosed by an internal medicine specialist or a gastroenterologist. Because diagnosing dyspepsia can be time consuming and expensive, all attempts are made to first rule out a structural cause of the pain to prevent the use of unnecessary tests. The diagnostic process would include a thorough medical history and physical examination.

The presence of *Helicobacter pylori*, a common cause of ulcers, in the stomach, would be determined. There is a higher risk for structural disease in persons older than 45 years; therefore, these persons would undergo upper gastrointestinal endoscopy (upper GI). Endoscopy is the use of a wand-like camera to visualize internal organs, including the stomach and intestinal tract.

If ulcer has been ruled out, then an upper GI (an x-ray study of the upper GI tract) and several blood tests would be performed. Ultrasound (visualization of internal organs using sound waves) may be performed to view the liver, pancreas, and gall bladder. More specific tests that may be conducted include lactose tolerance test, stomach-emptying study, gastroduodenal manometry (measures pressure and motility of the stomach and small intestine), electrogastrography (measures electrical activity of the stomach), and esophageal pH testing (measures the pH in the pipe running from the throat to the stomach).

Treatment

Alternative remedies can be effective in treating stomachache and associated digestive symptoms. Persons who experience chronic, unexplained stomach pain should consult a physician.

Herbals

The following herbal remedies help treat stomachaches:

- agave (*Agave americana*) tincture
- asafoetida (*Ferula asafoetida*) tincture
- cumin (*Cumin cyminum*) seed poultice

When gas is the reason for discomfort, these herbals can be used:

- angelica (*Angelica archangelica*) infusion
- anise (*Pimpinella anisum*) infusion
- catnip (*Nepeta cataria*) tea
- oatstraw (*Avena sativa*) tea

Indigestion accompanied by gas or due to increased stomach acid production can be soothed by the following herbals:

- arrowroot (*Maranta arundinacea*) infusion

- calendula (*Calendula officinalis*) and **comfrey** root tea

- cardamom (*Elettaria cardamomum*) powder

- **fennel** (*Foeniculum vulgare*) infusion

- galbanum (*Ferula gummosa*) infusion: acid indigestion

- Iceland moss (*Cetraria islandica*) infusion

- marsh mallow (*Althaea officinalis*) tea

- meadowsweet (*Filipendula ulmaria*) tea

- slippery elm (*Ulmus fulva*) powder or tea

Other disorders causing stomach pain and discomfort can be relieved with these herbals:

- Asian red ginseng (*Panax ginseng*) tea or tincture: stomach pain and bloating

- chamomile (*Chamomilla recutita*) tea: upset stomach, gas, and stomach spasm

- crab apple (flower remedy): stomachaches caused by bad food

- crampbark (*Viburnum opulus*) infusion: stomach spasm

- dandelion (*Taraxacum officinale*) root tea or tincture: heartburn, stomachache, and gas

- elderberry (*Sambucus nigra*) tea: stomach pain

- **ginger** (*Zingiber officinale*) raw or tea

- lemon balm (*Melissa officinalis*) tea: stomach spasm, gas, and bloating

- licorice (*Glycyrrhiza glabra*) root tea or tincture: heartburn and acid reflux

- **peppermint** (*Mentha piperita*) tea: upset stomach, gas, and stomach spasm

- thyme (*Thymus vulgaris*) tea: upset stomach

Homeopathy

Homeopathic remedies are chosen based upon the specific set of symptoms displayed by the patient. **Bryonia** is indicated for stomach pain that is worsened by motion. Colocynthis or Magnesia phosphorica is recommended for pain that is relieved by doubling up. Cuprum is indicated for violent, cramping pain. Dioscorea is chosen for pain that is lessened by standing up and worsened by doubling up. **Lycopodium** is indicated for persons who get bloated after eating or whose pain is worsened by pressure. Magnesia phosphorica is recommended for pain that is relieved by pressure. **Nux vomica** is indicated for stomach pain that occurs after eating rich or spicy foods or too much alcohol. **Pulsatilla** is chosen for persons who experience digestive symptoms after eating fatty foods.

Chinese medicine

Traditional Chinese medicine (TCM) treats stomachaches with **acupuncture**, ear acupuncture, **cupping**, herbs, and patent medicines. Common syndromes that cause abdominal pain include: Damp-heat stagnation, retention of cold, retention of food, deficiency and coldness of Zang Fu, and stagnation of qi and blood.

Abdominal pain caused by deficiency and cold is treated with Fu Zi Li Zhong Wan (prepared **Aconite** pill to regulate the middle). Abdominal pain caused by cold is treated with Liang Fu Wan (Galagal and **Cyperus** pill). All causes of abdominal pain (except damp-heat) may be treated with a mixture of Yan Hu Suo (*Rhizoma corydalis*), Chen Xiang (*Lignum aquilariae resinatum*), and Rou Gui (*Cortex cinnamomi*).

Ayurveda

Ayurvedic practitioners believe that indigestion is due to weak or insufficient agni (digestive fire). To enhance digestion, the patient can take fresh ginger; a mixture of **garlic** powder (one quarter teaspoon), trikatu (one half teaspoon), and rock salt (pinch); or a mixture of garlic (one clove), cumin powder (one quarter teaspoon), rocksalt (pinch), trikatu (pinch), and lime juice (one teaspoon) before meals. Bay leaf tea drunk after meals can enliven agni. Digestion may be enhanced with Shatavari or Teak tree (*Tectona grandis*) wood or bark.

Chronic indigestion and stomachaches may be relieved by taking a mixture of trikatu (one part), chitrak (two parts), and kutki (one part) with honey and ginger juice before meals. Common stomachaches may be relieved by taking a shankavati or lasunadivati pill twice daily; ajwan (one half teaspoon) and baking soda (one quarter teaspoon) in water; a mixture of cumin powder (one third teaspoon), asafetida (pinch), and rock salt (pinch) in water; or chewing one half teaspoon of roasted fennel, cumin, and coriander seeds.

Other treatments

Other treatments for stomachaches are:

- Acupressure. Pressing both Sp 16 points (located below the bottom of the rib cage) can relieve stomachaches.

- Aromatherapy. Sucking on a sugar cube containing one drop of the essential oil of peppermint can ease stomachaches. Taking honey containing one drop of essential oil of tarragon, marjoram, or **rosemary** reduces digestive tract spasms.

- Hydrotherapy. Stomachache can be relieved by drinking water containing **activated charcoal** powder. A hot water bottle or hot compress placed over the abdomen can help relieve stomach pains.

• Juice therapy. Digestion can be improved and gas dispelled by drinking fresh apple juice with mint, fennel, and ginger.

Allopathic treatment

Stomachaches may be treated with over the counter antacids (Tums, Pepto-Bismol) and antigas products (Gas-X). An *H. pylori* infection is treated with a combination of tetracycline, bismuth subsalicylate (Pepto-Bismol), and metronidazole (Metizol). Nonulcer dyspepsia may be treated with the proton pump inhibitors omeprazole (Prilosec) and lansoprazole (Prevacid); the H_2 receptor antagonists ranitidine (Zantac), cimetidine (Tagamet), famotidine (Pepcid), and nizatidine (Axid); or the prokinetic drug cisapride.

Stomachaches that are caused by diseases such as cancer, diabetes, pancreatitis, etc. would be treated using the specific medications and procedures recommended for the particular disease.

Expected results

Stomachaches may resolve spontaneously. Medical treatment of stomachaches can relieve symptoms temporarily but a cure is not expected.

Prevention

Common stomachaches can be prevented by avoiding the following: overeating, excessive alcohol consumption, problem foods, and smoking. Stomachaches may be prevented by enhancing digestion by taking fresh ginger or Draksha (Ayurvedic herbal wine) before meals. Ginger or bay leaf tea or lassi (yogurt with cumin and ginger powders in water) taken after meals can aid digestion and prevent stomachaches. Drinking warm drinks during meals aids digestion as does chewing food thoroughly. Persons should eat only when hungry and leave space in the stomach for proper digestion. Obesity can increase problems like reflux, and a 2001 study found a strong connection between obesity and severity of reflux.

Resources

BOOKS

Reichenberg-Ullman, Judyth, and Robert Ullman. *Homeopathic Self-Care: The Quick and Easy Guide for the Whole Family.* Rocklin, CA: Prima Publishing, 1997.

Talley, Nicholas J., and Gerald Holtmann. "Approach to the Patient With Dyspepsia and Related Functional Gastrointestinal Complaints." *Textbook of Gastroenterology.* 3rd ed. Edited by Tadataka Yamada, et al. Philadelphia: Lippincott Williams & Wilkins, 1999.

Ying, Zhou Zhong, and Jin Hui De. "Abdominal Pain." *Clinical Manual of Chinese Herbal Medicine and Acupuncture.* New York: Churchill Livingston, 1997.

PERIODICALS

Cavalli, Ellen. "Relief for Holiday Pigouts." *Vegetarian Times* (November 1999): 94+.

"Fast Lives Bring on the Burn." *Chemist and Druggist* (November 10, 2001): 37.

Levine, Beth. "How to Treat Any Kind of Tummyache." *Redbook* 190 (April 1998): 145+.

Sullivan, Karin Horgan. "Oh, What a Relief it is: Herbs to Soothe an Upset Stomach." *Vegetarian Times* (November 1996): 94+.

Wajed, Shahjehan A. "Elevated Body Mass Disrupts the Barrier to Gastroesophageal Reflux." *The Journal of the American Medical Association* (December 5, 2001): 2650.

ORGANIZATIONS

The American Gastroenterological Association (AGA). 7910 Woodmont Ave., 7th Floor, Bethesda, MD 20814. (310) 654-2055. <http://www.gastro.org/index.html>.

Belinda Rowland
Teresa G. Odle

Stomatitis *see* **Cantharis**

Stone massage

Definition

Stone massage is a form of bodywork that involves the application of heated or cooled stones (thermotherapy) to the body during deep tissue massage.

Origins

The use of materials of different temperatures on the body to bring about healing is an ancient technique. Stones have been used in many cultures, such as in the Native American sweat lodge, to adjust the temperature of the healing environment. Traditional **lomilomi** (Hawaiian massage) goes further and applies heated stones directly to the body.

Although stones have been used for many years as an adjunct to bodywork, their use was formalized in 1993 by Mary Nelson-Hannigan of Tucson, Arizona. Nelson-Hannigan developed a form of massage using a system of 54 hot stones, 18 frozen stones, and one room-temperature stone, which she calls LaStone Therapy. In addition to the use of stones as an extension of the therapist's hands in deep tissue massage, LaStone Therapy involves a spiritual element that opens energy channels (chakras) in the body, unblocks memories, and brings about spiritual healing.

Benefits

Stone therapy has benefits for both the client and the massage therapist. For the client the application of heat and cold on the body:

- Stimulates the circulatory system and promotes self-healing.
- Softens and relaxes the muscles.
- Helps to release toxins from the muscles.
- Induces a state of deep **relaxation** that washes away **stress**.
- Helps relieve **pain** and muscle spasms.
- Creates a feeling of peacefulness and spiritual well-being.

Stone therapy also benefits the massage therapist. It reduces stress and strain on the therapist's hands, wrists, and arms so that the therapist can work longer and more efficiently. The stones do the heavy work, so that the possibility of repetitive stress injuries to the therapist's thumbs and wrists is decreased.

Description

In many ways a stone massage session is similar to any other type of massage. The stones are heated (usually to about 130°F or 34°C) or frozen prior to the client's arrival. Massage oil is spread on the client's back and legs. The stones are then worked over the body. The client turns over and the process is repeated on the arms, hands, and fingers. The final parts to be massaged are the neck, head, and face.

Preparations

The client needs no special preparation before receiving a stone massage. The therapist prepares the stones in advance and maintains them at the proper temperatures.

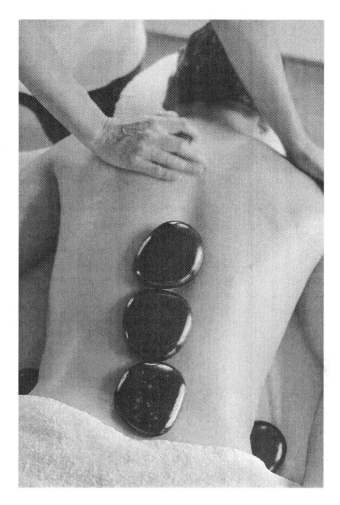

Man receiving hot stone massage. *(© Royalty-free/Corbis.)*

Precautions

No special precautions are necessary in having a stone massage session. This type of massage is suitable for almost everyone.

Side effects

Generally a stone massage produces only the positive side effects of a feeling of peacefulness and spiritual renewal. No negative side effects have been reported.

Research & general acceptance

The use of stones to alter body temperature has been used for centuries. Little modern research has been done on its effectiveness, although it is a generally accepted technique.

Training & certification

LaStone Therapy offers its own certification for people already trained as massage therapists who complete specific courses in LaStone Therapy. Many of these courses are recognized for credit by the American **Massage Therapy** Association, the International Myomassethics Federation, Inc., the National Certification Board for Therapeutic Massage & Bodywork, and the Associated Bodywork and Massage Professionals.

Resources

ORGANIZATIONS

American Massage Therapy Association. 820 Davis Street, Suite 100. Evanston, IL 60201. (847) 864-0123.

LaStone Therapy. 2919 E. Broadway Blvd., Suite 224. Tucson, AZ 85716. (520) 319-6414. http://www.lastonetherapy.com.

OTHER

Alaska Wellness. http://www.alaskawellness.com *The Original Hot Stone Massage.*

Tish Davidson

Strep throat

Definition

Strep throat is a contagious infection caused by the bacterium *Streptococcus pyogenes*.

Description

Strep throat primarily affects children, especially those between the ages of five and 15. Adults whose immune systems have been weakened by **stress** or other **infections** are also at risk. Most sore throats are associated with viral infections such as the **common cold** or the flu. Strep throat is responsible in only about 10%–15% of cases. Many people carry *Streptococcus pyogenes* in their systems without even knowing it. It can survive in the lining of the throat or nose for years without producing symptoms. Almost 20% of people in general good health may be harboring this bacterium unsuspectingly, according to one statistic.

Strep throat is often mistaken for a cold or the flu. It is important, however, to identify strep throat because if left untreated it can lead to serious health problems. In rare cases, untreated strep throat may increase the risk of developing scarlet or **rheumatic fever**. Rheumatic **fever**, in turn, is associated with **meningitis** and diseases affecting the heart, skin, kidneys, and joints. Strep throat may return repeatedly if not treated effectively the first time.

Another reason for getting treatment for strep throat is that *Streptococcus pyogenes* belongs to a group of disease-causing bacteria that produce superantigens. Superantigens are a group of toxins that have the ability to trigger excessive and abnormal activation of the body's T cells. T cells are produced in the thymus gland and regulate the human immune system's response to infection. Superantigens are being studied intensively for their roles in causing disease. *Streptococcus pyogenes* and *Staphylococcus aureus* together produce 19 different superantigens.

Causes & symptoms

Most people develop strep throat through close contact with someone who has an untreated strep infection. Infected mucus from the nose or throat is often spread via **sneezing** or coughing. Carriers of *Streptococcus pyogenes* who do not show symptoms of strep throat are less likely to infect others, as are people with strep throat who have received antibiotic therapy for 24 hours or more. Strep throat is not usually transmitted through casual contact. In rare cases, strep can develop after exposure to infected food, dairy products, or water.

People with weakened immune systems are more likely to become infected with strep throat. This infection can occur when the body is battling a cold or the flu. **Stress** or physical exhaustion can also weaken the immune system and increase the risk of bacterial infection. Strep throat usually strikes during the winter months. Symptoms develop two to four days after being infected.

While cold or flu symptoms often develop gradually over a period of several days, the symptoms associated with strep throat occur with little warning. Classic symptoms of strep include **sore throat** and fever. Other tell-tale signs may include swollen and tender lymph glands in the neck, redness on the inside of the throat, inflamed tonsils or gray/white patches on the tonsils, and **headache**. Trouble swallowing can also occur, and red specks may be visible on the roof of the mouth. **Nausea** and stomach **pain** are more likely in children infected with strep. Unlike a cold or the flu, strep throat does not usually produce **cough** or a stuffy, runny nose.

Diagnosis

Most doctors who suspect strep throat recommend a rapid strep test to confirm the diagnosis. This painless

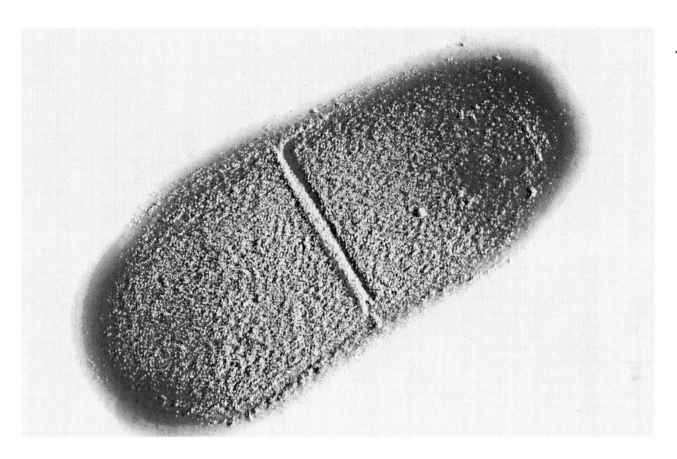

Group A *Streptococcus* bacterium. *(J.L. Carson. Custom Medical Stock Photo. Reproduced by permission.)*

test involves using a swab to remove a specimen from the throat of the infected person. The results of the test are available in 10–20 minutes. In addition, the doctor may send a similar specimen to a laboratory to have a throat culture performed, which takes a day or two to complete. A negative strep test or culture usually indicates that the cause is viral in nature, in which case antibiotics are of no help.

Treatment

Conventional medicine is very successful in treating strep throat. However, several alternative therapies may help to resolve the disease or relieve symptoms. Herbal remedies such as **echinacea** (*Echinacea* spp.), **goldenseal** (*Hydrastis canadensis*), and **garlic** (*Allium sativum*) are believed to strengthen the immune system and combat bacterial infections.

Goldenseal

One of its active agents is a chemical called berberine. This alkaloid is believed to have antibiotic effects against streptococci bacteria. It may also help to prevent *Streptococcus pyogenes* from attaching itself to the throat lining, according to a study published in the journal *Antimicrobial Agents and Chemotherapy* in 1988. Goldenseal is also believed to increase the activity of disease-fighting white blood cells.

Echinacea

This popular herb fights viral and bacterial infections by boosting the immune system, according to herbalists. Echinacea may also combat strep throat by interfering with the production of hyaluronidase, an enzyme that helps the offending bacterium to grow and spread.

Garlic

The focus of hundreds of medical studies and papers, garlic is believed to be an antibiotic as well as an antiviral. As an added benefit, garlic may also prevent **atherosclerosis**, lower **cholesterol** levels, and act as an antioxidant.

Zinc and **ginger** (*Zingiber officinale*) are sometimes recommended to help treat symptoms of sore throat. In addition to strengthening the immune system, zinc may reduce throat inflammation and pain regardless of the cause. Ginger may have analgesic properties and ease throat irritation.

In the practice of **homeopathy**, **belladonna**, **lachesis**, and mercurius are usually the remedies of choice for strep throat and other causes of throat irritation. Which remedy to use depends on the exact nature of the symptoms. These homeopathic treatments are not recommended for more than a few days or symptoms may actually return.

Vitamin C may also help to boost the immune system. In some studies, it has been shown to shorten the duration of colds.

Allopathic treatment

Antibiotics, the conventional treatment of choice, are very effective in curing strep throat. They also ease symptoms and are generally believed to reduce the risk of serious complications such as rheumatic fever. Ten days of oral penicillin is a typical course of therapy. People allergic to this drug usually take erythromycin instead. In some cases, a single injection of antibiotics may be preferred. It is important to complete the full course of antibiotic therapy (even if symptoms begin to subside earlier) in order to resolve the disease and prevent the development of complications. To further alleviate symptoms, acetaminophen or ibuprofen may also be used.

Studies of bacterial resistance to various drugs indicate that the strains of *S. pyogenes* found most commonly in the United States have developed some resistance to erythromycin as of 2002. As a result, doctors are more likely to prescribe antibiotics that belong to a newer group of drugs called quinolones. It is important to take quinolone antibiotics exactly as directed, as they have a number of side effects.

Expected results

The symptoms associated with strep throat usually begin to disappear within several days even without treatment. When antibiotics are used, fever may subside within 24 hours, and the course of the illness may be shortened by two days.

People who use alternative remedies in the absence of antibiotics should consult a doctor if symptoms do not subside within a week. In these cases, the use of antibiotics is strongly recommended.

Prevention

Washing the hands frequently can help to prevent strep throat. Exposure to infected people should also be avoided. In order to prevent transmission of the disease within households, consult a doctor if any family member suddenly develops a sore throat (especially if it is accompanied by fever).

KEY TERMS

. . . .

Analgesic—Pain reliever.

Antioxidant—An agent that helps to protect cells from damage caused by free radicals, the destructive fragments of oxygen produced as a byproduct during normal metabolic processes.

Echinacea—A popular herbal remedy used to treat colds, the flu, and urinary tract infections.

Meningitis—An inflammation of the lining of the brain.

Scarlet fever—A childhood disease characterized by a red skin rash appearing on the chest, neck, elbows, and thighs. Scarlet fever, which may also be accompanied by sore throat and fever, is caused by the bacterium *Streptococcus pyogenes*.

Superantigen—A type of bacterial toxin that triggers abnormal activation of T-cells, which regulate the body's response to infected or malignant cells. *Streptococcus pyogenes* is responsible for the production of a number of different superantigens.

Boosting the immune system is also important to help prevent the development of strep throat. Vitamin C and zinc are often recommended for this purpose, as are goldenseal, echinacea, and garlic. Reducing stress and getting proper sleep can also strengthen the body's defenses against infection.

Resources

BOOKS

Bennett, Claude J., and Fred Plum. *Cecil Textbook of Medicine.* Philadelphia, PA: W.B. Saunders Company, 1996.

Murray, Michael T., and Joseph Pizzorno. *Encyclopedia of Natural Medicine.* Rocklin, CA: Prima Publishing, 1998.

PERIODICALS

Barros, M.G. "Soothing Sore Throats Gingerly." *Cortlandt Forum* 67 (1995): 86-16.

Critchley, I. A., D. F. Sahm, C. Thornsberry et al. "Antimicrobial Susceptibilities of *Streptococcus pyogenes* Isolated from Respiratory and Skin and Soft Tissue Infections: United States LIBRA Surveillance Data from 1999." *Diagnostic Microbiology and Infectious Disease* 42 (February 2002): 129-135.

Llewelyn, M., and J. Cohen. "Superantigens: Microbial Agents That Corrupt Immunity." *Lancet Infectious Diseases* 2 (March 2002): 156-162.

Sun, D., H.S. Courtney, and E.H Beachey. "Berberine sulfate blocks adherence of *Streptococcus pyogenes* to epithelial cells, fibronectin,and hexadecane." *Antimicrob Agents Chemother* 32, no. 9 (1988): 1370-4.

ORGANIZATIONS

National Institute of Allergy and Infectious Disease. 31 Center Drive MSC 2520, Building 31, Room 7A-50, Bethesda, MD 20892- 2520.

OTHER

Discovery Health. http://www.discoveryhealth.com.
National Institute of Allergy and Infectious Disease. http://www.niaid.nih.gov.

Greg Annussek
Rebecca J. Frey, PhD

TOP TEN STRESSFUL EVENTS

Death of spouse
Divorce
Marital separation
Jail term or death of close family member
Personal injury or illness
Marriage
Loss of job due to termination
Marital reconciliation or retirement
Pregnancy
Change in financial state

Source: "What are the Leading Causes of Stress?" In *Science and Technology Desk Reference.* Edited by The Carnegie Library of Pittsburgh Science and Technology Department. Detroit: Gale Research, Inc., 1993, p. 415. (Electronic Illustrators Group. Reproduced by permission.)

Stress

Definition

Stress is an individual's physical and mental reaction to environmental demands or pressures.

Description

When stress was first studied, the term was used to denote both the causes and the experienced effects of these pressures. More recently, however, the word stressor has been used for the stimulus that provokes a stress response. One recurrent disagreement among researchers concerns the definition of stress in humans. Is it primarily an external response that can be measured by changes in glandular secretions, skin reactions, and other physical functions, or is it an internal interpretation of, or reaction to, a stressor; or is it both?

Stress was first studied in 1896 by Walter B. Cannon (1871–1945). Cannon used an x-ray instrument called a fluoroscope to study the digestive system of dogs. He noticed that the digestive process stopped when the dogs were under stress. Stress triggers adrenal hormones in the body and the hormones become unbalanced. Based on these findings, Cannon continued his experimentation and came up with the term homeostasis, a state of equilibrium in the body.

Hans Selye, a Canadian scientist (1907–1982), noticed that people who suffered from chronic illness or disease showed some of the same symptoms. Selye related this to stress and he began to test his hypothesis. He exposed rats to different physical stress factors such as heat, sound, poison, and shock. The rats showed enlarged glands, shrunken thymus glands and lymph nodes, and gastric ulcers. Selye then developed the Three Stage Model of Stress Response. This model consisted of alarm, resistance, and exhaustion. Selye also showed that stress is mediated by cortisol, a hormone that is released from the adrenal cortex. This increases the amount of glucose in the body while under stress.

Stress in humans results from interactions between persons and their environment that are perceived as straining or exceeding their adaptive capacities and threatening their well-being. The element of perception indicates that human stress responses reflect differences in personality, as well as differences in physical strength or general health.

Risk factors for stress-related illnesses are a mix of personal, interpersonal, and social variables. These factors include lack or loss of control over one's physical environment, and lack or loss of social support networks. People who are dependent on others (e.g., children or the elderly) or who are socially disadvantaged (because of race, gender, educational level, or similar factors) are at greater risk of developing stress-related illnesses. Other risk factors include feelings of helplessness, hopelessness, extreme fear or anger, and cynicism or distrust of others.

Causes & symptoms

Causes

The causes of stress can include any event or occurrence that a person considers a threat to his or her coping strategies or resources. Researchers generally agree that a certain degree of stress is a normal part of a living organism's response to the inevitable changes in its physical or social environment, and that positive as well as negative events can generate stress. Stress-related disease, however, results from excessive and prolonged demands on an organism's coping resources. It is now believed that 80–90% of all disease is stress-related.

Recent research indicates that some vulnerability to stress is genetic. Scientists at the University of Wisconsin and King's College, London, discovered that people who inherited a short, or stress-sensitive, version of the serotonin transporter gene were almost three times as likely to experience **depression** following a stressful event as people with the long version of the gene. Further research is likely to identify other genes that affect susceptibility to stress.

One cause of stress that has affected large sectors of the general population around the world since 2001 is terrorism. The events of September 11, 2001, the sniper shootings in Virginia and Maryland, the Bali nightclub bombing in 2002, and the suicide bombings in the Middle East in 2003 have all been shown to cause short-term symptoms of stress in people who read about them or watch television news reports as well as those who witnessed the actual events. Stress related to terrorist attacks also appears to affect people in countries far from the location of the attack as well as those in the immediate vicinity. It is too soon to tell how stress related to episodes of terrorism will affect human health over long periods of time, but researchers are already beginning to investigate this question.

Symptoms

The symptoms of stress can be either physical and/or psychological. Stress-related physical illnesses, such as **irritable bowel syndrome**, heart attacks, and chronic headaches, result from long-term overstimulation of a part of the nervous system that regulates the heart rate, blood pressure, and digestive system. Stress-related emotional illness results from inadequate or inappropriate responses to major changes in one's life situation, such as marriage, completing one's education, the death of a loved one, divorce, becoming a parent, losing a job, or retirement. Psychiatrists sometimes use the term adjustment disorder to describe this type of illness. In the workplace, stress-related illness often takes the form of burnout—a loss of interest in or ability to perform one's job due to long-term high stress levels.

Diagnosis

When the doctor suspects that a patient's illness is connected to stress, he or she will take a careful history that includes stressors in the patient's life (family or employment problems, other illnesses, etc.). Many physicians will evaluate the patient's personality as well, in order to assess his or her coping resources and emotional response patterns. There are a number of personality inventories and psychological tests that doctors can use to help diagnose the amount of stress that the patient experi-

ences and the coping strategies that he or she uses to deal with them. Stress-related illness can be diagnosed by primary care doctors as well as by those who specialize in psychiatry. The doctor will need to distinguish between adjustment disorders and **anxiety** or mood disorders, and between psychiatric disorders and physical illnesses (e.g. thyroid activity) that have psychological side effects.

Treatment

Relaxation training, **yoga**, **t'ai chi**, and **dance therapy** help patients relieve physical and mental symptoms of stress. **Hydrotherapy**, **massage therapy**, and **aromatherapy** are useful to some anxious patients because they can promote general relaxation of the nervous system. **Essential oils** of **lavender**, **chamomile**, neroli, sweet marjoram, and ylang-ylang are commonly recommended by aromatherapists for stress relief.

Meditation can also be a useful tool for controlling stress. **Guided imagery**, in which an individual is taught to visualize a pleasing and calming mental image in order to counteract feelings of stress, is also helpful. Many individuals may find activities such as **exercise**, art, music, and writing useful in reducing stress and promoting relaxation.

Sometimes the best therapy for alleviating stress is a family member or friend who will listen. Talking about stressful situations and events can help an individual work through his or her problems and consequently reduce the level of stress related to them. Having a social support network to turn to in times of trouble is critical to everyone's mental and physical well-being. **Pet therapy** has also been reported to relieve stress.

Herbs known as adaptogens may also be prescribed by herbalists or holistic healthcare providers to alleviate stress. These herbs are thought to promote adaptability to stress, and include **Siberian ginseng** (*Eleutherococcus senticosus*), ginseng (*Panax ginseng*), **wild yam** (*Dioscorea villosa*), borage (*Borago officinalis*), **licorice** (*Glycyrrhiza glabra*), **chamomile** (*Chamaemelum nobile*), **milk thistle** (*Silybum marianum*), and **nettle** (*Urtica dioica*).

Practitioners of Ayurvedic, or traditional Indian, medicine might prescribe root of winter cherry, fruit of emblic myrobalan, or the traditional formulas geriforte or mentat to reduce stress and fix the imbalance in the vata dosha.

It is also said that stress reduces the body's immune response, therefore vitamin supplementation can be helpful in counteracting the depletion. Diet is also important—coffee and other caffeinated beverages in high doses produce jitteriness, restlessness, anxiety, and **in-**

somnia. High-protein foods from animal sources elevate brain levels of dopamine and norepinephrine, which are associated with higher levels of anxiety and stress. Whole grains promote production of the brain neurotransmitter serotonin for a greater sense of well-being.

Allopathic treatment

Recent advances in the understanding of the many complex connections between the human mind and body have produced a variety of mainstream approaches to stress-related illness. Present treatment regimens may include one or more of the following:

• Medications. These may include drugs to control blood pressure or other physical symptoms of stress as well as drugs that affect the patient's mood (tranquilizers or antidepressants).

• Stress management programs. These may be either individual or group treatments, and usually involve analysis of the stressors in the patient's life. They often focus on job- or workplace-related stress. A number of studies have found that good stress management programs significantly reduce absenteeism from work and visits to the doctor. They also improve immune system function and overall well-being in patients with such chronic disorders as HIV infection and diabetes.

• Behavioral approaches. These strategies include relaxation techniques, breathing exercises, and physical exercise programs including walking.

• **Biofeedback**. Biofeedback is a technique in which patients are taught to interpret and respond to signals from their own bodies. It can be taught by doctors, dentists, nurses, and physical therapists as well as by psychologists or psychiatrists. Biofeedback is often recommended as a treatment for chronic tension-type headaches.

• Massage. Therapeutic massage relieves stress by relaxing the large groups of muscles in the back, neck, arms, and legs. It is particularly helpful for people who tend to convert stress into muscle tension.

• Cognitive therapy. These approaches teach patients to reframe or mentally reinterpret the stressors in their lives in order to modify the body's physical reactions.

Expected results

The prognosis for recovery from a stress-related illness is related to a wide variety of factors in a person's life, many of which are genetically determined (race, sex, illnesses that run in families) or beyond the individual's control (economic trends, cultural stereotypes and prejudices). It is possible, however, for humans to learn new responses to stress and change their experiences of it. A person's ability to remain healthy in stressful situations is sometimes referred to as stress hardiness. Stress-hardy people have a cluster of personality traits that strengthen their ability to cope. These traits include believing in the importance of what they are doing; believing that they have some power to influence their situation; and viewing life's changes as positive opportunities rather than as threats.

Prevention

Complete prevention of stress is neither possible nor desirable because stress is an important stimulus of human growth and creativity, as well as an inevitable part of life. In addition, specific strategies for stress prevention vary widely from person to person, depending on the nature and number of the stressors in an individual's life, and the amount of control he or she has over these factors. In general, however, a combination of attitudinal and behavioral changes work well for most patients. The best form of prevention appears to be parental modeling of healthy attitudes and behaviors within the family.

Resources

BOOKS

Clark, R. Barkley. "Psychosocial Aspects of Pediatrics and Psychiatric Disorders." *Current Pediatric Diagnosis &Treatment*. Edited by William W. Hay, Jr., et al. Stamford, CT: Appleton & Lange, 1997.

Eisendrath, Stuart J. "Psychiatric Disorders." *Current Medical Diagnosis & Treatment*. Edited by Lawrence M. Tierney, Jr., Stephen J. McPhee, and Maxine A. Papadakis. Stamford, CT: Appleton &Lange, 1997.

Pelletier, Kenneth R., MD. *The Best Alternative Medicine*, Part I, "Spirituality and Healing." New York: Simon & Schuster, 2002.

"Psychiatry in Medicine." Section 15, Chapter 185 in *The Merck Manual of Diagnosis and Therapy*, edited by Mark H. Beers, MD, and Robert Berkow, MD. Whitehouse Station, NJ: Merck Research Laboratories, 1999.

Selye, Hans, MD. *The Stress of Life*. New York, Toronto, and London: McGraw-Hill Book Company, 1956.

PERIODICALS

Antoni, M. H., D. G. Cruess, N. Klimas, et al. "Stress Management and Immune System Reconstitution in Symptomatic HIV-Infected Gay Men Over Time: Effects on Transitional Naive T Cells (CD4(+)CD45RA(+)CD29(+))." *American Journal of Psychiatry* 159 (January 2002): 143-145.

Blumenthal, J. A., M. Babyak, J. Wei, et al. "Usefulness of Psychosocial Treatment of Mental Stress-Induced Myocardial Ischemia in Men." *American Journal of Cardiology* 89 (January 15, 2002): 164-168.

Cardenas, J., K. Williams, J. P. Wilson, et al. "PSTD, Major Depressive Symptoms, and Substance Abuse Following September 11, 2001, in a Midwestern University Population" *International Journal of Emergency Mental Health* 5 (Winter 2003): 15–28.

KEY TERMS

. . . .

Adjustment disorder—A psychiatric disorder marked by inappropriate or inadequate responses to a change in life circumstances.

Biofeedback—A technique in which patients learn to modify certain body functions, such as temperature or pulse rate, with the help of a monitoring machine.

Burnout—An emotional condition, marked by tiredness, loss of interest, or frustration, that interferes with job performance. Burnout is usually regarded as the result of prolonged stress.

Stress hardiness—A personality characteristic that enables persons to stay healthy in stressful circumstances. It includes belief in one's ability to influence the situation; being committed to or fully engaged in one's activities; and having a positive view of change.

Stress management—A category of popularized programs and techniques intended to help people deal more effectively with stress.

Stressor—A stimulus or event that provokes a stress response in an organism. Stressors can be categorized as acute or chronic, and as external or internal to the organism.

Gallo, L. C., and K. A. Matthews. "Understanding the Association Between Socioeconomic Status and Physical Health: Do Negative Emotions Play a Role?" *Psychological Bulletin* 129 (January 2003): 10–51.

Hawkley, L. C., and J. T. Cacioppo. "Loneliness and Pathways to Disease." *Brain, Behavior, and Immunity* 17 (February 2003) (Supplement 1): S98–S105.

Latkin, C. A., and A. D. Curry. "Stressful Neighborhoods and Depression: A Prospective Study of the Impact of Neighborhood Disorder." *Journal of Health and Social Behavior* 44 (March 2003): 34–44.

Ottenstein, R. J. "Coping with Threats of Terrorism: A Protocol for Group Intervention." *International Journal of Emergency Mental Health* 5 (Winter 2003): 39–42.

Rahe, R. H., C. B. Taylor, R. L. Tolles, et al. "A Novel Stress and Coping Workplace Program Reduces Illness and Healthcare Utilization." *Psychosomatic Medicine* 64 (March-April 2002): 278-286.

Solomon, G. D. "Chronic Tension-Type Headache: Advice for the Viselike-Headache Patient." *Cleveland Clinic Journal of Medicine* 69 (February 2002): 173-174.

Surwit, R. S., M. A. van Tilburg, N. Zucker, et al. "Stress Management Improves Long-Term Glycemic Control in Type 2 Diabetes." *Diabetes Care* 25 (January 2002): 30-34.

West, P., and H. Sweeting. "Fifteen, Female and Stressed: Changing Patterns of Psychological Distress Over Time."

Journal of Child Psychology and Psychiatry 44 (March 2003): 399–411.

ORGANIZATIONS

The American Institute of Stress. 124 Park Avenue, Yonkers, NY 10703 (914) 963-1200. Fax: (914) 965-6267. <http://www.stress.org.>.

National Institute of Mental Health (NIMH). 6001 Executive Boulevard, Room 8184, MSC 9663, Bethesda, MD 20892-9663. (301) 443-4513. <www.nimh.nih.gov.>.

Stress and Anxiety Research Society (STAR). STAR is an international multidisciplinary organization of researchers that began in the Netherlands in 1980. <http://www.star-society.org.>.

OTHER

National Center for Post-Traumatic Stress Disorder, Department of Veterans Affairs. *Fact Sheet: Survivors of Human-Caused and Natural Disasters* . <http://www.ncptsd.org/facts/disasters/fs_survivors_disaster.html>.

National Institute of Mental Health (NIMH) news release, July 17, 2003. "Gene More Than Doubles Risk of Depression Following Life Stresses." < http://www.nimh.nih.gov/events/prgenestress.cfm>.

Paula Ford-Martin
Rebecca J. Frey, PhD

Stroke

Definition

Stroke is the common name for the injury to the brain that occurs when the flow of blood to brain tissue is interrupted by a clogged or burst artery. Arterial blood carries oxygen and **nutrition** to the cells of the body. When arteries are unable to carry out this function due to rupture, constriction, or obstruction, the cells nourished by these arteries die. The medical term for stroke is the acronym CVA, or cerebral vascular accident. It is estimated that four of every five families in the United States will be affected by stroke in their lifetime, and it is the top cause of adult disability worldwide. Stroke is ranked third in the leading causes of death in the United States, has left three million Americans permanently disabled, and costs the United States 30 billion dollars each year in terms of health care costs and lost productivity.

The most common type of stroke is classified as *ischemic* , or occurring because the blood supply to a portion of the brain has been cut off. Ischemic strokes account for approximately 80% of all strokes, and can be further broken down into two subtypes: thrombotic, also called cerebral thrombosis; and embolic, termed cerebral embolism.

Thrombotic strokes are by far the more prevalent, and can be seen in nearly all **aging** populations worldwide. As people grow older, **atherosclerosis**, or hardening of the arteries, occurs. This results in a buildup of a waxy cholesterol-laden substance in the arteries, which eventually narrows the interior space, or lumen, of the artery. This arterial narrowing occurs in all parts of the body, including the brain. As the process continues, the occlusion, or shutting off of the artery, eventually becomes complete, so that no blood supply can pass through. Usually the presentation of the symptoms of a thrombotic stroke are much more gradual and less dramatic than that of other strokes due to the slow ongoing process that produces it. Transient ischemic attacks, or TIAs, are one form of thrombotic stroke, and usually the least serious. TIAs represent the blockage of a very small artery or arteriole, or the intermittent or temporary obstruction of a larger artery. This blockage affects only a small portion of brain tissue and does not leave noticeable permanent ill effects. These transient ischemic attacks last only a matter of minutes, but are a forewarning that part of the brain is not receiving its necessary supply of blood, and thus oxygen and nutrition. Thrombotic strokes account for 40-50% of all strokes.

Embolic strokes are more acute and rapid in onset. They take place when the heart's rhythm is changed for a number of different reasons, and blood clot formation occurs. This blood clot can move through the circulatory system until it blocks a blood vessel and stops the blood supply to cells in a specific portion of the body. If it occludes an artery that nourishes heart muscle, it causes myocardial infarction, or **heart attack**. If it blocks off a vessel that feeds brain tissue, it is termed an embolic stroke. Embolisms account for 25-30% percent of all strokes. Normally these blockages occur in the brain itself when arteries directly feeding portions of brain tissue are blocked by a clot. But occasionally the obstruction is found in the arteries of the neck, especially the carotid artery.

Approximately 20% of cerebral vascular accidents are termed hemorrhagic strokes. Hemorrhagic strokes occur when an artery to the brain has a weakness and balloons outward, producing what is called an aneurysm. Such aneurysms often rupture due to this inflation and thinning of the arterial wall, causing a hemorrhage in the affected portion of the brain.

Both ischemic and hemorrhagic strokes display similar symptoms, depending on which portion of the brain is cut off from its supply of oxygen and nourishment. The brain is divided into left and right hemispheres. These hemispheres are responsible for bodily movement on the opposite side of the body from the brain hemisphere. For example, the left hemisphere of the brain is responsible for both motor control and sensory discrimination for the

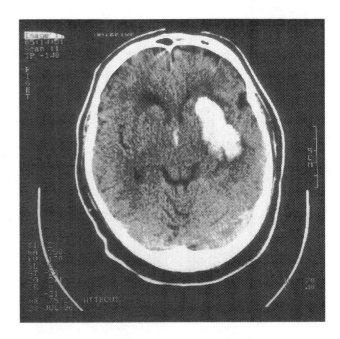

CAT scan of a brain showing a stroke resulting in hemorrhage (white area). *(Custom Medical Stock Photo. Reproduced by permission.)*

right side of the body, just as the right hemisphere is responsible for left body movements and feeling. Deeper brain tissue in the left hemisphere of the brain directs muscle tone and coordination for both the right arm and leg. As the communication and speech centers for the brain are also located in the left hemisphere of the brain, interruption of blood supply to that area can also typically affect the person's ability to speak.

Description

Strokes are always considered a medical emergency, and every minute is important in initiating treatment. With the possible exception of transient ischemic attacks, all other types of stroke are life-threatening events. Stroke is a leading cause of death in all nations of the Western world and the more affluent Asian countries. One-quarter of all strokes are fatal. Cerebral vascular accidents are typically a condition of the elderly, and more often happen to men than women. In the United States, strokes occur in roughly one of every 500 people, and the likelihood of becoming a stroke victim rises sharply as a person ages. The incidence of strokes among people ages 30-60 years is less than 1%. This figure triples by the age of 80 years.

Causes & symptoms

Along with the typical risk factors for **heart disease,** the most common risk factor for thrombotic stroke is age. Some buildup of material along the inner lumen

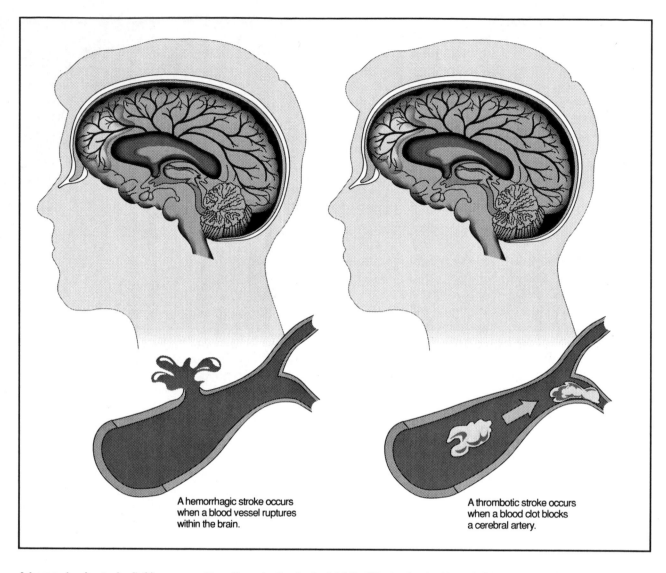

A hemorrhagic stroke (left) compared to a thrombotic stroke (right). (Illustration by Hans & Cassady, Inc. The Gale Group.)

of the artery, or atherosclerosis, is a normal part of growing older. **Hypertension**, or high blood pressure, can result from this buildup, as the heart attempts to pump blood through these narrowed arteries. High blood pressure is one of the foremost causes of stroke. Aside from aging and hypertension, heart disease, **obesity**, diabetes, **smoking**, oral contraceptives in women, polycythemia, and a condition called **sleep apnea** are all risk factors for stroke, as is a diet high in **cholesterol** or fatty foods.

The risk factors for hemorrhagic stroke are those that can weaken arteries supplying blood to the brain. They include high blood pressure, which can over a period of time cause the ballooning of arteries known as aneurysm, and hereditary malformations that produce defective and weakened veins and arteries. Substance abuse also is a major cause. It has been demonstrated for years that co-

caine and stimulants such as amphetamine drugs are culprits, and chronic **alcoholism** can cause a weakening of blood vessels that also can result in hemorrhagic stroke.

Exactly what triggers the actual ischemic stroke event continues to puzzle clinicians. Researchers refer to these triggers as "short-term risk" vs. "long-term risk" factors. If researchers can help identify the triggers for stroke in those with high risk factors, they might be able to help prevent the stroke from occurring. One 2002 report found that abrupt changes in body position caused by sudden loud noises or other unexpected events might trigger a stroke. These events occurred during a two-hour period before the stroke.

Diagnosis

As noted previously, the symptoms of stroke observed depend upon the part of the brain that is affected, and how large a portion of brain tissue has been damaged by the CVA. Unconsciousness and even seizures can be initial components of a stroke. Other effects materialize over a time period ranging from minutes to hours, and even, in some rare instances, over several days. **Headache** (often described as "the worst **headache** I've ever had" in hemorrhagic stroke); mental confusion; vertigo; vision problems, aphasia, or difficulty speaking and communicating, including slurring of words are major symptoms. Hemiplegia, or weakness or paralysis of one side of the body, is a symptom that is frequently seen. This one-sided weakness is often first noticed in the person's face. Stroke victims often have facial drooping, or slackness of the facial muscles on the affected side, as well as difficulty swallowing. The severity of these symptoms will depend upon the amount of brain tissue that has died and its location in the brain.

Computed tomography (CT) brain scans, angiography, lumbar puncture, and magnetic resonance imaging (MRI) are all used to rule out any other possible causes of the symptoms seen. Other possible causes of these symptoms could be brain tumor, brain **abscess**, subdural hematoma, encephalitis, and **meningitis**.

Treatment

There are many applications of alternative and complementary medicine in the treatment and prevention of stroke. Alternative therapies are also used in rehabilitation of stroke victims. **Acupuncture** and **acupressure** are commonly used for stroke patients, as is massage. Movement and **meditation** programs such as **t'ai chi** are also helpful. Herbs with antioxidant properties may be prescribed by a practitioner. Many therapies aid in blood pressure control, including meditation, **guided imagery** , **biofeedback** and t'ai chi.

Allopathic treatment

Much of the needed care immediately following a stroke will be to prevent damage beyond that which has already occurred. Paralysis requires prevention of contractures or tightening up of paralyzed limbs. This is done through physiotherapy, and may include the use of supportive braces for arms or hands, footboards or wearing sneakers when in bed to prevent foot drop. The severely ill stroke patient will need to be repositioned frequently to prevent complications such as **pneumonia** and venous or pulmonary embolism.

Because of difficulty in swallowing, the person who has suffered a stroke may need a temporary or permanent feeding tube inserted into the stomach to ensure adequate nutrition. Such tubes can be placed through the nose, into the esophagus, and into the stomach, or gastrically, with a wider-lumen tube surgically implanted into the stomach.

A severe stroke that results in coma or unconsciousness will require medical monitoring and support, including oxygen and even possibly intubation to assure an adequate airway and facilitate breathing. Provision of fluids that the person may not be able to take by mouth due to swallowing difficulties will be necessary, as will possibly the administration of such blood-thinning or clot-dissolving medications as Coumadin or heparin. A five-year clinical trial completed in 1995 and reported by the *New England Journal of Medicine* showed that stroke patients treated with t-PA, a clot-dissolving medication, within three hours of the stroke were one-third more likely to be left with no permanent residual difficulty. The trauma of the brain caused by stroke may result in **edema,** or swelling, which may have to be reduced by giving the patient diuretic or steroid medications. Sometimes surgical removal of a clot obstructing an artery is necessary. Hemorrhagic stroke can cause a buildup of pressure on the brain that must be relieved as quickly as possible to prevent further brain damage. In extreme cases, this may require incision through the skull to relieve that pressure.

Expected results

Studies reported by the National Institute of Neurological Disorders and Stroke report that 25% of people who suffer a stroke recover completely and 20% die within three months after the stroke. Of the remaining 55% percent, 5% will require long-term (nursing home) care, and for the rest — roughly half of all stroke patients — rehabilitative and restorative services will be necessary to regain as much of their former capabilities as possible. It has been estimated that the most common irreversible damage from stroke is the loss of intellectual functions.

Prevention

Control of blood pressure is the single most important factor in preventing stroke. People should have their blood pressure checked regularly, and if consistently elevated, (diastolic, or lower blood pressure beat above 90 to 100, systolic or top beat above 140 to 150), a physician should be consulted.

The American Heart Association recommends that cigarette smokers break the habit to reduce stroke risk. Current cigarette use can increase risk of cerebral infarction to nearly double, and **smoking** is associated with other risk factors of stroke. The AHA also recommends that those at risk for stroke avoid secondhand tobacco smoke if possible.

Diet, including reduction of **sodium** (salt) intake, **exercise** and weight loss, if overweight, are all non-drug treatments for lowering blood pressure. Other natural remedies include eating artichokes, which lowers the fat content of the blood; **garlic**, now believed to lower cholesterol and blood pressure as well as to reduce the clotting ability of the blood; and ginkgo, which improves circulation and strengthens arteries and veins. The use of **folic acid, lecithin**, vitamins B_6 and B_{12}, vitamins C and E are all recommended as supportive measures in reducing blood pressure. Two new Harvard studies found that eating a diet high in fruits and vegetables (particularly leafy green vegetables and cruciferous ones like broccoli, cauliflower, and cabbage) can reduce the risk of ischemic stroke. When fruits and vegetables were not only added to the diet, but replaced meat and trans fats, they further reduced stroke risk.

Avoiding substances that can cause stroke is another preventive measure. A 2002 report revealed that the popular herbal supplement ephedrine can cause stroke, heart attack, and sudden death.

Multiple studies have found that aspirin acts as a blood-thinning or clot-reducing medication when taken in small doses. One baby aspirin tablet per day provides this anticoagulant protection.

If necessary, a physician may also order medication to lower blood pressure. These medications include the following categories of drugs:

- *Beta blockers* reduce the force and speed of the heartbeat.

- *Vasodilators* dilate the blood vessels.

- *Diuretics* reduce the total volume of circulating blood and thus the heart's work by removing fluid from the body.

- *Lipid-lowering drugs* increase the loss of cholesterol from the body or prevent the conversion of fatty acids to cholesterol. This lowers fat levels in the blood stream.

A preliminary report out of France in 2002 stated that getting a flu shot might reduce risk of stroke. Previous research has also suggested that flu shots might stimulate a response in the immune system that helps reduce inflammation throughout the body. If true, those most likely to benefit would be people age 75 and older.

Resources

BOOKS

Clayman, Charles B., MD. *The American Medical Association Home Medical Encyclopedia*. New York: Random House, 1989.

Landis, Robyn, and Karta Purkh Singh Khalsa. *Herbal Defense: Positioning Yourself to Triumph Over Illness and Aging*. New York: Warner Books, 1997.

Sammons, James H., MD, John T. Baker, MD, Frank D. Campion, Heidi Hough, James Ferris, Brenda A. Clark. *The American Medical Association Guide to Prescription and Over-the-Counter Drugs*. New York: Random House, 1988.

Thomas, Clayton L. *Taber's Cyclopedic Medical Dictionary.* F.A.Davis Co., 1998.

PERIODICALS

"Abrupt Changes in Body Position Can Trigger Stroke." *Heart Disease Weekly* (March 24, 2002):15.

"Flu Shots May Prevent Strokes." *Medical Update* (February 2002):5.

Hall, Zach W., Ph.D. *New England Journal of Medicine* (December 14, 1995).

Samenuk, David. "Adverse Cardiovascular Events Temporarily Associated with Ma Huang, an Herbal Source of Ephedrine." *JAMA, Journal of the American Medical Association* (March 27, 2002):1506.

"Strategies Identified to Prevent Primary Stroke." *Clinician Reviews* (March 2002):89.

"Vegetables and Fruits Cut Stroke Risk." *Health Science* (Winter 2002):7.

ORGANIZATIONS

National Institute of Neurological Disorders and Stroke. National Institutes of Health, Building 31, Room 8A-16, P.O. Box 5801, Bethesda, MD 20824. (301) 496-5751.

National Stroke Association. 1-800-STROKES. http://www.stroke.org.

OTHER

Dr. Rappa. "What Is a Stroke?" http://www.medhealthsolution.com.

Joan Schonbeck
Teresa G. Odle

Structural integration *see* **Rolfing**

Substance abuse and dependence

Definition

Substance abuse is the continued compulsive use of mind-altering substances despite personal, social, and/or physical problems caused by the substance use. Abuse may lead to dependence, in which increased amounts are needed to achieve the desired effect or level of intoxication and the patient's tolerance for the drug increases.

Description

Substance abuse and dependence cut across all lines of race, culture, education, and socioeconomic status, leaving no group untouched by their devastating effects. Substance abuse is an enormous public health problem with far-ranging effects throughout society. In addition to the toll substance abuse can take on one's physical

FREQUENCY OF SUBSTANCE ABUSE BY GENDER AND AGE	
Men	
Ages 18 to 29	17 to 24 percent
Ages 30 to 44	11 to 14 percent
Ages 45 to 64	6 to 8 percent
Over age 65	1 to 3 percent
Women	
Ages 18 to 29	4 to 10 percent
Ages 30 to 44	2 to 4 percent
Ages 45 to 64	1 to 2 percent
Over age 65	less than 1 percent

health, it is considered an important factor in a wide variety of social problems, affecting rates of crime, domestic violence, sexually transmitted diseases (including HIV/AIDS), unemployment, homelessness, teen **pregnancy**, and failure in school. One study estimated that 20% of the total yearly cost of health care in the United States is spent on treating the effects of drug and alcohol abuse.

A wide range of substances can be abused. The most common classes include:

• alcohol

• cocaine-based drugs

• opioids (including such prescription **pain** killers as morphine and Demerol as well as such illegal substances as heroin)

• benzodiazapines (including prescription drugs used for treating **anxiety**, such as valium)

• sedatives or "downers" (including prescription barbiturate drugs commonly referred to as tranquilizers)

• stimulants or "speed" (including prescription amphetamine drugs used as weight loss drugs and in the treatment of attention deficit disorder) and Ecstasy (which in 2001 had been tried by more than 12% of teens, up 71% over 1999 figures)

• cannabinoid drugs obtained from the hemp plant (including **marijuana** and hashish).

• hallucinogenic or "psychedelic" drugs (including LSD, PCP or angel dust, and other PCP-type drugs)

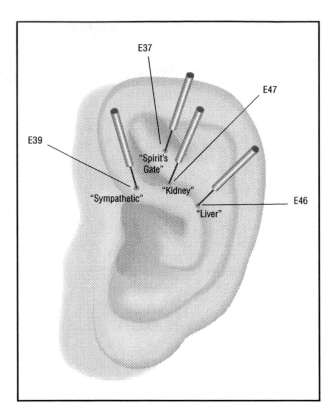

Acupuncture points associated with the relief of substance abuse problems. *Illustration by GGS Information Services, Inc. The Gale Group.*

• inhalants (including gaseous drugs used in the medical practice of anesthesia, as well as such common substances as paint thinner, gasoline, and glue). A 2002 study found that inhalant use among youths was even higher than that of Ecstasy

Over time, the same dosage of an abused substance will produce fewer of the desired feelings. This is known as drug tolerance. In order to continue to feel the desired effect of the substance, the person must take progressively higher drug doses.

Substance dependence is a phenomenon whereby a person becomes physically addicted to a substance. A substance-dependent person must have a particular dose or concentration of the substance in his or her bloodstream at any given moment in order to avoid the unpleasant symptoms associated with withdrawal from that substance. The common substances of abuse tend to exert either a depressive (slowing) or a stimulating (speeding up) effect on such basic bodily functions as respiratory rate, heart rate, and blood pressure. When a drug is stopped abruptly, the person's body will respond by overreacting to the substance's absence. Functions slowed by the abused substance will suddenly speed up, while previously stimulated functions will slow down.

This results in very unpleasant effects, known as withdrawal symptoms.

Addiction refers to the mental-state of a person who reaches a point where he/she must have a specific substance, even though the social, physical, and/or legal consequences of substance use are clearly negative (e.g., loss of relationships, employment, housing). Craving refers to an intense hunger for a specific substance, to the point where this need essentially directs the individual's behavior. Craving is usually seen in both dependence and addiction and can be so strong that it overwhelms a person's ability to make any decisions that will possibly deprive him/her of the substance. Drug possession and use becomes the most important goal, and other forces (including the law) have little effect on changing the individual's substance-seeking behavior.

Causes & symptoms

It is generally believed that there is not one single cause of substance abuse, though scientists are increasingly convinced that certain people possess a genetic predisposition that can affect the development of addictive behaviors. One theory holds that a particular nerve pathway in the brain (dubbed the "mesolimbic reward pathway") holds certain chemical characteristics that may increase the likelihood that substance use will ultimately lead to substance addiction. Certainly, however, other social factors are involved, including family problems and peer pressure. Primary mood disorders (bipolar), personality disorders, and learned behaviors can be influential on the likelihood that a person will become substance dependent.

The symptoms of substance abuse may be related to its social as well as its physical effects. The social effects of substance abuse may include dropping out of school or losing a series of jobs, engaging in fighting and violence in relationships, and legal problems (ranging from driving under the influence to the commission of crimes designed to obtain the money needed to support an expensive drug habit).

Physical effects of substance abuse are related to the specific drug being abused:

• Opioid drug users may appear slowed in their physical movements and speech, may lose weight, exhibit mood swings, and have constricted (small) pupils.

• Benzodiazapine and barbiturate users may appear sleepy and slowed, with slurred speech, small pupils, and occasional confusion.

• Amphetamine users may have excessively high energy, inability to sleep, weight loss, rapid pulse, elevated blood pressure, occasional psychotic behavior, and dilated (enlarged) pupils.

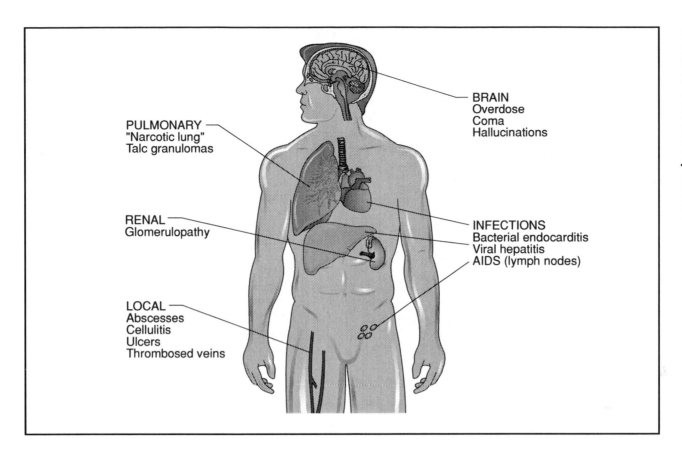

PULMONARY
"Narcotic lung"
Talc granulomas

RENAL
Glomerulopathy

LOCAL
Abscesses
Cellulitis
Ulcers
Thrombosed veins

BRAIN
Overdose
Coma
Hallucinations

INFECTIONS
Bacterial endocarditis
Viral hepatitis
AIDS (lymph nodes)

Substance abuse often causes a variety of medical abnormalities and conditions throughout the body, as shown in the illustration above. *(Illustration by Electronic Illustrators Group. The Gale Group.)*

• Marijuana users may be sluggish and slow to react, exhibiting mood swings and red eyes with dilated pupils.

• Cocaine users may have wide variations in their energy level, severe mood disturbances, psychosis, paranoia, and a constantly runny nose. Crack cocaine use may cause aggressive or violent behavior.

• Hallucinogenic drug users may display bizarre behavior due to hallucinations (hallucinations are imagined sights, voices, sounds, or smells which seem completely real to the individual experiencing them) and dilated pupils. LSD can cause flashbacks.

Other symptoms of substance abuse may be related to the form in which the substance is used. For example, heroin, certain other opioid drugs, and certain forms of cocaine may be injected using a needle and a hypodermic syringe. A person abusing an injectable substance may have "track marks" (outwardly visible signs of the site of an injection, with possible redness and swelling of the vein in which the substance was injected). Furthermore, poor judgment brought on by substance use can result in the injections being made under dirty conditions. These unsanitary conditions and the use of shared needles can cause **infections** of the injection sites, major infections of the heart, as well as infection with HIV (the virus which causes **AIDS**), certain forms of **hepatitis** (a liver infection), and **tuberculosis**.

Cocaine is often taken as a powdery substance that is "snorted" through the nose. This method of use can result in frequent **nosebleeds**, sores in the nose, and even erosion (an eating away) of the nasal septum (the structure that separates the two nostrils). Other forms of cocaine include smokable or injectable forms such as freebase and crack cocaine.

Overdosing on a substance is a frequent complication of substance abuse. Drug overdose can be purposeful (with suicide as a goal), or result from carelessness. It may also be the result of the unpredictable strength of substances purchased from street dealers, mixing of more than one type of substance or of a substance and alcohol, or as a result of the ever-increasing doses the person must take of those substances to which he or she has become tolerant. Substance overdose can be a life-threatening emergency, with the specific symptoms dependent on the type of substance used. Substances with depressive effects may dangerously slow the breathing and heart rate, lower the body temperature, and result in general unresponsiveness. Substances with stimulatory effects may dangerously increase the heart rate and blood pressure, increase body temperature, and cause bizarre behavior. With cocaine, there is a risk of **stroke**.

Still other symptoms may be caused by unknown substances mixed with street drugs in order to "stretch" a batch. A healthcare worker faced with a patient suffering extreme symptoms will have no idea what other substance that person may have unwittingly put into his or her body. Thorough drug screening can help with diagnosis.

Diagnosis

The most difficult aspect of diagnosis involves overcoming the patient's denial. Denial is a psychological trait whereby a person is unable to allow him- or herself to acknowledge the reality of a situation. This may lead a person to completely deny his or her substance use, or may cause the person to greatly underestimate the degree of the problem and its effects on his or her life.

One of the simplest and most common screening tools practitioners use to begin the process of diagnosing substance abuse is the CAGE questionnaire. CAGE refers to the first letters of each word that forms the basis of each of the four questions of the screening exam:

- Have you ever tried to *cut* down on your substance use?

- Have you ever been *annoyed* by people trying to talk to you about your substance use?

- Do you ever feel *guilty* about your substance use?

- Do you ever need an *eye opener* (use of the substance first thing in the morning) in order to start your day?

Other lists of questions may be used to assess the severity and effects of a person's substance abuse. Certainly, it is also relevant to determine whether anybody else in the user's family has ever suffered from substance or alcohol addiction.

A physical examination may reveal signs of substance abuse in the form of needle marks, tracks, trauma to the inside of the nostrils from snorting drugs, or unusually large or small pupils. With the person's permission, substance use can also be detected by examining an individual's blood, urine, or hair in a laboratory. Drug testing is limited by sensitivity, specificity, and the time elapsed since the person last used the drug.

Treatment

Treatment has several goals, which include helping a person deal with the uncomfortable and possibly life-threatening symptoms associated with withdrawal from an addictive substance (called **detoxification**), helping an abuser deal with the social effects that substance abuse has had on his or her life; and efforts to prevent relapse (resumed use of the substance). Individual or group **psychotherapy** may be helpful.

Ridding the body of toxins is believed to be aided by **hydrotherapy** (bathing regularly in water containing baking soda, sea salt, or Epsom salts). Hydrotherapy can include a constitutional effect where the body's vital force is stimulated and all organ systems are revitalized. Herbalists or naturopathic physicians may prescribe such herbs as **milk thistle** (*Silybum marianum*), burdock (*Arctium lappa*, a blood cleanser), and **licorice** (*Glycyrrhiza glabra*) to assist in detoxification. Anxiety brought on by substance withdrawal is thought to be lessened by using other herbs, which include **valerian** (*Valeriana officinalis*), vervain (*Verbena officinalis*), **skullcap** (*Scutellaria baicalensis*), and kava (*Piper methysticum*).

Other treatments aimed at reducing the **stress** a person suffers while attempting substance withdrawal and throughout an individual's recovery process include **acupuncture**, **hypnotherapy**, **biofeedback**, **guided imagery**, and various meditative arts (including **yoga** and **t'ai chi**).

Use of **acupuncture** to treat addiction is becoming more common. In 2002, a study was undertaken in Maine to treat substance abuse users who were dually diagnosed with chronic mental illness and substance abuse problems with ear acupuncture. The technique appears to cleanse organs and to aid in **relaxation**, which eases many of the stresses believed to lead these patients to maintain their reliance on the drugs. Another clinical trial in the same year, however, found that acupuncture was not effective alone for treating cocaine-dependent adults. However, the study did conclude that acupuncture may be effective for these patients when used in combination with other treatments. New research also suggests that **qigong** therapy may be an effective alternative for patients with heroin addiction.

Allopathic treatment

Detoxification may take from several days to many weeks. Detoxification can be accomplished "cold turkey," by complete and immediate cessation of all substance use, or by slowly decreasing (tapering) the dose which a person is taking, to minimize the side effects of withdrawal. Some substances absolutely must be tapered, because "cold turkey" methods of detoxification are potentially life-threatening. Alternately, a variety of medications may be utilized to combat the unpleasant and threatening physical symptoms of withdrawal. A substance (such as methadone in the case of heroin addiction) may be substituted for the original substance of abuse, with gradual tapering of this substituted drug. In practice, many patients may be maintained on methadone and lead a reasonably normal life. Because of the rebound effects of wildly fluctuating blood pressure, body temperature, heart and breathing rates, as well as the potential for bizarre behavior and hallucinations, a person undergoing withdrawal must be carefully monitored.

Expected results

After a person has successfully withdrawn from substance use, the even more difficult task of recovery begins. Recovery refers to the lifelong efforts of a person to avoid returning to substance use. The craving can be so strong even years and years after initial withdrawal that a previously addicted person is in danger of slipping back into substance use. Triggers for such a relapse include any number of life stresses (problems on the job or in the marriage, loss of a relationship, death of a loved one, financial stresses), in addition to seemingly mundane exposure to a place or an acquaintance associated with previous substance use. While some people remain in counseling indefinitely as a way of maintaining contact with a professional who can help monitor behavior, others find that various support groups or 12-step programs such as Alcoholics Anonymous (AA) and Narcotics Anonymous (NA) are most helpful in monitoring the recovery process and avoiding relapse.

Another important aspect of treatment for substance abuse concerns the inclusion of close family members in treatment. Because substance abuse has severe effects on the functioning of the family, and because research shows that family members can unintentionally develop behaviors that inadvertently serve to support a person's substance habit, most good treatment will involve all family members.

Prevention

Prevention is best aimed at teenagers, who are at very high risk for substance experimentation. Education regarding the risks and consequences of substance use, as well as teaching methods of resisting peer pressure, are both important components of a prevention program. Furthermore, it is important to identify children at higher risk for substance abuse (including victims of physical or sexual abuse; children of parents who have a history of substance abuse, especially alcohol; and children with school failure and/or attention deficit disorder). These children will require a more intensive prevention program. A 2002 report demonstrated that prevention programs worked with high-risk youth in reducing rates of alcohol, tobacco, and marijuana use.

Resources

BOOKS

American Psychiatric Association. *Diagnostic and Statistical Manual of Mental Disorders.* Washington, DC: American Psychiatric Association, 1994.

O'Brien, C.P. "Drug Abuse and Dependence." In *Cecil Textbook of Medicine,* edited by J. Claude Bennett and Fred Plum. Philadelphia: W.B. Saunders, 1996.

PERIODICALS

Imperio, Winnie A. "Substance Abuse Prevention Works." *Clinical Psychiatry News* (March 2002):41.

"Inhalant Use More Popular than Ecstasy, OxyContin." *Alcoholism & Drug Abuse Weekly* (March 25, 2002):8.

Margolin, Arthur, et al. "Acupuncture for the Treatment of Cocaine Addiction: A Randomized Controlled Trial." *JAMA, The Journal of the American Medical Association* (January 2, 2002):55–59.

Monroe, Judy. "Recognizing Signs of Drug Abuse." *Current Health* (September 1996):16+.

O'Brien, Charles P. and A. Thomas McLellan. "Addiction Medicine." *Journal of the American Medical Association* (18 June 1997): 1840+.

"Qigong Therapy Evaluated for Detoxification." *The Brown University Digest of Addiction Theory and Application* (March 2002):S1.

Rivara, et al. "Alcohol and Illicit Drug Abuse and the Risk of Violent Death in the Home." *Journal of the American Medical Association* (20 August 1997): 569+.

Savage, Lorraine. "Grant to Study Acupuncture's Effectiveness on Patients Suffering from Substance Abuse." *Healthcare Review* (March 19, 2002): 16.

KEY TERMS

Addiction—The state of being both physically and psychologically dependent on a substance.

Dependence—A state in which a person requires a steady concentration of a particular substance in order to avoid experiencing withdrawal symptoms.

Detoxification—A process in which an addict is withdrawn from a substance.

High—The altered state of consciousness that a person seeks when abusing a substance.

Street drug—A substance purchased from a drug dealer. It may be a legal substance, sold illicitly (without a prescription, and not for medical use), or it may be a substance which is illegal to possess.

Tolerance—A phenomenon whereby a drug user becomes physically accustomed to a particular dose of a substance and requires ever-increasing dosages in order to obtain the same effects.

Withdrawal—Those side effects experienced by a person who has become physically dependent on a substance, upon decreasing the substance's dosage, or discontinuing its use.

"Survey Finds Rise in Ecstasy Use Among Teens." *Alcoholism & Drug Abuse Weekly.* (February 25, 2002): 3.

ORGANIZATIONS

Al-Anon, Alanon Family Group, Inc. P.O. Box 862, Midtown Station, New York, NY 10018-0862. (800) 356-9996. http://www.recovery.org/aa.
Alcoholics Anonymous. World Service Organization. P.O. Box 459, New York, NY 10163. (212) 870-3400. http://www.aa.org.
National Alliance On Alcoholism and Drug Dependence, Inc. 12 West 21st St., New York, NY 10010. (212) 206-6770.

OTHER

National Clearinghouse for Alcohol and Drug Information. http://www.health.org.
Parent Resources and Information for Drug Education (PRIDE). 10 Park Place South, Suite 340, Atlanta, GA 30303. (800) 853-7867 or (404) 577-4500.

Paula Ford-Martin
Teresa G. Odle

Sugar diabetes *see* **Diabetes mellitus**

Sulfur

Description

Sulfur is a homeopathic remedy that is used to treat a variety of chronic or acute ailments. Elemental sulfur is present in all living tissues. Sulfur is often referred to as brimstone or flowers of sulfur.

Sulfur was used during biblical times as a remedy for skin disorders such as **acne** and **scabies**. Flowers of sulfur were burned to disinfect the rooms of persons with infectious disease. Sulfur was also taken with molasses as an internal cleanser, and was used to treat chronic **bronchitis**, **constipation**, and rheumatism. In the early 2000s the element is used in the manufacture of dyes, gunpowder, insecticides, fungicides, sulfuric acid, and rubber (as a hardening agent).

General use

Sulfur is known as the king of homeopathic remedies because it has such a wide range of use. It works well with almost every other remedy and it acts on many different maladies and ailments. This polychrest has a deep, long-lasting effect on the body and is often used to bring out symptoms for further treatment. For this reason, sulfur is generally used to treat chronic ailments, although it is also used for acute conditions such as fevers and colds. Sulfur stimulates the body's natural healing powers, causing a general improvement of symptoms and sometimes causing new symptoms.

Homeopaths prescribe sulfur to treat skin ailments such as herpes, **rashes**, **psoriasis**, **eczema**, and acne. Other conditions helped by this remedy include arthritis, colds, coughs, flatulence, gastrointestinal disturbances, and headaches.

Ailments are caused by loss of vital fluids, drug abuse, overeating, becoming chilled, a change from cold to warm weather, effects of a debilitating disease, or from suppression of skin eruptions, **hemorrhoids**, or bodily discharges.

Typical sulfur patients are fair-haired, blue-eyed persons with red faces and lips that become cracked when they are ill. Their tongues often have a white coating and are red around the edges and on the tip. They are lean, stoop shouldered, lazy, averse to bathing, untidy, and disorderly. They don't pay attention to what they are wearing and often walk around with unmatched socks or missing ties. Patients are oversensitive to odors, especially their own, which are usually smelly.

Sulfur patients have often been called the "ragged philosopher," referring to the patient's disorderly ways. For instance, a sulfur type might be an inventor or scholar who is so absorbed in his project that he forgets to wash or change clothes. Patients are very bright but they spend a lot of time wandering about and studying strange subjects. They are dreamers and philosophers who lack perseverance to see their dreams through to fruition. They start many projects but complete few.

Physical symptoms include excessive thirst, swollen glands, profuse sweat, sensitivity to heat, burning pains, hot feet, **boils**, and acne. Symptoms generally appear on the left side. Bodily discharges are hot, burning, and sour smelling. The patient is extremely intolerable of the cold and other weather conditions. Arthritis, coughing, and hoarseness of the throat are all caused by damp weather or a change in weather. Skin conditions are often caused by a change in weather.

These patients are very sensitive to food and the times they eat. If a meal is delayed they may become nauseous and weak. At 10 A.M. or 11 A.M. they get an empty feeling in their stomachs and feel an intense hunger. Patients generally suffer from **indigestion** and other gastrointestinal disorders. They crave alcohol, sweets, spicy foods, fatty foods, and stimulants, but dislike milk and meat. Bread, cold food or drinks, fats, milk, and sweets aggravate their systems.

Mentally, patients are irritable, critical, discontented, impatient, depressed, quarrelsome, restless, hurried, anxious, easily offended, fearful, timid, absent-minded, sad, and weepy. They would rather not work; their symptoms often occur as a result of physical or mental exertion. The patient is always tired and lacks endurance. If made to stand for long periods of time he may feel faint.

Symptoms are aggravated by bathing, cold air, motion, **itching**, **fasting**, heat, milk, or standing. They are worse from 10-11 A.M., after eating, or in a stuffy room. Symptoms such as headaches may recur on a regular basis, i.e. every seven or ten days. Patients are worse after a long sleep and may not want to get up. All sulfur symptoms are better from fresh air and warm drinks.

Specific indications

The backache typical of sulfur is aching, sore, and stiff. The back feels weak, tired, and bruised. It is worse from standing or walking, after sitting for long periods, during **menstruation**, or at night.

Sulfur patients catch colds easily and often. They cannot become overheated, remain in a cold place, or overexert themselves without catching a cold. The sulfur cold is accompanied by smelly nasal discharge, congestion, **sneezing**, eye inflammations, and an itchy, dry nose that, when blown, may bleed.

The sulfur **cough** is generally dry in the evening and loose in the morning. The chest is congested and the sides hurt from coughing. There is a feeling of dust in the throat. The discharge that is expectorated from the cough is of a greenish color. Patients may often awake from coughing. The cough is better when the patient is exposed to open air.

Diarrhea that occurs early in the morning around 5 A.M. is indicative of sulfur. The diarrhea is painless, slimy, watery, and foul smelling. It is accompanied by flatulence and is somewhat relieved by expulsion of the **gas**.

Earaches are accompanied by aching and lacerating pains. The **earache** is worse in the left ear. There is a ringing or roaring noise in the ear. The ears are frequently plugged and itchy.

Eye inflammations often accompany a cold. The eyes are itchy, watery, burning, dry, and sensitive to light. The eyelids itch in the daytime only. The patient may wake up with his eyes glued shut. Washing them, however, aggravates the condition.

Fatigue is worse in the evening or from talking. It is caused by sun exposure, hunger, or walking.

Fevers are hot and are accompanied by **chills**, shivering, and sweating. They are worse in the evening, after waking, or from mental exertion. The feet become extremely hot; therefore, the patient may stick his feet out from under the bedcovers to cool them.

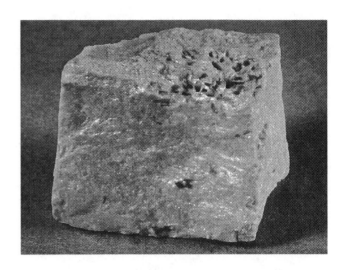

Sample of sulfur. *(JLM Visuals. Reproduced by permission.)*

The patient is very gassy and suffers from gas that smells like rotten eggs. The stomach is bloated and rumbles in irritation. The gas is often accompanied by a burning sensation and offensive-smelling stools.

Headaches are confined to the forehead or top of the head. They are hot and burning with hammering pains. These congestive headaches are caused by damp weather and are accompanied by **nausea** and **vomiting**. They often occur on Sunday and recur periodically. They are aggravated by motion, cold drinks, eating, bending over, blowing the nose, coughing, rising in the morning, and sneezing. Sometimes stars, zigzags, or other shapes will appear before the eyes.

Indigestion is common in sulfur patients. The patient can digest almost nothing, but he can't go long without eating. He has a weak stomach and a slow digestion. Stomach pains are sensitive to touch and a heavy feeling is present in the stomach. The patient is hungry at 10 A.M. and may need to eat to avoid feeling faint or weak. She may get a **headache** if she doesn't eat at that time. Indigestion is accompanied by sour belches, gas that smells rotten, bloating, and burning pains. It is worse after eating or from drinking milk.

Insomnia is caused by frequent waking in the early morning hours (3-5 A.M.). For this reason, the patient has a tendency to sleep late. However, no matter how much sleep the patient has, he always wakes up feeling tired. Short catnaps taken throughout the day refresh the patient. Patients are often unable to sleep before midnight.

Skin conditions are itchy, intense, and worse at night or in warm beds. The skin is itchy and burning and chaps easily. Ailments include herpes, rashes, acne, eczema, psoriasis, and **dermatitis**.

The **sore throat** is accompanied by swollen tonsils, burning pains, and a hoarse voice upon waking. The throat is dry and raw and may feel dusty. The throat is worse from coughing and swallowing.

Preparations

The homeopathic remedy is created by adding pure sulfur powder to a water/alcohol mixture or by grinding it with milk sugar. The mixture is then diluted and succussed to create the final preparation.

Sulfur is available at health food and drug stores in various potencies in the form of tinctures, tablets, and pellets.

Precautions

If symptoms do not improve after the recommended time period, a homeopath or health care practitioner should be consulted.

The recommended dose should not be exceeded.

Side effects

There are no side effects but individual aggravations may occur.

Interactions

When taking any homeopathic remedy, use of **peppermint** products, coffee, or alcohol is discouraged. These products may cause the remedy to be ineffective.

Sulfur should not be taken immediately before **lycopodium**.

Resources

BOOKS

Cummings, Stephen, M.D., and Ullman Dana, M.P.H., *Everybody's Guide to Homeopathic Medicines.* New York, NY: Jeremy P. Tarcher/Putnam, 1997.

Kent, James Tyler. *Lectures on Materia Medica.* Delhi, India: B. Jain Publishers, 1996.

Jennifer Wurges

Suma

Description

Suma is the common name for a tropical ground vine native to the Amazon rain forest of Central and South America. Its botanical name is *Pfaffia paniculata*, and it belongs to the Amaranthaceae family. Referred to by the people of the rain forest as *para todo*, which can be translated "for all things," the herb has been used for 300 years in the Amazon for many different ailments. It is sometimes called Brazilian ginseng. Aside from suma's reputation as an energy booster, aphrodisiac, and wound healer, it has also been used to treat a wide range of medical conditions such as diabetes, **cancer**, and various skin conditions. Despite suma's traditional use as a folk remedy, its medicinal properties are not widely recognized around the world. While suma is on the list of about 600 Brazilian medicinal plants published by Brazil's Department of Health in the early 1980s, the herb is not included in most of the well-known compilations of herbs outside of South America. Only the dried root of the suma plant is used as a drug. According to tradition, the root is also used in cooking and has a mild flavor resembling that of vanilla.

Suma is often marketed to the public as Brazilian ginseng, which is misleading because the two herbs are not related in any way. *Panax ginseng*, which is cultivated in several parts of the globe outside of South America, is a popular herbal stimulant and adaptogen in the United States, Asia, and Europe. Like ginseng, suma is described as an adaptogen. This drug class was first defined over 50 years ago by a Russian scientist to describe Siberian ginseng's broad therapeutic effects. In simple terms, an adaptogen acts nonspecifically to optimize function and help the body to adapt to physical and mental **stress** (infection, hot or cold temperatures, physical exertion, and emotional distress). In order to meet the stricter definition of this concept, an adaptogen should lack side effects, be effective against a wide range of diseases or disorders, and restore the body to a healthy equilibrium regardless of the cause of the disruption.

While it is not known exactly how suma produces its effects, researchers have identified some of the herb's chemical constituents. These include pfaffosides A, B, C, D, E, and F; sitosterol; stigmasterol; allantoin; and germanium. As of 2000 a significant amount of research is still required to confirm suma's indications and mechanisms of action, as well as safety data. The ideal dosage of the herb has also yet to be determined.

General use

While not approved as a medication by the Food and Drug Administration (FDA), suma has been reported to have a number of beneficial effects. There is, however, little scientific evidence to support these claims. Aside from its use as an energy booster, some people use the herb to treat **chronic fatigue syndrome**, ulcers, **anxiety**, menstrual problems, **impotence**, and menopausal symptoms. Olympic competitors from Russia have used suma in conjunction with other adaptogens to enhance athletic performance. The herb is also used to strengthen the immune system and fight infection. Like *Panax ginseng,* suma is purported to be an aphrodisiac.

While suma's effectiveness is based mainly on its history as a folk remedy, a few preliminary studies suggest that it may have potential as a cancer drug and anti-inflammatory. In one *in vitro* investigation, several chemicals in suma (pfaffosides) blocked the growth of melanoma tumors. These findings do not prove, however, that suma is effective in preventing or treating cancer in people. Even if certain chemicals in suma have the ability to fight cancer, it is not known if these can distinguish cancerous cells from healthy ones. Further studies are required to determine whether suma can shrink tumors safely without harming normal tissue. In a pharmacological study conducted by Italian researchers, an extract made from suma appeared to have mild anti-inflammatory and pain-relieving effects. Interestingly, suma did not seem to alleviate **pain** that was unrelated to inflammation.

Some of the most intriguing research regarding suma is difficult to verify. At the center of this research is Dr. Milton Brazzach of Sao Paulo University in Brazil, who has reportedly treated several thousand patients with suma after his wife was cured of **breast cancer** using the herb. He has prescribed suma in dosages as high as 28 g daily for periods of months and years to treat diabetes and various cancers such as **leukemia** and **Hodgkin's disease**. While Brazzach has reported that he achieved good results with suma, the full details of his research have not been published in peer-reviewed journals. Until these studies have been published and reviewed by other experts, the evidence of suma's effectiveness in the treatment of these diseases cannot be authenticated.

Not all practitioners of alternative medicine agree when it comes to the virtues and possible dangers of suma. In *The Way of Herbs,* Dr. Michael Tierra compares the herb to **Siberian ginseng** and **Korean ginseng** in terms of effectiveness. He reports that suma increased the sense of overall well-being in one elderly patient with cancer and had beneficial effects on a teenager with leukemia. Suma appears to have the most consistent effect in people who suffer from chronic fatigue syndrome or lack of energy, states Tierra. By contrast, prominent pharmacologist Dr. Varro Tyler emphasizes safety concerns in *Tyler's Honest Herbal.* Even without extensive scientific testing, many folk remedies are considered relatively safe due to the fact that they have been used with-

KEY TERMS

Adaptogen—A substance that acts in nonspecific ways to improve the body's level of functioning and its adaptations to stress.

Aphrodisiac—An agent that stimulates or enhances sexual function or arousal.

In vitro—A Latin phrase that literally means "in the glass." It refers to an entity or process developed in a laboratory or similar controlled nonliving environment.

Panax ginseng—A popular longevity herb cultivated in Asia, Russia, and the United States. Described by some herbalists as an adaptogen, it is purported to strengthen the immune system and have a number of other beneficial effects.

out apparent harm for centuries or even millennia, according to Tyler. It is not certain, however, that suma falls into the category of time-proven natural remedies. The claims that suma has been used for centuries in the Amazon are mainly derived from marketing material as opposed to recognized herbal literature. Due to concerns regarding the safety and effectiveness of suma, Tyler does not recommend using the herb for any purpose.

Preparations

The optimum daily dosage of suma has not been established with any certainty. The typical dosage is 1000 mg daily, taken in divided doses. Much higher dosages have also been recommended.

Precautions

Suma is not known to be harmful when taken in recommended dosages, though it is important to remember that the effects of taking the herb (in any amount) are unknown. According to a report published in the *Journal of Allergy and Clinical Immunology* in 1991, one person who inhaled powdered suma root (for use in the making of suma capsules) developed **asthma**. This case, however, does not necessarily mean that swallowing suma in recommended dosages will produce similar problems.

Due to lack of sufficient medical study, suma should be used with caution in children, women who are pregnant or breast-feeding, and people with liver or kidney disease.

Side effects

When taken in recommended dosages, suma is not associated with any bothersome or significant side effects.

Interactions

As of 2004, Suma is not known to interact adversely with any drugs or dietary supplements.

Resources

BOOKS

Foster, Steven and Varro E. Tyler. *Tyler's Honest Herbal.* Binghampton, NY: Haworth Herbal Press, 1999.

ORGANIZATIONS

American Botanical Council. PO Box 144345, Austin, TX 78714-4345.

OTHER

Discovery Health. http://www.discoveryhealth.com.

Greg Annussek

Sunburn

Definition

A sunburn is an inflammation or blistering of the skin caused by overexposure to the sun.

Description

Sunburn is caused by excessive exposure to the ultraviolet (UV) rays of the sun. There are two types of ultraviolet rays, UVA and UVB. UVA rays penetrate the skin deeply and can cause melanoma in susceptible people. UVB rays, which don't penetrate as deeply, cause sunburn and wrinkling. Most UVB rays are absorbed by sunscreens, but only about half the UVA rays are absorbed.

Skin **cancer** from sun overexposure is a serious health problem in the United States, affecting almost one million Americans each year. One person out of 87 will develop malignant melanoma, the most serious type of **skin cancer**, and 7,300 of them will die each year. The Environmental Protection Agency (EPA) reported in 2000 that the rate of malignant melanoma is rising faster in the United States than the rates of all other preventable cancers except **lung cancer**. One reason for this high rate is the popular belief that suntanned skin is healthy and attractive. Many people spend more time in the sun than is good for their skin trying to achieve a fashionable tan.

People with fair skin are most susceptible to sunburn, because their skin produces only small amounts of the protective black or dark brown pigment called melanin. However, people of any race can get sunburned if they do not protect their skin against overexposure. People trying to get a tan too quickly in strong sunlight are also more vulnerable to sunburn.

Repeated sun overexposure and burning can prematurely age the skin, causing yellowish, wrinkled skin. Overexposure, especially a serious burn in childhood, can increase the risk of skin cancer.

Causes & symptoms

The ultraviolet rays in sunlight destroy cells in the outer layer of the skin, damaging tiny blood vessels underneath. When the skin is burned, the blood vessels dilate and leak fluid. Cells stop making protein. Their DNA is damaged by the ultraviolet rays. Repeated DNA damage can lead to cancer.

When the sun **burns** the skin, it triggers immune defenses which identify the burned skin as foreign. At the same time, the sun transforms a substance on the skin which interferes with this immune response. While this substance keeps the immune system from attacking a person's own skin, it also means that any malignant cells in the skin will be able to grow freely.

Sunburn causes skin to turn red and blister. Several days later, the dead skin cells peel off. In severe cases, the burn may occur with sunstroke (**vomiting, fever**, and fainting).

While overexposure to the sun is harmful, even fatal, no exposure means the body can't manufacture **vitamin D**, which is the only vitamin whose biologically active form is a hormone. Vitamin D is produced in the skin from the energy of the sun's UV rays. People at risk for vitamin D deficiency include alcoholics, non-milk drinkers, and those who do not receive much sunlight—especially those who live in regions that get little natural light. Dr. Sheldon Saul Hendles says that as more people use sunscreens and decrease exposure to the sun, they should make sure to have adequate dietary and supplementary sources of vitamin D. Sunscreen prevents the synthesis of the vitamin.

Diagnosis

Symptoms of sunburn may not appear until several hours after exposure. A deep pink skin color accompanied by a sensation of heat and burning indicates a mild sunburn. A red color with visible clothing lines, burning, **itching**, and stinging indicates a moderate burn. Bright red skin with **blisters**, fever, **chills**, and **nausea** indicates severe burn and medical help should be sought quickly.

Treatment

Over-the-counter preparations containing **aloe** (*Aloe barbadensis*) are an effective treatment for sunburn, easing

pain and inflammation while also relieving dryness of the skin. A variety of topical herbal remedies applied as lotions, poultices, or compresses may also help relieve the effects of sunburn. **Calendula** (*Calendula officinalis*) is one of the most frequently recommended to reduce inflammation.

Other natural remedies include:

• Applying compresses dipped in cold water, one part skim milk mixed with four parts cold water, aluminum acetate antiseptic powder mixed with water, **witch hazel**, white vinegar, or baking soda mixed with water.

• Making a paste out of cornstarch and water, and applying directed to affected areas.

• Placing thin, cold slices of raw cucumber, potato, or apple on the burned areas.

• Making a soothing solution by boiling lettuce in water, strain, cool the water for several hours in the refrigerator, then use cotton balls to pat the liquid onto the skin.

• Applying tea bags soaked in cold water to burned eyelids.

• Soothing the burn with cool yogurt, then rinsing with a cold shower.

Another natural remedy that has been proposed for treating sunburn is gingko biloba extract. A Turkish study published in 2002 reported that gingko biloba appears to heal sunburned skin after exposure as well as protect against ultraviolet radiation before exposure. These findings, however, await confirmation by other researchers.

Allopathic treatment

Aspirin can ease pain and inflammation. Tender skin should be protected against the sun until it has healed.

In addition, people suffering from sunburn may apply:

• calamine lotion

• sunburn cream or spray

• cool tap-water compresses

• colloidal oatmeal (Aveeno) baths

• dusting powder to reduce chafing

People who are severely sunburned should see a doctor, who may prescribe corticosteroid cream to speed healing and prescription pain medication. Topical corticosteroids that have been shown to be safe as well as effective in treating sunburn include methylprednisolone aceponate and hydrocortisone 17-butyrate.

Expected results

Moderately burned skin should heal within a week. While the skin will heal after a sunburn, the risk of skin

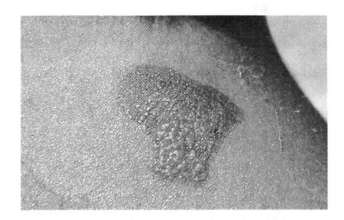

This person has a second-degree sunburn on the back of the neck. *(Custom Medical Stock Photo. Reproduced by permission.)*

cancer increases with exposure and subsequent burns. Even one bad burn in childhood carries an increased risk of skin cancer.

Prevention

Sun protection education

Concern about the rising rate of melanoma in Europe, Australia, and the United States has led public health experts to recommend adding instruction about the importance of sun protection to elementary and junior high school programs. A 1999 cross-sectional study of boys and girls in all 50 states found that 83% of the students had at least one sunburn during the previous summer, with 36% reporting three or more episodes of sunburn. Only 34% used sunscreen. As of 1998, only 3.4% of schools in the United States had sun protection policies to protect students from excessive sun exposure during recess or athletic practice. A standardized program of sun protection education developed by the EPA in 2000 has been reported to be effective in changing students' attitudes toward tanning and the importance of using sunscreen.

Specific preventive measures

To prevent sunburn, everyone over the age of six months should use a water-resistant sunscreen with a sun protective factor (SPF) of at least 15. Apply at least an ounce of sunscreen 15–30 minutes before going outside. It should be reapplied every two hours (more often after swimming). Babies should be kept completely out of the sun for the first six months of life, because their skin is thinner than the skin of older children. Sunscreens have not been approved for infants. Some people are allergic to para-aminobenzoic acid (PABA), a major ingredient in sunscreen products. They should check all labels or consult a doctor prior to application.

In addition, people should follow these guidelines:

- Limit sun exposure to 15 minutes the first day, even if the weather is hazy; then slowly increase exposure daily.

- Reapply sunscreen every two hours (more often if swimming or perspiring heavily).

- Reapply waterproof sunscreen after swimming more than 80 minutes, after toweling off, or after perspiring heavily.

- Avoid exposure to the sun between 10 A.M. and 3 P.M.

- Use waterproof sunscreen on legs and feet, since sun rays can burn even through water.

- Wear an opaque shirt in water, because reflected rays are intensified.

Patients using a sunscreen rated lower than SPF 15 should note that simply applying more of the same SPF won't prolong allowed time in the sun. Instead, patients should use a higher SPF in order to safely lengthen their exposure time. A billed cap protects 70% of the face; a wide-brimmed hat is better. People at very high risk for skin cancer can wear clothing that blocks almost all UV rays, but most people can simply wear white cotton summer-weight clothing with a tight weave. As of 2001, the U.S. Food and Drug Administration requires all sunscreen makers to label their products as providing minimum, moderate, or high levels of sun protection.

Resources

BOOKS

Blumenthal, Mark. *The Complete German Commission E Monographs: Therapeutic Guide to Herbal Medicine.* Boston: Integrative Medicine Communications, 1999.

Orkin, Milton, Howard Maibach, and Mark Dahl. *Dermatology.* Norwalk, CT: Appleton & Lange, 1992.

PERIODICALS

Buller, D. B., A. C. Geller, M. Cantor, et al. "Sun Protection Policies and Environmental Features in US Elementary Schools." *Archives of Dermatology* 138 (June 2002): 771-774.

Duteil, L., C. Queille-Roussel, B. Lorenz et al. "A Randomized, Controlled Study of the Safety and Efficacy of Topical Corticosteroid Treatments of Sunburn in Healthy Volunteers." *Clinical and Experimental Dermatology* 27 (June 2002): 314-318.

Geller, A. C., M. Cantor, D. R. Miller, et al. "The Environmental Protection Agency's National SunWise School Program: Sun Protection Education in US Schools (1999-2000)." *Journal of the American Academy of Dermatology* 46 (May 2002): 683-689.

Geller, A. C., G. Colditz, S. Oliveria, et al. "Use of Sunscreen, Sunburning Rates, and Tanning Bed Use Among More Than 10 000 US Children and Adolescents." *Pediatrics* 109 (June 2002): 1009-1014.

KEY TERMS

Gingko biloba—A shade tree native to China that has fan-shaped leaves and fleshy seeds. Gingko extract is being studied as a sunburn remedy and preventative.

Malignant melanoma—The most deadly of the three types of skin cancer.

Melanin—A biological pigment that gives color to skin, hair, and the iris of the eye.

Sunscreen—Products that block the damaging rays of the sun. Good sunscreens contain either para-aminobenzoic acid (PABA) or benzophenone, or both. Sunscreen protection factors range from 2-45.

Topical—A type of medication that is applied to the external surface of the skin.

Ozkur, M. K., M. S. Bozkurt, B. Balabanli, et al. "The Effects of EGb 761 on Lipid Peroxide Levels and Superoxide Dismutase Activity in Sunburn." *Photodermatology, Photoimmunology and Photomedicine* 18 (June 2002): 117-120.

Tyler, Varro. "Aloe: Nature's Skin Soother." *Prevention* 50 (April 1, 1998): 94-96.

ORGANIZATIONS

American Academy of Dermatology. 930 East Woodfield Rd., PO Box 4014, Schaumburg, IL 60168. (847) 330-0230. <www.aad.org>.

Environmental Protection Agency. Ten regional offices with region-specific addresses and phone numbers. <www.epa.gov>.

Ken R. Wells
Rebecca J. Frey, PhD

Sun's soup

Description

Sun's soup is a packaged food product made by Sun Farm Corporation (Milford, Connecticut) that contains vegetables and herbs. The soup's ingredients are said to possess anticancer and immune-building properties. Named for its creator, the biochemist Alexander Sun, Ph.D., who began work on the soup formula during the 1980s, it is also known as Dr. Sun's soup. Two versions are available: freeze-dried and frozen. It may be ordered online and by phone.

According to a National Cancer Institute report, the original soup formula contained shiitake mushrooms (*Lentinus edodes*), mung bean (*Phaseolus aureus*), and the Chinese herbs *Bai Hua She She Cao* (*Hedyotis diffusa*) and *Ban Zhi Lian* (*Scutellaria barbata*). The Institute report also included two other Sun Farm products, Selected Vegetables (SV) and Frozen Selected Vegetables (FSV), which are believed to contain:

- soybean (*Glycine max*)
- shiitake mushroom
- mung bean
- red date (*Ziziphus zizyphus*)
- scallion (*Allium cepa*)
- garlic (*Allium tuberosum*)
- leek (*Allium porrum*)
- lentil (seed of the *Lens esculenta* plant)
- **hawthorn** fruit (*Crataegus pinnatifida fructus*)
- onion (*Allium x proliferum*)
- ginseng (*Panax ginseng*)
- **angelica** root (*Dahurica*)
- licorice (*Glycyrrhiza glabra*)
- dandelion root (*Taraxacum officinale*)
- senega root (*Polygala senega*)
- ginger (*Zingiber officinale*)
- olive (*Bucida spinosa*)
- sesame seed (*Sesamum indicum*)
- parsley (*Petroselinum sativum* or *crispum*).

General use

When Alexander Sun's mother was diagnosed with non-small cell **lung cancer**, the Taiwanese biochemist began studying the research about treatments for her condition. According to an article on the Sun Farm Web site, Sun's mother underwent surgery to remove a tumor. During treatment that included chemotherapy, a new tumor was discovered. Sun then began researching **traditional Chinese medicine**, looking for herbal remedies that would help boost his mother's immune system and cause her tumor to shrink.

Based on his studies of Chinese medical textbooks, Sun developed an herb-and-vegeta ble soup, which his mother ate daily. According to the article, her condition was improved three months later, and doctors removed the remaining tumor. Sun's mother was reported to be cancer-free 13 years later, according to a citation in "Selected Vegetables/Sun's soup," a 13-page summary from the National Cancer Institute of the National Institutes of Health.

In 1992, Sun filed a patent application for his soup product, described as an "herbal treatment of malignancy." He received the patent three years later, and conducted clinical trials involving cancer patients who consumed the soup. Sun classified his product as a dietary supplement. In the United States, dietary supplements are categorized as foods rather than drugs. Companies planning to market new drugs must have their products evaluated by the United States Food and Drug Administration (FDA). The federal agency must approve the new drug before it is sold to the public as a medical treatment. No pre-market evaluation and approval is required for dietary supplements. However, the FDA may remove a supplement from the market if the product is determined to be unsafe.

As of 2004, Sun's soup is marketed as a food. The National Cancer Institute report noted that the FDA had not approved any formulation of Sun's soup for the treatment of cancer or any other medical condition. Clinical trials have been conducted on the soup, and the Sun Farm Web site contains references to those studies.

The National Cancer Institute report provided more in-depth analysis of two studies. The Institute cited research findings that Dr. Sun published in 1999 and 2001. While Sun's research indicated "improved survival" of cancer patients who consumed the soup, the Institute pointed out that only 18 people participated in the trials. That small number was among the "major weaknesses" of the research, according to the report. The Institute noted that different soup formulas were used in the studies, making it difficult to compare results.

Some of the known ingredients in Sun's soup may be effective as anticancer agents. The National Cancer Institute report described the potential benefits and uses of some ingredients in the various formulas of the herbal vegetable soup:

- Shiitake mushrooms are known to contain anticancer substances including lentinan.
- Mung bean may have an anticancer effect.
- *Bai Hua She She Cao* is a Chinese herb used to boost the immune system. It may have an anticancer effect.
- *Ban Zhi Lian* (barbat **skullcap**) may have an anticancer effect.
- Red date is the fruit of the jujube plant. It has been used to treat medical problems in some cultures.
- Hawthorn fruit is the fruit of the hawthorn tree or bush. It has been used to treat conditions such as heart and gastrointestinal disorders.

- Ginseng may have an anticancer effect.
- Angelica root is the root of the angelica herb. It is used to treat gastrointestinal conditions such as **gas**, appetite loss, and feelings of fullness.
- Senega root is the root of the *Polygala senega* herb. It is used to treat respiratory difficulties and other conditions.

Preparations

The original Sun's soup was prepared by adding it to hot water or another soup. The package contents may also be served on a salad.

The Sun Farm Web site lists daily recommended dosages for the supplement. For the freeze-dried product, the dosage is two 0.7-oz (20-g) pouches. The frozen soup is sold in 10-oz (0.3 kg) containers. The recommended dosage is one container per day.

Precautions

A diet rich in vegetables may reduce the risk of cancer. However, the FDA has not approved Sun's soup formula as a cancer treatment as of 2004, and the soup is marketed as a food product. On the Sun Farm Web site, the business has a disclaimer regarding any medical effect of its products. While the site contains information about clinical trials, Internet visitors are advised to check with their doctors regarding their medical condition.

The National Cancer Institute report concluded that there was little evidence that Sun's soup is effective as a cancer treatment. The Institute maintained that data are "limited" and "weak." The report called for larger, better-designed clinical studies to determine if the soup could be used to treat cancers, such as non-small cell lung cancer.

Sun's soup is said to be expensive, costing as much as hundreds of dollars per month, according to a 2001 report on the Cancer Guide Web site. The Sun Farm Web site in 2004 listed no prices for online ordering.

Side effects

According to the National Cancer Institute report, consumption of Sun's soup did not cause any adverse side effects. Some people reported feelings of fullness or bloating after consuming the soup.

Interactions

There are no published reports of drug interactions from consuming Sun's soup.

KEY TERMS

. . . .

Non-small cell lung cancer—A group of lung cancers: squamous cell carcinoma, adenocarcinoma, and large cell carcinoma.

OTHER

American Cancer Society. [cited April 30, 2004]. <http://www.cancer.org>.

Dunn, Steve. "Sun Soup." October 7, 2001. *Cancer Guide* [cited April 30, 2004.<http://wwww.cancerguide. org/sun_soup.html>.

Dupach, Etieune, Jr. "Cure for Cancer in a Bowl of Soup?" March 6,2000. [cited April 30, 2004). <http://www.sun-farmcorp.com/title-miami.htm>.

National Cancer Institute. (800) 4-CANCER. "Selected Vegetables/Sun's soup." July 24, 2003. [cited April 30, 2004]. <http://www.nci.nhi.gov/cancerinfo/pdq/cam/vegetables-sun-soup>.

Sun Farm Corporation. [cited April 30, 2004]. <http:// www. sunfarmcorp.com>.

Liz Swain

Swedish massage

Definition

Swedish massage is the most popular type of massage in the United States. It involves the use of hands, forearms or elbows to manipulate the superficial layers of the muscles to improve mental and physical health. Active or passive movement of the joints may also be part of the massage. The benefits of Swedish massage include increased blood circulation, mental and physical **relaxation**, decreased **stress** and muscle tension, and improved range of motion.

Origins

Swedish massage was invented by a Swedish fencing instructor named Per Henrik Ling in the 1830s. When he was injured in the elbows, he reportedly cured himself using tapping (percussion) strokes around the affected area. He later developed the technique currently known as Swedish massage. This technique was brought to the United States from Sweden by two brothers, Dr. Charles and Dr. George Taylor in the 1850s. The specific techniques used in Swedish massage involve the application of long gliding strokes, friction, and kneading and tapping movements on the soft tissues of the body. Sometimes passive or active joint movements are also used.

Benefits

Unlike drug therapy, which is often associated with many systemic and long-term side effects, **massage therapy** is relatively safe and has few contraindications. It also provides many benefits.

Physical benefits

There are numerous physical benefits associated with the use of Swedish massage:

- loosening tight muscles and stretching connective tissues
- relieving cramps and muscle spasms and decreasing muscle fatigue
- loosening joints and improving range of motion
- increasing muscle strength
- calming the nervous system
- stimulating blood circulation
- firming up muscle and skin tone
- relieving symptoms of such disorders as **asthma**, arthritis, **carpal tunnel syndrome**, chronic and acute **pain** syndromes, myofacial pain, **headache**, temporomandibular joint (TMJ) dysfunction, and athletic injuries
- speeding up healing from injury and illness
- improving **lymphatic drainage** of metabolic wastes

Mental and emotional benefits

Mental benefits associated with massage therapy include the following:

- mental relaxation
- improvement in length and quality of sleep
- relief of stress, **depression**, **anxiety** and irritation
- increased ability to concentrate
- improved sense of well-being

Description

In Swedish massage, the person to be massaged lies on a massage table and is draped with a towel or sheet. It is a full-body massage treatment, except in areas that are contraindicated or where the client requests not to be touched. Aromatic or unscented oil or lotion is used to facilitate the massage movements. Each session usually lasts 30-60 minutes. Depending on the client's preferences, a massage session may involve the use of several or all of the following basic techniques: effleurage, petrissage, friction, vibration, and tapotement.

Effleurage

Effleurage is the most common **stroke** in Swedish massage. It is a free-flowing and gliding movement towards the heart, tracing the contours of the body using the palm of one or both hands. Oil is applied with this stroke to begin the first stage of massage. The therapist applies a light or medium constant pressure. This stroke is used to warm up the muscles, relax the body, calm the nerves, improve blood circulation and heart function, and improve lymphatic drainage.

Pétrissage

This technique resembles kneading dough. It involves lifting, rolling, and squeezing the flesh under or between the hands. Pétrissage is designed to release muscle tension, improve blood flow, and increase lymphatic drainage.

Friction

Friction strokes work on deeper muscles than the techniques previously described. The friction technique is a pressure stroke and is the deepest that is used in Swedish massage. The massage therapist applies pressure by placing the weight of his or her body on the flat of the hand and the pads of the thumbs, knuckles, fingers, or the back of the forearms, and then releases the pressure slowly and gently. This movement should be a continuous sliding motion or a group of alternating circular motions.

Vibration

To effect vibration, the massage therapist gently shakes or trembles the flesh with the hand or fingertips, then moves on to another spot and repeats this stroke. Vibration is designed to release muscle tension in small muscle areas, such as those on the face or along the spine.

Tapotement

Tapotement, or tapping and percussion, is a quick choppy rhythmic movement that has a stimulating or toning effect. The following are variations of tapotement:

- **Cupping**: The therapist forms the hands into a cup shape with fingers straight but bending only at the lower knuckles; the thumbs are kept close to the palms. The therapist strikes the flesh with the flat of the hands one after another in quick succession.
- **Hacking**: This technique is similar to cupping. The therapist uses the sides of the hands with palms facing one another to make a chopping movement.

- Pummeling: For this stroke, the therapist makes loose fists in both hands and applies them rapidly in succession over the thighs and buttocks.

Tapotement techniques are invigorating to most people but may be too intense for some. When prolonged, tapotement leads to overstimulation and even exhaustion of the nerves and muscles. In addition, it should not be used over **varicose veins** or directly above bony structures.

Preparations

Swedish massage requires the following equipment:

- Massage surface: This may be a professional massage table or any firm but well-padded surface.

- A clean sheet to cover the part of the body that is not massaged.

- Cushions: These may be needed, depending on the client's wishes, to prevent lower back pain. The cushions may be placed under the head and the knees.

- Oils: The base oil should be a vegetable oil, cold pressed, unrefined, and free of additives. These oils contain such nutrients as vitamins and minerals in addition to fatty acids. They do not clog the pores as mineral oils often do. Essential (aromatic) oils may be added to provide additional relaxation or other therapeutic effects. Massage oil should be warmed in the therapist's hands before it is applied to the client's skin.

Precautions

Swedish massage should not be given to patients with the following physical disorders or conditions:

- nausea, **vomiting** or diarrhea
- fever
- broken bones, **fractures**, dislocations, or severe sprains
- contagious diseases
- open or unhealed sores or wounds
- body areas that are inflamed, swollen or bruised
- varicose veins
- recent surgery
- severe pain
- jaundice
- frostbite
- kidney disease
- large hernias
- hemorrhaging
- torn ligaments, tendons, or muscles

- high blood pressure or heart problems
- certain kinds of cancer
- history of **phlebitis** or thrombosis (These patients may have **blood clots** that may become dislodged and travel to the lungs, with potentially fatal results.)
- drug treatment with blood thinners (These medications increase the risk of bleeding under the skin.)

Some clients with histories of physical violence or abuse may feel uncomfortable about removing their clothing or other aspects of massage. A brief explanation of what happens in a massage session and how they can benefit from massage is usually helpful.

Side effects

There have been few reported side effects associated with massage of low or moderate intensity. Intense massage, however, may increase the risk of injury to the body. Vigorous massage has been associated with muscle pain and such injuries as bleeding in the liver or other vital organs, and the dislodgment of blood clots.

Research & general acceptance

Swedish massage is now gaining acceptance from the medical community as a complementary treatment. Studies have shown that massage can relax the body, decrease blood pressure and heart rate, and reduce stress and depression. It may also provide symptomatic relief for many chronic diseases. Many doctors now prescribe massage therapy as symptomatic treatment for **headache**, facial pain, carpal tunnel syndrome, arthritis, other chronic and acute conditions, stress, and athletic injuries. Many insurance companies now reimburse patients for prescribed massage therapy. As of 2000, however, Medicare and Medicaid do not pay for this form of alternative treatment.

Training & certification

There are 58 training programs accredited by the Commission for Massage Therapy Accreditation/Approval in the United States. They provide a minimum of 500 hours of massage training. Certified therapists have graduated from these programs and passed the national certification examination for therapeutic massage. They are also required to participate in continuing education programs to keep their skills current.

There are several national associations for massage therapists in the United States, including the American Massage Therapy Association and the National Association of Nurse Massage Therapists. Persons interested in massage therapy should contact these organizations for referral to local certified therapists.

KEY TERMS

Cupping—A type of percussion stroke in which the massage therapist strikes or thumps the muscles with cupped hands.

Effleurage—A massage technique that involves light stroking with the palms or thumbs.

Pétrissage—A massage technique in which the therapist kneads or squeezes the muscles with both hands.

Tapotement—A group of massage techniques in which the therapist strikes the soft tissues with the sides of the hands or with loose fists. It is intended to invigorate and tone the body.

Resources

BOOKS

Beck, Mark F. *Milady's Theory and Practice of Therapeutic Massage,* 3rd ed. Albany, NY: Milady Publishing, 1994.

Claire, Thomas. *Bodywork: What Type of Massage to Get and How to Make the Most of It.* New York: William Morrow and Company, Inc., 1995.

PERIODICALS

Trotter, James F. "Hepatic Hematoma after Deep Tissue Massage." *New England Journal of Medicine* 341 (1999): 2019-2020.

ORGANIZATIONS

American Massage Therapy Association. 820 Davis St., Suite 100. Evanston, IL 60201. (847) 864-0123. Fax: (847) 864-1178. http://wwww.amtamassage.org.

National Association of Nurse Massage Therapists. 1710 East Linden St. Tucson, AZ 85719.

National Certification Board of Therapeutic Massage and Bodywork. 8201 Greensboro Dr., Suite 300. McLean, VA 22102. (703) 610-9015. (800) 296-0664.

Mai Tran

Sweet clover

Definition

Sweet clover (*Melilotus officinalis*) is a biennial plant that grows to heights of 2-4 ft (0.6-1.2 m) and produces small yellow flowers emitting a fragrance resembling that of hay or vanilla. It is a member of the legume, or Leguminosae, family. During its first year of growth, most of its energy goes into developing its root system. In the sec- ond year it flowers between May and September, sets its seeds, and dies. Its seeds may remain viable for over 30 years. The plant is also called hart's tree, hay flower, king's clover, melilot, sweet lucerne, or wild laburnum. Sweet clover grows in North America, Europe, Australia, and the temperate regions of Asia. In the early 1900s, sweet clover was grown for forage and to build up the soil, since its roots help to keep nitrogen in the soil. In the twenty-first century it is used to support honey production. In some agricultural areas of the United States, however, sweet clover is now considered a nuisance because it spreads rapidly and can take over open fields or prairies.

General use

Sweet clover is valued for its medicinal uses because the flower contains coumarinic acids. Coumarin is the active ingredient in prescription anticoagulants (blood-thinning medications). Its presence in sweet clover allows it to reduce inflammation and swelling by increasing the flow of blood between the heart and the veins. As an herbal remedy, sweet clover is used in the treatment of **bruises, hemorrhoids**, and **varicose veins**. Its wound-healing properties have been confirmed in tests conducted on animals.

Taken internally as a tea or as a tisane, sweet clover relieves discomfort in the legs, particularly night cramps, **itching**, and swelling. The herb also supports the traditional medical treatments of vein inflammation, **blood clots**, and congestion of the lymph nodes. Applied externally as a poultice, sweet clover speeds the healing of bruises and eases the swelling of hemorrhoids.

Preparations

Commercial preparations of sweet clover are available as dried crushed herb, as ointments, and as suppositories.

To prepare a sweet clover infusion, boiling water is poured over 1-2 tsp of the crushed flowers and stems. The infusion is allowed to steep for 5-10 minutes, then strained into a cup. For the treatment of varicose veins, 2-3 cups per day is recommended.

To prepare as a poultice, the crushed herb is mixed with a small amount of boiling water, then spread on a soft cloth. The cloth is applied to the affected area until the cloth is cold. The poultice is applied as needed.

Precautions

The sale of herbal products is not regulated in the United States. They are sold as dietary supplements without proof of safety or a standard of quality control. In addition, the lack of comprehensive scientific research leaves the consumer without a standard to follow. There-

KEY TERMS

. . . .

Coumarin—A chemical compound found in sweet clover that has blood-thinning properties.

Poultice—A warm mass of moist cloth or other soft material, used as a healing treatment. Poultices may contain crushed herbs or they may be moistened with herbal preparations.

Tisane—A decoction of herbs, usually drunk for medicinal purposes.

fore, persons interested in using sweet clover or any other herbal remedy should always consult a physician or pharmacist before beginning a program of herbal therapy.

Side effects

Long-term ingestion of high doses of sweet clover can cause **headache** and stupor. In isolated cases, temporary liver damage can result. These side effects disappear when the treatment is halted.

Interactions

Although sweet clover does not have any identified interactions, prescription drugs containing coumarin have been known to interact adversely with other prescription drugs, especially blood thinners, aspirin, and heart medications. Persons taking prescription drugs of any type should check with their physicians before begining a regimen of sweet clover.

Coumarin can also cause birth defects and bleeding in the fetus. Therefore, the use of sweet clover should be avoided during **pregnancy**.

Resources

BOOKS

PDR for Herbal Medicines. Montvale, NJ: Medical Economics Company, 1998.

Mary McNulty

Swelling *see* **Edema**

Swimmer's ear

Definition

Swimmer's ear, also known as otitis externa, is an inflammation of the outer ear canal. Although it is most prevalent among young adults and children, who often contract the condition from frequent swimming, swimmer's ear can affect anyone.

Description

Swimmer's ear is an inflammation of the outer ear that may lead to a painful and often itchy infection. It begins with the accumulation of excess moisture from swimming or daily showering. The skin inside the ear canal may flake due to moisture. This flaking may cause persistent **itching** that may lead to a break in the skin from scratching. Broken skin allows bacteria or a fungus to infect the tissues lining the ear canal. Swimming in polluted water can easily bring harmful bacteria into the outer ear.

Causes & symptoms

Causes

In swimmer's ear, the patient nearly always has a history of recent exposure to water combined with mild injury to the skin of the inner ear. This injury is typically caused by scratching or excessive and improper attempts to clean wax from the ears. Wax is one of the best defense mechanisms the ear has against infection due to the protection it offers from excess moisture and the environment it provides for friendly bacteria. Earwax should not be removed by such sharp objects as fingernails or hairpins. If the wax is scratched away, it becomes easier for an infection to occur.

The infection itself is usually caused by gram-negative bacilli (*Pseudomonas aeruginosa* or *Proteus*) or by fungi (*Aspergillus*) or even yeasts that thrive in moist environments. There are a surprisingly large number of different organisms that can cause otitis externa; one study of 2039 patients diagnosed with swimmer's ear found that 202 different species of bacteria, 32 species of yeast, and 17 species of mold could be identified as the infectious agents in this group of patients.

In recent years, some of the organisms most likely to cause otitis externa have developed resistance to antibiotics; the resistant organisms vary from country to country. One Asian study found that *Staphylococcus aureus* is responsible for more cases of swimmer's ear in East Asia than *Pseudomonas aeruginosa*, and that methicillin-resistant *S. aureus*, or MRSA, is an increasingly worrisome problem in these countries. A study done in Texas, however, found that *Staphylococcus epidermidis* was responsible for the largest number of antibiotic-resistant cases.

In a minority of cases, otitis externa is caused by an allergic reaction. The most common allergens in chronic otitis externa are topical medications used in the ear, particularly preparations containing neomycin; nickel and other metals used in inexpensive earrings; and some materials used to make hearing aids.

Symptoms

The symptoms of swimmer's ear include swelling, redness, heat, and **pain**. The inflammation may produce a foul-smelling, yellowish, or watery discharge from the ear. The skin inside the ear canal may swell to the point that the examiner cannot see the patient's eardrum.

The patient may also experience itching inside the ear and a temporary minor **hearing loss** due to the blockage of the ear canal. The severe pain and tenderness associated with the condition may intensify when the patient's head is moved, or if the examiner gently pulls the earlobe.

Diagnosis

The diagnosis of swimmer's ear is made from clinical observation. The doctor looks inside the ear with an instrument called an otoscope. The otoscope allows him or her to see whether there is swelling, redness, and a discharge. The doctor may also take a specimen of the discharge by swabbing just inside the ear. This specimen is then sent to a laboratory to identify the bacterium or fungus.

Treatment

Swimmer's ear is not usually a dangerous infection and often heals itself within a few days. If the infection is mild, alternative methods of treatment may be beneficial.

Herbal remedies

Native Americans used **mullein** (*Verbascum thapsus*) oil to treat minor inflammations. To ease the discomfort of swimmer's ear, 1–3 drops of a mullein preparation may be placed in the ear every three hours.

Garlic (*Allium sativum*) has been shown to be effective in treating swimmer's ear. As a natural antibiotic, garlic is a useful herb for inflammation of the outer ear. Equal parts of garlic juice and glycerin are added to a carrier oil, such as olive or sweet almond. One to three drops of this mixture may be placed in the infected ear every three hours.

Homeopathy

Specific homeopathic remedies for swimmer's ear may include *Aconite*, *Apis*, *Graphites*, or *Pulsatilla*. A homeopathic practitioner should always be consulted for specific treatment recommendations.

A 1997 German study found that homeopathic treatments reduced the duration of pain in children with ear **infections** more quickly than those treated with conventional drugs. The homeopathic-treated group was also found to have a greater resistance to recurrence of the infection within one year after treatment.

Home remedies

The inflammation and pain of otitis externa may be eased with the following home remedies:

- The infected ear canal may be washed with an over-the-counter topical antiseptic. A homemade solution using equal parts white vinegar and isopropyl alcohol may be placed, a few drops at a time, into the ear every two to three hours. The vinegar-alcohol drops should be kept in the ear for at least 30 seconds.

- A warm heating pad or compress may be placed on the ear to relieve pain.

- Pain may also be eased by taking aspirin or another analgesic.

- To assist the healing process, the infected ear canal should be kept dry. When showering, the patient should use earplugs or a shower cap.

Allopathic treatment

A doctor will use conventional medicine to treat swimmer's ear. The ear is typically cleaned with a cotton-tipped probe or a suction device to relieve irritation and pain. Ear drops containing a combination of hydrocortisone to help relieve the itching and an antibiotic to fight infection (usually neomycin sulfate and polymyxin B sulfate) may be prescribed.

For severe pain, doctors may recommend aspirin, acetaminophen, or some other over-the-counter pain medication. To assist the healing process, the infected ear must be kept dry. An infection typically begins to improve within three to four days. If the pain persists or becomes worse, the doctor may prescribe an oral antibiotic or an anti-inflammatory drug.

If the doctor prescribes an oral antibiotic to treat the infection, it is important for the patient to finish taking the entire course of medication even if he or she feels better fairly quickly. The reason is that a single antibiotic can kill off most of the bacteria causing the infection, but a few organisms may survive that have a higher degree of natural resistance to the drug. If the patient stops taking the antibiotic too soon, not all the bacteria will be killed off, and those that survive may develop resistance to the particular drug that was used.

If the otitis externa is caused by an allergic reaction, a patch test is necessary in order to identify the substance or object that is causing the reaction. Treatment consists of avoiding further contact with the allergen; or switching medications if the patient has developed an allergic sensitivity to a topical ear medication.

Expected results

Swimmer's ear is usually a minor inflammation of the outer ear canal that may even heal itself within a few days. It usually responds to many alternative treatments as well as to the conventional methods prescribed by doctors.

Rapidly spreading redness and swelling of the outer ear or nearby skin, or **fever**, are indications of an aggressively spreading infection. These symptoms require immediate medical attention.

Prevention

Prevention is the key component in avoiding swimmer's ear. Patients should be careful when cleaning the ears—never dig into the ear canal; wear earplugs when swimming and avoid swimming in dirty water; and use earplugs or a shower cap when showering.

Additional methods to ensure the prevention of swimmer's ear include: putting a dropperful of isopropyl alcohol or white vinegar into the ear after swimming or showering to dry out the ear and help kill germs; before swimming, create a protective coating by squirting a dropperful of mineral oil, baby oil, or lanolin into the ear; and when wearing a hearing aid, remove it often to allow the ear an opportunity to dry out completely.

Resources

BOOKS

Cummings, Stephen, MD, and Dana Ullman, MPH. *Everybody's Guide to Homeopathic Medicines.* New York: G. P. Putnam's Sons, 1991.

The Editors of Time-Life Books. *The Medical Advisor: The Complete Guide to Alternative & Conventional Treatments.* Richmond, VA: Time-Life Inc., 1996.

The Merck Manual of Diagnosis and Therapy, edited by Mark H. Beers, MD, and Robert Berkow, MD. Whitehouse Station, NJ: Merck Research Laboratories, 1999.

PERIODICALS

Berenholz, L., U. Katzenell, and M. Harell. "Evolving Resistant *Pseudomonas* to Ciprofloxacin in Malignant Otitis Externa." *Laryngoscope* 112 (September 2002): 1619-1622.

Hwang, J. H., C. K. Chu, and T. C. Liu. "Changes in Bacteriology of Discharging Ears." *Journal of Laryngology and Otology* 116 (September 2002): 686-689.

Ramsey, A. M. "Diagnosis and Treatment of the Child with a Draining Ear." *Journal of Pediatric Health Care* 16 (July-August 2002): 161-169.

> ## KEY TERMS
> ....
> **Analgesic**—A medication given to relieve pain.
>
> **Mullein**—A plant related to the figwort, used by Native Americans to treat inflammations. It is still recommended by naturopaths to reduce the discomfort of swimmer's ear.
>
> **Otitis externa**—Inflammation of the outer ear. Otitis externa is the medical term for swimmer's ear.
>
> **Otoscope**—An instrument that allows doctors to examine the inside of a patient's ear.
>
> **Topical**—A type of medication that is applied to the skin or other outer surface of the body.

Roland, P. S., and D. W. Stroman. "Microbiology of Acute Otitis Externa." *Laryngoscope* 112 (July 2002): 1166-1177.

Sood, S., D. R. Strachan, A. Tsikoudas, and G. I. Stables. "Allergic Otitis Externa." *Clinical Otolaryngology* 27 (August 2002): 233-236.

ORGANIZATIONS

American Academy of Otolaryngology-Head and Neck Surgery. 1 Prince Street. Alexandria, VA 22314. (703) 836-4444.

American Academy of Pediatrics (AAP). 141 Northwest Point Boulevard, Elk Grove Village, IL 60007. (847) 434-4000. <www.aap.org>.

International Foundation for Homeopathy. 2366 Eastlake Avenue East, Suite 329. Seattle, WA 98102. (206) 324-8230.

Beth Kapes
Rebecca J. Frey, PhD

Swollen testicles *see* **Epididymitis**

Syntonic optometry

Definition

Syntonic optometry uses colored light shone into a patient's eyes to treat visual and other dysfunctions.

Origins

The founding father of syntonic optometry is Dr. Harry Riley Spitler, who developed the discipline during the 1920s and 1930s. Building on the work of earlier investigators including Edwin Babbit, Spitler studied the effects of light on human health and performance. Illness, he concluded, is largely caused by imbalances in the body's endocrine and nervous systems. Balance could be restored and healing achieved, he decided, by exposing the eyes to visible frequencies of light. Spitler founded the College of Syntonic Optometry in 1933, and eight years later he wrote a book titled *The Syntonic Principle.*

Benefits

Practitioners of syntonic optometry claim to be able to treat or support treatment of asthenopia (eye **fatigue**), strabismus (crossed eyes), amblyopia (unclear vision), ametropia (defective refraction of light), problems with focusing or converging the eyes, and visual field constrictions related to brain trauma, visual/emotional **stress**, or degenerative eye disorders. They also claim to be able to help correct visual attention deficit, and learning and behavior problems related to vision.

Description

In syntonic optometry, the patient is exposed to one or more colors of light for a fixed period of time. This is done in a darkened room, with colors generated by a machine known as a syntonizer. In a typical session, a patient might absorb one color for 10 minutes, then another for an additional 10 minutes. Alternatively, just one color might be absorbed for 20 minutes. Treatment typically could involve between three and five sessions a week, for a period of four to eight weeks. In most cases, syntonics is used in conjunction with other therapeutic procedures.

Precautions

The usefulness of syntonic optometry is a contentious issue, and a medical opinion should be sought in all cases of serious illness. The application of syntonic optometry to treating behavioral and **learning disorders** is especially controversial. Because the aftereffects of these problems can affect a child for a lifetime, it is prudent to obtain a second opinion from a university-affiliated practitioner.

Side effects

Conducted properly, syntonic optometry is thought to be generally free of adverse side effects, although it is expensive.

Research & general acceptance

The American Academy of Ophthalmology, an association of medical eye specialists, states that "as with other forms of vision therapy, there is no scientifically verified evidence to support claims for syntonic optome-

try." The College of Syntonic Optometry acknowledges that "researchers and other professionals are still a step away from understanding the clinical methods and practice of light stimulation which syntonists have used with positive results for over a half a century." There is, however, growing acceptance in medical circles of the therapeutic effects of light, especially its usefulness in treating **seasonal affective disorder**.

Training & certification

The College of Syntonic Optometry, an international group based in the United States, offers training, research grants, and membership to registered optometrists. The college also offers associate memberships to licensed educators and health care practitioners who employ phototherapy techniques. Practitioners of syntonic optometry are most common in the United States but can also be found in numerous other countries.

Resources

ORGANIZATIONS

College of Syntomic Optometry. (717) 387-0900. http:\\www. syntonicphototherapy.com.

David Helwig

Syphilis

Definition

Syphilis is an infectious systemic disease that may be either congenital or acquired through sexual contact or contaminated needles.

Description

Syphilis has both acute and chronic forms that produce a wide variety of symptoms affecting most of the body's organ systems. The range of symptoms makes it easy to confuse syphilis with less serious diseases and ignore its early signs. Acquired syphilis has four stages (primary, secondary, latent, and tertiary) and can be spread by sexual contact during the first three of these four stages.

Syphilis, which is also called lues (from a Latin word meaning "plague"), has been a major public health problem since the sixteenth century. The disease was treated with mercury or other ineffective remedies until World War I, when effective treatments based on arsenic or bismuth were introduced. These were succeeded by antibi-

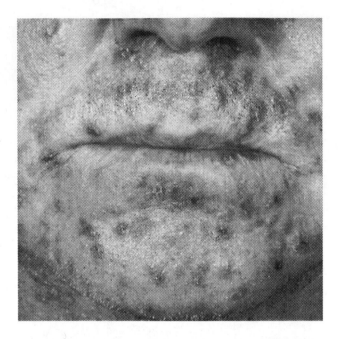

This patient has secondary syphilis, which is characterized by the appearance of lesions on the skin. *(Custom Medical Stock Photo. Reproduced by permission.)*

otics after World War II. At that time, the number of cases in the general population decreased, partly because of aggressive public health measures. This temporary decrease, combined with the greater amount of attention given to **AIDS** in recent years, leads some people to think that syphilis is no longer a serious problem. In fact, the number of cases of syphilis in the United States rose between 1980 and 2001. This increase affected both sexes, all races, all parts of the nation, and all age groups, including adults over 60. The number of women of childbearing age with syphilis is the highest that has been recorded since the 1940s. About 25,000 cases of infectious syphilis in adults are reported annually in the United States. It is estimated, however, that 400,000 people in the United States need treatment for syphilis every year, and that the annual worldwide total is 50 million persons.

In 1999, the Centers for Disease Control and Prevention (CDC) joined several other federal agencies in announcing the "National Plan to Eliminate Syphilis in the United States." Eliminating the disease was defined as the absence of transmission of the disease; that is, no transmission after 90 days following the report of an imported index case. The national goals for eliminating syphilis include bringing the annual number of reported cases in the United States below 1000, and increasing the number of syphilis-free counties to 90% by 2005. In November 2002, the CDC released figures for 2000–2001, which indicate that the number of reported cases of primary and secondary syphilis rose slightly. This rise, however, occurred only among men who have sex with other men. The CDC also stated that the number of new cases of syphilis has actually declined among women as well as among non-Hispanic blacks.

The increased incidence of syphilis since the 1970s is associated with drug abuse as well as changes in sexual behavior. The connections between drug abuse and syphilis include needle sharing and exchanging sex for drugs. In addition, people using drugs are more likely to engage in risky sexual practices. As of 2002, the risk of contracting syphilis is particularly high among those who abuse crack cocaine.

With respect to changing patterns of conduct, a sharp increase in the number of people having sex with multiple partners makes it more difficult for public health doctors to trace the contacts of infected persons. Women are not necessarily protected by having sex only with other women; in the past few years, several cases have been reported of female-to-female transmission of syphilis through oral-genital contact. In addition, the incidence of syphilis among men who have sex with other men continues to rise. Several studies in Latin America as well as in the United States reported in late 2002 that unprotected sexual intercourse is on the increase among gay and bisexual men.

Changing patterns of sexual behavior have led to a striking increase in the number of cases of syphilis in eastern Europe since the collapse of the Soviet Union; Slovenia reported an 18-fold increase in reported cases of syphilis just between 1993 and 1994. Over half of the new cases were linked to a source of infection in another European country.

In general, high-risk groups for syphilis in the United States and Canada include:

- sexually active teenagers
- people infected with another sexually transmitted disease (STD), including AIDS, herpes, and **gonorrhea**
- sexually abused children
- women of childbearing age
- prostitutes of either sex and their customers
- prisoners
- persons who abuse drugs or alcohol

The chances of contracting syphilis from an infected person in the early stages of the disease during unprotected sex range from 30–50%.

Causes & symptoms

Syphilis is caused by a spirochete, *Treponema pallidum.* A spirochete is a thin spiral- or coil-shaped bacterium that enters the body through the mucous membranes or breaks in the skin. In 90% of cases, the spirochete is transmitted by sexual contact. Transmission by blood transfusion is possible but rare, not only because blood products are screened for the disease, but also because the spirochetes die within 24 hours in stored blood. Other methods of transmission are highly unlikely because *T. pallidum* is easily killed by heat and drying.

Primary syphilis

Primary syphilis is the stage of the organism's entry into the body. The first signs of infection are not always noticed. After an incubation period ranging from 10–90 days, the patient develops a chancre, which is a small blister-like sore about 0.5 in (13 mm) in size. Most chancres are on the genitals, but may also develop in or on the mouth or on the breasts. Rectal chancres are common in male homosexuals. Chancres in women are sometimes overlooked if they develop in the vagina or on the cervix. The chancres are not painful and disappear in three to six weeks even without treatment. They resemble the ulcers of lymphogranuloma venereum, herpes simplex virus, or skin tumors.

About 70% of patients with primary syphilis also develop swollen lymph nodes near the chancre. The nodes may have a firm or rubbery feel when the doctor touches them but are not usually painful.

Secondary syphilis

Syphilis enters its secondary stage ranging from six to eight weeks to six months after the infection begins. Chancres may still be present but are usually healing. Secondary syphilis is a systemic infection marked by the eruption of skin **rashes** and ulcers in the mucous membranes. The skin rash may mimic a number of other skin disorders such as drug reactions, **rubella** ringworm, **mononucleosis**, and **pityriasis rosea**. Characteristics that point to syphilis include:

• a coppery color

• absence of **pain** or itching

• occurrence on the palms of hands and soles of feet

The skin eruption may resolve in a few weeks or last as long as a year. The patient may also develop condylomata lata, which are weepy pinkish or gray areas of flattened skin in the moist areas of the body. The skin rashes, mouth and genital ulcers, and condylomata lata are all highly infectious.

About 50% of patients with secondary syphilis develop swollen lymph nodes in the armpits, groin, and neck areas; about 10% develop inflammations of the eyes, kidney, liver, spleen, bones, joints, or the meninges (membranes covering the brain and spinal cord). They may also have a flulike general illness with a low **fever**, **chills**, loss of appetite, headaches, runny nose, **sore throat**, and aching joints.

Latent syphilis

Latent syphilis is a phase of the disease characterized by relative absence of external symptoms. The term latent does not mean that the disease is not progressing or that the patient cannot infect others. For example, pregnant women can transmit syphilis to their unborn children during the latency period.

The latent phase is sometimes divided into early latency (less than two years after infection) and late latency. During early latency, patients are at risk for spontaneous relapses marked by recurrence of the ulcers and skin rashes of secondary syphilis. In late latency, these recurrences are much less likely. Late latency may either resolve spontaneously or continue for the rest of the patient's life.

Tertiary syphilis

Untreated syphilis progresses to a third or tertiary stage in about 35–40% of patients (only those who go untreated). Patients with tertiary syphilis cannot infect others with the disease. It is thought that the symptoms of this stage are a delayed immune hypersensitivity reaction to the spirochetes. Some patients develop so-called benign late syphilis, which begins between three and 10 years after infection and is characterized by the development of gummas. Gummas are rubbery tumor-like growths that are most likely to involve the skin or long bones but may also develop in the eyes, mucous membranes, throat, liver, or stomach lining. Gummas are increasingly uncommon since the introduction of antibiotics for treating syphilis. Benign late syphilis is usually rapid in onset and responds well to treatment.

CARDIOVASCULAR SYPHILIS. Cardiovascular syphilis occurs in 10–15% of patients who have progressed to tertiary syphilis. It develops between 10 and 25 years after infection and often occurs together with neurosyphilis. Cardiovascular syphilis usually begins as an inflammation of the arteries leading from the heart and heart attacks, scarring of the aortic valves, congestive heart failure, or the formation of an aortic aneurysm.

NEUROSYPHILIS. About 8% of patients with untreated syphilis will develop symptoms in the central nervous system that include both physical and psychiatric symptoms. Neurosyphilis can appear at any time from five to 35 years after the onset of primary syphilis. It affects men more frequently than women and Caucasians more frequently than African Americans.

Neurosyphilis is classified into four types:

- Asymptomatic. In this form of neurosyphilis, the patient's spinal fluid gives abnormal test results but there are no symptoms affecting the central nervous system.

- Meningovascular. This type of neurosyphilis is marked by changes in the blood vessels of the brain or inflammation of the meninges (the tissue layers covering the brain and spinal cord). The patient develops headaches, irritability, and visual problems. If the spinal cord is involved, the patient may experience weakness of the shoulder and upper arm muscles.

- Tabes dorsalis. Tabes dorsalis is a progressive degeneration of the spinal cord and nerve roots. Patients lose their sense of perception of body position and orientation in space (proprioception), resulting in difficulties walking and loss of muscle reflexes. They may also have shooting pains in the legs and periodic episodes of pain in the abdomen, throat, bladder, or rectum. Tabes dorsalis is sometimes called locomotor ataxia.

- General paresis. General paresis refers to the effects of neurosyphilis on the cortex of the brain. The patient has a slow but progressive loss of memory, decreased ability to concentrate, and less interest in self-care. Personality changes may include irresponsible behavior, **depression**, delusions of grandeur, or complete psychosis. General paresis is sometimes called **dementia** paralytica, and is most common in patients over 40.

Special populations

NEWBORNS. Congenital syphilis has increased at a rate of 400–500% over the past decade, on the basis of criteria introduced by the Centers for Disease Control (CDC) in 1990. In 1994, more than 2,200 cases of congenital syphilis were reported in the United States. The prognosis for early congenital syphilis is poor: about 54% of infected fetuses die before or shortly after birth. Those who survive may look normal at birth but show signs of infection between three and eight weeks later.

Infants with early congenital syphilis have systemic symptoms that resemble those of adults with secondary syphilis. There is a 40–60% chance that the child's central nervous system will be infected. These infants may have symptoms ranging from **jaundice**, enlargement of the spleen and liver, and **anemia** to skin rashes, condylomata lata, certain congenital bone abnormalities, inflammation of the lungs, "snuffles" (a persistent runny nose), and swollen lymph nodes.

CHILDREN. Children who develop symptoms after the age of two years are said to have late congenital syphilis. The characteristic symptoms include facial deformities (saddle nose), Hutchinson's teeth (abnormal upper incisors), saber shins, dislocated joints, deafness, mental retardation, paralysis, and seizure disorders.

PREGNANT WOMEN. Syphilis can be transmitted from the mother to the fetus through the placenta at any time during **pregnancy**, or through the child's contact with syphilitic ulcers during the birth process. The chances of infection are related to the stage of the mother's disease. Almost all infants of mothers with untreated primary or secondary syphilis will be infected, whereas the infection rate drops to 40% if the mother is in the early latent stage and 6–14% if she has late latent syphilis.

Pregnancy does not affect the progression of syphilis in the mother; however, pregnant women should not be treated with tetracyclines.

HIV PATIENTS. Syphilis has been closely associated with HIV infection since the late 1980s. Syphilis sometimes mimics the symptoms of AIDS. Conversely, AIDS appears to increase the severity of syphilis in patients suffering from both diseases, and to speed up the development or appearance of neurosyphilis. Patients with HIV are also more likely to develop lues maligna, a skin disease that sometimes occurs in secondary syphilis. Lues maligna is characterized by areas of ulcerated and dying tissue. In addition, HIV patients have a higher rate of treatment failure with penicillin than patients without HIV.

ADULT MALES. A recent study indicates that infection with syphilis increases a man's risk of developing **prostate cancer** in later life. It is thought that infection may represent one mechanism among several through which prostate **cancer** may develop.

Diagnosis

Patient history and physical diagnosis

The diagnosis of syphilis is often delayed because of the variety of early symptoms, the varying length of the incubation period, and the possibility of not noticing the initial chancre. Patients do not always connect their symptoms with recent sexual contact. They may go to a dermatologist when they develop the skin rash of secondary syphilis rather than to their primary care doctor. Women may be diagnosed in the course of a gynecological checkup. Because of the long-term risks of untreated syphilis, certain groups of people are now routinely screened for the disease:

- pregnant women
- sexual contacts or partners of patients diagnosed with syphilis
- children born to mothers with syphilis
- patients with HIV infection
- persons applying for marriage licenses

When the doctor takes the patient's history, he or she will ask about recent sexual contacts in order to determine whether the patient falls into a high-risk group. Other symptoms, such as skin rashes or swollen lymph nodes, will be noted with respect to the dates of the patient's sexual contacts. Definite diagnosis, however, depends on the results of laboratory blood tests.

Blood tests

There are several types of blood tests for syphilis presently used in the United States. Some are used in follow-up monitoring of patients as well as diagnosis.

NONTREPONEMAL ANTIGEN TESTS. Nontreponemal antigen tests are used as screeners. They measure the presence of reagin, which is an antibody formed in reaction to syphilis. In the Venereal Disease Research Laboratory (VDRL) test, a sample of the patient's blood is mixed with cardiolipin and **cholesterol**. If the mixture forms clumps or masses of matter, the test is considered reactive or positive. The serum sample can be diluted several times to determine the concentration of reagin in the patient's blood.

The rapid plasma reagin (RPR) test works on the same principle as the VDRL. It is available as a kit. The patient's serum is mixed with cardiolipin on a plastic-coated card that can be examined with the naked eye.

Nontreponemal antigen tests require a doctor's interpretation and sometimes further testing. They can yield both false-negative and false-positive results. False-positive results (test shows a positive result when the patient does not have the disease) can be caused by other infectious diseases, including mononucleosis, **malaria**, leprosy, **rheumatoid arthritis**, and lupus. HIV patients have a particularly high rate (4%, compared to 0.8% of HIV-negative patients) of false-positive results on reagin tests. False negative results (patient does have the disease, but test comes back negative) can occur when patients are tested too soon after exposure to syphilis; it takes about 14–21 days after infection for the blood to become reactive.

TREPONEMAL ANTIBODY TESTS. Treponemal antibody tests are used to rule out false-positive results on reagin tests. They measure the presence of antibodies that are specific for *T. pallidum*. The most commonly used tests are the microhemagglutination-*T. pallidum* (MHA-TP) and the fluorescent treponemal antibody absorption (FTA-ABS) tests. In the FTA-ABS, the patient's blood serum is mixed with a preparation that prevents interference from antibodies to other treponemal **infections**. The test serum is added to a slide containing *T. pallidum*. In a positive reaction, syphilitic antibodies in the blood coat the spirochetes on the slide. The slide is then stained with fluorescein, which causes the coated spirochetes to fluoresce when the slide is viewed under ultraviolet (UV) light. In the MHA-TP test, red blood cells from sheep are coated with *T. pallidum* antigen. The cells will clump if the patient's blood contains antibodies for syphilis.

A newer treponemal antibody test developed in Belgium, the INNO-LIA, uses recombinant and peptide antigens derived from *T. pallidum* proteins. Preliminary testing in Europe indicates that the INNO-LIA is the most accurate of the available treponemal antibody tests for syphilis.

Treponemal antibody tests are more expensive and more difficult to perform than nontreponemal tests. They are therefore used to confirm the diagnosis of syphilis rather than to screen large groups of people. These tests are, however, very specific and very sensitive; false-positive results are relatively unusual.

INVESTIGATIONAL BLOOD TESTS. As of 1998, ELISA, Western blot, and PCR testing are being studied as additional diagnostic tests, particularly for congenital syphilis and neurosyphilis.

Other laboratory tests

MICROSCOPE STUDIES. The diagnosis of syphilis can also be confirmed by identifying spirochetes in samples of tissue or lymphatic fluid. Fresh samples can be made into slides and studied under darkfield illumination. A newer method involves preparing slides from dried fluid smears and staining them with fluorescein for viewing under UV light. This method is replacing darkfield examination because the slides can be mailed to professional laboratories.

SPINAL FLUID TESTS. Testing of cerebrospinal fluid (CSF) is an important part of patient monitoring as well as a diagnostic test. The VDRL and FTA-ABS tests can be performed on CSF as well as on blood. An abnormally high white cell count and elevated protein levels in the CSF, together with positive VDRL results, suggest a possible diagnosis of neurosyphilis. CSF testing is not used for routine screening. It is used most frequently for infants with congenital syphilis, HIV-positive patients, and patients of any age who are not responding to penicillin treatment.

Treatment

It is difficult to obtain information about alternative treatments for syphilis. The disease has a high profile as a public health issue and few alternative practitioners want to risk accusations of minimizing its dangers. One respected resource for alternative therapies states bluntly, "Syphilis should not be treated only with natural therapies." Most naturopathic practitioners agree that antibiotics are essential for the treatment of syphilis. Others would add that recovery from the disease can be assisted by dietary changes, sleep, **exercise**, and **stress** reduction, and immune support measures.

Homeopathy

Homeopathic practitioners are forbidden by law in the United States to claim that homeopathic treatment can cure syphilis. Given the high rate of syphilis in HIV-positive patients, however, some alternative practitioners who are treating AIDS patients with homeopathic remedies maintain that they are beneficial for syphilis as well. The remedies suggested most frequently are *Medorrhinum*, *Syphilinum*, *Mercurius vivus*, and *Aurum*. The use of *Mercurius vivus* as a homeopathic remedy reflects the past use of mercury to treat syphilis prior to the discovery of penicillin. *Syphilinum* represents a class of homeopathic remedy called nosodes. A nosode is a homeopathic medicine made from diseased material, such as bacteria, viruses, or pus. Its effect is based on the homeopathic law of similars, in which a substance that causes a specific set of symptoms in a healthy person is determined curative when given to a sick person with the same symptoms. *Syphilinum* is a nosode made from a dilution of killed *Treponema pallidum*. The historical link between **homeopathy** and syphilis is Hahnemann's theory of miasms, which he defined as fundamental predispositions toward disease that were transmitted from one generation to the next. He thought that the syphilitic miasm was the second oldest cause of constitutional weakness in humans.

Other

Traditional Chinese medicine (TCM) and other alternative methods emphasize the mental aspects of conditions and diseases such as syphilis. Mind-body medicine, **guided imagery** and affirmations are often used to help support a person through such a disease. New thought holds that humans can control physical as well as mental or spiritual events through the power of thinking itself. Some alternative therapies reflect new thought beliefs by maintaining that humans make themselves ill through harmful thought patterns, and that they can heal themselves by affirming positive beliefs. The affirmation suggested for healing syphilis is "I decide to be me." Most alternative practitioners would recommend this or similar new thought affirmations only as adjuncts to conventional medical treatment for syphilis.

One interesting recent historical development is that outdated or discredited treatments for syphilis have resurfaced as alternative treatments for AIDS or cancer. One study of alternative treatments for HIV infection notes that **hyperthermia**, which involves treating a disease by giving the patient a fever, originated as a treatment for syphilis. Syphilis patients were given malaria in the belief that the resultant fever would kill the spirochetes that cause syphilis.

Another example is the so-called Hoxsey treatment for cancer, which was started in the 1920s by an Illinois practitioner named Harry Hoxsey. The treatment is no longer legally available in the United States but is offered through a clinic in Tijuana, Mexico. The treatment consists of several chemical mixtures applied externally and a formula of nine herbs taken internally. The Hoxsey herbal formula is almost identical to a remedy that was listed in the 1926 and 1936 editions of the United States National Formulary called "Compound Fluidextract of Trifolium." It was recommended as a treatment for secondary and tertiary syphilis. One of the external Hoxsey compounds contains both arsenic and antimony, which were used to treat syphilis before the use of antibiotics. The internal formula includes *Phytolacca americana*, or pokeweed, which was used by Native Americans to treat syphilitic chancres; and *Stillingia sylvatica*, or queens-root, which has also been used to treat syphilis. There is no demonstrated data to support the therapy's effectiveness for syphilis.

It should be noted that many alternative medicine therapies that claim to help such infectious diseases as syphilis have little data supporting their effectiveness.

Allopathic treatment

Medications

Syphilis is treated with antibiotics given either intramuscularly (benzathine penicillin G or ceftriaxone) or orally (doxycycline, minocycline, tetracycline, or azithromycin). Neurosyphilis is treated with a combination of aqueous crystalline penicillin G, benzathine penicillin G, or doxycycline. It is important to keep the levels of penicillin in the patient's tissues at sufficiently high levels over a period of days or weeks because the spirochetes have a relatively long reproduction time. Penicillin is more effective in treating the early stages of syphilis than the later stages.

In the fall of 2000, the CDC convened a group of medical advisors to discuss backup medications for treating syphilis. Although none of the newer drugs will displace penicillin as the primary drug, the doctors recommended azithromycin and ceftriaxone as medications that should have a larger role in the treatment of syphilis than they presently do.

Doctors do not usually prescribe separate medications for the skin rashes or ulcers of secondary syphilis.

The patient is advised to keep them clean and dry, and to avoid exposing others to fluid or discharges from condylomata lata.

Pregnant women should be treated as early in pregnancy as possible. Infected fetuses can be cured if the mother is treated during the second and third trimesters of pregnancy. Infants with proven or suspected congenital syphilis are treated with either aqueous crystalline penicillin G or aqueous procaine penicillin G. Children who acquire syphilis after birth are treated with benzathine penicillin G.

Jarisch-Herxheimer reaction

The Jarisch-Herxheimer reaction, first described in 1895, is a reaction to penicillin treatment that may occur during the late primary, secondary, or early latent stages. The patient develops chills, fever, **headache**, and muscle pains within two to six hours after the penicillin is injected. The chancre or rash gets temporarily worse. The Jarisch-Herxheimer reaction, which lasts about a day, is thought to be an allergic reaction to toxins released when the penicillin kills massive numbers of spirochetes.

Expected results

The expected results of alternative therapies used as adjuncts to conventional antibiotic treatment, for stress reduction or similar purposes, would include improvements in the patient's emotional and spiritual quality of life. The effectiveness of homeopathic treatment for syphilis has not been evaluated in clinical trials, although there are anecdotal reports of successful treatment of syphilis by homeopathic methods.

Analysis of the Hoxsey formulae, however, indicate that they should not be used to treat syphilis or other venereal diseases. Two ingredients in the internal formula have toxic effects: queensroot contains an irritant that can cause inflammation or swelling of the skin and mucous membranes, while pokeweed can cause potentially fatal respiratory paralysis. In addition, the arsenic and antimony in the external formula could potentially cause heavy metal toxicity.

Prevention

Immunity

Patients with syphilis do not acquire lasting immunity against the disease. As of 2002, no effective vaccine for syphilis has been developed even though the genome of *T. pallidum* was completely sequenced in 1998. The sequencing may, however, speed up the process of developing an effective vaccine. Prevention depends on a combination of personal and public health measures.

Lifestyle choices

The only reliable methods for preventing transmission of syphilis are sexual abstinence or monogamous relationships between uninfected partners. Condoms offer some protection but protect only the covered parts of the body.

Public health measures

CONTACT TRACING. United States law requires reporting of syphilis cases to public health agencies. Sexual contacts of patients diagnosed with syphilis are traced and tested for the disease. Tracing includes all contacts for the past three months in cases of primary syphilis and for the past year in cases of secondary disease. Neither the patients nor their contacts should have sex with anyone until they have been tested and treated.

Because of the rising incidence of syphilis abroad, a growing number of public health physicians are recommending routine screening of immigrants, refugees, and international adoptees for syphilis as of late 2002.

All patients who test positive for syphilis should be tested for HIV infection at the time of diagnosis.

PRENATAL TESTING OF PREGNANT WOMEN. Pregnant women should be tested for syphilis at the time of their first visit for prenatal care, and again shortly before delivery. Proper treatment of secondary syphilis in the mother reduces the risk of congenital syphilis in the infant from 90% to less than 2%.

As of late 2002, many obstetricians and gynecologists are recommending routine screening of nonpregnant as well as pregnant women for syphilis. At present, only about half of obstetricians and gynecologists in the United States screen nonpregnant women for **chlamydia** and gonorrhea, while fewer than a third screen them for syphilis.

EDUCATION AND INFORMATION. Patients diagnosed with syphilis should be given information about the disease and counseling regarding sexual behavior and the importance of completing antibiotic treatment. It is also important to inform the general public about the transmission and early symptoms of syphilis, and provide adequate health facilities for testing and treatment.

Resources

BOOKS

Burton Goldberg Group. *Alternative Medicine: The Definitive Guide.* Fife, WA: Future Medicine Publishing, Inc., 1995.

Fiumara, Nicholas J. "Syphilis." In *Conn's Current Therapy,* edited by Robert E. Rakel. Philadelphia: W.B. Saunders Company, 1998.

Jacobs, Richard A. "Infectious Diseases: Spirochetal." In *Current Medical Diagnosis & Treatment 1998,* edited by

KEY TERMS

Chancre—The initial skin ulcer of primary syphilis, consisting of an open sore with a firm or hard base.

Condylomata lata—Highly infectious patches of weepy pink or gray skin that appear in the moist areas of the body during secondary syphilis.

Darkfield—A technique of microscopic examination in which light is directed at an oblique angle through the slide so that organisms look bright against a dark background.

General paresis—A form of neurosyphilis in which the patient's personality, as well as his or her control of movement, is affected. The patient may develop convulsions or partial paralysis.

Gumma—A symptom that is sometimes seen in tertiary syphilis, characterized by a rubbery swelling or tumor that heals slowly and leaves a scar.

Index case—The first case of a contagious disease in a group or population that serves to call attention to the presence of the disease.

Jarisch-Herxheimer reaction—A temporary reaction to penicillin treatment for syphilis that includes fever, chills, and worsening of the skin rash or chancre.

Lues maligna—A skin disorder of secondary syphilis in which areas of ulcerated and dying tissue are formed. It occurs most frequently in HIV-positive patients.

Miasm—In homeopathy, an inherited weakness or predisposition to disease. One of the most powerful miasms is the so-called syphilitic miasm.

Nosode—A homeopathic remedy made from microbes, pus, or other diseased matter. The nosode called *Syphilinum* is made from a diluted solution of killed spirochetes.

Spirochete—A type of bacterium with a long, slender, coiled shape. Syphilis is caused by a spirochete.

Tabes dorsalis—A progressive deterioration of the spinal cord and spinal nerves associated with tertiary syphilis.

Lawrence M. Tierney Jr. et al. Stamford, CT: Appleton & Lange, 1998.

Ramin, Susan M., et al. "Sexually Transmitted Diseases and Pelvic Infections." In *Current Obstetric & Gynecologic Diagnosis & Treatment,* edited by Alan H. DeCherney and Martin L. Pernoll. Norwalk, CT: Appleton & Lange, 1994.

Sigel, Eric J. "Sexually Transmitted Diseases." In *Current Pediatric Diagnosis & Treatment,* edited by William W. Hay Jr., et al. Stamford, CT: Appleton & Lange, 1997.

"Syphilis." Section 13, Chapter 164 in *The Merck Manual of Diagnosis and Therapy,* edited by Mark H. Beers, MD, and Robert Berkow, MD. Whitehouse Station, NJ: Merck Research Laboratories, 1999.

Wolf, Judith E. "Syphilis." In *Current Diagnosis 9,* edited by Rex B. Conn, et al. Philadelphia: W.B. Saunders Company, 1997.

PERIODICALS

Augenbraun, M. H. "Treatment of Syphilis 2001: Nonpregnant Adults." *Clinical Infectious Diseases* 35 (October 15, 2002) (Suppl. 2): S187–S190.

Campos-Outcalt, D., and S. Hurwitz." Female-to-Female Transmission of Syphilis: A Case Report." *Sexually Transmitted Diseases* 29 (February 2002): 119–120.

Centers for Disease Control. "Primary and Secondary Syphilis—United States, 2000-2001." *Morbidity and Mortality Weekly Report* 51 (November 1, 2002): 971–973.

Dennis, L. K., and D. V. Dawson. "Meta-Analysis of Measures of Sexual Activity and Prostate Cancer." *Epidemiology* 13 (January 2002): 72–79.

Gibbs, R. S. "The Origins of Stillbirth: Infectious Diseases." *Seminars in Perinatology* 26 (February 2002): 75–78.

Grgic-Vitek, M., I Klavs, M. Potocnik, and M. Rogl-Butina. "Syphilis Epidemic in Slovenia Influenced by Syphilis Epidemic in the Russian Federation and Other Newly Independent States." *International Journal of STD and AIDS* 13 (December 2002) (Suppl. 2): 2–4.

Hagedorn, H. J., A. Kraminer-Hagedorn, K. de Bosschere, et al. "Evaluation of INNO-LIA Syphilis Assay as a Confirmatory Test for Syphilis." *Journal of Clinical Microbiology* 40 (March 2002): 973–978.

Hogben, M., J. S. Lawrence, D. Kasprzyk, et al. "Sexually Transmitted Disease Screening by United States Obstetricians and Gynecologists." *Obstetrics and Gynecology* 100 (October 2002): 801–807.

Kolivras, A., J. de Maubeuge, M. Song, et al. "A Case of Early Congenital Syphilis." *Dermatology* 204 (2002): 338–340.

Pao, D., B. T. Goh, and J. S. Bingham. "Management Issues in Syphilis." *Drugs* 62 (2002): 1447–1461.

Ross, M. W., L. Y. Hwang, C. Zack, et al. "Sexual Risk Behaviours and STIs in Drug Abuse Treatment Populations Whose Drug of Choice is Crack Cocaine." *International Journal of STD and AIDS* 13 (November 2002): 769–774.

Stauffer, W. M., D. Kamat, and P. F. Walker. "Screening of International Immigrants, Refugees, and Adoptees." *Primary Care* 29 (December 2002): 879–905.

Sutmoller, F., T. L. Penna, C. T. de Souza, et al. "Human Immunodeficiency Virus Incidence and Risk Behavior in the 'Projeto Rio': Results of the First 5 Years of the Rio de Janeiro Open Cohort of Homosexual and Bisexual Men, 1994–98." *International Journal of Infectious Diseases* 6 (December 2002): 259–265.

Whittington, W. L., T. Collis, C. Dithmer-Schreck, et al. "Sexually Transmitted Diseases and Human Immunodeficiency Virus-Discordant Partnerships Among Men Who Have Sex With Men." *Clinical Infectious Diseases* 35 (October 15, 2002): 1010–1017.

ORGANIZATIONS

Centers for Disease Control and Prevention. 1600 Clifton Road NE, Atlanta, GA, 30333. (404) 639-3534.

Rebecca J. Frey, PhD

Systemic lupus erythematosus

Definition

Systemic lupus erythematosus (also called lupus or SLE) is a disease in which a person's immune system attacks and injures the body's own organs and tissues. Almost every system of the body can be affected.

Description

The body's immune system is a network of cells and tissues responsible for clearing the body of invading organisms, like bacteria, viruses, and fungi. Antibodies are special immune cells that recognize these invaders, and begin a chain of events to destroy them. In an autoimmune disorder like SLE, a person's antibodies begin to identify the body's own tissues as foreign. Cells and chemicals of the immune system damage the tissues of the body. The reaction that occurs in tissue is called inflammation. Inflammation includes swelling, redness, increased blood flow, and tissue destruction.

In SLE, some of the common antibodies that normally fight diseases are thought to be out of control. These include antinuclear antibodies, which are directed against the cell structure that contains genetic material (the nucleus), and anti-DNA antibodies, which are directed against genetic material (DNA).

SLE can occur in both males and females of all ages, but 90% of patients are women. The majority of these women are in their childbearing years. African Americans are more likely than Caucasians to develop SLE.

Occasionally, such medications as hydralazine and procainamide can cause symptoms very similar to SLE. This condition is called drug-induced lupus. Drug-induced lupus usually disappears after the patient stops taking the particular medication.

Causes & symptoms

The cause of SLE is unknown. Because the vast majority of patients are women, some research is being done to determine what (if any) link the disease has to female hormones. Susceptibility to SLE is known to have a genetic basis, although more than one gene is believed to be involved in disease development. As of 2002, notable progress has been made in narrowing the location of these genes. Because SLE patients may suddenly have worse symptoms (called a flare) after exposure to sunlight, such foods as **alfalfa** sprouts, and certain medications, environmental factors may also be at work.

The severity of symptoms varies over time, with periods of mild or no symptoms followed by a flare. During a flare, symptoms increase in severity and new organ systems may become affected.

Many SLE patients have fevers, **fatigue**, muscle **pain**, weakness, decreased appetite, and weight loss. The spleen and lymph nodes are often swollen and enlarged. Recurrent **infections**, particularly those caused by bacteria, are common in patients with SLE. The development of other symptoms in SLE varies depending on the organs affected.

• Joints. Joint pain and problems, including arthritis, are very common. About 90% of all SLE patients have these types of problems.

• Skin. A number of skin rashes may occur, including a red butterfly-shaped rash that spreads across the face. The "wings" of the butterfly appear across the cheekbones, and the "body" appears across the bridge of the nose. A discoid, or coin-shaped, rash causes red scaly bumps on the cheeks, nose, scalp, ears, chest, back, and the tops of the arms and legs. The roof of the mouth may develop sore, irritated pits (ulcers). **Hair loss** is common. SLE patients tend to be very easily sunburned (photosensitive).

• Lungs. Inflammation of the tissues that cover the lungs and line the chest cavity causes pleuritis, with fluid accumulating in the lungs. The patient frequently experiences coughing and shortness of breath.

• Heart and circulatory system. Inflammation of the tissue surrounding the heart causes pericarditis; inflammation of the heart itself causes myocarditis. These heart problems may result in abnormal heartbeat (arrhythmias), difficulty pumping the blood strongly enough (heart

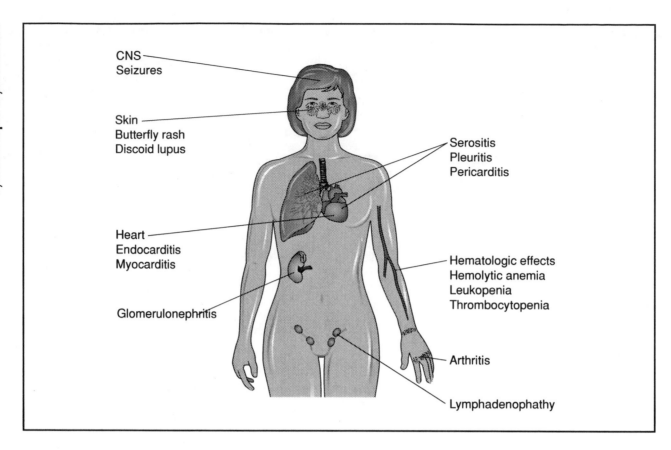

CNS
Seizures

Skin
Butterfly rash
Discoid lupus

Serositis
Pleuritis
Pericarditis

Heart
Endocarditis
Myocarditis

Hematologic effects
Hemolytic anemia
Leukopenia
Thrombocytopenia

Glomerulonephritis

Arthritis

Lymphadenophathy

Systemic lupus erythematosus (SLE) is an autoimmune disease in which the individual's immune system attacks, injures, and destroys the body's own organs and tissues. Nearly every system of the body can be affected by SLE, as depicted in the illustration above. *(Illustration by Electronic Illustrators Group. The Gale Group.)*

failure), or even sudden death. **Blood clots** often form in the blood vessels and may lead to complications.

• Nervous system. Headaches, seizures, changes in personality, and confused thinking (psychosis) may occur. The molecular mechanism responsible for brain dysfunction in lupus was identified in 2001.

• Kidneys. The kidneys may suffer significant destruction, with serious life-threatening effects. They may become unable to adequately filter the blood, leading to kidney failure.

• Gastrointestinal system. Patients may experience **nausea, vomiting, diarrhea,** and abdominal pain. The lining of the abdomen may become inflamed (peritonitis).

• Eyes. The eyes may become red, sore, and dry. Inflammation of one of the nerves responsible for vision may cause vision problems, and blindness can result from inflammation of the blood vessels (vasculitis) that serve the retina.

Diagnosis

Diagnosis of SLE can be somewhat difficult. There are no definitive tests for diagnosing SLE. Many of the

symptoms and laboratory test results of SLE patients are similar to those of patients with other diseases, including **rheumatoid arthritis, multiple sclerosis,** and various nervous system and blood disorders.

Laboratory tests that are helpful in diagnosing SLE include several tests for a variety of antibodies commonly elevated in SLE patients (including antinuclear antibodies, anti-DNA antibodies, etc.). A blood test called the lupus erythematosus cell preparation (or LE prep) test is also performed. The LE prep is positive in 70–80% of all patients with SLE. SLE patients tend to have low numbers of red blood cells (**anemia**) and low numbers of certain types of white blood cells. The erythrocyte sedimentation rate (ESR), a measure of inflammation in the body, tends to be quite elevated. Samples of tissue (biopsies) from affected skin and kidneys show characteristics of the disease.

The American Rheumatism Association developed a list of symptoms used to diagnose SLE. Research supports the idea that people who have at least four of the 11 criteria (not necessarily simultaneously) are extremely likely to have SLE. The criteria are:

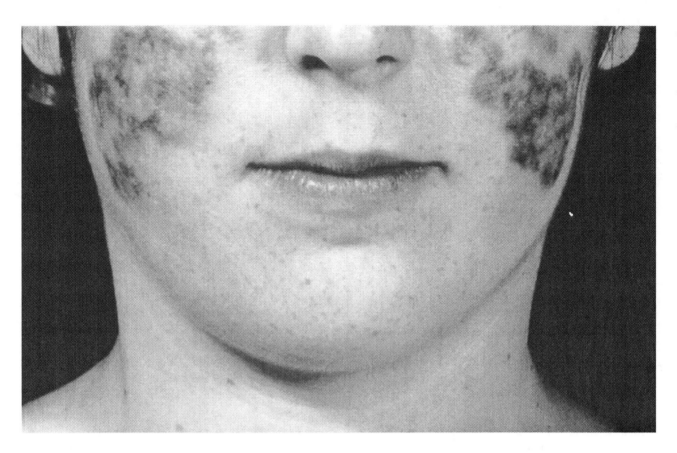

Lupus can cause skin rashes on any part of the body. One that often occurs on the face is called the butterfly rash. *(NMSB/Custom Medical Stock Photo. Reproduced by permission.)*

- butterfly rash

- discoid rash

- photosensitivity

- mouth ulcers

- arthritis

- inflammation of the lining of the lungs or the lining around the heart

- kidney damage, as noted by the presence of protein or other abnormal substances called casts in the urine

- seizures or psychosis

- the presence of certain types of anemia and low counts of particular white blood cells

- the presence of certain immune cells, anti-DNA antibodies, or a falsely positive test for syphilis

- the presence of antinuclear antibodies

Treatment

Although there is no cure for SLE, a number of alternative treatments may help reduce symptoms.

- Acupuncture can relieve pain in joints and muscles.

- Chinese herbals are chosen based on treatment principles and the patients specific symptoms. A simple decoction for the treatment of SLE joint and kidney problems is Lei Gong Teng (*Caulis tripterygii*), Ji Xue Teng (*Caulis spatholobi*), and Gan Cao (*Radix glycyrrhizae*). Chinese patent medicines for SLE include Qin Jiao Wan (**Gentiana** Macrophylla Pill) and Kun Ming Shan Hai Tang Pian (Tripterygii Tablet).

- DHEA (dehydroepiandrosterone) treatment, in a small study, led to disease improvement and reduction in the use of corticosteroids.

- Diet. The SLE patient should drink plenty of water and eat a well balanced diet of whole, unprocessed foods that are low in fat and high in fiber. Mackerel, sardines, and salmon contain the beneficial fatty acid omega-3. **Caffeine**, sugar, alcohol, red meats, and alfalfa sprouts should be avoided. Because food **allergies** can be associated with SLE, an elimination/change in diet can help identify the offending foods (often wheat, dairy products, and/or soy).

- Enzyme therapy treats SLE with 10X U.S.P. of **digestive enzymes**, protease, lipase, amylase, and cellulase to improve digestion of foods, based on the theory that a leaky gut causes SLE.

- Exercise can reduce fatigue, reduce muscle weakness, speed weight loss, and increase energy, stamina, and confidence.

- Herbals remedies include capsaicin (*Capsicum* species) cream, **pau d'arco** (*Tabebuia* species), pine (*Pinus* species) extract, **wheat grass** (*Triticum aestivum*), *Bupleurum falcatum*, **licorice** (*Glycyrrhiza glabra*), wild **Mexican yam** (*Dioscorea villosa*), stinging **nettle** (*Urtica dioica*), **flaxseed** (*Linus usitatissimum*) oil, **turmeric** (*Curcuma* species), and borage (*Borago officinalis*) oil.

- Massage can relieve pain and reduce **stress**.

- Probiotic treatment using *Lactobacillus* species to restore a healthy balance of bacteria in the intestines.

- Stress management techniques, such as **guided imagery**, **meditation**, **hypnotherapy**, and **yoga**, can reduce stress that exacerbates SLE.

- Supplements commonly recommended for SLE patients include vitamins B, C, and E, beta-carotene, **bioflavonoids**, **selenium**, **zinc**, **magnesium**, a complete trace mineral supplement, **glutamine**, gamma-oryzanol, 1-butyrate, fructooligosaccharides (FOS), and **omega-3 fatty acids** (**fish oil**). **Vitamin A** is believed to help improve discoid skin rashes.

- Support groups for SLE patients can provide emotional and social help.

Allopathic treatment

Treatment depends on the organ systems affected and the severity of the disease. Patients with a mild form of SLE can be treated with nonsteroidal anti-inflammatory drugs, or NSAIDs, like ibuprofen (Motrin, Advil) and aspirin. More severely ill patients with potentially life-threatening complications (including kidney disease, pericarditis, or nervous system complications) will require treatment with more potent drugs, including steroid medications and possibly other drugs that decrease the activity of the immune system (immunosuppressant drugs).

Kidney failure may require the blood to be filtered by a machine (dialysis) or even a kidney transplantation.

Expected results

The prognosis for patients with SLE varies, depending on the organ systems most affected and the severity of inflammation. Some patients have long periods of remission with mild or no symptoms. About 90–95% of patients are still living after two years with the disease, 82–90% after five years, 71–80% after 10 years, and 63–75% after 20 years. The most likely causes of death during the first 10 years include infections and kidney failure. During years 11–20 of the disease, the development of abnormal blood clots is the most common cause of death.

For pregnant SLE patients, about 30% of the pregnancies end in miscarriage and about 25% of all babies are born prematurely. Most babies born to mothers with SLE are normal. Rarely, babies develop a condition called neonatal lupus, which is characterized by a skin rash, liver or blood problems, and a serious heart condition.

Prevention

There are no known ways to avoid developing SLE. However, it is possible for a patient who has been diagnosed with SLE to prevent flares of the disease. Recommendations to prevent flares include decreasing sun exposure, getting sufficient sleep, eating a healthy diet, decreasing stress, and exercising regularly.

Resources

BOOKS

Aaseng, Nathan. *Autoimmune Diseases*. New York: F. Watts, 1995.

Hahn, Bevra Hannahs. "Systemic Lupus Erythematosus." In *Harrison's Principles of Internal Medicine*. 15th ed., edited by Anthony S. Fauci, et al. New York: McGraw-Hill, 2001.

Long, James W. *The Essential Guide to Chronic Illness*. New York: HarperPerennial, 1997.

Ravel, Richard. "Systemic Lupus Erythematosus (SLE)." In *Clinical Laboratory Medicine: Clinical Application of Laboratory Data*. St. Louis: Mosby, 1995.

Wallace, Daniel J. *The Lupus Book*. New York: Oxford University Press, 1995.

Ying, Zhou Zhong, and Jin Hui De. "Lupus Erythematosus." In *Clinical Manual of Chinese Herbal Medicine and Acupuncture*. New York: Churchill Livingston, 1997.

PERIODICALS

Graham, R. R., W. A. Ortmann, P. M. Gaffney, et al. "Localization of the Human SLE Susceptibility Genes Within the HLA Using a Recombinant Ancestral Haplotype Approach. *American Journal of Human Genetics* 69 (October 2001): 507.

"Lupus Brain Damage Pathway Identified Through Molecular Mechanism." *Immunotherapy Weekly* (December 12, 2001): 7.

Mann, Judy. "The Harsh Realities of Lupus." *The Washington Post* 120 (October 8, 1997): C12.

Noel, V., O. Lortholary, P. Casassus, et al. "Risk Factors and Prognostic Influence of Infection in a Single Cohort of 87

KEY TERMS

. . . .

Autoimmune disorder—A disorder in which the body's antibodies mistake the body's own tissues for foreign invaders. The immune system then attacks and causes damage to these tissues.

Immune system—The system of specialized organs, lymph nodes, and blood cells throughout the body that work together to prevent foreign organisms (bacteria, viruses, fungi, etc.) from invading the body.

Psychosis—Extremely disordered thinking with a poor sense of reality; may include hallucinations (seeing, hearing, or smelling things that are not really there).

Adults with Systemic Lupus Erythematosus." *Annals of the Rheumatic Diseases* 60 (December 2001): 1141–1144.

Umansky, Diane. "Living with Lupus." *American Health for Women* 16 (June 1997): 92+.

Yap, Hui-Kim, Siau-Gek Ang, Yee-Hing Lai, Vinod Ramgolam, and Stanley C. Jordan. "Improvement in Lupus Nephritis Following Treatment with a Chinese Herbal Preparation." *Archives of Pediatric and Adolescent Medicine* 153 (August 1999): 850–852.

ORGANIZATIONS

American College of Rheumatology. 1800 Century Place, Suite 250, Atlanta, GA 30345. (404) 633-3777. acr@rheumatology.org. <http://www.rheumatology.org>.

Lupus Foundation of America, Inc. 1300 Piccard Dr., Suite 200, Rockville, MD 20850. (800) 558-0121. <http://www.lupus.org>.

OTHER

Balch, T. Stephen. "Living Well with Lupus." January 1, 2001 [cited October 2002]. <http://www.hamline.edu/~lupus/articles/living_well_with_lupus.html>.

Hoffman, David L. "The Use of Herbs in the Treatment of Systemic Lupus Erythematosus." *HealthWorld Online.* [cited October 2002]. <http://www.healthy.net>.

Belinda Rowland
Rebecca J. Frey, PhD

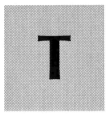

T

Taheebo *see* **Pau d'arco**

T'ai chi

Definition

T'ai chi is an ancient Chinese exercise with movements that originate in **martial arts** practice. While used as a type of self-defense in its most advanced form, t'ai chi is practiced widely for its health and **relaxation** benefits. Those in search of well being and a way to combat **stress** have made what has also been called "Chinese shadow boxing" one of the most popular low-intensity workouts around the world.

Origins

Also known as t'ai chi ch'uan (pronounced *tie-jee chu-wan*), the name comes from Chinese characters that translated mean "supreme ultimate force." The concept of t'ai chi, or the "supreme ultimate," is based on the Taoist philosophy of yin and yang, or the attraction of opposites. Yin and yang combine opposing but complementary forces to create harmony in nature. By using t'ai chi, a person can bring this principle of harmony into their own life. A disturbance in the flow of ch'i (qi), or the life force, is what **traditional Chinese medicine** regards as the cause of all diseases in the body. By enhancing the flow of ch'i, practitioners of t'ai chi believe that the exercise can promote physical health. Students of t'ai chi also learn how to use the exercise in the form of **meditation** and mental exercise by understanding how to center and focus their cerebral powers.

In the traditional Chinese understanding of health and well-being, t'ai chi is not regarded as a self-sufficient compartment of a person's life, as physical exercise often is viewed by Westerners. Instead, t'ai chi is considered part of an overall way of healthful living that includes massage, proper diet, **meditation,** and herbal medicines as needed.

The origins of t'ai chi are rooted deep in the martial arts and Chinese folklore, causing its exact beginnings to be based on speculation. The much-disputed founder of t'ai chi is Zhang San-feng (Chang San-feng), a Daoist (Taoist) monk of the Wu Tang Monastery, who, according to records from the Ming-shih (the official records of the Ming dynasty), lived sometime during the period from 1391–1459. Legend states that Zhang happened upon a fight between a snake and a crane, and, impressed with how the snake became victorious over the bird through relaxed, evasive movements and quick counterstrikes, he created a fighting form that copied the snake's strongest attributes. With his experience in the martial arts, Zhang combined strength, balance, flexibility, and speed to bring about the earliest form of t'ai chi.

Historians also link Zhang to joining yin-yang from Taoism and "internal" aspects together into his exercises. This feeling of inner happiness, or as a renowned engineering physicist and t'ai chi master, Dr. Martin Lee, states in his book *The Healing Art of t'ai Chi*, of becoming one with nature," remains a primary goal for those who practice t'ai chi. Although its ancient beginnings started as a martial art, t'ai chi was modified in the 1930s to the relaxing low-intensity exercise that continues to have the potential to be transformed into a form of self-defense, similar to karate or kung-fu.

Benefits

The art of t'ai chi is many things to the many who practice it. To some, it is a stretching exercise that incorporates a deep-breathing program. To others, it is a martial art—and beyond this, it is often used as a dance or to accompany prayer. While the ways in which it is used may vary, one of the main benefits for those who practice it remains universal—t'ai chi promotes good health. This sense of well-being complements t'ai chi's additional benefits of improved coordination, balance, and body awareness, while it also calms the mind and reduces stress. Those in search of harmony between the mind and the body practice "dynamic relaxation."

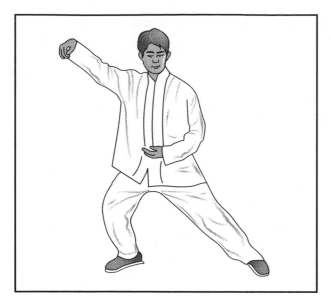

T'ai chi is a Chinese exercise system that uses slow, smooth body movements to achieve a state of relaxation . The posture above is part of the single whip sequence of t'ai chi motions. (Illustration by Electronic Illustrators Group.) *The Gale Group.*

Dr. Martin Lee believes that the ancient art also holds healing powers. In his book, *The Healing Art of T'ai Chi,* he states: "By practicing t'ai chi and understanding chi and its breathing techniques, I was able to heal my **allergies** and other ailments." Lee contends that stress is the culprit of much of the **pain** and suffering that are a part of everyday life. The growing evidence that stress contributes to devastating physical and mental ailments has led Lee to teach a systematic, effective, and manageable way to restore both body and mind to a natural stress-free state. As of 1996, Lee had been teaching t'ai chi for 20 years to help his students with physical ailments that have been caused by stress. He believes that illness can be overcome through understanding the body as a mental and physical system, which is accomplished through t'ai chi.

While the martial arts offer very vigorous physical workouts and often result in injuries, the practice of t'ai chi is a good alternative to these sports without overstraining the body. Those with bad backs have also found t'ai chi to ease their discomfort.

Description

Zhang, the notable originator of t'ai chi, created a combination of movements and beliefs that led to the formation of the fundamental "Thirteen Postures" of his art. Over time, these primary actions have transformed into soft, slow, relaxed movements, leading to a series of movements known as the form. Several techniques linked together create a form. Proper posture is a key el-

ement when practicing t'ai chi to maintain balance. All of the movements used throughout the exercise are relaxed with the back straight and the head up.

Just as the movements of t'ai chi have evolved, so have the various styles or schools of the art. As the form has grown and developed, the difference in style along with the different emphasis from a variety of teachers has as well. A majority of the different schools or styles of t'ai chi have been given their founder's surname.

The principal schools of t'ai chi include:

- Chen style
- Hao (or Wu Shi) style
- Hu Lei style
- Sun style
- Wu style
- Yang style
- Zhao Bao style.

Many of the most commonly used groupings of forms are based on the Yang style of t'ai chi developed by Yang Pan-Hou (1837–1892). Each of the forms has a name, such as "Carry the Tiger to the Mountain," and as the progression is made throughout the many forms, the participant ends the exercise almost standing on one leg. While most forms, like "Wind Blows Lotus Leaves," has just one movement or part, others, like "Work the Shuttle in the Clouds," have as many as four. While the form is typically practiced individually, the movement called "Pushing Hands" is a sequence practiced by two people together.

Preparations

Masters of t'ai chi recommend that those who practice the art begin each session by doing a warm-up of gentle rotation exercises for the joints and gentle stretching exercises for the muscles and tendons. Some other suggestions to follow before beginning the exercise include: gaining a sense of body orientation; relaxation of every part of the body; maintaining smooth and regular breathing; gaining attention or feeling; being mindful of each movement; maintaining proper posture; and moving at the same pace throughout each movement. The main requirement for a successful form of t'ai chi is to feel completely comfortable while performing all of the movements.

Precautions

Although t'ai chi is not physically demanding, it requires close attention to one's posture. Those who want to practice the exercise should notify their physician before beginning. The physician will know whether the person is taking medications that might interfere with balance, or has a condition that could make a series of t'ai chi movements unwise to attempt.

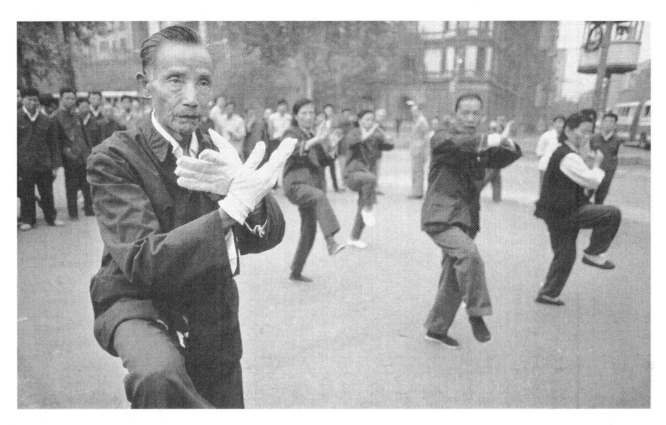

Group of people practicing t'ai chi in the streets of Shanghai, China. *(Kelly-Mooney Photography. Corbis Images. Reproduced by permission.)*

Research & general acceptance

While the reasons why t'ai chi is practiced vary, research has uncovered several reasons why it may help many medical conditions. For example, people with **rheumatoid arthritis** (RA) are encouraged to practice t'ai chi for its graceful slow sweeping movements. Its ability to combine stretching and range-of-motion exercises with relaxation techniques work well to relieve the stiffness and weakness in the joints of RA patients. An ongoing research program at Stanford University in California is evaluating the beneficial effects of t'ai chi on patients with **fibromyalgia**. A study of fibromyalgia patients in Georgia reported in 2003 that t'ai chi brought about significant improvement in the patients' control of their symptoms.

T'ai chi has also been shown to benefit patients with **osteoarthritis** (OA). A group of Korean researchers found that women diagnosed with OA showed significant improvement in their balance and abdominal muscle strength after a 12-week program of Sun-style t'ai chi.

In 1999, investigators from Johns Hopkins University in Baltimore, Maryland, studied the effects of t'ai chi on patients with elevated blood pressure. Sixty-two sedentary adults with high-normal blood pressure or stage I **hypertension** who were aged 60 or older began a 12-week aerobic program or a light-intensity t'ai chi program. The exercise sessions both consisted of 30-minute sessions, four days a week. The study revealed that while the aerobics did lower the systolic blood pressure of participants, the t'ai chi group systolic level was also lowered by an average of seven points—only a point less than the aerobics group. Interestingly, t'ai chi hardly raises the heart rate while still having the same effects as an intense aerobics class.

In addition to lowering blood pressure, research suggests that t'ai chi improves heart and lung function. The exercise is linked to reducing the body's level of a stress hormone called cortisol, and to the overall effect of higher confidence for those who practice it. As a complementary therapy, t'ai chi is also found to enhance the mainstream medical care of **cancer** patients who use the exercise to help control their symptoms and improve their quality of life.

Physical therapists investigated the effects of t'ai chi among 20 patients during their recovery from coronary artery bypass surgery. The patients were placed into either the t'ai chi group or an unsupervised control group. The t'ai chi group performed classical Yang exercises each morning for one year, while the control group walked three times a week for 50 minutes each session. In 1999, the study reported that after one year of training, the t'ai chi group showed significant improvement in their cardiorespiratory function and their work rate,

LAO TZU

Lao Tzu (sixth century B.C.) is believed to have been a Chinese philosopher and the reputed author of the *Tao te ching*, the principal text of Taoist thought. He is considered the father of Chinese Taoism.

The main source of information on Lao Tzu's life is a biography written by the historian Ssu-ma Ch'ien (145-86 B.C.) in his *Records of the Historian*. Actually, Lao Tzu is not really a person's name and is only an honorific designation meaning "old man." It was common in this period to refer to respected philosophers and teachers with words meaning "old" or "mature." It is possible that a man who assumed the pseudonym Lao Tzu was a historical person, but the term Lao Tzu is also applied as an alternate title to the supreme Taoist classic, *Tao te ching* (Classic of the Way and the Power).

An important quality of the tao is its "weakness," or "submissiveness." Because the tao itself is basically weak and submissive, it is best for a person to put himself in harmony with the tao. Thus, the *Tao te ching* places strong emphasis on nonaction (*wu wei*), which means the absence of aggressive action. One does not strive for wealth or prestige, and violence is to be avoided. This quietist approach to life was extremely influential in later periods and led to the development of a particular Taoist regimen that involved special breathing exercises and special eating habits that were designed to maintain quietude and harmony with the tao.

but the unsupervised control group displayed only a slight decrease in both areas.

T'ai chi has also shown to keep people from falling— something that happens to one in three people over age 65 each year. Researchers from Emory University in Atlanta, Georgia, had dozens of men and women in their 70s and older learn the graceful movements of t'ai chi. The study discovered that those who learned to perform t'ai chi were almost 50% less likely to suffer falls within a given time frame than subjects who simply received feedback from a computer screen on how much they swayed as they stood. Those who suffer falls experience greater declines in everyday activities than those who do not fall, and are also at a greater risk of requiring placement in a nursing home or other type of assisted living. Researchers recommend the use of t'ai chi for its ability to help people raise their consciousness of how their bodies are moving in the environment around them. By raising awareness of how the body moves, people can focus on their relationship to their physical environment and situations they encounter everyday.

In addition to studying the cardiovascular and range-of-motion benefits of t'ai chi, researchers are also investigating its positive effects on the immune system. A team of scientists in California reported in 2003 that t'ai chi boosts the resistance of older people to the **shingles** virus— a virus that is both more common and more severe in the elderly.

Some research done in the United States focuses on the emotional and psychological benefits of t'ai chi. One recently discovered advantage of t'ai chi is its ability to hold people's interest longer than many other forms of exercise. One study in Oregon found that only 20% of people enrolled in a six-month t'ai chi program dropped out before the end, compared to an average of 55% for other forms of exercise. With regard to **depression**, a study of college students found that those who were taking t'ai chi classes had a lower rate of depression than students enrolled in other fitness programs.

One interesting recent change in the acceptance of t'ai chi in the United States and Canada is its growing popularity among men. In the 1970s and 1980s, many adult males regarded t'ai chi as a form of exercise that was not challenging enough for "real men." Since the late 1990s, however, more men have begun practicing t'ai chi in order to relieve stress or as a form of cross-training with another sport.

While the additional benefits of t'ai chi remain to be studied in the United States, it continues to be widely practiced in this and other Western countries. The ancient art maintains its prominence in China, where many people incorporate it into their daily routines at sunrise.

Training & certification

Masters of t'ai chi are trained extensively in the various forms of the art by grandmasters who are extremely skillful of the exercise and its origins. For those who wish to learn t'ai chi from a master, classes are taught throughout the world in health clubs, community centers, senior citizen centers, and official t'ai chi schools. Before entering a class, the instructor's credentials should be reviewed, and they should be questioned about the form of t'ai chi they teach. Some of the more rigorous forms of the art may be too intense for older people, or for those who are not confident of their balance. Participants are encouraged to get a physician's approval before beginning any t'ai chi program.

There is no age limitation for those who learn t'ai chi, and there is no special equipment needed for the exercise. Participants are encouraged to wear loose clothing and soft shoes.

Resources

BOOKS

Lee, Martin, Emily Lee, Melinda Lee, and Joyce Lee. *The Healing Art of T'ai Chi.* New York: Sterling Publishing Company, Inc., 1996.

KEY TERMS

Aerobics—Any of various forms of sustained vigorous exercise, such as jogging, calisthenics, or jazz dancing, intended to stimulate and strengthen the heart and respiratory system.

Cortisol—A steroid hormone released by the cortex (outer portion) of the adrenal gland when a person is under stress.

Fibromyalgia—A chronic disease syndrome characterized by fatigue, widespread muscular soreness, and pain at specific points on the body.

Qi—The traditional Chinese term for vital energy or the life force. The word is also spelled "ki" or "chi" in English translations of Japanese and Chinese medical books.

Taoism—A Chinese religion and philosophy based on the doctrines of Laotse, which advocates simplicity and selflessness.

Pelletier, Kenneth R., MD. *The Best Alternative Medicine,* Part I: Sound Mind, Sound Body. New York: Simon & Schuster, 2002.

Reid, Daniel. *Chinese Herbal Medicine.* Boston, MA: Shambhala, 1996.

PERIODICALS

Christou, E. A., Y. Yang, and K. S. Rosengren. "Taiji Training Improves Knee Extensor Strength and Force Control in Older Adults." *Journals of Gerontology, Series A: Biological Sciences and Medical Sciences* 58 (August 2003): 763–766.

Cooper, Bob. "An Exercise in Vitality: Put Away Your Prejudices—T'ai Chi Ain't Just for Senior Citizens and Vegans." *Men's Fitness* 18 (September 2002): 86-91.

Filusch-Betts, Elaine. "The Effect of T'ai Chi on Cardiorespiratory Function in Patients with Coronary Artery Bypass Surgery." *Physical Therapy* (September 1999).

Irwin, M. R., J. L. Pike, J. C. Cole, and M. N. Oxman. "Effects of a Behavioral Intervention, T'ai Chi Chih, on Varicella-Zoster Virus Specific Immunity and Health Functioning in Older Adults." *Psychosomatic Medicine* 65 (September-October 2003): 824–830.

Li, F., K. J. Fisher, P. Harmer, and E. McAuley. "Delineating the Impact of T'ai Chi Training on Physical Function Among the Elderly." *American Journal of Preventive Medicine* 23 (August 2002): 92-97.

Song, R., E. O. Lee, P. Lam, and S. C. Bae. "Effects of T'ai Chi Exercise on Pain, Balance, Muscle Strength, and Perceived Difficulties in Physical Functioning in Older Women with Osteoarthritis: A Randomized Clinical Trial." *Journal of Rheumatology* 30 (September 2003): 2039–2044.

Taggart, H. M., C. L. Arslanian, S. Bae, and K. Singh. "Effects of T'ai Chi Exercise on Fibromyalgia Symptoms and Health-Related Quality of Life." *Orthopaedic Nursing* 22 (September-October 2003): 353–360.

ORGANIZATIONS

American Association of Oriental Medicine. 909 22nd St. Sacramento, CA 95816. (916) 451-6950. <www.aaom.org>.

Canadian Taijiquan Federation. P.O. Box 421, Milton, Ontario L9T 4Z1. <www.canadiantaijiquanfederation.ca>.

Patience T'ai Chi Association. 2620 East 18th Street, Brooklyn, NY 11235. (718) 332-3477. <www.patiencetaichi.com>.

OTHER

WebMD. http://WebMD.com.

"Yang Style T'ai Chi Ch'uan." http://www.chebucto.ns.ca/Philosophy/Taichi/styles.html.

Beth Kapes
Rebecca J. Frey, PhD

T'ai chi ch'uan *see* **T'ai chi**

Tang shen *see* **Codonopsis root**

Tangerine peel

Description

This popular widely known fruit goes by a variety of names, creating some possible confusion at times as to which plant one is dealing with. Commonly known as mandarin in much of the world (in Japan it goes by satsuma), the fruit is most often called tangerine in the United States. Generally listed under the botanical name *Citrus reticulata*, it is also known as *C. nobilis, C. madurensis, C. unshiu, C. deliciosa, C. tangerina* or *C. erythrosa*.

A native of Asia, the plant was introduced into Europe early in the nineteenth century. By midcentury, it had spread to the United States, where it was rechristened tangerine. Today, the easily cultivated plant is grown around the Mediterranean, in north Africa, and in both North and South America. Tangerines are generally bigger, rounder, and have more of a yellow-colored skin; mandarins, on the other hand, are smaller, more angular, and deeper orange in color.

The oils produced from the many different cultivars of this plant can vary significantly in chemical composition, reflecting both the particular variety, the country of origin, and the local growing environment.

This small evergreen tree reaches a height of up to about 20 ft (6 m). It has glossy pointed leaves and produces fragrant white flowers. The round fleshy fruit is green when young but ripens to a bright orange or yellow-orange. It was traditionally presented as a gift to the Mandarins of China.

General use

Tangerine peel—called *Chen Pi* or, sometimes, *Ju Hong,* meaning red tangerine peel—has a lengthy history of use in **traditional Chinese medicine**. It is commonly used to treat **indigestion**, **diarrhea**, **vomiting** and other forms of digestive weakness or upset, as well as **hiccups** and certain types of coughs (specifically, wet coughs involving excessive production of phlegm). It is said to settle, regulate, and normalize the flow of qi (in traditional Chinese medicine, the term for life force), and to break up congestion. In addition, it is believed to enhance the flow of liquids through the body.

The peel of young green tangerines is called *Qing Pi* and is used to treat pain—particularly in the side and the breast, as well as **pain** from hernia. In addition, the green peel has been used in the treatment of low blood pressure and (in combination with other herbs) breast inflammation.

C. reticulata is also an ingredient in many traditional Chinese tonics. Among these are the Great Orange Peel Decoction used to treat **gout**, the Two Cure Decoction used to control **morning sickness** in pregnant women, and the Five Seed Decoction used to treat male sexual problems, including low sperm count, **impotence**, and premature ejaculation. A related fertility-and-longevity formula, the Duke of Chou's Centenarian Liquor, is said to have been prescribed for the founder of the Chou Dynasty more than 3,000 years ago. Tangerine peel is also used to make Dr. Huang's Internal Injury Poultice, which is said to promote healing and ease inflammation in connection with pulled muscles, sprains, twisted tendons, and other sports injuries.

The other primary application for *C. reticulata* is in **aromatherapy**, where it is used to treat a wide variety of conditions. Some of these uses parallel those in traditional Chinese medicine: for digestive and intestinal complaints (as well as hiccups), to stimulate the lymph system, to eliminate excess fluid, to boost the flow of urine, and to combat **obesity**. In France and other parts of Europe, it is known particularly as a remedy for children and the elderly—both for digestive problems and to soothe overwrought young minds. One of the gentler citrus oils, tangerine is also used frequently by pregnant women, and is generally said to be a calmative and tranquilizer, helpful in treating nervous tension, emotional **stress**, **depression**, and sleep-related difficulties.

Mirroring its use in cosmetics, the oil is also used to treat various skin conditions (such as healing scars, stretch marks, and even **acne**), and to discourage excessively oily skin.

Tangerine peel is also an ingredient in certain herbal formulas for pets, particularly to treat excess **gas**.

A 2002 study aimed to test the effect of aromatherapy on pain perception. One of the pleasant odors included orange water, while medicinal odors included vinegar and a dental product. The study found that pleasant odors reduced pain perception in women, but not in men. The study suggested that in clinical settings, smells like disinfectants might promote the perception of pain in some patients.

Preparations

In traditional Chinese medicine, the dried peel of the fruit is used, often aged (sometimes until it turns black in color) and sometimes even toasted in a wok. *Chen Pi* means aged peel. A decoction is then made from the peel in combination with other herbs. Both the outermost peel (exocarp) and the inner peel (pericarp) are used for different specific medicinal purposes. *C. reticulata* is also used to make poultices—a paste of finely powdered herbs that is applied externally to help heal internal injuries. Tangerine peel is also available in pill form.

Aromatherapy, on the other hand, relies on the essential oil extracted from the peel. Depending on the precise type of fruit used, the oil can range from yellow-orange to orange in color, and its chemical properties and uses will also vary. Among the primary chemical constituents of the oil are limonene (as much as 90%), geraniol, citral, and citronella. Several of these (most prominently limonene) have been investigated in the laboratory, showing some potential as **cancer** inhibitors. Mandarin oil also contains nitrogen compounds such as methyl methyl-anthranilate, which may not be present in tangerine oil.

All of these oils are cold-pressed. In addition, yet another type of mandarin oil is made from the plant's twigs and leaves, using steam distillation. Mandarin oil is widely used in beverages for its intensely orange flavor, as well as in the production of cosmetics and soaps. It blends readily with other oils. Tangerine oil, on the other hand, is not commonly used in cosmetics.

The oil can be applied in a variety of ways: in therapeutic massage, in healing baths, in compresses, or in unguents (healing salves or ointments). It can also be taken in food or drink, put in a diffuser or inhaler, or used in pillows.

Precautions

Because of the potential confusion over which variety of the plant is called for in a given situation, extra caution is advised to avoid compromising the therapeutic action, introducing unwanted elements, or provoking unintentional interactions. This is particularly true in the context of traditional Chinese medicine in which many different kinds of citrus fruits are used, often for overlapping but not identical purposes. In aromatherapy too, however, care should be taken to determine which oil is required for the desired formula or use.

Side effects

Occasional allergic reactions to tangerine peel have been noted in the form of prolonged **sneezing**, **cough**, chest discomfort, and restlessness.

Interactions

There are no known interactions with prescription drugs as of 2004.

Resources

BOOKS

Lawless, Julia. *The Illustrated Encyclopedia of Essential Oils.* Rockport, Mass.: Element Books, 1995.
Reid, Daniel. *A Handbook of Chinese Healing Herbs.* Boston: Shambhala Publications, 1995.

PERIODICALS

Berger, Joanne M. "Smells Like Relief (Indications)." *Internal Medicine News* (August 1, 2002): 39.

Peter Gregutt
Teresa G. Odle

TB *see* **Tuberculosis**
TCM *see* **Traditional Chinese medicine**

Tea tree oil

Description

Tea tree oil (*Melaleuca alternifolia*) is a multi-purpose herb that traces its roots to the Aboriginal people of Australia. For thousands of years, they used the leaves as an antiseptic and antifungal by crushing the leaves and making a mudpack. However, the plant didn't receive the name "tea tree" until 1770, when the name was given by the British explorer Captain James Cook and his crew. Although Cook's crew first used the leaves for tea, they later mixed them with spruce leaves as a beer. The plant's medicinal properties remained a secret with the Australian aboriginal people until the early 1920s, when a Sydney, Australia chemist, Dr. Arthur Penfold, researched its antiseptic properties. In 1929, along with F.R. Morrison, Penfold published "Australian Tea Trees of Economic Value." This study started a flurry of research into tea tree oil. The Australian government con-

sidered tea tree oil a World War II essential for their armed forces' first aid kits. After the war, increased use of pharmaceutical antibiotics decreased tea tree oil's appeal everywhere except in Australia. Tea tree oil started to regain its popularity in 1960, with a recharge in its research around the world. Today, *Melaleuca alternifolia* is also grown in California.

Properties of tea tree oil

Tea tree oil's properties are contained in the oils of its leaves. The oil is steam-distilled from the leaves and then tested for chemical properties, which can number between 50 and 100. The number of components may explain tea tree oil's many beneficial uses. The main active components are terpinen-4-ol, 1,8-cineole, gamma-terpinene, p-cymene and other turpenes. Its aroma is one of a healthy pleasant disinfectant.

General use

Antibacterial

The most promising new function of tea tree oil is to counter methicillin-resistant *Staphylococcus aureus* (MRSA), also called the hospital super bug. In United States and European hospitals, MRSA grew from under 3% in the 1980s to 40% in the late 1990s. This super bug attacks people who have **wounds**, such as post-operative **infections**, and a depressed immune system. MRSA resists conventional antibiotics, except Vancomycin. A Thursday Plantation *in vitro* study, at East London University, comparing Vancomycin and tea tree oil, shows the latter as a powerful alternative. This study corroborated the University of Western Australia study by Thomas Riley and Christine Carson. Because the spread of MRSA occurs mainly by hands, one London hospital uses tea tree oil soap for staff and patient hygiene.

Research reported on in 2002 reported that tea tree oil performed better than certain antibiotics in fighting MRSA, but the sample size of the study was small. Later studies involving herpes simplex and orthopedic **infections** also showed promising results for tea tree oil, but again failed to show enough statistical significance to prove tea tree oil works better than antibiotics.

Tea tree oil works as an expectorant when inhaled or taken internally and has a soothing effect; therefore, it can be used for throat and chest infections, and clearing up mucus. It is also effective against earaches, cystitis, and gingivitis. Inhaling steaming hot water with 5 drops of tea tree essential oil added can not only soothe coughing and plugged noses, but doing so at the start of the infection might stop it from spreading. Gargling with 6 drops of tea tree oil in a glass of warm water may soothe sore throats.

Antiseptic

Tea tree essential oil is an excellent natural antiseptic for skin infections. The oil immediately penetrates outer skin layers and mixes with body oils to treat such conditions as insect bites, cuts, **burns, acne**, infected wounds, **bruises, boils, scabies**, lice, chillblains, **diaper rash, hives**, poison ivy and **oak, prickly heat**, and **sunburn** .

A study published in the *Medical Journal of Australia* , in 1990 outlined the results of using 5% tea tree oil gel versus 5% benzoyl peroxide lotion for **acne**. The 124 participants showed improvement with both treatments. Benzoyl peroxide worked better with non-inflamed acne while the tea tree gel caused only 44% of side effects such as dryness and red skin compared to benzoyl peroxide's 79%.

The simplest methods to treat acne with tea tree oil are to wash the face with soap containing tea tree essential oil or swab pure tea tree oil on the acne twice daily. (Too high a percentage or direct application of essential oil can cause irritation and blistering.) Applying tea tree oil cream can also prevent blistering from sunburns.

Anti-inflammatory

Tea tree oil has pain-numbing properties and can be used topically for sprains, arthritis, bunions, **bursitis, eczema, gout, carpal tunnel syndrome**, and **hemorrhoids**. It is best to use products containing essential tea tree oil, since the pure essential oil would be irritating to sensitive areas.

A study at the Flinders University of Adelaide researched tea tree oil's effects on various inflammations in the body to discover if the essential oil reduces the inflammation besides killing the microorganisms causing it.

For relief from **pain** caused by the various arthritic afflictions (**rheumatoid arthritis, osteoarthritis**, etc.), 18 drops of tea tree oil can be combined with 1/8 cup of almond oil, then put in a dark bottle and shaken before applying topically two to four times a day as a massage oil. It can also be used to massage the wrists for **carpal tunnel syndrome**. A dozen drops of tea tree oil can be added to bath water.

Anti-fungal

Tea tree oil is an excellent antifungal agent and can be employed to treat *Candida albicans,* **athlete's foot, jock itch**, ringworm, thrush, and onychomycosis (nail infections).

A study published in the *Journal of Family Practice* in 1994 compared the treatment of onychomycosis with a pharmaceutical clotrimazole solution at 1% to tea tree oil at 100% on 117 patients. After six months, the two groups had similar results, with the culture from the clotrimazole group showing 11% infection and that of the tea tree oil group, 18%.

For ringworm and nail infections, besides applying a tea tree gel, cream, or essential oil, bath and laundry water can be disinfected by adding a few drops of tea tree essential oil to the tub and washing machine.

Preventative

Tea tree oil can boost suppressed immune systems and help those with chronic illnesses such as **chronic fatigue syndrome**. Surgeons in Australian hospitals treat patients in these situations with tea tree oil before surgery.

To increase the power of the immune system, several drops of tea tree oil can be added to the bath or weekly massages. A few drops of tea tree oil can also be added to vaporizers.

Personal hygiene

To fight plaque, brushing with toothpaste containing tea tree oil or adding some to regular toothpaste is advised, as is adding a few drops of tea tree oil to mouthwash. The latter helps both teeth and gums. For sore gums, a few drops of the oil can be swabbed on the sore area.

Household cleaning

Tea tree oil's natural solvent properties make it an excellent biodegradable cleaning product. It can be used for washing cotton diapers; as a deodorizer, or disinfectant; to remove mold; and to treat houseplants for molds, fungus, and **parasitic infections**.

Animal care

Because pets also suffer many of the same diseases as humans, tea tree oil can also be used as treatment for such diseases as arthritis, fleas, **bad breath, gum disease**, abscesses, **dermatitis**, lice, parasites, ringworm, **rashes** and sprains. Dogs in particular are susceptible to mange, a hard-to-eliminate skin disorder causing **hair loss** and **itching**. Washing a dog or cat using a mild soap and water, then clipping or shaving excess hair before soaking a cotton puff with tea tree oil and saturating specific areas twice daily will help treat mange. For overall application, mixing 1 teaspoon tea tree oil with 1/3 cup of water and spraying the mixture from a plant mister onto the mangy areas is advised.

When using tea tree oil for animals, it should always be diluted, as full strength can cause such reactions as muscle **tremors** and poor coordination. The oil should be kept away from the eyes.

Precautions

It is wise to check with your health care practitioner when using tea tree oil internally. Some people might be allergic to the cineole in tea tree oil, although studies show that the 1,8-cineole part improves the skin's absorption of the oil. Dr. Ian Southwell, Research Scientist at the New South Wales Department of Australia suggests the **allergies** could be from alcoholic tea tree oil substances. In 1998-99, skin sensitivity studies conducted at the University of Western Australian Centre for Pathology and Medical Research showed that only three out of 219 volunteers had an allergic reaction to only one or two tea tree oil ingredients. Pure tree oil is also contraindicated for babies, young children, pregnant women, and some pets.

Australian Standard No. AS 2782-1985 requires tea tree oil to contain a minimum of terpinen-4-ol over 30% and cineole content of 15%. Tea tree oil is not to be used for daily hygiene, and is toxic to the liver and kidneys in high or chronic doses. High doses can also be irritating to the skin and provoke an allergic reaction in some people.

Resources

BOOKS

Ali, Dr. Elivs, Dr. George Grant, and Ken Vegotsky. *The Tea Tree Oil Bible*. Niagra Falls, NY: AGES Publications, Inc., 1999.

Murray, Michael. *The Healing Power of Herbs*. Rocklin, CA: Prima Publishing, 1995.

Rothenberg, Mikel A., and Charles F. Chapman. *Barron's Dictionary of Medical Terms* third edition. New York Barron's Education Series, Inc., 1994.

PERIODICALS

"Ti-tree Oil and Chickenpox." *Aromatherapy Quarterly* (Summer 1986):12.

Walsh, Nancy. "Tea Tree Oil for Infections." *Internal Medicine News* (July 1, 2002):16–21.

OTHER

"Antimicrobial activity of Tea Tree Oil." http://www.pharminfo.com/pubs/msb/teaoil240.html.

Australian Tea Tree Oil—Product Safety and recent progress in Research and Development. Courtesy of Robert Riedl, Technical Manager, Regional Affairs, from his lecture in London, England, September, 1999, Thursday Plantation Laboratories Limited, New South Wales, Australia.

The Tea Tree Oil Information Site. http://www.teatree.co.uk.

Thursday Plantation. http://www.thursdayplantation.com.

Sharon Crawford
Teresa G. Odle

Teen nutrition

Definition

Teen **nutrition** involves making sure that teens eat healthy foods to help them grow and develop normally, as well as to prevent **obesity** and future disease. Following dietary guidelines recommended by research and medical professionals supports proper nutrition. The guidelines include selections from different food groups to provide the vitamins and minerals teens need as they grow through puberty and into adulthood. The U.S. Department of Agriculture's (USDA) Food Guide Pyramid recommends how many servings a day an adolescent should eat of each food group, such as milk, vegetables, fruits, fats, and meats. By sticking closely to the guidelines, parents can ensure their teens get a well-balanced diet that supplies the vitamins and calories they need to stay healthy and support growing bodies and active lifestyles.

Origins

Humans, unlike plants, cannot manufacture the nutrients they need to function. Each culture over centuries has developed its own traditional diet. In Western civilization, many of these **diets** have developed into convenient, fatty and sugary foods, leading to obesity even in children and teens.

Advice on nutritional choices predates recorded language, but the first science-based approach to a healthy diet probably began just over 100 years ago. W. O. Atwater, the first director of the Office of Experiment Stations in the USDA and a pioneer in the field of nutrition investigation, developed some of the components needed for a food guide. He created food tables with data on protein, fat, carbohydrate, mineral matter, and fuel value for common foods.

Food guides with food groups similar to those used today first appeared in USDA publications in 1916 and were developed by the nutrition specialist Caroline L. Hunt. The first daily food guide was published under the title *Food for Young Children*. In the early 1930s, the Depression caused economic restraints on families and the USDA responded with advice on how to select healthy foods more cheaply. In 1941, the Food and Nutrition Board of the National Academy of Sciences released the first recommended dietary allowances (RDAs) for calories and essential nutrients. The nine nutrients included on the list were protein, **iron**, **calcium**, vitamins A, C, and D, thiamin, **riboflavin**, and **niacin**.

Throughout the years following the release of the first guidelines, recommendations were debated and revised. The new food guide was first presented in 1984 as a *food wheel*. The USDA first used a pyramid to represent the food groups in 1992 after intensive research on the most effective way to visually communicate healthy eating by portion and food choice. Although it has been modified over the years, the pyramid has continued to represent the food groups. A new revision of the guidelines has been planned for 2005.

Benefits

The Food Guide Pyramid and other healthy eating recommendations generally apply to children age two and older. When used as a starting point for planning family meals and snacks, applying these sensible recommendations to teenagers' daily diets can encourage good eating habits before adulthood. This will help teens develop mentally and physically and prevent obesity or eating disorders. Many nutritional experts agree that if teens eat a balanced diet that includes all of the recommended food groups, they will not need to take any vitamin supplements. Eating a balanced diet with a variety of foods will give teens the energy they need to stay physically active—which is important to their growth, mental health, and to keeping obesity in check.

Description

In spite of recommendations, the quality of most teens' food intake is not what it should be. Today, about nine million U.S. children ages six to 19 are overweight. The number of teens age 12 to 19 with weight problems has tripled since the 1980s. Body mass index (BMI) is a measurement system used to assess if a child (or adult) is underweight, overweight, or at risk for becoming overweight. Pediatricians use height and weight measurements taken at a child's regular checkups to determine his or her BMI. Anyone who weighs more than 85% of teens the same height, age, and sex is considered overweight. The Centers for Disease Control (CDC) considers anyone in the 95th percentile obese. To help guide teens, their families, schools, and others in making healthy nutritional choices, the USDA guidelines suggest the following daily food selections:

• Six to 11 servings of breads, cereals, rice, and pasta

• Three to five servings of vegetables

• Two to four servings of fruit

• Two to three servings of dairy products

• Two or three servings of meat, fish, poultry, and legumes

Fats, oils, and sweets are at the top of the pyramid, but are not considered an actual food group. They occur in many foods from other groups and should be used only sparingly. The USDA says only about 30% of daily calories should come from fat.

Calcium requirements are particularly important for teens, yet studies show that about 60% of teenage boys and more than 85% of teenage girls fail to get the recommended daily allowance of calcium. Calcium not only helps strengthen bones and make for healthier teeth, it also is important in the teen years to prevent future **os-**teoporosis, a painful condition that causes weakened, less dense bones in later adult years. Teens should consume 1,200–1,500 mg of calcium per day. Some excellent sources of calcium include:

• lowfat milk: 300 mg per cup

• white beans: 115 mg per 0.5 cup

• lowfat yogurt: 300 mg per 8 oz

• orange: 40–50 mg per medium-sized orange

Iron requirements are also very important for adolescent health and growth. Teens need 12–15 mg of iron per day. A variety of iron sources come from each food group. Some include:

• peanut butter

• whole grain bread

• spinach

• green beans and lima beans

• beef, poultry, or fish

• strawberries

For both calcium and iron, female teens need the higher recommended amount per day in order to build strong bone and muscle that will prevent against osteoporosis and other conditions associated with postmenopausal women. Teen males need at least the minimum requirement.

Preparations

Getting teenagers to eat the right foods is easier if they have begun good eating habits at a young age and if they are offered a variety of healthy foods. Many books, magazines, and web sites offer tips on making healthy foods interesting. Many of these resources are geared to teens and include recipes. Some selections for each food group include:

• Breads, cereals, and pastas include whole grain breads, bagels, unsweetened cereals, rice, whole grain crackers, cornbread, English muffins, and rice cakes.

• Vegetable servings can come from cooked or raw vegetables such as asparagus, beets, broccoli, carrots, corn, green and red peppers, green beans, kale, peas, pumpkin, squash, sweet potato, tomato, zucchini, or vegetable juice.

• Good fruit choices include such whole fruits as apples, applesauce, bananas, cantaloupe, apricots, peaches, fruit cocktail, plums, grapefruit, kiwi, nectarines, strawberries, and watermelon.

• In addition to milk, lowfat yogurts and cheeses are good dairy sources, as are lowfat cottage cheese, custard, ice milk, and occasional ice cream servings.

• Meat, fish, poultry, and legumes choices include lean meats, dried beans, peanut butter, shellfish, dried peas, lentils, and tofu.

To reduce fat in a teen's diet, parents and their teenage children can switch to low-fat or nonfat milk, remove skin from poultry or trim fat from red meat, reduce use of margarine and butter, use lowfat cooking methods such as baking, broiling, and steaming, and serve foods rich in fiber. Fresh salads can improve fiber in diet, as can adding oat or wheat bran to baked foods. Milk, cheeses, tofu, and salmon are good sources of calcium. Fruit smoothies are good replacements for milk shakes.

It is important that teens eat three meals a day and not skip breakfast. Studies have shown that children and teens that skip breakfast have more trouble concentrating and do not perform as well in school. Skipping breakfast in childhood and adolescence also is related to later health problems such as obesity and **heart disease**.

While the obesity problem in today's youth can be blamed on a number of factors, including larger food portions for adults and children, convenient salty snack foods, and cheap and convenient fast food, much attention has been focused on the nation's schools. There are fewer physical education classes because of more emphasis on academic classes. Those gym classes that remain have too much standing around and not enough activities that interest the students, say some experts. School lunches generally offer balanced nutrition, but many schools also offer "snack bars" or vending machines that dispense sodas and sugary, fatty, or salty snacks. Many teens have been choosing these snacks over the prepared school lunches.

To counter the problem in schools, the Healthy Schools Summit was held in October 2002. It consisted of representatives from more than 30 national education, fitness, nutrition, and health organizations, as well as 450 school administrators, government leaders, food service directors, counselors, dietitians, nurses, and health and fitness teachers. Since that time, many school districts around the country have been working to improve their physical education programs and to remove or change the selections offered in vending machines and snack bars on school campuses. Educating teens and helping them choose healthy alternatives from home, school, or away from campus can help solve the problem as well.

At home, parents also choose convenient snack and fast foods because, both parents often work long hours. Along with bigger portions and increased time spent in front of the television instead of out being physically active, today's youth are becoming obese. They are receiving and growing accustomed to less nutritional food choices. Many experts say that getting teens up off the couch and stocking healthy snack choices helps. Also, many sources can help parents find healthier alternatives to fast food meals for their families. Suggestions include cooking meals on weekends and freezing them for busy weekdays, and looking for cookbooks or online sources of quick and healthy recipes. Simply cooking with less fat by using cooking sprays and baking, roasting, or poaching methods instead of frying helps teens and adults. Also, offering teens healthy snacks to last them until mealtime will keep them from reaching for poor snack choices and make them less likely to overeat at the evening meal.

Teens who are very active and participate in organized sports need a particularly healthy diet. Many teens hear of ideas such as loading up on carbohydrates or proteins to train for sports, often the night before a competition. In reality, the best training is to stick to the Food Pyramid, say nutrition experts. Athletic teens may eat extra helpings of complex carbohydrates, such as whole grain rice, pasta, bread, and cereal. Some extra protein is good to help build strong muscles, but eating too much of just one food group rather than a balanced diet is not recommended for athletes or anyone else. An active male teen needs approximately 2,800 calories per day. They should eat the higher suggested number of servings in each food group. Active female teens require 2,200 calories per day. They should eat the average number of suggested servings per food group. Teens that are not as active and are overweight should eat the lower number of suggested servings per food group and cut back on their daily ingestion of fats, oils, and sugars.

While all teens need to drink plenty of water, those who participate in sports need to drink even more. Some experts say an easy formula to remember is one cup of fluid for every one-half hour of physical activity. Another telltale sign of thirst is the color of a teen's urine. If a teen's urine is clear or the color of pale lemonade, he/she is drinking enough fluids. Dark urine the color of apple juice indicates too little hydration and the teen is in danger of dehydration or heatstroke.

For a variety of reasons, some teenagers follow vegetarian diets. Some people are concerned that a vegetarian diet is harmful for children and teens, but generally, if the teen still follows the recommended Food Guide Pyramid and makes good food choices, a vegetarian diet can be healthy. About 2% of children ages six to 17 never eat meat, fish, or poultry. A survey in early 2003 found that vegetarian adolescents drank fewer sodas and ate less fast food than non-vegetarian teens. Vegetarian teens may need vitamin supplements to make up for some of the vitamins normally obtained in meats or meat products; a physician or professional nutritionist can help determine the proper level of supplement needed.

Precautions

Many teens and their parents have been cautioned not to turn to fad diets for teenage weight problems. Many of the diets and diet products on the market have not been proven by clinical studies as effective in the long term for adults; they certainly have not been proven safe or effective as a solution to weight problems in children and teens. Often, teenagers are more susceptible to claims made about diet plans and parents should help them research these diets or to speak with a physician or other licensed practitioner to determine their effectiveness.

The best solution for obesity is a combination of activity, a balanced diet that follows the USDA guidelines for food groups and portions, and involvement of a physician, dietitian, or other trained professional as needed. Further, adolescents who worry too much about weight and appearance can develop social anxieties and eating disorders such as anorexia and bulimia. Over one third of American teenaged females have used such unhealthy methods as self-induced **vomiting**, laxative abuse, diet pills, and water pills to control their weight.

Eating disorders

Anorexia usually occurs in teenage girls and young women who have a greater than normal fear of being fat. People with anorexia hardly eat at all, and they obsess over the food they do eat. A teenage girl with anorexia might weigh every bit of food she eats, compulsively count all calories, or **exercise** to the extreme to work off calories she has consumed. The difference between anorexia and normal dieting is the obsession with weight loss and the desire to go beyond being fit and trim to being as thin as possible, no matter the cost. Warning signs for anorexia are a weight drop to abut 20% below normal, a teen who denies feeling hungry, excessive exercise, feeling fat, and withdrawal from social activities.

Teens with bulimia binge on food for a few hours, then get rid of it quickly by vomiting or taking laxatives. This binge and purge behavior is more difficult to spot than anorexia, because the teenager may be of average weight. The warning signs for bulimia include frequent excuses to go to the restroom immediately after meals, eating huge amounts of food without gaining weight, and using laxatives or diuretics.

Side effects

Only the fat-soluble (capable of being dissolved in fat or oil) vitamins A, D, K and E have side effects that are potentially, though rarely, toxic (poisonous).

In their book *The Real Vitamin & Mineral Book,* Sheri Lieberman and Nancy Bruning state, "The facts are that only a few vitamins and minerals have any known toxicities, all of which are reversible, with the exception of vitamin D. Anything can be harmful if you take enough of it—even pure water. But vitamins and minerals are among the safest substances on earth. The amounts needed to become toxic are enormous." They add that being on medication or having a medical condition can influence vitamin/mineral requirements and indicate that when one's physician is not well-versed in nutrition, it is ideal to have him work with a qualified nutritionist.

With regard to vitamin D, they indicate, "According to several studies, up to 1,000 IU per day of vitamin D appears to be safe. Both the beneficial and adverse effects of exceeding this amount are controversial. Overdosing of vitamin D is *irreversible and may be fatal.* Symptoms of too much vitamin D are nausea, loss of appetite, headache, **diarrhea**, fatigue, restlessness, and calcification of the soft tissues (insoluble lime salts in tissue) of the lungs and the kidneys, as well as the bones." Vitamin D (400 IU) is usually sold with vitamin A (5,000 IU) in a tiny tablet or capsule.

Lieberman and Bruning say that active vitamin A from fish liver oil or synthetic palmitate is stored in the liver; that 15,000 IU would cause problems in infants; but that 100,000 IU of active vitamin A would have to be taken daily for months before any signs of toxicity (state of being poisonous) appear. Vitamin A in the form of beta-carotene can be taken without any risk of toxicity.

At doses of 800–1,200 IU per day, Lieberman/Bruning found no well-documented toxicity of vitamin E. At doses of over 1,200 IU per day, adverse effects such as flatulence, diarrhea, **nausea**, headache, heart palpitations, and fainting have been reported, but were completely reversible when dosage was reduced.

Vitamin K is easily obtained by the body from a healthy diet and deficiencies are rare, especially in children. It is given prophylactically to newborn infants to prevent hemorrhage and before surgery to people with blood-clotting problems. Lieberman/Bruning describe the major effect of too much vitamin K as an anemia where red blood cells die more quickly than usual and cannot be replaced by the body.

Eating disorders

If a teen weighs less than 15% of the normal weight for his/her height, he/she may not have enough body fat to keep vital organs functioning. When a person is undernourished the body slows down as if it is starving and blood pressure, pulse rate, and breathing slow. Girls with anorexia often stop menstruating. Anorexics can also experience lack energy and concentration, as well as lightheadedness. They become anemic, their bones can become brittle, and they can damage their heart, liver, and kidneys. In the most severe cases, they can suffer malnutrition or even death.

The repeated vomiting of bulimia causes constant stomach **pain**. It also can damage the stomach and kidneys. Acids from the stomach that come up into the mouth when vomiting can cause tooth decay. Teenage girls with bulimia also may stop having menstrual cycles. Constant vomiting may also cause bulimics to lose too much of a mineral called **potassium**, which can lead to heart problems and even death.

Research & general acceptance

The American Medical Association (AMA) has based many of its food choices on the Dietary Guidelines for Americans, which were developed through research by the U.S. Department of Agriculture and the U.S. Department of Human Services. Input for the guidelines comes from a number of resources, including national surveys from the Centers for Disease Control (CDC).

As for teens, accepting the importance of nutrition is another story. A 2000 report from the CDC showed that many teens know the basics of healthy eating but few actually follow the recommendations. They simply prefer unhealthy foods most of the time. In focus groups, some teens in the eighth and ninth grades said they would eat healthy foods right before participating in a sport, but most thought their current behaviors could not affect their health at this time in their lives.

Training & certification

Qualified dieticians and nutritionists may have a bachelor's, master's or doctoral degree in nutrition and dietetics from an accredited college. They also are required to constantly update their knowledge with continuing education. Through the American Dietetic Association, these professionals can gain certification in their fields, including a certificate of training in childhood and adolescent weight management. Pediatricians obtain M.D. or D.O degrees and some specialize in childhood diseases and treatment. In the field of alternative medicine, parents may choose to seek treatment from naturopaths and homeopaths.

Andrew Weil, M.D. points out the benefits of naturopathic medicine by saying that naturopaths go beyond the impression that they are 'New Age.' "Naturopathy comes from the old tradition of European health spas with their emphasis hydro (water) therapy, massage, and nutritional and herbal treatment." Naturopaths are well trained in the sciences and have more experience with nutritional and herbal medicine that allopathic physicians may not have. Naturopathy is based on a general philosophy that focuses on the body's natural healing potential in an attempt to circumvent the use of drugs and surgery; however, naturopathic physicians may focus on different styles, using such therapies as acupuncture, bodywork, herbalism, and **homeopathy**. They are licensed in only a few states in the United States, mostly in the West. According to Dr. Weil, "Good naturopaths are worth consulting for childhood illnesses, recurrent upper respiratory infections and sinusitis, gynecological problems, and all ailments for which conventional doctors have only suppressive treatments. Naturopaths can be valuable as advisors to help people design healthy lifestyles." To find a naturopathic physician in their area, parents can contact the American Association of Naturopathic Physicians, 601 Valley Street, Suite 105, Seattle, Washington 98109, (206) 298-0126.

With regard to homeopathy, Dr. Weil also has positive feedback for the discipline. Homeopathy is a system that has a two-hundred-year-old history. Homeopaths use diluted natural remedies work on the body's energy field to encourage healing. Homeopathic physicians can be M.D.s, osteopaths, naturopaths, chiropractors, or lay persons. If a parent wishes to consult an alternative practitioner for homeopathic advice, the National Center for Homeopathy can be contacted at 801 North Fairfax Street, Suite 306, Alexandria, Virginia 22314, (703) 548-7790.

Resources

PERIODICALS

Berler, Ron. "The Problem is Big: More Kids than Ever are Overweight. We'll Tell You About the Crisis, Offer Some Solutions, and Explain Why Controlling Your Weight Can Make You a Better Athlete." *Sports Illustrated for Kids* (October 1, 2003):60.

"Food Insecurity." *Pediatrics* (February 2003):357–358.

"Kids Don't Think Obesity is a Health Problem." *Nutrition Today* (July-August 2003): 115–116.

Perry, Cheryl L, et al. "Adolescent Vegetarians: How Well do Their Dietary Patterns Meet the Healthy People 2010 Objectives?." *American Academy of Child and Adolescent Psychiatry* (February 2003): 252–253.

ORGANIZATIONS

The American Academy of Pediatrics. 141 Northwest Point Boulevard, Elk Grove Village, IL 60007-1098. (888) 227-1770. <http://www.aap.org/family>.

International Food Information Council. 1100 Connecticut Avenue, NW, Suite 430, Washington, DC, 20036. (202) 296-6540. <http://www.ific.org>.

KidsHealth/Nemours Foundation. 4600 Touchton Road East, Building 200, Suite 500, Jacksonville, FL 32246. <http://www.kidshealth.org/teen/>.

National Eating Disorders Association. 603 Stewart Street, Suite 803, Seattle, WA 98101. (800)931-2237. <http://www.nationaleatingdisorders.org>.

U.S. Department of Agriculture and U.S. Department of Health and Human Services. (888)878-3256. <http://www.usda.gov/FoodAndNutrition>.

OTHER

"BMI For Children and Teens." National Center for Chronic Disease Prevention and Health Promotion. [cited June 18, 2004]. <http://www.cdc.gov/nccdphp/dnpa/bmi/bmi-for-age.htm>.

"Eating Disorders: Anorexia and Bulimia." TeenHealth/ Nemours Foundation. [cited June 18, 2004]. <http://www.kidshealth.org>.

"Healthy Weight, Physical Activity, and Nutrition: Focus Group Research With African American, Mexican American and White Youth. Executive Summary." Centers for Disease Control. <http://www.cdc.gov>.

Teresa G. Odle

Teeth clenching *see* **Bruxism**

Teething problems

Definition

Teething is the eruption of the primary set of teeth (baby teeth) through the gums.

Description

Humans are born with two sets of teeth under the gums. Twenty of these are primary, or baby teeth. Occasionally a child is born with some primary teeth already visible, but more commonly, they begin to erupt around the middle of the first year. The timing of eruption is quite variable but tends to be similar among members of the same family. Generally, all 20 primary teeth have come in by two and a half years of age. Lower teeth usually come in before their upper counterparts. Incisors often erupt first (centrals, then laterals), followed by first molars, canines, and then two-year molars. An early or late pattern of getting baby teeth will sometimes correspond with a similar pattern of losing the baby teeth and getting the permanent teeth. Issues of spacing and orientation of these first teeth do not necessarily indicate that there will be a problem with the permanent teeth. Gaps and crookedness will often resolve.

Causes & symptoms

Many symptoms of teething are nonspecific and can occur for weeks or even months before the teeth actually appear. The teething child may be more irritable, particularly at night. Drooling is likely to become heavier when teeth are coming through, which can also cause the stools to become looser. The excess saliva may cause a rash around the mouth and chin, and produce coughing. Some children will run a low-grade **fever**, typically about 101°F (38.3°C). Commonly the baby will chew on fingers or other objects to relieve the discomfort. This may also include biting during nursing. The areas where teeth are coming through may appear swollen and red. Sucking can be painful for some babies, who may find nursing uncomfortable at the height of teething.

Occasionally, a small, dark blue area will form on the gums where a tooth is about to emerge. This is the result of a small amount of bleeding beneath the surface of the gums, and is not a cause for concern. It will generally resolve without any special treatment, but cold compresses may be used for comfort and to reduce swelling.

Babies may sail through teething with very little apparent discomfort, or may particularly struggle with certain circumstances. Sometimes the first teeth to erupt seem the most bothersome. The parents of other babies find that it is the large molars which cause the most problem, or groups of teeth coming in simultaneously.

Diagnosis

Swollen gums combined with irritability are good clues to teething **pain**, but serious or long lasting symptoms warrant a visit to the health care provider. If the baby has a fever over 101 °F (38.3deg;C), teething is unlikely to be the cause. Even lower fevers that persist for three days or more should prompt a call to ask whether the baby needs to be seen. Teething is not usually associated with nasal discharge. Although babies that are cutting teeth sometimes pull at their ears, a combination of ear pulling, cold symptoms, and increased nighttime fussing could indicate an **ear infection**. If the child seems to be getting worse or there is any doubt that the symptoms are attributable to teething, professional advice should be sought.

Treatment

Pressure on the areas where teeth are coming through can provide comfort for teething babies. Some babies appear to get relief from a gentle gum massage, or they may enjoy chewing on different textures of teething toys. Some types can be chilled or frozen, which can numb the tender gums a little. A clean damp washcloth placed in the freezer is an inexpensive substitute for a freezable toy and may be dampened with **chamomile** tea. Chilled foods or drinks can also do the trick, but parents should not use items that could become choking hazards.

Drool **rashes** are treated by keeping the affected area as free from saliva as possible, and using a mild skin cream. A diaper or wash cloth placed under the crib sheet where the baby's head rests will help to absorb the excess saliva and keep the face from being as wet.

Be sure to take care of primary teeth as they come in. A piece of moist gauze is an effective cleanser for baby's first teeth. To prevent dental caries, avoid letting children sleep with a bottle of anything but water. Milk and juice can pool in the mouth, coat the teeth in sugar, and result in decay. Sticky foods and other processed sugars also put teeth at higher risk for damage. A toothbrush will be a more effective cleaner than gauze once the molars come in, and can be used with plain water. Children who aren't yet able to spit out toothpaste residue can get an overdose of fluoride from swallowing fluoridated toothpaste.

Homeopathic treatment

Homeopathic tablets and gels, typically combination homeopathic remedies, are available for teething **pain**. They are nontoxic, and some find them invaluable in treating teething pain. Individual homeopathic remedies are also available based on the specific symptoms the baby is having. Consult a practitioner for assistance with the correct remedy and dose.

Herbal treatment

Slippery elm powder and infusion of German chamomile can be made into a paste to be applied to swollen gums. Some babies have also been permitted to teethe on peeled root of **marsh mallow** (no relation to the

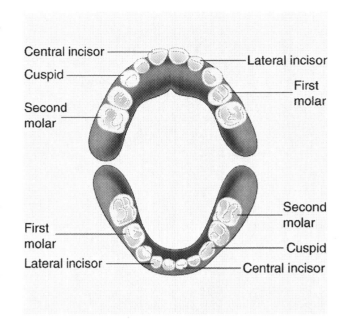

Babies begin teething in the first year of life. By age two, they have a full set of 20 primary teeth. *(Illustration by Electronic Illustrators Group. The Gale Group)*

confection) to soothe inflammation. Chamomile tea in double strength can be very soothing, especially at night.

Allopathic treatment

Acetaminophen (Tylenol) or ibuprofen (Motrin, Advil) can be given to alleviate the swelling and discomfort of teething, particularly at night to allow less interruption of sleep. A healthcare provider can outline the appropriate dose and frequency. Topical gels with anesthetic ingredients are available, but they work only for a brief time and occasionally cause allergic reactions. They also cause numbness, which may be unpleasant to the baby.

Expected results

Teething is an experience that every baby goes through, either with periodic discomfort or none at all. Fortunately, once all the primary teeth come in, it is over.

Prevention

Teething pain cannot be completely prevented, but parental attentiveness to comfort measures can help the baby get through it with less distress.

Resources

BOOKS

Eisenberg, Arlene, Heidi Murkoff and Sandee Hathaway. *What to Expect the First Year.* New York: Workman Publishing, 1989.

Sears, William and Martha Sears. *The Baby Book*. Boston: Little, Brown and Company, 1993.

OTHER

Greene, Alan. *Dr. Greene's HouseCalls: Dealing with teething pain*. http://drgreene.com/990703.asp (1999).

Judith Turner

Temporomandibular joint syndrome

Definition

Temporomandibular joint syndrome (TMJ) is the name given to a group of symptoms that cause pain in the head, face, and jaw. The symptoms include headaches, soreness in the chewing muscles, and clicking or stiffness of the joints.

Description

TMJ syndrome, which is also sometimes called TMJ disorder, results from pressure on the facial nerves due to muscle tension or abnormalities of the bones in the area of the hinge joint between the lower jaw and the temporal bone. This hinge joint is called the temporomandibular joint. There are two temporomandibular joints, one on each side of the skull just in front of the ear. The temporal bone is the name of the section of the skull bones where the jawbone (the mandible) is connected. The jawbone is held in place by a combination of ligaments, tendons, and muscles. The temporomandibular joint also contains a piece of cartilage called a disc, which keeps the temporal bone and the jawbone from rubbing against each other. The jaw pivots at the joint area in front of the ear. The pivoting motion of the jaw is complicated because it can move downward and from side to side as well as forward. Anything that causes a change in shape or functioning of the temporomandibular joint will cause pain and other symptoms.

Causes & symptoms

TMJ syndrome has several possible physical causes:

- Muscle tension. Muscle tightness in the temporomandibular joint usually results from overuse of muscles. This overuse in turn is often associated with psychological **stress** and clenching or grinding of the teeth (**bruxism**).

- Injury. A direct blow to the jaw or the side of the head can result in bone fracture, soft tissue bruising, or a dislocation of the temporomandibular joint itself.

- Arthritis. Both **osteoarthritis** and **rheumatoid arthritis** can cause TMJ.

- Internal derangement. Internal derangement is a condition in which the cartilage disk lies in front of its proper position. In most cases of internal derangement, the disc moves in and out of its correct location, making a clicking or popping noise as it moves. In a few cases, the disc is permanently out of position, and the patient's range of motion in the jaw is limited.

- Hypermobility. Hypermobility is a condition in which the ligaments that hold the jaw in place are too loose and the jaw tends to slip out of its socket.

- Birth abnormalities. These are the least frequent causes of TMJ but do occur in a minority of patients. In some cases, the top of the jawbone is too small; in others, the top of the jawbone outgrows the lower part.

- Oral habits. Some dentists think that such habits as wide yawning, lip or tongue biting, or mouth breathing can contribute to TMJ by putting the jaw in an abnorml position for long periods of time.

- Dental work. Some people develop TMJ following dental work that requires the dentist to hold the patient's jaw open wide for extended periods of time. Other patients develop TMJ following removal of the wisdom teeth.

In addition to the physical causes of TMJ, dentists are increasingly recognizing the importance of psychosocial factors in the disorder. One recent finding is the importance of the patient's concept of pain itself. People who are already suffering from **depression** or an **anxiety** disorder, people who have little social support in their lives, and people who feel that they have little control over their lives are at greater risk of developing chronic pain syndromes, including TMJ.

In many cases TMJ results from a combination of psychological, anatomical, and functional factors rather than a single abnormality.

The symptoms of TMJ depend in part on its cause or causes. The most common symptoms are facial pain in front of the ears; headaches; sore jaw muscles; a clicking sound when chewing; a grating sensation when opening and closing the mouth; and temporary locking of the jaw. Some patients also report a sensation of buzzing or ringing in the ears. Usually, the temporomandibular joint itself is not painful. Most cases of TMJ are seen in women between 20–50 years of age.

Diagnosis

TMJ syndrome is most frequently diagnosed by dentists. The dentist can often diagnose TMJ based on physical examination of the patient's face and jaw. The examination might include pressing on (palpating) the jaw muscles for soreness or asking the patient to open and close the jaw in order to check for misalignment of the teeth in the upper and lower jaw. This condition is called malocclusion. The dentist might also gently move the patient's jaw in order to check for loose ligaments.

Imaging studies are not usually necessary to diagnose TMJ. In most cases, x rays and MRI scans of the temporomandibular joint will be normal. Consequently, these two tests are not commonly used to diagnose TMJ. If the dentist suspects that the patient has internal derangement of the disc, a technique called arthrography can be used to make the diagnosis. In an arthrogram, a special dye is injected into the joint, which is then x-rayed. Arthrography can be used to evaluate the movement of the jaw and the disc as well as size and shape, and to evaluate the effectiveness of treatment for TMJ.

Another aid to diagnosing TMJ is a new questionnaire designed to discriminate between facial pain related to TMJ and myogenic facial pain, a chronic condition that is caused by trigger points in the muscles of the face and neck. The McGill Pain Questionnaire has been reported to have a high degree of reliability in distinguishing between patients with TMJ and patients with myogenic facial pain.

Treatment

In many cases, the cause of pain in the TMJ area is temporary and disappears without treatment. About 80% of patients with TMJ will improve in six months without medications or physical treatments.

Biofeedback, which teaches an individual to control muscle tension and any associated pain through thought and visualization techniques, is also a treatment option for TMJ. In biofeedback treatments, sensors placed on the surface of the jaw are connected to a special machine that allows the patient and healthcare professional to monitor a visual and/or audible readout of the level of tension in the jaw muscles. Through **relaxation** and visualization exercises, the patient learns to relieve the tension and can actually see or hear the results of his or her efforts instantly through the sensor readout on the biofeedback equipment. Once the technique is learned and the patient is able to recognize and differentiate between the feelings of muscle tension and muscle relax-

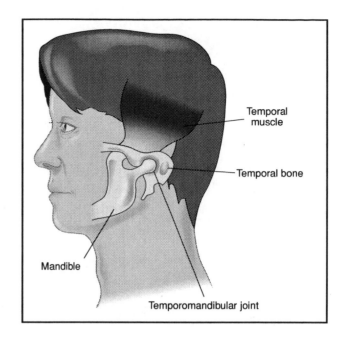

Temporomandibular joint syndrome (TMJ) is caused by any misalignment of the joint that connects the mandible to the temporal bone. Muscle tension, misaligned bite, or head injury can cause the pain associated with TMJ. *(Illustration by Electronic Illustrators Group. The Gale Group)*

ation, the electromyographic biofeedback equipment itself is no longer needed and the patient has a powerful, portable, and self-administered treatment tool to deal with pain and tension.

Stress management and relaxation techniques may be useful in breaking the habit of jaw clenching and teeth grinding. Tight jaw muscles are often relaxed by applying warm compresses to the sides of the face. **Acupuncture** may relieve the jaw tension associated with TMJ. **Massage therapy** and deep tissue realignment can also assist in releasing the clenching pattern. Extra **calcium** and **magnesium** can also help relax jaw muscles.

Allopathic treatment

Allopathic practitioners are increasingly recommending more conservative treatments for TMJ, on the grounds that the majority of patients can be successfully treated with noninvasive, reversible approaches. These include patient education and eating softer foods as well as medication and the use of bite plates.

Patients with TMJ can be given muscle relaxants if their symptoms are related to muscle tension. Some patients may be given aspirin or nonsteroidal anti-inflammatory drugs (NSAIDs) for minor discomfort. If the TMJ is related to rheumatoid arthritis, it may be treated with corticosteroids, methotrexate (MTX, Rheumatrex) or gold **sodium** (Myochrysine).

Patients who have difficulty with bruxism may be treated with splints. A plastic splint called a nightguard is given to the patient to place over the teeth before going to bed. Splints can also be used to treat some cases of internal derangement by holding the jaw forward and keeping the disc in place until the ligaments tighten. The splint is adjusted over a period of two to four months.

TMJ can also also be treated with ultrasound, stretching exercises, transcutaneous electrical nerve stimulation (TENS), stress management techniques, or friction massage. A 2002 study done at the University of Maryland found that all of these treatments are helpful to patients with TMJ, but none appears to be clearly superior to the others.

Surgery is ordinarily used only to treat TMJ caused by birth deformities or certain forms of internal derangement caused by misshapen discs.

Expected results

The prognosis for recovery from TMJ is excellent for almost all patients. Most patients do not need any form of long-term treatment. Surgical procedures to treat TMJ are quite successful. In the case of patients with TMJ caused by arthritis or infectious diseases, the progression of the arthritis or the success of eliminating infectious agents determines whether TMJ can be eliminated.

Resources

BOOKS

"Disorders of the Temporomandibular Joint." In *Merck Manual of Medical Information: Home Edition,* edited by Robert Berkow, et al. Whitehouse Station, NJ: Merck Research Laboratories, 1997.

Murphy, William A., Jr., and Phoebe A. Kaplan. "Temporomandibular Joint." In *Diagnosis of Bone and Joint Disorders,* edited by Donald Resnick. Philadelphia: W. B. Saunders Company, 1995.

PERIODICALS

Grace, E. G., E. Sarlani, and B. Read. "The Use of an Oral Exercise Device in the Treatment of Muscular TMD." *Cranio Clinics International* 20 (July 2002): 204-208.

Mongini, F., F. Raviola, and M. Italiano. "The McGill Pain Questionnaire in Patients with Myogenic Facial Pain and TMJ Disorders." *Journal of Oral Rehabilitation* 29 (September 2002): 875.

Nilges, P. "Psychosocial Factors in Patients with Temporomandibular Pain." [in German] *Schmerz* 16 (September 2002): 365-372.

Syrop, S. B. "Initial Management of Temporomandibular Disorders." *Dentistry Today* 21 (August 2002): 52-57.

Vanderas, A. P., and L. Papagiannoulis. "Multifactorial Analysis of the Aetiology of Craniomandibular Dysfunction in Children." *International Journal of Paediatric Dentistry* 12 (September 2002): 336-346.

Yamakawa, M., T. Ansai, S. Kasai, et al. "Dentition Status and Temporomandibular Joint Disorders in Patients with Rheumatoid Arthritis." *Cranio Clinics International* 20 (July 2002): 165-171.

ORGANIZATIONS

American Dental Association. 211 East Chicago Avenue, Chicago, IL 60611. (312)440–2500. <www.ada.org>.

National Institute of Dental and Craniofacial Research (NIDCR). National Institutes of Health, Bethesda, MD 20892. (301) 496-4261. <www.nidr.nih.gov>.

TMJ Association, Ltd. <www.tmj.org>.

Paula Ford-Martin
Rebecca J. Frey, PhD

Tendinitis

Definition

Tendinitis is a condition caused by the tearing of tendon fibers and subsequent inflammation in the tendon. Tendons are the strong connective tissue that connect muscle to bone.

Description

When a muscle contracts, it pulls on the tendon, which is composed of tissue that cannot stretch. The tendon then transmits that pulling force to the bone and moves the bone, producing movement. Tendinitis usually results from excessive repeated demands placed on the tendon by the muscle. Tendinitis is not usually caused by a sudden injury; it is more commonly a result of a long period of overuse. Tendinitis occurs frequently with active individuals and those whose occupational tasks require repetitive motion.

Tendons that commonly become inflamed include:

- tendons of the hand
- tendons of the upper arm that affect the shoulder
- tendons of the forearm at the elbow
- the tendon of the quadriceps muscle group at the knee
- the Achilles tendon at the ankle

Causes & symptoms

Repeated overuse of the tendon will cause small tears to develop in the tendon fibers. As a result, the body will initiate the injury repair process in the area and lay down scar tissue. Inflammation will develop in the area as part of the injury repair process. Inflammation increases the blood supply, bringing nutrients to the damaged tissues along with infection-fighting agents. The result is swelling, tenderness, **pain**, and heat. Redness may occur if the injury is close to the skin. Since many cases of tendinitis result from chronic inflammatory conditions that develop from long periods of overuse, the inflammatory process is not as exaggerated as with an acute injury. Therefore swelling, heat, and redness are not always visible in a tendinitis complaint because the inflammation is really at a low level.

Recent research has found that tendinitis sometimes develops as a side effect of treatment with quinolones, which are a group of antibiotics frequently used to treat bacterial **infections**. The tendon most likely to be affected by these drugs is the Achilles tendon, and the tendinitis usually develops within the first few weeks of antibiotic treatment.

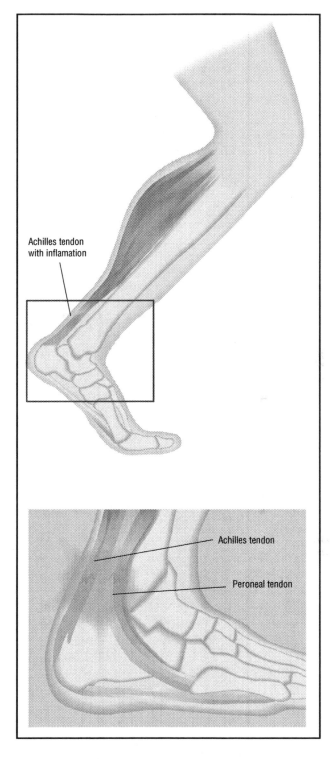

Achilles tendon with inflamation

Achilles tendon

Peroneal tendon

(Illustration by GGS Information Services, Inc. The Gale Group.)

Diagnosis

Some common tendon injuries are superficial and easy to identify. These include lateral epicondylitis (commonly referred to as **tennis elbow**) and Achilles' tendinitis, which affects the tendon just above the heel of the foot. While tennis elbow occurs more often in workers than in athletes (in spite of its name), tendinitis affecting the Achilles tendon is almost always related to sports. Tendinitis in the shoulder area is almost always found in workers who frequently carry heavy loads as part of their job.

Tendinitis is most often diagnosed by evaluating factors in the patient's history that indicate muscular overuse. Tendinitis will often develop when an individual suddenly increases his or her level of activity without adequate training or conditioning. This occurs frequently in occupational and recreational settings.

In addition to evaluating factors in the patient's history that are likely to lead to tendinitis, the clinician may use several physical examination procedures. Most tendons are near the surface of the skin and therefore can be easily palpated (touched or pressed in order to make a diagnosis), especially by practitioners of manual therapy who have highly developed palpation skills. Pressure placed directly on these tendons is likely to cause discomfort. In addition, the practitioner may ask the patient to contract the muscle attached to the tendon, usually against resistance, to see if this maneuver causes pain.

Treatment

Ice is often advocated for tendinitis when the tendon is in an irritated state. Ice is particularly useful for limiting inflammation in the tendon. Ice may be applied by placing a bag of ice on the skin. It may also be applied directly to the skin using an ice cube wrapped in a paper towel or ice frozen in a paper cup with the top portion of the cup peeled away to expose the ice. An ice massage—rubbing the skin and underlying tissue with ice in a slow, circular, or back-and-forth motion—will cool the injured area quickly. If ice is applied to the skin without a barrier between the ice and the skin, the patient should be carefully monitored so that frostbite does not occur. Generally no more than about five minutes of treatment in one area is necessary with ice massage.

Compression wraps, such as elastic bandages, may be used to help provide mechanical support for the tendon during active movement. These compression wraps can be helpful, but they may also slow the healing process in the tendon if left on for long periods because they decrease blood supply in the area.

Various types of soft tissue manipulation are very effective for treating tendinitis and may be employed by a variety of practitioners, including chiropractors, massage therapists, physical therapists, and osteopaths. One of the most common methods of soft tissue treatment for tendinitis is a vigorous friction massage to the damaged tendon. This friction massage will stimulate the healing of tissue in the area. It is also thought to help produce a healthy and strong scar-tissue repair of the damaged tendon fibers. Practitioners of manual therapy are also likely to advocate a regular stretching program to help decrease tension in those muscles that may be pulling excessively on the tendon.

Acupuncture and **traditional Chinese medicine** are quite effective in treating tendinitis. Acupuncture may be used in the immediate vicinity of the tendinitis to help address muscular dysfunction. Acupuncture treatment may also use more distant points along the energy meridians to help address pain and reduce inflammation. Acupuncture may also have significant benefits in creating an optimum environment for healing of the tendon fiber to take place.

Topical liniments and herbal preparations are often used to treat tendinitis. They have anti-inflammatory properties and will help heal the torn tendon fibers. If the condition is chronic, treatment with **moxibustion** (burning a small amount of **mugwort** near the skin) may hasten the healing process. Some oral herbal preparations may also be used in order to create the optimal healing environment for the tendon and address any underlying problems. Practitioners of traditional Chinese medicine may also use a special form of **acupressure** massage called *tui-na*.

Allopathic treatment

Pain and anti-inflammatory medications (aspirin, naproxen, and ibuprofen) will help and are often used to treat tendinitis along with ice, compression wraps, and activity modification, as mentioned earlier. Sometimes the inflammation lingers and requires additional treatment. Injections of anti-inflammatory medication, such as cortisone, often relieve chronic tendinitis, but they should be used with caution. Research has indicated that cortisone may have detrimental effects on the healing of connective tissues and may, in fact, weaken them in the long run. This side effect would make the person susceptible to a greater injury in the future.

If tendinitis is persistent and unresponsive to nonsurgical treatment, the afflicted portion of the tendon can be removed through surgery. Surgery is also performed to remove the **calcium** buildup that comes with persistent tendinitis.

Expected results

Generally, tendinitis will heal if the activity that provokes it is stopped. Various kinds of treatments may accelerate the healing process. Some tendinitis complaints

KEY TERMS

Moxibustion—A treatment in which crushed leaves of the mugwort, or moxa, plant (*Artemisia vulgaris*) are shaped into a cigar-like form that is lit and held directly over the skin of the area being treated.

Palpation—A diagnostic technique in which the organ or tissue is examined or explored by pressing lightly on the skin above the injury.

Quinolones—A group of antibiotics, often used to treat bacterial infections, that sometimes cause tendinitis.

Tendon—A band or cord of thick white fibrous tissue that connects a muscle to bone.

may last for a long time because they are not given adequate healing time before the individual returns to a vigorous level of activity.

Prevention

If given enough time, tendons will strengthen to meet the demands placed on them. The blood supply to tendons is poor, which means that tendons grow slowly. Therefore, adequate time is required for good conditioning. Stretching the muscles that are associated with problematic tendon will also help decrease overuse of the tendon.

Resources

BOOKS

Beinfield, Harriet, and Efrem Korngold. *Between Heaven and Earth: A Guide to Chinese Medicine.* New York: Ballantine, 1991.

Hammer, Warren I. *Functional Soft Tissue Examination and Treatment by Manual Methods: New Perspectives.* 2nd ed. Gaithersburg, MD: Aspen, 1999.

Kaptchuk, Ted J. *The Web That Has No Weaver.* Chicago: NTC Publishing Group, 1999.

Pelletier, Kenneth R. *The Best Alternative Medicine: What Works? What Does Not?* New York: Simon & Schuster, 2000.

Malone, Terry R., Thomas G. McPoil, and Arthur J. Nitz, eds. *Orthopedic and Sports Physical Therapy.* St. Louis: Mosby, 1997.

Weintraub, William. *Tendon and Ligament Healing: A New Approach Through Manual Therapy.* Berkeley, Calif.: North Atlantic Books, 1999.

PERIODICALS

Fenwick, S. A., B. L. Hazleman, and G. P. Riley. "The Vasculature and Its Role in the Damaged and Healing Tendon." *Arthritis Research* 4 (March 2002): 252-260.

Frost, P., J. P. Bonde, S. Mikkelsen, et al. "Risk of Shoulder Tendinitis in Relation to Shoulder Loads in Monotonous Repetitive Work." *American Journal of Industrial Medicine* 41 (January 2002): 11-18.

Oliphant, C. M., and G. M. Green. "Quinolones: A Comprehensive Review." *American Family Physician* 65 (February 2002): 455-464.

Schepsis, A. A., H. Jones, and A. L. Haas. "Achilles Tendon Disorders in Athletes." *American Journal of Sports Medicine* 30 (March-April 2002): 287-305.

Stahlmann, R. "Clinical Toxicological Aspects of Fluoroquinolones." *Toxicology Letter* 127 (February 28, 2002): 269-277.

Whitney Lowe
Rebecca J. Frey, PhD

Tennis elbow

Definition

Tennis elbow is an inflammation of several structures of the elbow. These include muscles, tendons, bursa, periosteum, and epicondyle (bony projections on the outside and inside of the elbow, where muscles of the forearm attach to the bone of the upper arm). This condition is also called epicondylitis, lateral epicondylitis, medial epicondylitis, or golfer's elbow, where **pain** is present at the inside epicondyle.

Description

The classic tennis elbow is caused by repeated forceful contractions of wrist muscles located on the outer forearm. The stress, created at a common muscle origin, causes microscopic tears leading to inflammation. This is a relatively small surface area located at the outer portion of the elbow (the lateral epicondyle). Medial tennis elbow, or medial epicondylitis, is caused by forceful repetitive contractions from muscles located on the inside of the forearm. All of the forearm muscles are involved in tennis serves, when combined motions of the elbow and wrist are employed. This overuse injury is common in adults between ages 20–40.

People at risk for tennis elbow are those in occupations that require strenuous or repetitive forearm movement. Such jobs include mechanics, assembly line work, house painting, or carpentry. Sport activities that require individuals to twist the hand, wrist, and forearm, such as tennis, throwing a ball, bowling, golfing, and skiing, can cause tennis elbow. Individuals in poor physical condition who are exposed to repetitive wrist and forearm movements for long periods of time may also be prone to tennis elbow.

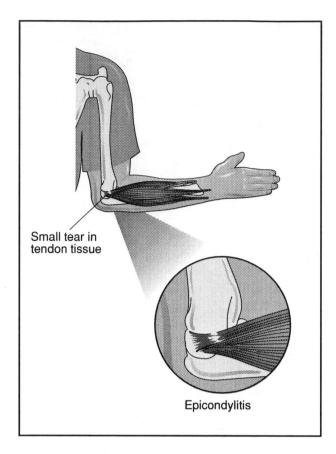

Epicondylitis

Small tear in tendon tissue

The classic tennis elbow is caused by repeated forceful contractions of wrist muscles located on the outer forearm. The stress created at a common muscle origin causes microscopic tears leading to inflammation. Persons who are most at risk of developing tennis elbow are those whose occupations requires strenuous or repetitive forearm movement.
(Illustration by Electronic Illustrators Group. The Gale Group.)

Causes & symptoms

Tennis elbow pain originates from a partial tear of the tendon and the attached covering of the bone. It is caused by chronic stress on tissues attaching a group of forearm muscles known as extensor muscles to the elbow area. Individuals experiencing tennis elbow may complain of pain and tenderness over either of the two epicondyles. This pain increases with gripping or rotation of the wrist and forearm. If the condition becomes long-standing and chronic, a decrease in grip strength can develop.

Diagnosis

Diagnosis of tennis elbow includes the individual observation and recall of symptoms, a thorough medical history, and physical examination by a physician. Diagnostic testing is usually not necessary unless there may be evidence of nerve involvement from underlying caus-

es. X rays are usually always negative because the condition is primarily soft tissue in nature, in contrast to a disorder of the bones. However, magnetic resonance imaging (MRI) has been shown to be helpful in diagnosing cases of early tennis elbow because it can detect evidence of swelling and tissue tears in the common extensor muscle group.

Treatment

Heat or ice is helpful in relieving tennis elbow pain. Once acute symptoms have subsided, heat treatments are used to increase blood circulation and promote healing. The physician may recommend physical therapy to apply **diathermy** or ultrasound to the inflamed site. These are two common modalities used to increase the thermal temperature of the tissues in order to address both pain and inflammation. Occasionally, a tennis elbow splint may be useful to help decrease stress on the elbow throughout daily activities. Routine exercises are very important to improve flexibility to all forearm muscles, and will aid in decreasing muscle and tendon tightness that has been creating excessive pull at the common attachment of the epicondyle.

Massage therapy also has been found to be beneficial if symptoms are mild. Massage techniques are based primarily on increasing circulation to promote efficient reduction of inflammation. Manipulation, **acupuncture**, and **acupressure** have been used as well. Contrast **hydrotherapy** (alternating hot and cold water or compresses, three minutes hot, 30 seconds cold, repeated three times, always ending with cold) applied to the elbow can help bring nutrient-rich blood to the joint and carry away waste products. **Botanical medicine** and **homeopathy** may also be effective therapies for tennis elbow. For example, **cayenne** (*Capsicum frutescens*) ointment or **arnica**, **wintergreen**, or rue oil applied topically may help to increase blood flow to the affected area and speed healing.

Allopathic treatment

The physician may also prescribe nonsteroidal anti-inflammatory drugs (NSAIDs) to reduce inflammation and pain. Injections of cortisone or anesthetics are often used if physical therapy is ineffective. Cortisone reduces inflammation, and anesthetics temporarily relieve pain. Physicians are cautious regarding an excessive number of injections as they have been found to weaken the tendon's integrity. In addition, a significant number of patients experience a temporary increase in pain following corticosteroid injections.

A newer method of treatment for tennis elbow is shock wave therapy, in which pulses of high-pressure sound are directed at the injured part of the tendon. The "shock" refers to the high pressure, which breaks down scar tissue and stimulates the regrowth of blood vessels in healthy tissue. Shock wave therapy sessions take about 20 minutes and have been reported to have a success rate of 80%. Shock wave therapy has very few side effects; one group of German physicians found that temporary reddening of the skin or small **bruises** were the most commonly reported side effects.

Botulinum toxin, or Botox, is also being tried as a treatment for tennis elbow as of late 2003. Although further research needs to be done, Botox appears to relieve pain in chronic tennis elbow by relaxing muscles that have gone into spasm from prolonged inflammation.

Surgery

If conservative methods of treatment fail, surgical release of the tendon at the epicondyle may be a necessary form of treatment. Although surgical intervention is relatively rare in the treatment of tennis elbow, it is completely succesful in about 70% of cases.

Expected results

Tennis elbow is usually curable; however, if symptoms become chronic, it is not uncommon for treatment to continue for three to six months.

Prevention

Until symptoms of pain and inflammation subside, activities requiring repetitive wrist and forearm motion should be avoided. Once pain decreases to the point that return to activity can begin, the playing of such sports as tennis for long periods should not occur until excellent condition returns. Many times, choosing a different size or type of tennis racquet or tool may help. Frequent rest periods are important despite what the wrist and forearm activity may be. Compliance to a stretching and strengthening program is very important in helping prevent recurring symptoms and exacerbation. In some cases, the patient may be advised to change his or her occupation to prevent further injury.

Resources

BOOKS

Hertling, Darlene, and Randolph M. Kessler. *Management of Common Musculoskeletal Disorders: Physical Therapy Principles and Methods.* 2d ed. Philadelphia: J.B. Lippincott Company, 1990.

Norkin, Cynthia C., and Pamela K. Levangie. *Joint Structure and Function: A Comprehensive Analysis.* Philadelphia: F.A. Davis Company, 1992.

KEY TERMS

Epicondyle—A projection on the surface of a bone; often an area for muscle and tendon attachment.

Epicondylitis—A painful and sometimes disabling inflammation of the muscle and surrounding tissues of the elbow caused by repeated stress and strain on the forearm near the lateral epicondyle of the humerous (arm bone).

Extensor muscles—A group of muscles in the forearm that serve to lift or extend the wrist and hand. Tennis elbow results from overuse and inflammation of the tendons that attach these muscles to the outside of the elbow.

Periosteum—A fibrous vascular membrane that covers bones.

Shock wave therapy—A method of treating tennis elbow and other musculoskeletal injuries that involves directing bursts of high-pressure sound waves at the affected area.

PERIODICALS

Altay, T., I. Gunal, and and H. Ozturk. "Local Injection Treatment for Lateral Epicondylitis." *Clinical Orthopedics* 398 (May 2002): 127-130.

Das, D., and N. Maffulli. "Surgical Management of Tennis Elbow." *Journal of Sports Medicine and Physical Fitness* 42 (June 2002): 190-197.

de Seze, M. P., M. de Seze, P. Dehail, et al. "Botulinum Toxin A and Musculoskeletal Pain." [in French] *Annales de réadaptation et de médecine physique* 46 (July 2003): 329–332.

Haake, M., I. R. Boddeker, T. Decker, et al. "Side-Effects of Extracorporeal Shock Wave Therapy (ESWT) in the Treatment of Tennis Elbow." *Archives of Orthopaedic and Trauma Surgery* 122 (May 2002): 222-228.

Mackay, D., A. Rangan, G. Hide, et al. "The Objective Diagnosis of Early Tennis Elbow by Magnetic Resonance Imaging." *Occupational Medicine (London)* 53 (August 2003): 309–312.

Melikyan, E. Y., E. Shahin, J. Miles, and L. C. Bainbridge. "Extracorporeal Shock-Wave Treatment for Tennis Elbow. A Randomised Double-Blind Study." *Journal of Bone and Joint Surgery, British Volume* 85 (August 2003): 852–855.

Rompe, J. D., M. Buch, L. Gerdesmeyer, et al. "Musculoskeletal Shock Wave Therapy— Current Database of Clinical Research." [in German] *Zeitschrift Orthopädische Ihre Grenzgebiet* 140 (May-June 2002): 267-274.

Smith, A. M., J. A. Castle, and D. S. Ruch. "Arthroscopic Resection of the Common Extensor Origin: Anatomic Considerations." *Journal of Shoulder and Elbow Surgery* 12 (July-August 2003): 375–379.

Walther, M., S. Kirschner, A. Koenig, et al. "Biomechanical Evaluation of Braces Used for the Treatment of Epicondylitis." *Journal of Shoulder and Elbow Surgery* 11 (May-June 2002): 265-270.

Wang, A. A., E. Whitaker, D. T. Hutchinson, and D. A. Coleman. "Pain Levels After Injection of Corticosteroid to Hand and Elbow." *American Journal of Orthopedics* 32 (August 2003): 383–385.

ORGANIZATIONS

American College of Occupational and Environmental Medicine (ACOEM). 1114 North Arlington Heights Road, Arlington Heights, IL 60004. (847) 818-1800. <www.acoem.org>.

American College of Sports Medicine. PO Box 1440, Indianapolis, IN 46206–1440 or 401 W. Michigan St., Indianapolis, IN 46202. (317) 637–9200. Fax: (317) 634–7817. <www.acsm.org>.

Kathleen D. Wright
Rebecca J. Frey, PhD

Tetanus

Definition

Tetanus is a rare but often fatal disease that affects the central nervous system by causing painful and often violent muscular contractions. The earliest descriptions of the disease can be found in the medical papyri of ancient Egypt. The disease begins when the tetanus bacterium (*Clostridium tetani*) enters the body, usually through a wound or cut that has come in contact with the spores of the bacterium. Tetanus spores are commonly found in soil, dust, and animal manure. Tetanus is a noncommunicable disease, meaning that it cannot be passed directly from one person to another.

Description

Tetanus is uncommon in the United States, with nearly all cases occurring in adults who were not vaccinated as children, or in those who have not had a booster vaccination in 10 years.

In the United States, there are between 50 and 100 reported cases of tetanus a year. About 30% of cases are fatal. Most people who die of tetanus **infections** are over 50 years old.

Tetanus causes convulsive muscle spasms and rigidity that can lead to respiratory paralysis and death. It is sometimes called "lockjaw" because one of the most common symptoms is a stiff jaw that cannot be opened.

Sometimes tetanus is localized, that is; it affects only the part of the body where the infection began. However, in almost all reported cases, tetanus spreads to the entire body. The incubation period from the time of the injury until the first symptoms appear ranges from five days to three weeks. Symptoms usually occur within eight to 12 days. The chance of death is increased when symptoms occur early.

Causes & symptoms

Tetanus is caused by a bacterium called *Clostridium tetani*, whose spores (the dormant form) are found in soil, street dust, and animal feces. The bacteria enter the body through cuts and abrasions but will multiply only in an environment that is anaerobic, or oxygen-free. Deep puncture **wounds** and wounds with a lot of dead tissue provide an oxygen-free environment for the bacteria to grow.

As *C. tetani* grows, it excretes a highly poisonous toxin called tetanospasmin into the bloodstream, spreading it throughout the nervous system. The infection is usually transmitted through deep puncture wounds or through cuts or scratches that are not cleaned well. Many people associate tetanus with rusty nails and other dirty objects, but any wound can be a source. Less common ways of getting tetanus are animal scratches and bites; surgical wounds; dental work; punctures caused by glass, thorns, needles, and splinters; and therapeutic abortion. Rare cases have been reported in people with no known wound or medical condition.

Neonatal tetanus in newborns can be caused by cutting the umbilical cord with an unsterile instrument or by improper care of the umbilical stump. Neonatal tetanus is less common in developed countries.

Tetanus toxin affects the nerve endings, causing a continuous stimulation of the muscles. Initial symptoms may include restlessness, irritability, a stiff neck, and difficulty swallowing. In about half of all cases, the first symptom is a stiff or "locked" jaw, which prevents patients from opening their mouths or swallowing. This symptom is also called *trismus* and results in a facial expression called *risus sardonicus*, which is a Latin phrase meaning "sardonic smile." Trismus is often followed by stiffness of the neck and other muscles throughout the body as well as uncontrollable spasms. Sometimes these convulsions, known as *opisthotonos*, are severe enough to cause broken bones. Other symptoms of tetanus include loss of appetite and drooling. People with localized tetanus experience **pain** and tingling only at the wound site and spasms in nearby muscles.

In the underdeveloped world, neonatal tetanus accounts for about one-half of tetanus deaths and is related to infection of the umbilical stump in a baby born of an unimmunized mother. In many cases the risk is increased by the mother's giving birth on a floor made of hard-packed soil. Worldwide, 800,000 children die of tetanus each year.

Diagnosis

Tetanus is diagnosed by the clinical symptoms and a medical history that shows no tetanus immunization. Early diagnosis and treatment is crucial for recovery.

In general, the shorter the incubation period, the more severe the disease.

Treatment

As traditional medical treatment revolves around drug therapy, **traditional Chinese medicine** herbal remedies are the most common alternative treatment for tetanus. Herbs that have sedative effects should be given to reduce the frequency of convulsions, along with herbs to fight the bacteria.

Tetanus and convulsions can be treated with a concoction made from the dried body of a long-nosed pit viper, called this drug Qi She in Mandarin. Chan Tui, or **cicada** slough (the skin the cicada sheds) is also helpful. Also helpful are the dried root of the *Saposhnikovia divaricata,* called divaricate saposhnikovia root, and jack-in-the-pulpit tuber, if it is treated to remove toxins.

There are several alternative treatments aimed at prevention of the disease.

Allopathic treatment

Tetanus is a life-threatening disease. Patients diagnosed with it are usually hospitalized, usually in an intensive care ward. Treatment can take several weeks and includes antibiotics to kill the bacteria and shots of antitoxin to neutralize the toxin. It also includes antianxiety drugs to control muscle spasms or barbiturates for sedation. In severe cases, patients are placed on an artificial respirator. Recovery can take six weeks or more. After recovery, since the levels of circulating toxin are quite low, the patient must still be adequately immunized against this disease.

Expected results

Full recovery is common in patients who can be kept alive during the most violent portion of the attacks. Yet up to 30% of tetanus victims in the United States die. Early diagnosis and treatment improves the prognosis. Neonatal tetanus, however, has a mortality rate of more than 90%.

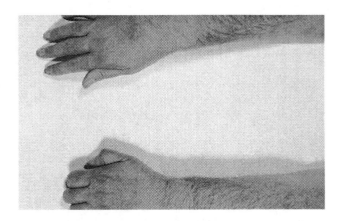

One characteristic of tetanus toxin is the recurrent contracture of a muscle. Here, the patient's left hand is affected. *(Custom Medical Stock Photo. Reproduced by permission.)*

Prevention

Castor oil is a natural remedy that can be used to clean out a wound and prevent tetanus. When a wound is sustained, a cotton ball dunked in castor oil should be placed on the wound, and then fixed on the wound with a bandage. Castor oil has tremendous drawing power and can pull out rust and other infectious agents. The dressing should be changed every two hours the first day of treatment and twice a day for the next three days.

Tetanus is easily preventable through vaccination. All children should have a series of five doses of DTaP, a combined vaccine that offers protection against diphtheria, tetanus, and pertussis, before the age of seven. This measure is supported by numerous organizations, including the World Health Organization, the Centers for Disease Control and Prevention, the Advisory Committee on Immunization Practices, the Committee on Infectious Diseases of the American Academy of Pediatrics, and the American Academy of Family Physicians. Children in the United States will not be admitted to school without proof of this and other immunizations.

The DTaP vaccine should be given at ages two months, four months, six months, 15-18 months, and four to six years. DTaP is the preferred vaccine for children up to the age of seven in the United States; it has fewer side effects than DTP and can be used to complete a vaccination schedule begun with DTP. DTaP was first approved by the Food and Drug Administration in September 1996. In December 1996, it was approved for use in infants. Between age 11 and 13, children should have a booster, called Td, for diphtheria and tetanus.

Adults should have a Td booster every 10 years. Statistics from the Centers for Disease Control and Prevention show that fewer than half of Americans aged 60 and older have antibodies against tetanus. The Centers for Disease Control and Prevention suggests that adults be revaccinated at mid-decade birthdays (for example, at 45). Adults who have never been vaccinated against tetanus should get a series of three injections of Td over six to 12 months and then follow the 10-year booster shot schedule.

Side effects of the tetanus vaccine are minor: soreness, redness, or swelling at the site of the injection that appear any time from a few hours to two days after the vaccination and disappear in a day or two. Rare but serious side effects that require immediate treatment by a doctor are serious allergic reactions or deep, aching pain and muscle wasting in the upper arms. These symptoms could start from two days to four weeks after the shot and could continue for months.

For those who are averse to immunizations, tetanus immunity can be boosted naturally by taking **vitamin E**, according to a study from Tufts University in Medford, Massachusetts. To get the most benefit, 200 mg should be taken daily.

Keeping wounds and scratches clean is important in preventing infection. Since *C. tetani* grows only in the absence of oxygen, the wounds must be adequately cleaned of dead tissue and foreign substances. Run cool water over the wound and wash it with a mild soap. Dry it with a clean cloth or sterile gauze. To help prevent infection, apply an antibiotic cream or ointment and cover the wound with a bandage. Try the castor oil remedy. The longer a wound takes to heal, the greater the chance of infection. Consult a doctor if the wound doesn't heal, if it is red or warm, or if it drains or swells.

If the wounded individual does not have an adequate history of immunization, a doctor may administer a specific antitoxin (human tetanus immune globulin, TIG) to produce rapid levels of circulating antibody. The antitoxin is given at the same time as a dose of vaccine but at a separate site.

Some persons will report a history of significant allergy to "tetanus shots." In most cases, the reaction occurred in the remote past and was probably caused by antitoxin derived from horse serum. More recently, however, the use of aluminum as an adjuvant, or substance added to a vaccine to increase the body's immune response, has been associated with skin eruptions and swelling in hypersensitive individuals. In some cases, these persons can be safely vaccinated for tetanus with a graduated series of shots. Adverse reactions of any kind to tetanus vaccine should be reported to the Center for Biologics Evaluation and Research (CBER) of the Food and Drug Administration (FDA).

KEY TERMS

Adjuvant—A substance added to a vaccine to stimulate a stronger immune response. Aluminum is commonly used as an adjuvant in tetanus vaccines.

Anaerobe—A type of bacterium that does not require oxygen to live. The tetanus bacterium is an anaerobe.

Clostridium—A genus of deadly bacteria that are responsible for tetanus and other serious diseases, including botulism and gangrene from war wounds. It thrives without oxygen.

DTaP—Diphtheria and tetanus toxoids and accellular pertussis combination vaccine.

DTP—Diphtheria, tetanus, and whole-cell pertussis vaccine.

Lockjaw—A common name given to the disease taken from its most pervasive symptom.

Td—The abbreviation for tetanus and diptheria vaccine.

Toxin—A poisonous substance, often produced by bacteria, that flows through the body.

Resources

BOOKS

Evelyn, Nancy. *The Herbal Medicine Chest.* Trumansburg, N.Y.: The Crossing Press, 1986.

Magill's Medical Guide, edited by Tracy Irons-Georges. Englewood Cliffs, N.J.: Salem Press, 1998.

PERIODICALS

Baylor, N. W., W. Egan, and P. Richman. "Aluminum Salts in Vaccines—US Perspective." *Vaccine* 20 (May 31, 2002)(Supplement 3): S18-S23.

Quddus, A., et al. "Neonatal Tetanus: Mortality Rate and Risk Factors in Loralai District, Pakistan." *International Journal of Epidemiology* 31 (June 2002): 648-653.

Rennels, M. B., M. A. Deloria, M. E. Pichichero, et al. "Lack of Consistent Relationship Between Quantity of Aluminum in Diphtheria-Tetanus-Acellular Pertussis Vaccines and Rates of Extensive Swelling Reactions." *Vaccine* 20 (May 31, 2002)(Supplement 3): S44-S47.

Shin, D. H., J. H. Park, P. J. Jung, et al. "A Case of Maternal Tetanus in Korea." *Journal of Korean Medical Science* 17 (April 2002): 260-262.

Williams, A. N., et al. "Tetanus Immunisation in Hypersensitive Individuals." *Journal of the Royal Army Medical Corps* 148 (June 2002): 148-150.

ORGANIZATIONS

Food and Drug Administration (FDA), Center for Biologics Evaluation and Research (CBER), 1401 Rockville Pike, Suite 200-N, Rockville, MD 20852. <www.fda.gov/cber>.

OTHER

Centers for Disease Control and Prevention. "Tetanus & Diphtheria (Td) Vaccine." *Healthtouch Online.* http://www.healthtouch.com/bin/EContent_HT/showAllLfts.asp.

"Shots for Safety." *National Institute on Aging Age Page.* www.nih.gov/nia/health/pubpub/shots.htm.

"TCM Herbal Database." *China-Med.net.* http://www.china-med.net/herb_search.html.

Lisa Frick
Rebecca J. Frey, PhD

Thai massage

Definition

Thai massage, also known as Nuad Bo-Rarn in its traditional form, is a type of Oriental bodywork therapy that is based on the treatment of the human body, mind, and spirit. The therapy includes treating the electromagnetic or energetic field which surrounds, infuses and brings the body to life through pressure and/or manipulative massage.

Origins

The origins of traditional Thai massage reportedly began over 2,000 years ago along with the introduction of Buddhism. It is one of four branches of traditional medicine in Thailand, the others being herbs, **nutrition**, and spiritual practice. The legendary historical creator of Thai medicine is Dr. Jivaka Kumar Bhaccha, known as Shivago Komarpaj in Thailand. Bhaccha was from the north of India and said to be a close associate of the Buddha and chief to the original community gathered around the Buddha. The movement of medicine into Thailand accompanied migration of monks from India to Thailand, possibly around the second century B.C.E. Thai medicine developed within the context of Buddhist monasteries and temples, where Thai have traditionally sought relief from all kinds of suffering.

While the recorded history of Thai massage was lost during the Burmese attack on the royal capital of Ayutthia in 1767, the surviving records are now inscribed in stone and can be found at the Sala Moh Nuat (massage pavilion) within the temple of Pra Chetuphon in Bangkok, known as Wat Po, the temple of the reclining Buddha. Its spiritual aspect also remains as teachers

of the therapy begin classes with the practice of *wai-kru,* a series of prayers and recitations dedicated to Shivago Komarpaj, the father of Thai massage and the Goddess of Healing, and teachers of the tradition through the centuries.

Benefits

The benefits of Thai massage are numerous, with the most predominant being the maintenance of good health and the ability to treat a wide spectrum of health concerns. Traditional Thai massage is known for its ability to clear the energy pathways.

The following are some of the benefits of traditional Thai massage.

• increases flexibility and range of movement

• eliminates muscle **pain** and muscle spasms

• improves postural alignment

• calms the nervous system and promotes a deep sense of **relaxation** with an increased energy level

• allows for a significant release of deep, emotional distress

• stimulates blood circulation and lymph drainage

• stimulates internal organs

• relieves **fatigue**, swollen limbs, painful joints, and headaches

Description

Thai massage looks like a cross between **acupressure**, **yoga**, and zen **shiatsu** and is inspired by Buddhist teachings. The actual massage consists of slow, rhythmic compressions and stretches along the body's energy lines, also called sen in Thai. Over 70,000 *sen* are said to exist within the body, and Thai massage concentrates on applying pressure along 10 of the most important sen, using the palms of the hands, thumbs, elbows, and feet. The effort from the practitioner works to free tension within the body. Practitioners also position the body into yoga-like poses and gently rock the body to open the joints and facilitate limbering.

A thorough Thai massage includes the following four basic positions:

• from the front with the client lying supine

• from the side with the client alternately lying on either side

• from the back with the client lying prone

• in a sitting position

One of the most important principles of Thai massage is the continuous flow of sequential movements that

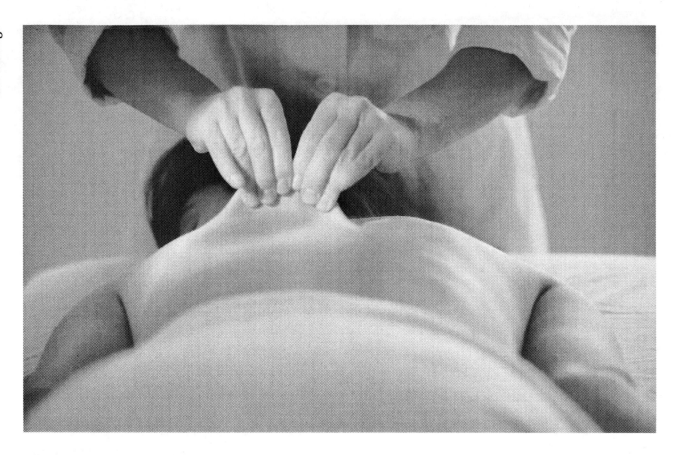

Thia massage therapist using techniques designed to alter the flow of qi, or energy, in the body. *(Photo Researchers, Inc. Reproduced by permission.)*

prepares the client for the next step in the massage. The practitioner is always aware of his position so that an uninterrupted slow rhythm is maintained. Deep, sustained pressure ensures that the myofascia, or the muscle's connective tissue, soften and relax in order to release the flow of energy along the sen, and to prepare the client for the large-scale stretches that follow.

There are two styles of practice, Northern (*Chiangmai*) and Southern (Bangkok). The former is considered gentler. The latter is faster and sometimes more intense. The Southern style is more widely used in Thailand, while the Northern style has become popular in the United States.

Preparations

The preparation needed before receiving a Thai massage is minimal. A Thai massage is typically performed on a floor mat-enabling practitioners to use their body weight and to incorporate the many movements that would not be possible with a massage table. Normally, the client remains fully clothed, and lubricant for the skin is rarely used. A Thai massage usually lasts one to two hours, but may be three hours or more if needed.

Precautions

While some of the pressure techniques used in Thai massage may seem too penetrating to many, most can adjust to it quickly. For those who are frail or stiff, a skilled practitioner will be able to adjust all of the soft tissue and manipulation work to their level of comfort.

Research & general acceptance

The practice of Thai massage is multinational. While a unique modality, Thai massage is slowly spreading into the western world. Knowledge of therapeutic benefits comes from anecdotal evidence rather than research in the Western scientific mode.

Training & certification

Thai massage can be strenuous for the practitioner. To become a Thai master, it is said that the best place to learn is where the therapy originates. The well known school at Wat Po in Bangkok and in Chiang Mai, The Institute of Thai Massage, both in Thailand, are famous for their teaching of the ancient art. It is also possible to re-

KEY TERMS

Buddhism—A philosophy founded in India in the sixth century B.C. and based on the teachings of the historical Buddha, born Siddartha Gautama.

Lymph—An alkaline fluid found in the lymphatic vessels that is usually clear, transparent fluid, unless it is draining from the intestines when it then appears milky.

ceive instruction in the United States from teachers who studied in Thailand, as well as from Thai instructors who came over to offer classes in American massage schools.

Practitioners of Thai massage are taught the most important aspects of the meditative spirit—awareness, mindfulness, and concentration. Correct body positioning and posture control while giving a massage are of vital importance to the practitioner in order to avoid injury, especially to the back.

Resources

PERIODICALS

Kallenbach, Laurel. "In Good Hands: Five hands-on therapies offer a combination of energy, reduced tension and a healing touch." *Delicious! Your magazine of Natural Living* (January 31, 2000).

Mercati, Maria. "The Healing Benefits of Oriental Massage." *Positive Health* (May 31, 1999).

Simpson, Ian. "Traditional Thai Massage." *Journal of the Australian Traditional-Medical Society* (June 30, 1998).

OTHER

American Oriental Bodywork Therapy Association. http://www.aobta.org.

Beth Kapes

The Zone diet *see* **Zone diet**

Therapeutic touch

Definition

Therapeutic touch, or TT, is a noninvasive method of healing derived from an ancient laying-on of hands technique. In TT, the practitioner alters the patient's energy field through a transfer of energy from the hands of the practitioner to the patient.

Origins

Therapeutic touch was developed in 1972 by Dora Kunz, a psychic healer, and Dolores Krieger, PH.D., R.N, a nurse and professor of nursing at New York University. In 1971, when Krieger had been working as a registered nurse in a hospital, she became very frustrated when one of her patients, a 30-year-old female, lay dying from a gallbladder condition. In desperation, she tried what she was learning from Kunz. After one treatment, the patient's condition began to mend; and she lived, surprising the other hospital staff. Krieger and Kunz met during the study of Oskar Estebany, a world renowned healer. They had invited Estebany to form a study group for three years, observing his work with patients. In this study, Estebany practiced healing on various patients using the laying-on of hands. Using her psychic and intuitive abilities, Kunz would observe and assist in the healing, while Krieger recorded the activities of the healing session and compiled profiles of the patients.

As the study progressed, Kunz began teaching Krieger how to heal, based on her perceptions of Estebany's healing techniques. During her research of ancient healing methods, Krieger concluded that the energy transfer between the healer and the recipient that takes place in a TT session is *prana*, an Eastern Indian word that means energy, vitality, and vigor. Krieger then combined her research with Kunz's techniques to develop TT.

TT was initially developed for use by persons in the health professions, but is currently taught worldwide to anyone who is interested in learning the technique. As of 1998, an estimated 100,000 people around the world have been trained in TT; 43,000 of those persons are healthcare professionals, many of whom use TT in conjunction with traditional medicine, as well as osteopathic, **chiropractic**, naturopathic, and homeopathic therapies. TT is taught in over 100 colleges, universities, and medical schools.

Benefits

The major effects of TT are **relaxation**, **pain** reduction, accelerated healing, and alleviation of psychosomatic symptoms. Studies have shown that TT has a beneficial effect on the blood, as it has the ability to raise hemoglobin values. It also affects brain waves to induce a relaxed state. TT can induce the relaxation response often within five minutes.

Krieger has said that it is not individual illnesses that validate the effectiveness of TT, but rather the body systems that are most sensitive to TT. She and others have found that the most sensitive body system is the autonomic nervous system (ANS), which, for example,

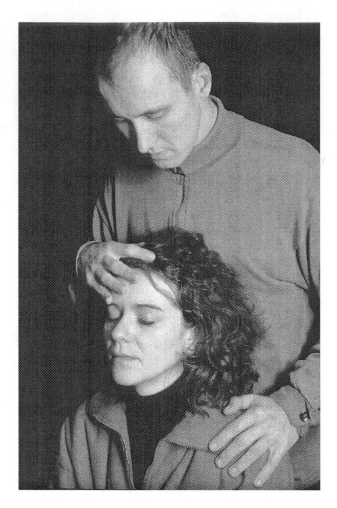

Man placing his hands on a woman's head and shoulder during touch, hand or therapeutic touch healing. *Photography by Cordelia Molloy/SPL/ Photo Researchers, Inc. Reproduced by permission.*

controls urination. Next in order of sensitivity are the lymphatic and circulatory systems, and then finally the musculoskeletal system. In addition, the female endocrine system is more sensitive to TT than the corresponding male system. Thus, TT helps with **dysmenorrhea**, amenorrhea, problems with conception, and the course of **pregnancy**.

TT is reported to have a positive effect on the immune system and thus accelerates the healing of **wounds**. Nurses use therapeutic touch in operating rooms to calm patients before surgery and in recovery rooms on postoperative patients to help speed the healing process. TT is used in the treatment of such terminally ill patients as those with **cancer** and acquired immune deficiency syndrome (**AIDS**), to relieve **anxiety** and **stress**, create peace of mind, and reduce pain.

Many nurses use TT in the nursery. The conditions of many premature babies who received TT have report-

edly improved rapidly. TT has been used to calm colicky infants, assist women in **childbirth**, and increase milk let-down in breast-feeding mothers.

Other claims made for TT include relief of acute pain, **nausea**, **diarrhea**, tension and migraine headaches, **fever**, and joint and tissue swelling. TT has been used to treat thyroid imbalances, ulcers, psychosomatic illnesses, **premenstrual syndrome**, **Alzheimer's disease**, **stroke** and coma, **multiple sclerosis**, **measles**, **infections**, **asthma**, and bone and muscle injuries.

Therapeutic touch is performed in many different locations, including healing centers, delivery rooms, hospitals, hospice settings, accident scenes, homes, and schools.

Description

Therapeutic touch treats the whole person: relaxes the mind, heals the body, and soothes the spirit. The principle behind it is that it does not stop at the skin. The human body has an energy field or aura that extends several inches to several feet from the body. When illness occurs, it creates a disturbance or blockage in the vital energy field. The TT practitioner uses her/his hands to sense the blockage or disturbance. In a series of gentle strokes, the healer removes the disturbance and rebalances the energy to restore health.

The TT session generally lasts about 20–30 minutes. Although the technique is called "therapeutic touch," there is generally no touching of the client's physical body, only his or her energetic body or field. TT is usually performed on fully clothed patients who are either lying down on a flat surface or sitting up in a chair.

Each session consists of five steps. Before the session begins, the practitioner enters a state of quiet **meditation** where he/she becomes centered and grounded in order to establish intent for the healing session and to gain access to the compassion necessary to heal.

The second step involves an assessment of the person's vital energy field. During this step, the practitioner places the palms of his/her hands 2–3 in (5–8 cm) from the patient's body and sweeps them over the energy field in slow, gentle strokes beginning at the head and moving toward the feet. The practitioner might feel heat, coolness, heaviness, pressure, or a prickly or tingling sensation. These cues, as they are called, signal blockages or disturbances in the field.

To remove these blockages and restore balance to the body, the practitioner then performs a series of downward sweeping movements to clear away any energy congestion and smooth the energy field. This is known as the unruffling process and is generally performed from the head toward the feet. To prevent any energy from clinging to him/her, the practitioner shakes his/her hands after each stroke.

During the next phase, the practitioner acts as a conduit to transfer energy to the patient. The energy used is not solely the energy of the practitioner. The practitioner relies on a universal source of energy so as not to deplete his/her own supply. In short, the healer acts as an energy support system until the patient's immune system is able to take over.

The practitioner then smoothes the field to balance the energy and create a symmetrical flow. When the session is over, it is recommended that the patient relax for 10–15 minutes in order for the energies to stabilize.

Side effects

The side effects reported occur when an excess of energy enters the body for an extended period of time creating restlessness, irritability, and hostility, or increasing anxiety and pain. **Burns** are sensitive to therapeutic touch, and it is recommended that TT be performed on burned tissue for short periods, generally two to three minutes at a time.

Research & general acceptance

Therapeutic touch is not generally accepted by Western medical professionals, although it has been studied by researchers at the Office of Alternative Medicine of the National Institutes of Health. Anecdotal research has been performed on TT since its development in 1972, but little quantitative research has been carried out. In April 1998 therapeutic touch became national news, however, when an elementary-school student carried out research for a science project that questioned the claims made for TT. Twenty-one TT practitioners with experience ranging from one to 27 years were blindfolded and asked to identify whether the investigator's hand was closer to their right hand or their left. Placement of the investigator's hand was determined by flipping a coin. The TT practitioners were able to identify the correct hand in only 123 (44%) of 280 trials, a figure that could result from random chance alone.

On the other side of the debate, one frequently cited study was designed to determine the effect TT would have on wounds that resulted from a biopsy of the upper arm. Forty-four patients placed their injured arms through a hole in a door. Twenty-two of them received TT on their arms. The other half received no treatment. The wounds treated with TT healed more quickly than the wounds that received no treatment.

In 1998, a study was performed on 27 patients with **osteoarthritis** in at least one knee. For six weeks, the patients were treated with therapeutic touch, mock thera-

DOLORES KRIEGER 1935–

Dolores Krieger, a prominent professor of nursing at the New York University Division of Nursing, conceived of therapeutic touch as a healing technique in the early 1970s and introduced the therapy in 1972. Therapeutic touch rarely consists of physical contact with the patient. The practitioner focuses positive energy through their hands, which are held or waved two to three inches away from the patient, and directs it towards the patient's energy field. Krieger developed the technique along with a colleague, Dora Van Gelder Kunz, who is believed to be clairvoyant. They initially taught the system to graduate students at the nursing school, and it evolved from that basis. Since the introduction of therapeutic touch, Krieger traveled the world in teaching the technique before she retired as professor emerita at the university. An estimated 70,000 nurses were trained by Krieger and Kunz.

In 1981 Dr. Krieger published *Foundations for Holistic Health Nursing Practices*. She later published a manual, *The Therapeutic Touch: How to Use Your Hands to Help or to Heal,* in 1992.

Krieger became embroiled in controversy over the potential benefits of therapeutic touch technique between 1996-98, when nine-year-old schoolgirl Emily Rosa challenged the validity of the therapy with a simple experiment. She gathered 21 practitioners and through a covered box held her hand over one of the practitioner's own to test whether they could sense her energy field. Only 44% of the time were the practitioners able to determine which of their hands that Rosa's was hovering over. Although Rosa contacted Krieger in 1997, Krieger refused to meet with her, refused to participate in Rosa's experiment, and disputed the relevancy of an elementary school student's observations. Krieger holds both an R.N. and a Ph.D. degree and dismissed the validity of the experiment due to the student's and practitioners' lack of experience.

Krieger continues to promote her technique. Her latest book, *Therapeutic Touch As Transpersonal Healing,* was published in 2002.

Gloria Cooksey

peutic touch, or standard care. According to *The Journal of Family Practice*, the results showed that the patients who had received TT had "significantly decreased pain and improved function as compared with both the placebo and control groups."

Therapeutic touch can be combined with a number of different therapies, including **acupressure**, massage, mental imagery, physical therapy, and **yoga**. When combined with massage and physiotherapy, TT may reduce tension headaches, back pain, stress-related problems, circulatory problems, and **constipation**. **Shiatsu** and TT may help sinusitis, digestive disorders, muscle cramps, menstrual difficulties, and **insomnia**. Yoga and TT may be beneficial in the treatment of **bronchitis**, asthma, blood pressure, **fatigue**, and anxiety.

TT is practiced in over 70 countries worldwide: by Egyptians and Israelis during fighting in the Gaza Strip; in South Africa to reduce racial strife; and in Poland, Thailand, and the former Soviet Union.

Training & certification

Therapeutic touch is taught at over 100 universities and nursing and medical schools around the United States and Canada. Although the technique was developed primarily for nurses, anyone can learn TT.

State laws vary regarding the practice of TT. In general, laypersons are allowed to practice TT within their families. Therapeutic touch is considered an extension of health care skills, so most health care professionals are covered under state medical practice acts.

Many hospitals have established policies allowing nurses and staff to perform TT on patients at no extra charge. The American Nurse's Association often holds workshops on TT at national conventions. Therapeutic touch classes are often held for the general public through community education, healing clinics, and holistic schools.

Resources

BOOKS

Krieger, Dolores, Ph.D., R.N. *Accepting Your Power to Heal. The Personal Practice of Therapeutic Touch.* Rochester, VT: Bear & Company, 1993.

Krieger, Dolores, Ph.D., R.N. *The Therapeutic Touch. How to Use Your Hands to Help or to Heal.* Saddle River, NJ: Prentice Hall Press, 1979.

Macrae, Janet, Ph.D., R.N. *Therapeutic Touch: A Practical Guide.* New York: Knopf, 1998.

PERIODICALS

Baird, Carol L. "First-line Treatment for Osteoarthritis: Part 2: Nonpharmacologic Interventions and Evaluation." *Orthopaedic Nursing* 20 (November-December 2001): 13–20.

Gordon, A., J. H. Merenstein, et al. "The Effects of Therapeutic Touch on Clients with Osteoarthritis of the Knee." *Journal of Family Practice* 47 (1998): 271–277.

Rosa, Linda, MSN, Emily Rosa, Larry Sarner, and Stephen Barrett, MD. "A Close Look at Therapeutic Touch." *Journal of the American Medical Association* 279 (April 1, 1998): 1005–11.

OTHER

The Nurse Healers Professional Associates International (NH-PAI), the Official Organization of Therapeutic Touch. 3760 S. Highland Drive, Salt Lake City, UT 84106. (801) 273-3399. nhpai@therapeutic-touch.org. <http://www.therapeutic-touch.org>.

Jennifer Wurges
Rebecca J. Frey, PhD

Thiamine

Description

Thiamine, also known as vitamin B_1, was the first of the water-soluble B-vitamin family to be discovered. It is an essential component of an enzyme, thiamine pyrophosphate, that is involved in metabolizing carbohydrates. Thiamine works closely with other B vitamins to assist in the utilization of proteins and fats as well, and helps mucous membranes and the heart to stay healthy. The brain relies on thiamine's role in the conversion of blood sugar (glucose) into biological energy to function properly. Thiamine is also involved in certain key metabolic reactions occurring in nervous tissue, the heart, in the formation of red blood cells, and in the maintenance of smooth and skeletal muscle.

General use

The recommended daily allowance (RDA) of thiamine is 0.3 mg for infants less than six months old, 0.4 mg for those from six months to one year old, 0.7 mg for children ages one to three years, 0.9 mg for those four to six years, and 1.0 mg for those seven to 10 years. Requirements vary slightly by gender after age 10. Males need 1.3 mg from 11 to 14 years, 1.5 mg from 15 to 50 years, and 1.2 mg when over age 50 years. Females require 1.1 mg from 11 to 50 years of age, and 1.0 mg if older than 50 years. The RDA is slightly higher for women who are pregnant (1.5 mg) or lactating (1.6 mg). Adults need a minimum of 1.0 mg of thiamine a day, but the requirement is increased by approximately 0.5 mg for each 1,000 calories of daily dietary intake over a 2,000-calorie base.

Thiamine has limited therapeutic use apart from supplements for people who are deficient or have significant risk factors for deficiency, such as **alcoholism**. High doses are used to treat some metabolic disorders, including certain enzyme deficiencies, Leigh's disease, and maple syrup urine disease. People suffering from diabetic neuropathy may sometimes benefit from additional thiamine. This supplementation should be taken only on the advice of a healthcare provider. Claims have been made that it can also help people with **Alzheimer's disease**, **epilepsy**, **canker sores**, **depression**, **fatigue**, **fibromyalgia**, and **motion sickness**. Improvement of these conditions based on supplementation with thiamine is unsubstantiated. Although a deficiency of thiamine may cause canker sores, taking extra amounts of the vitamin after they appear does not seem to help them heal.

Preparations

Natural sources

While all plant and animal foods have thiamine, higher levels of thiamine are found in many nuts, seeds, brown rice, seafood, and whole-grain products. Sunflower seeds are a particularly good source. Grains are stripped of the B vitamin content during processing, but it is often added back to breads, cereals, and baked goods. Legumes, milk, beef liver, and pork are other foods with high vitamin B_1 content. Thiamine is destroyed by prolonged high temperatures, but not by freezing. Food should be cooked in small amounts of water so that thiamine and other water-soluble vitamins don't leach out. Baking soda should not be added to vegetables, and fresh foods should be eaten to avoid sulfite preservatives. Both of these chemicals will break down the thiamine content found in foods. Drinking tea or alcohol with a meal will also drastically decrease the amount of thiamine that is absorbed by the body.

Supplemental sources

Thiamine is available in oral, intramuscular injectable, and intravenous formulations. Injectable formulas are usually preserved for persons who are severely thiamine deficient. Supplements should always be stored in a cool dry place, away from direct light, and out of the reach of children.

Deficiency

A deficiency of thiamine leads to a condition known as beriberi. Once common in sailors, it has become rare in the industrialized parts of the world except in cases of alcoholism and certain disease conditions. Beriberi is, however, frequently found in refugee camps and similar shelters for displaced persons. Infantile beriberi is presently the leading cause of death among the children of ethnic minority groups in southeast Asia. The syndrome typically causes poor appetite, abdominal **pain**, heart enlargement, **constipation**, weakness, swelling of limbs, muscle spasms, **insomnia**, and **memory loss**. Under treatment, the condition can resolve very quickly. Untreated beriberi will lead eventually to Wernicke-Korsakoff syndrome. These patients experience confusion, disorientation, inability to speak, gait difficulties, numbness or tingling of extremities, **edema**, **nausea**, **vomiting**, visual difficulties, and may progress to psychosis, coma, and death. Even in advanced states, this condition can be reversible if thiamine is given, nutritional status is improved, and use of alcohol is stopped.

Risk factors for deficiency

The leading risk factor for developing a deficiency of thiamine is alcoholism. Generally, alcoholics eat poorly, and therefore have a low dietary intake of thiamine and other vitamins to begin with. Alcohol also acts directly to destroy thiamine and increases the excretion of it. People with **cirrhosis** of the liver, malabsorption syndromes, diabetes, kidney disease, chronic **infections**, or hypermetabolic conditions also have increased susceptibility to thiamine deficiency. The elderly are more prone to poor nutritional status as well as difficulties with absorption, and may need a supplement. Others with nutritionally inadequate **diets**, or an increased need as a result of **stress**, illness, or surgery may benefit from additional vitamin B_1 intake since utilization is higher under these conditions. Those who diet or fast frequently may also be at risk for low levels of thiamine. Use of tobacco products, or carbonate and citrate food additives can impair thiamine absorption. A shortage of vitamin B_1 is likely to be accompanied by a shortage of other B vitamins, and possibly other nutrients as well. A supplement containing a balance of B complex and other vitamins is usually the best approach unless there is a specific indication for a higher dose of thiamine, or other individual vitamins.

Precautions

Thiamine should not be taken by anyone with a known allergy to B vitamins, which occurs rarely.

Side effects

In very unusual circumstances, large doses of thiamine may cause **rashes**, **itching**, or swelling. These reactions are more common with intravenous injections than oral supplements. Most people do not experience any side effects from oral thiamine.

KEY TERMS

Beriberi—A deficiency disease caused by insufficient thiamine in the diet. Its symptoms include abdominal cramps, muscle spasms, and memory loss.

Hypermetabolic—Conditions that increase the rate of metabolism, such as fever and hyperthyroidism.

Neuropathy—Abnormality of the nerves that may be manifested as numbness, tingling, or weakness of the affected area.

Wernicke-Korsakoff syndrome—A disorder of the central nervous system resulting from long-term thiamine deficiency. It is characterized by amnesia, confusion, visual problems, and unsteady gait; and is most commonly seen in alcoholics.

Interactions

Oral contraceptives, antibiotics, sulfa drugs, and certain types of diuretics may lower thiamine levels in the body. Consult a health care professional about the advisability of supplementation. Taking this vitamin may also intensify the effects of neuromuscular blocking agents that are used during some surgical procedures. B vitamins are best absorbed as a complex, and **magnesium** also promotes the absorption of thiamine.

Resources

BOOKS

Bratman, Steven, and David Kroll. *Natural Health Bible.* Rocklin, CA: Prima Publishing, 1999.

Griffith, H. Winter. *Vitamins, Herbs, Minerals & Supplements: The Complete Guide.* Arizona: Fisher Books, 1998.

Jellin, Jeff, Forrest Batz, and Kathy Hitchens. *Pharmacist's Letter/Prescriber's Letter Natural Medicines Comprehensive Database.* California: Therapeutic Research Faculty, 1999.

Pressman, Alan H., and Sheila Buff. *The Complete Idiot's Guide to Vitamins and Minerals.* New York: Alpha Books, 1997.

PERIODICALS

McGready, Rose, Julie A. Simpson, Thein Cho, et al. "Postpartum Thiamine Deficiency in a Karen Displaced Population." *American Journal of Clinical Nutrition* 74 (December 2001): 808–813.

OTHER

American Society for Nutritional Sciences. <http://www.nutrition.org>.

Judith Turner
Rebecca J. Frey, PhD

Thrombophlebitis *see* **Phlebitis**
Thrombus *see* **Blood clots**
Thrush *see* **Yeast infection**

Thuja

Description

Thuja is a general term for trees of the genus *Thuja*, which belongs to the Cupressaceae or cypress family. The most common species in North America are *Thuja occidentalis*, whose common names include arbor vitae or tree of life, white cedar, yellow cedar, American cedar, hackmatack, Thuia du Canada, swamp cedar, and Lebensbaum; and *Thuja plicata*, the Western **red cedar**. The species of cedar found in China and Japan is *Thuja orientalis*, and is known as ce bai ye or ya bai shu in Chinese.

Thujas are evergreen conifers, or cone-bearing trees. The name "Thuja" was given to this group of trees by the Swedish botanist Linnaeus in 1753; it comes from the Greek word *thuo*, which means "to sacrifice," as cedar wood was often burned with animal sacrifices by the ancients to add a pleasing aroma to the fire.

Thuja occidentalis is native to North America and grows in dense forests in southeastern Canada and the northeastern United States. American cedar trees grow to a height of about 60 ft (18.2 m), with trunks between 12 and 24 in (31 and 61 cm) in diameter. They are slow-growing trees, and prefer wet soils. American cedars are some of the oldest trees in northern woods; some are estimated to be at least 800 years old. *Thuja occidentalis* is conical in shape, with the lower branches almost horizontal to the ground and the upper branches more nearly vertical, forming a dense cone at the top of the tree. The leaves of the American cedar are bright green, opposite leaves that resemble overlapping scales, and give off a fragrant odor when crushed. The tiny yellow or greenish flowers appear between April and July. American cedar cones are pale green when young but turn a pale reddish-brown color as they mature.

The Western red cedar, or *Thuja plicata*, which is found from Alaska southward to the Pacific Northwest, Montana and Idaho, Alberta, and British Columbia, is similar in shape to *Thuja occidentalis*, except that it is a much taller tree, growing to a height of 150–200 ft (46–61 m). *Thuja orientalis*, on the other hand, is a short tree growing to a height of only 12–20 ft (4–6 m), and is sometimes used to form hedges, as it tolerates pruning. The Chinese cedar, however, is not as hardy as its North American counterparts.

Thuja is also the name for a homeopathic remedy made from *Thuja occidentalis*.

General use

Cedar trees in general have a long history of use for furniture and buildings as well as in various herbal remedies and **aromatherapy** preparations. According to the Old Testament, King Hiram of Tyre sent cedar wood from Lebanon to King Solomon for the construction of the Temple in Jerusalem. Cedar wood has also been used for centuries to line closets or make chests to protect clothing from moths. The fragrant wood was also used by Native Americans as well as the ancient Egyptians, Greeks, and Romans as an ingredient in incense blends.

In Western herbal medicine, cedar leaf oil was used as an emmenagogue, abortifacient, vermifuge, diuretic, and digestive aid. It was applied externally to relieve the pains of arthritis and rheumatism, to treat external **fungal infections** of the skin (ringworm and thrush), and to remove anal or **genital warts**. Native Americans used cedar leaf preparations to relieve **headache** and to prevent scurvy. Cedar leaves and twigs are in fact rich in **vitamin C**, and it was their effectiveness in preventing or treating scurvy that led to the tree's being called arbor vitae or tree of life. In addition, recent research has shown that extracts prepared from either *Thuja occidentalis* or *Thuja plicata* do in fact have antiviral, anti-inflammatory, and antibacterial properties. A group of German researchers reported in 2002 that an extract prepared from cedar leaf, alcohol, and water inhibits the reproduction of **influenza** virus type A, while a team of researchers in Japan found that an extract of Western red cedar was effective in treating **eczema**. Lastly, another group of Japanese researchers reported in 2003 that several compounds isolated from the stem bark of Japanese cedar appear to have significant antitumor activity.

In **traditional Chinese medicine**, the leaves and stems of *Thuja orientalis* are used to treat nervous disorders, **insomnia**, and heart palpitations, as well as to stop hemorrhages and bring down fevers. Traditional Chinese physicians also make a preparation of fresh cedar leaves steeped for seven days in a 60% alcohol solution to promote hair growth. The mixture is rubbed on the bald spots three times daily.

The homeopathic preparation known as *Thuja* is made from the leaves of *Thuja occidentalis*, and is given to treat soft or bleeding **warts** on the chin, genitals, or anus. The most widely used homeopathic *materia medica*, or reference book, also recommends *Thuja* for headaches that feel like a nail is being driven into the head; vertigo brought on by standing up; emotional **depression** and restlessness; **pain** or **itching** in the scalp; painful swallowing or a feeling of obstruction in the throat; intense thirst at night or early in the morning; stomach cramps that are worse in the evening; difficulty in breathing combined with a violent thirst for cold water; frequent need to urinate, with frothy or cloudy urine; insomnia or restless sleep; or **fever** and **chills** that grow worse toward evening.

In **aromatherapy**, cedar leaf oil is classified as a base note, which means that it has a very long-lasting scent when added to a perfume or incense blend. One Canadian producer of essential oil advises, "… the scent is strong and should be used sparingly. One small application is all you need!" It is considered to have a sedative or calming effect, and is recommended for treating **anxiety** states as well as **asthma**, **bronchitis**, and head colds. Some aromatherapists also recommend cedar leaf oil for treating **acne** and **dandruff**.

Cedar leaf oil is still used in some mainstream over-the-counter (OTC) preparations to relieve congestion in the upper respiratory tract. The best-known of these cold remedies is Vicks VapoRub™, which can be applied directly to the chest and covered with a hot towel, or added to a vaporizer to produce fragrant steam. Cedar leaf oil is also added to pest repellant sprays and paints to protect against mites, moths, and rodents. It is used to scent some brands of shoe polish, and is blended into some men's colognes, including Hugo Boss and Ralph Lauren's Safari.

Preparations

Most products used in Western medicine and aromatherapy that contain cedar oil are made with oil from the leaves and twigs of *Thuja occidentalis*. These parts of the tree yield about 1% volatile oil, which is about 65% thujone. The other components include fenchone, borneol, limonene, pinene, camphor, myrcene, a flavonoid known as thujin, and tannin. The essential oil is either clear or pale yellow in color. Most of the cedar leaf oil used in North America is made in Quebec by small family businesses; about 80% of their production is sold in the United States. The oil is extracted from the leaves by a process of steam distillation, cooled in an indirect contact heat exchanger, filtered, and stored in barrels for distribution to wholesalers.

According to a Canadian producer, essential oil from American cedar can be applied directly to picnic tables or outdoor furniture as a natural insect repellant, or to wooden drawers or closets to repel moths. A few drops of cedar leaf oil can also be added to a pail of warm water for damp-mopping hardwood floors. When the oil is used in aromatherapy, a few drops are mixed with several ounces of safflower or another vegetable oil for massages, or added to bath water for **hydrotherapy**.

Essential cedar leaf oil should never be applied directly to the skin, as it can cause irritation. It should be mixed with softened beeswax or a mild cream if used externally to treat aching muscles or joints. A 1/2-oz bottle of the oil costs about $10 in health food stores.

For internal use as a diuretic or expectorant, Western herbalists recommend taking 1/4-tsp of liquid extract of cedar leaf in a glass of water three to six times a day. Alternately, an infusion can be prepared by adding 1 ounce of fresh cedar leaves to a pint of boiling water. The infusion is taken cold in 1-tbsp doses every three to six hours.

Homeopathic preparations of *Thuja* include pills, granules, and liquid dilutions, in potencies ranging from 3X to 50M. The cost of these preparations ranges from $5.99 for a half-ounce container of 3X pills to $43.69 for a 1-oz (28-g) bottle of 50M liquid dilution. Tinctures of *Thuja* are sold only to homeopathic practitioners, and cost around $8 for a 1-oz bottle. Boiron, a well-known manufacturer of homeopathic remedies, also offers a *Thuja* ointment for the treatment of external warts; a 1-oz (28-g) tube costs between $5.05 and $7.24, depending on the supplier.

Incense made from pure cedar or containing a mixture of cedar and other fragrances is available in stick or cone form for prices ranging between $1.49 and $5 for two to four ounces of incense.

Precautions

Herbal preparations for internal use that contain cedar leaf oil should not be used by pregnant women, as the oil may cause contractions of the uterus. In addition, anyone using the essential oil for external applications is advised to consult either a professional aromatherapist or their physician beforehand, as the high content of thujone in cedar leaf oil is a health concern. Thujone in pure form is a neurotoxin, which means that it affects the central nervous system in humans and other mammals. Absinthe, a liqueur containing thujone derived from **wormwood**, can cause convulsions, hallucinations, and psychotic episodes. Absinthe has been banned in the United States, as have flavoring agents containing thujone. In addition to products containing thujone derived from wormwood, products made with cedar leaf oil have been investigated by the U. S. National Toxicology Program to make certain that workers involved in the manufacture of perfumes or other products scented with the oil were not at risk. The agency reported that the oil does not appear to be harmful to the skin or respiratory system under ordinary workplace conditions; all known instances of thujone poisoning since 1968 have been caused by drinking absinthe or undiluted **essential oils** of wormwood, **sage**, or cedar. With one exception, all these poisonings took place in France.

KEY TERMS

Abortifacient—A drug or preparation given to induce abortion.

Conifer—Any of several families of trees and shrubs, mostly evergreen, belonging to the order Coniferales, distinguished by bearing seeds and pollen in the form of dry scales arranged in a cone.

Emmenagogue—A medication or herbal preparation given to bring on a woman's menstrual period.

Expectorant—A medication or herbal preparation given to promote coughing, in order to bring up phlegm or other secretions from the upper respiratory tract.

Diuretic—A medication or preparation given to increase the body's output of urine.

Thujone—A natural compound found in the essential oils of cedar, wormwood, sage, mugwort, and clary. It is banned as a flavoring agent in the United States because of its neurotoxicity. Thujone is classified as a monoterpene ketone. It is insoluble in water, but can be dissolved in alcohol or chloroform.

Vermifuge—A medication or preparation given to expel worms and other intestinal parasites.

Volatile oil—Any plant oil that evaporates at room temperature and retains the odor of the plant from which it comes. Volatile oils are also called essential oils.

Side effects

No side effects have been reported as of 2004 from the use of perfumes, incense, aromatherapy products, pest repellants, or OTCs for external use that contain cedar leaf oil when used as directed. In addition, no side effects have been reported for homeopathic preparations containing *Thuja*.

Interactions

No interactions between products containing cedar oil and prescription medications have been reported as of early 2004.

Resources

BOOKS

Cummings, Stephen, MD, and Dana Ullman, MPH. *Everybody's Guide to Homeopathic Medicines*, revised ed. NY: G. P. Putnam's Sons, 1991.

Grieve, M., and C. F. Leyel, ed. *A Modern Herbal*, vol. 2. Mineola, NY: Dover Publications, Inc., 1971.

Price, Shirley. *Practical Aromatherapy*, 2nd ed. London: Thorsons, 1994.

Reid, Daniel P. *Chinese Herbal Medicine* . Boston: Shambhala, 1993.

PERIODICALS

Arima, Y., Y. Nakai, R. Hayakawa, and T. Nishino. "Antibacterial Effect of Beta-Thujaplicin on Staphylococci Isolated from Atopic Dermatitis: Relationship Between Changes in the Number of Viable Bacterial Cells and Clinical Improvement in an Eczematous Lesion of Atopic Dermatitis." *Journal of Antimicrobial Chemotherapy* 51 (January 2003): 113–122.

Bodinet, C., R. Mentel, U. Wegner, et al. "Effect of Oral Application of an Immunomodulating Plant Extract on Influenza Virus Type A Infection in Mice." *Planta Medica* 68 (October 2002): 896–900.

Iwamoto, M., T. Minami, H. Tokuda, et al. "Potential Antitumor Promoting Diterpenoids from the Stem Bark of *Thuja standishii*." *Planta Medica* 69 (January 2003): 69–72.

ORGANIZATIONS

Cèdres Recyclés. 60 Adrien Robert, Hull, Quebec, Canada J8Y 3S2. (819) 771-3446. Fax: (819) 771-0067. <http://cedarleaf.org>.

National Toxicology Program (NTP) Liaison and Scientific Review Office. P. O. Box 12233, MD A3-01, Research Triangle Park, NC 27709. (919) 541-0530. <http://ntp-server.niehs.nih.gov>.

Valley Cedar Leaf Oil. RR #5, Eganville, Ontario, Canada K0J 1T0. (613) 628-2892. <http://www.valleycedarleafoil.com>.

OTHER

National Toxicology Program (NTP). *Summary of Data for Chemical Selection Alpha-Thujone 546-80-5*. <http://ntp-server.niehs.nih.gov/htdocs/Chem_Background/ExecSumm/Thujone.html>.

Rebecca J. Frey, PhD

Thuja occidentalis see **Thuja**

Thunder god vine

Description

Thunder god vine (*Tripterygium wilfordii*) is the English translation of the Chinese name for the perennial plant *lei gong teng*. The plant grows in the mountains of China, as well as Taiwan and Myanmar (formerly Burma). It is a deciduous climbing vine that sheds its leaves, and produces white flowers and red fruit with three "wings." The plant's leaves, flowers, and outer skin of the root are poisonous. In fact, honey taken from the plant's pollen is also poisonous. The root pulp is the nonpoisonous part, which is used medicinally. There is a risk of poisoning if the herb is not extracted properly.

The potentially dangerous aspects of this plant are reflected in two of its Chinese folk names, "Walk Seven Steps and Die" and "Intestine-Breaking Plant." In Asia, the plant is also called "three-wing-nut."

In ancient China, practitioners carefully extracted the portion of the thunder god vine used for treatment. They gathered roots in the summer or early fall. The poisonous bark was removed and the inner portion of the root was utilized. In past centuries, this procedure may have involved grinding the root into a powder. The remedy usually was applied topically to the skin, since there was a risk of poisoning if thunder god vine was taken orally.

General use

Use of thunder god vine in **traditional Chinese medicine** dates back thousand of years. Ancient Chinese practitioners used the root of thunder god vine to treat a range of conditions including **rheumatoid arthritis**, swelling, skin **infections** and leprosy, **fever**, **boils**, and **chills**. However, practitioners were aware that the plant could be deadly. In fact, it was likely used as a murder weapon. Farmers in Asia also used thunder god vine as an insecticide.

In the latter half of the twentieth century, interest again turned to the healing potential of thunder god vine. Research of the remedy included a double-blind trial performed in China during the 1980s. Among the researchers was the physician Xue-Lian Tao, a former post-doctoral fellow at University of Texas Southwestern Medical Branch (UTSMB). In the study, the scientists and the research subjects (over 2,000 patients) did not know whether participants received the extract or a placebo. Patients reported that the remedy reduced the symptoms of rheumatoid arthritis.

Tao returned to the United States and continued research with Dr. Peter Lipsky, then-director of the Harold C. Simmons Arthritis Center at the University of Texas. Research in the United States focused on finding a safe dosage of thunder god vine and locating the part of the plant that appeared to ease arthritis **pain**. Lipsky reported that in 1994 the team evaluated the toxicity of the vine, and found "very little" toxicity, thus reducing the possibility of poisoning. They also saw the potential in the herbal remedy.

During the 1990s, researchers at UTSMB studied the plant's effectiveness in treating the symptoms of inflammatory conditions such as rheumatoid arthritis (RA). If thunder god vine is proven safe and effective for medical treatment of RA, researchers hope it may also be approved to treat other autoimmune conditions. These include lupus (a rheumatic condition that affects the skin and tissue, producing symptoms of rash, joint pain, and inflammation) and psoriasis—this inflammatory condition causes portions of the skin to raise, turn red, and scale. By 1998, the research team had developed a root extract from the plant that could be studied for its effectiveness in providing relief of arthritis symptoms. They named the extract "Texas Ethyl Acetate" (TEA), and applied to the United States Food and Drug Administration (FDA) for permission to test the extract on arthritis patients.

The FDA issued permission for the thunder god vine research using root extract. Studies were done through UTSMB and the National Institutes of Health (NIH). In 1999, Lipsky was named scientific director of NIH's National Institute of Arthritis and Muscoskeletal and Skin Diseases (NIAMS).

In 2002, NIAMS announced the results of a 20-week study involving 21 rheumatoid arthritis patients. Patients received a high-dose extract, low-dose extract, or a placebo. After four weeks, rapid improvement in symptoms was reported by 80% of those in the high-dose group, and in 40% of low-dose participants. No change was reported by people who took placebos. Lipsky rated the results as promising, saying that the extract slowed down an overactive immune system.

Response to the NIAMS study was generally positive. However, some scientists noted that the test group was small and the trial lasted only 20 weeks. Lipsky announced in 2002 that additional research was planned, using thunder god vine to treat RA and conditions such as lupus.

Prior to the NIAMS study, researchers imported thunder god vine root extract from China, where its medicinal use stretches back thousands of years. In 2002, after news of the NIAMS study was released, it was announced that Phytomedics Inc., a New Jersey biopharmaceutical company, was growing thunder god vine. Phytomedics Inc. renamed the extract "PMI-001," and announced plans to develop a botanical drug for the treatment of arthritis. The New Jersey-based company partnered with Pfizer, another pharmaceutical company, to manufacture the drug. As of 2004, the PMI-001 product had not been brought to the FDA.

Preparations

The remedy portion of thunder god vine is the vascular part of the root, the interior section consisting of cells that carry water and food to the plant. The plant interior is dried and cut into pieces for processing.

Thunder god vine is available in the United States, where it has been advertised as a Chinese herb that may offer temporary relief for conditions such as aches, joint pain, colds, **fatigue**, **insomnia**, **stress**, and **anxiety**. The herbal remedy has been sold on the Internet, where a California business offers thunder god vine in pill form. The business recommended a daily dosage of two pills taken with warm water.

After UTSMB received approval from the FDA, researchers extracted the active ingredient from the plant. The process involved extracting ethanol and acetate from the root. The extract powder was then packaged into capsules.

According to the Arthritis Foundation, some research participants took a daily dosage of 30 milligrams of thunder god vine extract.

Precautions

As of 2004, no standard safe dosage of thunder god vine had been established. The herb's use as a diet supplement has not been evaluated for safety or content of the product. Herbal supplements are not regulated by the FDA; therefore, ordering this product carries risks. The consumer has no assurance about the strength of the dosage or the portion of the plant used to make the supplement.

In the United States, thunder god vine cannot be marketed as a drug until it receives FDA approval, a process that includes evaluation of a product for safety and effectiveness. This preliminary review is not required for herbs marketed as diet supplements. However, the FDA can stop the sale of supplements determined to be unsafe.

The leaves and flowers of thunder god vine are very toxic and may cause death. Extreme caution in purchasing is advised to ascertain that the supplement is a proper extraction made only from the interior of the plant root.

Side effects

Thunder god vine is toxic and could be lethal if not properly extracted.

In the Chinese 1980s double-blind trial, some people experienced **diarrhea** and related gastrointestinal disturbances. Tao reported that those side effects disappeared as people continued treatment. Moreover, side effects in the NIAMS study were described as "minor."

According to the Arthritis Foundation, possible side effects of thunder god vine include upset stomach and skin reactions. Men may experience temporary **infertility**, while women may stop having menstrual periods (amenorrhea).

Interactions

People taking immunosuppressive drugs such as prednisone should not use thunder god vine.

Resources

PERIODICALS

Balick, Michael J., and Roberta Lee. "Digging in the Herb Garden: Responding to a Patient's Query About Thunder God Vine." *Alternative Therapies* (November/December 2001): 100–3.

OTHER

DeNoon, Daniel. "Chinese Herb May Ease Arthritis." (August 13, 2002. *WebMD* [cited April 30, 2004]. <http:// www.my. webmd.com>.

Freeman, Elizabeth. "Chinese Thunder God Vine Gives Relief from Rheumatoid Arthritis Symptoms." National Institute of Arthritis and Musculoskeletal and Skin Diseases. October 2002. [cited April 30, 2004]. <http://www.niams.nih. gov/ne/highlights/spotlight/2002/thunder.htm>.

National Institute of Arthritis and Musculoskeletal and Skin Diseases. [cited April 30, 2004]. <http://www.niams.nih.gov>.

Phytometics Inc. [cited April 30, 2004]. <http://www.phy-tometics.com>.

United States Food and Drugs Administration. [cited April 30, 2004]. <http://www.fda.gov>.

University of Texas Southwestern Medical Center. [cited April 30, 2004] <http://www.swmed.edu>.

Liz Swain

Thyme

Description

Thyme (*Thymus vulgaris L.*), known as garden thyme, and *T. serpyllum*, known as creeping thyme, mother of thyme, wild thyme, and mountain thyme, are two similarly beneficial evergreen shrubs of the Lamiaceae or mint family. The aromatic thyme is a perennial native of southern Europe and the western Mediterranean. Thyme is extensively culti-vated, both commercially and in home gardens, as a culinary and medicinal herb. There are hundreds of species of thyme.

Garden thyme grows from a woody, fibrous root to produce thin, erect, stems up to 15 in (38 cm) high. It is most commonly cultivated for its culinary uses. Wild thyme is found growing on heaths, in sheep pastures, and mountainous areas in temperate regions. It was probably introduced to North America by European colonists, and has escaped cultivation. Wild thyme produces long, low-lying, sprawling and creeping stems. This habit inspired the designation *serpyllum* referring to the serpent-like growth of the species. Thyme has tiny narrow gray-green leaves that grow in opposite pairs on the square woody stems. The edges of the stalkless, and slightly hairy leaves are rolled inward. The blossoms may be white to rose-colored or a blue to purple hue, depending on the species and variety. Flowers are tiny and tubular and grow in terminal clusters up to 6 in (15.2 cm) long. Flowering time is mid-summer. Seeds are minuscule and abundant. Thyme thrives in sunny locations on dry stony banks and heaths. The aromatic herb attracts bees that produce a uniquely flavored honey from the herb. It also acts to repel whiteflies.

Thyme has been known since ancient times for its magical, culinary, and medicinal virtues. Tradition held that an infusion of thyme taken as a tea on midsummer's eve would enable one to see the fairies dancing. Young women wore a corsage of blossoming thyme to signal their availability for romance. The generic name may have been inspired by one of thyme's traditional attributes. Greek folk herbalists believed that thyme would impart courage (*thumus* in Greek) to those who used the herb, particularly soldiers. Greek men particularly liked the pungent scent of thyme and would rub the herb on their chests. The Romans believed that adding thyme to bath water would impart energy. They also included thyme in bedding to chase melancholy and to prevent nightmares. The strong scent of thyme was employed as a moth repellent, and burned as fumigating incense. The philosopher-herbalist Pliny the **Elder** recommended burning the dried herb in the house to "put to flight all venomous creatures." In the kitchen thyme has been used for centuries to season sauces, soups, stuffing, and soups. Thyme has long been recognized for its antiseptic properties. The Egyptians used the herb in formulas for embalming the dead. The herb was among those burned in sickrooms to help stop the spread of disease. Oil of thyme was used on surgical dressings and in times of war as recently as World War I, to treat battle **wounds**.

General use

The fresh and dried leaf, and the essential oil extracted from the fresh flowering herb, are medicinally potent. Thyme is one of the most versatile herbs for use in home remedies. It is aromatic, antiseptic, diaphoretic (increases

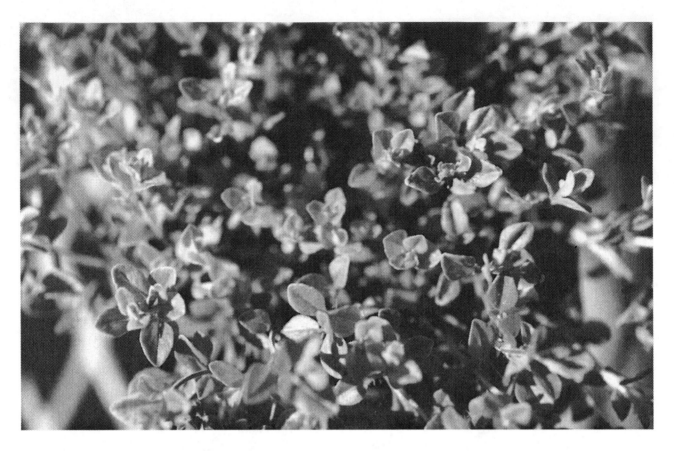

Thyme plant. *(Photo by Kelly Quinn. Reproduced by permission.)*

perspiration), analgesic, antispasmodic, and diuretic. It acts as an emmenagogue (brings on the menstrual discharge), carminative (expels **gas**), and stimulant. Thyme's essential oil contains a crystalline phenol known as thymol, a powerful and proven antibiotic and disinfectant that enhances the immune system and fights infection. The aromatic and medicinal strength of the essential oil varies with the species harvested. The essential oil exerts a swift and effective action against bacteria. With external application, the essential oil is especially good for maintaining the health of the teeth and gums and relieving **toothache**. An ointment made with the essential oil is used to disinfect cuts and wounds, and is effective against the fungi that cause athletes' foot. As a massage oil, thyme can relieve rheumatism, **gout**, and **sciatica** (**pain** along the course of a sciatic nerve, especially in the back of the thigh). As an ingredient in a lotion used as a chest rub, thyme will help break up catarrh (inflammation of the mucous membrane) of the upper respiratory tract. A strong decoction of the leaves and flowers, added to the bath water, will stimulate circulation. When used as a hair rinse, combined with a scalp massage, the herb decoction may help to prevent **hair loss**.

Taken internally as an infusion or syrup, thyme is an effective remedy for ailments of the respiratory, digestive, and genitourinary systems. The herb relaxes the bronchial muscles, helping to quell dry coughs. The warm infusion can relieve migraine **headache**, **colic**, and flatulence, promote perspiration, and expel **worms**. A strong decoction, sweetened with honey, is good for easing the spasms of whooping **cough** and expelling catarrh. The infused herb can be used as a gargle for **sore throat**. Taken warm, thyme tea will bring relief for menstrual pain, and relieve **diarrhea**. Thyme has an antioxidant effect and is a good tonic and digestive tea. The phytochemicals (plant chemicals) in thyme include tannins, **bitters**, essential oil, terpenes, flavonoids, and saponins.

Preparations

The aerial parts of thyme can be harvested before and during flowering. The leaves should be removed from the woody stems and placed in single layers on a paper-lined tray in a warm airy room out of direct sunlight, or hung to dry in bunches in a shady location. The dried leaf should be stored in dark glass, tightly sealed, and clearly labeled containers. Thyme can also be frozen for later use.

Infusion: Two ounces of fresh thyme leaf (less if dried) are placed in a warmed glass container, and 2.5

cups of fresh nonchlorinated boiling water are added to the herbs. Twice as much herb is used in preparing an infusion for use as a gargle or bath additive. The tea should be covered and infused from 10-30 minutes, depending on the strength desired. After straining, the prepared tea will store for about two days in the refrigerator. Thyme tea may be enjoyed by the cupful as a tonic beverage taken after meals up to three times a day.

Tincture: Four ounces of finely-cut fresh or powdered dry herb are combined with 1 pt of brandy, gin, or vodka in a glass container. There should be enough alcohol to cover the plant parts and have a 50:50 ratio of alcohol to water. The mixture is stored away from light for about two weeks, and needs to be shaken several times each day. The mixture is strained and then stored in a tightly-capped, dark glass bottle. A standard dose is one-half to one teaspoon of the tincture, taken in hot water, up to three times a day.

Essential oil: Commercial extracts of essential oil of thyme are available. These are not to be taken internally. The essential oil must be diluted in water or vegetable oil, such as almond or sunflower oil, before applying to minimize the toxicity. The oil contains thymol, a component in many commercially available antiseptics, mouthwash, toothpaste, and gargle preparations. It is antibacterial and antifungal.

Precautions

Very small amounts of thyme used in culinary preparations are generally safe. In large amounts, thyme acts as a uterine stimulant. Pregnant women should not use the herb, tincture, or essential oil of thyme.

Excessive use of undiluted essential oil is toxic. If the oil is ingested, it may cause gastrointestinal distress such as diarrhea, **nausea**, and **vomiting**. Other adverse toxic effects may include headache, muscular weakness, and **dizziness**. The oil of thyme may act to slow the heartbeat, depress respiration, and lower body temperature. Applied externally in undiluted form the essential oil may cause skin irritation. The oil should be diluted before use.

Side effects

The U. S. Food and Drug Administration (FDA) has rated thyme as "food safe." The *PDR For Herbal Medicine* lists "No health hazards or side effects" when the herb is properly administered in designated therapeutic dosages.

Interactions

None reported as of 2004.

Resources

BOOKS

Duke, James A., Ph.D. *The Green Pharmacy.* PA: Rodale Press, 1997.

Elias, Jason, and Shelagh Ryan Masline. *The A to Z Guide to Healing Herbal Remedies.* New York: Lynn Sonberg Book Associates, 1996.

Foster, Steven, and James A. Duke. *Peterson Field Guides, Eastern/Central Medicinal Plants.* Boston-New York: Houghton Mifflin Company, 1990.

Gibbons, Euell. *Stalking The Healthful Herbs, Field Guide Edition.* New York: David McKay Company, Inc., 1974

Hutchens, Alma R. *A Handbook Of Native American Herbs.* Boston: Shambhala Publications, Inc., 1992.

Kowalchik, Claire, and William H.Hylton. *Rodale's Illustrated Encyclopedia of Herbs.* PA: Rodale Press, 1987

Lust, John. *The Herb Book* New York: Bantam Books, 1974.

Magic And Medicine of Plants. Pleasantville, NY: the Reader's Digest Association, Inc. 1986.

McIntyre, Anne. *The Medicinal Garden.* New York: Henry Holt and Company, Inc., 1997.

Meyer, Joseph E. *The Herbalist.* Glenwood, IL: Clarence Meyer, 1973.

Ody, Penelope. *The Complete Medicinal Herbal.* New York: Dorling Kindersley, 1993.

PDR for Herbal Medicines. NJ: Medical Economics Company, 1998.

Phillips, Roger, and Nicky Foy. *The Random House Book of Herbs.* New York: Random House, Inc., 1990.

Polunin, Miriam, and Christopher Robbins. *The Natural Pharmacy.* New York: Macmillan Publishing Company, 1992.

Prevention's 200 Herbal Remedies. Pennsylvania: Rodale Press, Inc., 1997.

Schar, Douglas. *The Backyard Medicine Chest, An Herbal Primer.* Washington, DC: Elliott & Clark Publishing, 1995.

Thomson, M.D., William A. R. *Medicines From The Earth, A Guide to Healing Plants.* San Francisco: Harper & Row, 1978.

Tyler, Varro E., Ph.D. *Herbs of Choice, The Therapeutic Use of Phytomedicinals.* NY: The Haworth Press, Inc., 1994

ORGANIZATIONS

National Association of Holistic Aromatherapy. 836 Hanley Industrial Court, St. Louis, MO 63144. 888-ASK-NAHA. http://www.naha.org.

Clare Hanrahan
Teresa G. Odle

TIA *see* **Stroke**

Tibetan medicine

Definition

Tibetan medicine differs from allopathic medicine in that it has no concept of illness as such, but rather the concept is of disharmony of the organism. Accordingly, this system of medicine, like many alternative therapies, seeks to achieve a harmony of the self.

Medicine is one of five branches of Tibetan science, and is known to the Tibetans as *gSoba Rig-pa*—the science of healing. The Tibetan pharmacopoeia utilizes many different elements in the treatment of disease, such as trees, rocks, resins, soil, precious metals, sap, and so on, but like Chinese medicine, to which it is related, it mainly relies on herbs for treatment.

Origins

Tibetan medicine, like its relative Chinese medicine, is an ancient art that has become associated with many legends and is surrounded by a cloud of mysticism. Although Tibetan culture is more recent, Tibetan medical practices can be traced back over 2,500 years. It is now practiced in secret or by those in exile since Communist rule has suppressed it in its country of origin.

The treatise of Tibetan medicine, which can be described as a manual compiled over thousands of years, is called the *Chzud-shi*. In addition to the medical theory, this manual also incorporates the Tibetan pharmacopoeia.

Benefits

Tibetan medicine has been particularly successful at treating chronic conditions such as rheumatism, arthritis, **ulcers, digestive** problems, **asthma**, **hepatitis, eczema**, liver disorders, sinus problems, emotional disorders and nervous system problems. Like many alternative therapies, it is a holistic therapy that treats the whole person and encourages a healthy way of life that will promote well-being at all levels.

Description

Harmony and the balance of all aspects of the human organism are the concepts that form the basis for Tibetan medicine. The three elements that must be kept in harmony are known collectively as the *Nyipa sum*, and they are *rLung, mKhris-pa,* and *Bad-kan.* It is said that the Tibetan words describing their medicine are very difficult to translate, rather an explanation of the meaning is attempted. Desire, hatred, and delusion are considered to be very harmful influences affecting this harmony, and illustrate the close connection between the Tibetan medical art and Buddhist teachings.

rLung is considered to be a "subtle flow of energy" that is most closely connected with the "air" element. However, since all five elements; earth, water, fire, air and space, in addition to the concepts of heat and cold play a complex role in the health of the individual, this is no simple matter. All elements and aspects are held to be interdependent.

Types of rLung:

- *Srog-'dzin* (life-grasping rLung). Located in the brain, this energy governs swallowing of food, breathing, spitting, **sneezing**, and the clearing and steadying of the mind.
- *Gyen-rgyu* (rLung moving upwards). Located in the chest, it governs speech, physical vigor, general health, and appearance of skin.
- *Khyab-byed* (all pervading rLung). Located in the stomach, it governs digestion, metabolism, and the seven physical sustainers referred to as lus-zung dhun.
- *Thur-sel* (downward cleansing rLung). Located in the rectum, it governs the elimination of waste products and reproductive fluids in addition to the birth process (for women).

Types of mKhris-pa:

- *mKhris-pa* is the heat of human nature, related to fire, described as oily, sharp, hot, light, pungent and moist. Its major function is to balance body temperatures. It governs hunger and thirst, and regulates skin condition. There are five types of mKhris-pa:
- *Ju-byed.* This is located between the stomach and the intestine. Governs digestion and assimilation, providing heat and energy.
- *SGrub-byed.* Located in the heart. Responsible for anger, aggression, and hatred, and is considered to lead to desire, achievement, and ambition.
- *mDangs-sgur.* Located in the liver, it is responsible for maintaining and promoting color and essential components of blood.
- *mThong-byed.* Located in the eye, it governs vision.
- *mDog-sel.* Located in the skin, it governs skin appearance and texture.

Types of Bad-kan:

- *rTen-byed* (supporting Bad-kan). Located in the chest, plays a supporting role to the other four types of Bad-kan.

- *Myag-byed* (mixing Bad-kan). Located in the upper half of the body. Mixes nutrients (liquids and solids).

- *Myong-byed* (experiencing Bad-kan). Located in the tongue, governs experience of taste.

- *Tsim-byed* (satisfaction Bad-kan). Located in the head. Governs the five senses and responsible for heightening their power.

- *Byor-byed* (joining Bad-kan). Located in the joints, it is considered responsible for their flexibility.

When these components of *Nyipa sum* are balanced, the seven bodily sustainers will also be in harmony. They are essential nutrients, blood, muscle tissue, fat, bone, marrow, and reproductive fluids.

Diagnosis

A practitioner of Tibetan medicine will employ several diagnostic tools. Chief of these is a very complicated system of pulse reading, which involves 13 different positions with a possibility of over 300 different readings. This is similar to **traditional Chinese medicine** and **Ayurvedic medicine**. The pulse is likened to a messenger between doctor and patient. For this diagnosis to be effective, it is necessary for the patient to be rested and relaxed.

Another tool of diagnosis is observation, which consists of urinalysis and examining the tongue. To examine the urine, a physician will assess the color, vapor, odor, bubbles, sediments, and albumin content. The color of urine is determined by food and drink, the seasons, and whatever diseases the patient suffers from.

The final tool of diagnosis is questioning. The physician will ask specific questions of his patient, and will include such questions as how and when the illness started, where **pain** is felt, and if the condition is affected by foods eaten.

Treatment

Treatment is divided into four categories, which are dietary advice, lifestyle recommendations, the prescription of medicine, and if necessary, surgical procedures, according to the type of patient. Treatment proceeds in this order according to the seriousness of the disorder. For example, minor problems are considered to need merely a reassessment of dietary habits, but only in the most serious cases will surgery be considered.

Preparations

A Tibetan physician prescribes medicines and recommends surgery as a last resort. When it is necessary, the prescription is likely to be made up from certain herbs in the form of a decoction, powder, or pills. The prescription will be made up at one of the branches of the Tibetan Medical Institute specifically for each patient.

Precautions

The qualifications of any Tibetan physician should be checked before treatment proceeds.

Side effects

As a natural therapy, Tibetan medicine, if administered correctly, is not known to be associated with any side effects. According to the primary Tibetan medical treatise, one of the criteria for medical prescriptions is that they should be absolutely harmless.

Research & general acceptance

The Tibetan system of medicine has roots in medical practices over 2,500 years old, so it can be considered well researched. Despite the Communist crackdown in Tibet, and the oppression and persecution of their physicians, the Tibetan people still prefer to seek the advice of a traditional physician rather than take advantage of "new" systems of medicine.

In 1994, the Natural Medicine Research Unit, (NMRU) of Hadassah University Hospital in Jerusalem began a double-blind randomized clinical trial of Tibetan herbal formulas which had been on sale in Switzerland for more than seventeen years. Previous trials had already demonstrated the harmlessness of these formulas. The aim of the unit is to compile a database of Tibetan formulas.

Training & certification

The headquarters of the main Tibetan medical institute is now in Dharamsala in northern India. Tibetan medicines are also manufactured there. The minimum period of training for a Tibetan physician is seven years. The first five years mainly consist of theoretical training, and for the sixth and seventh years, medical students are sent for a period of practical training under a senior physician at one of the Institute's branches, of which there are over 30 in India and Nepal.

Resources

BOOKS

Clark, Barry, ed. *The Quintessence Tantras of Tibetan Medicine.* Ithaca, NY: Snow Lion Publications, 1995.

Donden, Yeshi. *Healing from the Source.* Ithaca, NY: Snow Lion Publications, 2000.

ORGANIZATIONS

The official website of the exiled Tibetan government. http://www.tibet.com/Med_Astro/tibmed.html.

OTHER

World around BaiKal. http://www.pitt.edu/~jpc7/baikal/5.htm.

Patricia Skinner

Tinea pedis *see* **Athlete's foot**

Tinnitus

Definition

Tinnitus is a condition where the patient hears ringing, buzzing, or other sounds without an external cause. Patients may experience tinnitus in one or both ears or in the head.

Description

Tinnitus affects as many as 40 million adults in the United States. It is defined as either objective or subjective. In objective tinnitus, the doctor can hear the sounds as well as the patient. Objective tinnitus is typically caused by tumors, turbulent blood flow through malformed vessels, or by rhythmic muscular spasms. Most cases of tinnitus are subjective, which means that only the patient can hear the sounds.

Causes & symptoms

Subjective tinnitus is frequently associated with **hearing loss** and damage to the cochlea, or the inner ear. About 90% of patients have sensorineural hearing loss; 5% suffer from conductive hearing loss; and 5% have normal hearing.

The causes of subjective tinnitus include:

- impacted ear wax
- ear **infections**
- hardening of the structures of the inner ear
- hearing loss related to age
- prolonged exposure to excessive noise
- ototoxic medications, including aspirin, quinine, some diuretics, heavy metals, alcohol, and certain antibiotics
- Ménière's syndrome
- head trauma
- systemic diseases, including **syphilis**, **hypertension**, **anemia**, or hypothyroidism
- tumors of the ear

Diagnosis

Diagnosis of tinnitus includes a physical examination of the patient's head and neck. The doctor will use an instrument called an otoscope to examine the ears for wax, infection, or structural changes. He or she will also use a stethoscope to listen to the blood vessels in the neck.

The patient's doctor may also refer him or her to an audiologist, who is a health care professional trained to perform diagnostic testing of hearing problems.

In some cases, tinnitus is a symptom of **temporo-mandibular joint disorder**, or TMJ, which is caused by dysfunction of the temporomandibular joint in the jaw. The muscles and nerves in the jaw are located very close to the nerves that control hearing, which is why TMJ can cause tinnitus. Patients with tinnitus may be referred to a dentist or orthodontist for assessment of their jaw muscles or a misaligned bite.

Additional tests may include the following:

Tuning fork tests

The Rinne and Weber tests are commonly used to evaluate the type and severity of hearing loss. In the Weber test, the doctor holds a tuning fork against the patient's forehead or front teeth. If the hearing loss is sensorineural, the sound radiates to the ear with better hearing; if the hearing loss is conductive, the sound will be louder in the damaged ear. In the Rinne test, the tuning fork is placed alternately on the mastoid bone, which is behind the ear, and then in front of the ear. In conductive hearing loss, bone conduction (BC) is greater than air conduction (AC). In sensorineural hearing loss, AC is greater than BC.

Diagnostic imaging

Magnetic resonance angiography or venography (MRA and MRV) can be used to evaluate malformations of the blood vessels. Computed tomography scans (CT scans) or magnetic resonance imaging scans (MRIs) can be used to locate tumors or abnormalities of the brain stem.

Blood tests

The doctor may order a complete blood count (CBC) with specific antibody tests to rule out syphilis or immune system disorders.

Treatment

Dietary adjustments, including the elimination of coffee and other stimulants, may be useful in treating tinnitus. In addition, reducing the amount of fat and **cholesterol** in the diet can help improve blood circulation to the ears. Nutritional supplementation with **vitamin C**, **vitamin E**, B vitamins, **calcium**, **magnesium**, **potassium**, and **essential fatty acids** is also recommended.

In particular, **zinc** supplements have been recommended for patients diagnosed with tinnitus. A recent Turkish study has confirmed that older people whose **diets** have been deficient in zinc may benefit from supplements of this mineral as a treatment for tinnitus, but that younger patients eating well-balanced diets do not find that their symptoms improve when they take zinc supplements. The American Tinnitus Association comments that zinc supplements "… generally carry little risk to health and some people find them helpful."

Gingko biloba, an herbal extract, has been shown to decrease tinnitus symptoms in controlled animal studies and may be helpful in treating humans, since it is believed to enhance circulation to the brain in situations where reduced circulation is the cause. Individuals taking such blood thinners as coumadin or heparin should not take *Ginkgo biloba,* as the herb can interfere with platelet activating factor, the chemical that enables blood to clot.

Acupuncture treatments may help decrease the level of tinnitus sounds the patient hears, and constitutional homeopathic treatment may also be effective. Some Chinese herbal treatments can be effective, as well.

Tinnitus Retraining Therapy, or TRT, has been successful in treating some subjective tinnitus patients. This therapy is based on the assumption that the severity of tinnitus is determined not by the patient's auditory system, but by the parts of the brain that control emotion (the limbic system) and body functions (autonomic nervous system). TRT focuses on habituating the patient to his or her tinnitus, retraining the brain to, in effect, "become used to" the tinnitus so that it does not perceive it as an annoyance.

Allopathic treatment

Some cases of tinnitus can be treated by removal of the underlying cause. These include surgical treatment of impacted ear wax, tumors, head injuries, or malformed blood vessels; discontinuance of ototoxic medications; and antibiotic treatment of infections.

Patients whose tinnitus is related to TMJ usually experience improvement in or complete disappearance of the tinnitus when the dental problem is corrected.

Subjective tinnitus, especially that associated with age-related hearing loss, can be treated with hearing **aids**, noise generators or other masking devices, **biofeedback**, antidepressant medications, or lifestyle modifications.

One mainstream form of **psychotherapy** that is recommended to patients with tinnitus is cognitive-behavioral therapy, or CBT. CBT works by changing the patient's emotional reaction to the tinnitus. The patient keeps a symptom diary and works on an individual basis with a counselor to identify negative thought patterns and behaviors related to the tinnitus and then changes them. The latest innovation in CBT for tinnitus is therapy via the Internet. According to a 2002 study by a group of Swedish researchers, 31% of patients who participated in a CBT program via the Internet reported significant relief from tinnitus at 1-year follow-up.

Expected results

The prognosis depends on the cause of the tinnitus and the patient's emotional response. Most patients with subjective tinnitus do not find it seriously disturbing, but about 5% have strong negative feelings. These patients are frequently helped by instruction in **relaxation** techniques.

Studies indicate that CBT is most effective as a treatment for tinnitus when it is combined with masking techniques or medication.

Prevention

One preventive measure is to wear earplugs when operating loud machinery or spending extended periods in such noisy environments as rock concerts. Prolonged exposure to noises of 90 decibels (about as loud as a running blender) or higher can cause permanent hearing loss and tinnitus. In some cases a change of occupation may be advisable; a recent British study found that as many as 266,000 men and 84,000 women in the United Kingdom between the ages of 35 and 64 suffer from tinnitus resulting from work-related noise.

More detailed information and advice on dealing with tinnitus associated with noise-induced hearing loss is available from the National Institute on Deafness and Communication Disorders (NIDCD), listed under Resources below.

Resources

BOOKS

House, John W. "Tinnitus." In *Conn's Current Therapy,* edited by Robert E. Rakel. Philadelphia: W. B. Saunders, 1998.

Jackler, Robert K., and Michael J. Kaplan. "Ear, Nose, & Throat." In *Current Medical Diagnosis & Treatment 1998*, edited by Lawrence M. Tierney, Stephen J. McPhee, and Maxine Papadakis. Stamford, CT: Appleton & Lange, 1997.

Pelletier, Kenneth R., MD. *The Best Alternative Medicine*, Part II, "CAM Therapies for Specific Conditions: Tinnitus." New York: Simon & Schuster, 2002.

"Tinnitus." Section 7, Chapter 82 in *The Merck Manual of Diagnosis and Therapy*, edited by Mark H. Beers, MD, and Robert Berkow, MD. Whitehouse Station, NJ: Merck Research Laboratories, 2001.

PERIODICALS

Andersson, G., T. Stromgren, L. Strom, and L. Lyttkens. "Randomized Controlled Trial of Internet-Based Cognitive Behavior Therapy for Distress Associated with Tinnitus." *Psychosomatic Medicine* 64 (September-October 2002): 810–816.

Delb, W., R. D'Amelio, C. J. Boisten, and P. K. Plinkert. "Evaluation of the Tinnitus Retraining Therapy as Combined with a Cognitive Behavioral Group Therapy" [in German] *HNO* 50 (November 2002): 997–1004.

Henry, J. A., M. M. Jastreboff, P. J. Jastreboff, et al. "Assessment of Patients for Treatment with Tinnitus Retraining Therapy." *Journal of the American Academy of Audiology* 13 (November-December 2002): 523–544.

Jastreboff, P.J., W.C. Gray, and S.L. Gold. "Neurophysiological Approach to Tinnitus Patients." *American Journal of Otology* 17 (1996): 236–240.

Palmer, K. T., M. J. Griffin, H. E. Syddall, et al. "Occupational Exposure to Noise and the Attributable Burden of Hearing Difficulties in Great Britain." *Occupational and Environmental Medicine* 59 (September 2002): 634–639.

Schechter, M. A., and J. A. Henry. "Assessment and Treatment of Tinnitus Patients using a 'Masking Approach.'" *Journal of the American Academy of Audiology* 13 (November-December 2002): 545–558.

Yetiser, S., F. Tosun, B. Satar, et al. "The Role of Zinc in Management of Tinnitus." *Auris Nasus Larynx* 29 (October 2002): 329–333.

ORGANIZATIONS

American Academy of Audiology. 11730 Plaza America Drive, Suite 300, Reston, VA 20190. (703) 790-8466. <www.audiology.org>.

American Tinnitus Association. P.O. Box 5, Portland, Oregon 97207-0005. (800) 634-8978 or (503) 248-9985. <www.ata.org>.

Better Hearing Institute. 515 King Street, Suite 420, Alexandria, VA 22314. (703) 684-3391.

National Institute on Deafness and Other Communication Disorders (NIDCD), National Institutes of Health. 31 Center Drive, MSC 2320. Bethesda, MD 20892-2320. <www.nidcd.nih.gov>.

Vestibular Disorders Association (VEDA). PO Box 4467, Portland, OR 97208-4467. (800) 837-8428. <www.vestibular.org>.

OTHER

National Institute on Deafness and Other Communication Disorders (NIDCD). *Noise-Induced Hearing Loss* . Bethesda, MD: NIDCD, 2002. NIH Publication No. 97-4233. <www.nidcd.nih.gov/health/hearing/noise/asp>.

Paula Ford-Martin
Rebecca J. Frey, PhD

Tonsillitis

Definition

Tonsillitis is an infection and swelling of the tonsils, which are oval-shaped masses of lymph gland tissue located on both sides of the back of the throat.

Description

The tonsils normally help to prevent **infections**. They act like filters to trap bacteria and viruses entering

KEY TERMS

Audiologist—A healthcare professional who performs diagnostic testing of impaired hearing.

Cochlea—The hearing part of the inner ear. This snail-shaped structure contains fluid and thousands of microscopic hair cells tuned to various frequencies, in addition to the organ of Corti (the receptor for hearing).

Conductive hearing loss—Hearing loss caused by loss of function in the external or middle ear.

Ménière's syndrome—A disease of the inner ear, marked by recurrent episodes of loss of balance (vertigo) and roaring in the ears lasting several hours. Its cause is unknown.

Ototoxic—Damaging to the nerves controlling the senses of hearing and balance.

Sensorineural hearing loss—Hearing loss caused by damage to the nerves or parts of the inner ear that control the sense of hearing.

the body through the mouth and sinuses. The tonsils also stimulate the immune system to produce antibodies which fight off infections. Anyone can have tonsillitis; however, it is most common in children between the ages of five and 10 years.

Causes & symptoms

Tonsillitis is caused by viruses or bacteria that cause the tonsils to swell and become inflamed. A mild or severe **sore throat** is one of the first symptoms of tonsillitis. Symptoms can also include **fever**, **chills**, lethargy, muscle aches, **earache**, **pain** or discomfort when swallowing, and swollen glands in the neck. Young children may be fussy and stop eating. When a doctor or nurse looks into the mouth with a otoscope, the tonsils may appear swollen and red. Sometimes they will have white or yellow spots and a thin mucous coating. Symptoms usually last four to six days.

Diagnosis

The diagnosis of tonsillitis is made from the visible symptoms and a physical examination of the patient. The doctor will examine the eyes, ears, nose, and throat, looking at the tonsils for signs of swelling, redness, or a discharge. A careful examination of the throat is necessary to rule out diphtheria and other conditions that may cause a sore throat. Since most sore throats in children are caused by viruses rather than bacteria, the doctor may take a throat culture or rapid diagnostic test in order to test for the presence of streptococcal bacteria. A throat culture is performed by wiping a cotton swab across the tonsils and back of the throat and sending the swab to a laboratory for culturing. *Streptococcus pyogenes*, the bacterium that causes **strep throat**, is the most common disease agent responsible for tonsillitis. Depending on what type of test is used for strep, the doctor may be able to determine within a few minutes if *S. pyogenes* is present. The quick tests for strep are not as reliable as a laboratory culture, which can take 24-48 hours. If the results of a quick test are positive, however, the doctor can prescribe antibiotics right away. If the quick test results are negative, the doctor can do a throat culture to verify the results and wait for the laboratory report before prescribing antibiotics. A blood test may also be done to rule out a more serious infection or condition, and to check the white blood cell count to see if the body is responding to the infection. In some cases, the doctor may order blood tests for **mononucleosis**, since about a third of patients with mononucleosis develop infections in the tonsils.

Treatment

Treatment of tonsillitis usually involves keeping the patient comfortable while the illness runs its course. This

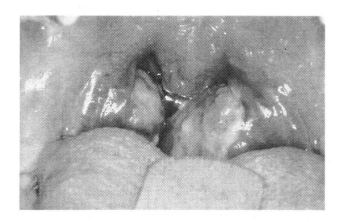

An examination of this patient's mouth reveals acute tonsillitis. *(Custom Medical Stock Photo. Reproduced by permission.)*

supportive care includes bed rest, drinking extra fluids, gargling with warm salt water, and taking pain relievers to reduce fever. Frozen juice bars and cold fruit drinks can bring some temporary relief of sore throat pain and drinking warm tea or broth can be soothing.

Strengthening the immune system is important whether tonsillitis is caused by bacteria or viruses. Naturopaths often recommend dietary supplements of **vitamin C**, **bioflavonoids**, and beta-carotenes—found naturally in fruits and vegetables—to ease inflammation and fight infection. A variety of herbal remedies also may be helpful in treating tonsillitis. **Calendula** (*Calendula officinalis*) and cleavers (*Galium aparine*) target the lymphatic system, while **echinacea** (*Echinacea spp.*) and **astragalus** (*Astragalus embranaceus*) stimulate the immune system. **Goldenseal** (*Hydrastis canadensis*), **myrrh** (*Commiphora molmol*), and bitter orange (*Citrus aurantium*) act as antibacterials. *Lomatium dissectum* and *Ligusticum porteri* have an antiviral action.

Some of the homeopathic medicines that may be used to treat symptoms of tonsillitis include *Belladonna, Phytolacca, Mercurius, Lycopodium, Lachesis, Hepar sulphuris, Arsenicum,* or *Rhus toxicodendron.* As with any condition, the treatment and dosage should be appropriate for the particular symptoms and age of the patient. Other demulcent herbs include teas made with **slippery elm** bark, **wild cherry**, and **licorice**.

Allopathic treatment

If the throat culture shows that *S. pyogenes* is present, penicillin or other antibiotics will be prescribed. An injection of benzathine or procaine penicillin may be most effective in treating the infection, but it is also painful. If an oral antibiotic is prescribed, it must be taken for the full course of treatment, which is usually 10-14 days.

Shaw, Michael. "Tonsillitis." In *Everything You Need to Know about Diseases*. Springhouse, PA: Springhouse Corporation, 1996.

Kathleen D. Wright

KEY TERMS

Streptococcus pyogenes—A common bacterium that causes strep throat and can also cause tonsillitis.

Tonsils—Oval-shaped masses of glandular tissue located on both sides at the back of the throat. Tonsils act like filters to trap bacteria and viruses.

Expected results

Tonsillitis is usually resolved within a few days with rest and supportive care. Treating the symptoms of sore throat and fever will make the patient more comfortable. If fever persists for more than 48 hours, however, or is higher than 102°F (39°C), the patient should be seen by a doctor. If antibiotics are prescribed to treat an infection, they should be taken as directed for the complete course of treatment, even if the patient starts to feel better in a few days. Prolonged symptoms may indicate that the patient has other upper respiratory infections, most commonly in the ears or sinuses. An **abscess** behind the tonsil (a peritonsillar abscess) may also occur. In rare cases, a persistent sore throat may point to more serious conditions such as **rheumatic fever** or **pneumonia**.

Prevention

The bacteria and viruses that cause tonsillitis are easily spread from person to person. It is not unusual for an entire family or several students in the same classroom to come down with similar symptoms, especially if *S. pyogenes* is the cause. The risk of transmission can be lowered by avoiding exposure to anyone who already has tonsillitis or a sore throat. Drinking glasses and eating utensils should not be shared and should be washed in hot, soapy water before reuse. Old toothbrushes should be replaced to prevent reinfection. People who are caring for someone with tonsillitis should wash their hands frequently, to prevent spreading the infection to others.

Resources

BOOKS

Berkow, Robert. "Tonsillitis." In *The Merck Manual of Diagnosis and Therapy*. Rahway, NJ: Merck Research Laboratories, 1992.

Eckman, Margaret, and Nancy Priff. "Ear, Nose, and Throat Disorders: Tonsillitis." In *Diseases*. Springhouse, PA: Springhouse Corporation, 1997.

Inlander, Charles B., ed., et al. "Tonsillitis." *The Consumer's Medical Desk Reference*. New York: A Stonesong Press Book, 1995.

Norris, June. "Tonsillitis." In *Professional Guide to Diseases*. Springhouse, PA: Springhouse Corporation, 1995.

Toothache

Definition

A toothache is any **pain** or soreness within or around a tooth, indicated by inflammation and infection.

Description

A toothache may feel like a sharp pain or a dull, throbbing ache. The tooth may be sensitive to pressure, heat, cold, or sweets. In cases of severe pain, identifying the problem tooth is often difficult. Any patient with a toothache should see a dentist at once for diagnosis and treatment. Most toothaches get worse if not treated.

Causes & symptoms

Toothaches may result from any of a number of causes:

- tooth decay (dental caries)
- inflammation of the tooth pulp (pulpitis)
- abscesses
- **gum disease**, including periodontitis
- loose or broken filling
- cracked or impacted tooth
- exposed tooth root
- food wedged between teeth or trapped below the gum line
- tooth nerve irritated by clenching or grinding of teeth (bruxism)
- pressure from congested sinuses
- traumatic injury

Diagnosis

Diagnosis includes identifying the location of the toothache, as well as the cause. The dentist begins by asking the patient specific questions including increased sensitivity or if the pain is worse at night. The patient's mouth is then examined for signs of swelling, redness, and obvious tooth damage. The presence of pus indicates

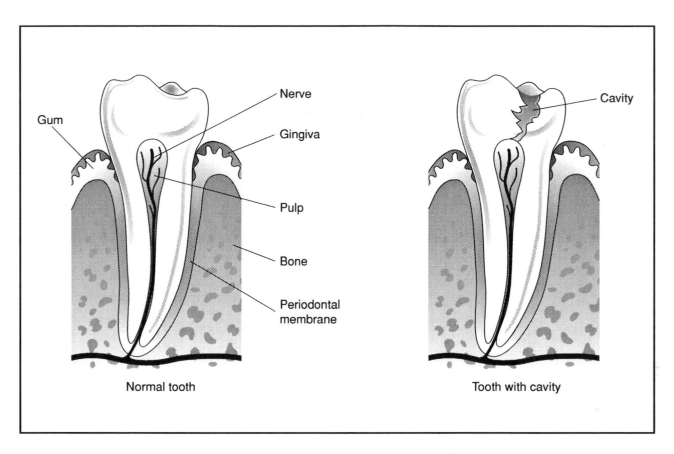

Tooth decay is the destruction of the outer surface, or enamel, of a tooth. It is caused by acid buildup from plaque bacteria, which dissolves the minerals in the enamel and creates cavities. *(Illustration by Electronic Illustrators Group. The Gale Group.)*

an **abscess** or gum disease. The sore area is flushed with warm water to dislodge any food particles and to test for sensitivity to temperature. The dentist may then dry the area with gauze to determine sensitivity to pressure. Finally, the dentist may take x rays, looking for evidence of decay between teeth, a cracked or impacted tooth, or a disorder of the underlying bone.

Treatment

Emergency self-care

Toothaches should always be professionally treated by a dentist. Some methods of self-treatment, however, may help manage the pain until professional care is available:

• Rinsing with warm salt water.

• Using dental floss to remove any food particles.

• Taking aspirin or acetaminophen (Tylenol) to relieve pain. The drug should be swallowed—*never* placed directly on the aching tooth or gum.

• Applying a cold compress against the outside of the cheek. Do not use heat, because it will tend to spread infection.

• Using clove oil (*Syzygium aromaticum*) to numb the gums. The oil may be rubbed directly on the sore area or used to soak a small piece of cotton and applied to the sore tooth.

• A washcloth soaked in **chamomile** tea and placed on the infected tooth or swished around in the mouth will help to ease the pain.

Toothaches caused by infection or tooth decay must be treated by a dentist. Several alternative therapies may be helpful for pain relief until dental treatment is available. The herb **corydalis** (*Corydalis yanhusuo*) may also help relieve toothache pain. Pain also may be reduced using **acupressure**, **acupuncture**, or **reiki**. Acupuncture should be done only by a licensed practitioner.

Allopathic treatment

Treatment will depend on the underlying cause of the toothache. If the pain is due to tooth decay, the dentist will remove the decayed area and restore the tooth with a filling of silver amalgam or composite resin. Loose or broken fillings are removed, decay cleaned out, and a new filling is placed. If the pulp of the tooth is damaged, root canal therapy is needed. The dentist or endodontist removes the decayed pulp, fills the space left behind with a soothing paste, and covers the tooth with a crown to protect and seal it. If the damage cannot be treated by these methods, the tooth must be extracted.

Expected results

Prompt dental treatment provides a positive outcome for a toothache. In the absence of active infection, fillings, root canal treatments, or extractions may be performed with minimal discomfort to the patient. When a toothache is left untreated, a severe infection may develop and spread to the sinuses or jawbone, and eventually cause **blood poisoning**.

Prevention

Maintaining proper oral hygiene is the key to the prevention of toothaches. The best way to prevent tooth decay is to brush at least twice a day, preferably after every meal and snack. Flossing once a day also helps prevent gum disease by removing food particles and bacteria at and below the gum line, as well as between teeth. People should visit their dentist at least every six months for oral examinations and professional cleaning.

Resources

ORGANIZATIONS

Academy of General Dentistry. Suite 1200, 211 East Chicago Avenue, Chicago, IL 60611. (312) 440-4300. http://www.agd.org.

Alliances, Inc. 2121 Eisenhower Avenue, Suite 603, Alexandria, VA 22314. (800) 463-6482. http://www.medsource.com.

American Dental Association. 211 East Chicago Avenue, Chicago, IL 60611. (312) 440-2500. http://www.ada.org.

Kathleen Wright

▌ Tourette syndrome

Definition

Tourette syndrome (TS) is an inherited disease of the nervous system, first described more than a century ago by a pioneering French neurologist, George Gilles de la Tourette. Before they are 18 years of age, patients with TS develop motor tics; that is, repeated, jerky, purposeless muscle movements in almost any part of the body. Patients also develop vocal tics, which occur in the form of loud grunting or barking noises, or in some cases words or phrases. In most patients, the tics come and go, and are often replaced by different sounds or movements. The tics may become more complex as the patient grows older.

Description

TS is three times more common in men than in women. The motor tics, which usually occur in brief episodes several times a day, may make it very hard for the patient to perform such simple acts as tying shoelaces, not to mention work-related tasks or driving. In addition, TS may have negative effects on the patient's social development. Some patients have an irresistible urge to curse or use offensive racial terms (a condition called coprolalia), although these impulses are not under voluntary control. Other people may not enjoy associating with TS patients. Even if they are accepted socially, TS patients live in fear of offending others and embarrassing themselves. In time, they may close themselves off from former friends and even relatives.

It is important to note, however, that the symptoms of Tourette syndrome are not always dramatic and are often overlooked in people with mild cases of the disorder. A 2001 report published in *Pain & Central Nervous System Week*, in fact, states that TS is much more common than doctors had thought. A study of 1,596 special-education children in Rochester, NY, found that 8% met the criteria for TS, and 27% had a tic disorder. In Rochester's general population, 3% were found to have Tourette syndrome, and 20% had a tic disorder. The rate of 3% in the general population is 50–75 times higher than the usual estimates given.

The tics of TS are often described as involuntary, meaning that patients cannot stop them. This description is not strictly true, however. A tic is a very strong urge to make a certain motion or sound. It is more like an itch that demands to be scratched. Some patients are able to control their tics for several hours, but once they are allowed expression, they are even stronger and last longer. Tics become worse when the patient is under **stress**, and usually are much less of a problem during sleep.

Some people with TS have trouble paying attention. They often seem grumpy and may have periods of **depression**. TS patients may think the same thoughts over and over, a mental tic known as an obsession. It is these features that place TS patients on the border between diseases of the nervous system and psychiatric illness. In fact, before research showed that the brains of TS patients undergo abnormal chemical changes, many doctors were convinced that TS was a mental disorder. It still is not clear whether these behaviors are a direct result of TS itself or a reaction to the stress of having to live with the disease.

Causes & symptoms

Causes

Tourette syndrome has been linked to parts of the brain known as the basal ganglia, which regulate movements and are involved in concentration, paying attention, and decision-making. Research has also demonstrated that in TS there is a malfunction in the brain's production or use of important substances called neurotransmitters. Neurotransmitters are chemicals that control the signals that are sent along the nerve cells. The neurotransmitters dopamine and serotonin have been implicated in TS; noradrenaline is thought to be the most important stimulant. Medications that mimic noradrenaline may cause tics in susceptible patients.

TS has a genetic component. If one parent has TS, each child has a 50% chance of getting the abnormal gene. Seven of every 10 girls who inherit the gene, and nearly all boys who inherit it, will develop symptoms of TS. Overall, about one in every 2,500 persons has full-blown TS. Three times as many will have some features, usually chronic motor tics or obsessive thoughts. Patients with TS are more likely to have trouble controlling their impulses, to have **dyslexia** or other learning problems, and to talk in

their sleep or wake frequently. Compulsive behavior, such as constantly washing the hands or repeatedly checking that a door is locked, is a common feature of TS. Compulsions are seen in 30–90% of all TS patients.

Recent research findings suggest that Tourette syndrome may also be related to an autoimmune response. A subset of TS patients have symptoms triggered by infection with Group A beta-hemolytic streptococci. In addition, blood serum antibodies against human basal ganglia have been found in patients with TS.

Symptoms

Motor tics in TS can be classified as simple or complex. Simple tics are sudden brief movements involving a single group of muscles or a few groups that may be repeated several times. Complex tics consist of a repeated pattern of movements that can involve several muscle groups and usually occur in the same order. For instance, a boy with TS may repeatedly move his head from side to side, blink his eyes, open his mouth, and stretch his neck. Vocal tics may be sounds or noises that lack all meaning, or repeated words and phrases that can be understood. Tics tend to get worse and better in cycles, and patients can develop new tics as they grow older. The symptoms of TS may get much better for weeks or months at a time, only to worsen later.

The following examples show why TS can be such a strange and dramatic disorder:

- Simple motor tics. These may include blinking the eyes, pouting the lips, shaking or jerking the head, shrugging the shoulders, and grimacing or making faces. Any part of the body may be tensed up or rapidly jerked, or a patient may suddenly kick. Rapid finger movements are common, as are snapping the jaws and clicking the teeth.

- Complex motor tics. These may include jumping, touching parts of the body or certain objects, smelling things over and over, stamping the feet, and twirling about. Some TS patients throw objects, others arrange things in a certain way. Biting, head-banging, writhing movements, rolling the eyes up or from side to side, and sticking out the tongue may all be seen. A child may write the same letter or word over and over, or may tear apart papers and books. Though they do not intend to be offensive, TS patients may make obscene gestures like "giving the finger," or they may imitate any movements or gestures made by others.

- Simple vocal tics. These include clearing the throat, coughing, snorting, barking, grunting, yelping, and clicking the tongue. Patients may screech or make whistling, hissing, or sucking sounds. They may repeat sounds such as "uh, uh," or "eee."

• Complex vocal tics and patterns. Older children with TS may repeat a phrase such as "Oh boy," "All right," or "What's that?" Or they may repeat everything they or others say a certain number of times. Some patients speak very rapidly or loudly, or in a strange tone or accent. Coprolalia (saying "dirty words" or suggestive or hostile phrases) is probably the best known feature of TS, but fewer than one-third of all patients display this symptom.

Behavioral abnormalities that may be associated with TS include attention deficit hyperactivity disorder (ADHD) and disruptive behaviors, including conduct disorder and oppositional defiant disorder, with aggressive, destructive, antisocial, or negativistic behavior. Academic disorders, **learning disorders**, and sleep abnormalities (such as sleepwalking and nightmares) are also seen in TS patients.

Diagnosis

There are no specific tests for TS. TS is diagnosed by observing the symptoms and asking whether relatives have had a similar condition. To qualify as TS, both motor and vocal tics should be present for at least a year and should begin before age 18 (or, some believe, age 21). Often, the diagnosis is delayed because the patient is misunderstood not only at home and at school, but in the doctor's office as well. It may take some time for the patient to trust the doctor enough not to suppress the strangest or most alarming tics. Blood tests may be done in some cases to rule out other movement disorders. A test of the brain's electrical activity (electroencephalograph or EEG) is often abnormal in TS, but not specific. A thorough medication history is very important in making the diagnosis as well, because stimulant drugs may provoke tics or aggravate the symptoms of TS.

Treatment

Although there is no cure for TS, many alternative treatments may lessen the severity and frequency of the tics. These include:

• **Acupuncture**. In one study, acupuncture treatment of 156 children with TS had a 92.3% effective rate.

• Behavioral treatments. Some of these can help TS patients control tics. A large variety of these methods exist, some with proven success.

• Cognitive **behavioral therapy**. This form of therapy helps the patient to change his or her ingrained response to a particular stimulus. It is somewhat effective in treating the obsessive-compulsive behaviors associated with TS.

• Neurofeedback (electroencephalographic **biofeedback**). In neurofeedback, the patient learns to control brain wave patterns; it may be effective in reducing the symptoms of TS. There are, however, no data on this modality as a treatment for TS.

• Psychotherapy. This form of treatment can help the TS patient, and his or her family, cope with depression, poor relationships, and other issues commonly associated with TS.

• **Relaxation** techniques. **Yoga** and progressive muscular relaxation are believed to help TS, especially when used in combination with other treatments, because they lower the patient's stress level. One small study found that relaxation therapy (awareness training, deep breathing, behavioral relaxation training, applied relaxation techniques, and biofeedback) reduced the severity of tics, although the difference between the treatment group and control group was not statistically significant.

• Stress reduction training. This training may help relieve the symptoms of TS because stress worsens the tics.

• Other alternative therapies. **Homeopathy**, hypnosis, **guided imagery**, and eliminating allergy-provoking foods from the diet have all been reported as helping some TS patients.

Allopathic treatment

Most TS patients do not need to take drugs, as their tics do not seriously interfere with their lives. Drugs that are used to reduce the symptoms of TS include haloperidol (Haldol), pimozide (Orap), clonidine (Catapres), guanfacine (Tenex), and risperidone (Risperdal). One interesting recent finding is that the transdermal nicotine patch, developed to help people quit **smoking**, improves the control of TS symptoms in children who take haloperidol. Use of the patch allows the haloperidol dosage to be cut in half without loss of effectiveness in symptom control.

Stereotactic treatment, which is high-frequency stimulation of specific regions of the brain, was reported to be successful in significantly reducing tics in a TS patient who had failed to respond to other treatments.

Expected results

Although there is no cure for TS, many patients improve as they grow older, often to the point where they can manage their lives without drugs. A few patients recover completely after their teenage years. Others learn to live with their condition. There is always a risk, however, that a patient who continues having severe tics will become more antisocial or depressed, or develop severe mood swings and panic attacks.

KEY TERMS

Basal ganglia (singular, ganglion)—Masses of gray matter in the cerebral hemispheres of the brain that are involved in the regulation of voluntary movements. Tourette syndrome has been linked to these areas of the brain.

Biofeedback—A method of learning to modify a body function, such as blood pressure, muscle tension, or rate of breathing, with the help of an electronic instrument.

Compulsion—A very strong urge to do or say something, usually something irrational or contrary to one's will. Compulsions are often experienced as irresistible.

Coprolalia—The involuntary use of vulgar or obscene language.

Dyslexia—Difficulty in reading, spelling, and writing words.

Neurotransmitters—Any of several chemical substances that transmit nerve impulses across the small gaps between nerve cells.

Tic—An involuntary sudden spasmodic muscle contraction.

Prevention

The only known way to prevent TS as of 2004 is for a couple not to have children when one of them has the condition. Any child of a TS parent has a 50% chance of inheriting the syndrome.

Resources

BOOKS

Landau, Elaine. *Tourette Syndrome*. Danbury, CT: Franklin Watts, 1998.

Leckman, James F., and Donald J. Cohen. *Tourette's Syndrome—Tics, Obsessions, Compulsions: Developmental Psychopathology and Clinical Care*. New York: John Wiley &Sons, Inc., 1998.

The Merck Manual of Diagnosis and Therapy. Edited by Mark H. Beers, MD, and Robert Berkow, MD. Whitehouse Station, NJ: Merck Research Laboratories, 1999.

PERIODICALS

"Nicotine Patch Could Help Against Condition's Tics." *Health & Medicine Week* (October 8, 2001).

"Rate of Disease Much Higher Than Had Been Thought." *Pain & Central Nervous System Week* (November 19, 2001): 9.

Trifiletti, Rosario. "Antistriatal Antibodies in Tourette Syndrome: Not a Simple Story." *Neurology Alert* 20 (October 2001): 14.

ORGANIZATIONS

National Institute of Neurological Disorders and Stroke. National Institutes of Health. P.O. Box 5801, Bethesda, MD 20824. (800) 352-9424. <http://www.ninds.nih.gov>.

Tourette Syndrome Association, Inc. 42-40 Bell Boulevard, Bayside, NY 11361-2820. (718) 224-2999. Fax: (718) 279-9596. ts@tsa-usa.org. <http://www.tsa-usa.org>.

OTHER

"Tourette Disorder." *Internet Mental Health*. [cited October 2002]. <http://www.mentalhealth.com/fr00.html>.

Belinda Rowland
Rebecca J. Frey, PhD

Toxemia *see* **Blood poisoning**

Toxic building syndrome *see* **Sick building syndrome**

Toxic shock syndrome

Definition

Toxic shock syndrome (TSS) is an uncommon but potentially serious illness that occurs when poisonous substances (toxins) produced by certain bacteria enter the bloodstream. The toxins cause a type of **blood poisoning** caused by staphylococcal, or less commonly streptococcal, **infections** in the lungs, throat, skin or bone, or from injuries. Women using super-absorbent tampons during **menstruation** were found to be most likely to get toxic shock syndrome.

Description

TSS first came to the attention of the public in the 1970s. Shortly after the introduction of a super-absorbent tampon, young women across the United States experienced an epidemic of serious but unexplained symptoms. Thousands went to emergency rooms with high **fever**, **vomiting**, peeling skin, low blood pressure, **diarrhea**, and a rash resembling **sunburn**. The only thing they had in common was that they all were menstruating at the time they felt sick, and all were using tampons—especially super-absorbent products.

At its height, the epidemic affected 15,000 people in the United States each year between 1980 and 1984; 15% of the women died. Since the offending products were taken off the market, the numbers of TSS cases have declined sharply. As of 1998, only about 5,000 cases are diagnosed annually in the United States, 5% of which are fatal. The decline is most likely due to the tampon manufacturers' discontinuing the use of some synthetic materials, and the removal from the market of the brand of tampon associated with most cases of TSS. As of the early 2000s, most of these products are made with rayon and cotton.

In spite of TSS's association with menstruating women, the disease can affect anyone of either sex or any age or race. The infection may occur in children, men, and non-menstruating women who are weakened from surgery, injury, or disease, and who cannot fight off a staphylococcal infection. New mothers are also at higher risk for TSS, particularly if they had a caesarean section or if they are breastfeeding their infants.

Most cases reported in Western countries still involve menstruating women under age 30. TSS still occurs in about 17 out of every 100,000 menstruating girls and women each year; more than half of these cases are related to tampons. Between 5% and 10% of patients with TSS die.

In the developing countries, however, toxic shock syndrome often affects children. A recent report of staphylococcal TSS from Saudi Arabia concerned a four-month-old infant. **Burns** appear to increase the risk of TSS in children in all countries.

Streptococcal toxic shock syndrome (STSS)

A new type of toxic shock syndrome is caused by a different bacterium, called Group A streptococcus. This form of TSS is called streptococcal toxic shock syndrome, or STSS. Officially recognized in 1987, STSS is related to the strain of streptococcus called the flesh-eating bacterium. STSS affects only one or two out of every 100,000 Americans. It almost never follows a simple **strep throat** infection.

In Europe and the United Kingdom, however, the incidence of streptococcal toxic shock syndrome has continued to rise through the 1990s. In one district in the United Kingdom, the annual rate rose from 1.1 cases per million population in 1990 to 9.5 cases per million by 1999. The fatality rate is 64%, even in healthy young adults.

Causes & symptoms

Transmission

STSS is caused by a strain of *Streptococcus pyogenes* found in the nose, mouth, and occasionally the vagina. The bacteria produce a characteristic toxin. In large enough quantities, the toxin can enter the bloodstream, causing a potentially fatal infection.

While experts know the name of the bacterium, more than 10 years after the 1980s epidemic scientists still do not fully understand the link between TSS and tampons. Most medical researchers today suspect that the absorbent tampons introduce oxygen into the vagina, which is normally an oxygen-free area of the body. Oxygen triggers bacterial growth, and the more absorbent the tampon, the more bacteria it can harbor. Some experts believe that the reason TSS is linked to tampons in particular is that bacteria can contaminate and multiply in a tampon. If left in place for a long time—as a woman could do with a super absorbent product—the bacteria have a better chance of multiplying and producing a large amount of toxin. It is also possible that the tampons or the chemicals they contain may irritate the vaginal lining, enabling the toxin to enter the bloodstream.

These type of bacteria are normally present either on hands or in the vagina, and it takes an amount of bacteria only the size of a grain of sand to start an infection. Of the 15% of women who carry *Staphylococcus aureus*, only about 5% have the strain that produces the TSS toxin.

Symptoms

TSS. TSS begins suddenly, with a high fever of 102°F (38.9°C) or above, vomiting and watery diarrhea, **headache**, and sunburn-like rash; together with a **sore throat** and body aches. Blood pressure may plummet a day or two after the first symptoms appear. When the blood pressure drops, a woman may become disoriented or go into shock and her kidneys may fail. After these developments, the skin on her hands and feet may peel.

STSS. STSS can occur after a streptococcal infection in the body, usually from an infected wound or even **chickenpox**. Typically, within 48-96 hours, the patient's blood pressure drops. There is also fever, **dizziness**, breathing problems, and a weak, rapid pulse. The area around the wound may swell, the liver and kidneys can fail, and bleeding problems may occur.

Diagnosis

Any woman who is wearing a tampon and begins to experience the symptoms of toxic shock syndrome should remove the tampon right away and seek medical care.

The doctor will probably examine the vagina for signs of inflammation and rule out common sexually transmitted diseases with similar symptoms. A variety of blood tests, tests of vaginal secretions, and a physical examination are needed to identify this condition.

Treatment

Toxic shock syndrome is a life-threatening condition. If it is suspected, emergency medical attention should be sought immediately. Treatment with antibiotic drugs and IV fluids will be necessary.

Goldenseal, **calendula**, and **echinacea** can be applied topically. A diet low in sugar, with an increase in the consumption of vegetables and fruit helps to build the immune system. Movement therapies and **exercise** are also beneficial.

Allopathic treatment

TSS

In a menstruating woman, the vagina is first cleansed with an antiseptic solution to eliminate some of the bacteria that produce the toxin. TSS is treated with antibiotics, together with other drugs and fluids to lower fever and control blood pressure.

STSS

Antibiotics are used to treat STSS. Surgery may be needed to remove dead skin and muscle.

Expected results

TSS lasts as long as three weeks, and may have a tendency to recur. About a third of the women who are treated for TSS have it again within six months. In addition, TSS can affect the liver, kidneys, lungs, and other organs, depending on the severity of the infection. Untreated toxic shock syndrome can be fatal.

Prevention

TSS

Women who wear tampons should change them often and use different brands and types of pads and tampons. If a woman really prefers tampons, experts recommend using the lowest possible absorbency product made of cotton and rayon, and wearing it only during the day. In the past, it was difficult to compare absorbency rates for different products. Today, the Food and Drug Administration (FDA) requires standardized absorbency measurements on all tampon boxes. Above all, women should wash their hands before inserting a tampon, and change the tampon every four to six hours.

Anyone who has had TSS even once should not use tampons again.

STSS

Doctors still are not sure how people can avoid STSS, but they advise patients to clean and bandage open **wounds** immediately. Anyone with a red, swollen, or tender wound, or a sudden fever should seek medical care.

KEY TERMS

Shock—A condition in which the amount of blood circulating in the body is inadequate to meet the body's needs. Shock can be caused by certain diseases, serious injury, or blood loss.

Staphylococcus—A genus of bacteria that is commonly found on human skin and mucous membranes.

Streptococcus—A genus of sphere-shaped bacteria that can cause a wide variety of infections.

Resources

BOOKS

Turkington, Carol A. *Infectious Disease A to Z*. New York: Facts on File, 1998.

PERIODICALS

Amir, L. "Breastfeeding and *Staphylococcus aureus*: Three Case Reports." *Breastfeeding Review* 10 (March 2002): 15-18.

Barnham, M. R., N. C. Weightman, A. W. Anderson, and A. Tanna. "Streptococcal Toxic Shock Syndrome: A Description of 14 Cases from North Yorkshire, UK." *Clinical Microbiology and Infection* 8 (March 2002): 174-178.

Ghazal, S. S., M. N. Al-Hawasi, S. A. Al-Mosallam, et al. "Staphylococcal Toxic Shock Syndrome in a Small Infant." *Saudi Medical Journal* 23 (February 2002): 229-231.

Johnson, D., and P. D. Panthirana. "Toxic Shock Syndrome Following Cessation of Prophylactic Antibiotics in a Child with a 2% Scald." *Burns* 28 (March 2002): 181-184.

"Toxic shock syndrome—United States." *Morbidity and Mortality Weekly Report* 46 (22) (June 6, 1997): 492-495.

Paula Ford-Martin
Rebecca J. Frey, PhD

Traditional African medicine

Definition

Traditional African medicine is a holistic discipline involving extensive use of indigenous herbalism combined with aspects of African spirituality.

Origins

Despite numerous attempts at government interference, this ancient system of healing continues to thrive in Africa and practitioners can be found in many other parts

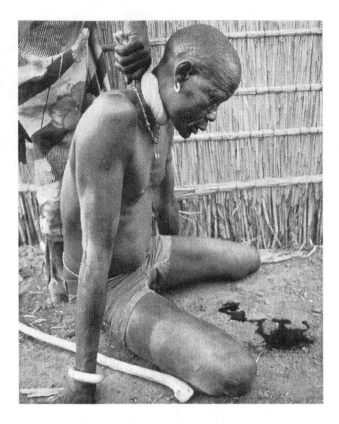

An African man has cut his forehead to relieve a headache.
(Photo Researchers, Inc. Reproduced by permission.)

of the world. Under colonial rule, many nations considered traditional diviner-healers to be practitioners of witchcraft and outlawed them for that reason. In some areas of colonial Africa, attempts were also made to control the sale of traditional herbal medicines. After Mozambique obtained independence in 1975, diviner-healers were sent to reeducation camps. Opposition to traditional medicine has been particularly vehement during times of conflict, when people have been more likely to call on the supernatural realm. More recently, interest has been expressed in integrating traditional African medicine with the continent's national health care systems. In Kwa-Mhlanga, South Africa, a 48-bed hospital combines traditional African medicine with **homeopathy**, **iridology**, and other Western healing methods, as well as traditional Asian medicine. Founded by a traditional African healer, the hospital is said to be the first of its kind in the country.

Benefits

Practitioners of traditional African medicine claim to be able to cure a wide range of conditions, including cancers, acquired immunodeficiency syndrome (**AIDS**), psychiatric disorders, high blood pressure, cholera, **infertility**, and most venereal diseases. Other applications include **epilepsy**, **asthma**, **eczema**, hayfever, **anxiety**, **depression**, benign prostatic hypertrophy, urinary tract **infections**, **gout**, and healing of **wounds** and **burns**.

Description

Traditional African medicine involves diviners, midwives, and herbalists. Diviners are responsible for determining the cause of illness, which in some causes are believed to stem from ancestral spirits and other influences. Traditional midwives make extensive use of indigenous plants to aid **childbirth**. Herbalists are so popular in Africa that an herb trading market in Durban is said to attract between 700,000 and 900,000 traders a year from South Africa, Zimbabwe, and Mozambique. Smaller herb markets exist in virtually every community.

There are strong spiritual aspects to traditional African medicine, with a widespread belief among practitioners that psychospiritual aspects must be addressed before medical aspects. Among traditional healers, the ability to diagnose an illness is considered a gift from both God and the practitioner's ancestors. A major emphasis is placed on determining the root cause underlying any sickness or bad luck. Illness is said to stem from a lack of balance between the patient and his or her social environment. It is this imbalance that determines the choice of the healing plant, which is valued as much for its symbolic and spiritual significance as for its medicinal effect. For example, the colors white, black, and red are considered especially symbolic or magical. Seeds, leaves, and twigs bearing these colors are deemed to possess special properties. Diviners may use plants not only for healing purposes but also to control weather and events. In addition to plants, traditional African healers may employ charms, incantations, and casting of spells.

One traditional African medicinal cure that has developed a wide following outside the continent is pygeum (*Prunus africana*), which has been sold in Europe since the 1970s as a treatment for mild-to-moderate benign prostatic hyperplasia. Each year, 2,000 metric tons of pygeum bark are harvested in Cameroon and another 600 tons are harvested in Madagascar. In Africa, the bark is made into a tea. Elsewhere in the world, it is sold in powders, tinctures, and pills, often combined with other herbs believed to help with prostate problems. Users report greater ease of urination, with reduced inflammation and **cholesterol** deposits.

A comparison between numbers of traditional healers and medical doctors demonstrates the importance of this healing modality in Africa. In the Venda area of South Africa, there is one traditional practitioner for every 700–1,200 people, compared to one physician for every 17,400 people. Swaziland has one traditional healer for every 110 people. Benin City, Nigeria has the same ratio. Urban Kenya has one traditional healer per 833 population.

Precautions

All cases of serious illness need to be examined by a medical doctor. Even though many prostate conditions are not serious, patients thinking of using pygeum should first undergo a medical examination to rule out more serious problems.

Concern has been expressed that increased demand for wild plants used in traditional African medicine is endangering local plant populations. For example, the Washington-based group Future Harvest says that a $220 million annual market for *Prunus africana* as a prostate remedy could lead to extinction of the slow-maturing evergreen tree in the African wilds.

Some Christian church officials express opposition to elements of witchcraft used by some African healers.

Side effects

Serious side effects, even death, can result from incorrect identification of healing plants. For example, species of the **aloe** plant are extensively used in traditional African medicine, but some forms, such as *Aloe globuligemma,* are toxic and can result in death if misidentified.

Convulsions and fatalities have been linked to the use of African herb concoctions known as *imbiza,* used for male erectile problems. Suppliers insist the problems occur only when too much of the concoction is consumed.

Research & general acceptance

Although many of the principles and methods of traditional African medicine are quite foreign to orthodox medical thinking, there is nonetheless considerable interest in exploiting Africa's ethnobotanical knowledge for drug-development purposes. For example, American researchers have expressed interest in using seed extracts from *Garcinia kola,* a common African tree used by traditional healers, to treat Ebola and Marburg disease.

Training & certification

The field is largely unregulated. In Africa, many traditional practitioners are simple, uneducated people who have nonetheless accumulated a great deal of knowledge about native plants and their actions on the human body. There is considerable interest in integrating traditional African medicine more fully with the continent's national medical systems. In Harare, Zimbabwe, a school of Traditional African

Medicine opened its doors in October, 1999. Students include both traditional healers and university graduates.

Resources

PERIODICALS

Kale, R. "Traditional healers in South Africa: a parallel health care system." *British Medical Journal* 310 (6988) (May 6 1995):1182-5.

David Helwig

Traditional Chinese Herbalism see **Herbalism, traditional Chinese**

Traditional Chinese medicine

Definition

Traditional Chinese medicine (TCM) is based on a set of interventions designed to restore balance to human beings. The therapies usually considered under the heading of classic Chinese medicine include:

• acupunture and **moxibustion**

• dietary regulation

• herbal remedies

• massage

• therapeutic **exercise**

These forms of treatments are based upon beliefs that differ from the disease concept favored by Western medicine. What is referred to as illness by Western medicine is considered in traditional Chinese medicine to be a matter of disharmony or imbalance.

The philosophy behind Chinese medicine is a melding of tenets from Buddhism, Confucianism, and the combined religious and philosophical ideas of Taoism. Although there are various schools of thought among practitioners of traditional Chinese medicine, five Taoist axioms form its basis:

• There are natural laws which govern the universe, including human beings.

• The natural order of the universe is innately harmonious and well-organized. When people live according to the laws of the universe, they live in harmony with that universe and the natural environment.

• The universe is dynamic, with change as its only constant. Stagnation is in opposition to the law of the universe and causes what Western medicine calls illness.

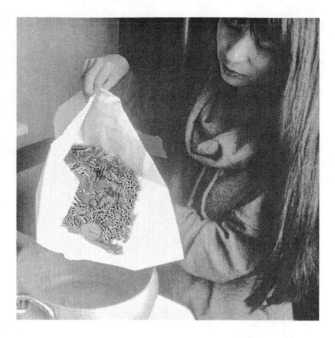

Chinese medicine practitioner preparing herbal medicines. *(Eric Nelson. Custom Medical Stock Photo, Inc. Reproduced by permission.)*

- All living things are connected and interdependent.

- Humans are intimately connected to and affected by all facets of their environment.

Origins

Historical background

Traditional Chinese medicine is over 2,000 years old. It originated in the region of eastern Asia that today includes China, Tibet, Vietnam, Korea, and Japan. The first written Chinese medical treatises (as the West understands the term) date from the Han dynasty (206 B.C.–A.D. 220). Tribal shamans and holy men who lived as hermits in the mountains of China as early as 3500 B.C. practiced what was called the "Way of Long Life." This regimen included a diet based on herbs and other plants; kung-fu exercises; and special breathing techniques that were thought to improve vitality and life expectancy.

After the Han dynasty, the next great age of Chinese medicine was under the Tang emperors, who ruled from A.D. 608-A.D. 906. The first Tang emperor established China's first medical school in A.D. 629. Under the Song (A.D. 960–1279) and Ming (A.D. 1368–1644) dynasties, new medical schools were established, their curricula and qualifying examinations were standardized, and the traditional herbal prescriptions were written down and collected into encyclopedias. One important difference between the development of medicine in China and in the West is the greater interest in the West in surgical procedures and techniques. In the nineteenth and early twentieth centuries, the opening of China to the West led to the establishment of Western-style medical schools in Shanghai and other large cities, and a growing rivalry between the two traditions of medicine. In 1929 a group of Chinese physicians who had studied Western medicine petitioned the government to ban traditional Chinese medicine. This move was opposed, and by 1933 the Nationalist government appointed a chief justice of the Chinese Supreme Court to systematize and promote the traditional system of medicine. In contemporary China, both traditional and Western forms of medicine are practiced alongside each other.

Philosophical background: the cosmic and natural order

In Taoist thought, the Tao, or universal first principle, generated a duality of opposing principles that underlie all the patterns of nature. These principles, yin and yang, are mutually dependent as well as polar opposites. They are basic concepts in traditional Chinese medicine. Yin represents everything that is cold, moist, dim, passive, slow, heavy, and moving downward or inward; while yang represents heat, dryness, brightness, activity, rapidity, lightness, and upward or outward motion. Both forces are equally necessary in nature and in human well-being, and neither force can exist without the other. The dynamic interaction of these two principles is reflected in the cycles of the seasons, the human life cycle, and other natural phenomena. One objective of traditional Chinese medicine is to keep yin and yang in harmonious balance within a person.

In addition to yin and yang, Taoist teachers also believed that the Tao produced a third force, primordial energy or *qi* (also spelled chi or ki). The interplay between yin, yang, and qi gave rise to the Five Elements of water, metal, earth, wood, and fire. These entities are all reflected in the structure and functioning of the human body.

The human being

Traditional Chinese physicians did not learn about the structures of the human body from dissection because they thought that cutting open a body insulted the person's ancestors. Instead they built up an understanding of the location and functions of the major organs over centuries of observation, and then correlated them with the principles of yin, yang, qi, and the Five Elements. Thus wood is related to the liver (yin) and the gall bladder (yang); fire to the heart (yin) and the small intestine (yang); earth to the spleen (yin) and the stomach (yang); metal to the lungs (yin) and the large intestine (yang); and water to the kidneys (yin) and the bladder (yang). The Chinese also believed that the body contains Five Essential Substances, which include blood, spirit, vital essence (a principle of growth and development produced by the body from qi and blood); fluids (all body fluids other than blood, such as saliva, spinal fluid, sweat, etc.); and qi.

A unique feature of traditional Chinese medicine is the meridian system. Chinese doctors viewed the body as regulated by a network of energy pathways called meridians that link and balance the various organs. The meridians have four functions: to connect the internal organs with the exterior of the body, and connect the person to the environment and the universe; to harmonize the yin and yang principles within the body's organs and Five Substances; to distribute qi within the body; and to protect the body against external imbalances related to weather (wind, summer heat, dampness, dryness, cold, and fire).

Benefits

Traditional Chinese medicine offers the following benefits:

- It is believed by some to treat certain chronic illnesses more effectively than Western medicine.

- It is holistic; all aspects of the person's being are taken into account.

- It treats the root cause of the disease as well as the manifest symptoms. Chinese practitioners distinguish between the root (*ben*) of an illness and its branches (*biao*). The root is the basic pattern of imbalance in the patient's qi; the branches are the evident symptoms.

- Traditional Chinese medicine does not rely on pharmaceutical products that often cause side effects.

- It improves a person's general health as well as treating specific diseases or disorders.

- It is often less expensive than standard allopathic treatment.

- It is not a self-enclosed system but can be used in combination with Western medicine.

- It can be used to treat the side effects of Western modalities of treatment.

Description

Acupuncture/moxibustion

Acupuncture is probably the form of treatment most familiar to Westerners. It is often used for **pain** relief, but has wider applications in traditional Chinese practice. It is based on a view of the meridians that regards them as conduits or pathways for the qi, or life energy. Disease is attributed to a blockage of the meridians; thus acupunc-

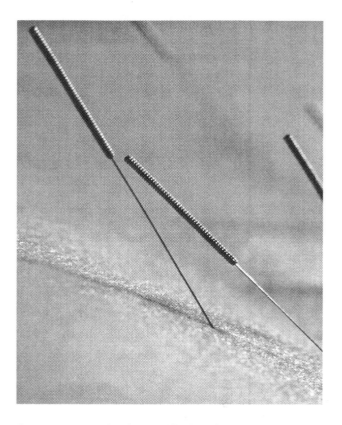

Acupuncture needles inserted in the skin. *(Photo Researchers, Inc. Reproduced by permission.)*

ture can be used to treat disorders of the internal organs as well as muscular and skin problems. The insertion of needles at specific points along the meridians is thought to unblock the qi. More than 800 acupuncture points have been identified, but only about 50 are commonly used. Acupuncture is usually used as a treatment together with herbal medicines.

Moxibustion refers to the practice of burning a moxa wick over the patient's skin at vital points. Moxa is a word derived from Japanese and means "burning herbs." The moxa wick is most commonly made from *Artemisia vulgaris*, or Chinese **wormwood**, but other herbs can also be used. Moxibustion is thought to send heat and nourishing qi into the body. It is used to treat a number of different illnesses, including **nosebleeds**, pulled muscles, **mumps**, arthritis, and vaginal bleeding.

Dietary regulation

Diet is regarded as the first line of treatment in Chinese medicine; acupuncture and herbal treatments are used only after changes in diet fail to cure the problem. Chinese medicine uses foods to keep the body in internal harmony and in a state of balance with the external environment. In giving dietary advice, the Chinese physician takes into account the weather, the season, the geography of the area, and the patient's specific imbalances (including emotional upsets) in order to select foods that will counteract excesses or supply deficient elements. Basic preventive dietary care, for example, would recommend eating yin foods in the summer, which is a yang season. In the winter, by contrast, yang foods should be eaten to counteract the yin temperatures. In the case of illness, yin symptom patterns (**fatigue**, pale complexion, weak voice) would be treated with yang foods, while yang symptoms (flushed face, loud voice, restlessness) would be treated by yin foods.

Chinese medicine also uses food as therapy in combination with exercise and herbal preparations. One aspect of a balanced diet is maintaining a proper balance of rest and activity as well as selecting the right foods for the time of year and other circumstances. If a person does not get enough exercise, the body cannot transform food into qi and Vital Essence. If they are hyperactive, the body consumes too much of its own substance. With respect to herbal preparations, the Chinese used tonics taken as part of a meal before they began to use them as medicines. Herbs are used in Chinese cooking to give the food specific medicinal qualities as well as to flavor it. For example, **ginger** might be added to a fish dish to counteract **fever**. Food and medical treatment are closely interrelated in traditional Chinese medicine. A classical Chinese meal seeks to balance not only flavors, aromas, textures, and colors in the different courses that are served, but also the energies provided for the body by the various ingredients.

Herbal remedies

Chinese herbal treatment differs from **Western herbalism** in several respects. In Chinese practice, several different herbs may be used, according to each plant's effect on the individual's qi and the Five Elements. There are many formulas used within traditional Chinese medicine to treat certain common imbalance patterns. These formulas can be modified to fit specific individuals more closely.

In 2002, a study in Texas showed that a traditional Chinese antirheumatic herb extract helped patients with **rheumatoid arthritis** by improving symptoms such as morning stiffness and tender, swollen joints. Side effects of decreased appetite and **nausea** were tolerable for those the herb helped. The researchers planned to move on to a more scientifically controlled clinical trial phase to further test the herb's effectiveness. Another scientific study that year reported new benefits for applying soy proteins, an ancient Chinese practice, to the skin. Scientists worked on a new preparation that showed benefits in re-

ducing age spots and ultraviolet ray damage, and smoothing and moisturizing the skin, among other benefits.

A traditional Chinese herbal formula typically contains four classes of ingredients, arranged in a hierarchical order: a chief (the principal ingredient, chosen for the patient's specific illness); a deputy (to reinforce the chief's action or treat a coexisting condition); an assistant (to counteract side effects of the first two ingredients); and an envoy (to harmonize all the other ingredients and convey them to the parts of the body that they are to treat).

Massage

Massage is recommended in traditional Chinese medicine to unblock the patient's meridians, stimulate the circulation of blood and qi, loosen stiff joints and muscles, and strengthen the immune system. It may be done to relieve symptoms without the need for complex diagnosis. **Chinese massage** is commonly used to treat back strain, pulled muscles, **tendinitis**, **sciatica**, rheumatism, arthritis, sprains, and similar ailments. In *Tui na* massage, the practitioner presses and kneads various qi points on the patient's body. The patient does not need to undress but wears thin cotton clothes. He or she sits on a chair or lies on a massage couch while the practitioner presses on or manipulates the soft tissues of the body. *Tui na* means "push and grasp" in Chinese. It is not meant to be relaxing or pampering but is serious treatment for sports injuries and chronic pain in the joints and muscles. *Tui na* is used to treat the members of Chinese Olympic teams.

Therapeutic exercise

Therapeutic exercise, or *qigong*, is an ancient Chinese form of physical training that combines preventive healthcare and therapy. *Qigong* relies on breathing techniques to direct the qi to different parts of the body. The literal translation of *qigong* is "the cultivation and deliberate control of a higher form of vital energy." Another form of therapeutic exercise is **t'ai chi**, in which the person moves through a series of 30–64 movements that require a relaxed body and correct rhythmic breathing. Many Chinese practice t'ai chi as a form of preventive medicine.

Preparations

Preparations for treatment in traditional Chinese medicine are similar to preparing for a first-time visit to a Western physician. The patient will be asked to give a complete and detailed medical history. The practitioner may touch the patient's acupuncture meridians to evaluate them for soreness or tightness. The major difference that the patient will notice is the much greater attention given in Chinese medicine to the tongue and the pulse. The Chinese practitioner will evaluate the patient's tongue for form, color, and the color and texture of the tongue fur. In taking the pulse, the Chinese therapist feels three pressure points along each wrist, first with light pressure and then with heavy pressure, for a total of 12 different pulses on both wrists. Each pulse is thought to indicate the condition of one of the 12 vital organs.

Precautions

There are no special precautions necessary for treatment with traditional Chinese medical techniques other than giving the practitioner necessary details about major or chronic health problems.

Side effects

Side effects with traditional Chinese medicine are usually minor. With herbal treatments, there should be no side effects if the patient has been given the correct formula and is taking it in the prescribed manner. Some people feel a little sore or stiff the day after receiving *Tui na* massage, but the soreness does not last and usually clears up with repeated treatments. Side effects from acupuncture or from therapeutic exercise under the guidance of a competent teacher are unusual. However, care should be taken in using herbal preparations and possible side effects or toxins within any preparations, as well as interactions with other drugs. Patients should consult with qualified practitioners.

Research & general acceptance

At present, there is renewed interest in the West in traditional Chinese medicine. Of the 700 herbal remedies used by traditional Chinese practitioners, over 100 have been tested and found effective by the standards of Western science. Several United States agencies, including the National Institutes of Health, the Office of Alternative Medicine, and the Food and Drug Administration (FDA) are currently investigating Chinese herbal medicine as well as acupuncture and *Tui na* massage. In general, however, Western studies of Chinese medicine focus on the effects of traditional treatments and the reasons for those effects, thus attempting to fit traditional Chinese medicine within the Western framework of precise physical measurements and scientific hypotheses.

As use of traditional Chinese medicine has increased steadily in the West, many allopathic physicians have needed to understand the intricacies of the practice and to know how to deal with adverse reactions to herbal remedies. In 2002, a project was undertaken to develop a Chinese herbal medicine toxicology database to share information about English and Chinese studies on Chinese

herbal medicines. The goal of the project was to help doctors in Western hospitals better manage poisonings or adverse reactions to Chinese medicines.

Training & certification

Traditional Chinese medicine practitioners can be either acupuncturists, herbalists, or both. At present, no schools accredited in the United States confer the degree of Doctor of Oriental Medicine because the standards for such a degree have not yet been established. More than half of the 50 states now have licensing boards for acupuncturists as of the early 2000s. There is no present independent licensing for herbalists. California has been the only state that has required (since 1982) acupuncture

---

KEY TERMS

Five Elements—The five basic substances (water, wood, earth, fire, and metal) that symbolize the fundamental qualities of the universe. In Chinese food cures, the five elements are correlated with the internal organs of the body and with the five basic food tastes.

Five Substances—The basic entities in the human body that serve its development and maintenance. They include qi, Vital Essence, Spirit, Blood, and Fluids.

Meridians—Pathways of subtle energy that link and regulate the various structures, organs, and substances in the human body.

Moxibustion—A technique of treatment in which the practitioner warms the skin over vital qi points by holding a burning herbal wick above the skin.

Qi—The universal life-force or energy. The quality, quantity, and balance of a person's qi determines their state of health and longevity.

Qigong—A form of therapeutic exercise that emphasizes breathing techniques to direct the qi to different parts of the body.

Taoism—The system of thought that shaped the view of creation underlying traditional Chinese medicine.

Tui na—A form of Chinese massage in which the therapist vigorously pushes and kneads the soft tissues of the patient's body. Its name means "push and grasp."

Yin and yang—In Taoist thought, the two primordial opposing yet interdependent cosmic forces.

practitioners to take licensing examinations in both acupuncture and herbal medicine.

There is also a national organization called the National Commission for the Certification of Acupuncture and Oriental Medicine (NCCAOM) that offers certification in acupuncture. This certification provides the basis for licensure in a number of states. The NCCAOM also offers a certificate in herbal medicine that does not lead to licensure at present but is beginning to be used in some states as a basis for practice.

Resources

BOOKS

Mills, Simon, M.A., and Steven Finando, PhD. *Alternatives in Healing.* New York: NAL Penguin, Inc., 1989.

Reid, Daniel P. *Chinese Herbal Medicine.* Boston: Shambhala, 1993.

Stein, Diane. "All Women Are Healers: A Comprehensive Guide to Natural Healing." *Chinese Healing and Acupressure.* Freedom, CA: The Crossing Press, 1996.

Svoboda, Robert, and Arnie Lade. *Tao and Dharma: Chinese Medicine and Ayurveda.* Twin Lakes, WI: Lotus Press, 1995.

PERIODICALS

Bensoussan, Alan, et al."Development of a Chinese Herbal Medicine Toxicology Database." *Journal of Toxicology: Clinical Toxicology* (March 2002): 159.

"Chinese Herbal Extract Safe and Effective for RA." *The Journal of Musculoskeletal Medicine* (January 2002): 43.

Liu, Jue-Chen, et al. "Applications of Soy in Skin Care." *The Journal of Nutrition* (March 2002): 574S.

ORGANIZATIONS

American Association of Oriental Medicine. 909 22nd St. Sacramento, CA 95816. <http://www.aaom.org>.

American Foundation of Traditional Chinese Medicine (AFTCM). 505 Beach Street. San Francisco, CA 94133. (415) 776-0502. Fax: (415) 392-7003. aftcm@ earthlink. net.

Florida Institute of Traditional Chinese Medicine. (800) 565-1246. fitcm@gte.net.

Joan Schonbeck
Teresa G. Odle

Trager psychophysical integration

Definition

Trager psychophysical integration therapy, also known as the Tragerwork system of physical integration, is a combination of hands-on tissue mobilization, **relaxation**, and movement reeducation called Mentastics. The underlying principle of psychophysical integration is that clients learn to be lighter, easier, and freer by experiencing lightness, ease, and freedom of movement in their bodies.

The Trager method is a psychologically grounded physical approach to muscle relaxation, which is induced when a practitioner and patient achieve a state of mind called hook-up. Hook-up is described as a connection to a state of grace or powerful and nourishing life force. It is the opposite of strain or effort.

Origins

Psychophysical integration therapy began with Dr. **Milton Trager** (1908–1977), who earned a medical degree in midlife after working out his approach to healing chronic **pain**. Trager was born with a spinal deformity and overcame it through practicing a variety of athletic exercises. At the time that he discovered his approach to bodywork, he was training to become a boxer. His therapy came to public attention when Esalen Institute in California, the famous center of the human potential movement, invited him to give a demonstration of his technique during the mid-1970s. Trager abandoned his private medical practice in 1977 to devote his full energy to the development and further understanding of psychophysical integration. The Trager Institute, which continues his work, was founded in 1980.

Benefits

Psychophysical integration therapy has been helpful in relieving muscle discomfort in patients afflicted with polio, muscular dystrophy, **Parkinson's disease, multiple sclerosis**, post-stroke trauma, and psychiatric disturbances. The therapy is useful in alleviating such chronic conditions as back and leg pain. Athletes may benefit from this system to increase resilience to injuries and to improve their mental attitudes. In addition, the Trager Institute maintains that Tragerwork helps clients achieve greater mental clarity through the release of "deep-seated physical and mental patterns."

Description

The Trager method consists of two parts, a passive aspect referred to as tablework and an active aspect called Mentastics, which is a self-care **exercise** program. Although the benefits of the Trager approach are said to be cumulative, practitioners and clients appear to be free to set their own schedules for a series of sessions. There is no minimum number of sessions that clients must agree to take.

Tablework

The tablework is performed on a comfortable padded table. Sessions last about 60-90 minutes. The practitioner moves the client in ways that he or she naturally moves in such a way that he or she experiences how it feels to move effortlessly and freely on one's own. The movements resemble general mobilization techniques, and incorporate some manual, cervical, and lumbar traction. The goal of tablework is to allow the client "slowly to give up muscular and mental control and sink into a very deep state of relaxation not unlike that experienced in hypnosis."

Mentastics

Mentastics are free-flowing dance-like movements intended to increase the client's self-awareness, as well as providing tools to help the client move through and control chronic pain. The client is encouraged to "let go," which means that they are asked to begin a movement, then release their muscle tension and allow the weight of the body part involved to complete the motion. By experiencing movement as something pleasurable and positive rather than painful or negative, clients begin to loosen up, learn new movements more easily, and even begin inventing their own. In the early stages of treatment, clients are advised to do Mentastic movements at home for 10–15-minute sessions, three times per day.

Preparations

Prior to a session of tablework, the client dresses for comfort, "with a minimum of swimwear or briefs," according to the Trager Institute. The client is also covered with a drape. No oils or lotions are used.

The practitioner prepares for the session by clearing his or her mind of everything but the client, until he or she achieves a state of hook-up. This attitude of "relaxed meditative awareness" on the part of the practitioner is one of the unique features of Tragerwork. It is described as allowing the therapist "to connect deeply with the recipient in an unforced way and enables the practitioner to perceive the slightest responses from the [client's] body."

Precautions

Because of the unusual sensitivity and heightened awareness that is associated with the practitioner's touch, pain should never result from tablework sessions. It is important for clients to alert the practitioner to any pain associated with either the tablework or the Mentastics program.

Although the movements used in Trager tablework are gentle and noninvasive, clients who have had recent injuries or surgery should wait to heal before undertaking a course of Tragerwork.

Side effects

The Trager method should not produce physical side effects when employed by a qualified practitioner. It is

MILTON TRAGER 1909–1997

Milton Trager was a medical doctor and a somatic educator, specializing in body learning. He was a contemporary of F. Matthias Alexander, Moshe **Feldenkrais**, and Ida Rolf.

As a young man in the 1920s, he occupied himself with gymnastics and boxing. Through his intensely physical pursuits, he arrived at his self-taught body learning theories. The techniques that he nurtured emphasized body control over strength, prowess, and endurance. For example, in striving to leap as high as possible, Trager focused his concentration on landing as softly as possible. He obtained a degree in physical medicine before serving in the military during World War II.

Upon his return, Trager funded his medical school education with his GI benefits. He established a private practice and spent the ensuing 50 years refining his body learning techniques and assisting afflicted individuals in the process. When Trager's father was stricken with sciatic **pain**, Trager learned to relieve the spasms by hand. In time he learned to alleviate the symptoms of polio victims and others who suffered from muscle spasms.

Trager established the Trager Institute in the 1970s to propagate the techniques that he developed. By the year 2000, an estimated 2,000 students and practitioners had embraced the Trager approach.

Trager lived with his wife Emily in Southern California at the time of his death in January 1997.

Gloria Cooksey

possible that some clients may have emotional reactions associated with the release of physical patterns acquired as a response to trauma, but such reactions are unusual.

Research & general acceptance

Tragerwork, like other forms of bodywork, has gained increasing acceptance as a form of treatment since the 1980s. In 2000 there were 1,200 certified psychophysical integration practitioners in 15 countries worldwide. The therapy has been reported as a commonly employed treatment for mainstream athletes. In addition, the National Institutes of Health lists psychophysical therapy as a mind-body form of complementary alternative medicine.

Training & certification

Practitioners of psychophysical therapy undergo classroom instruction as well as a directed practice (internship) where they apply the learned techniques. Psychophysical therapy is demanding, and proficiency in the practice results only after dozens of therapy sessions have been completed. As many as 100 sessions may be given before the student practitioner achieves the appropriate mental and physical state to communicate an effortless way of being.

Practitioner certification is available for Tragerwork. The curriculum at the Florida Institute of Psychophysical Integration involves a 15-day (150-hour) program of study. Course work progresses through three phases. The initial phase, independent study, is followed by a residential internship. A third phase of combined work and study brings the student to sufficient mastery of the Trager method for certification.

Guidelines for acceptance at the Florida Institute include a college degree and a background in counseling, touch, and massage. Also required are an understanding of the human muscular system and the completion of preliminary postural integration studies. Students must be at least 25 years of age.

Resources

BOOKS

Juhan, Deanne. *Job's Body.* Barrytown, NY: Station Hill Press, 1987.

Trager, Milton, M.D. *Trager Mentastics: Movements as a Way to Agelessness.* Barrytown, NY: Station Hill Press, 1987.

ORGANIZATIONS

Florida Institute of Psychophysical Integration: Quantum Balance. 5837 Mariner Drive. Tampa, FL 33609-3411. (813) 186-2273. Fax: (813) 287-2870. Dr.Joy@JohnsonMail.com.

Trager Institute. 21 Locust Avenue. Mill Valley, CA 94941-2806. (415) 388-2688. Fax: (415) 399-2710. admin@trager.com. http://www.trager.com.

Gloria Cooksey

Transcendental meditation *see* **Meditation**
Transient ischemic attack *see* **Stroke**
Trefoil *see* **Red clover**

Tremor

Definition

Tremor is an unintentional (involuntary), rhythmical alternating movement that may affect the muscles of any part of the body. Tremor is caused by the rapid alternating contraction and **relaxation** of muscles and is a common symptom of diseases of the nervous system (neurologic disease).

Description

Occasional tremor is felt by almost everyone, usually as a result of fear or excitement. However, uncontrollable tremor or shaking is a common symptom of disorders that destroy nerve tissue such as **Parkinson's disease** or **multiple sclerosis**. Tremor may also occur after **stroke** or head injury. Other tremor appears without any underlying illness.

Causes & symptoms

Tremor may be a symptom of an underlying disease or it may be caused by drugs. It may also exist as the only symptom (essential tremor).

Underlying disease

Some types of tremor are signs of an underlying condition. About 1.5 million Americans have Parkinson's disease, a disease that destroys nerve cells. Severe shaking is the most apparent symptom of Parkinson's disease. This coarse tremor features four to five muscle movements per second. These movements are evident at rest but decline or disappear during movement.

Other disorders that cause tremor are multiple sclerosis, Wilson's disease, mercury poisoning, thyrotoxicosis, and liver encephalopathy.

A tremor that gets worse during body movement is called an "intention tremor." This type of tremor is a sign that something is amiss in the cerebellum, a region of the brain concerned chiefly with movement, balance, and coordination.

Drugs and tremor

Several different classes of drugs can cause tremor as a side effect. These drugs include amphetamines, antidepressant drugs, antipsychotic drugs, **caffeine**, and lithium. Tremor also may be a sign of withdrawal from alcohol or street drugs.

Essential tremor

Many people have what is called "essential tremor," in which the tremor is the only symptom. This type of shaking affects between three and four million Americans.

The cause of essential tremor is not known, although it is an inherited problem in more than half of all cases. The genetic condition has an autosomal dominant inheritance pattern, which means that any child of an affected parent will have a 50% chance of developing the condition.

Essential tremor most often appears when the hands are being used, whereas a person with Parkinson's disease will most often have a tremor while walking or while the hands are resting. People with essential tremor will usually have shaking head and hands, but the tremor may involve other parts of the body. The shaking often begins in the dominant hand and may spread to the other hand, interfering with eating and writing. Some people also develop a quavering voice.

Essential tremor affects men and women equally. The shaking often appears at about age 45, although the disorder may actually begin in adolescence or early adulthood. Essential tremor that begins very late in life is sometimes called "senile tremor."

Diagnosis

Close attention to where and how the tremor appears can help provide a correct diagnosis of the cause of the shaking. The source of the tremor can be diagnosed when the underlying condition is found. Diagnostic techniques that make images of the brain, such as computed tomography scan (CT scan) or magnetic resonance imaging (MRI), may help form a diagnosis of multiple sclerosis or other tremor caused by disorders of the central nervous system. Blood tests can rule out metabolic causes such as thyroid disease. A family history can help determine whether the tremor is inherited.

Treatment

Neither tremor nor most of its underlying neurological causes can be cured. Tremor caused by medications or by drug withdrawal, can sometimes be lessened with herbs that relax the nerves and muscle tissue, such as **skullcap** (*Scutellaria laterifolia*), **valerian** (*Valeriana officinalis*), and Jamaican dogwood (*Piscidia piscipula*).

Patients suffering from Parkinson's disease-related tremors may benefit from mucuna seeds (*Mucuna pruriens*). Practitioners of Ayurveda, or traditional Indian medicine, have prescribed mucuna to treat Parkinson's disease (or *Kampavata*) for over 4,000 years. Mucuna contains a natural form of L-dopa, a powerful anti-Parkinson's drug.

Allopathic treatment

Most people with essential tremor respond to drug treatment, which may include propranolol, primidone, or a benzodiazepine. People with Parkinson's disease may respond to anti-Parkinson's drugs.

Research has shown that about 70% of patients treated with botulinus toxin (Botox) have some improvement in tremor of the head, hand, and voice. Botulinus is derived from the bacterium *Clostridium botulinum*. This bacterium causes botulism, a form of **food poisoning**. It is poisonous because it weakens muscles. A very weak solution of the toxin is used in cases of tremor and paralysis to force the muscles to relax. However, some patients experience unpleasant side effects with this drug and cannot tolerate effective doses. For other patients, the drug becomes less effective over time. Medications do not produce any tremor relief in about half of all patients.

Tremor control therapy

Tremor control therapy is a type of treatment that uses mild electrical pulses to stimulate the brain. These pulses block the brain signals that trigger tremor. In this technique, the surgeon implants an electrode into a large oval area of gray matter within the brain that acts as a relay center for nerve impulses and is involved in generating movement (thalamus). The area that is particularly targeted for relief of tremor associated with PD is called the ventralis intermedius nucleus of the thalamus. The electrode is attached to an insulated wire that runs through the brain and exits the skull where it is attached to an extension wire. The extension is connected to a generator similar to a heart pacemaker. The generator is implanted under the skin in the chest, and the extension is tunneled under the skin from the skull to the generator. The patient can control his or her tremor by turning on the generator with a hand-held magnet to deliver an electronic pulse to the brain.

Some patients experience complete relief with this technique, but others receive no benefit at all. About 5% of patients experience complications from the surgical procedure, including bleeding in the brain. The procedure causes some discomfort, because patients must be awake while the implant is placed. Batteries must be replaced by surgical procedure every three to five years.

Other surgical treatments

A patient with extremely disabling tremor may find relief with a surgical technique called thalamotomy, in which the surgeon destroys part of the thalamus. However, the procedure produces such side effects as numbness, balance problems, or speech problems in a significant number of cases.

Pallidotomy is another type of surgical procedure sometimes used to decrease tremors from Parkinson's disease. In this technique, the surgeon destroys part of a small structure within the brain called the globus pallidus internus. The globus is part of the basal ganglia, another part of the brain that helps control movement. This surgical technique also carries the risk of permanent disabling side effects.

Fetal tissue transplantation (also called a nigral implant) is a controversial experimental method to treat Parkinson's disease symptoms. This method implants fetal brain tissue into the patient's brain to replace malfunctioning nerves. Unresolved issues include how to harvest the fetal tissue and the moral implications behind using such tissue, the danger of tissue rejection; and the amount of tissue required. Although initial studies using this technique looked promising, there has been difficulty in consistently reproducing positive results. More promising is the development of dopamine-producing cells from neuronal stem cells for transplantation into the brains of patients with PD. A method for producing these dopaminergic cells was patented in 2001.

Small amounts of alcohol may temporarily (sometimes dramatically) ease the shaking. Some experts recommend a small amount of alcohol (especially before dinner). The possible benefits, of course, must be weighed against the risks of alcohol abuse.

Expected results

Essential tremor and tremor caused by neurologic disease (including Parkinson's disease) slowly get worse and can interfere with a person's daily life. While the condition is not life-threatening, it can severely disrupt a person's everyday experiences. One recent finding is that Parkinson's patients are more concerned about the limitations imposed on their functioning and social life by the tremor than they are by the symptom itself.

Prevention

Essential tremor and tremor caused by a disease of the central nervous system cannot be prevented. Avoiding

---

use of such stimulant drugs as caffeine and amphetamines can prevent tremor that occurs as a side effect of drug use.

Resources

BOOKS

Fauci, Anthony S. et al., eds. *Harrison's Principles of Internal Medicine.* New York: McGraw-Hill, 1998.

PERIODICALS

Eskandar, Emad N., G. Rees Cosgrove, Leslie A. Shinobu. "Surgical Treatment of Parkinson Disease. (Contempo Updates Linking Evidence and Experience). " *Journal of the American Medical Association* 286 (December 26, 2001): 3056-3059.

"Neuralstem Patents Methods for Generating Dopamine-Producing Neurons from Neural Stem Cells." *Stem Cell Week* (December 31, 2001): 13.

Whetten-Goldstein, K., et al. "Patients' Perceptions of Living with Parkinson's Disease." *Gerontologist* (October 15, 2001): 281.

ORGANIZATIONS

American Academy of Neurology. 1080 Montreal Ave., St. Paul, MN 55116. (612) 695-1940. http://www.aan.com/public/con.html.

American Parkinson Disease Association. 1250 Hylan Boulevard, Suite 4B, Staten Island, NY 10305-1946. (800) 223-2732. http://www.apdaparkinson.com/.

International Tremor Foundation. 7046 West 105th Street, Overland Park, KS 66212. (913) 341-3880.

National Parkinson Foundation. 1501 NW Ninth Avenue, Miami, FL 33136. (800) 327-4545. http://www.parkinson.org.

Paula Ford-Martin
Rebecca J. Frey, PhD

Trepanation

Definition

Trepanation is a surgical procedure in which a circular piece of bone is removed from the skull by a special saw-like instrument called a trephine or trepan. The operation is also known as trephination or trephining. The English word "trepan" comes from the Greek word *trypanon*, which means "auger" or "drill."

In standard medical practice, trepanation is occasionally performed by a neurosurgeon in order to relieve pressure on the brain caused by trauma, or to remove a blood clot from brain tissue. In recent years, however, trepanation has been touted by a small group of alternative practitioners as a way to expand one's consciousness through the increase of blood flow to the brain and opening the "third eye," also known as the inner eye or eye of the mind. Practitioners of kundalini **yoga** refer to the opening of the third eye, located in the middle of the forehead, as entry into a new and completely different dimension of reality.

Origins

Trepanation is the oldest surgical procedure known to humans; skulls of Cro-Magnon people estimated to be 40,000 years old have been discovered with circular holes as large as 2 in in diameter. The Incas of Peru are known to have performed trepanation as early as 2000 B.C. It is thought that these operations were performed to treat people suffering from psychotic disorders, **epilepsy,** or chronic migraine headaches by allowing demons to escape through the hole in the skull.

The oldest written reference to trepanation comes from Hippocrates (c. 400 B.C.), whose descriptions of head injuries refer to it as a necessary treatment for skull **fractures** with bone fragments pushed inward and compressing the brain. Celsus and Galen refer to Roman surgeons of the first century A.D. as performing trepanations with implements resembling carpenters' drills. Trephines were refined in various ways through the Middle Ages, the Renaissance, and the eighteenth and nineteenth centuries. It should be emphasized that trepanations were done by ancient, medieval, and early modern physicians to relieve pressure on brain tissue—not to perform surgery on the brain itself. Care was taken not to penetrate the dura mater, which is the outermost of the three meninges or membranes that lie beneath the skull and form a protective cover for the brain and spinal cord. Historians of medicine estimate, however, that as many as 40 percent of patients died from **infections** following the procedure rather than from the surgery itself.

Contemporary interest in trepanation as a path to expanded consciousness goes back only to the 1960s. Bart Huges, a Dutchman who was expelled from medical school in the early 1960s for failing his examinations and using **marijuana,** is generally considered the founder of alternative trepanation. Huges developed a theory that he called brainbloodvolume while he was **smoking** marijuana at a party on the island of Ibiza. He noticed another guest standing on his head to increase the intoxicating effects of the drug. Huges concluded that the expansion of consciousness associated with hallucinogens results from an increased volume of blood in the brain. He reasoned that the removal of a piece of the skull would allow an even larger amount of blood to enter the brain, speeding up the delivery of oxygen and glucose to the brain cells as well as the removal of toxins. Huges had also learned in medical school that infants are born with soft spots in the skull known as fontanelles, which are membrane-covered areas where the bone has not yet completely formed. He concluded that trepanation would help to return an adult's consciousness to the intense imagination and vivid dreams of a child.

Huges—who never obtained a medical degree—managed to convert several individuals to his brainbloodvolume theory—among them Peter Halvorson, who underwent trepanation and credits it with curing his

depression, increasing his energy level, and giving him a permanent drug-free high. As of 2004, Halvorson is the head of the International Trepanation Advocacy Group (ITAG), headquartered in Wernersville, Pennsylvania. The ITAG web site includes accounts of a pilot study of six volunteers who were trepanned in June 2002 as well as personal testimonials from others who have undergone the procedure.

Benefits

According to the testimonials collected by Halvorson, trepanation confers the following benefits:

• relief from **anxiety**, depression, and other mood disorders

• feelings of freedom and serenity

• a richer emotional life

• greater ability to recall dreams on awaking

• decrease in frequency and severity of chronic headaches

• higher energy levels

Other people who have undergone trepanation, however, maintain that these benefits are only temporary and may be due to the **placebo effect**. A man who performed trepanation on himself in 2000 reported to an interviewer from an online body modification journal that he had "come to the frustrating conclusion [four weeks after the procedure] that the trepanation has had no lasting effect… Trepanation has no more physiological effect than any other trauma… it does not do what many hope it will."

Description

Surgical trepanation

A standard trepanation—most commonly done to relieve pressure on the brain when a portion of the skull has been pushed inward—is performed with the patient under general anesthesia under sterile conditions. The neurosurgeon cuts the scalp over the injured area, pulls back a flap of skin, and bores a hole in the underlying skull with a trephine. After the depressed bone has been removed together with any **blood clots** that have formed, the surgeon carefully cleanses the area and closes the incision.

Alternative trepanation

Some alternative trepanations have been performed by people on themselves, with friends to assist with the procedure. In the early 1980s, several people in England performed the entire operation on themselves, with others present to help only if an emergency arose. The reason for this stipulation was to protect the others in the room from criminal prosecution for performing surgery without credentials. The trepanner typically shaved his or her head and injected a local anesthetic. He or she then made an incision in the scalp over the area to be trepanned. Next, a hole between 1/4 and 1/2 in in diameter was cut in the skull with a foot-powered dental drill. The trepanner then removed the piece of skull, cleaned the incision, and bandaged it. The scalp gradually grew back over the hole, leaving only a small permanent indentation. More recently, however, trepanners have allowed others to assist with the operation; the man who was interviewed for the online journal had three friends who covered the walls of his room with plastic sheeting, did part of the drilling, and rinsed out the incision from time to time with sterile saline solution. He reported that the entire procedure took about 3-1/2 hours.

The participants in the ITAG pilot study, however, went to a clinic in Monterrey, Mexico, for their trepanations. The ITAG web site states plainly that "Self-trepanation today is a very selfish act. It opens the door for no one and you'd always have to keep it a secret. The public mind can't handle this. You'd be labeled 'insane.'" According to the ITAG web site, the surgeon who presently performs the procedures for Halvorson's groups was trained in Texas and is board-certified in four countries (France, Spain, Mexico, and the United States). The trepanations take about 35 minutes to complete. The cost of the operation is $2400–$3600, not including travel and hotel fees.

Preparations

People who have performed trepanations on themselves have prepared by assembling the needed equipment and setting aside a room in their house to serve as the operating room.

ITAG requires persons interested in trepanation (who must be 18 or older) to go through a period of mental preparation known as engramming, which Halvorson defines idiosyncratically as "becom[ing] thoroughly acquainted with the terminology of conscious expansion." In addition, the volunteers must sign an informed consent form and a protocol that indicates that they understand the procedure is considered experimental. They are given MRIs before and after the trepanation.

Precautions

Mainstream medical professionals uniformly warn against alternative trepanation because it is an extremely risky procedure—particularly if done by amateurs—with no certain or permanent benefits. Because scalp incisions bleed profusely, people who attempt to trepan themselves are likely to find that the flow of blood obscures their field of vision, thus increasing the risk of self-injury.

KEY TERMS

Engram—A permanent trace left in nerve tissue by a stimulus; in psychology, a latent memory picture or lasting trace left in the psyche by any experience.

Fontanelle—A membrane-covered soft spot in an infant's skull where the bone has not yet completely formed.

Kundalini yoga—A type of yoga that focuses on the body's innate psychospiritual energy (*kundalini shakti* or "serpent power" in Sanskrit) through breathing exercises, meditation, yoga postures, and chanting. Its goal is to empower the individual's consciousness to merge with universal consciousness.

Meninges—The three layers of membranous tissue that form a protective cover for the brain and spinal cord. The outermost layer is the dura mater, the middle is the arachnoid mater, and the innermost is the pia mater. In trepanation, a piece of the skull is removed without cutting through the underlying meninges.

Third eye—A term used to refer to the inner eye or eye of the mind. Opening the third eye refers to admission to a new level of consciousness.

Trephine—A saw- or drill-like instrument used to remove a circular piece of bone from the skull. It is also called a trepan.

Side effects

The potential side effects of alternative trepanation are severe, even life-threatening; they include permanent injury or death from infections, **stroke**, direct damage to brain tissue, generalized encephalitis, epilepsy, or brain abscesses.

Research & general acceptance

Trepanation is not accepted as an alternative therapy by any mainstream physicians or surgeons in the United States or Canada. In addition to the dangers of the procedure itself, neurosurgeons who have studied the claims made for trepanation say that Huges' brainbloodvolume theory is anatomically impossible.

Training & certification

As of 2004, there are *no* reputable medical school courses, training institutions, or licensing procedures in the United States or Canada for trepanation performed as a means to altered or higher consciousness.

Resources

BOOKS

Michell, John. *Eccentric Lives and Peculiar Notions* . Secaucus, NJ: Citadel Press, 1984.

PERIODICALS

Clower, W. T., and S. Finger. "Discovering Trepanation: The Contribution of Paul Broca." *Neurosurgery* 49 (December 2001): 1417–1425.

Facchini, F., E. Rastelli, L. Ferrero, and E. Fulcheri. "Cranial Trepanation in Two Skulls of Early Medieval Italy." *Homo* 53 (2003): 247–254.

Van Alphen, H. A. "Elective Trepanation for Acute Epidural Hematoma by Dr. Nicolaes Tulp (1593–1674)." *Neurosurgery* 48 (February 2001): 401–404.

Weber, J., and A. Czarnetzki. "Trepanations from the Early Medieval Period of Southwestern Germany—Indications, Complications and Outcome." *Zentralblatt für Neurochirurgie* 62 (February 2001): 10–14.

ORGANIZATIONS

American Association of Neurological Surgeons (AANS). 5550 Meadowbrook Drive, Rolling Meadows, IL 60008. (888) 566-AANS or (847) 378-0500. Fax: (847) 378-0600. <http://www.aans.org>.

International Trepanation Advocacy Group (ITAG), Inc. P. O. Box 65, Wernersville, PA 19565. (610) 693-6869. Fax: (610) 693-3261. <http://www.trepan.com>.

OTHER

Henderson, Bryan. "Trepanation." Interview conducted for *Body Modification Ezine* (BME). <http://www.bm ezine.com/news/people/A10101/trepan>.

Rebecca J. Frey, PhD

Trichomoniasis

Definition

Trichomoniasis refers to an infection of the genital and urinary tract. It is the most common sexually transmitted disease, affecting about 120 million women worldwide each year.

Description

Trichomoniasis is caused by a protozoan (the smallest, single-celled members of the animal kingdom). *Trichomonas vaginalis* is almost always passed through sexual contact. Trichomoniasis is primarily an infection

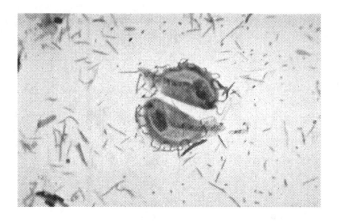

A close up image of *Trichomonas vaginalis*, the parasite that causes vaginitis in humans. *(Custom Medical Stock Photo. Reproduced by permission.)*

of women's vaginal and urinary tracts. A woman is most susceptible to infection just after having completed her menstrual period. Men may carry the organism unknowingly, since infection in men may cause mild or no symptoms. Men may also experience urethral discharge or persistent urethritis. Trichomoniasis is associated with HIV transmission and may be associated with adverse **pregnancy** outcomes.

Causes & symptoms

Because trichomoniasis is a sexually transmitted disease, it occurs more often in individuals who have multiple sexual partners. The protozoan is passed to an individual by contact within the body fluids of an infected sexual partner. It often occurs simultaneously with other sexually transmitted diseases, especially **gonorrhea**.

In women, the symptoms of trichomoniasis include an unpleasant vaginal odor, and a heavy, frothy, yellow discharge from the vagina. The genital area (vulva) is often very itchy, and there is frequently **pain** with urination or with sexual intercourse. The labia (lips) of the vagina, the vagina itself, and the cervix (the narrowed, lowest segment of the uterus that extends into the upper part of the vagina) will be bright red and irritated. Women may also experience lower abdominal discomfort.

In men, there may be no symptoms at all. Some men notice a small amount of yellowish discharge from the penis, usually first thing in the morning. There may be some mild discomfort while urinating, testicular pain or tenderness, or lower abdominal pain. Some men infected with trichomoniasis experience persistent urethritis.

The use of antibiotics is a contributing factor to recurrent trichomoniasis in some women because antibiotics affect the balance of bacteria in the vagina, allowing such organisms as *T. vaginalis* to multiply more rapidly.

Diagnosis

Diagnosis is easily made by taking a sample of the discharge from the woman's vagina or from the opening of the man's penis. The sample is put on a slide and viewed under a microscope. The protozoa, which are able to move about, are easily viewed.

Trichomoniasis tends to be underdiagnosed in men because of the relative mildness of symptoms in men and insufficiently sensitive diagnostic tests. The recent introduction of DNA amplification, however, indicates that the incidence of trichomoniasis in men is much higher than was previously thought.

Treatment

Cure of trichomoniasis may be difficult to achieve with alternative treatments. Some practitioners suggest eliminating sweets and carbohydrates from the diet and supplement with **antioxidants**, including vitamins A, C, and E, and **zinc**. Naturopaths may recommend treatment with two douches (a wash used inside the vagina), alternating one in the morning and one at bedtime. One douche contains the herbs **calendula** (*Calendula officinalis*), **goldenseal** (*Hydrastis canadensis*), and **echinacea** (*Echinacea* spp.); the other douche contains plain yogurt with live **acidophilus** cultures. The herbal douche helps to kill the protozoa while the yogurt reestablishes healthy flora in the vagina. **Tea tree oil** is another alternative remedy for trichomoniasis. Acidifying the vagina by douching with boric acid or vinegar may also be useful. Although not a cure, *The Gynecological Sourcebook* suggests inserting a **garlic** (*Allium sativum*) suppository (a peeled whole clove wrapped in gauze) every 12 hours for symptomatic relief.

Other remedies include vaginal suppositories that include the ingredient acidophilus once a day for three days. An alternative medicine practitioner can recommend the correct mixture. A vaginal douche consisting of **grapefruit seed extract** may also help relieve symptoms.

Allopathic treatment

The usual treatment is a single large dose of metronidazole (Flagyl) or split doses over the course of a week. Some sources suggest clotrimazole (Gyne-lotrimin, Mycelex) as an alternative treatment showing a lower cure rate. Application of Betadine, a concentrated antiseptic solution, is another recommendation, although Betadine is messy, stains, and should not be used by pregnant women. However, the Centers for Disease Control (CDC) states that there are no effective alternatives to therapy with metronidazole available. Topical treatment with metronidazole is not advised. Individual evaluations are recommended for those who are allergic to metronidazole or who experience treatment-resistant trichomoniasis. Sexual partners of an infected individual must all be treated, to prevent the infection from being passed back and forth. Sexual intercourse should be avoided until all partners are cured.

As of late 2003, the number of cases of metronidazole-resistant trichomoniasis appears to be increasing rapidly. Some success has been reported with the broad-spectrum anti-parasitic drug nitazoxanide, but further research needs to be done. A group of researchers in Thailand is currently investigating the effectiveness of a group of drugs known as bisquaternary quinolinium salt compounds in treating trichomoniasis.

Women who are taking antibiotics for other illnesses should speak to their health care provider about the possibile effects of the medication(s) on the balance of organisms in their vagina.

Expected results

Prognosis is excellent (90–95%) with appropriate treatment of the patient and all sexual partners. Without treatment, the infection can remain for a long time, and can be passed to all sexual partners.

Prevention

All sexually transmitted diseases can be prevented by using adequate protection during sexual intercourse. Effective forms of protection include male and female condoms. Other preventive measures are similar to those for other forms of vaginitis, including wearing loose cotton clothing and not using douches, vaginal deodorants, or sprays.

Resources

BOOKS

Nash, Theodore E., and Peter F. Weller. "Protozoal Intestinal Infections and Trichomoniasis." *Harrison's Principles of Internal Medicine, 14th ed.* Edited by Anthony S. Fauci, et al. New York: McGraw-Hill, 1998.

Pelletier, Kenneth R., MD. *The Best Alternative Medicine*, Part II, "CAM Therapies for Specific Conditions: Vaginitis." New York: Simon & Schuster, 2002.

Plorde, James J. "Introduction to Pathogenic Parasites: Pathogenesis and Chemotherapy of Parasitic Diseases." *Sherris Medical Microbiology: An Introduction to Infectious Diseases.* Edited by Kenneth J. Ryan. Norwalk, CT: Appleton and Lange, 1994.

Rosenthal, M. Sara. *The Gynecological Sourcebook.* Los Angeles, Lowell House. 1994.

PERIODICALS

Chavalitshewinkoon-Petmitr, P., M. Ramdja,S. Kajorndechaki-at, et al. "In vitro Susceptibility of *Trichomonas vaginalis*

to AT-Specific Minor Groove Binding Drugs" *Journal of Antimicrobial Chemotherapy* 52 (August 2003): 287–289.

Ching, Susanne, and Phuong H. Nguyen. "Vaginitis." *eMedicine*, 5 April 2002. <http://emedicine.com/med/topic2358.htm>.

Davis, Annabel. "*Trichomonas vaginalis*: Signs, Tests, and Treatment." *Nursing Times* 94 (November 25-December 1, 1998): 58-59.

Dunne, R. L., L. A. Dunn, P. Upcroft, et al. "Drug Resistance in the Sexually Transmitted Protozoan *Trichomonas vaginalis.*" *Cell Research* 13 (August 2003): 239–249.

Pirotta, M. V., J. M. Gunn, and P. Chondros. "'Not Thrush Again!' Women's Experience of Post-Antibiotic Vulvovaginitis." *Medical Journal of Australia* 179 (July 7, 2003): 47–49.

Schwebke, J. R., and E. W. Hook, 3rd. "High Rates of *Trichomonas vaginalis* Among Men Attending a Sexually Transmitted Diseases Clinic: Implications for Screening and Urethritis Management." *Journal of Infectious Diseases* 188 (August 1, 2003): 465–468.

OTHER

Centers for Disease Control and Prevention (CDC). "Fact Sheet:*Trichomonas* Infection. <http://www.cdc.gov/ncidod/dpd/parasites/trichomonas/factsht_trichomonas.htm>.

Kathy S. Stolley
Rebecca J. Frey, PhD

Trigger point therapy

Definition

Trigger point therapy is a bodywork technique that involves the application of pressure to tender muscle tissue in order to relieve **pain** and dysfunction in other parts of the body. It may also be called myofascial (*myo* meaning muscle, *fascial* meaning connective tissue) trigger point therapy. Trigger point therapy is sometimes regarded as one of a group of treatment aproaches called neuromuscular therapy or NMT. **Myotherapy**, developed by **Bonnie Prudden**, is a related type of trigger point therapy.

Origins

Trigger point therapy was developed by Dr. Janet Travell in the United States in the 1940s; she is credited with having first used the phrase "trigger point" in print in 1942. Through her work and events in her personal life, Travell advanced the theory that pain experienced in one part of the body is actually caused by an injury or dysfunction in another part of the body. Ultimately, she mapped what she termed the body's trigger points and the manner in which pain radiates to the rest of the body. Travell's work came to national attention when she treated President John F. Kennedy for his back pain.

Trigger points are thought to result from a variety of causes, including birth trauma, **hypoglycemia**, vitamin B$_6$ deficiency, food **allergies**, traumatic injuries, poor posture, skeletal asymmetry, overexertion, or such diseases of the digestive tract as ulcers and **irritable bowel syndrome**. During times of physical or emotional **stress**, the points cause muscles to spasm. Travell's therapy called for the injection of saline (a salt solution) and procaine (also known as Novocaine, an anesthetic) into the trigger point. Although beneficial in the relief of pain, the injections are a painful procedure for some people.

In the 1970s, Bonnie Prudden, a physical fitness and **exercise** therapist, found that applying sustained pressure to a trigger point also relieved pain. Prudden developed her techniques over a number of years and called the treatments myotherapy. Myotherapy is beneficial to patients who find that trigger point injections are too painful.

Benefits

Trigger point therapy is said to interrupt the neural signals that cause both the trigger point and the pain. The object is to eliminate pain and to reeducate the muscles into pain-free habits. In this manner, the swelling and stiffness of neuromuscular pain is reduced, range of motion is increased, and flexibility and coordination are improved. The therapy can also relieve tension and improve circulation.

The list of conditions that benefit from trigger point therapy include arthritis; **carpal tunnel syndrome**; chronic pain in the back, knees, and shoulders; headaches; menstrual cramps; **multiple sclerosis**; muscle spasms, tension, and weakness; postoperative pain; **sciatica**; **temporomandibular joint syndrome** (TMJ); **tendinitis**; and whiplash injuries.

Description

Typically, a health care professional refers a patient to a trigger point therapist. The therapist will take a history of injuries suffered, occupations held, and sports played. He or she will ask the individual to describe the pain and its location in detail.

The therapist will then probe the area of the coordinating trigger point. An injection of lidocaine, saline, or other medicines, or probing with a dry needle, may be done. In myotherapy, once the point is found, the therapist will apply sustained pressure using the fingers, knuckles, or elbows for several seconds.

Pain relief is often experienced immediately. Following the injection or pressure treatment, the therapist will then gently stretch the muscles of the trigger point. Finally, a series of exercises is taught to the individual to reeducate the muscles and to prevent the pain from returning.

Workbooks are now available to help patients maximize the benefits of trigger point therapy through self-treatment at home.

Preparation

Persons should consult a health care professional before beginning trigger point therapy to insure that the pain is not caused by fracture or disease. In fact, a certified trigger point therapist will not provide services to someone who is not referred by a health care professional.

The therapy is usually conducted on a padded table or treatment chair. The individual should wear comfortable loose-fitting clothing. An ongoing, honest interaction with the therapist will facilitate the sessions.

Treatment sessions can last 30 minutes to an hour. The range of cost is approximately $45–60 per session. Acute pain can be relieved in as little as one session. Chronic pain may require numerous treatments.

Precautions

Persons with infectious diseases, open sores, or recent injuries should wait until they have recovered before beginning trigger point therapy.

Persons taking anticoagulant prescription drugs may experience bruising after trigger point therapy.

Research & general acceptance

Research into the effects of trigger point therapy is sketchy, although the growing acceptance of **acupuncture** within the mainstream medical community has led to a few recent published studies of trigger point therapy. Interest in trigger point therapy is growing in Europe and

Asia as well as in the United States; one recent study by a group of Japanese researchers reported that trigger point therapy was superior to standard allopathic drugs in relieving the pain of renal colic.

The American Academy of Pain Management (AAPM) reports that studies of trigger point therapy on back pain and headaches have been conducted on groups of fewer than 10 people. The AAPM does, however, recognize trigger point therapy as a valid approach to the management and relief of pain.

In the traditional medical community, trigger point therapy is viewed as a complement to treatment. Patients are referred by a variety of health professionals including psychiatrists, orthopedic surgeons, and anesthesiologists.

Training & certification

The Pittsburgh School of Pain Management, formerly the Academy for Myofascial Trigger Point Therapy, is located in Pittsburgh, Pennsylvania. The school is licensed by the Commonwealth of Pennsylvania and offers a 650-hour program for persons seeking certification as myofascial trigger point therapists. Eligible entrants are those with such allied health backgrounds as nursing, dentistry, **massage therapy**, physical therapy, occupational therapy, exercise physiology, and sports training. Additionally, a background in biology, anatomy, **nutrition** and/or physiology are often accepted as qualifications. Graduates of the Academy are allowed to sit for certification by the National Certification Board for Trigger Point Myotherapy.

Practitioners carrying the Bonnie Prudden myotherapist certification will have completed a nine-month, 1,300-hour training program and passed the board examination. Therapists are re-certified with a 45-hour training program every other year.

Resources

BOOKS

Credit, Larry, Sharon G. Hartunian, and Margaret J. Nowak. *Your Guide to Complementary Medicine.* Garden City Park, New York: Avery Publishing Group, 1998.

Davies, Clair. *The Trigger Point Therapy Workbook: Your Self-Treatment Guide for Pain Relief.* Oakland, CA: New Harbinger Publications, 2001.

Prudden, Bonnie. *Myotherapy: Bonnie Prudden's Complete Guide to Pain-Free Living.* New York: Ballantine 1984.

Travell, Janet, M.D. *Office Hours: Day and Night.* Cleveland, OH: New American Library, 1968.

PERIODICALS

Baldry, P. "Superficial Versus Deep Dry Needling." *Acupuncture in Medicine* 20 (August 2002): 78-81.

KEY TERMS

. . . .

Bodywork—Any healing technique involving hands-on massage or manipulation of the body.

Myotherapy—A form of trigger point therapy that relies on deep massage of the trigger points rather than injections to relieve pain.

Trigger point—An area of intense irritability within soft tissue structures, characterized by local soreness and sometimes referred pain.

Iguchi, M., Y. Katoh, H. Koike, et al. "Randomized Trial of Trigger Point Injection for Renal Colic." *International Journal of Urology* 9 (September 2002): 475-479.

Irnich, D., N. Behrens, J. M. Gleditsch, et al. "Immediate Effects of Dry Needling and Acupuncture at Distant Points in Chronic Neck Pain: Results of a Randomized, Double-Blind, Sham-Controlled Crossover Trial." *Pain* 99 (September 2002): 83-89.

ORGANIZATIONS

American Academy of Pain Management. 13947 Mono Way #A, Sonora, CA 95370. (209) 533-9744. <www.aapainmanage.org>.

American Academy of Pain Medicine. 4700 W. Lake, Glenview, IL 60025. (847) 375-4731. <www.painmed.org>.

Bonnie Prudden Pain Erasure, LLC. P.O. Box 65240, Tucson, AZ 85728-5240. (800) 221-4634. <www. bonnieprudden.com>.

Pittsburgh School of Pain Management. 1312 E. Carson Street, Pittsburgh, PA 15203. (412) 481-2553. <www. painschool.com>.

Mary McNulty
Rebecca J. Frey, PhD

Triphala

Description

Triphala, an ancient herbal blend, is one of the most commonly used herbal remedies in the Ayurvedic system of healing. **Ayurvedic medicine** originated in ancient India, has developed over thousands of years, and is one of the oldest systems of healing. Thus triphala is one of the longest-used herbal remedies in the world. Triphala, meaning "three fruits," is made from the fruits of three trees that grow throughout India and the Middle East, including amalaki fruit (*Embelica officinalis*), bibhitaki fruit (*Terminalia belerica*), and haritaki fruit (*Terminalia chebula*). In preparing triphala, these fruits are dried, ground into powder, and then blended together according to the precise directions of Ayrurvedic tradition.

Amalaki fruit, also called amla or Indian gooseberry, is renowned as one of the best rejuvenating herbs in Ayurvedic medicine. It contains more **vitamin C** than almost any other fruit, consisting of nearly 3,000 mg of vitamin C per piece. It has been nicknamed the "nurse herb" in India, because of its widespread effectiveness against sickness and its cooling effects on the body. Haritaki is also considered one of the most useful of Ayurvedic herbs, particularly for its rejuvenating, warming, and balancing effects. Combined with bibhitaki fruit, another tonifying and warming herb, these three compounds are believed to have healing and balancing effects on all three of the principal body types or constitutions (termed doshas) in Ayurvedic medicine. As a balanced formula, triphala can be effectively used by most people and is prescribed for a variety of health conditions.

General Use

Triphala is taken as a general health tonic, useful for all body types and a variety of conditions. It is commonly prescribed to tone and strengthen the digestive system, particularly in cases of weak digestion and **constipation**. Triphala is a gentle laxative that can be used daily and is not habit-forming, and has no adverse effects on the intestinal flora (the microorganisms that aid digestion). It is said to improve the function of the stomach and intestines, and is also prescribed for cases of excess stomach acid. Triphala regulates and detoxifies the bowels, improves overall health by increasing the efficiency and absorption of digestion, and reduces **gas**. It has a balancing effect on the body's metabolism, and is prescribed to restore appetite. The herbal compound also helps the body to eliminate excess fat, by improving metabolism. Because of its gentle properties, triphala is recommended as a digestive aid for the elderly and for those with sensitive stomachs.

In addition to restoring the balance of the digestive tract, triphala is used as a blood builder and purifier, and may increase red blood cell count and hemoglobin levels. Some healers prescribe it for diabetes, for its balancing effect on blood sugar levels. It also has anti-cholesterol and anti-mucus properties in the body. Triphala is believed to strengthen the kidneys and liver, and is prescribed for **hepatitis** sufferers.

Triphala is a source of vitamin C and is believed to improve the function of the immune system. The herbs in triphala have anti-inflammatory properties. The remedy is prescribed for **gout**, a form of arthritis caused by excess uric acid in the body, and other inflammatory conditions. Triphala is said to have a calming and tonic effect on the nervous system, and is recommended for

Alzheimer's disease and other degenerative disorders of the nervous system.

Another use for triphala is to strengthen the eyes, particularly in cases of **cataracts**, **glaucoma**, and **conjunctivitis**. It can be used as an eyewash and may reduce soreness and redness in the eyes. Triphala can also be applied topically to the skin to speed the healing of **bruises** and **sunburn**.

Preparations

Triphala is available as a powder, and in tablets and capsules as well. For those who do not like very strong and bitter tastes, tablets or capsules are recommended. Triphala can be taken daily. As a digestive tonic and laxative, it is best taken in the evening, about two hours after eating, and at least 30 minutes before bedtime. No food should be eaten for one and a half hours after ingestion. Tablets and capsules can be swallowed, while the powder can be mixed thoroughly in a small amount of cold or warm water. The powder can also be simmered in water and drunk as a medicinal tea.

Individuals should start with small amounts of triphala, a quarter-teaspoon of the powder or one tablet, gradually increasing the dosage until finding the optimal dosage. No more than one teaspoon of the powder or four to six tablets or capsules should be taken per day. The dosage should be reduced in cases of stomach upset or **diarrhea**.

As triphala is not addictive, it can be taken over long periods of time. It is recommended that every ten weeks, users should stop taking the herbal compound for two to three weeks, to give the body a rest and to maintain the effectiveness of the remedy.

When used as an eyewash, one teaspoon of triphala powder can be added to one cup of boiled and cooled water. The solids should be removed by straining through a dense cloth. The eyewash can be applied to the eyes three times per day. For topical application to the skin, the powder can be mixed with a small amount of water to make an easily applied paste.

Precautions

Triphala is not recommended during **pregnancy** or nursing, and should not be used with cases of diarrhea and dysentery.

Side Effects

The use of triphala may increase intestinal gas at first, as a possible by-product of the cleansing and **detoxification** effects in the digestive tract. Loose stools or diarrhea may indicate too high a dosage, and the amount ingested should be reduced.

KEY TERMS

Dosha—One of the three physical constitution types (vata, pitta, and kapha) in Ayurvedic medicine.

Intestinal flora—The friendly bacteria that live in the digestive tract and aid digestion of food.

Interactions

There are no known interactions between triphala and standard Western prescription drugs as of 2004.

Resources

BOOKS

Frawley, Dr. David and Dr. Vasant Lad. *The Yoga of Herbs: An Ayurvedic Guide to Herbal Medicine.* Twin Lakes, WI: Lotus Press, 2001.

Morrison, Judith. *The Book of Ayurveda.* New York: Fireside Books, 1995.

Tierra, Michael. *The Way of Herbs.* New York: Pocket Books, 1998.

Tiwari, Maya. *Ayurvedic Secrets of Healing.* Twin Lakes, WI: Lotus Press, 1995.

ORGANIZATIONS

The Ayurvedic Institute. 11311 Menaul NE, Albuquerque, New Mexico 87112. (505)291-9698. <http://www.Ayurveda.com>.

Douglas Dupler

TSS *see* **Toxic shock syndrome**

Tuberculosis

Definition

Tuberculosis (TB) is a contagious and potentially fatal disease that can affect almost any part of the body but manifests mainly as an infection of the lungs. It is caused by a bacterial microorganism, the tubercle bacillus or *Mycobacterium tuberculosis*. TB infection can either be acute and short-lived or chronic and long-term.

Description

Although TB can be prevented, treated, and cured with proper treatment and medications, scientists have never been able to eliminate it entirely. The organism that causes tuberculosis, popularly known as consump-

tion, was discovered in 1882. Because antibiotics were unknown, the only means of controlling the spread of infection was to isolate patients in private sanatoria or hospitals limited to patients with TB—a practice that continues to this day in many countries. TB spread very quickly and was a leading cause of death in Europe. At the turn of the twentieth century more than 80% of the people in the United States were infected before age 20, and tuberculosis was the single most common cause of death. Streptomycin was developed in the early 1940s and was the first antibiotic effective against the disease. The number of cases declined until the mid- to late-1980s, when overcrowding, homelessness, immigration, decline in public health inspections, decline in funding, and the **AIDS** epidemic caused a slight resurgence of the disease. The increase in TB in the United States peaked in 1992, and new cases reported in the United States continue to decrease as of 2004. Yet the number of cases in foreign-born individuals is rising, and the number of deaths from TB has been rising, making TB a leading cause of death from infection throughout the world. It is estimated that in the next 10 years 90 million new cases of TB will be reported, with the result of 30 million deaths, or about 3 million deaths per year.

Several demographic groups are at a higher risk of contracting tuberculosis. Tuberculosis is more common in elderly persons. More than one-fourth of the nearly 23,000 cases of TB in the United States in 1995 were reported in people above age 65. TB also is more common in populations where people live under conditions that promote infection, such as homelessness and injection drug use. In the late 1990s, two-thirds of all cases of TB in the United States affected African Americans, Hispanics, Asians, and persons from the Pacific Islands. Finally, the high risk of TB includes people who have a depressed immune system. High-risk groups include alcoholics, people suffering from malnutrition, diabetics, and AIDS patients — and those infected by human immunodeficiency virus (HIV) — who have not yet developed clinical signs of AIDS. TB is the number one killer of women of childbearing age worldwide. In poor countries, women with TB often don't know they have the disease until symptoms become severe.

As of late 2002, TB is a major health problem in certain immigrant communities, such as the Vietnamese in southern California. One team of public health experts in North Carolina maintains that treatment for tuberculosis is the most pressing healthcare need of recent immigrants to the United States. In some cases, the vulnerability of immigrants to tuberculosis is increased by occupational exposure, as a recent outbreak of TB among Mexican poultry farm workers in Delaware indicates. Other public health experts are recommending tubercu-

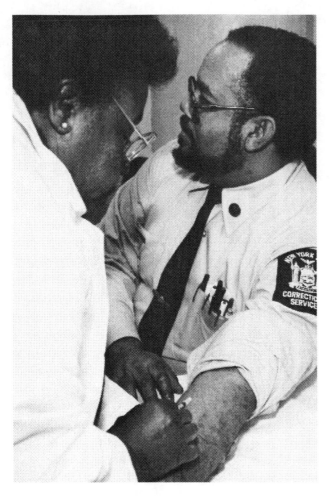

Nurse giving a tuberculosis skin test. *(AP/Wide World Photos. Reproduced by per)*

losis screening at the primary care level for all new immigrants and refugees.

Causes & symptoms

Transmission

Tuberculosis spreads by droplet infection, in which a person breathes in the bacilli released into the air when a TB patient exhales, coughs, or sneezes. However, TB is not considered highly contagious compared to other infectious diseases. Only about one in three people who have close contact with a TB patient, and fewer than 15% of more remote contacts, are likely to become infected. Unlike many other **infections**, TB is not passed on by contact with a patient's clothing, bed linens, or dishes and cooking utensils. Yet if a woman is pregnant, her fetus may contract TB through blood or by inhaling or swallowing the bacilli present in the amniotic fluid.

Once inhaled, water in the droplets evaporates and the tubercle bacilli may reach the small breathing sacs in the lungs (the alveoli), then spread through the lymph vessels to nearby lymph nodes. Sometimes the bacilli move through blood vessels to distant organs. At this point they may either remain alive but inactive (quiescent), or they may cause active disease. The likelihood of acquiring the disease increases with the concentration of bacilli in the air, and the seriousness of the disease is determined by the number of bacteria with which a patient is infected.

Ninety percent of patients who harbor *M. tuberculosis* do not develop symptoms or physical evidence of the disease, and their x rays remain negative. They are not contagious; however, these individuals may get sick at a later date and then pass on TB to others. Though it is impossible to predict whether a person's disease will become active, researchers surmise that more than 90% of cases of active tuberculosis come from this pool of people. An estimated 5% of infected persons get sick within 12-24 months of being infected. Another 5% heal initially but, after years or decades, develop active tuberculosis. This form of the disease is called reactivation TB, or post-primary disease. On rare occasions a previously infected person gets sick again after a second exposure to the tubercle bacillus.

Pulmonary tuberculosis

Pulmonary tuberculosis is TB that affects the lungs, and represents about 85% of new cases diagnosed. It usually presents with a **cough**, which may or may not produce sputum. In time, more sputum is produced that is streaked with blood. The cough may be present for weeks or months and may be accompanied by chest **pain** and shortness of breath. Persons with pulmonary TB often run a low-grade **fever** and suffer from nightsweats. The patient often loses interest in food and may lose weight. If the infection allows air to escape from the lungs into the chest cavity (pneumothorax) or if fluid collects in the pleural space (pleural effusion), the patient may have difficulty breathing. The TB bacilli may travel from the lungs to lymph nodes in the sides and back of the neck. Infection in these areas can break through the skin and discharge pus.

Extrapulmonary tuberculosis

Although the lungs are the major site of damage caused by tuberculosis, many other organs and tissues in the body may be affected. Abut 15% of newly diagnosed cases of TB are extrapulmonary, with a higher proportion of these being HIV-infected persons. The usual progression of the disease is to begin in the lungs and spread to locations outside the lungs (extrapulmonary sites). In some cases, however, the first sign of disease appears outside the lungs. The many tissues or organs that tuberculosis may affect include:

- Bones. TB is particularly likely to attack the spine and the ends of the long bones.

- Kidneys. Along with the bones, the kidneys are probably the most common site of extrapulmonary TB. There may, however, be few symptoms even though part of a kidney is destroyed.

- Female reproductive organs. The ovaries in women may be infected; TB can spread from them to the peritoneum, which is the membrane lining the abdominal cavity.

- Abdominal cavity. Tuberculous peritonitis may cause pain ranging from the mild discomfort of stomach cramps to intense pain that may mimic the symptoms of appendicitis.

- Joints. Tubercular infection of joints causes a form of arthritis that most often affects the hips and knees.

- Meninges. The meninges are tissues that cover the brain and the spinal cord. Infection of the meninges by the TB bacillus causes tuberculous **meningitis**, a condition that is most common in young children and the elderly. It is extremely dangerous. Patients develop headaches, become drowsy, and eventually comatose. Permanent brain damage can result without prompt treatment.

- Skin, intestines, adrenal glands, and blood vessels. All these parts of the body can be infected by *M. tuberculosis*. Infection of the wall of the body's main artery (the aorta), can cause it to rupture with catastrophic results. Tuberculous pericarditis occurs when the membrane surrounding the heart (the pericardium) is infected and fills up with fluid that interferes with the heart's ability to pump blood.

- Miliary tuberculosis. Miliary TB is a life-threatening condition that occurs when large numbers of tubercle bacilli spread throughout the body. Huge numbers of tiny tubercular lesions develop that cause marked weakness and weight loss, severe **anemia**, and gradual wasting of the body.

Diagnosis

TB is diagnosed through laboratory test results. The standard test for tuberculosis infection, the tuberculin skin test, detects the presence of infection, not of active TB. Skin testing has been done for more than 100 years. In this process, tuberculin is an extract prepared from cultures of *M. tuberculosis*. It contains substances belonging to the bacillus (antigens) to which an infected person has been sensitized. When tuberculin is injected into the skin of an infected person, the area around the injection becomes hard, swollen, and red within one to three days.

Today skin tests utilize a substance called purified protein derivative (PPD) that has a standard chemical composition and is therefore a good measure of the presence of tubercular infection. The PPD test, also called the Mantoux test, is not always 100% accurate; it can produce false positive as well as false negative results. The test may indicate that some people who have a skin reaction are not infected (false positive) and that some who do not react are in fact infected (false negative). The PPD test is, however, useful as a screener and can be used on people who have had a suspicious chest x ray, on those who have had close contact with a TB patient, and persons who come from a country where TB is common.

Because of the multiple and varied symptoms of TB, diagnosis on the basis of external symptoms is not always possible. TB is often discovered by an abnormal chest x ray or other test result rather than by a claim of physical discomfort by the patient. After an irregular x ray, a PPD test is always done to show whether the patient has been infected. To verify the test results, the physician obtains a sample of sputum or a tissue sample (biopsy) for culture. In cases where other areas of the body might be infected, such as the kidney or the brain, body fluids other than sputum (urine or spinal fluid, for example) can be used for culture.

One important new advance in the diagnosis of TB is the use of molecular techniques to speed the diagnostic process as well as improve its accuracy. As of late 2002, four molecular techniques are increasingly used in laboratories around the world. They include polymerase chain reaction to detect mycobacterial DNA in patient specimens; nucleic acid probes to identify mycobacteria in culture; restriction fragment length polymorphism analysis to compare different strains of TB for epidemiological studies; and genetic-based susceptibility testing to identify drug-resistant strains of mycobacteria.

Treatment

Because of the nature of tuberculosis, the disease should never be treated by alternative methods alone. Alternative treatments can help support healing, but treatment of TB must include drugs and will require the care of a physician. Any alternative treatments should be discussed with a medical practitioner before they are applied.

Supportive treatments include:

- Diet. Nutritionists recommend a whole food diet including raw foods, fluids, and particularly pears and pear products (pear juice, pear sauce), since pears may help heal the lungs. Other helpful foods include **fenugreek**, **alfalfa** sprouts, **garlic**, pomegranate, and yogurt or kefir. Four tablespoons of pureed steamed asparagus at breakfast and dinner taken for a few months may also be helpful.

- Nutritional therapy. Nutritionists may recommend one or many of the following vitamins and minerals: **vitamin A** at 300,000 IU for the first three days, 200,000 IU for the next two days, then 50,000 IU for several weeks; beta-carotene at 25,000-50,000 IU; **vitamin E** at up to 1,000 IU daily unless the patient is a premenopausal woman with premenstrual symptoms; lipotrophic formula (one daily); deglycerolized **licorice**; citrus seed extract; **vitamin C**; lung glandular; **essential fatty acids**; **vitamin B complex**; multiminerals; and zinc.

- Herb therapy may use the tinctures of **echinacea**, elecampane, and **mullein** taken three times per day, along with three garlic capsules three times per day.

- Hydrotherapy may be used up to five times weekly. Dr. **Benedict Lust**, the founder of naturopathy, supposedly cured himself of tuberculosis by using hydrotherapy.

- Juice therapy. Raw potato juice, may be taken three times daily with equal parts of carrot juice plus one teaspoon of olive or almond oil, one teaspoon of honey, beaten until it foams. Before using the potato juice, starch should be allowed to settle from the juice.

- Topical treatment may use **eucalyptus** oil packs, grape packs or grain alcohol packs.

Professional practitioners may also treat tuberculosis using **cell therapy**, magnetic field therapy, or **traditional Chinese medicine**. **Fasting** may be undertaken, but only with a doctor's supervision.

Allopathic treatment

Drug therapy

Five drugs are most commonly used today to treat tuberculosis: isoniazid (INH), rifampin, pyrazinamide, streptomycin, and ethambutol. Of the five medications, INH is the most frequently used drug for both treatment and prevention. The first three drugs may be given in the same capsule to minimize and treat active TB the number of pills in the dosage. As of 1998, many patients are given INH and rifampin together for six months, with pyrazinamide added for the first two months. Hospitalization is rarely necessary because many patients are no longer infectious after about two weeks of combination treatment. A physician must monitor side effects and conduct monthly sputum tests. In 2002, the Centers for Disease Control (CDC) worked with medical organizations to release new guidelines that better individualize the drug regimens received by TB patients depending on their disease symptoms and severity. Many can now receive once-weekly doses of rifapentine in the continuation phase of treatment.

The first large scale trial of a new agent to treat TB began in 2002. The promising new drug, called moxifloxacin, may mean a shorter treatment course for TB sufferers in the near future. It will also be tested in combination with rifapentine, and researchers believe that using the drugs together will mean a less frequent dosing schedule for patients.

Drug resistance has become a problem in treating TB. When patients do not take medication properly or for long enough periods of time, the TB organisms may become drug resistant. This makes the patient vulnerable to further infection and allows the TB organism to develop resistance.

Surgery

Surgical treatment of TB may be used if medications are ineffective. There are three surgical treatments for pulmonary TB: pneumothorax, in which air is introduced into the chest to collapse the lung; thoracoplasty, in which one or more ribs are removed; and removal of a diseased lung, in whole or in part. It is possible for patients to survive with one healthy lung.

Expected results

The prognosis for recovery from TB is good for most patients, if the disease is diagnosed early and given prompt treatment with appropriate medications on a long-term regimen. According to a 2002 Johns Hopkins study, most patients in the United States who die of TB are older—average age 62— and suffer from such underlying diseases as diabetes and kidney failure.

Modern surgical methods are usually effective when necessary. Miliary tuberculosis is still fatal in many cases but is rarely seen today in developed countries. Even in cases in which the bacillus proves resistant to all of the commonly used medications, other seldom-used drugs may be tried because the tubercle bacilli have not yet developed resistance to them.

Prevention

Vaccination is widely used as a prevention measure for TB. A vaccine called BCG (Bacillus Calmette-Guérin, named after its French developers) is made from a weakened mycobacterium that infects cattle. Vaccination with BCG does not prevent infection, but it does strengthen the immune system of first-time TB patients. As a result, serious complications are less likely to develop. BCG is used more widely in developing countries than in the United States. Though the vaccine has been proven beneficial and fairly safe, its use is still controversial. It is not clear whether the vaccine's effectiveness depends on the population in which it is used or on variations in its formulation. Recently, efforts have been focused on developing a new vaccine.

Generally, prevention focuses on the prevention of transmission, skin-testing high-risk persons and providing preventive drug therapy to people at risk. Measures such as avoidance of overcrowded and unsanitary conditions are necessary aspects of prevention. Hospital emergency rooms and similar locations can be treated with ultraviolet light, which has an antibacterial effect.

INH is also given to prevent TB, and decreases the incidence of TB by about 60% over the life of the patient. INH is effective when taken daily for 6 to 12 months by people in high-risk categories who are under 35 years of age. About 1% of patients in preventive treatment develop toxicity. Because INH carries the risk of side effects (liver inflammation, nerve damage, changes in mood and behavior), it is important for its use to be monitored and to give it only to persons at special risk.

Unfortunately, failure of TB patients to complete the full course of their drugs adds to TB incidence and encourages development of drug-resistant strains of the disease. As scientists try to develop drugs that require shorter courses, physicians must work with patients to encourage compliance with their treatments. Even if symptoms go away, patients often have to continue their drug treatment for six months to be sure to stop the spread of their TB infection to others.

Resources

BOOKS

Burton-Goldberg Group. *Alternative Medicine: The Definitive Guide.* Puyallup, WA: Future Medicine Publishing, Inc., 1994.

"Infectious Diseases Caused by Mycobacteria." Section 13, Chapter 157 in *The Merck Manual of Diagnosis and Therapy*, edited by Mark H. Beers, MD, and Robert Berkow, MD. Whitehouse Station, NJ: Merck Research Laboratories, 2001.

Merck Manual of Medical Information: Home Edition. Edited by Robert Berkow, et al. Whitehouse Station, NJ: Merck Research Laboratories, 1997.

Pelletier, Kenneth R., MD. *The Best Alternative Medicine*, Part II, "CAM Therapies for Specific Conditions: Tuberculosis." New York: Simon & Schuster, 2002.

Smolley, Lawrence A., and Debra F. Bryse. *Breathe Right Now: A Comprehensive Guide to Understanding and Treating the Most Common Breathing Disorders.* New York: W. W. Norton & Co., 1998.

PERIODICALS

"Changing Patterns of New Tuberculosis Infections." *Infectious Disease Alert* (August 15, 2002): 171–172.

KEY TERMS

Bacillus Calmette-Guérin (BCG)—A vaccine made from a damaged bacillus similar to the tubercle bacillus, which may help prevent serious pulmonary TB and its complications.

Miliary tuberculosis—A form of TB in which the bacillus spreads through all body tissues and organs, producing many thousands of tiny tubercular lesions. Miliary TB is often fatal unless promptly treated.

Mycobacteria—A group of bacteria that includes *Mycobacterium tuberculosis*, the bacterium that causes tuberculosis, and other forms that cause related illnesses.

Pneumothorax—Air inside the chest cavity, which may cause the lung to collapse. Pneumothorax is both a complication of pulmonary tuberculosis and a means of treatment designed to allow an infected lung to rest and heal.

Purified protein derivative (PPD)—An extract of tubercle bacilli that is injected into the skin to find out whether a person presently has or has ever had tuberculosis.

Sputum—Secretions produced in a patient's infected lung and coughed up. Sputum is routinely used as a specimen for culturing the tubercle bacillus in the laboratory.

"'Drug of Dreams' Preps for First Large-Scale Trail: Study to Begin this Year; Moxifloxacin to Debut Soon in Study 27." *TB Monitor* (July 2002): 73.

Efferen, Linda S. "Tuberculosis: Practical Solutions to Meet the Challenge." *Journal of Respiratory Diseases* (November 1999): 772.

Fielder, J. F., C. P. Chaulk, M. Dalvi, et al. "A High Tuberculosis Case-Fatality Rate in a Setting of Effective Tuberculosis Control: Implications for Acceptable Treatment Success Rates." *International Journal of Tuberculosis and Lung Disease* 6 (December 2002): 1114–1117.

"Guidelines Roll Out Two New Variations: Experts Give Both a Thumbs Up." *TB Monitor* (August 2002): 85.

Houston, H. R., N. Harada, and T. Makinodan. "Development of a Culturally Sensitive Educational Intervention Program to Reduce the High Incidence of Tuberculosis Among Foreign-Born Vietnamese." *Ethnic Health* 7 (November 2002): 255–265.

Kim, D. Y., R. Ridzon, B. Giles, and T. Mireles. "Pseudo-Outbreak of Tuberculosis in Poultry Plant Workers, Sussex County, Delaware." *Journal of Occupational and Environmental Medicine* 44 (December 2002): 1169–1172.

Moua, M., F. A. Guerra, J. D. Moore, and R. O. Valdiserri. "Immigrant Health: Legal Tools/Legal Barriers." *Journal of Law and Medical Ethics* 30 (Fall 2002) (3 Suppl.): 189–196.

"New Drugs Sought for Top Killer of Young Women Worldwide." *Women's Health Weekly* (July 25, 2002): 20.

"Poor Patient Compliance Key to Drug Resistance in Tuberculosis." *Pulse* (July 1, 2002): 18.

Stauffer, W. M., D. Kamat, and P. F. Walker. "Screening of International Immigrants, Refugees, and Adoptees." *Primary Care* 29 (December 2002): 879–905.

Su, W. J. "Recent Advances in the Molecular Diagnosis of Tuberculosis." *Journal of Microbiology, Immunology, and Infection* 35 (December 2002): 209–214.

ORGANIZATIONS

American Lung Association. 432 Park Avenue South, New York, NY 10016. (800) LUNG-USA. <www.lungusa.org>.

National Heart, Lung, and Blood Institute (NHLBI). P. O. Box 30105, Bethesda, MD 20824-0105. (301) 592-8573. <www.nhlbi.nih.gov>.

OTHER

New York State Department of Health. Communicable Disease Fact Sheet. nyhealth@health.state.ny.us.

University of Wisconsin-Madison Health Sciences Libraries. "Pulmonary Medicine" Healthweb. http://www.biostat.wisc.edu/chslib/hw/pulmonar.

Amy Cooper
Teresa G. Odle
Rebecca J. Frey, PhD

Tui na *see* **Traditional Chinese medicine**

Turmeric

Description

Turmeric is a member of the *Curcuma* botanical group, which is part of the **ginger** family of herbs, the Zingiberaceae. Its botanical name is *Curcuma longa*. Turmeric is widely grown both as a kitchen spice and for its medicinal uses. Two closely related plants, *Curcuma petolata* and *Curcuma roscoeana*, are natives of Cambodia and are grown for their decorative foliage and blossoms. All curcumas are perennial plants native to southern Asia. They grow in warm, humid climates and thrive only in temperatures above 60°F (29.8°C). India, Sri Lanka, the East Indies, Fiji, and Queensland (Australia) all have climates that are conducive to growing turmeric.

The turmeric plant is identifiable by both its characteristic tuberous root and the leaves that extend upward from erect, thick stems arising from the root. Turmeric root is actually a fleshy oblong tuber 2–3 in (5–10 cm) in length, and close to 1 in (2.54 cm) wide. It is tapered at each end, and its exterior can be yellow, tan, or olive-green in color. The interior of the root is hard, firm, and either orange-brown or deeply rust-colored, with transverse resinous parallel rings. M. Grieve, in *A Modern Herbal*, states that the root is dense and breaks into a powder that is lemon yellow in color. Turmeric root has a fragrant aroma and a somewhat bitter, peppery, biting taste reminiscent of ginger. When eaten, it colors the saliva yellow and leaves a warm sensation in the mouth.

The root contains a bitter volatile oil, brown coloring matter, gum, starch, **calcium** chloride, woody fiber and a yellowish coloring material that is known as cucurmin. In addition to the root, the turmeric plant produces rhizomes, which are underground stems growing parallel to the ground that produce roots below and new shoots from their upper surface. Turmeric rhizomes have also been used for medicinal purposes. The plant's leaves are divided, lance-shaped and narrower at each end. They are close to 2 ft (61 cm), lustrous and deep green. The flowers arise from those leaves, and are a pale yellow color, growing in groupings of three to five.

General use

Powdered turmeric root is perhaps best known as a popular spice, frequntly used in Eastern cooking. It is an ingredient of curry powders, and is also used to give mustard its characteristic color. It is sometimes used as a substitute for **saffron**. The addition of turmeric to such oils as olive or **sesame oil** extends their shelf life due to its antioxidant properties. In addition, some orange and lemon drinks are now colored with turmeric, which is considered safer than artificial colorings derived from coal tar.

The powdered root of turmeric has been used for making a deep yellow dye for fabrics for hundreds of years, though it does not produce an enduring color-fast tint. It is also used as a coloring for medicines at times. A less familiar use of turmeric is in chemistry, in the making of papers to test for alkaline solutions. White paper soaked in a tincture of turmeric turns reddish-brown and dries to a violet color when an alkaline solution is added.

Though its use in Western herbal medicine has declined over the years, turmeric has long been used and continues in use in Eastern medicine, both Oriental herbal medicine and Ayurveda, the traditional system of medicine from India. R.C. Srimal, in *Turmeric: A Brief Review of Medicinal Properties*, describes the herb as having the ability to protect the liver against toxic substances, especially such heavy metals as lead; to prevent the formation of **gallstones** or decrease the size of stones already formed; and to increase the flow of bile.

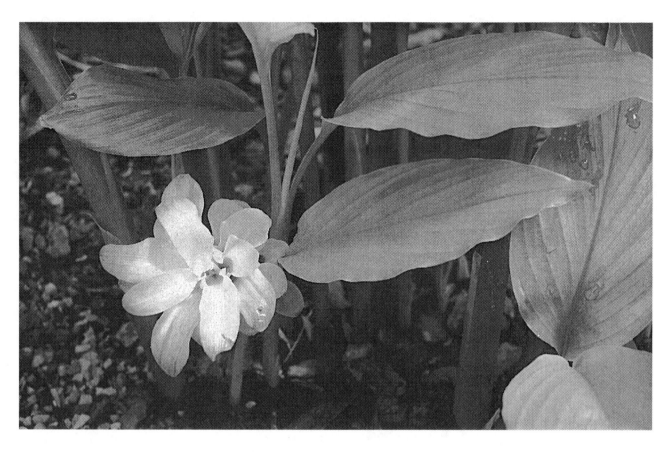

Turmeric blossom. (© *PlantaPhile, Germany. Reproduced by permission.*)

Some studies have demonstrated that turmeric exhibits anti-inflammatory properties that are useful in the treatment of both **osteoarthritis** and **rheumatoid arthritis**. Alcohol extracts of turmeric have been found to reduce blood sugar, which could eventually affect the treatment of diabetes. In addiion, clinical trials in China have demonstrated that simply using turmeric as a food seasoning can reduce serum **cholesterol levels**. The World Health Organization has recommended the use of this spice.

A substance known as a lipopolysaccharide isolated from the turmeric root has shown a capacity to stimulate and increase the activity of the immune system. In addition, research has shown turmeric to be effective in destroying gram-positive salmonella bacteria *in vitro*. Turmeric also demonstrates antifungal properties.

Turmeric has long been used as an Eastern folk remedy for eye discharges and as a cooling, soothing skin lotion. In Chinese herbal medicine, under the name of *jiang huang*, the turmeric rhizome is used in many different formulas as an anti-inflammatory **pain** reliever, especially for shoulder pain. It is believed to invigorate and improve the movement of blood and stimulate **menstruation**. The turmeric tuber, which is called *yu jin* in Chinese

medicine, also has many important uses. It is given for **jaundice**, pain in the liver area, agitation, and **insomnia**.

The cucurmin found in turmeric is being studied as a possible treatment to prevent **cancer**. Cucurmin appears to lower the rate of genetic mutations in experimental animals. It has also been shown to induce apoptosis, or cell self-destruction, in **leukemia** cells. In addition, recent studies done on tissue samples from the human digestive tract indicate that cucurmin may help to prevent colon cancer.

Preparations

Turmeric root is cleaned, boiled, and dried in the oven before being powdered. This pulverized root can then be dissolved in either water or alcohol. It is usually dissolved in boiling alcohol and filtered to make a medicinal tincture.

In India and Pakistan, turmeric is dissolved in water for use as an eyewash, and in milk to make a soothing skin lotion.

Precautions

Practitioners of Chinese herbal medicine advise against using turmeric during **pregnancy**.

KEY TERMS

Antifungal—A type of medication prescribed to treat infections caused by fungi.

Anti-inflammatory—A type of medication or substance that reduces the symptoms of fever and inflammation.

Apoptosis—A form of cell death in which a damaged cell shuts down and in effect commits suicide. Cucurmin induces apoptosis in some kinds of cancer cells.

Cucurmin (sometimes spelled Curcumin)—A yellow material that gives turmeric root its characteristic color.

Gram-positive bacteria—Bacteria that retain a dark violet stain when treated with an iodine-based stain known as Gram's iodine, named for a Danish bacteriologist. Common examples of gram-positive bacteria include several species of streptococci, staphylococci, and *Clostridia*.

In vitro—A term used to describe research carried out in laboratory equipment rather than in a living organism.

Lipopolysaccharide—A complex carbohydrate with lipids (organic fats and waxes) attached to its molecule.

Rhizome—An underground stem of a plant, usually horizontal, that sends roots from its lower surface and new shoots from the upper surface.

Tuber—A thick, fleshy underground stem that produces buds that can give rise to new plants.

Side effects

Like other anti-inflammatory agents, turmeric has been found to contribute to the formation of stomach ulcers.

Resources

BOOKS

Grieve, M., and C. F. Leyel. *A Modern Herbal: The Medical, Culinary, Costmetic and Economic Properties, Cultivation and Folklore of Herbs, Grasses, Fungi, Shrubs and Trees With All of Their Modern Scientific Uses.* New York: Barnes and Noble Publishing, 1992.

Molony, David, and Ming Ming Pan Molony. *The American Association of Oriental Medicine's Complete Guide to Chinese Herbal Medicine.* New York: Berkley Publishing, 1999.

Phillips, Ellen, and C. Colston Burrell. *Rodale's Illustrated Encyclopedia of Perennials.* Emmaus, PA: Rodale Press, Inc., 1993.

Srimal, R. C. *Turmeric: A Brief Overview of Medicinal Properties* . London: Filoterapia, 1997.

PERIODICALS

Anto, R. J., A. Mukhopadhyay, K. Denning, and B. B. Aggarwal. "Curcumin (Diferuloylmethane) Induces Apoptosis Through Activation of Caspase-8, BID Cleavage and Cytochrome C Release: Its Suppression by Ectopic Expression of Bcl-2 and Bcl-xl." *Carcinogenesis* 23 (January 2002): 143-150.

Ireson, C. R., D. J. Jones, S. Orr, et al. "Metabolism of the Cancer Chemopreventive Agent Curcumin in Human and Rat Intestine." *Cancer Epidemiology and Biomarkers* 11 (January 2002): 105-111.

Shukla, Y., A. Arora, and P. Taneja. "Antimutagenic Potential of Curcumin on Chromosomal Aberrations in Wistar Rats." *Mutation Research* 25 (March 2002): 197-202.

Joan Schonbeck
Rebecca J. Frey, PhD

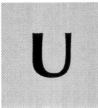

Ulcerative colitis *see* **Inflammatory bowel disease**

Ulcers, digestive

Definition

An ulcer is an eroded area of skin or mucous membrane. In common usage, however, ulcer usually refers to disorders in the upper digestive tract. The terms ulcer, gastric ulcer, and peptic ulcer are often used interchangeably. Peptic ulcers can develop in the lower part of the esophagus, the stomach, the first part of the small intestine (the duodenum), and the second part of the small intestine (the jejunum).

Description

It is estimated that 2% of the adult population in the United States has active digestive ulcers, and that about 10% will develop ulcers at some point in their lives. There are about 500,000 new cases in the United States every year, with as many as 4 million recurrences. The male/female ratio for digestive ulcers is 3:1.

The most common forms of digestive ulcer are duodenal and gastric. About 80% of all digestive ulcers are duodenal ulcers. This type of ulcer may strike people in any age group but is most common in males between the ages of 20 and 45. The incidence of duodenal ulcers has dropped over the past 30 years. Gastric ulcers account for about 16% of digestive ulcers. They are most common in males between the ages of 55 and 70. The most common cause of gastric ulcers is the use of nonsteroidal anti-inflammatory drugs, or NSAIDs. The current widespread use of NSAIDs is thought to explain why the incidence of gastric ulcers in the United States is rising.

Causes & symptoms

Causes of ulcers

There are three major causes of digestive ulcers: infection; certain medications; and disorders that cause oversecretion of stomach juices.

HELICOBACTER PYLORI INFECTION. *Helicobacter pylori* is a bacterium that lives in the mucous tissues that line the digestive tract. Infection with *H. pylori* is the most common cause of duodenal ulcers. About 95% of patients with duodenal ulcers are infected with *H. pylori*, as opposed to only 70% of patients with gastric ulcers.

USE OF NONSTEROIDAL ANTI-INFLAMMATORY DRUGS (NSAIDS). Nonsteroidal anti-inflammatory drugs, or NSAIDs, are painkillers that many people use for headaches, sore muscles, arthritis, and menstrual cramps. Many NSAIDs are available without prescriptions. Common NSAIDs include aspirin, ibuprofen (Advil, Motrin), flurbiprofen (Ansaid, Ocufen), ketoprofen (Orudis), and indomethacin (Indacin). Chronic NSAID users have 40 times the risk of developing a gastric ulcer as nonusers. Users are also three times more likely than nonusers to develop bleeding or fatal complications of ulcers. Aspirin is the most likely NSAID to cause ulcers.

Other Risk Factors

- Hypersecretory syndromes, including Zollinger-Ellison syndrome, secrete excessive amounts of digestive juices into the digestive tract. Fewer than 5% of digestive ulcers are due to these disorders.

- **Smoking** increases a patient's chance of developing an ulcer, decreases the body's response to therapy, and increases the chances of dying from complications.

- Blood type. Persons with type A blood are more likely to have gastric ulcers, while those with type O are more likely to develop duodenal ulcers.

- Attitudes toward **stress**, rather than the presence of stress, puts one at risk for ulcers.

- Having a critical illness. Patients who are very sick are at increased risk of developing stress-related ulcers.

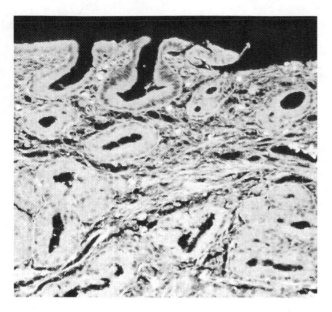

A light microscopy image of a stomach ulcer. *(Photograph by J.L. Carson, Custom Medical Stock Photo. Reproduced by permission.)*

The consumption of high-fat or spicy foods is not a significant risk factor.

Symptoms

Not all digestive ulcers produce symptoms; as many as 20% of ulcer patients have so-called painless or silent ulcers. Silent ulcers occur most frequently in the elderly and in chronic NSAID users.

The symptoms of gastric ulcers include feelings of **indigestion** and **heartburn**, weight loss, and repeated episodes of gastrointestinal bleeding. Ulcer **pain** is often described as gnawing, dull, aching, or resembling hunger pangs. The patient may be nauseated and suffer loss of appetite. About 30% of patients with gastric ulcers are awakened by pain at night. Many patients have periods of chronic ulcer pain alternating with symptom-free periods that last for several weeks or months. This characteristic is called periodicity.

The symptoms of duodenal ulcers include heartburn, stomach pain relieved by eating or taking antacids, weight gain, and a burning sensation at the back of the throat. The patient is most likely to feel discomfort two to four hours after meals, or after having citrus juice, coffee, or aspirin. About 50% of patients with duodenal ulcers awake during the night with pain, usually between midnight and 3 A.M. A regular pattern of ulcer pain associated with certain periods of day or night or a time interval after meals is called rhythmicity.

Complications

Between 10%–20% of peptic ulcer patients develop complications at some time during the course of their illness. All of these are potentially serious conditions. Complications are not always preceded by diagnosis of or treatment for ulcers; as many as 60% of patients with complications have not had prior symptoms.

Bleeding is the most common complication of ulcers. It may result in **anemia**, **vomiting** blood, or the passage of bright red blood through the rectum. The mortality rate from ulcer hemorrhage is 6-10%.

About 5% of ulcer patients develop perforations, which are holes through which the stomach contents can leak out into the abdominal cavity. The incidence of perforation is rising because of the increased use of NSAIDs, particularly among the elderly. The signs of an ulcer perforation are severe pain, **fever**, and tenderness when the doctor touches the abdomen. Most cases of perforation require emergency surgery. The mortality rate is about 5%.

Ulcer penetration is a complication in which the ulcer erodes through the intestinal wall without digestive fluid leaking into the abdomen. Instead, the ulcer penetrates into an adjoining organ, such as the pancreas or liver. The signs of penetration are more severe pain *without* rhythmicity or periodicity, and the spread of the pain to the lower back.

Obstruction of the stomach outlet occurs in about 2% of ulcer patients. It is caused by swelling or scar tissue formation that narrows the opening between the stomach and the duodenum (the pylorus). Over 90% of patients with obstruction have recurrent vomiting of partly digested or undigested food; 20% are seriously dehydrated.

Diagnosis

Physical examination and patient history

The diagnosis of peptic ulcers is rarely made on the basis of a physical examination alone. The only significant finding may be mild soreness in the area over the stomach when the doctor presses (palpates) it. The doctor is more likely to suspect an ulcer if the patient has one or more of the following risk factors:

- member of the male sex
- age over 45
- recent weight loss, bleeding, recurrent vomiting, **jaundice**, back pain, or anemia
- history of using aspirin or other NSAIDs
- history of heavy smoking
- family history of ulcers or stomach **cancer**

Endoscopy and imaging studies

An endoscopy is considered the best procedure for diagnosing ulcers and taking tissue samples. An endoscope is a slender tube-shaped instrument used to view the tissues lining the stomach and duodenum. If the ulcer is in the stomach, then a tissue sample will be taken because 3-5% of gastric ulcers are cancerous. Duodenal ulcers are rarely cancerous. Radiological studies are sometimes used instead of endoscopy because they are less expensive, more comfortable for the patient, and are 85% accurate in detecting cancer.

Laboratory tests

Blood tests usually give normal results in ulcer patients without complications. They are useful, however, in evaluating anemia from a bleeding ulcer or a high white cell count from perforation or penetration. Serum gastrin levels can be used to screen for Zollinger-Ellison syndrome.

It is important to test for *H. pylori* because almost all ulcer patients who are not taking NSAIDs are infected. Noninvasive tests include blood tests for immune response and a breath test. In the breath test, the patient is given an oral dose of radiolabeled urea. If *H. pylori* is present, it will react with the urea and the patient will exhale radiolabeled carbon dioxide. Invasive tests for *H. pylori* include tissue biopsies and cultures performed from fluid obtained by endoscopy.

Treatment

Alternative treatments can relieve symptoms and promote healing of ulcers. A primary goal of these treatments is to rebalance the stomach's hydrochloric acid output and to enhance the mucosal lining of the stomach.

Food **allergies** have been considered a major cause of stomach ulcers. An elimination/challenge diet can help identify the allergenic food(s) and continued elimination of these foods can assist in healing the ulcer.

Ulcer patients should avoid aspirin, stop smoking, avoid antacids, and reduce stress. Dietary changes include avoidance of sugar, **caffeine**, and alcohol, and reducing milk intake.

Supplements

Dietary supplements that help to control ulcer symptoms include:

- vitamin A
- B-complex vitamins
- vitamin C
- vitamin E
- glutamine
- rice bran oil (gamma oryzanol)
- selenium
- deglycyrrhizinated **licorice** (DGL)
- zinc picolinate

Herbals

Botanical medicine offers the following remedies that may help treat ulcers:

- Bilberry (*Vaccinium myrtillus*): heals ulcers.
- Cabbage: heals ulcers.
- Calendula (*Calendula officinalis*): heals duodenal ulcers.
- Chamomile tea: speeds healing, reduces mucosal reaction, reduces stress, and lessens gas.
- Comfrey (*Symphytum officinale*) root: soothes the stomach, lessens bleeding, and speeds healing, however, the patient must take caution, in that prolonged or excessive use can be harmful to the liver.
- Geranium (*Pelargonium odoratissimum*): lessens bleeding.
- Licorice (*Glycyrrhiza glabra*): heals ulcers.
- **Marsh mallow** (*Althaea officinalis*) root: soothes the stomach.
- Meadowsweet: soothes the stomach.
- Plantain (*Plantago major*): soothes the stomach.
- Slippery elm (*Ulmus fulva*): lessens bleeding and heals mucous membrane.
- Wheat grass (*Triticum aestivum*): heals ulcers.

Chinese medicines

Chinese herbal treatment principles are based upon specific groups of symptoms. Chinese patent medicines are also based upon specific symptoms and include:

- Wu Bei San (cuttlefish bone and **fritillaria**): acid reflux and bleeding
- Wu Shao San (cuttlefish bone and paeonia): acid reflux and bleeding
- Liang Fu Wan (galangal and **cyperus** pill): pain
- 204 Wei Tong Pian (204 epigastric pain tablet): pain, acid reflux, and bleeding
- Xi Lei San (tin-like powder): ulcer with tarry stool

Other treatments

Other treatments for ulcers are:

- Essence therapy. **Dandelion** essence can help reduce tension, and pink **yarrow** essence can help the patient distinguish between his or her problems and those of others.

- Reflexology. For ulcers, the practitioner work the solar plexus and stomach points on the feet and the solar plexus, stomach, and top of shoulder points on the hands.

- **Biofeedback**. Thermal biofeedback can help protect and heal the stomach.

- Sound therapy. Music with a slow, steady beat can promote **relaxation** and reduce stress.

- Ayurveda. Ayurvedic treatment is individualized to each patient but common ulcer remedies include: **aloe vera** natural gel, **arrowroot** powder with hot milk, and tea prepared from cumin, coriander, and **fennel** seeds.

- Acupuncture. Ulcers can be treated using target points for stress, **anxiety**, and stomach problems.

- Relaxation techniques. Stress reduction and involvement in stress management programs may help relieve ulcer symptoms.

Allopathic treatment

Medications

Most drugs that are used to treat ulcers work by either lowering the rate of stomach acid secretion or protecting the mucous tissues that line the digestive tract.

Medications that lower the rate of stomach acid secretions fall into two major categories: proton pump inhibitors and H_2 receptor antagonists. The proton pump inhibitors, which have been in use since the early 1990s, include omeprazole (Prilosec) and lansoprazole (Prevacid). The H_2 receptor antagonists include ranitidine (Zantac), cimetidine (Tagamet), famotidine (Pepcid), and nizatidine (Axid).

Drugs that protect the stomach tissues are sucralfate (Carafate), bismuth preparations, and misoprostol (Cytotec).

Most doctors presently recommend treatment to eliminate *H. pylori* to prevent ulcer recurrences. Without such treatment, ulcers recur at the rate of 80% per year. The drug combination used to eliminate the bacterium is tetracycline, bismuth subsalicylate (Pepto-Bismol), and metronidazole (Metizol). Eradication is not always successful, however, for reasons that are unclear.

Surgery

Surgical treatment of ulcers is generally used only for complications and suspected cancer. The introduction of a newer technique for repairing perforated ulcers using a laparoscope rather than opening the patient's abdomen may reduce some of the risks associated with surgical treatment of ulcers. The most common surgical procedures are vagotomies, in which the connections of the vagus nerve to the stomach are cut to reduce acid secretion; and antrectomies, which involve the removal of part of the stomach.

Expected results

The prognosis for recovery from ulcers is good for most patients. Very few ulcers fail to respond to the medications that are currently used to treat them. Recurrences can be cut to 5% by eradication of *H. pylori*. Most patients who develop complications recover without problems even when emergency surgery is necessary.

Prevention

Strategies for the prevention of ulcers or their recurrence include the following:

- giving misoprostol to patients who must take NSAIDs
- participating in integrated stress management programs
- avoiding unnecessary use of aspirin and NSAIDs
- improving the nutritional status of critically ill patients
- quitting smoking
- cutting down on alcohol, tea, coffee, and sodas containing caffeine
- eating high-fiber foods

Resources

BOOKS

Miller, David K. "Chronic Abdominal Pain." In *Current Diagnosis 9*. Edited by Rex B. Conn, et al. Philadelphia: W. B. Saunders Company, 1997.

Viggiano, Thomas R. "Peptic Ulcer Disease." In *Current Diagnosis 9*. Edited by Rex B. Conn, et al. Philadelphia: W. B. Saunders Company, 1997.

Way, Lawrence W. "Stomach and Duodenum." In *Current Surgical Diagnosis & Treatment*. Edited by Lawrence W. Way. Stamford, CT: Appleton & Lange, 1994.

Ying, Zhou Zhong, and Jin Hui De. "Gastrointestinal Diseases." In *Clinical Manual of Chinese Herbal Medicine and Acupuncture*. New York: Churchill Livingston, 1997.

PERIODICALS

Bown, R. L. "An Overview of the Pharmacology, Efficacy, Safety and Cost-Effectiveness of Lansoprazole." *International Journal of Clinical Practice* 56 (March 2002): 132-139.

Chen, M. H., M. S. Wu, W. C. Lee, et al. "A Multiple Logistic Regression Analysis of Risk Factors in Different Subtypes of Gastric Ulcer." *Hepatogastroenterology* 49 (March-April 2002): 589-592.

Fagerstrom, K. "The Epidemiology of Smoking: Health Consequences and Benefits of Cessation" *Drugs* 62 (2002): Supplement 2: 1-9.

Flannery, J., and D. A. Tucker. "Pharmacologic Prophylaxis and Treatment of Stress Ulcers in Critically Ill Patients." *Critical Care Nursing Clinics of North America* 14 (March 2002): 39-51.

Han, K. "The Effect of an Integrated Stress Management Program on the Psychologic and Physiologic Stress Reactions

KEY TERMS

. . . .

Bismuth—A metallic element used to make medications that soothe the stomach lining. Bismuth appears to have some antimicrobial effectiveness against *Helicobacter pylori*.

Duodenum—The first of the three segments of the small intestine that connects the stomach and the jejunum. Most peptic ulcers are in the duodenum.

Helicobacter pylori—A bacterium that causes inflammation of the stomach lining.

Laparoscope—An instrument that allows a surgeon to look into the abdominal cavity through a small incision and perform surgery on a small area.

Zollinger-Ellison syndrome—A disorder characterized by the presence of tumors (gastrinomas) that secrete a hormone (gastrin), which stimulates the production of digestive juices.

of Peptic Ulcer in Korea." *Journal of Holistic Nursing* 20 (March 2002): 61-80.

Siu, W. T., H. T. Leong, B. K. Law, et al. "Laparoscopic Repair for Perforated Peptic Ulcer: A Randomized Controlled Trial." *Annals of Surgery* 235 (March 2002): 320-321.

Wermeille, J., M. Cunningham, J. P. Dederding, et al. "Failure of *Helicobacter pylori* Eradication: Is Poor Compliance the Main Cause?" *Gastroenterology and Clinical Biology* 26 (March 2002): 207-209.

ORGANIZATIONS

American College of Gastroenterology. 4900-B South Thirty-First Street, Arlington, VA 22206–1656. (703) 820–7400. http://www.acg.cgi.gi.org/acghome/html.

Digestive Health Initiative. 7910 Woodmont Avenue, #914, Bethesda, MD 20814. (800) 668–5237. http://www.gastro.org./dhi.html.

OTHER

Hoffman, David L. "Peptic Ulceration." *HealthWorld Online.* http://www.healthy.net/library/books/hoffman/digestive/ulcerati.htm.

Belinda Rowland
Rebecca J. Frey, PhD

Unani-tibbi

Definition

Unani-tibbi denotes Arabic or Islamic medicine, also known as prophetic medicine. It traditionally makes use of a variety of techniques including diet, herbal treatments, manipulative therapies, and surgery. Unani-tibbi is a complete system, encompassing all aspects and all fields of medical care, from **nutrition** and hygiene to psychiatric treatment.

Origins

The name **unani-tibbi** is something of a misnomer, as literally translated from the Arabic, it means Greek medicine. This is because the early Arab physicians took their basic knowledge from the Greeks. At the time, Greek medical knowledge was the best to be had, particularly from Galen, the renowned second-century Greek physician who treated the gladiators and Emperor Marcus Aurelius.

However, from that point onwards, Islamic medical scholars were responsible for many developments and advancements that, at the time, placed Arabic medicine firmly in the vanguard of medical science. There followed a steady stream of Muslim medical scholars, who not only upheld the high standards that came to be known of unani-tibbi, but carried on adding to and improving the basic pool of knowledge.

Some notable scholars of the science of unani-tibbi include:

- Al Tabbari (838–870)
- Al Razi (Rhazes) (841–926)
- Al Zahrawi (930–1013)
- Avicenna (980–1037)
- Ibn Al Haitham (960–1040)
- Ibn Sina (Avicenna), (980–1037)
- Ibn Al Nafees (1213–1288)
- Ibn Khaldun (1332–1395)

Medical innovations introduced by unani-tibbi physicians included:

- Avicenna was the first to describe **meningitis**, so accurately and in such detail, that it has scarcely required additions after 1,000 years.

- Avicenna was the first to describe intubation (surgical procedure to facilitate breathing)—Western physicians began to use this method at the end of the eighteenth century.

- The use of plaster of Paris for **fractures** by the Arabs was standard practice—it was "rediscovered" in the West in 1852.

- Surgery was used by the Arabs to correct cataracts.

- Ibn Al Nafees discovered pulmonary blood circulation.

- A strict system of licensing for medical practitioners was introduced in Baghdad in 931, which included taking the Hippocratic oath, and specific periods of training for doctors.

- There was a system of inspection of drugs and pharmaceuticals—the equivalent of the Federal Drug Administration (FDA)—in Baghdad 1,000 years ago.

- The European system of medicine was based on the Arabic system, and even as recently as the early nineteenth century, students at the Sorbonne had to read the canon of Avicenna as a condition to graduating.

- Unani-tibbi hospitals were, from the beginning, free to all without discrimination on the basis of religion, sex, ethnicity, or social status.

- Their hospitals allocated different wards for each classification of disease.

- Hospitals had unlimited water supplies and bathing facilities.

- Before the advent of the printing press, there were extensive handwritten libraries in Baghdad, (80,000 volumes), Cordova, (600,000 volumes), Cairo, (two million volumes), and Tripoli, (three million volumes).

- All Unani-tibbi hospitals kept patient records.

- A hospital was established for lepers.

- In 830, nurses were brought from Sudan to work in the Qayrawan hospital in Tunisia.

- A system of fountain-cooled air was devised for the comfort of patients suffering from fever.

- Avicenna described the contamination of the body by "foreign bodies" prior to infection, and Ibn Khatima also described how "minute bodies" enter the body and cause disease—well in advance of Pasteur's discovery of microbes.

- Al Razi was the first to describe smallpox and **measles**. He was accurate to such a degree that nothing has been added since.

- Avicenna described **tuberculosis** as being a communicable disease.

- Avicenna devised the concept of anesthetics. The Arabs developed a "soporific sponge," (impregnated with aromatics and narcotics and held under the patient's nose), which preceded modern anesthesia.

- The Arab surgeon, Al Zahrawi was the first to describe hemophilia.

- Al Zahrawi was also the first surgeon in history to use cotton, which is an Arabic word, as surgical dressings for the control of hemorrhage.

- Avicenna accurately described surgical treatment of **cancer**, saying that the excision must be radical and remove all diseased tissue, including amputation and the removal of veins running in the direction of the tumor.

He also recommended cautery of the area if needed. This observation is relevant even today.

- Avicenna, Al Razi, and others formed a medical association for the purpose of holding conferences so that the latest developments and advancements in the field of medicine could be debated and passed on to others.

Benefits

What began as an advanced medical system that set world standards, has now come to be regarded as a system of folk medicine. This decline coincided with the decline of the Islamic Empire and the dissolution of the caliphate (spiritual head of Islam), as these were directly responsible for the direction and impetus of Islamic scientific scholars in all fields.

Unani-tibbi practitioners still treat people with herbal remedies and manipulation, for a variety of illnesses. In the Islamic world, many of the poorer people who cannot afford allopathic medicine still resort to this traditional medicine. There are also people who prefer unani-tibbi to allopathic medicine, as indeed, the traditional unani-tibbi remedies do not bring with them the side effects commonly experienced with allopathic drugs.

Description

Similar to Greek humoral theory, unani-tibbi considers the whole human being, spiritual, emotional, and physical. Basic to the theory is the concept of the "four humors." These are Dum (blood), Bulghum (phlegm), Sufra (yellow bile), and Sauda (black bile). Each is further categorized as being hot and moist (blood), cold and moist (phlegm), hot and dry (yellow bile), and cold and dry (black bile). Every individual has his/her own unique profile of humors, which must be maintained in harmony to preserve health. If the body becomes weak, and this harmony is disrupted, a physician can be called upon to help restore the balance.

This restoration may be done using correct diet and nutrition and/or the unani-tibbi system of botanical therapy, **cupping**, bleeding, manipulation, and massage, among others, as treatments for all disease and ailments. Herbs or substances used to treat a patient will be matched to his humor type.

Unani-tibbi employs a detailed system of diagnosis, including observation of urine and stools, palpation of the body and pulse, and observation of the skin and eyes.

It also employs a system of prophylactics in order to preserve health and ward off disease. This includes the adherence to strict hygiene rules, protection of air, food and water from contamination or pollution, sufficient rest and **exercise**, and attention to spiritual needs. Certain herbs are also taken on a prophylactic basis, such as black cumin and **sage**.

In general, unani-tibbi treatment is not expensive, and it is certainly less expensive than allopathic medicine. However, charges vary according to area and practitioner. Fees should be discussed with a practitioner before treatment begins.

Preparations

Remedies are often provided by the practitioner or are obtained from a specialized herbalist. The ingredients are mainly herbs and honey. It must be noted that the honey used will be raw and unadulterated, rather than the type found in supermarkets, which is usually heat-treated.

A famous and widely used medicinal herb is black cumin (*Nigella sativa*), also known as Hab Al Baraka in Arabic, which means blessed seed. Black cumin has been cultivated since Assyrian times and it is beneficial for a very long list of ailments. It is widely mixed with other herbs for greater beneficial effect and is said to strengthen the immune system when taken over a period of time. Research has proved that it has the ability to slow the division of cancer cells.

Precautions

The achievements of the unani-tibbi practitioners of today bear little resemblance to those of their illustrious predecessors, and some of those claiming to practice traditional medicine are woefully ill-equipped to practice. However, many Arab and Muslim doctors, after qualifying in allopathic medicine, are still treating their patients with traditional remedies and are taking the trouble to educate themselves in this ancient art.

In India, where Islamic medicine is primarily known as unani-tibbi, the government has set up a Central Council for Research in Unani Medicine (CCRUM), which also has a licensing system for these traditional practitioners.

In the Arab countries, it is known as tibb-nabawi, or prophetic medicine, and mainly utilizes herbal remedies, honey, and other bee products.

Side effects

There are no known side effects of this form of treatment.

Research & general acceptance

The herbal remedies employed by unani-tibbi are chosen for their non-toxicity and absence of side effects.

Although unani-tibbi has not been the subject of a great deal of research by modern-day scientists, it still

***

KEY TERMS

Excision—Surgical removal of tissue.

Hemophilia—Any of several x-linked genetic disorders characterized by the lack of clotting factors in the blood.

Intubation—A surgical procedure in which a tube is inserted into the windpipe of a seriously ill patient to facilitate breathing.

Tibb nabawi—Prophetic medicine (another name for unani-tibbi).

***

enjoys great popularity in Muslim countries. The records left by Islamic medical scholars become more remarkable in the light of modern medicine, when their achievements and theories still hold their own next to the latest in medical technology.

The CCRUM in India is conducting research into aspects of unani-tibbi that are likely to be of particular benefit to modern society. To cite one example, an examination of the substances that were originally used as safe forms of contraception, with none of the side effects of present-day chemical contraception.

Training & certification

There are two classifications of practitioners of unani-tibbi. There are the simple folk practitioners, dispensers of herbal remedies and so on, and the highly qualified doctors and scholars who are still conducting research. Research is currently being conducted at the King Abdul Azeez University in Riyadh, Saudi Arabia, and the Sultan Qaboos University in Oman, among others, into the efficacy of traditional herbal remedies.

The CCRUM in India issues licenses to unani-tibbi practitioners and provides funds for research.

Resources

BOOKS

Shealy, Norman C., M.D., Ph.D. *Alternative Medicine, An Illustrated Encyclopedia of Natural Healing.* London: Element Books, 1996.

ORGANIZATIONS

International Institute of Islamic Medicine & The Islamic Medical Association of North America. http://www.iiim.org/.

Unani Tibbi Herbal Healing. 311 North Robertson Blvd., PMB 396, Beverly Hills, CA 90211. (310) 308-9881 or (310) 284-3626. Fax: (561)325-6252. Consult-free@unanitibb.com.http://unanitibb.com/.

Patricia Skinner

Urinary incontinence

Definition

Urinary incontinence is unintentional loss of urine that is sufficient enough in frequency and amount to cause physical and/or emotional distress in the person experiencing it.

Description

Approximately 13 million Americans suffer from urinary incontinence. Women are affected by the disorder more frequently than are men; one in 10 women under age 65 suffers from urinary incontinence. A study published in late 2002 found that between 21% and 29% of adult women in the workforce reported at least one episode of urinary incontinence each month. Older Americans, too, are more prone to the condition. Twenty percent of Americans over age 65 are incontinent. In general, the condition is underrecognized and undertreated.

There are five major categories of urinary incontinence: overflow, stress, urge, functional, and reflex:

- Overflow incontinence. Overflow incontinence is caused by bladder dysfunction. Individuals with this type of incontinence have an obstruction to the bladder or urethra, or a bladder that doesn't contract properly. As a result, their bladders do not empty completely, and they have problems with frequent urine leakage.

- Stress incontinence. Stress incontinence occurs when an individual involuntarily loses urine after pressure is placed on the abdomen (i.e., during **exercise**, sexual activity, sneezing, coughing, laughing, or hugging).

- Urge incontinence. Urge incontinence occurs when a person feels a sudden need to urinate and cannot control the urge to do so. As a consequence, urine is involuntarily lost before the individual can get to the toilet.

- Functional incontinence. Individuals who have control over their own urination and have a fully functioning urinary tract, but cannot make it to the bathroom in time due to a physical or cognitive disability, are functionally incontinent. These individuals may suffer from arthritis, **Parkinson's disease**, **multiple sclerosis**, or Alzheimer's disease.

- Reflex incontinence. Individuals with reflex incontinence lose control of their bladder without warning. They typically suffer from neurological impairment.

In some cases, an individual may develop short-term or *acute incontinence*. Acute incontinence may occur as a symptom or byproduct of illness, as a side effect of medication, or as a result of dietary intake. The condition is typically easily resolved once the cause is determined and addressed.

Causes & symptoms

Urinary incontinence can be caused by a wide variety of physical conditions, including:

- **Childbirth**. Childbirth can stretch the pelvic muscles and cause the bladder to lose some support from surrounding muscles, resulting in stress incontinence.

- Dysfunction of the bladder and/or the urinary sphincter. In a continent individual, as the bladder contracts, the outlet that releases urine into the urethra (bladder sphincter) opens and urine exits the body. In individuals with overflow incontinence, bladder contractions and dilation of the sphincter do not occur at the same time.

- Enlarged prostate. In men, an enlarged prostate gland can obstruct the bladder, causing overflow incontinence.

- Hysterectomy or other gynecological surgery. Any surgery involving the urogenital tract runs the risk of damaging or weakening the pelvic muscles and causing incontinence.

- Menopause. The absence of estrogen in the postmenopausal woman can cause the bladder to drop, or prolapse.

- Neurological conditions. The nervous system sends signals to the bladder telling it when to start and stop emptying. When the nervous system is impaired, incontinence may result. Neurological conditions such as multiple sclerosis, **stroke**, spinal cord injuries, or a brain tumor may cause the bladder to contract involuntarily, expelling urine without warning, or to cease contractions completely, causing urinary retention.

- Obesity. Persons who are overweight have undue pressure placed on their bladder and surrounding muscles.

- Obstruction. A blockage at the bladder outlet may permit only small amounts of urine to pass, resulting in urine retention and subsequent overflow incontinence. Tumors, calculi, and scar tissue can all block the flow of urine. A urethral stricture, or narrow urethra caused by scarring or inflammation, may also result in urine retention.

Acute incontinence is a temporary condition caused by a number of factors, including:

- Bladder irritants. Substances in the urine that irritate the bladder may cause the bladder muscle to malfunction. The presence of a urinary tract infection and the ingestion of excess **caffeine** can act as irritants. Highly concentrated urine resulting from low fluid intake may also irritate the bladder.

TYPES OF INCONTINENCE	
Type	**Description**
Overflow	The bladder never empties and signal to void is lost. Urine overflows in small amounts and bladder remains partially full.
Stress	Prevalent in women, stress incontinence occurs when the pelvic floor muscles are weakened and cannot support increased bladder pressure. Coughing, sneezing, exercising, and laughing can trigger urine flow.
Urge	The bladder contracts when full and urine flows. The patient as no control over the urge to void.

- **Constipation**. Constipation can cause incontinence in some individuals. Stool that isn't passed presses against the bladder and urethra, triggering urine leakage.

- Illness or disease. Diabetes can greatly increase urine volume, making some individuals prone to incontinence. Other illnesses may temporarily impair the ability to recognize and control the urge to urinate, or to reach the toilet in time to do so.

- Medications and alcohol. Medications that sedate, such as tranquilizers and sleeping pills, can interfere with the proper functioning of the urethral nerves and bladder. Both sedatives and alcohol can also impair an individual's ability to recognize the need to urinate, and act on that need in a timely manner. Other medications such as diuretics, muscle relaxants, and blood pressure medication can also affect bladder function.

- Surgery. Men who undergo prostate surgery can suffer from temporary stress incontinence as a result of damage to the urethral outlet.

Diagnosis

Urinary incontinence may be diagnosed by a general practitioner, urologist, or gynecologist. If the patient is over age 65, a gerontologist may diagnose and treat the condition. A thorough medical history and physical examination is typically performed, along with specific diagnostic testing to determine the cause of the incontinence. Diagnostic testing may include x rays, ultrasound, urine tests, and a physical examination of the pelvis. It may also include a series of exams that measure bladder pressure and capacity and the urinary flow (urodynamic testing). The patient may also be asked to keep a diary to record urine output, frequency, and any episodes of incontinence over a period of several days or a week.

Treatment

Adjusting dietary habits and avoiding acidic and spicy foods, alcohol, caffeine, and other bladder irritants can help to prevent urinary leaking. The patient should eat recommended amounts of whole grains, fruits, and vegetables to avoid constipation. Bladder training, used to treat urge incontinence, can also be a useful treatment tool. The technique involves placing a patient on a toileting schedule. The time interval between urination is then gradually increased until an acceptable time period between bathroom breaks is consistently achieved.

Therapies designed to strengthen the pelvic muscles are also recommended for the treatment of urinary incontinence. Pelvic toning exercises, known as Kegel or PC muscle exercises, can alleviate stress incontinence in both men and women. These exercises involve repeatedly tightening the muscles of the pelvic floor.

Biofeedback techniques can teach incontinent patients to control the urge to urinate. Biofeedback uses sensors to monitor temperature and muscle contractions in the vagina to help incontinent patients learn to increase their control over the pelvic muscles.

An infusion, or tea, of **horsetail** (*Equisetum arvense*), agrimony (*Agrimonia eupatoria*), and sweet sumac (*Rhus aromatica*) may be prescribed by an herbalist or naturopath to treat stress and urge incontinence. These herbs are natural astringents and encourage toning of the digestive and urinary tracts. Other herbs, such as urtica or stinging **nettle** (*Urtica urens*), **plantain** (*Plantago major*), or maize (*Zea mays*) may be helpful. Homeopathic remedies may include **pulsatilla** and causticum. Chinese herbalists might recommend golden lock tea, a mixture of several herbs that helps the body retain fluids.

Allopathic treatment

There are numerous invasive and noninvasive treatment options for urinary incontinence:

- Behavior modification therapy. Behavior modification is a psychological approach to the treatment of urinary incontinence in which patients gradually increase the length of the time interval between voidings and "retrain" the bladder in other ways. It is reported to be highly effective in treating urge incontinence.

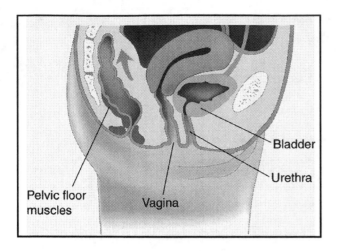

Strengthening the pelvic floor muscles by performing Kegel exercises helps to alleviate stress incontinence in women. Contract the pelvic floor muscles as if stopping an imaginery flow of urine. Hold for 10 seconds and repeat. *(Illustration by Electronic Illustrators Group. The Gale Group.)*

- Collagen injections. Collagen injected in the tissue surrounding the urethra can provide urethral support for women suffering from stress incontinence.

- External occlusive devices. A new single-use disposable urethral cap is available without a prescription as of late 2002 for women suffering from stress urinary incontinence. The cap is noninvasive and appears to be quite effective in managing incontinence.

- Inflatable urethral insert. Sold under the tradename Reliance, this disposable incontinence balloon for women is inserted into the urethra and inflated to prevent urine leakage.

- Intermittent urinary catheterization. This procedure involves the The periodic insertion of a catheter into a patient's bladder to drain urine from the bladder into an attached bag or container.

- Medication. Estrogen hormone replacement therapy can help improve pelvic muscle tone in post-menopausal women. Other medications, including flurbiprofen, capsaicin and botulinum toxin, are sometimes prescribed to relax the bladder muscles or to tighten the urethral sphincter. As of late 2002, newer medications for the treatment of urinary incontinence are undergoing clinical trials. One of these drugs, duloxetine, differs from present medications in targeting the central nervous system's control of the urge to urinate rather than the smooth muscle of the bladder itself.

- Perineal stimulation. Perineal stimulation is used to treat stress incontinence. The treatment uses a probe to deliver a painless electrical current to the perineal area muscles. The current tones the muscle by contracting it.

- Permanent catheterization. A permanent, or indwelling, catheter may be prescribed for chronic incontinence that doesn't respond to other treatments.

- Sacral nerve stimulation (SNS). Also known as sacral neuromodulation, SNS is a procedure in which a surgeon implants a device that sends continuous stimulation to the sacral nerves that control the urinary sphincter. The FDA approved sacral nerve stimulation for the treatment of urinary urge incontinence in 1997 and for urinary frequency in 1999.

- Surgery. Bladder neck suspension surgery is used to correct female urinary stress incontinence. Bladder enlargement surgery may be recommended to treat incontinent men and women with unusually small bladders.

- Urinary sphincter implant. An artificial urinary sphincter may be used to treat incontinence in men and women with urinary sphincter impairment.

- Vaginal inserts. Devices constructed of silicone or other pliable materials can be inserted into a woman's vagina to support the urethra.

Expected results

Left untreated, incontinence can cause physical and emotional upheaval. Individuals with long-term incontinence suffer from urinary tract **infections**, and skin **rashes** and sores. Incontinence can also affect their self-esteem and cause **depression** and social withdrawal. They frequently stop participating in physical activities they once enjoyed because of the risk of embarrassing "accidents." However, with the wide variety of treatment options for incontinence available today, the prognosis for incontinent patients is promising. If incontinence cannot be stopped, it can be improved in the majority of cases.

Prevention

Women who are pregnant or who have gone through childbirth can reduce their risk for stress incontinence by strengthening their perineal area muscles with Kegel exercises. Men who have undergone prostate surgery may also benefit from pelvic muscle exercises. Men and women should consult with their doctor before initiating any type of exercise program.

Resources

BOOKS

Blaivas, Jerry. *Conquering Bladder and Prostate Problems: The Authoritative Guide for Men and Women.* New York, NY: Plenum, 1998.

"Urinary Incontinence." Section 17, Chapter 215 in *The Merck Manual of Diagnosis and Therapy*, edited by Mark H. Beers, MD, and Robert Berkow, MD. Whitehouse Station, NJ: Merck Research Laboratories, 1999.

PERIODICALS

Amundsen, C. L., and G. D. Webster. "Sacral Neuromodulation in an Older, Urge-Incontinent Population." *American Journal of Obstetrics and Gynecology* 187 (December 2002): 1462–1465.

Bachmann, G., and B. Wiita. "External Occlusive Devices for Management of Female Urinary Incontinence." *Journal of Women's Health (Larchmont)* 11 (November 2002): 793–800.

Burgio, K. L. "Influence of Behavior Modification on Overactive Bladder." *Urology* 60 (November 2002): (5 Suppl. 1): 72–76.

Burgio, K. L., P. S. Goode, J. L. Locher, et al. "Behavioral Training With and Without Biofeedback in the Treatment of Urge Incontinence in Older Women: A Randomized Controlled Trial." *Journal of the American Medical Association* 288 (November 13, 2002): 2293–2299.

Haeusler, G., H. Leitich, M. van Trotsenburg, et al. "Drug Therapy of Urinary Urge Incontinence: A Systematic Review." *Obstetrics and Gynecology* 100 (November 2002) (5 Pt 1): 1003–1016.

Palmer, M. H., and S. Fitzgerald. "Urinary Incontinence in Working Women: A Comparison Study." *Journal of Women's Health (Larchmont)* 11 (December 2002): 879–888.

Sandroff, Ronni. "Urgent Matters: Incontinence is Treatable, If Only Women Would Talk About It." *American Health for Women* 16, no. 8 (Oct 1997): 28–30.

Viktrup, L. "Female Stress and Urge Incontinence in Family Practice: Insight Into the Lower Urinary Tract." *International Journal of Clinical Practice* 56 (November 2002): 694–700.

Yoshimura, N., and M. B. Chancellor. "Current and Future Pharmacological Treatment for Overactive Bladder." *Journal of Urology* 168 (November 2002): 1897–1913.

ORGANIZATIONS

American Foundation for Urologic Disease. 1128 North Charles Street, Baltimore, MD 21201. (800) 242-2383. http://www.afud.org/.

American Urological Association (AUA). 1120 North Charles Street, Baltimore, MD 21201. (410) 727-1100. <www.auanet.org>.

Center for Biologics Evaluation and Research (CBER), U. S. Food and Drug Administration (FDA). 1401 Rockville Pike, Rockville, MD 20852-1448. (800) 835-4709 or (301) 827-1800. <www.fda.gov/cber>.

National Association for Continence. 2650 East Main Street, Spartanburg, SC 29307. (800) 252-3337. http://www.nafc.org.

National Kidney and Urologic Diseases Information Clearinghouse. 3 Information Way, Bethesda, MD 20892-3580. (800) 891-5390.

Paula Ford-Martin
Rebecca J. Frey, PhD

Urinary tract infection *see* **Bladder infection**

KEY TERMS

Bladder neck—The place where the urethra and bladder join.

Bladder sphincter—The outlet that releases urine into the urethra.

Calculi (singular, calculus)—Mineral deposits that can form a blockage in the urinary system.

Occlusive—Closing off. One of the newest treatments for stress urinary incontinence in women is an external occlusive single-use cap that covers the urethral opening.

Perineal area—The genital area between the vulva and anus in a woman, and between the scrotum and anus in a man.

Sacral nerves—The five pairs of nerves that arise from the lowermost segments of the spinal cord and control bladder, bowel, and pelvic functions. Stimulation of the sacral nerves by an implanted device is a newer treatment for urinary incontinence.

Urine therapy

Definition

Urine therapy is the use of one's urine, internally or externally, to heal **wounds** or alleviate disease symptoms and/or for overall well-being. It is also called uropathy, auto-urine therapy, amaroli, or shivambu.

Origins

References to the use of urine for medicinal purposes can be traced to ancient Egyptian, Chinese, Aztec, and Hindu histories. Proponents also point to Proverbs 5:15 in the Old Testament of the Bible: "Drink water from thy own cistern, and the streams of thy own well."

As an integral part of the ayurvedic tradition of **yoga**, urine therapy is known as amaroli. Ayurvedic yogis are encouraged to drink their own urine between 4 and 6 A.M. in the morning in the belief that the hormones ingested will facilitate a meditative state.

The rationale of the therapy is that urine is a by-product of blood filtration, not excess water from consumed food and liquid. In fact, the medical term for urine is plasma ultrafiltrate. Blood filled with nutrients passes through the liver where toxins are filtered out and excreted as solid waste matter. This purified blood then travels to the kidneys where any excess elements form urine and are then eliminated from the body. As urine passes through the urethra, it is a sterile solution. Ninety-five percent of it is water; the remaining five percent is a combination of urea, vitamins, minerals, enzymes, hormones, proteins, and antibodies. Urine therapy advocates argue that the presence of these nutrients are proof of urine's medicinal powers.

Urea is an antibacterial, antifungal, and antiviral agent that forms when the body balances its ratio of **sodium** chloride to water. Urea is often used to make ointments and lotions for its properties of reducing inflammation and ability to kill bacteria. It can be duplicated under laboratory conditions by dissolving **calcium** cyanamid in water, and then heated under high pressure to produce a compound of urea and calcium hydroxide.

Benefits

Urine therapy has been touted as a remedy for a long list of ailments, including **multiple sclerosis**, colitis, lupus, **rheumatoid arthritis**, **cancer**, **hepatitis**, hyperactivity, **psoriasis**, **eczema**, diabetes, herpes, **mononucleosis**, and adrenal failure. It is a commonly used treatment for snakebites and bee and jellyfish stings. Childhood illnesses such as acute flu, colds, viral **infections**, **mumps**, chicken pox, and **allergies** are also said to be alleviated by urine therapy. Urine is an ingredient in Pergonal, a fertility drug, and in pharmaceuticals used to dissolve **blood clots**.

Description

Urine therapy can be applied internally or externally. For internal use, a sample of the morning's first urine is collected in a sterile container. Using a clean medicine dropper, the patient places an amount between one to ten drops under the tongue. Usually, one to five drops are applied on the first day; 5-10 drops on the second day; 5-10 drops on the morning of the third day, followed by 5-10 drops that evening.

In homeopathic urine therapy, drops of urine are diluted in quantities of distilled water. Drops of the dilution are placed under the tongue hourly until a noticeable improvement in illness or the temporary worsening of the condition occurs. Then drops are applied at lengthening intervals for three days.

Only fresh urine should be used when taken orally. The genital area should be washed before collecting a specimen. The best time to collect urine is first thing in the morning, and collecting the sample mid-stream. Individuals should refrain from eating for a half hour after ingesting the urine.

For external use, new or old urine can be applied. Old urine has a higher ammonia content that is more effective on skin such **rashes** as eczema and psoriasis. To store urine for later use, one should pour it into a dark glass bottle and close it tightly. Keep the bottle in a cool, dark place for at least four days.

A small amount is applied to the affected area with a cotton ball or pad. Continue massaging 5-10 applications to the area until it is soaked. Tape a clean, soaked pad to the area for several hours. The urine can also be sprayed onto the skin. For cosmetic purposes, fresh or 1-2 day-old urine can be lightly massaged into the skin or added in small amounts to moisturizing cream. Some practitioners recommend avoiding the use of soap or lotion after applying urine to the skin. Dryness can be alleviated with **sesame oil**.

Injections of urine are not advised. One of the key components of therapy is the gradual introduction of urine into the body. The abrupt introduction of urine into the bloodstream could exacerbate possible side effects.

Preparation

Because any food, liquids, drugs, and/or medications consumed will affect the urine, an examination of one's diet is recommended before starting urine therapy. Keeping a daily **nutrition** journal will help to chart the body's reaction to different foods and the body's digestive patterns. High consumption of meat, for example, is thought to elevate the body's acid levels, particularly just before **fasting** or undergoing an intensive regime of urine therapy.

Users of urine therapy often keep regular measurements of their acid and alkaline levels, glucose levels, and blood pressure. Monitoring the body's acid and alkaline is accomplished by keeping track of the pH level in the saliva or urine. The ideal pH range for saliva is 6.4 to 7.2; below 6.4 too acidic, above 7.2 too alkaline. Urine pH normally varies from 5.0 in the morning to 8.0 in the evening.

Glucose tests measure the level of sugar in the blood, by millimoles per litres (mmol/l). Normal levels range from 4 to 8 mmol/l during the day, with the lowest levels occurring in the morning and higher measures occurring after meals.

At-home testing kits for pH levels, glucose levels, and blood pressure are available in most stores that carry over-the-counter (OTC) medical products.

Precautions

Urine that will be taken orally should never be heated or boiled. On the other hand, some advocates suggest that boiled urine is best for massage purposes. Boiling should be done in a stainless steel pot.

PHOTO GALLERY

Entries with this symbol 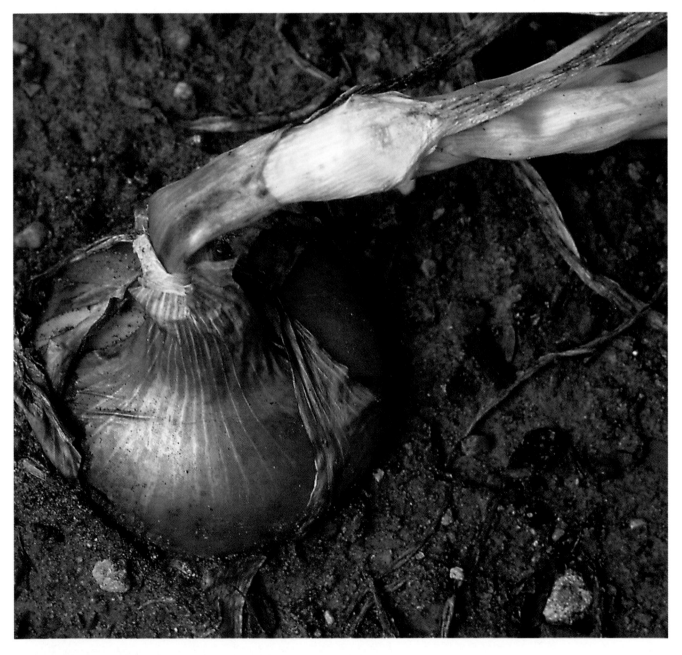 *in the main body have corresponding photographs in this alphabetically arranged color section.*

Onion plant *(**Allium cepa**).* *(PlantaPhile Germany. Reproduced by permission.)*

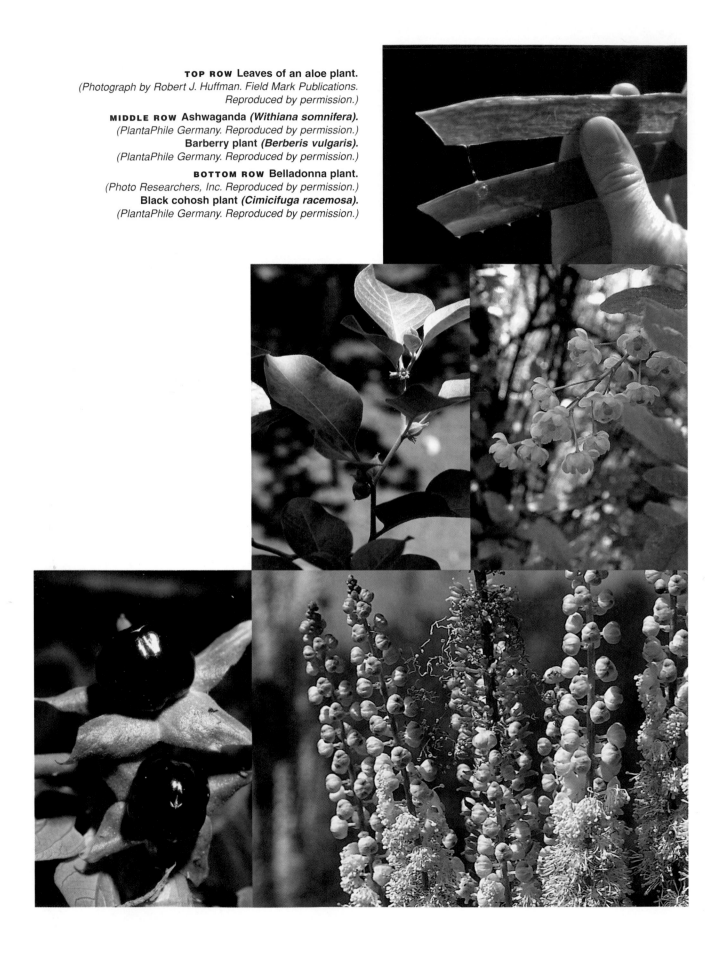

TOP ROW Leaves of an aloe plant.
(Photograph by Robert J. Huffman. Field Mark Publications. Reproduced by permission.)
MIDDLE ROW Ashwaganda *(Withiana somnifera).*
(PlantaPhile Germany. Reproduced by permission.)
Barberry plant *(Berberis vulgaris).*
(PlantaPhile Germany. Reproduced by permission.)
BOTTOM ROW Belladonna plant.
(Photo Researchers, Inc. Reproduced by permission.)
Black cohosh plant *(Cimicifuga racemosa).*
(PlantaPhile Germany. Reproduced by permission.)

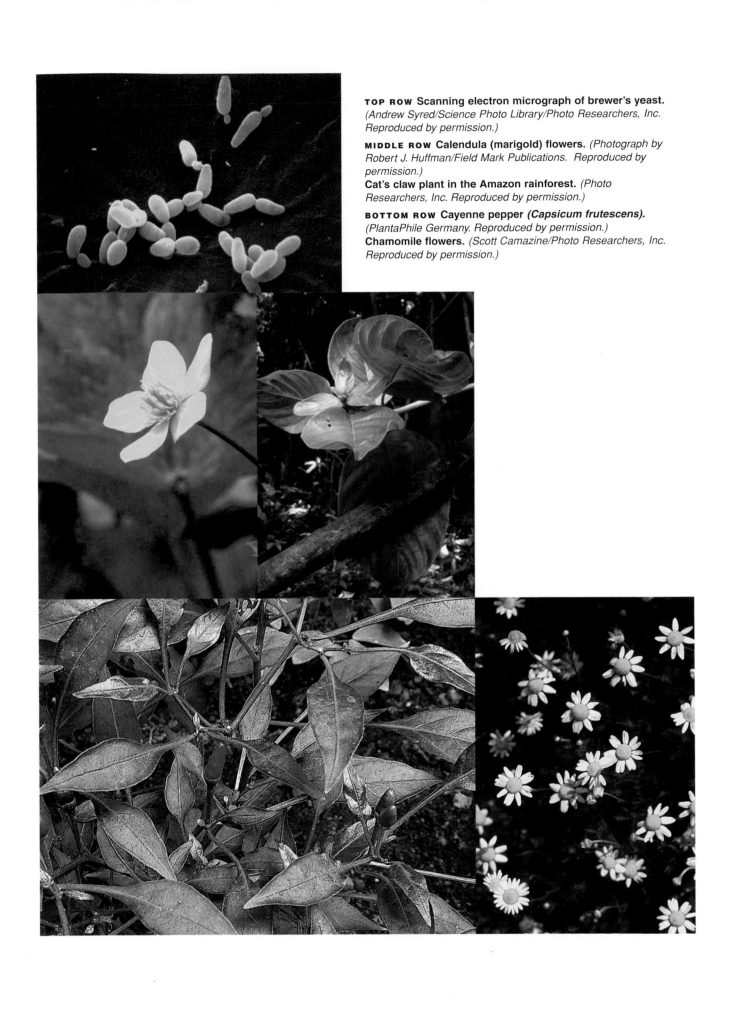

TOP ROW Scanning electron micrograph of brewer's yeast. *(Andrew Syred/Science Photo Library/Photo Researchers, Inc. Reproduced by permission.)*

MIDDLE ROW Calendula (marigold) flowers. *(Photograph by Robert J. Huffman/Field Mark Publications. Reproduced by permission.)*
Cat's claw plant in the Amazon rainforest. *(Photo Researchers, Inc. Reproduced by permission.)*

BOTTOM ROW Cayenne pepper *(Capsicum frutescens).* *(PlantaPhile Germany. Reproduced by permission.)*
Chamomile flowers. *(Scott Camazine/Photo Researchers, Inc. Reproduced by permission.)*

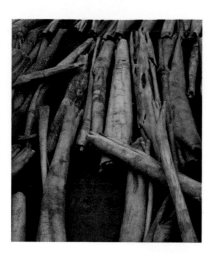

Cinnamon bark drying by a road in Sumatra. *(Photo Researchers, Inc. Reproduced by permission.)*

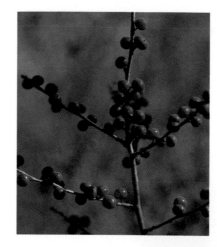

High-bush cranberry in Michigan. *(Photograph by Robert J. Huffman/Field Mark Publications. Reproduced by permission.)*

A dandelion plant with flower. *(Photograph by Robert J. Huffman/Field Mark Publications. Reproduced by permission.)*

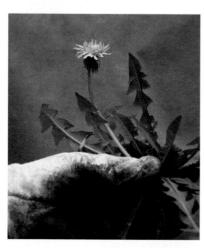

Echinacea flowers, also called purple coneflowers. *(Photo Researchers, Inc. Reproduced by permission.)*

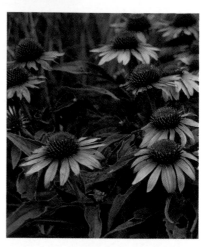

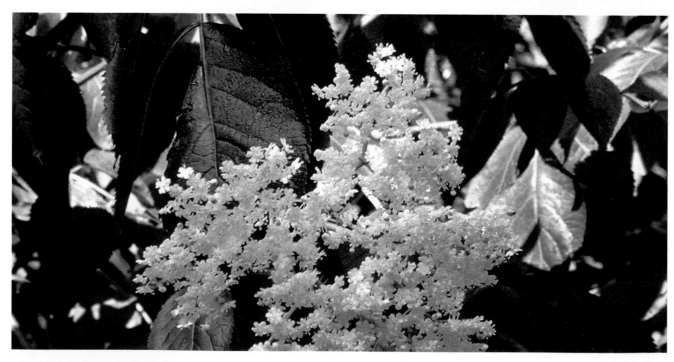

Elder *(Sambuccus nigra).* *(PlantaPhile Germany. Reproduced by permission.)*

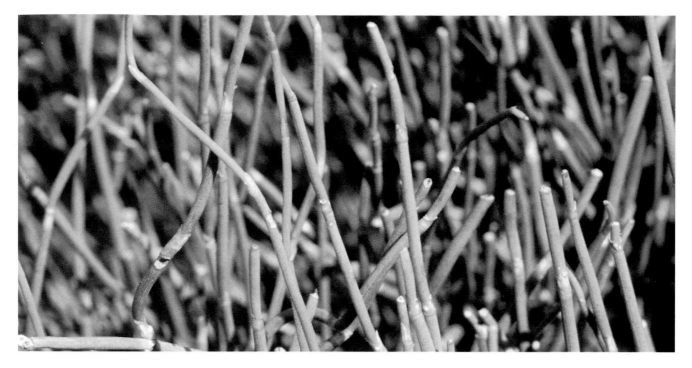

Ephedra *(Ephedra sinica)*. *(PlantaPhile Germany. Reproduced by permission.)*

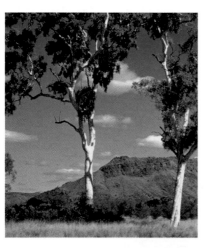

Eucalyptus trees in Australia. *(JLM Visuals. Reproduced by permission.)*

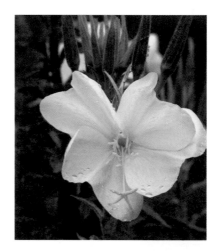

Evening primose flower. *(Photo Researchers, Inc. Reproduced by permission.)*

Whole, cloved, and minced garlic. *(Photograph by Robert J. Huffman. Field Mark Publications. Reproduced by permission.)*

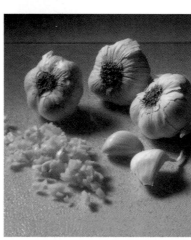

Ginger plant. *(JLM Visuals. Reproduced with permission.)*

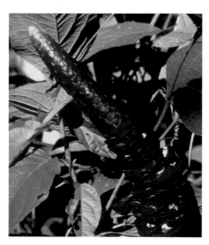

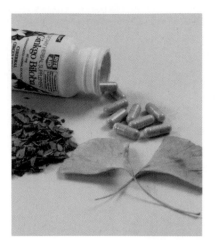

Various forms of ginko biloba. *(Photograph by Robert J. Huffman. Field Mark Publications. Reproduced by permission.)*

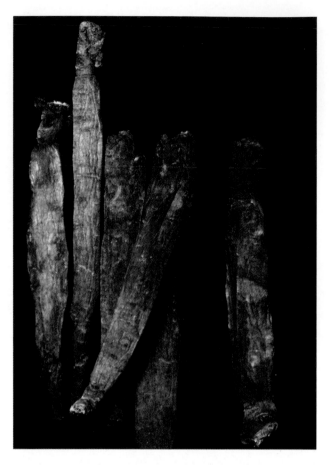

Cultivated American ginseng. *(JLM Visuals. Reproduced with permission.)*

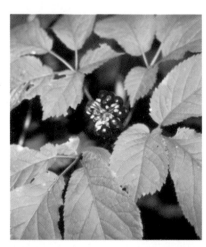

Dried Korean ginseng. *(Custom Medical Stock Photo. Reproduced by permission.)*

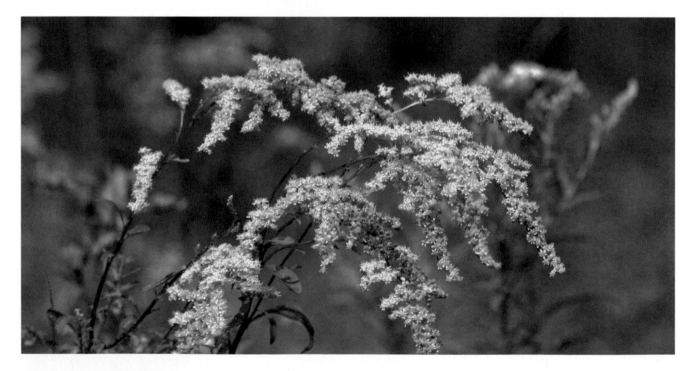

Flowering goldenrod plant. *(John Dudak/Phototake NYC. Reproduced with permission.)*

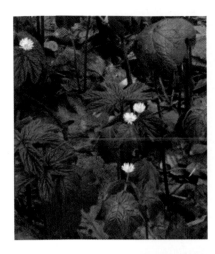

Cluster of goldenseal plants. *(Photo Researchers, Inc. Reproduced by permission.)*

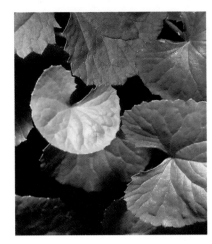

Gotu kola (*Centella asiatica*). *(PlantaPhile Germany. Reproduced by permission.)*

Purple grapes. *(Photograph by James Lee Sikkema. Reproduced by permission.)*

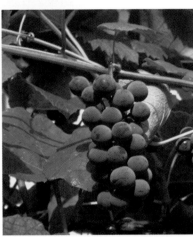

Green tea plant (*Camellia sinensis*). *(PlantaPhile Germany. Reproduced by permission.)*

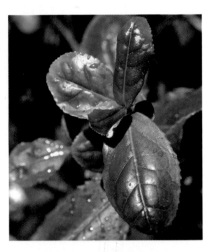

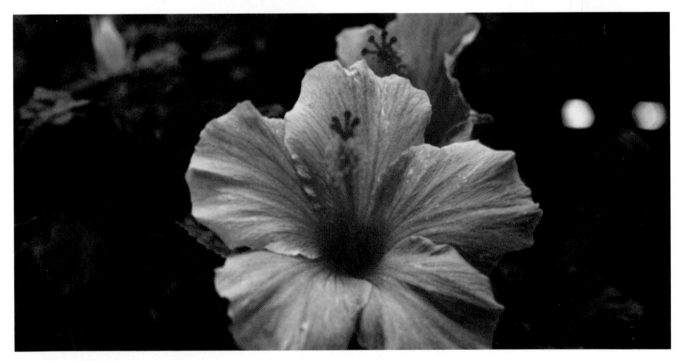

Hibiscus flower. *(Photo by Kelly Quinn. Reproduced by permission.)*

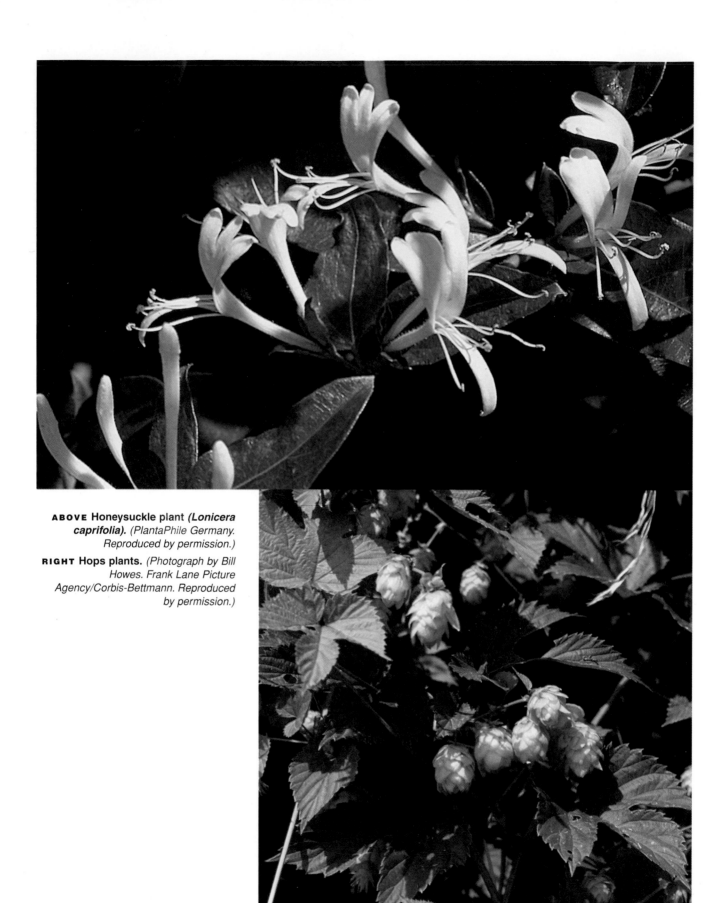

ABOVE Honeysuckle plant *(Lonicera caprifolia)*. *(PlantaPhile Germany. Reproduced by permission.)*

RIGHT Hops plants. *(Photograph by Bill Howes. Frank Lane Picture Agency/Corbis-Bettmann. Reproduced by permission.)*

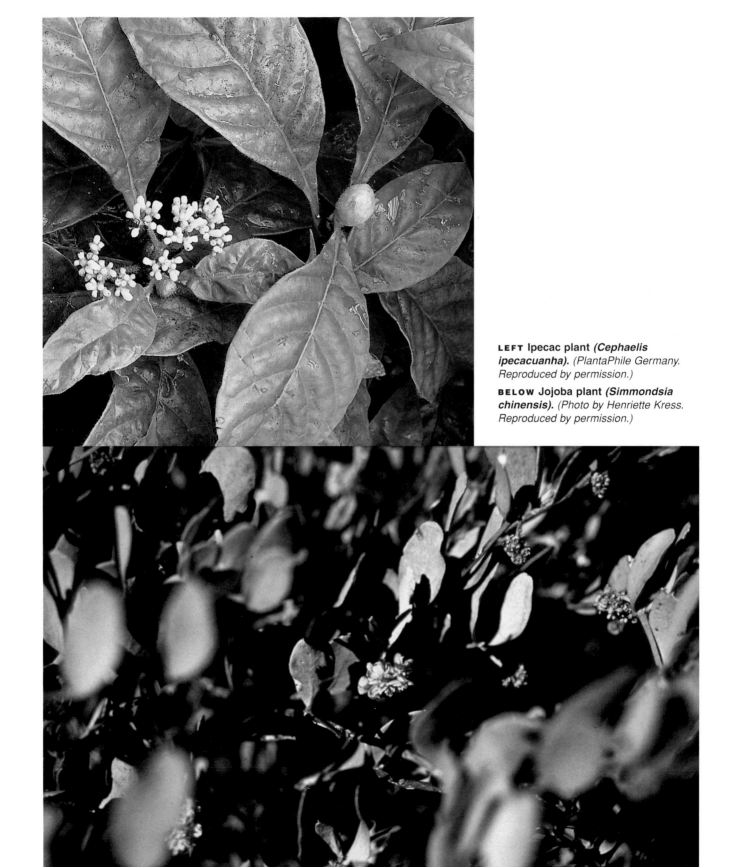

LEFT Ipecac plant *(Cephaelis ipecacuanha).* (PlantaPhile Germany. Reproduced by permission.)

BELOW Jojoba plant *(Simmondsia chinensis).* (Photo by Henriette Kress. Reproduced by permission.)

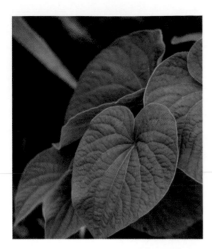

Kava kava leaves. *(Photo Researchers, Inc. Reproduced by permission.)*

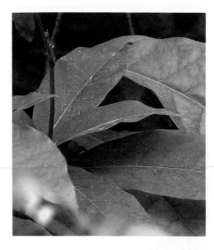

Kola nut *(Cola acuminata).* *(PlantaPhile Germany. Reproduced by permission.)*

Lavender *(Lavendula officinalis).* *(Photo by Henriette Kress. Reproduced by permission.)*

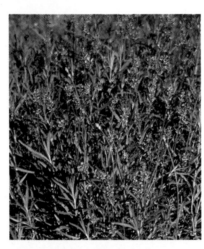

Lemongrass plant *(Cymbopogon citratus).* *(PlantaPhile Germany. Reproduced by permission.)*

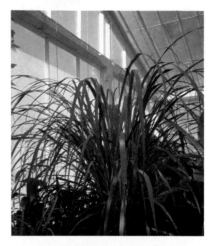

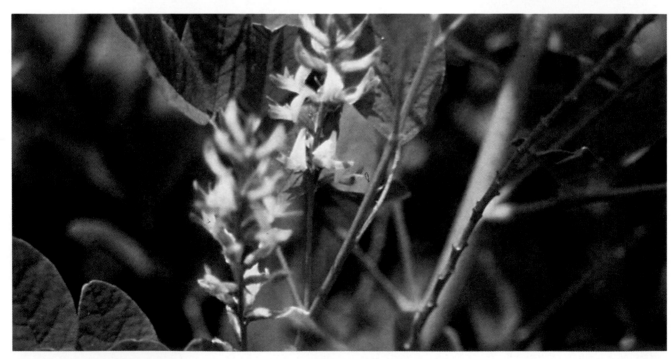

Licorice plant *(Glycyrrhiza glabra).* *(Photo by Henriette Kress. Reproduced by permission.)*

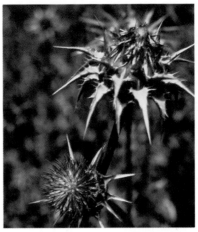

Milk thistle *(Silybum marianum). (Photo by Henriette Kress. Reproduced by permission.)*

Mistletoe plant on a tree. *(JLM Visuals. Reproduced by permission.)*

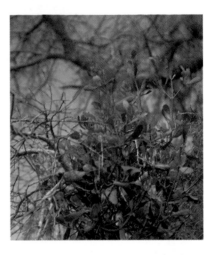

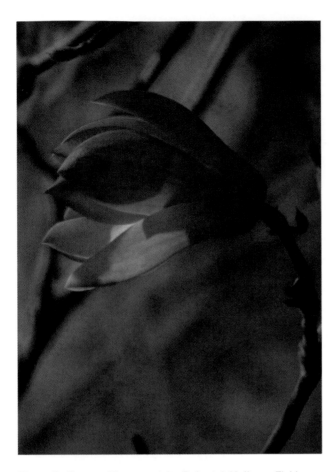

Magnolia flower. *(Photograph by Robert J. Huffman. Field Mark Publications. Reproduced by permission.)*

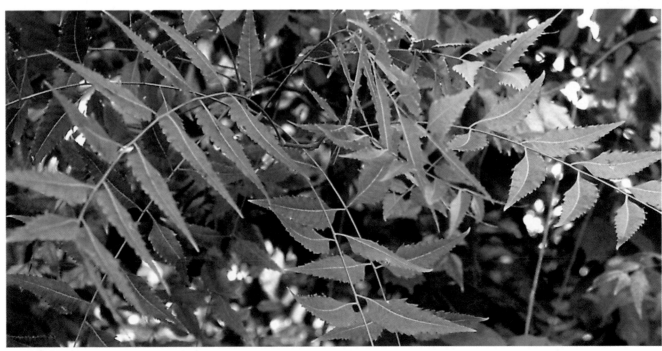

Neem *(Antelaea azadirachtu). (PlantaPhile Germany. Reproduced by permission.)*

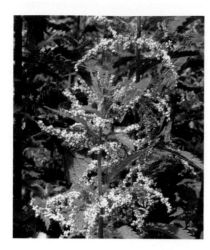

Nettles (Urtica diocia). *(PlantaPhile Germany. Reproduced by permission.)*

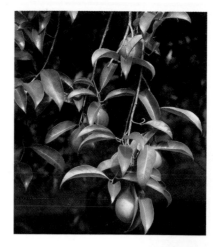

Nutmeg (Myristica fragrans). *(PlantaPhile Germany. Reproduced by permission.)*

Passionflower (Passiflora incarnata). *(PlantaPhile Germany. Reproduced by permission.)*

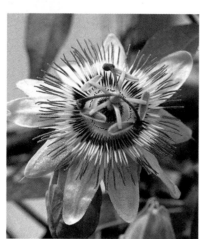

Peppermint plants in Oregon. *(Photo Researchers, Inc. Reproduced by permission.)*

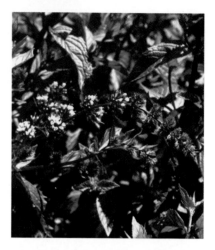

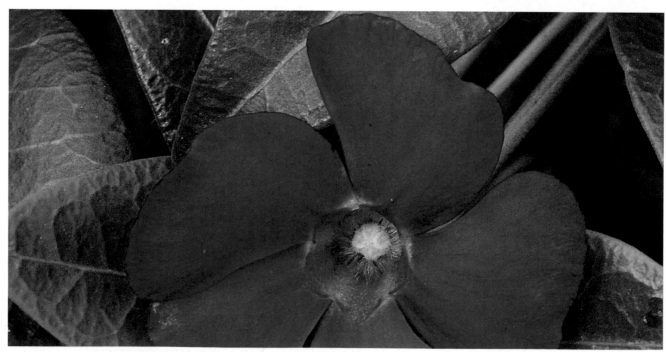

Periwinkle (Vinca minor). *(PlantaPhile Germany. Reproduced by permission.)*

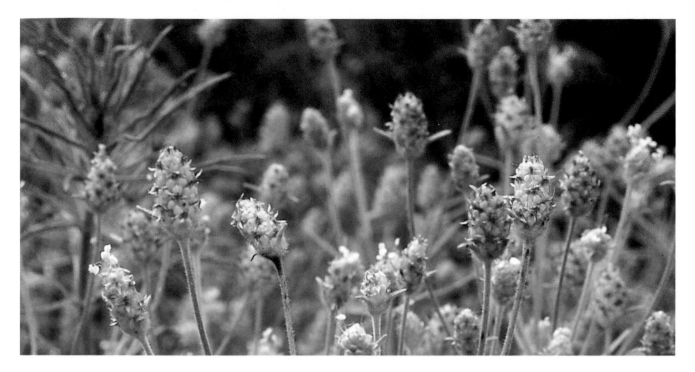

Psyllium *(Plantago afra)*. *(PlantaPhile Germany. Reproduced by permission.)*

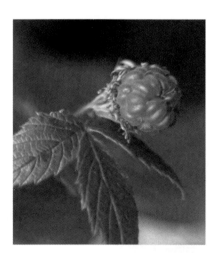

Raspberry on a bush. *(Photograph by Robert J. Huffman. Field Mark Publications. Reproduced by permission.)*

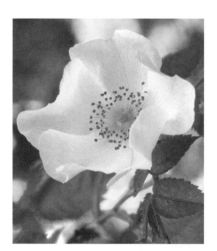

Rose hip plant *(Rosa canina)*. *(PlantaPhile Germany. Reproduced by permission.)*

Rosemary *(Rosmarinus officinalis)*. *(Photo by Henriette Kress. Reproduced by permission.)*

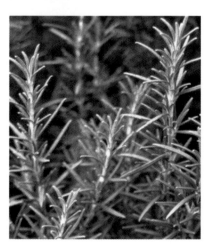

Saffron *(Crocus sativus)*. *(PlantaPhile Germany. Reproduced by permission.)*

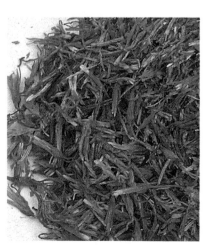

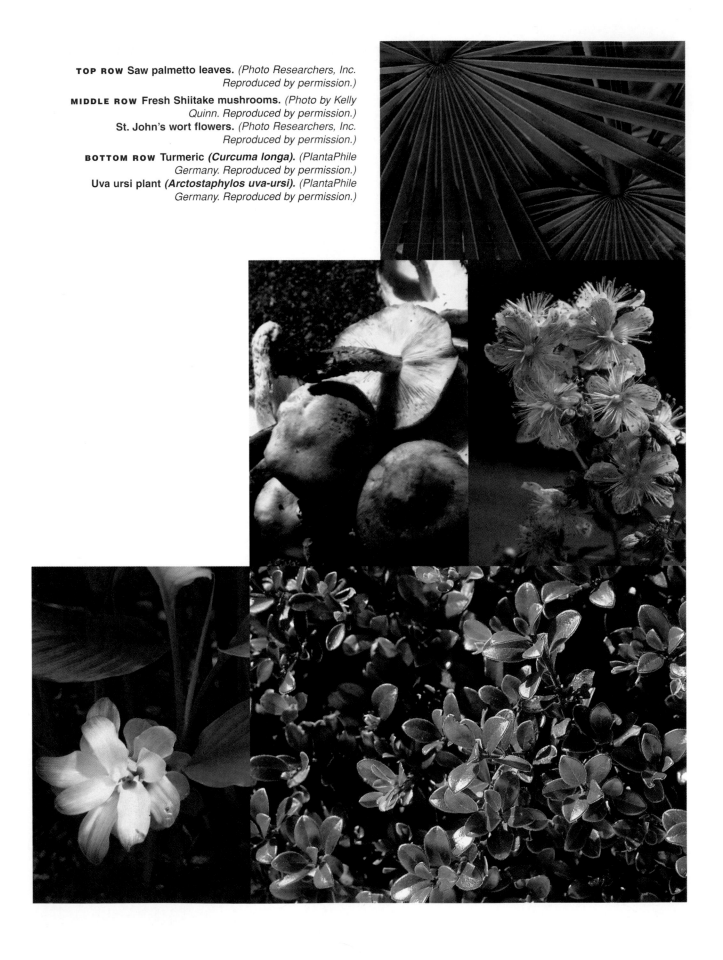

TOP ROW Saw palmetto leaves. *(Photo Researchers, Inc. Reproduced by permission.)*

MIDDLE ROW Fresh Shiitake mushrooms. *(Photo by Kelly Quinn. Reproduced by permission.)*
St. John's wort flowers. *(Photo Researchers, Inc. Reproduced by permission.)*

BOTTOM ROW Turmeric *(Curcuma longa)*. *(PlantaPhile Germany. Reproduced by permission.)*
Uva ursi plant *(Arctostaphylos uva-ursi)*. *(PlantaPhile Germany. Reproduced by permission.)*

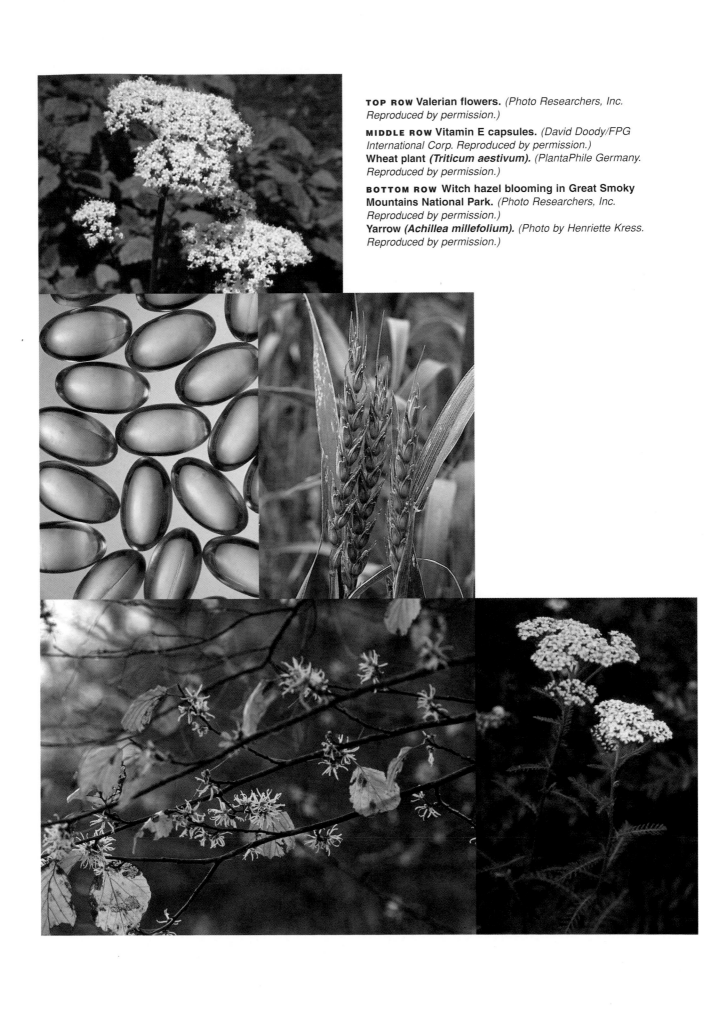

TOP ROW Valerian flowers. *(Photo Researchers, Inc. Reproduced by permission.)*

MIDDLE ROW Vitamin E capsules. *(David Doody/FPG International Corp. Reproduced by permission.)*
Wheat plant *(Triticum aestivum).* *(PlantaPhile Germany. Reproduced by permission.)*

BOTTOM ROW Witch hazel blooming in Great Smoky Mountains National Park. *(Photo Researchers, Inc. Reproduced by permission.)*
Yarrow *(Achillea millefolium).* *(Photo by Henriette Kress. Reproduced by permission.)*

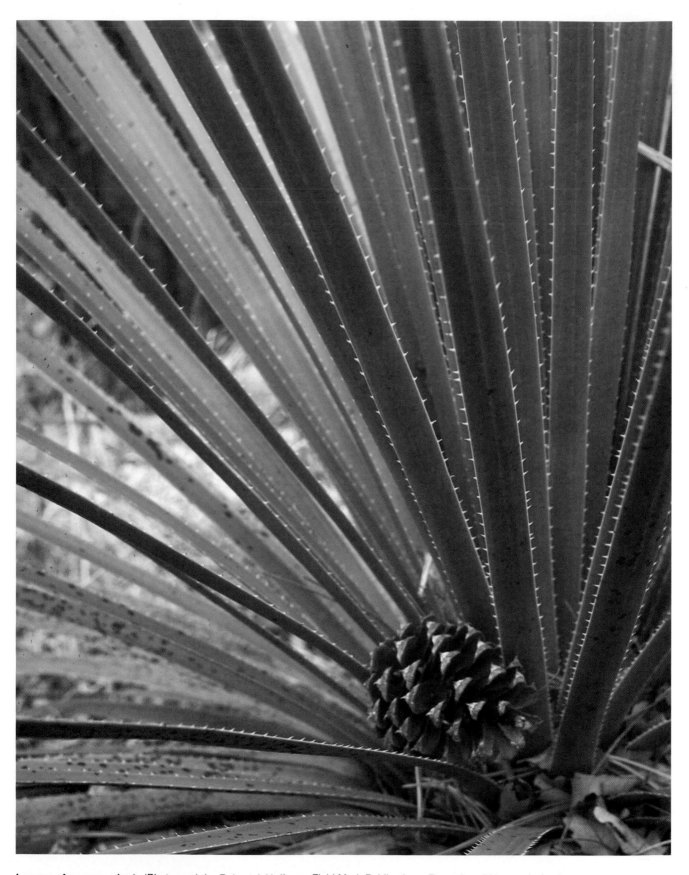

Leaves of a yucca plant. *(Photograph by Robert J. Huffman. Field Mark Publications. Reproduced by permission.)*

Proponents are divided on whether or not pregnant women should practice urine therapy. Some believe that it is beneficial for both the mother and the growing fetus. Others advise against it. Because of the fertility properties of urine, birth control pills may be less effective.

Several pre-existing conditions preclude the use of urine therapy. Heavy smokers and people taking therapeutic or recreational drugs should not use their own urine. Those suffering from bladder infections or venereal disease are also advised against ingesting their urine.

Side Effects

Side effects can include **headache**, **diarrhea**, itch and rashes, **pain**, **fatigue**, soreness of the shoulder, and **fever**. An increase in symptoms of the specific illness may also occur. These symptoms can last from a week to six months. Starting the therapy with small doses can alleviate some of these side effects.

Research & general acceptance

Much of the current research is based on anecdotal evidence from users of urine therapy. Nonetheless, its popularity is growing worldwide. The first World Conference on Urine Therapy was held in 1996 in India. Two more conferences were convened at three-year intervals: in 1999 in Germany and in 2003 in Brazil. In the United States, urine therapy advocates cite the works of John W. Armstrong, *The Water of Life: A Treatise on Urine Therapy*, Martha M. Christy, *Your Own Perfect Medicine*, and Coen Van Der Kroon, *The Golden Fountain*.

Although components of urine are extracted to create a number of topical creams and fertility drugs, the drinking of urine is not generally accepted by the Western medical establishment. Dr. **Andrew Weil**, a noted physician, self-healing expert, and author of *Natural Health, Natural Medicine,* posits that reports of positive results experienced by users have more to do with placebo effects than with the actual healing properties of urine. According to Weil, treatments that elicit negative emotional charges can be result in benefits when the treatment "mobilizes attention and belief." In other words, adhering to urine therapy in spite of one's loathing for it increases its **placebo effect**.

Training & certification

No training or certification is required.

Resources

BOOKS

Christy, Martha M. *Your Own Perfect Medicine.* Mesa, Arizona: Wishland Publishing, 2000.

KEY TERMS

....

Blood pressure—The force applied to the walls of the arteries as the heart pumps blood through the body.

Placebo—A medication prescribed more for the mental relief of the patient than for its actual effect on the individual's disorder.

Placebo effect—Improvement in a illness or symptom that occurs in response to treatment but cannot be credited to the specific treatment used .

Urea—A colorless compound that is the primary component of urine in mammals and that results from the oxidation of proteins.

Urethra—The canal carrying urine from the bladder

PERIODICALS

Bouaravong, Natalie. "Urine Therapy" *Berkeley Medical Journal Issues* [cited June 18, 2004]. <http://www.ocf.berkeley.edu/~issues/fall02/urine.html>.

ORGANIZATIONS

Chinese Association of Urine Therapy. 72 Wu Kon Lio Road, Wuku Industrial Park, Taipei Hsien, Taiwan, Republic of China. 886-2-22988446. <http://www.everlifepharm.com/urine/>.

OTHER

"Urine Therapy." Biomedx.com/ [cited April 13, 2004]. <http://biomedx.com/urine/>.

Mary McNulty

Usnea

Description

Usnea is a unique species of herb because it is created through a symbiotic relationship between lichens and algae. Symbiosis refers to the living together of two different organisms. In the case of lichens, both the alga and the fungus benefit from the relationship. Other names for usnea include lichen moss and old man's beard. Usnea can be found in forests in northern North America and are also found in Europe.

Some usnea are able to keep growing even after being broken off from the parent organism. Usnea are very sensitive to the air quality and may be killed by absorbing pollutants. In fact, usnea are used as indicators of regional pollution levels.

When a fungus and an alga combine, the resulting organism does not resemble either component. The fungal component has the main influence over the appearance and is the determinant for the species name of each lichen. The local environment also influences the appearance of the lichen. In general, usnea appear as long, hairy or fuzzy strings that hang from trees, rocks, and decomposing wood. The fibers (branches) of usnea are round and contain a slender white cord at the core. During wet conditions, the white cord has elastic properties. Lichens are usually gray or green in color that varies depending upon the algal component. For instance, green lichens have a green algal component. Some usnea are able to keep growing even after being broken off from the parent organism. Usnea are very sensitive to the air quality and may be killed by absorbing pollutants. In fact, usnea are used as indicators of regional pollution levels.

The primary active ingredient in usnea is usnic acid. Usnic acid protects the lichen from overexposure to light and its bitter taste prevents invertebrates (creatures that lack a spinal cord) from eating it. Usnic acid has antibacterial and antitumor activities. Against certain bacteria, usnic acid is stronger than the antibiotic penicillin. Usnic acid is effective against gram-positive bacteria including *Streptococcus*, *Staphylococcus*, and *Pneumococcus* but, unlike many antibiotics, does not harm the gram-negative bacteria that live in the gut and vagina. It is also effective against the bacterium that causes **tuberculosis** and may be effective against certain fungi and protozoans (simple, single-celled organisms such as trichomonas). It is believed that usnic acid works by disrupting the metabolism (the chemical and physical processes of an organism) of bacteria while leaving human cells unharmed.

Usnea contains mucilage, which can help ease coughing. It also has expectorant (brings up lung mucous) activity. Mucilage is a thick slimy substance produced by plants that has a soothing effect on mucous membranes. Herbalists consider usnea a muscle relaxant and an immune system stimulant.

Other constituents of usnea species may include barbatolic, evernic, lobaric, tartaric, thamnolic, stictinic, and usnaric acids.

General use

Usnea was historically used to treat **indigestion** because of its bitter taste and activity as a digestive system stimulant. The peoples of ancient China, Egypt, and Greece used usnea to treat **infections**. In the fourteenth century, it was believed that usnea could strengthen hair because of its hair-like appearance.

Usnea is used to treat abscesses, colds, **cough**, cystitis, **fungal infections** (such as athletes foot or ring-

worm), gastrointestinal (stomach and intestine) irritations, **influenza**, sore throats (including **strep throat**), respiratory infections (sinusitis, **bronchitis**, **pneumonia**, etc.), skin ulcers, urinary tract infections, and vaginal infections. Extracts of lichens have been used in deodorants and soaps. Usnea is also used to promote healthy teeth and gums and to treat oral infections. It is used by naturopathic physicians to treat mild **cervical dysplasia** (abnormal growth of cells on the cervix).

Usnea barbata is a homeopathic remedy for headaches and sunstroke. *Usnea hirta* is used as an antibiotic as is *Usnea florida*, which can also be an antituberculosis agent. *Usnea longissima* is used as an expectorant.

Because of the absorbent quality of usnea, it has been used in baby diapers, wound dressings, and feminine napkins (sanitary pads).

Preparations

Usnea is commercially available in bulk form or as a powder, capsule, or tincture.

The tincture should be diluted in water before ingesting or using externally. Usnea tincture may be taken every two hours to treat bacterial infections. Other sources recommend taking 3-4 ml of tincture three times daily.

A usnea tea can be prepared by steeping 2-3 tsp of dried lichen or 1-2 tsp of powdered lichen in 1 cup of boiling-hot water. The tea may be taken three times a day.

In the capsule form, the patient should take 100 mg of usnea three times a day.

Usnea is used externally to treat fungal infections and skin ulcers. It can also be used as a douche to treat cystitis, urinary tract infections, and vaginal infections. Usnea is generally used as a vaginal suppository to treat mild cervical dysplasia. It is taken by mouth to treat colds, strep throat, influenza, sore throats, respiratory infections, and gastrointestinal disorders.

Precautions

Usnea should not be used for more than three weeks in a row. Pregnant women should not use usnea because it may promote uterine contractions.

Side effects

Usnea may cause gastrointestinal disorders in some persons.

Interactions

As of 2004, there are no reports of interactions between usnea and other drugs or herbal medicines.

Resources

BOOKS

"Usnea." In *The Alternative Advisor: The Complete Guide to Natural Therapies and Alternative Treatments.* Alexandria VA: Time-Life Books, 1997.

OTHER

"Lichen Information Sheet: Some Types of Lichen." http://www.alaskascreensavers.com/gallery/lichens/ak/lichinfo.htm.

"Usnea Lichens." http://www.nature.ca/English/treasures/trsite/trplant/tr3/tr3amaze.html.

Willis, Cindy. "Herb to Know: Usnea." http://www.wisetouch.com/usnea.html.

Belinda Rowland

Uterine cancer

Definition

Uterine **cancer** can be divided into two primary forms, cervical and endometrial. Cancer of the cervix most often affects the neck of the cervix or the opening or the opening into the uterus from the vagina. Endometrial cancer affects the inside lining of the uterus.

Description

Cervical cancer is much more prevalent than cancer of the endometrium; some estimate the incidence ratio as 3:1. Statistics from the year 2000 indicated cervical cancer was the second leading cause of cancer deaths in women ages 20-39 years, and the fifth leading cause of cancer death in women from 40-59 years old. Unlike many other cancers, early cancer of the cervix can be identified as much as 10 or more years before the cancer invades other tissues. These visible changes in the structure and activity of the cervical cells are seen under the microscope with Papanicolaou (Pap) tests and are referred to as mild dysplasia. Over a time period of five to 10 years, these abnormal cells may disappear without treatment, or may invade into deeper tissues and progress into a true cancer. The cancerous cells then may spread to endometrium, lymph glands, and nerves in the pelvic region.

As the population ages, cancer of the endometrium is becoming more common. Statistics indicate that approximately 50% of women with postmenopausal bleeding are diagnosed with endometrial cancer. This early symptom of irregular vaginal bleeding often allows removal of the uterus to result in cure of the disease, as endometrial cancer progresses and spreads slowly.

While all women are at risk for developing uterine cancer, specific risk factors for cervical cancer include sexual activity at an early age, and sex with multiple partners. **Infertility**, diabetes, **obesity**, and estrogen therapy place a woman at high risk for endometrial cancer. Other risk factors for uterine cancer include: endometrial hyperplasia, sexual inactivity, undergoing **menopause** after age 59 years, and never having had children.

Causes & symptoms

An important factor linked to cervical cancer is infection with one of the most common sexually transmitted diseases—human papillomavirus (HPV). Some strains of HPV can cause **genital warts** while others have no observable symptoms. Individuals infected with the herpes simplex virus, human immunodeficiency virus (HIV) or acquired immune deficiency syndrome (**AIDS**) are at increased risk for developing cancer of the cervix; the associated suppression of the immune system allows the HPV to more easily invade. Other chronic **infections** and erosions of the cervix also may increase the risk of cervical cancer.

While some women who have precancerous cervical changes experience no symptoms, others notice heavier or longer menstrual periods or vaginal bleeding after douching, intercourse or between periods. Symptoms of more advances stages of uterine cancer may include a foul-smelling vaginal discharge, rectal pressure or **constipation**, loss of appetite, **fatigue**, and back or leg **pain**.

Diagnosis

An annual Pap test and pelvic examination beginning as soon as young woman becomes sexually active, or between the age 17-20 years, are the most important diagnostic steps for early detection of uterine cancer. The Pap smear can pick up cervical dyplasia and the conventional physican may then perform a colposcopy and biopsy of the cervix to give a better understanding of the abnormalities. If only a small area of the cervix is affected, the recommendation may be made for more frequent Pap tests (about every three to six months) to monitor for changes in the cells of the cervix. Additional diagnostic tests for uterine cancer may include laparoscopy, laparotomy, or vaginosonography.

In 2002, a Food and Drug Administration (FDA) advisory panel suggested adding a screening test for HPV in addition to Pap smears since HPV is such a high risk factor for cervical cancer. The screening test could help separate women at high risk for more frequent screening than women not at high risk.

Treatment

After **cervical dysplasia** has been found, several herbal remedies and supplements may be helpful. Practitioners of herbal medicine refer to this class of herbs as *emmenagogues*. It includes supplements such as **squawvine**, **motherwort**, true unicorn, false unicorn, **black cohosh**, and **blessed thistle**. Studies have shown that as many as 67% of women with cervical dysplasia are deficient in various nutrients, including folate, beta-carotene, **selenium**, and vitamins B_6 and C. While these studies make no claim that taking a multivitamin or mineral supplement can reverse advanced cervical dysplasia, taking these supplements preventively may make sense.

The woman with uterine cancer will also benefit from nutritional supplements and a diet aimed at strengthening the immune system. **Echinacea** and **garlic** supplements may not only have positive effects on immunities, but also counteract the side effects of cancer treatment. Many trace elements, flavonoids, and other phytochemicals are provided by eating a well balanced diet that may not be provided in a pill. Even with relatively low levels of dietary intake, shiitake mushrooms, lentinus edodes, laminaria sea vegetables, and kombu **kelp** are believed to have anti-cancer properties. The use of any supplements or specific dietary modification should be discussed with the physician treating the cancer in order to avoid any undesirable drug interactions or side effects.

Research emphatically supports the mind-body connection when considering the health of the individual with cancer. Studies have also shown the positive effects of imagery on boosting immunities and natural killer cells. Visualization of the dominant white blood cells successfully attacking weak cancer cells can not only have a positive effect on the mood and mental status, but may also shrink tumors and extend the life of a patient with cancer. Laughter has also been found to enhance immunities and stimulate the sympathetic nervous system, pituitary gland, and the hormones that reduce **stress**, inflammation, and pain.

In addition to the well known effects of massage for **relaxation** and stress reduction, there are other physiologic effects that may help the individual with cancer. Massage may slow the body's release of the stress hormone cortisol, decreasing **anxiety** and allowing for more effective periods of sleep and regeneration. Massage has also been found to increase the production of serotonin, which can improve overall mood and immune status.

Allopathic treatment

Early stages of cervical dysplasia may require only frequent reevaluation to monitor progression or regression of the abnormal cells. Regression of abnormal cells may occur due to the immune response or lifestyle changes, such as discontinuing **smoking** or oral contraceptive use. In more advanced cases, the cervical lining may be removed via cautery, freezing or laser procedures.

Age, overall health status, and the presence of other abnormal findings will impact on the selection of most appropriate treatment plan for uterine cancer. Surgery may be presented as a treatment option for invasive cancer. Extent of the surgical procedures will depend upon the stage of the cancer. A hysterectomy, lymphadenectomy, or total pelvic exenteration may be recommended. Radiation therapy may be offered instead of or in addition to surgical removal of the affected tissues. Depending on the individual's disease stage, and the response and tolerance to the radiation, treatment may be provided by external beams directed over the pelvis, or by the insertion of radium tubes into the uterus and/or vagina. Chemotherapy may also be recommended, involving the infusion of tumor-fighting drugs directly into the circulatory system.

Expected results

The outcomes for the individual with uterine cancer are significantly related to the stage of the disease when cancer is found and treatment initiated. Early interventions can result in nearly 100% cure rates, while those individuals whose cancer is not discovered until abnormal tissue growth has invaded surrounding organs may have less positive outcomes. Those with advanced disease may experience pain, vaginal bleeding and/or foul smelling discharge, and intestinal obstruction.

KEY TERMS

Endometrium—The tissue that lines the uterus.

Hyperplasia—An overgrowth of cells that results in increased size of a body organ.

Hysterectomy—Surgical removal of the uterus and proximal vagina.

Laparoscopy—An examination of the interior of the abdomen with a lighted tube called a laparoscope.

Laparotomy—Surgical operation performed to open the abdomen for inspection of the internal organs, or as a preliminary step to additional surgery.

Pelvic lymphadenectomy—Surgical removal of the lymph nodes and passageways within the pelvis.

Total pelvic exenteration—Surgical procedure involving removal of the rectum, lower portion of the large intestine, the urinary bladder, the pelvic reproductive organs, lymph nodes, pelvic muscles, and perineum. Both urinary and fecal diversions are required for this surgery.

Prevention

The best preventive measure against uterine cancer is an annual pelvic examination and Pap test. In fact, a 2002 report from the College of American Pathologists stated that 80 percent of the women who die from cervical cancer had not had a Pap test in the five years preceding their diagnosis. Recognition of risk factors for uterine cancer, along with an awareness of the early signs and symptoms of cervical dysplasia, can promote the early detection of changes in the cervical cells.

Resources

BOOKS

Fugh-Berman, Adriane. *Alternative Medicine: What Works.* Baltimore, MD: Williams and Wilkins, 1997.

Gottlieb, James. *New Choices in Natural Healing.* Emmaus, PA: Rodale Press, Inc., 1995.

PERIODICALS

Bence, Sharlene. "Stop Cervical Cancer in Its Tracks." *Nursing Management* (April 2000): 40-43.

"College of American Pathologists Applauds New Pap Test Guidelines." *Women's Health Weekly* (May 30, 2002):12.

Frieden, Joyce. "FDA Advisory Panel; Backs HPV Test as Pap Smear Adjunct (Identifies High-Risk Strains)." *Family Practice News* (June 15, 2002):30–31.

Kathleen Wright
Teresa G. Odle

Uterine fibroids

Definition

Uterine fibroids (also called leiomyomas or myomas) are benign growths of the muscle inside the uterus. They are not cancerous, nor are they related to **cancer**. Fibroids can cause a wide variety of symptoms, including heavy menstrual bleeding and pressure on the pelvis.

Description

Uterine fibroids are extremely common. About 25% of women in their reproductive years have noticeable fibroids. There are probably many more women who have tiny fibroids that are undetected.

Fibroids develop in women between the ages of 30–50. They are never seen in women younger than 20 years old. After **menopause**, if a woman does not take estrogen, fibroids shrink. It appears that African American women are much more likely to develop uterine fibroids.

Fibroids are divided into different types, depending on the location. Submucous fibroids are found in the uterine cavity; intramural fibroids grow on the wall of the uterus; and subserous fibroids are located on the outside of the uterus. Many fibroids are so large that they fit into more than one category. The symptoms caused by fibroids are often related to their location.

Causes & symptoms

No one knows exactly what causes fibroids. The growth of fibroids, however, appears to depend on the hormone estrogen. Fibroids often grow larger when estrogen levels are high, as in **pregnancy**. Medications that lower the estrogen level can cause the fibroids to shrink.

The signs and symptoms of fibroids include:

- Heavy uterine bleeding. This is the most common symptom, occurring in 30% of women who have fibroids. The excess bleeding usually happens during the menstrual period. Flow may be heavier, and periods may last longer. Women who have submucous or intramural fibroids are most likely to have heavy uterine bleeding.

- Pelvic pressure and **pain**. Large fibroids that press on nearby structures such as the bladder and bowel can cause pressure and pain. Larger fibroids tend to cause more severe symptoms.

- **Infertility**. This is a rare symptom of fibroids. It probably accounts for less than 3% of infertility cases. Fibroids can cause infertility by compressing the uterine cavity. Submucous fibroids can fill the uterine cavity and interfere with implantation of the fertilized egg.

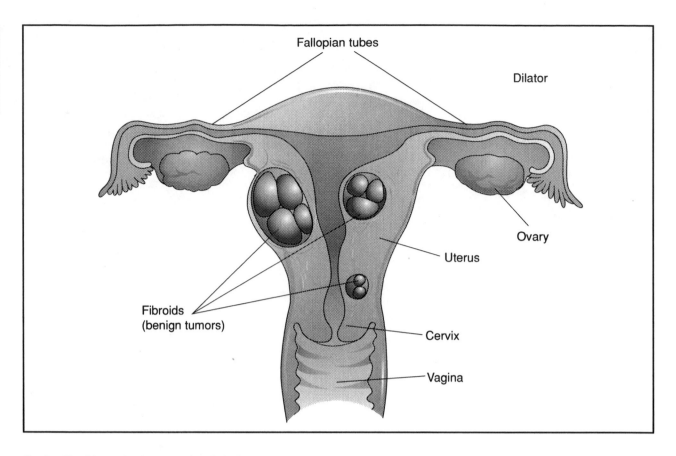

Fallopian tubes

Dilator

Ovary

Uterus

Fibroids
(benign tumors)

Cervix

Vagina

Uterine fibroids are benign growths of uterine muscle and are very common. They are divided into three types, depending on the location. Submucous fibroids are found in the uterine cavity; intramural fibroids grow on the wall of the uterus; and subserous fibroids are located on the outside of the uterus. *(Illustration by Electronic Illustrators Group. The Gale Group.)*

• Miscarriage. This is also an unusual symptom of fibroids, probably accounting for only a tiny fraction of the miscarriages that occur.

• Pregnancy complications. Fibroids can greatly increase in size during pregnancy, because of increased levels of estrogen. They can cause pain, and even lead to premature labor.

Diagnosis

A healthcare provider can usually feel fibroids during a routine pelvic examination. Ultrasound can be used to confirm the diagnosis, but this is not generally necessary.

Treatment

There are several natural treatments that help lower estrogen levels and slow the growth of the benign tumors. One study of alternative and complementary treatments for uterine fibroids found, however, that the cost of the alternative remedies was significantly higher than the cost of conventional treatments.

Nutritional therapy

There are several things women can do nutritionalwise to avoid having fibroids or prevent them from getting bigger:

• Eat more fruits, green or sea vegetables, whole grains, nuts, and seeds.

• Eat more soy foods such as tofu, tempeh, miso, or soy burger. Soy products contain isoflavones, which help reduce high levels of estrogens in the body.

• Avoid foods with high fat or sugar content, **caffeine**, or alcohol.

• Avoid eating produce sprayed with insecticides.

Nutritional supplements

The following supplements may be helpful in lowering estrogen levels and controlling fibroids:

• Bromelain: reduces inflammation.

• Choline: may improve liver function.

• Flaxseed: helps reduce excessive production of estrogens and other hormones.

- Vitamin E and **evening primrose oil**: help to regulate hormone production and may even shrink the fibroids.

- Vitamin C and **bioflavonoids**: have antiinflammatory and antioxidant effects.

Herbal treatment

Kuei-chih-fu-ling-wan (Keishi-bukuryo-gan; KBG) is a traditional Chinese herbal preparation that can effectively shrink fibroid tumors in 60% of patients, according to one study conducted by Japanese scientists. KBG is a mixture of the following herbs: cassia bark (*Keihi*), herbaceous peony roots (*Shakuyaku*), peach kernels (*Tounin*), herbaceous fungus (*Bukuryo*), and root bark of peony (*Botanpi*). In addition to reducing fibroid size, KBG also successfully alleviated fibroid symptoms such as severe menstrual bleedings or menstrual pain in 90% of the women in the study. These researchers suggest that KBG may work by inhibiting the production of sex hormones including estrogen. Unlike many other presently available herbal preparations that may be effective but lack scientific evidence to support their uses, KBG is proven safe as well as having few side effects. Women with fibroids, therefore, have one more alternative treatment to hysterectomy.

There are many herbal formulas that can be used depending on specific symptoms and body types. Another herbal treatment that may also be effective is **wild yam** progesterone cream. However, these are potent drugs and patients should consult their doctors before trying any of these treatments.

Homeopathy

A homeopathic physician may prescribe patient-specific homeopathic remedies to control fibroid symptoms.

Allopathic treatment

Not all fibroids cause symptoms. Even fibroids that do cause symptoms may not require treatment. In the majority of cases, the symptoms are inconvenient and unpleasant, but do not result in health problems.

Occasionally, fibroids lead to such heavy menstrual bleeding that the woman becomes severely anemic. In these cases, treatment of the fibroids may be necessary. Very large fibroids are much harder to treat. Therefore, many doctors recommend treatment for moderately-sized fibroids, in order to prevent them from growing into large fibroids that cause worse symptoms.

The following are possible treatment plans:

- Observation (watchful waiting). Most women already have symptoms at the time their fibroids are discovered, but feel that they can tolerate their symptoms. Therefore, no active treatment is given, but the woman and her physician stay alert for signs that the condition might be getting worse.

- Hysterectomy. This procedure involves surgical removal of the uterus, and it is the only definitive cure for fibroids. In fact, 25% of hysterectomies are performed because of symptomatic fibroids. A gynecologist can remove a fibroid uterus during either an abdominal or a vaginal hysterectomy. The choice depends on the size of the fibroids and other factors such as previous births and previous surgeries.

- Myomectomy. In this surgical procedure only the fibroids are removed; the uterus is repaired and left in place. This is the surgical procedure many women choose if they are not finished with childbearing. At first glance, it seems that this treatment is a middle ground between observation and hysterectomy. However, myomectomy is actually a difficult surgical procedure, more difficult than a hysterectomy. Myomectomy often causes significant blood loss, and blood transfusions may be required. In addition, some fibroids are so large, or buried so deeply within the wall of the uterus, that it is not possible to save the uterus, and a hysterectomy must be done, even though it was not planned.

- Lowering estrogen levels. Since fibroids are dependent on estrogen for their growth, medical treatments that lower estrogen levels can cause fibroids to shrink. A group of medications known as GnRH antagonists can dramatically lower estrogen levels. Women who take these medications for three to six months find that their fibroids shrink in size by 50% or more. They usually experience dramatic relief of their symptoms of heavy bleeding and pelvic pain.

- Uterine artery embolization (UAE). Embolization is a newer alternative to hysterectomy that shrinks fibroids by cutting off their blood supply. In UAE, the surgeon inserts a catheter into the uterine arteries. Small particles of polyvinyl foam or other inert substances are injected through the catheter into the arteries. The particles form an embolus, or clump, that blocks the blood supply to the fibroids and causes them to shrink. UAE is still controversial, however, because it has been associated with significant complications.

Unfortunately, GnRH antagonists cause unpleasant side effects in over 90% of women. The therapy is usually used for only three months, and should not be used for more than six months because the risk of developing brittle bones (osteoporosis)begins to rise. Once the treatment is stopped, the fibroids begin to grow back to their original size. Within six months, most of the old symptoms return. Therefore, GnRH agonists cannot be used as long-term solution. At the moment, treatment with GnRH antagonists is used mainly in preparation for surgery (myomectomy or hysterectomy). Shrinking the size of the fibroids makes surgery much easier, and reducing the heavy bleeding allows a woman to build up her blood count before surgery.

Fibroids can cause problems during pregnancy because they often grow in size. Large fibroids can cause pain and lead to premature labor. Fibroids cannot be removed during pregnancy because of the risk of injury to the uterus and hemorrhage. GnRH antagonists cannot be used during pregnancy. Treatment is limited to pain medication and medication to prevent premature labor, if necessary.

Expected results

Many women who have fibroids have no symptoms or have only minor symptoms of heavy menstrual bleeding or pelvic pressure. However, fibroids tend to grow over time, and gradually cause more symptoms. Many women ultimately decide to have some form of treatment. Currently, hysterectomy is the most popular form of treatment.

Prevention

Eating a healthful diet, reducing **stress**, and exercising regularly is the preferred preventive treatment regimen of many diseases including fibroids.

Resources

BOOKS

Bruce, Debra F. "Fibroids." In *The Unofficial Guide to Alternative Medicine.* New York, NY: McMillan General Reference, 1998, pp. 278-281.

Fetrow, Charles W., and Juan R. Avila. "Wild Yam." In *The Complete Guide to Herbal Medicines.* Springhouse, PA: Springhouse Corporation, 2000.

Friedman, Andrew J. "Uterine Fibroids." *Primary Care of Women.* edited by Karen J. Carlson and Stephanie A. Eisenstat. St. Louis, Missouri: Mosby-Year Book, Inc., 1995, pp. 275-278.

Muto, Michael G., and Andrew J. Friedman. "Leiomyomas." In *Kistner's Gynecology* . Sixth edition. Edited by Kenneth J. Ryan, Ross S. Berkowitz, and Robert L. Barbieri, St. Louis, MO: Mosby, 1995, pp. 147-149.

Zand, Janet, Allan N. Spreen, and James B. LaValle. "Fibroids, Uterine." In *Smart Medicine for Healthier Living: A Practical A-to-Z Reference to Natural and Conventional Treatments for Adults.* Garden City Park, NY: Avery Publishing Group, 1999: 282-285.

PERIODICALS

Lumsden, M. A. "Embolization versus Myomectomy versus Hysterectomy: Which Is Best, When?" *Human Reproduction* 17 (February 2002): 253-259.

Mehl-Madrona, L. "Complementary Medicine Treatment of Uterine Fibroids: A Pilot Study." *Alternative Therapies in Health and Medicine* 8 (March-April 2002): 34-6, 38-40, 42, 44-6.

Sakamoto, Shinobu, Haruno Yoshino, and Yaeko Sharahata. "Pharmacotherapeutic Effects of Kuei-chih-fu-ling-wan (Keishi-bukuryo-gan) on Human Uterine Myomas." *American Journal of Chinese Medicine* (1991): 313-317.

Todd, A. "An Alternative to Hysterectomy." *RN* 65 (March 2002): 30-34.

Watson, G. M., and W. J. Walker. "Uterine Artery Embolisation for the Treatment of Symptomatic Fibroids in 114 Women: Reduction in Size of the Fibroids and Women's Views of the Success of the Treatment." *British Journal of Obstetrics and Gynecology* 109 (February 2002): 129-135.

Mai Tran
Rebecca J. Frey, PhD

Uva ursi

Description

Uva ursi is a Latin name which means bear's grape. Its botanical name is *Arctostaphylos* and it is of the Ericaceae family. Other common names include bearberry, kinnikinnick (the name given to it by native Americans), whortleberry, spreng, mountain **cranberry** , and meal-berry. It is a low-growing evergreen plant, usually reaching no more than 16 in (41 cm) in height.

Growing in the cooler, northern climates, uva ursi likes well-drained sandy soil and a sunny location. It can be found in the mountainous areas of Europe, Asia and America, where it is commonly used for ornamental purposes, mostly as shrubbery or hedging. It is widely found in Canada and the United States, but no further south than Wisconsin and New Jersey. In the British Isles, it is common in the Highlands of Scotland, the hilly areas of Ireland, and as far south as Yorkshire in England.

Uva ursi bears many pink or white flowers, which may be tinged with red, and grow in clusters. Bears are known to be fond of its red berries, hence the common name. The leaves, which are the part of the plant used for medicinal purposes, are smooth-edged, leathery, small, (between half an inch to an inch long), and oval. They are dark green in color and have lighter undersides. The leaves have no odor but are to be distinguished by their exceedingly bitter taste. They are attached to the branch by a very short stem. The branches tend to trail, are covered with a light brown bark, and are inclined to form a thick mass one to two feet long. Shoots rise obliquely from the stems and have soft hairs.

The chemical constituents of uva ursi include:

- arbutin (a glycoside) up to 10%, which is converted to hydroquinone in alkaline urine, thus releasing its active ingredient

- methyl arbutin

- flavonoids

- tannins, which can irritate stomach lining if taken in large quantities or over a long period of time

- alantoin

- phenolic acids (gallic and ellacic)

- volatile oil

- resin

- ursolic acid, which is known to be an effective diuretic

- quercetin and myricetin (coloring)

On incineration, the leaves yield approximately 3% ash. uva ursi also contains the following nutrients:

- vitamin A

- iron

- manganese

- selenium

- silicon

General use

Uva ursi, which is generally categorized as a treatment for the urinary and glandular systems, was commonly included in all the old pharmacopoeias, where it was sometimes mistakenly named Arbutas, and classified as such.

It has also been included in the modern pharmacopoeias due to its many medicinal uses and the fact that modern research has not detracted from the high esteem in which it is held in alternative health circles. The leaves of uva ursi are used mainly for kidney and urinary **infections** , for which it is exceptionally effective, having both anti-inflammatory and antiseptic properties. It is a famous herbal cure for cystitis, from which most women suffer at some time or another. It is also effective for the treatment of **kidney stones**, as it acts on these by softening them and has muscle relaxant properties, which may be beneficial in patients with this disorder.

Other illnesses for which it has been used include Bright's disease, dysentery, nephritis, **gonorrhea** and **syphilis**, excessive **menstruation**, stimulation of the spleen, liver and pancreas, **hemorrhoids**, **menopause**, and diabetes. Research has indicated that the herb is more effective in its whole state than when broken down into components.

Some of the other uses for which uva ursi is also known include the following:

- Some native Americans combined it with tobacco and smoked it.

- Its astringent properties make it useful for **infections** (it dries them up).

- The tea may be used as an antiseptic for cuts and abrasions.

- It is sometimes used as a weight loss aid because it promotes production of urine, being an effective diuretic.

- In some places, notably Russia, it is drunk as a tea.

- Uva ursi is one of the rare herbs that can be helpful in cases of bedwetting.

- Uva ursi has such a high tannin content that the leaves have actually been used to tan leather in Russia and Scandinavia.

- In Scandinavia, an ash-colored dye is made from the plant.

- Uva ursi berries are used as food for grouse.

Preparations

The leaves of the uva ursi plant may be harvested at any time, although traditionally this precious medicinal

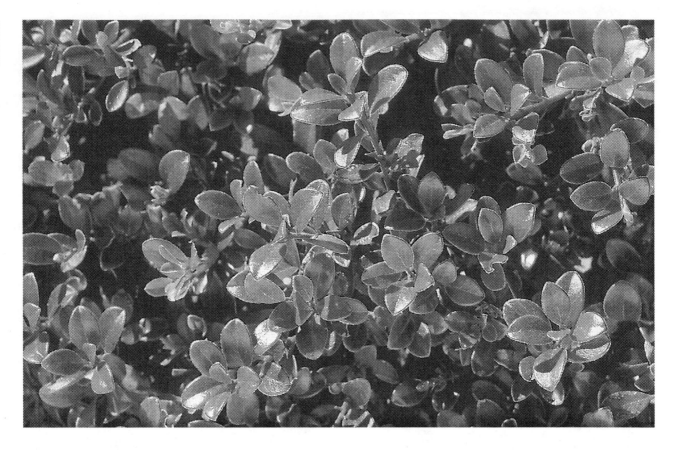

Uva ursi. (© *PlantaPhile, Germany. Reproduced by permission.*)

herb is gathered in late summer or autumn. The leaves should be picked in the morning after the dew has dried. They should then be left in a well-aired place to dry naturally and then stored in an airtight container (preferably glass or stainless steel, as these won't react with the volatile oils) to keep them dry, as they have a tendency to reabsorb moisture from the atmosphere. The hairs, which are present in growing uva ursi leaves, are absent once the herb is dried because they drop off in the drying process.

A guide to dosages of uva ursi preparations is as follows:

• Herbal extracts, as capsules or tablets, 250-500 mg three times daily.

• Tinctures, (which are alcohol-based), 5ml three times daily.

• For the purpose of treating urinary tract infections, 6-8 g of bicarbonate of soda in a glass of water should also be taken. This combination ensures alkalinity of the urine, thus releasing the active ingredient from the uva ursi. Another way to ensure alkalinity of the urine is to adhere to a vegetarian diet with lots of raw fruits and vegetables for a period.

• The leaves may be wrapped in gauze and added to bath water for the treatment of hemorrhoids, inflammations and skin infections.

• Uva ursi should not be taken for more than two weeks at a time and individuals with high blood pressure should not take it at all. Some practitioners assert that this herb should not be used for more than three days at a time, as it can irritate mucous membranes.

• Uva ursi may be taken as a tea (infusion) for the treatment of minor vaginal irritations, menstrual bloating, and diabetes.

Uva ursi tea should not be boiled, as it becomes bitter and unpalatable and poisonous compounds may result. It is sufficient to prepare an infusion by soaking the leaves for a few hours in cold water. This mode of preparation inhibits the release of tannins that may irritate the stomach lining. Alternatively, boiling water may be added to the leaves, (one pint of water to 1 oz of leaves), which should then be allowed to steep for a while.

Some practitioners recommend always combining uva ursi with marsh mallow root or other mucilaginous diuretics.

Although high doses of uva ursi are not recommended for long periods, one cup of the tea is permissible as a prophylactic in cases of recurring cystitis. However, it is preferable to discontinue even prophylactic treatment from time to time.

Precautions

Occasionally, uva ursi is adulterated with other herbs, most notably cowberry and box, which will render the remedy less effective. Care must be taken to obtain the remedy from a reputable dealer.

Pregnant women should not take uva ursi. It should not be given to small children unless under the supervision of a health care practitioner.

Long-term use of uva ursi is not recommended as hydroquinone (produced in the body in response to uva ursi) is poisonous in large amounts. Practitioners recommend that it be taken for no more than two weeks at a time.

Despite the powerful antiseptic/antibiotic properties of uva ursi, a natural health practitioner should be consulted if it is being used to treat infection.

It should be noted that practitioners recommend all alternative treatments should be used in conjunction with a healthy lifestyle.

Side effects

Uva ursi has been known to cause mild **nausea**. Fruit juice, **vitamin C**, and other acidic foods should not be taken with uva ursi preparations, in order to promote a pH balance in the body, thus preserving effectiveness of the remedy. If a patient develops any of the following toxic reactions that may be provoked by uva ursi, such as nausea and **vomiting**, shortness of breath, convulsions, ringing in the ears or even delirium and faintness, medical help should be sought immediately.

KEY TERMS

Astringent—Drying effect.

Infusion—To make a tea.

Prophylactic—Preventative measure.

The bicarbonate of soda, which is recommended to be taken with uva ursi in cases of urinary tract infection, is unsuitable for those who suffer from high blood pressure, and in any case should not be taken for more than two weeks.

Uva ursi is not recommended for use during **pregnancy** as it may restrict blood supply to the fetus, due to its astringent properties.

Interactions

Uva ursi should not be taken in conjunction with the herb **buchu**, and should also not be taken with **cranberry** or anything containing cranberries. It should also not be used in conjunction with any drugs, which induce acid urine. Uva ursi may temporarily turn the urine green, which is a harmless side effect.

Arbutin, which is a constituent of uva ursi, is known to increase the anti-inflammatory effect of synthetic cortisone. This interaction may require a change in dosage.

Resources

OTHER

HealthNotes. http://www.healthnotes.com.

Snowbound Herbals. http://www.sbherbals.com/021999HotM.html.

MotherNature.com. http://www.mothernature.com/ency/Herb/Uva_Ursi.asp.

Patricia Skinner

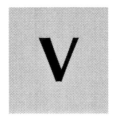

Vaginitis

Definition

Vaginitis is a condition characterized by inflammation of the vagina and vulva, most often caused by a bacterial, fungal, or parasitic infection.

Description

Vaginitis, vulvitis, and vulvovaginitis are general terms that refer to the inflammation of the vagina and/or vulva (the external genital organs of a woman). These conditions can be caused by bacterial, fungal, or parasitic **infections**; or by any type of allergic or irritation reaction to such things as spermicidal products, condoms, soaps, and bubble bath. A type of vaginitis that is caused by a low estrogen level is called atrophic vaginitis.

In general, vaginitis causes one or more of these symptoms: vaginal discharge; irritation; a burning sensation; and **itching**. One of the most common reasons women visit their doctor is because of a change in their vaginal discharge. It is completely normal for a woman to have a vaginal discharge, with the amount and consistency varying during the course of the menstrual cycle. The three most common types of vaginitis are bacterial vaginosis, candida vulvovaginitis, and **trichomoniasis**. Each will be discussed separately.

Bacterial vaginosis

Bacterial vaginosis is the most common cause of vaginitis during the childbearing years. Forty percent to 50% of vaginitis cases are caused by bacterial vaginosis. The occurrence of bacterial vaginosis is difficult to determine, but studies have proposed that 10–41% of women have had it at least once. The occurrence of bacterial vaginosis in the United States is highest among African-American women and women who have had multiple sexual partners, and is lowest among Asian women and women with no history of sexual contact with men. Bacterial vaginosis is not considered a sexually transmitted disease although it can be acquired through sexual intercourse. Recent findings indicate that bacterial vaginosis can be transmitted among women who have sex only with women, if vaginal secretions are exchanged.

Bacterial vaginosis is not caused by a particular organism but by a change in the balance of normal vaginal bacteria or by a change in the pH balance. Ninety percent of the bacteria found in a healthy vagina belong to the genus *Lactobacillus*. For various reasons, there is a shift in the bacterial population that results in overgrowth of other bacteria. Patients suffering from bacterial vaginosis have very high numbers of such bacteria as *Gardnerella vaginalis*, *Mycoplasma hominis*, *Bacteroides* species, and *Mobiluncus* species; and these bacteria can be found at numbers 100–1,000 times greater than are found in the healthy vagina. In contrast, *Lactobacillus* bacteria are very low in number or completely absent from the vagina of women with bacterial vaginosis.

Candida vulvovaginitis

Candida vulvovaginitis also has been called vulvovaginal candidiasis, candidal vaginitis, monilial infection, or vaginal **yeast infection**. Twenty to 25% of the vaginitis cases are candida vulvovaginitis. It has been estimated that about 75% of all women get a vaginal yeast infection at least once. In 80–90% of the cases, candida vulvovaginitis is caused by an overgrowth of the yeast *Candida albicans*. The remaining cases are caused by other species of *Candida*. It is not known what causes the yeast overgrowth. However, it is known that antibiotics can inadvertently kill normal bacteria in the vagina and cause an overgrowth of *Candida*.

Candida vulvovaginitis is not considered a sexually transmitted disease because *Candida* species are commonly found in the healthy vagina. It is rare to find this disease in girls before puberty and in celibate women. Vaginal yeast **infections** tend to occur more frequently in women who are pregnant; diabetic and not controlling their disease; taking birth control pills, steroid drugs, or antibiotics; and those with the human immunodeficiency virus (HIV). The occurrence of four or more attacks per year is called recurrent vaginal candidiasis.

Trichomoniasis

Trichomoniasis, which is sometimes called "trich," accounts for 15–20% of the cases of vaginitis. It is estimated that two million to three million American women get trichomoniasis each year. Unlike the previous two types of vaginitis, trichomoniasis is primarily a sexually transmitted disease in that the disease is passed from person-to-person primarily by sexual contact. Trichomoniasis occurs in both men and women and is caused by an infection with the single-celled parasite *Trichomonas vaginalis*. Infection with *Trichomonas vaginalis* is frequently associated with other sexually transmitted diseases and helps spread the **AIDS** virus.

Causes & symptoms

Vaginitis is most often caused by a bacterial, fungal, or parasitic infection as described above. Other microorganisms may cause vaginitis, or it may be caused by allergic reaction, irritation, injury, low estrogen levels, and certain diseases. Common causes of bacterial vaginosis include:

- Repeated sexual intercourse over a short period of time, which raises vaginal pH and results in growth of bacteria and infection-like symptoms.

- Chronic vulvar dampness, aggravated by **stress** or restrictive, nonabsorbent synthetic clothing.

- Chemical irritants.

- Antibiotics, which disrupt the natural vaginal (and bowel) bacterial environment.

Additional risk factors for bacterial vaginosis include stress; a poor diet; use of an intrauterine device (IUD); being a member of a non-white race; a history of at least one prior **pregnancy**; first sexual activity at an early age; having multiple sex partners, and a history of sexually transmitted diseases.

Persons at an increased risk for candida vulvovaginitis include those who have had previous candida infections, have **AIDS**, or are diabetic; women who use douches, perfumed feminine hygiene sprays, vaginal sponges, or an IUD; those taking birth control pills, antibiotics, or corticosteroids; and those who wear tight clothing, are pregnant, or engage in frequent sexual intercourse.

The typical symptoms of vaginitis are vaginal discharge, itching, burning sensation, and irritation. Some women have few or no symptoms, while others may have pronounced symptoms. The main symptom of bacterial vaginosis is a fishy-smelling, thin, milky-white or gray vaginal discharge.

Itching and burning may also be present. The fishy smell is stronger after sexual intercourse. The symptoms of *candida vulvovaginitis* are itching, soreness, painful sexual intercourse, and a thick, white, curdy (like cottage cheese) vaginal discharge. Trichomoniasis symptoms in women range from none at all to painful urination; painful sexual intercourse; and a yellow-green to gray, foul-smelling, sometimes frothy, vaginal discharge. In men, trichomoniasis may present no symptoms, or it may be associated with urethral discharge or persistent urethritis (inflammation of the urethra).

Diagnosis

Vaginitis can be diagnosed and treated by a nurse practitioner or physician. Most insurance companies cover the costs of diagnosis and treatment. To diagnose vaginitis, the doctor will examine the vagina (using a speculum to keep the vagina open) and take a sample of the vaginal discharge for tests and microscopic analysis. Laboratory culture results should be available in two to three days, but the microscopic examination of the vaginal discharge may be performed immediately in the doctor's office. Diagnosis may be difficult because there are many different causes of vaginitis. Women who think that they have vaginitis should always visit their doctor to get an accurate diagnosis. Many women assume that they have a yeast infection and take over-the-counter medicines without first consulting their doctors.

To make a diagnosis of bacterial vaginosis, the doctor will check for four signs, called Amsel's criteria. These signs are: a thin, milky-white discharge that clings to the walls of the vagina; presence of a fishy odor; a vaginal pH of greater than 4.5; and the presence of "clue cells" in the vagina. Clue cells are vaginal cells that are covered with small bacteria. A diagnosis of candida vulvovaginitis is made after finding a normal vaginal pH (4–4.5) as well as the presence of many yeast cells in the sample of vaginal discharge or growth of yeast on laboratory media. A trichomoniasis diagnosis is made when the parasites are found in the vaginal discharge either by microscopic examination or in laboratory cultures. The newest system for testing for trichomoniasis is the In-Pouch test, which is more accurate than the older wet-mount method and easier to perform.

Treatment

Herbal remedies for vaginal infections are being aggressively investigated as of 2002 in hopes of lowering the rates of sexually transmitted diseases in developing countries that cannot afford Western allopathic treatments. Chinese, Ayurvedic, naturopathic, and homeopathic treatments for vaginitis are all being studied.

One of the primary focuses of alternative treatment for vaginal conditions including vaginitis is rebalancing the normal vaginal flora. To assist with this rebalancing, *Lactobacillus acidophilus* and *L. bifidus* are recommended, either taken internally or introduced directly into the vagina. Plain yogurt with live **acidophilus** cultures or **acidophilus** powder or capsules may be eaten. Yogurt can be inserted directly into the vagina or a tampon can be soaked in yogurt and inserted. **Garlic** (*Allium sativum*), taken both internally and inserted into the vagina (a peeled whole clove wrapped in gauze), may be helpful due to its antibacterial and antifungal actions. A variety of other herbs can be used as douches or in suppository form to help treat acute flare-ups of vaginal symptoms. For example, one remedy for reducing inflammation is a douche made by adding 1–2 tsp of **calendula** (*Calendula officinalis*) to boiling water, steeping the mixture, and letting it cool before using.

Herbal remedies for yeast also include a variety of antifungal, antiseptic, or immune-strengthening agents such as **tea tree oil** (inserted via a soaked tampon, douche, or suppository), **black walnut** (*Juglans nigra*), pau d'arco (*Tabebuia impestiginosa*), **echinacea** (*Echinacea* species), and **goldenseal** (*Hydrastis canadensis*). Echinacea and **goldenseal** should be taken only for a limited time. As with many herbs, medical supervision may be advised for those with certain health conditions. Persons with specific **allergies** may not be able to use some remedies. For example, **echinacea** should not be used by anyone allergic to plants in the sunflower family, and goldenseal should not be used during pregnancy or by anyone allergic to ragweed.

A boric acid douche can help to acidify the vaginal pH so that unwanted bacteria cannot survive and multiply. Because some women may be sensitive to this douche, a health professional should oversee this treatment. Also, care must be taken to keep boric acid away from children. Vaginal pH may also be lowered by using Summer's Eve medicated douche, which contains **potassium** iodide, or a vinegar douche (1 tbsp of vinegar per quart of warm water).

The Gynecological Sourcebook recommends Betadine and gentian violet for treating candida vulvovaginitis. Betadine, an antiseptic **iodine** solution, should not be used by pregnant women. Gentian violet is an antifungal stain. Both solutions are messy and leave stains, and some women may be allergic to either or both of them. *Oxygen Healing Therapies* reports successful treatment of candidiasis with intravenous hydrogen peroxide. Various homeopathic treatments are available over the counter or prepared for individual cases by homeopaths. Commonly cited ingredients are **pulsatilla** and **sepia**. For atrophic vaginitis, especially in menopausal women, topical application of progesterone cream can help symptoms abate by slowing the thinning of the tissue.

Dietary modification and nutritional supplementation may also be helpful in the treatment of vaginitis. Antioxidant vitamins, including A, C, and E, as well as B complex vitamins and **vitamin D** are recommended. *Prescriptions for Nutritional Healing* notes that if atrophic vaginitis is treated with prescription estrogen ointments, the body's need for vitamin B_6 is increased. Topical application of **vitamin E** from prepared creams or from torn vitamin E capsules may help relieve itching. Other home remedies for itching from *The Gynecological Sourcebook* include **witch hazel** or cottage cheese compresses; or baths with epsom salts or baking soda followed by blow-drying the vagina and dusting the vagina with cornstarch.

Allergy tests may be useful for women with yeast infections. Additionally, foods that yeast organisms thrive on should be avoided. These foods include cheese, alcohol, chocolate, soy sauce, sugar, vinegar, fruits, and any fermented foods or foods containing molds (e. g., blue cheese). Wearing cotton underwear and loose-fitting clothes and avoiding pantyhose can help keep the vagina cool and dry, thus helping to prevent some forms of vaginitis. For recurrent yeast infections, alternative treatments recommended in *The Gynecological Sourcebook* include boric acid douches in declining doses; oral ingestion of acidophilus with meals; and caprylic acid and myocidin, which are fatty acids derived from antifungal oils. Cases of chronic vaginitis should be addressed on systemic level by an alternative practitioner.

Allopathic treatment

Both bacterial vaginosis and trichomoniasis require prescription medication for treatment. Candidal vulvovaginitis may be treated with either prescription or over-the-counter medicines. It is not advisable to take over-the-counter medications for vaginal yeast infections if one does not in fact have a yeast infection. A survey of 390 gynecologists found that 44% of the women who were diagnosed with bacterial vaginosis had first treated themselves with over-the-counter yeast infection medications.

Bacterial vaginosis should be treated daily for one week with the antibiotics metronidazole (Flagyl, Protostat) or clindamycin (Cleocin), either as pills taken orally or in a gel or cream form inserted into the vagina. Trichomoniasis is treated with either a large single dose of metronidazole or with a smaller dose taken twice daily for one week. Male sexual partners of women with trichomoniasis also must be treated, and intercourse should be avoided until both partners are cured. Possible side effects of the oral antibiotics include **nausea** and adverse reactions to drinking alcohol during the treatment period. Following treatment, natural flora need to be built up again through introduction of acidophilus and other lactobacilli.

Candida vulvovaginitis is most often treated by the application of medicated gels, creams, or suppositories applied directly to the vagina. The antifungal drugs used to treat candida vulvovaginitis include oral fluconazole (Diflucan); butoconazole (Femstat); clotrimazole (Gynelotrimin, Mycelex); miconazole (Monistat); ticonazole (Vagistat), and nystatin (Mycostatin, Nilstat, Nystex). Most require only one or a few days of therapy to be effective. Women who have recurrent candidal infections may receive treatment for several weeks followed by some form of a long-term preventative treatment. Ketoconazole (Nizoral) may be used to treat recurrent vaginitis.

Normal allopathic treatment of atrophic vaginitis includes either estrogen creams or low-dosage estrogen tablets. Tibolone, a synthetic steroid, is also given for the treatment of atrophic vaginitis. It appears to prevent bone loss as well as improving the condition of the vaginal lining.

Expected results

Vaginitis is a disease with minor symptoms, and most women respond well to medications. It is believed, however, that certain vaginal infections left untreated can lead to more serious conditions, such as **pelvic inflammatory disease**; endometritis; postsurgical infections; and spread of the AIDS virus. Bacterial vaginosis has been identified as a risk factor in certain complications of pregnancy, including early pregnancy loss, preterm labor, and low birth weight infants. In addition, recurrent trichomonal infection appears to be associated with an increased risk of cervical **cancer**.

Prevention

Women may avoid vaginal infections by following these suggestions:

• Do not take over-the-counter yeast infection treatments unless the woman has been diagnosed with candidiasis before and recognizes the symptoms.

• Avoid douching because it may disturb the balance of organisms in the vagina and may spread them higher into the reproductive system.

• Do not use vaginal deodorants or sprays because they can also disturb the vagina's natural balance.

• Thoroughly dry oneself after bathing and remove a wet bathing suit promptly.

• Avoid wearing tight clothing and wear cotton underwear. Change underwear often and avoid pantyhose made from synthetic fibers.

• Clean diaphragms, cervical caps, and spermicide applicators after every use. Use condoms to avoid sexually transmitted diseases.

KEY TERMS

Atrophic vaginitis—An inflammation of the vagina that develops when the estrogen levels in the body drop. It is usually associated with normal menopause or with surgical removal of the ovaries, but can occur with breast-feeding or premature menopause.

Parasite—An animal or plant that can only survive by living inside or upon another animal or plant.

pH—A measurement of the acidity or alkalinity (basicity) of a solution. A low pH indicates an acid solution; a high pH indicates a base, or alkaline, solution. The normal vaginal pH is 4-4.5.

Vaginosis—Bacterial infection of the vagina, caused by an overgrowth of bacteria that normally live in the vagina.

Vulva—The external genital organs of a woman, including the outer and inner lips, clitoris, and opening of the vagina.

• After a bowel movement, wipe the area around the anus from front to back to avoid spreading intestinal bacteria into the vagina.

Resources

BOOKS

Rosenthal, M. Sara. *The Gynecological Sourcebook.* Los Angeles: Lowell House, 1994.

PERIODICALS

Barenfanger, J., C. Drake, and C. Hanson. "Timing of Inoculation of the Pouch Makes No Difference in Increased Detection of *Trichomonas vaginalis* by the InPouch TV method." *Journal of Clinical Microbiology* 40 (April 2002): 1387-1389.

Cullins, Vanessa E., et al. "Treating Vaginitis." *Nurse Practitioner* 24 (October 1999): 46–65.

Davis, S. R. "The Effects of Tibolone on Mood and Libido." *Menopause* 9 (May-June 2002): 153-155.

Marrazzo, J. M., L. A. Koutsky, D. A. Eschenbach, et al. "Characterization of Vaginal Flora and Bacterial Vaginosis in Women Who Have Sex with Women." *Journal of Infectious Diseases* 185 (May 1, 2002): 1307-1313.

Pumpradit, W., and M. Augenbraun. "Bacterial Vaginosis Complicating Pregnancy and Gynecologic Surgery." *Current Infectious Diseases Report* 4 (April 2002): 141-143.

Sayed el-Ahl, S. A., H. S. el-Wakil, N. M. Kamel, and M. S. Mahmoud. "A Preliminary Study on the Relationship Between *Trichomonas vaginalis* and Cervical Cancer in Egyptian Women." *Journal of the Egyptian Society of Parasitology* 32 (April 2002): 167-178.

Sobel, Jack D. "Vaginitis." *New England Journal of Medicine* 337 (December 1997): 1896–1903.

Vermani, K., and S. Garg. "Herbal Medicines for Sexually Transmitted Diseases and AIDS." *Journal of Ethnopharmacology* 80 (April 2002): 49-66.

Williams, Pamela A. "Nonscientifically Validated Herbal Treatments for Vaginitis." *Nurse Practitioner* 24 (August 1999): 101–4.

ORGANIZATIONS

National Institutes of Health, Office of Research on Women's Health. <www4.od.nih.gov/orwh>.

National Vaginitis Association. 117 South Cook Street, Suite 315, Barrington, IL 60010. (800) 909-8745. VagAssoc@aol.com. <www.vaginalinfection.com>.

OTHER

JAMA Women's Health STD Information Center. <www.ama-assn.org/special/std>.

Patricia Skinner

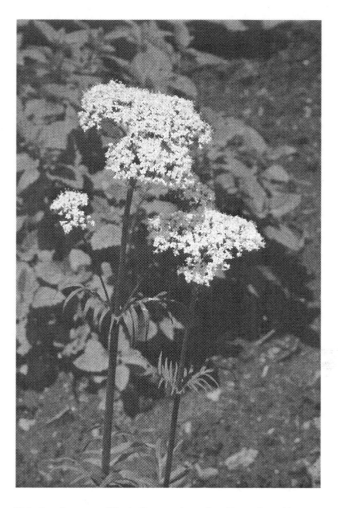

Valerian flowers. *(Photo Researchers, Inc. Reproduced by permission.)*

Valerian

Description

Valerian (*Valeriana officinalis*) is one of about 200 members of the Valerianaceae family. This plant is native to Europe and west Asia; it is naturalized throughout North America. A common name for this hardy perennial is garden heliotrope. Valerian has been valued for its soothing qualities for at least a millennium. The name valerian may have come from the Latin *valere* meaning "to be strong" or "to be in good health." Chaucer called the herb setewale. Other common names include all-heal, vandal root, and Capon's tail. The Greek doctor Galen called a particularly odorous species of valerian "phu," referring to the distinctively unpleasant smell of the dried root. The strong odor appeals to earthworms, intoxicates cats, and attracts rats. According to legend, the Pied Piper of Hamlin, with the assistance of the odorous valerian root, lured the town's rats to the river to drown. Some Asian species of valerian have a more pleasant aroma and may have included spikenard (the biblical name for valerian), which was known as a perfume from the East.

In ancient times, valerian was believed to be under the influence of the god Mercury. The herb grows in lime-rich soil near streams, or in damp, low meadows where it may reach a height of 5 ft (1.5 m). It is also found in drier environments at higher elevations, where it grows to just 2 ft (0.6 m). Roots harvested from the drier environment may be more medicinally potent. This variety is sometimes known as sylvestus.

Valerian's short vertical rhizome is dark yellow-brown in color and has round rootlets. These rootlets produce hollow, fluted stems with opposite leaves and a single leaflet at the tip, and as many as eight to 10 pairs of toothed leaflets. The upper leaves are attached at their base and emerge from a white sheath along the stem. The stems remain erect and unbranched until the very top, were the small, white flowers, tinged with pink, bloom in clusters in the middle of summer. Seeds are winged with tufts of white hair, and they scatter on the wind.

General use

As of 2003, researchers have identified some of the active ingredients in valerian that are responsible for its medicinal properties. A team of pharmacologists in Argentina reported in the spring of 2003 that they had isolated two new flavonoids, 6-methylapigenin and hesperidin, as compounds with sedative and sleep-enhancing properties. In addition to these flavonoids, valerian contains volatile oil, valepotriates, glycosides, alkaloids, choline, tannins, and resins. Valerian's rhizome and root are the medicinal part of this herb. Fresh root will produce the highest quality of medicinal extract.

Valerian acts as a **pain** reliever, antispasmodic, sedative, carminative, and can help support nerve tissue. A British study published in 2002 suggests that valerian's effectiveness in relieving **stress** is related to its ability to lower the body's reactivity in stressful situations. Valerian can also help to promote menstrual flow. As a natural tranquilizer, valerian can soothe **anxiety**, nervous tension, **insomnia**, and **headache**. It acts on the peripheral nerves and relaxes both the smooth and skeletal muscle tissue to reduce tension. It also strengthens the heart and provides relief from menstrual cramps, stomach cramps, irritable bowel, and upset stomach caused by nerves. Valerian has also been shown to lower blood pressure. One study found that valerian tends to sedate the agitated person and stimulate the fatigued person, bringing about a balancing effect on the system. Externally, a lotion prepared with valerian extract will ease irritation of skin **rashes** and soothe swollen joints.

The plant has been used as a medicinal herb for more than a thousand years, especially for mild cases of insomnia. Research shows that proper use of valerian promotes sleep, reduces night awakenings, and increases dream recall in most people. Historically, valerian has been highly regarded as a tranquilizer that acts without narcotic effects. It is particularly popular with women; a recently introduced herbal formula for menopausal women contains valerian along with **hops** and **black cohosh** as an active ingredient. The herb has also been used to treat illnesses as diverse as **epilepsy** and the plague. In the sixteenth century, valerian was reported to have cured a case of epilepsy. It was also used to treat hysteria, migraine, and vertigo. Culpeper recommended the herb for "driving away splinters or thorns from the flesh." Valerian was listed in the *United States Pharmacopoeia* from the early seventeenth century until the mid-twentieth century. During World War I, soldiers traumatized by the constant bombing and those suffering from "shell shock" were treated with valerian. The herb was listed in the *U.S. National Formulary* until 1950, and continues to be listed in the official pharmacopoeias of Germany, Belgium, and France.

More recently, valerian is being studied as a possible chemopreventive for **cancer**. Further research is necessary, however, to determine its effectiveness in this regard.

Preparations

Valerian root should be harvested in the autumn of its second year. Valerian works well in combination with other tranquilizing herbs such as **passionflower** (*Passiflora in-carnata*) to safely induce sleep, or **skullcap** (*Scutellaria laterifolia*) to relieve nervous tension. The somewhat bitter, unpleasant taste of the tea may be masked by adding **peppermint** oil, or the user can take the herb in capsule form. Combinations contain equal parts of each herb. The herb may be drunk as an herbal tea, used as a tincture, or swallowed in capsule form one hour before bedtime.

Precautions

Valerian should not be used in large doses or for an extended period. People should not take it continuously for more than two to three weeks. Users of valerian may become tolerant to its effects with prolonged use. Increasing the dose of the herb to achieve desired effects may result in negative side effects. Prolonged use, according to some research, could result in liver damage and central nervous system impairment.

Side effects

Large doses of valerian may occasionally cause headache, muscle spasm, heart palpitations, **dizziness**, gastric distress, sleeplessness, and confusion. Uninterrupted use may cause **depression**.

Interactions

Although valerian has been regarded as a relatively safe herb because few interactions with prescription medications have been reported, newer research indicates that it should be used cautiously following surgery. Like St. Johní's wort, valerian can interact with anesthetics and other medications given to patients after surgery. Because valerian has a mild sedative effect, it should not be taken together with alcoholic beverages, benzodiazepines, barbiturates, or antihistamines. Long-term safety studies of valerian have not been done as of early 2003.

Resources

BOOKS

McIntyre, Anne. *The Medicinal Garden*. New York: Henry Holt and Company, 1997.

Ody, Penelope. *The Complete Medicinal Herbal*. New York: Dorling Kindersley, 1993.

PDR for Herbal Medicines. NJ: Medical Economics Company, 1998.

Pelletier, Kenneth R., MD. *The Best Alternative Medicine*, Part I: Western Herbalism. New York: Simon & Schuster, 2002.

Prevention's 200 Herbal Remedies, 3rd edition. Excerpted from *The Complete Book of Natural & Medicinal Cures*. Pennsylvania: Rodale Press, Inc., 1997.

Tyler, Varro E., Ph.D. *The Honest Herbal*. New York: Pharmaceutical Products Press, 1993.

KEY TERMS

Carminative—A medication or preparation that prevents the formation of intestinal gas or allows it to be expelled.

Flavonoid—Any of a group of plant compounds with an aromatic nucleus, often found as a pigment. Two new flavonoids identified in valerian may be the source of its sedative effects.

Rhizome—A fleshy plant stem that grows horizontally under or along the ground; roots are sent out below this stem and leaves or shoots are sent out above it.

OTHER

PERIODICALS

Ang-Lee, Michael, et al. " Herbal Medicines and Perioperative Care." *Journal of the American Medical Association* 286 (July 11, 2001): 208.

Cropley, M., Z. Cave, J. Ellis, and R. W. Middleton. "Effect of Kava and Valerian on Human Physiological and Psychological Responses to Mental Stress Assessed Under Laboratory Conditions." *Phytotherapy Research* 16 (February 2002): 23–27.

Hadley, S., and J. J. Petry. "Valerian." *American Family Physician* 67 (April 15, 2003): 1755–1758.

Kapadia, G. J., M. A. Azuine, H. Tokuda, et al. "Inhibitory Effect of Herbal Remedies on 12-o-Tetradecanoylphorbol-13-Acetate-Promoted Epstein-Barr Virus Early Antigen Activation." *Pharmacological Research* 45 (March 2002): 213–222.

Marder,M., H. Viola, C. Wasowski, et al. "6-Methylapigenin and Hesperidin: New Valeriana Flavonoids with Activity on the CNS." *Pharmacology, Biochemistry, and Behavior* 75 (June 2003): 537–545.

Sun, J. "Morning/Evening Menopausal Formula Relieves Menopausal Symptoms: A Pilot Study." *Journal of Alternative and Complementary Medicine* 9 (June 2003): 403–409.

Tesch, B. J. "Herbs Commonly Used by Women: An Evidence-Based Review." *American Journal of Obstetrics and Gynecology* 188 (May 2003) (Suppl 5): S44–S55.

ORGANIZATIONS

National Center for Complementary and Alternative Medicine (NCCAM) Clearinghouse. P.O. Box 7923, Gaithersburg, MD 20898-7923. (888) 644-6226. <http://nccam.nih.gov>.

U. S. Food and Drug Administration (FDA). 5600 Fishers Lane, Rockville, MD 20857. (888) 463-6332. <http://www.fda.gov>.

Clare Hanrahan
Rebecca J. Frey, PhD

Vanadium

Description

Named after the Scandinavian goddess of youth and beauty, vanadium is a trace element that has gained attention in recent years as a possible aid in controlling diabetes. While such macrominerals as **calcium** , **magnesium**, and **potassium** have become household names because they make up over 98% of the body's mineral content, certain trace minerals are also considered essential in very tiny amounts to maintain health and ensure proper functioning of the body.They usually act as coenzymes, working as a team with proteins to facilitate important chemical reactions. Even without taking vanadium supplements, people have about 20–25 micrograms (mcg) of the mineral in their bodies, which is derived from an average balanced diet. Despite the fact that vanadium has been studied for over 40 years, it is still not known for certain if the mineral is critical for optimal health. Whether taking extra amounts of vanadium is therapeutic or harmful is even more controversial. Like **chromium**, another trace mineral, vanadium has become the focus of study as a possible aid in lowering blood sugar levels in people with diabetes. Vanadium has also been touted as a potential treatment for **osteoporosis**. Some athletes and weight lifters take it to build muscle or improve performance.

Studies in animals suggest that vanadium may be necessary for the formation of bones, teeth, and cartilage. The mineral may also play a role in growth and reproduction as well as affect the processing of **cholesterol** and insulin in the body. In one animal study, goat kids whose mothers received a diet deficient in vanadium showed skeletal damage; they died within days of their birth. In studies of mice, vanadium has been shown to lower blood sugar and levels of low-density lipoprotein (LDL) cholesterol and triglyceride. It is not certain, however, that such study results as these confirm the nutritional importance of the mineral for human beings. The effects of a vanadium-free diet have not been studied in people. Even if vanadium supplements prove to be effective for certain purposes, such as helping to control diabetes, animal studies suggest that the high dosages of vanadium necessary to produce results may be harmful. High dosages are often necessary because vanadium is not well absorbed by the body. As of 2000, a significant amount of research is still required to determine if vanadium can in fact produce significant health benefits safely and effectively. The proper dosage of the mineral supplement has also yet to be determined.

General use

Vanadium has been investigated most often as a possible aid in controlling diabetes. Studies in animals with type 1 (insulin-dependent) and type 2 (non-insulin-dependent) diabetes indicate that vanadium can help to improve blood sugar levels. Studies using human subjects have produced encouraging if preliminary results. Vanadium is used by some athletes and weight lifters to build muscle despite the fact that it does not appear to be effective for this purpose. Moreover, the potential usefulness of vanadium in treating osteoporosis is considered highly speculative. All of the human studies discussed below were conducted in small numbers of people for short periods of time and involved relatively high dosages of the mineral.

Diabetes

Several studies conducted in people suggest that vanadium may help to control blood sugar levels in diabetics. The mineral appears to work by mimicking the effects of insulin or by increasing the body's sensitivity to the hormone. This mechanism could allow diabetics to effectively control their blood sugar while using lower dosages of insulin medication. In a placebo-controlled study published in 1996 in the medical journal *Metabolism*, eight people with type 2 diabetes received vanadium for one month. Researchers found that vanadium was moderately successful in lowering blood sugar levels and had few side effects. Six of the eight patients taking vanadium during the study experienced gastrointestinal side effects during the first week of treatment, but these disappeared with continued use. In another small study of vanadium involving people with type 2 diabetes, published in the *Journal of Clinical Investigation* in 1995, researchers from the Albert Einstein College of Medicine reported that three weeks of treatment with the mineral improved the body's sensitivity to insulin. The effects of vanadium in lowering blood sugar levels persisted for up to two weeks after the drug was discontinued. A study published in the journal *Diabetes* in 1996, which involved seven people with type 2 diabetes as well as six nondiabetics, reported that vanadium improved insulin sensitivity in the diabetic subjects. Interestingly, the mineral did not improve sensitivity in the subjects who did not have the disease.

Sports medicine

The use of vanadium by body builders appears to stem from a misunderstanding of the mineral's effects. Because insulin is a hormone that plays a role in increasing muscle mass, some weight lifters have taken vanadium in high dosages because they believe it will act like insulin and make them stronger. The problem is that vanadium does not appear to mimic insulin or increase its efficiency in healthy people, only in diabetics. For people considering vanadium as an aid in strengthening muscles,

the scientific evidence is not very convincing. In one double-blind, placebo-controlled study published in the *International Journal of Sport Nutrition* in 1996, high dosages of vanadium were given to a few dozen weight trainers for 12 weeks. The bench press and leg extension weight-training exercises were used to measure results. Researchers found that there was no difference in body composition between those who took vanadium and those in the placebo group. Vanadium appeared to slightly enhance performance during the leg extension aspect of the study, but this advantage can be explained by other factors and cannot be attributed to the mineral itself with any certainty.

Osteoporosis

It is important not to confuse vanadium with **calcium**. Calcium is considered an essential building block of bone, and calcium supplements are often an important part of a bone-strengthening program in women with osteoporosis. Studies in mice indicating that vanadium is also deposited in bone have led to suggestions that the mineral may be effective as a potential treatment for osteoporosis. It is known, however, that minerals can be added to bones without actually making them stronger. There is no evidence that taking vanadium supplements can increase bone density in humans.

Preparations

The estimated dosage of vanadium, which is available as an over-the-counter dietary supplement, generally ranges from 10–30 mcg a day. It is important to remember, however, that safe and effective dosages for the mineral have not yet been established. Some practitioners of complementary medicine, such as Dr. Robert Atkins, have recommended dosages as high as 25–50 mg (milligrams, not micrograms) daily for people with diabetes. The long-term health risks associated with taking dosages in this range are unknown.

Even without taking supplements, most adults get anywhere between 10–60 mcg of vanadium through a normal diet. Some authorities believe it is safer for people to avoid vanadium supplements altogether and increase their intake of foods known to contain the mineral. These include meat, seafood, whole grains, vegetable oil, canned fruit juices, soy products, and such vegetables as green beans, corn, carrots, and cabbage. Alcoholic beverages such as wine and beer also contain vanadium. Overdosing on the vanadium contained in food is not considered a significant risk because the mineral is present only in very small amounts in plants and animals.

Precautions

It is important not to exceed the recommended intake of vanadium without medical supervision. Studies

KEY TERMS

Diabetes—A disease in which the body either cannot produce adequate amounts of insulin (type 1) or properly metabolize the hormone (type 2).

Insulin—A hormone produced by the pancreas that helps to regulate blood sugar levels.

Osteoporosis—An age-related disease in which bones become fragile and prone to debilitating fractures.

Placebo—A sugar pill or inactive agent often used in the control group of a medical study.

Triglyceride—A term referring to the total amount of fat in the blood. Triglyceride should not be confused with cholesterol, which is technically classified as a steroid and not as a fat.

conducted in rats suggest that high dosages of vanadium can be harmful. This results from the fact that the mineral tends to build up in the body, reaching dangerously high levels when taken in excess. The reader should keep in mind that high dosages of vanadium have not yet been proven to have significant health benefits. The long-term health risks associated with taking vanadium supplements (in any dosage) are unknown.

Side effects

When taken in recommended dosages, vanadium has not been associated with any significant or bothersome side effects. At high dosages, vanadium has been known to cause stomach cramping and **diarrhea** as well as a green tongue.

Interactions

No drugs are known to interact adversely with vanadium. Smokers may absorb less of the mineral.

Resources

BOOKS

Atkins, Robert C. *Dr. Atkins' Vita-Nutrient Solution.* New York: Simon & Schuster, 1998.

Miller, Lucinda G., and Wallace J. Murray. *Herbal Medicinals: A Clinician's Guide.* New York: Pharmaceutical Products Press, 1998.

Sifton, David W. *PDR Family Guide to Natural Medicines and Healing Therapies.* New York: Three Rivers Press, 1999.

ORGANIZATIONS

Herb Research Foundation. 1007 Pearl Street, Suite 200. Boulder, CO 80302.

National Diabetes Information Clearinghouse. 1 Information Way. Bethesda, MD 20892-3560.

OTHER

Discovery Health. http://www.discoveryhealth.com.

National Institute of Diabetes and Digestive and Kidney Diseases. http://www.niddk.nih.gov.

Greg Annussek

Varicella *see* **Chickenpox**

Varicose veins

Definition

Varicose veins are dilated, tortuous, elongated superficial veins that appear most often in the legs.

Description

Varicose veins, also called varicosities, are seen most often in the legs, although they can be found in other parts of the body. Most often, they appear as lumpy, winding vessels just below the surface of the skin. There are three types of veins: superficial veins that are just beneath the surface of the skin; deep veins that are large blood vessels found deep inside the muscles; and perforator veins that connect the superficial veins to the deep veins. The superficial veins are the blood vessels most often affected by this condition and are the veins that are visible when the varicose condition has developed.

The inside walls of veins have valves that open and close in response to the blood flow. When the left ventricle of the heart pushes blood out into the aorta, it produces the high pressure pulse of the heartbeat and pushes blood throughout the body. Between heartbeats, there is a period of low blood pressure. During this period blood in the veins is affected by gravity and wants to flow downward. The valves in the veins prevent this from happening. Varicose veins start when one or more valves fail to close. The blood pressure in that section of vein increases, causing additional valves to fail. This allows blood to pool and stretch the veins, further weakening the walls of the veins. The walls of the affected veins lose their elasticity in response to increased blood pressure. As the vessels weaken, more and more valves are unable to close properly. The veins become larger and wider over time and begin to appear as lumpy, winding chains underneath the skin. Varicosities can also develop in the deep veins. Varicose veins in the superficial veins are called primary varicosities, while varicose veins in the deep veins are called secondary varicosities.

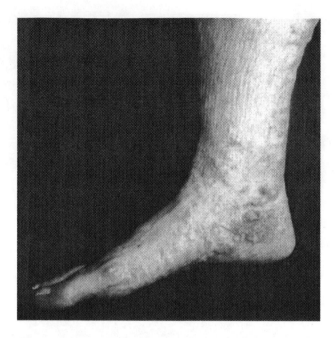

Varicose veins on a man's leg. *(Photograph by Keith, Custom Medical Stock Photo. Reproduced by permission.)*

Causes & symptoms

Varicose veins have a number of different causes; lifestyle and hormonal factors play a role. Some families seem to have a higher incidence of varicose veins, indicating that there may be a genetic component to this disease. Varicose veins are progressive; as one section of a vein weakens, it causes increased pressure on adjacent sections of the vein. These sections often develop varicosities. Varicose veins can appear following **pregnancy**, thrombophlebitis, congenital blood vessel weakness, or **obesity**, but they are not limited to these conditions. **Edema** of the surrounding tissue, ankles, and calves is not usually a complication of primary (superficial) varicose veins. When edema develops, it usually indicates that the deep veins may have varicosities or clots.

Varicose veins are a common problem. More than 80 million Americans experience the symptoms and complications of varicose veins, including 10%–15% of men and 20%–25% of women. The symptoms can include aching, **pain**, itchiness, or burning sensations, especially when standing. In some cases, with chronically bad veins, there may be a brownish discoloration of the skin or ulcers (open sores) near the ankles. A condition that is frequently associated with varicose veins is spider-burst veins. Spider-burst veins are very small veins that are enlarged. They may be caused by back-pressure from varicose veins, but can be caused by other factors. They are frequently associated with pregnancy and there may be hormonal factors associated with their develop-

ment. They are primarily of cosmetic concern and do not present any medical concerns.

Diagnosis

Varicose veins can usually be seen. In cases where varicose veins are suspected, a physician may frequently detect them by palpation (pressing with the fingers). The physician will examine the veins while the patient is first in a standing position and a second time while the patient is lying down. X rays or ultrasound tests can detect varicose veins in the deep and perforator veins and rule out **blood clots** in the deep veins. A handheld Doppler instrument is now the preferred diagnostic tool for evaluating the leg veins.

Treatment

There is no cure for varicose veins. Treatment falls into two classes: relief of symptoms and removal of the affected veins. Symptom relief includes such measures as wearing support stockings, which compress the veins and hold them in place. This pressure keeps the veins from stretching and limits pain. Other measures include sitting down, using a footstool to support the feet when sitting, avoid standing for long periods of time, and raising the legs whenever possible. These measures work by reducing the blood pressure in leg veins. Prolonged standing allows the blood to collect under high pressure in the varicose veins. **Exercise** such as walking, biking, and swimming, is beneficial. When the legs are active, the leg muscles help pump the blood in the veins. This limits the amount of blood that collects in the varicose veins and reduces some of the symptoms but does not stop the disease.

Herbal therapy can be helpful in the treatment of varicose veins. **Essential oils** of cypress and geranium or extracts from **horse chestnut** seeds (*Aesculus hippocastanum*) are massaged into the legs, stroking upwards toward the heart. Application to broken skin and massage directly on the varicose veins should be avoided. Horse chestnut may also be taken orally and biothavenoids are used to increase vascular stability. In late 2001 a new product derived from aescinate, a chemical found in horse chestnut, was approved by the Food and Drug Administration (FDA) for topical use in the treatment of varicose and spider veins. The new product, sold under the name of Essaven gel, reduces edema. It can be applied underneath support hosiery if desired.

Drinking fresh fruit juices, particularly those of dark colored berries (cherries, blackberries, and blueberries) can help tone and strengthen the vein walls. The enzyme **bromelain**, found in pineapple juice, can aid in the prevention of blood clots associated with the pooling of blood in the legs.

Deep breathing exercises performed while lying down with the legs elevated can assist gravity in circulating blood from the legs. The flow of fresh blood into the legs can help relieve any pain.

Allopathic treatment

Surgery can be used to remove varicose veins from the body. It is recommended for varicose veins that are causing pain or are very unsightly, and when hemorrhaging or recurrent thrombosis appear. Surgery involves making an incision through the skin at both ends of the section of vein being removed. A flexible wire is inserted through one end and extended to the other. The wire is then withdrawn, pulling the vein out with it. This is called "stripping" and is the most common method to remove superficial varicose veins. As long as the deeper veins are still functioning properly, a person can live without some of the superficial veins. Because of this, stripped varicose veins are not replaced.

Injection therapy is an alternate therapy used to seal varicose veins. This prevents blood from entering the sealed sections of the vein. The veins remain in the body, but no longer carry blood. This procedure can be performed on an out-patient basis and does not require anesthesia. It is frequently used if people develop more varicose veins after surgery to remove the larger varicose veins and to seal spider-burst veins for people concerned about cosmetic appearance. Injection therapy is also called sclerotherapy. At one time, a method of injection therapy was used that did not have a good success rate. Veins did not seal properly and blood clots formed. Modern injection therapy is improved and has a much higher success rate.

Two new allopathic treatments have been developed since 1999 that are much less invasive than stripping the veins. One is called radio frequency closure, or the closure technique. In radio frequency closure, the surgeon inserts a catheter into the varicose vein through a small puncture. The catheter is used to deliver radio frequency energy to the wall of the vein, which causes the vein to contract and seal itself shut. The nearby veins then take over the flow of venous blood from the legs.

The second new treatment is called the endovascular laser procedure. The doctor uses a diode laser wire or fiber that is inserted directly into the vein. Energy transmitted from a laser heats the varicose vein and seals it shut. The patient can go back to work the next day, although a support stocking must be worn for two weeks after the laser procedure.

Expected results

Untreated varicose veins become increasingly large and more obvious with time. Surgical stripping of vari-

KEY TERMS

Aescinate—A chemical found in horse chestnut that is effective in relieving the tissue swelling associated with varicose veins.

Congenital—Existing at or before birth; a condition that developed while the fetus was in utero or as a consequence of the birth process.

Edema—Swelling caused by the collection of fluid in a tissue or body cavity.

Hemorrhage—Rapid high-volume loss of blood.

Palpation—A diagnostic technique in which the examiner gently presses, or palpates, a specific area of the patient's body. Palpation is used in the diagnosis of varicose veins.

Topical—A form of medication that is applied to the external surface of the affected part of the body.

cose veins is successful for most patients. Most do not develop new, large varicose veins following surgery. Surgery does not decrease a person's tendency to develop varicose veins. Varicose veins may develop in other locations after stripping.

Prevention

While genetic factors play a significant role in the development of varicose veins, swimming and other exercises to increase circulation in the legs help to prevent varicose veins. Preventive measures are especially important during pregnancy, when the additional weight of the fetus and placenta can exert pressure on the mother's legs and feet.

Resources

BOOKS

Alexander, R.W., R. C. Schlant, and V. Fuster, eds. *The Heart,* 9th ed. New York: McGraw-Hill, 1998.

Berkow, Robert, ed. *Merck Manual of Medical Information.* Whitehouse Station, NJ: Merck Research Laboratories, 1997.

Larsen, D.E., ed. *Mayo Clinic Family Health Book.* New York: William Morrow and Company, Inc., 1996.

PERIODICALS

Altizer, James W. "Varicose Veins: A Primary Care Update." *Patient Care* 35 (October 30, 2001): 33.

Belcaro, G., A. N. Nicolaides, G. Geroulakis, et al. "Essaven Gel: Review of Experimental and Clinical Data." *Angiology* 52 (December 2001): S1-S4.

"New Noninvasive Procedures Treat Leg Veins Problems." *Medical Devices & Surgical Technology Week* (December 9, 2001): 16.

Kathleen D. Wright
Rebecca J. Frey, PhD

Veganism

Definition

Veganism is a system of dietary and lifestyle practices that seeks to promote health and peace while reducing the suffering of both people and animals. Vegans (pronounced vee-guns) are vegetarians who do not eat any foods (eggs, dairy products, meat, etc.) derived from animal sources. Most vegans also do not use products that require for their production the death or suffering of animals, such as leather, fur, wool, and certain cosmetics.

Origins

The word "vegetarian" was coined in England in 1847 by the founders of the Vegetarian Society of Great Britain. "Vegetarian" has been used to describe people who do not eat meat, but do consume dairy products and eggs. The Vegan Society was founded in England in 1944 by Donald Watson and others who believed that vegetarians should strive to exist without eating or using any animal products at all. Watson stated that the crisis of World War II may have been a motivation behind his founding of the Vegan Society, because he saw so much turmoil and suffering in the world around him. The Vegan founders believed that the first step to creating a better world would be to develop a diet that did not cause the death or suffering of any living beings. The term "vegan" is derived from the Latin word *vegetus*, which means "full of life," which the founders hoped their system would be. "Vegan" also starts with the same three letters as "vegetarian," and ends with the last two, as its founders believed they were starting with vegetarian ideas and taking them to their logical conclusion.

The American Vegan Society (AVS) was founded in 1960 by Jay Dinshah. The same year, the AVS began to publish a journal called *Ahimsa*, which is a Sanskrit word that means "not causing harm" and "reverence for life." Dinshah and others conceived veganism to be a philosophy of living that has nonviolence, peace, harmony, honesty, service to the world, and knowledge as its goals. In 1974, the AVS became affiliated with the North American Vegetarian Society, which was formed to bring together all of the vegetarian groups in North America.

Since the 1970s, there has been a vast amount of research concerning **nutrition** and diet. It has been discovered that **diets** that are centered around meat and dairy products, such as the typical American diet, are high in **cholesterol** and saturated fat but low in fiber. These diets have been linked to many health problems, including **heart disease**, strokes, and diabetes, which together cause 68% of all the deaths in the United States. Thus, the interest in diets that reduce or eliminate foods that contribute to these conditions has grown considerably. In 1992, the *Vegetarian Times* magazine took a poll that estimated that 13 million Americans, or 5% of the population, consider themselves vegetarian. Of the vegetarians, 4% are vegans, which amounts to nearly 520,000 Americans.

Benefits

Vegan diets are often recommended as dietary therapy for heart disease, high cholesterol, diabetes, strokes, **cancer**, **obesity**, arthritis, **allergies**, **asthma**, environmental illness, **hypertension**, **gout**, **gallstones**, **kidney stones**, ulcers, colitis, digestive disorders, **premenstrual syndrome**, **anxiety**, and **depression**. At present, however, no studies exist that define the efficacy of vegan diets in treating these conditions. Nevertheless, a well-designed vegan diet is an effective weight-loss diet, and is an economical and easy preventive health practice.

Description

Veganism can be better understood by considering the ethical, ecological, and health reasons that motivate vegans.

Ethical considerations

A vegan lifestyle seeks to promote awareness, compassion, and peace. Veganism is an ethical system as well as a diet. Ethics refers to rules of conduct or the ways in which people interact with others and the world. One poll in England showed that 83% of vegans listed ethical reasons as their main consideration in their practices. Vegans believe that health encompasses not only individuals' bodies, but also includes healthy relationships between people and their actions towards other living things, the earth, and the environment. Vegans believe that as long as animals are treated cruelly and are killed for meat, then the world's ethical and spiritual health will suffer. Vegans believe that people should become aware of how their food choices are creating suffering and affecting the health of the world as a whole. For instance, it has been estimated that the grain that goes to feed livestock in America could feed 1.3 billion people, which would relieve a large measure of the **pain** and suffering in the world.

Vegans claim that egg and dairy production may cause animals just as much suffering as killing them for meat, because modern factory farming treats animals as unfeeling machines instead of as living beings. Eggs are produced by keeping chickens in small cages and in painful and unsanitary conditions. Vegans claim that dairy cattle are subjected to cruel treatment as well, being bred artificially and caged for much of their lives. Dairy cattle are also injected with hormones that make them produce unnaturally high quantities of milk while weakening their immune systems and making them sick and unhealthy. Large amounts of antibiotics need to be used on weakened cows, which in turn affects the health of humans and creates diseases that are resistant to medicine. Dairy farming causes death to cows as well because undesirable or old cows are slaughtered for meat.

Other animal products are avoided by vegans as well. Leather, wool, and fur are not used because they result in the suffering of animals from their production. Some vegans do not use honey because they believe that the collection of honey is harmful to bees. Many vegans avoid using sugar, because some sugar is made by using charcoal made from the bones of dead cattle. Vegans also do not use products that have been tested on animals, and vegans are active in resisting the use of animals for dissection and medical experiments. Vegans are typically outspoken against hunting and the cruel treatment of animals in zoos or for entertainment (e.g., cockfighting and bullfighting).

Helping the Earth

Vegans believe that their dietary and lifestyle practices would contribute to a healthier world ecology. Vegans can cite many statistics that show that the American meat-centered diet is contributing to environmental problems. The main thrust of vegans' ecological position is that it takes many more resources to produce meat than it does to provide a grain-based diet, and people can be fed better with grain than with meat. For instance, it takes 10 lbs (4.5 kg) of grain to make 1 lb (0.45 kg) of beef. On one acre of land, 20,000 lbs (9,000 kg) of potatoes can be grown compared to 125 lbs (57 kg) of beef during the same time. In America, livestock consume six and a half times as much grain as the entire population. Different dietary habits here could improve the world, vegans argue. Environmental problems caused by the inefficient production of livestock include topsoil loss, water shortages and contamination, deforestation, toxic waste, and air pollution.

Health considerations

People who eat vegetarian diets are at lower risk for many conditions, including heart disease, certain can-

cers, diabetes, obesity, high blood pressure, gallstones, and kidney stones. A vegan diet contains no cholesterol, because cholesterol is found only in animal products. Diets high in cholesterol and saturated fat are responsible for heart disease. American men overall have a 50% risk of having a **heart attack**, while vegans have only a 4% risk. Vegans consume as much as four times the amount of fiber as the average person, and high fiber intake is believed to reduce the risk of heart disease, diabetes, cancer, and digestive tract problems. Vegan diets are also high in protective nutrients that are found in fruits and vegetables, such as **antioxidants**.

A vegan diet can also reduce exposure to chemicals that are found in meat and dairy products, such as pesticides and synthetic additives such as hormones. Chemicals tend to accumulate in the tissue of animals that are higher in the food chain, a process called bioaccumulation. By not eating animal products, vegans can avoid the exposure to these accumulated toxins, many of which are believed to influence the development of cancer. It is important, however, for vegans to eat organically produced vegetables and grains, as vegans who eat nonorganic food get high doses of pesticides. One study showed that DDT, a cancer-causing pesticide, was present in significant levels in mother's milk for 99% of American women, but only 8% of vegetarian women had significant levels of the pesticide. The risks of women getting **breast cancer** and men contracting **prostate cancer** are nearly four times as high for frequent meat eaters as for those who eat meat sparingly or not at all. High consumption of dairy products has been linked to diabetes, **anemia**, **cataracts**, and other conditions.

Vegan diets may also be beneficial for those with allergic or autoimmune disorders such as asthma, allergies, and **rheumatoid arthritis**. Animal products cause allergic reactions in many people, and studies have shown that allergic responses and inflammation may be improved by eliminating animal products from the diet. Furthermore, vegan diets are effective weight loss diets, because the high levels of fiber and low levels of fat make it possible for dieters to eat until they are full and still take in lower calories than other diets.

Preparations

Those considering veganism may wish to adopt the diet gradually to allow their bodies and lifestyles time to adjust to different eating habits. Some nutritionists have recommended "transition" diets to help people change from a meat-centered diet in stages. Many Americans eat meat products at nearly every meal, and the first stage of a transition diet is to substitute just a few meals a week with wholly vegetarian foods. Then, particular meat products can be slowly reduced and eliminated from the diet and replaced with vegetarian foods. Red meat can be reduced and then eliminated, followed by poultry and fish. For vegans, the final step would be to substitute eggs and dairy products with other nutrient-rich foods. Individuals should be willing to experiment with transition diets, and be patient when learning how combine veganism with such social activities as dining out.

Vegans should become informed on healthful dietary and nutrition practices as well. Sound nutritional guidelines include decreasing the intake of fat, increasing fiber, and emphasizing fresh fruits, vegetables, legumes, and whole grains in the diet while avoiding processed foods and sugar. Vegans can experiment with meat substitutes, foods that are high in protein and essential nutrients. Tofu and tempeh are soybean products that are high in protein, **calcium**, and other nutrients. There are "veggie-burgers" that can be grilled like hamburgers, and vegan substitutes for turkey and sausage with surprisingly realistic textures and taste. Furthermore, there are many vegan cookbooks on the market, as cooking without meat or dairy products can be challenging for some people.

Vegans should also become familiar with food labels and food additives, because there are many additives derived from animal sources that are used in common foods and in such household items as soap. Vegans may also find social support at local health food stores or food cooperatives.

Precautions

Vegans should be aware of particular nutrients that may be lacking or need special attention in non-animal diets. These include protein, **vitamin B$_{12}$**, **riboflavin**, **vitamin D**, calcium, **iron**, **zinc**, and **essential fatty acids**. Furthermore, pregnant women, growing children, and people with certain health conditions have higher requirements for these nutrients.

Vegans should be sure to get complete proteins in their diets. A complete protein contains all of the essential **amino acids**, which are essential because the body cannot make them. Meat and dairy products generally contain complete proteins, but most vegetarian foods such as grains and legumes contain incomplete proteins since they lack one or more of the essential amino acids. Vegans can easily obtain complete proteins by combining particular foods. For instance, beans are high in the amino acid **lysine** but low in tryptophan and **methionine**. Rice is low in lysine and high in tryptophan and methionine. Thus, a combination of rice and beans makes a complete protein. In general, combining legumes such as soy, lentils, beans, and peas with grains like rice, wheat, or oats forms complete proteins. Nuts or peanut butter with grains such as whole wheat bread also forms complete proteins. Proteins do not necessarily need to be combined in the same meal, but should generally be combined over a period of a few days.

Getting enough vitamin B$_{12}$ is an issue for vegans because meat and dairy products are its main sources. Vegans are advised to take vitamin supplements containing B$_{12}$. **Spirulina**, a nutritional supplement made from algae, is used as a vegetarian source of this vitamin, as are fortified soy products and nutritional yeast. The symptoms of vitamin B$_{12}$ deficiency include muscle twitching and irreversible nerve damage; weakness; numbness and tingling in the extremities; and a sore tongue.

Riboflavin (vitamin B$_2$) is also generally found in high amounts in animal sources, so vegans should be aware of this fact and take a supplement if necessary. Vegetable sources of riboflavin include **brewer's yeast**, almonds, mushrooms, whole grains, soybeans, and green leafy vegetables.

Vitamin D can be obtained from vitamin supplements, fortified foods, and sunshine. Calcium can be obtained from enriched tofu, seeds, nuts, legumes, and dark green vegetables, including broccoli, kale, spinach, and collard greens. Iron is found in raisins, figs, legumes, tofu, whole grains (particularly whole wheat), potatoes, and dark green leafy vegetables, and by cooking with iron skillets. Iron is absorbed more efficiently by the body when iron-containing foods are eaten with foods that contain **vitamin C**, such as fruits, tomatoes, and green vegetables. Zinc is abundant in nuts, pumpkin seeds, legumes, whole grains, and tofu. Getting enough omega-3 essential fatty acids may be an issue for vegans. These are found in walnuts, canola oil, and such supplements as **flaxseed** oil. Vegans should consider purchasing organically grown food when possible, to avoid exposure to pesticides and to contribute to sound agricultural practices.

Research & general acceptance

Scientists have analyzed **vegetarianism** more frequently, mainly because there are higher numbers of lacto-ovo vegetarians around the world than there are vegans. Studies have repeatedly shown many benefits of plant-based diets.

A significant study of veganism was published in 1985 in the *Journal of Asthma*, which used a vegan diet to treat asthma. After one year, 92% of patients exhibited significant improvement in asthma symptoms and in such measurements as lung capacity and cholesterol levels. People on the diet also experienced fewer episodes of colds and **influenza**. Researchers concluded that the vegan diet was helpful for asthma because it reduced

KEY TERMS

. . . .

Bioaccumulation—The process in which toxic chemicals collect in the tissues of humans and other animals toward the top of the food chain.

Cholesterol—A steroid fat found in animal foods that is also produced in the body from saturated fat for several important functions. Excess cholesterol intake is linked to many diseases.

Complex carbohydrates—Carbohydrates that are broken down by the body into simple sugars for energy. They are found in grains, fruits and vegetables. Complex carbohydrates are generally recommended by nutritionists over refined sugar and honey, because they are a better source of energy and often contain fiber and nutrients as well.

Legume—A group of plant foods that includes beans, peas, and lentils. Legumes are high in protein, fiber, and other nutrients.

Organic food—Food grown without the use of synthetic pesticides and fertilizers.

Saturated fat—A fat that is usually solid at room temperature. Saturated fats are found mainly in meat and dairy products but also in such vegetable sources as some nuts, seeds, and avocados.

Unsaturated fat—A type of fat found in plant foods that is typically liquid at room temperature. Unsaturated fats can be monounsaturated or polyunsaturated, depending on their chemical structure. They are the most frequently recommended dietary fats.

food allergies, which are commonly caused by animal products. Scientists theorized that the animal-free diet also may have altered the patients' prostaglandin levels. Prostaglandins are hormone-like substances responsible for many body processes including allergic reactions. Finally, researchers proposed that the high quantity of antioxidants and plant nutrients in the vegan diet may have contributed to strengthened immune systems.

Resources

BOOKS

Barnard, Neal, M.D. *Food For Life.* New York: Harmony, 1993.
Stepaniak, Joanne. *The Vegan Sourcebook.* Los Angeles: Lowell House, 1998.

PERIODICALS

Ahimsa. American Vegan Society (AVS). 56 Dinshah Lane. PO Box H. Malaga, NY 08328. (609) 694-2887.

Vegetarian Journal. Vegetarian Resource Group (VRG). PO Box 1463. Baltimore, MD 21203.

ORGANIZATIONS

Vegan Outreach. 211 Indian Drive. Pittsburgh, PA 15238. (412) 968-0268.

Douglas Dupler

Vegetarianism

Definition

Vegetarianism refers to voluntary abstinence from eating meat. Vegetarians refrain from eating meat for various reasons, including religious, health, and ethical ones. Lacto-ovo vegetarians supplement their diet with dairy (lactose) products and eggs (ovo). Vegans (pronounced vee-guns) do not eat any animal-derived products at all.

Origins

The term vegetarian was coined in 1847 by the founders of the Vegetarian Society of Great Britain, but vegetarianism has been around as long as people have created **diets**. Some of the world's oldest cultures advocate a vegetarian diet for health and religious purposes. In India, millions of Hindus are vegetarians because of their religious beliefs. One of the ancient mythological works of Hinduism, the *Mahabharata*, states that, "Those who desire to possess good memory, beauty, long life with perfect health, and physical, moral and spiritual strength, should abstain from animal foods." The **yoga** system of living and health is vegetarian, because its dietary practices are based on the belief that healthy food contains *prana*. Prana is the universal life energy, which yoga experts believe is abundant in fresh fruits, grains, nuts and vegetables, but absent in meat because meat has been killed. Yogis also believe that spiritual health in influenced by the practice of *ahimsa*, or not harming living beings. The principle of *ahimsa* (non-violence) appears in the Upanishads (Vedic literature) from c. 600–300 B.C. Taking of animal life or human life under any circumstances is sinful and results in rebirth as a lower organism. It became a fundamental element of Jainism, another religion of India. Some Buddhists in Japan and China are also vegetarian because of spiritual beliefs. In the Christian tradition, the Trappist Monks of the Catholic Church are vegetarian, and some vegetarians argue that there is evidence that Jesus and his early followers were vegetarian. Other traditional cultures,

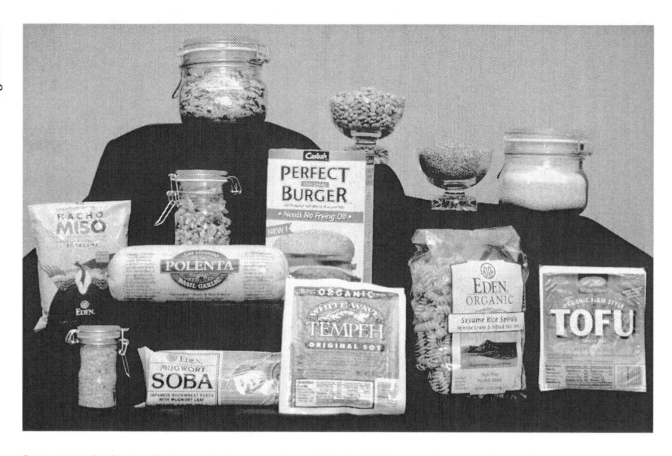

Some vegetarian foods. *(Photograph by Robert J. Huffman. Field Mark Publications. Reproduced by permission.)*

such as those in the Middle East and the Mediterranean regions, have evolved diets that frequently consist of vegetarian foods. The **Mediterranean diet**, which a Harvard study declared to be one of the world's healthiest, is primarily, although not strictly, vegetarian.

The list of famous vegetarians forms an illustrious group. The ancient Greek philosophers, including Socrates, Plato, and Pythagoras, advocated vegetarianism. In modern times, the word to describe someone who likes to feast on food and wine is "epicure," but it is little known that Epicurus, the ancient philosopher, was himself a diligent vegetarian. Other famous vegetarians include Leonardo da Vinci, Sir Isaac Newton, Leo Tolstoy, Ralph Waldo Emerson, and Henry Thoreau. This century's celebrated vegetarians include Gandhi, the physician Albert Schweitzer, writer George Bernard Shaw, musician Paul McCartney, and champion triathlete Dave Scott. Albert Einstein, although not a strict vegetarian himself, stated that a vegetarian diet would be an evolutionary step for the human race.

Vegetarianism in America received a lot of interest during the last half of the nineteenth century and the beginning of the twentieth century, during periods of experimentation with diets and health practices. Vegetari-

anism has also been a religious practice for some Americans, including the Seventh-day Adventists, whose lacto-ovo vegetarian diets have been studied for their health benefits. Vegetarianism has been steadily gaining acceptance as an alternative to the meat-and-potatoes bias of the traditional American diet. In 1992, *Vegetarian Times* magazine performed a poll that showed that 13 million Americans, or 5% of the population, identified themselves as vegetarians.

Several factors contribute to the interest in vegetarianism in America. Outbreaks of **food poisoning** from meat products, as well as increased concern over the additives in meat such as hormones and antibiotics, have led some people and professionals to question meat's safety. There is also an increased awareness of the questionable treatment of farm animals in factory farming. But the growing health consciousness of Americans is probably the major reason for the surge in interest in vegetarianism. **Nutrition** experts have built up convincing evidence that there are major problems with the conventional American diet, which is centered around meat products that are high in **cholesterol** and saturated fat and low in fiber. **Heart disease, cancer**, and diabetes, which cause 68% of all deaths in America, are all be-

DR. JOHN HARVEY KELLOGG 1852–1943

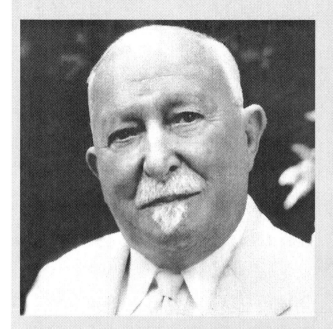

(AP/Wide World Photos. Reproduced by permission.)

John Harvey Kellogg is known as the father of modern breakfast cereal. He was born in Tyrone Township, Michigan, on February 26, 1852, into a Seventh Day Adventist family. At age 12, he became an apprentice at the Review and Herald Press, a publishing company run by the church. He attended school in Battle Creek, Michigan. He attended Bellevue Hospital Medical College in New York where he received his medical degree in 1875. In 1876, at the age of 24, Kellogg became an abdominal surgeon and superintendent of the Western Health Reform Institute, which he renamed the Battle Creek Sanitarium. There, he began applying his theories about natural living to his medical practice. Himself a vegetarian, he first advocated a diet high in whole grains, fruits, nuts, and legumes. He later included all types of vegetables in the diet. His controversial health regimen included morning calisthenics, open-air sleeping, cleansing enemas, chewing food hundreds of times before swallowing, and drinking plenty of water.

In the 1890s, Kellogg established a laboratory at the sanitarium to develop more nutritious foods. His brother, Will Keith Kellogg, joined in his research. In 1895 they developed a breakfast cereal of wheat flakes called Granose. The cereal quickly grew in popularity and was soon sold by mail order. This was followed by rice flakes and corn flakes. The brothers established the Sanitas Food Company. But philosophical differences led them to split into two companies. Will founded the W. K. Kellogg Company, which retained the rights to the cereal products. John set up the Battle Creek Food Company, which produced coffee substitutes and soymilk. John Kellogg also edited *Good Health Magazine*, which promoted vegetarianism, for 60 years. In 1904, he published a book, *The Miricle of Life*. He continued to promote his version of healthy living and radical techniques until his death in 1943.

Ken R. Wells

lieved to be influenced by this diet. Nutritionists have repeatedly shown in studies that a healthy diet consists of plenty of fresh vegetables and fruits, complex carbohydrates such as whole grains, and foods that are high in fiber and low in cholesterol and saturated fat. Vegetarianism, a diet that fulfills all these criteria, has become part of many healthy lifestyles. In alternative medicine, vegetarianism is a cornerstone dietary therapy, used in **Ayurvedic medicine**, **detoxification** treatments, macrobiotics, the **Ornish diet** for heart disease, and in therapies for many chronic conditions.

Benefits

Vegetarianism is recommended as a dietary therapy for a variety of conditions, including heart disease, high cholesterol, type 2 diabetes, and **stroke**. Vegetarianism is a major dietary therapy in the alternative treatment of cancer. Other conditions treated with a dietary therapy of vegetarianism include **obesity**, **osteoporosis**, arthritis, **aller-**gies, **asthma**, environmental illness, **hypertension**, **gout**, **gallstones**, **hemorrhoids**, **kidney stones**, ulcers, colitis, **premenstrual syndrome**, **anxiety**, and **depression**. Vegetarians often report higher energy levels, better digestion, and mental clarity. Vegetarianism is an economical and easily implemented preventative practice as well.

Preparations

Some people, particularly those with such severe or chronic conditions as heart disease or cancer, may be advised by a health practitioner to become vegetarian suddenly. For most people, nutritionists recommend that a vegetarian diet be adopted gradually, to allow people's bodies and lifestyles time to adjust to new eating habits and food intake.

Some nutritionists have designed transition diets to help people become vegetarian in stages. Many Americans eat meat products at nearly every meal, and the first stage of a transition diet is to substitute just a few meals a week with wholly vegetarian foods. Then, particular meat products can be slowly reduced and eliminated from the diet and replaced with vegetarian foods. Red meat can be reduced and then eliminated, followed by pork, poultry, and fish. For those wishing to become strict vegetarians or vegans, the final step would be to substitute eggs and dairy products with other nutrient-rich foods. Individuals should be willing to experiment with transition diets, and should have patience when learning how to combine vegetarianism with such social activities as dining out. Fortunately, the number of restaurants that offer vegetarian dishes, or even all-vegetarian menus, is growing in the United States, particularly along the West Coast.

The transition to vegetarianism can be smoother for those who make informed choices with dietary practices. Sound nutritional guidelines include decreasing the intake of fat, increasing fiber, and emphasizing fresh fruits, vegetables, legumes, and whole grains in the diet while avoiding processed foods and sugar. Everyone can improve their health by becoming familiar with recommended dietary and nutritional practices, such as reading labels and understanding such basic nutritional concepts as daily requirements for calories, protein, fat, and nutrients. Would-be vegetarians can experiment with meat substitutes, foods that are high in protein and essential nutrients. Thanks to the growing interest in vegetarianism, many meat substitutes are now readily available. Tofu and tempeh are products made from soybeans that are high in protein, **calcium**, and other nutrients. There are "veggie-burgers" that can be grilled like hamburgers, and vegetarian substitutes for turkey and sausage with surprisingly authentic textures and taste. There are many vegetarian cookbooks on the market as well.

A set of guidelines for North American vegetarian diets, updated for 2004, is available from the American Dietetic Association and the Dietitians of Canada. The new guidelines are intended to promote variety within vegetarian diets and to meet the needs of different stages in the life cycle as well as incorporate the most recent findings of medical research.

One remaining drawback to the widespread practice of vegetarianism is the unpleasant taste or smell of many vegetables. A number of phytonutrients have a bitter, astringent, or acrid taste that they impart to products made from vegetables that contain them. Some experts think that people tend to reject such strong-smelling or bitter-tasting vegetables as turnips, cabbage, brussels sprouts, or broccoli because humans have been programmed in the course of evolution to associate bitter taste with poisonous plants. It is increasingly recognized that the major barrier to dietary change for the sake of health is

taste. One recommendation for improving the taste appeal of vegetarian diets is more frequent use of spices. In addition to pleasing the human palate, spices derived from plants have been shown to have chemoprotective effects, boosting the immune system, reducing inflammation, and fighting harmful bacteria and viruses.

Precautions

In general, a well-planned vegetarian diet is healthful and safe; in the summer of 2003, a position paper endorsed by the American Dietetic Association and the Dietitians of Canada referred to vegetarian diets as "healthful, nutritionally adequate, and [able to] provide health benefits in the prevention and treatment of certain diseases." However, vegetarians, and particularly vegans who eat no animal products, should be aware of particular nutrients that may be lacking in non-animal diets. These are **amino acids**, **vitamin B$_{12}$**, **vitamin D**, calcium, **iron**, **zinc**, and **essential fatty acids**. Furthermore, pregnant women, growing children, and those with health conditions have higher requirements for these nutrients.

Vegetarians should be aware of getting *complete protein* in their diets. A complete protein contains all of the essential amino acids, which are the building blocks for protein essential to the diet because the body cannot make them. Meat and dairy products generally contain complete proteins, but most vegetarian foods such as grains and legumes contain incomplete proteins, lacking one or more of the essential amino acids. However, vegetarians can easily overcome this by combining particular foods in order to create complete proteins. For instance, beans are high in the amino acid **lysine** but low in tryptophan and **methionine**, but rice is low in lysine and high in tryptophan and methionine. Thus, combining rice and beans makes a complete protein. In general, combining legumes such as soy, lentils, beans, and peas with grains like rice, wheat, or oats forms complete proteins. Eating dairy products or nuts with grains also makes proteins complete. Oatmeal with milk on it is complete, as is peanut butter on whole wheat bread. Proteins do not necessarily need to be combined in the same meal, but generally within four hours.

Getting enough vitamin B$_{12}$ may be an issue for some vegetarians, particularly vegans, because meat and dairy products are the main sources. Vitamin supplements that contain vitamin B$_{12}$ are recommended, particularly for older vegetarians. **Spirulina**, a nutritional supplement made from algae, is also a vegetarian source, as are fortified soy products and nutritional yeast.

Vitamin D can be obtained by vitamins, fortified foods, and sunshine. Calcium can be obtained in enriched tofu, seeds, nuts, legumes, dairy products, and dark green vegetables including broccoli, kale, spinach, and collard greens. Iron is found in raisins, figs, legumes, tofu, whole grains (particularly whole wheat), potatoes, and dark green leafy vegetables. Iron is absorbed more efficiently by the body when iron-containing foods are eaten with foods that contain **vitamin C**, such as fruits, tomatoes, and green vegetables. Zinc is abundant in nuts, pumpkin seeds, legumes, whole grains, and tofu. For vegetarians who don't eat fish, getting enough omega-3 essential fatty acids may be an issue, and supplements such as **flaxseed** oil should be considered, as well as eating walnuts and canola oil.

Vegetarians do not necessarily have healthier diets. Some studies have shown that some vegetarians consume large amounts of cholesterol and saturated fat. Eggs and dairy products contain cholesterol and saturated fat, while nuts, oils, and avocados are vegetable sources of saturated fat. To reap the full benefits of a vegetarian diet, vegetarians should be conscious of cholesterol and saturated fat intake. Vegetarians may also consider buying organic foods, which are grown without the use of synthetic chemicals, as another health precaution. Lastly, consuming large quantities of vegetables without other carbohydrates and sources of protein can produce its own kind of dietary imbalance. Cases have been reported of carotenemia, which is a yellowish discoloration of the skin caused by high levels of carotene, a fat-soluble plant pigment turned into **vitamin A** in the liver. In one instance, the patient developed blood carotene levels nine times higher than normal values after putting himself on a diet that involved eating 2–3 pounds of vegetables every day. While carotenemia resulting from high vegetable intake has no known lasting consequences to health, it is still an indication of the importance of balance in vegetarian diets.

Research & general acceptance

A vegetarian diet has many well-documented health benefits. It has been shown that vegetarians have a higher life expectancy, as much as several years, than those who eat a meat-centered diet. The U.S. Food and Drug Administration (FDA) has stated that data have shown vegetarians to have a strong or significant probability against contracting obesity, heart disease, **lung cancer**, colon cancer, **alcoholism**, hypertension, diabetes, gallstones, gout, kidney stones, and ulcers. However, the FDA also points out that vegetarians tend to have healthy lifestyle habits, so other factors may contribute to their increased health besides diet alone.

Vegetarianism has been associated with for many decades with abstinence from other habit-forming substances, including alcohol and tobacco. There is evidence, however, that this long-standing connection between vegetarianism and other health-conscious practices is breaking down. A recent study of Scandinavian teenage vegetarians found that there was no difference between their lifestyles and those of meat-eating peers with regard to **smoking**, alcohol consumption, **exercise**, or weight. Partly because of this trend, physicians in family practice as well as those in sports medicine are increasingly recommending nutritional counseling for vegetarian teens.

A vegetarian diet, as prescribed by Dr. Dean Ornish, has been shown to improve heart disease and reverse the effects of **atherosclerosis**, or hardening of the arteries. It should be noted that Dr. Ornish's diet was used in conjunction with exercise, **stress** reduction, and other holistic methods. The Ornish diet is lacto-ovo vegetarian, because it allows the use of egg whites and nonfat dairy products.

Vegetarians have a resource of statistics in their favor when it comes to presenting persuasive arguments in favor of their eating habits. Vegetarians claim that a vegetarian diet is a major step in improving the health of citizens and the environment. Americans eat over 200 lbs (91 kg) of meat per person per year. The incidence of heart disease, cancer diabetes, and other diseases has increased along with a dramatic increase in meat consumption during the past century. Many statistics show significantly smaller risks for vegetarians contracting certain conditions. The risks of women getting **breast cancer** and men contracting prostrate cancer are nearly four times as high for frequent meat eaters as for those who eat meat sparingly or not at all. For heart attacks, American men have a 50% risk of having one, but the risk drops down to 15% for lacto-ovo vegetarians and to only 4% for vegans. For cancer, studies of populations around the world have implied that plant-based diets have lower associated risks for certain types of cancer.

Vegetarians claim other reasons for adopting a meat-free diet. One major concern is the amount of pesticides and synthetic additives such as hormones that show up in meat products. Chemicals tend to accumulate in the tissue of animals that are higher in the food chain, a process called *bioaccumulation*. Vegetarians, by not eating meat, can avoid the exposure to these accumulated toxins, many of which are known to influence the development of cancer. One study showed that DDT, a cancer-causing pesticide, was present in significant levels in mother's milk for 99% of American women, but only 8% of vegetarian women had significant levels of the pesticide. Women who eat meat had 35 times higher levels of particular pesticides than vegetarian women. The synthetic hormones and antibiotics added to American cattle has led some European countries to ban American beef altogether. The widespread use of antibiotics in livestock has made many infectious agents more resistant to them, making some diseases harder to treat.

Vegetarians resort to ethical and environmental arguments as well when supporting their food choices. Much of U.S. agriculture is dedicated to producing meat, which is an expensive and resource-depleting practice. It has been estimated that 1.3 billion people could be fed with the grain that America uses to feed livestock, and starvation is a major problem in world health. Producing meat places a heavy burden on natural resources, as compared to growing grain and vegetables. One acre of land can grow approximately 40,000 lbs (18,000 kg) of potatoes or 250 lbs (113 kg) of beef, and it takes 50,000 gal (200,000 l) of water to produce 1 lb (0.45 kg) of California beef but only 25 gal (100 l) of water to produce 1 lb (0.45 kg) of wheat. Half of all water used in America is for livestock production. Vegetarians argue that the American consumption of beef may also be contributing to global warming, by the large amounts of fossil fuels used in its production. The South American rainforest is being cleared to support American's beef consumption, as the United States yearly imports 300 million lbs (136 million kg) of meat from Central and South America. The production of meat has been estimated as causing up to 85% of the loss of topsoil of America's farmlands. A German researcher in the field of nutrition ecology hs summarized the environmental benefits of vegetarian diets: "Research shows that vegetarian diets are well suited to protect the environment, to reduce pollution, and to minimize global climate changes."

Despite the favorable statistics, vegetarianism does have its opponents. The meat industry in America is a powerful organization that has spent millions of dollars over decades advertising the benefits of eating meat. Vegetarians point out that life-long eating habits are difficult to change for many people, despite research showing that vegetarian diets can provide the same nutrients as meat-centered diets.

Resources

BOOKS

Akers, Keith. *A Vegetarian Sourcebook*. New York: Putnam, 1993.

Null, Gary. *The Vegetarian Handbook*. New York: St. Martins, 1987.

Pelletier, Kenneth R., MD. *The Best Alternative Medicine*, Part I: Food for Thought. New York: Simon & Schuster, 2002.

Robbins, John. *Diet for a New America*. Walpole, NH: Stillpoint, 1987.

PERIODICALS

American Dietetic Association; Dietitians of Canada. "Position of the American Dietetic Association and Dietitians of

---

> ## KEY TERMS
>
> **Cholesterol**—A steroid fat found in animal foods that is also produced in the body from saturated fat for several important functions. Excess cholesterol intake is linked to many diseases.
>
> **Complex carbohydrates**—Complex carbohydrates are broken down by the body into simple sugars for energy, are found in grains, fruits and vegetables. They are generally recommended in the diet over refined sugar and honey, because they are a more steady source of energy and often contain fiber and nutrients as well.
>
> **Legume**—Group of plant foods including beans, peas, and lentils, which are high in protein, fiber, and other nutrients.
>
> **Organic food**—Food grown without the use of synthetic pesticides and fertilizers.
>
> **Saturated fat**—Fat that is usually solid at room temperature, found mainly in meat and dairy products but also in vegetable sources such as some nuts, seeds, and avocados.
>
> **Tempeh**—A fermented cake of soybeans and other grains; it is a staple food in Indonesia.
>
> **Tofu**—A soft cheeselike food made from curdled soybean milk.
>
> **Unsaturated fat**—Fat found in plant foods that is typically liquid (oil) at room temperature. They can be monounsaturated or polyunsaturated, depending on the chemical structure. Unsaturated fats are the most recommended dietary fats.
>
> **Vegan**—A vegetarian who omits all animal products from the diet.

Canada: Vegetarian Diets." *Canadian Journal of Dietetic Practice and Research* 64 (Summer 2003): 62–81.

Berger, Joanne M. "Curiously Yellow." *Family Practice News* 32 (September 1, 2002): 47.

Fornell-Barratt, Anne, and Adam Drewnowski. "The Taste of Health: Nature's Bitter Gifts." *Nutrition Today* 37 (July-August 2002): 144-150.

Greydanus, D. E., and D. R. Patel. "Sports Doping in the Adolescent Athlete: The Hope, Hype, and Hyperbole." *Pediatric Clinics of North America* 49 (August 2002): 829-855.

Jenkins, D. J., C. W. Kendall, A. Marchie, et al. "Type 2 Diabetes and the Vegetarian Diet." *American Journal of Clinical Nutrition* 78 (September 2003) (3 Suppl): 610S–616S.

Kwok, E., G. Cheng, J. Woo, et al. "Independent Effect of Vitamin B_{12} Deficiency on Hematological Status in Older Chinese Vegetarian Women." *American Journal of Hematology* 70 (July 2002): 186-190.

Lampe, J. W. "Spicing Up a Vegetarian Diet: Chemopreventive Effects of Phytochemicals." *American Journal of Clinical Nutrition* 78 (September 2003) (Suppl 3): 579S–583S.

Larsson, C. L., K. S. Klock, A. Nordrehaug-Astrom, et al. "Lifestyle-Related Characteristics of Young Low-Meat Consumers and Omnivores in Sweden and Norway." *Journal of Adolescent Health* 31 (August 2002): 190-198.

Leitzmann, C. "Nutrition Ecology: The Contribution of Vegetarian Diets." *American Journal of Clinical Nutrition* 78 (September 2003) (Suppl 3): 657S–659S.

Messina, V., V. Melina, and A. R. Mangels. "A New Food Guide for North American Vegetarians." *Canadian Journal of Dietetic Practice and Research* 64 (Summer 2003): 82–86.

ORGANIZATIONS

American Dietetic Association. 216 West Jackson Blvd., Chicago, IL 60606. (312) 899-0040. <www.eatright.org>.

Dietitians of Canada/Les diététistes du Canada. 480 University Avenue, Suite 604, Toronto, ON M5G IV2. (416) 596-0857. <http://www.dietitians.ca/>.

North American Vegetarian Society (NAVS). PO Box 72, Dolgeville, NY 13329. (518) 568-7970.

OTHER

Vegetarian Journal. Vegetarian Resource Group (VRG). PO Box 1463, Baltimore, MD 21203.

Vegetarian Times. 4 High Ridge Park, Stamford, CT 06905. (877) 321-1796.

Vegetarian Nutrition and Health Letter. 1707 Nichol Hall, Loma Linda, CA 92350. (888) 558-8703.

Douglas Dupler
Rebecca J. Frey, PhD

Venom immunotherapy

Definition

Venom immunotherapy is the process of injecting venom to treat various conditions. The most common form of venom immunization is bee venom therapy (BVT), with honeybee venom or stingers used to treat conditions. BVT is one form of **apitherapy**, which is the therapeutic use of products made by honeybees. Other products used in apitherapy include **bee pollen** and **royal jelly**.

Origins

Apitherapy is thousands of years old. In ancient Egypt, venom from bee stings was used to treat arthritis. Hippocrates, the Greek physician known as the "father of medicine," used bee stings for treatments several cen-

turies before the birth of Christ. Descriptions of apitherapy are found in 2,000-year-old Chinese writings, the Bible, and the Koran.

Bee venom therapy has remained part of folk medicine throughout the centuries. The modern study of apitherapy is said to have started in 1888, with Austrian physician Phillip Terc's research titled "Report about a Peculiar Connection between the Beestings and Rheumatism."

Benefits

Although a bee sting is painful for most people, the sting can be fatal to some. Approximately 15% of the population is allergic to the sting of such insects as bees and wasps. Allergic reactions range from mild to life-threatening.

In mainstream allopathic medicine, honeybee venom is used to treat people who are allergic to bee stings. A small amount of venom is injected during desensitization treatments to help patients develop a tolerance to stings.

Honeybee venom immunotherapy is used to treat many other conditions in alternative medicine. BVT is regarded as an effective treatment for arthritis, **multiple sclerosis** (MS), acute and chronic injuries, migraine headaches, **gout**, acute **sore throat**, **psoriasis**, **irritable bowel syndrome**, Bell's palsy, **depression**, **AIDS**, scar tissue, and **asthma**.

Bee venom is also said to relieve **premenstrual syndrome** (PMS) and conditions related to **menopause**. However, BVT is most commonly used as an anti-inflammatory remedy for arthritis and MS. Advocates maintain that it will provide relief for **rheumatoid arthritis** when injected into the joints. Bee venom is also used to lessen the **pain** and swelling of **osteoarthritis** as well as such inflammations and injuries as **tendinitis** and **bursitis**. Furthermore, people diagnosed with MS say that BVT significantly reduces symptoms that include muscle spasms and tiredness.

Description

Bee venom therapy involves the injection of venom by a needle, insertion of the stinger, or stinging by live bees. While a licensed physician must give injections, other treatments can be done by a bee venom therapist, a beekeeper, the patient, or a friend or relative.

The cost and length of treatment depends on the condition, as well as when and where a person is treated. If a physician provides the treatment, the doctor's appointment may be covered by health insurance. Rates for other therapies are set by beekeepers and bee venom therapists. Information about these providers can be found through organizations such as the American Apitherapy Society. The society's resources include an extensive web site with information about BVT. Apitherapy resources include books and videos about home treatment. Live bees can be ordered by mail; one business in June 2000 charged $50 for four boxes, each containing about 60 bees.

When live bees are utilized, tweezers are used to remove one bee from a container such as a box, jar, or hive. The bee is held over the area to be treated until it stings the patient. The stinger is removed after three to five minutes.

Patients receive an average of two to five stings per session. The number of stings and the number of sessions varies with the condition treated. Tendinitis might require two to three stings per session for two to five sessions. Arthritis is sometimes treated with several stings per session at two to three weekly sessions. MS may take months to treat. While BVT advocates say MS patients are more energetic after several sessions, they maintain that treatment should be done two to three times weekly for six months.

Preparations

Before beginning venom immunotherapy, a person should be tested for **allergies**. If a relative or friend plans to help with the therapy, that person should be tested too. Bee venom may cause a severe allergic reaction called anaphylaxis. The symptoms of anaphylaxis include shock, respiratory distress, and in some cases, death. Even if tests indicate that a person isn't allergic to bee stings, it is important to obtain an emergency bee-sting allergy kit before beginning treatment.

Precautions

People should check with their doctor or practitioner before beginning bee venom immunotherapy. The therapy is not recommended for pregnant women, diabetics, people with heart conditions, **tuberculosis**, or **infections**.

An allergy test is a must before starting bee venom therapy. A person who is allergic to bee stings should not start venom treatment. In some cases, scarring and infections have resulted when the stinger was left in too long.

Side effects

If there is an allergic reaction to bee venom therapy, emergency treatment should be started. Such symptoms as minor **itching** and swelling, however, are not causes for alarm. They are signs of the healing process.

KEY TERMS

Anaphylaxis—An allergic hypersensitivity reaction to such allergens as bee stings. Anaphylaxis can result in shock, difficulty in breathing, and even death.

Apitherapy—A form of alternative therapy based on the use of honey and other bee products.

Research & general acceptance

During the late 1990s, researchers in countries including the United States, France, and Russia began researching the effect of bee venom immunotherapy on humans. Before that, research with such animals as mice indicated that venom could be beneficial for treating inflammatory conditions.

Anecdotal reports by people with MS indicated that venom immunotherapy is effective. Those supporting the study of this therapy include the Multiple Sclerosis Association of America and the American Apitherapy Society. As of June 2000, it remains to be seen whether bee venom immunotherapy is effective.

Training & certification

Although a doctor can administer bee venom therapy, no specific training or certification is required to perform the therapy. Training in handling bees is recommended. Organizations such as the American Apitherapy Society can provide information about training and therapy providers.

Resources

BOOKS

The Editors of Time-Life Books. *The Alternative Advisor.* Alexandria, VA: Time-Life Books, 1997.

Gottlieb, Bill. *New Choices in Natural Healing.* Emmaus, PA: Rodale Press, Inc., 1995.

Rosenfeld, Isadore. *Dr. Rosenfeld's Guide to Alternative Medicine.* New York: Random House, 1996.

ORGANIZATIONS

American Apitherapy Society (AAS). 5370 Carmel Road. Hillsboro, OH 45133. (937) 466-9214. Fax: (937) 466-9215. http://www.beesting.com

Arthritis Foundation. 1330 W. Peachtree St. Atlanta, GA 30309. http://www.arthritis.org.

Multiple Sclerosis Association of America. 706 Haddonfield Road. Cherry Hill, NJ 08002. (800) 833-4672.

Liz Swain

Vertigo *see* **Dizziness**

Vision disorders *see* **Hyperopia; Macular degeneration; Myopia; Night blindness; Retinal detachment**

Vision therapy *see* **Bates method**

Visualization *see* **Guided imagery**

Vitamin A

Description

Vitamin A is one of four fat-soluble vitamins necessary for good health. It serves an important role as an antioxidant by helping to prevent free radicals from causing cellular damage. Adequate levels are important for good eyesight, and poor night vision may be one of the first symptoms of a deficiency. It is also necessary for proper function of the immune, skeletal, respiratory, reproductive, and integumentary (skin) systems.

General use

An adequate level of vitamin A unquestionably contributes to good health. It is essential for the proper function of the retina, where it can act to prevent **night blindness**, as well as lower the odds of getting age-related **macular degeneration** (AMD), which is the most common cause of blindness in the elderly. There is also evidence that good levels of vitamin A in the form of **carotenoids** may decrease the risk of certain cancers, heart attacks, and strokes. The immune system is also strengthened. It is unclear, however, if supplemental forms of vitamin A have the same benefit as consuming the nutrient in natural foods in the case of a person without deficiency. Taking high levels of vitamin A in any supplemental form is not advisable without the counsel of a healthcare professional.

Preparations

Natural sources

There are two basic forms of vitamin A. Retinoids, the active types, are contained in animal sources, including meat, whole milk, and eggs. Liver is particularly rich in vitamin A, since it is one of the storage sites for excess. Precursor forms of the vitamin (carotenoids) are found in orange and leafy green produce such as sweet potatoes, carrots, collard greens, spinach, winter squash, kale, and turnip greens. Very fresh foods have the highest levels, followed by frozen foods. Typically, canned produce has little vitamin A. Preparing vegetables by steaming, baking, or grilling helps them to release the carotenes they contain. Alpha and **beta carotene**, as well

as some of the other lesser-known carotenoids, can be converted to vitamin A in the small intestine. This is done by the body on an as-needed basis, so there is no risk of overdose as there is with the active form.

Supplemental sources

Supplements may contain either the active or precursor forms of vitamin A. The active form may be more desirable for those who may have some difficulty in converting the carotenoids into the active vitamin. This is more often true in those over age 55 or who have a condition that impairs the absorption of fat. There is a water-soluble form of the vitamin, retinyl palmitate, which may be better utilized in the latter case. Carotenes are also available either as oil-based or natural water-based formulas. Be sure to store both away from light and heat, which will destroy them.

Units

There are several units that can express the amount of vitamin A activity in a product. Many supplements are still labeled with the old International Unit (IU), although the more current and most accurate unit is the Retinol Equivalent (RE). The new measurement distinguishes between the differences in absorption of retinol and beta carotene. One RE is equal to one microgram (MICROg) of retinol, or six MICROg of beta carotene.

Dose limits

Adults should take no more than 25,000 IU (5,000 RE) per day of vitamin A in its active form, except in the case of women who are pregnant or may become pregnant. The latter group should not exceed 10,000 IU (2,000 RE) per day in order to avoid potential toxic effects to the fetus. The best way to get vitamins is in the natural food form, as the complexities are not always either known or reproducible in a supplement. A diet rich in foods containing carotenoids is optimal, but in the event of nutritional deficiencies, supplements may be needed. Mixed carotenoids are preferable to either large doses of vitamin A or pure beta carotene supplements to avoid toxicity and maximize healthful benefits. Some of the minor carotenoids appear to have beneficial effects that are still being explored. A good mixture will contain alpha and beta carotene, as well as **lycopene** and xanthophylls. Eating foods high in many carotenoids may confer some benefits—such as a lower risk of **cancer**, heart attacks, and strokes—which a supplement may not.

Deficiency

Levels of vitamin A low enough to cause symptomatic deficiency are uncommon in people of normal health in industrialized nations. Symptoms of deficiency may include, but are not limited to, loss of appetite, poor immune function causing frequent **infections** (especially respiratory), **hair loss, rashes**, dry skin and eyes, visual difficulties including night blindness, poor growth, and **fatigue**. Generally symptoms are not manifested unless the deficiency has existed for a period of months. Deficiencies are more likely in people who are malnourished, including alcoholics, the chronically ill, and those with impaired fat absorption. Another group at increased risk of vitamin A deficiency are persons with type 1 diabetes whose disorder is poorly controlled. People with normal health and nutritional status have a considerable vitamin A reserve.

In countries where nutritional status tends to be poor and deficiency is more common, vitamin A has been found to reduce the mortality rate of children suffering from a number of different viral infections.

Experts in plant genetics have been working on a strain of rice that contains beta carotene, hoping to help people in developing countries avoid the risk of vitamin A deficiency. Known as Golden Rice, the new strain is being sent to research institutes in developing countries for further study.

Risk factors for deficiency

Taking the RDA level of a nutrient will prevent a deficiency in most people, but under certain circumstances, an individual may require higher doses of vitamin A. Those who consume alcoholic beverages may be more prone to vitamin A deficiency. People taking some medications, including birth control pills, methotrexate, cholestyramine, colestipol, and drugs that act to sequester bile will also need larger amounts. Those who are malnourished, chronically ill, or recovering from surgery or other injuries may also benefit from a higher than average dose. Patients undergoing treatments for cancer, including radiation and chemotherapy, typically have compromised immune systems that may be boosted by judicious supplementation with vitamin A. Other conditions that may impair vitamin A balance include chronic **diarrhea**, cystic fibrosis, and kidney or liver disease. Diabetics are often deficient in vitamin A, but may also be more susceptible to toxicity. Any supplementation for these conditions should be discussed with a healthcare provider. Supplements are best taken in the form of carotenoids to avoid any potential for toxicity. There is not an established RDA for beta carotene. Recommendations for how much to take vary between 6 and 30 mg a day, but the middle range—around 15 mg—is a reasonable average.

Precautions

Overdose can occur when taking megadoses of the active form of this vitamin. Amounts above what is being utilized by the body accumulate in the liver and fatty tissues. Symptoms may include dry lips and skin, bone and joint **pain**, liver and spleen enlargement, diarrhea, **vomiting**, headaches, blurry or double vision, confusion, irritability, fatigue, and bulging fontanel (soft spot on the head) in infants; these are most often reversible, but a doctor should be contacted if a known overdose occurs. Very high levels of vitamin A may also create deficiencies of vitamins C, E, and K. Symptoms will generally appear within six hours following an acute overdose, and take a few weeks to resolve after ceasing the supplement. Children are more sensitive to high levels of vitamin A than adults are, so instructions on products designed for children should be followed with particular care. Vitamin supplements should always be kept out of reach of children.

It is especially important to avoid overdoses in **pregnancy**, as it may cause miscarriage or fetal malformations. Using supplements that provide carotenoids will avoid the potential of overdose. Those with kidney disease are also at higher risk for toxicity due to either vitamin A or beta carotene, and should not take these supplements without professional healthcare advice.

There is some evidence that taking beta carotene supplements puts smokers at a higher risk of lung cancers. The CARET (Beta Carotene and Retinol Efficacy Trial) study is one that demonstrated this effect. Clarification through more study is needed, as evidence also exists showing that beta carotene, along with other **antioxidants**, can be a factor in cancer prevention. For example, a team of American researchers has recently reviewed evidence that vitamin A protects against **bladder cancer**, and a group in Germany is testing an aerosol form of vitamin A to prevent **lung cancer**. Some of the lesser-known carotenoids may be key factors in the relationship between vitamin intake and cancer. Whole sources of vitamin A are better obtained from foods than from supplements. Smokers should consult with a healthcare provider before taking supplemental beta carotene.

Side effects

Very high levels of carotenoids (carotenemia) may cause an orange discoloration of the skin, which is harmless and transient.

Interactions

Vitamin A supplements should not be taken in conjunction with any retinoid medications, including isotretinoin (Accutane), a drug used to treat **acne**. There is a higher risk of toxicity.

A very low fat diet or use of fat substitutes impairs absorption of all the fat-soluble vitamins, including A. Mineral oil and aluminum-containing antacids may also inhibit absorption, as do the cholesterol-lowering drugs cholestyramine and colestipol. Vitamin A reserves of the body are depleted by a number of substances, including alcohol, barbiturates, **caffeine**, cortisone, tobacco, and very high levels of **vitamin E**. Overuse of alcohol and vitamin A together may increase the possibility of liver damage.

Taking appropriate doses of **vitamin C**, vitamin E, **zinc**, and **selenium** optimizes absorption and use of vitamin A and carotenoids. As vitamin A is fat-soluble, a small amount of dietary fat is also helpful.

Studies of both children and pregnant women with **iron** deficiency **anemia** show that this condition is better treated with a combination of iron supplements and vitamin A than with iron alone.

Resources

BOOKS

Bratman, Steven, and David Kroll. *Natural Health Bible.* Prima Publishing, 1999.

Feinstein, Alice. *Prevention's Healing with Vitamins.* Rodale Press, 1996.

Griffith, H. Winter. *Vitamins, Herbs, Minerals & Supplements: The Complete Guide.* Fisher Books, 1998.

Jellin, Jeff, Forrest Batz, and Kathy Hitchens. *Pharmacist's letter/Prescriber's Letter Natural Medicines Comprehensive Database.* Therapeutic Research Faculty, 1999.

PERIODICALS

Baena, R. M., C. Campoy, R. Bayes, et al. "Vitamin A, Retinol-Binding Protein and Lipids in Type 1 Diabetes Mellitus." *European Journal of Clinical Nutrition* 56 (January 2002): 44–50.

Beyer, P., S. Al-Babili, X. Ye, et al. "Golden Rice: Introducing the Beta-Carotene Biosynthesis Pathway Into Rice Endosperm by Genetic Engineering to Defeat Vitamin A Deficiency." *Journal of Nutrition* 132 (March 2002): 506S–510S.

Kamat, A. M., and D. L. Lamm. "Chemoprevention of Bladder Cancer." *Urology Clinics of North America* 29 (February 2002): 157–168.

Kohlhaufl, M., K. Haussinger, F. Stanzel, et al. "Inhalation of Aerosolized Vitamin A: Reversibility of Metaplasia and Dysplasia of Human Respiratory Epithelia— A Prospective Pilot Study." *European Journal of Medical Research* 7 (February 21, 2002): 72–78.

Miksad, R., V. de Ledinghen, C. McDougall, et al. "Hepatic Hydrothorax Associated with Vitamin A Toxicity." *Journal of Clinical Gastroenterology* 34 (March 2002): 275–279.

van den Berg, H., M. van der Gaag, and H. Hendriks. "Influence of Lifestyle on Vitamin Bioavailability." *International Journal of Vitamin and Nutrition Research* 72 (January 2002): 53–59.

Yeum, K. J., and R. M. Russell. "Carotenoid Bioavailability and Bioconversion." *Annual Review of Nutrition* 22 (2002): 483–504.

Judith Turner
Rebecca J. Frey, PhD

Antioxidant—Any substance, such as vitamin A, that blocks the destructive action of free radicals.

Carotenoids—Any of a group of over 600 orange or red substances which are found primarily in vegetables, many of which are vitamin A precursors.

Free radical—Highly reactive atoms that are very reactive as a result of having one or more unpaired electrons. They form through exposure to smoke and other environmental pollutants, as well as radiation and other sources. They have great potential to cause cellular damage, and may even be a factor in aging.

Retinoids—Any of the group of substances which comprise active vitamin A, including retinaldehyde, retinol, and retinoic acid.

Vitamin B$_{12}$

Description

Cobalamin, also known as B$_{12}$, is a member of the water-soluble family of B vitamins. It is a key factor in the body's proper use of **iron** and formation of red blood cells. The nervous system also relies on an adequate supply of cobalamin to function appropriately, as it is an essential component in the creation and maintenance of the myelin sheath that lines nerve cells. Other roles of cobalamin include working with **pyridoxine** (vitamin B$_6$ and **folic acid** to reduce harmful homocysteine levels, participating in the metabolization of food, and keeping the immune system operating smoothly.

General use

Very small amounts of cobalamin are needed to maintain good health. The RDA value is 0.3 micrograms (mcg) for infants under 6 months, 0.5 mcg for those 6 months to 1 year old, 0.7 mcg for children 1-3 years old, 1.0 mcg for children 4-6 years old, 1.4 mcg for children 7-10 years old, and 2 mcg for those 11 years of age and older. Requirements are slightly higher for pregnant (2.2 mcg) and lactating (2.6 mcg) women.

The primary conditions that benefit from supplementation with cobalamin are megaloblastic and pernicious **anemia**. Megaloblastic anemia is a state resulting from an inadequate intake of cobalamin, to which vegans are particularly susceptible because of the lack of animal food sources. Vegans, who do not consume any animal products including meat, dairy, or eggs, should take at least 2 mcg of cobalamin per day in order to prevent this condition. In the case of pernicious anemia, intake may be appropriate but absorption is poor due to a lack of normal stomach substance, called intrinsic factor, that facilitates absorption of vitamin B$_{12}$. Large doses are required to treat pernicious anemia, which occurs most commonly in the elderly population as a result of decreased production of intrinsic factor by the stomach. Supplements are generally effective when taken orally in very large amounts (300-1000 mcg/day) even if no intrinsic factor is produced. These supplements require a prescription, and should be administered with the guidance of a health care provider. Injections, instead of the supplements, are often used.

Those who have **infections**, **burns**, some types of **cancer**, recent surgery, illnesses that cause decay or loss of strength, or high amounts of **stress** may need more than the RDA amount of B$_{12}$ and other B vitamins. A balanced supplement is the best approach.

Male **infertility** can sometimes be resolved through use of cobalamin supplements. Other conditions that may be improved by cobalamin supplementation include: **asthma**, **atherosclerosis** (hardening of the arteries caused by plaque formation in the arteries), **bursitis** (inflammation of a bodily pouch, especially the shoulder or elbow), **Crohn's disease** (chronic recurrent inflammation of the intestines), **depression**, diabetes, high **cholesterol**, **osteoporosis**, and vitiligo (milky-white patches on the skin). There is not enough evidence to judge whether supplementation for these diseases is effective.

Preparations

Natural sources

Usable cobalamin is only found naturally in animal source foods. Fresh food is best, as freezing and exposure to light may destroy some of the vitamin content. Clams and beef liver have very high cobalamin levels. Other good sources include chicken liver, beef, lamb, tuna, flounder, liverwurst, eggs, and dairy products. Some plant foods may contain cobalamin, but it is not in a form that is usable by the body.

Supplemental sources

Cobalamin supplements are available in both oral and injectable formulations. A nasal gel is also made. Generally a balanced B-complex vitamin is preferable to taking high doses of cobalamin unless there is a specific indication for it, such as megaloblastic anemia. Strict vegetarians will need to incorporate a supplemental source of B$_{12}$ in the diet. Cyanocobalamin is the form

most commonly available in supplements. Two other, possibly more effective, types are hydrocobalamin and methyl-cobalamin. As with all supplements, cobalamin should be stored in a cool, dry, dark place and out of the reach of children.

Deficiency

Cobalamin deficiency may be manifested as a variety of symptoms since cobalamin is so widely used in the body. Severe **fatigue** may occur initially. Effects on the nervous system can be wide-ranging, and include weakness, numbness and tingling of the limbs, **memory loss**, confusion, delusion, poor balance and reflexes, hearing difficulties, and even **dementia**. Severe deficiency may appear similar to **multiple sclerosis**. **Nausea** and **diarrhea** are possible gastrointestinal signs. The anemia that results from prolonged deficiency may also be seen as a pallor, especially in mucous membranes such as the gums and the lining of the inner surface of the eye.

Megaloblastic anemia is a common result of inadequate cobalamin. This condition can also result if a person stops secreting enough intrinsic factor in the stomach, a substance essential for the absorption of cobalamin. Inadequate intrinsic factor leads to pernicious anemia, so called because it persists despite iron supplementation. Long-term deficiencies of cobalamin also allow homocysteine levels to build up. Negative effects of large amounts of circulating homocysteine include **heart disease**, and possibly brain toxicity. Taking high levels of folic acid supplements can mask cobalamin deficiency and prevent the development of megaloblastic anemia, but neurological damage can still occur. This damage may become permanent if the cobalamin deficiency persists for a long period of time.

Risk factors for deficiency

The primary groups at risk for cobalamin deficiency are vegans who are not taking supplements, and the elderly. Older adults are more likely to have both insufficient intrinsic factor secreted by the stomach and low levels of stomach acid, causing cobalamin to be poorly absorbed. Malabsorptive diseases and stomach surgery can also predispose to a deficiency.

Precautions

People who are sensitive to cobalamin or cobalt should not take cobalamin supplements. Symptoms of hypersensitivity may include swelling, **itching**, and shock. Adverse effects resulting from B$_{12}$ supplementation are rare. Cobalamin should also be avoided by those who have a type of hereditary optic nerve atrophy known as Leber's disease.

KEY TERMS

Homocysteine—An amino acid produced from the metabolization of other amino acids. High levels are an independent risk factor for heart disease.

Megaloblastic anemia—A condition caused by cobalamin deficiency, which is characterized by red blood cells which are too few, too fragile, and abnormally large. Also known as macrocytic anemia.

Pernicious anemia—Megaloblastic anemia resulting from a cobalamin deficiency that is the result of poor absorption due to inadequate production of intrinsic factor in the stomach.

Vegan—A person who doesn't eat any animal products, including dairy and eggs.

Side effects

Very high doses of cobalamin may sometimes cause **acne**.

Interactions

Large amounts of **vitamin C** taken within an hour of vitamin B supplements will destroy the cobalamin component. Absorption of cobalamin is also impaired by deficiencies of folic acid, iron, or **vitamin E**. Improved absorption occurs when it is taken with other B vitamins or **calcium**. Some medications may also cause an increased use or decreased absorption of this vitamin. Those on colchicine, corticosteroids, methotrexate, metformin, phenformin, oral contraceptives, cholestyramine, colestipol, clofibrate, epoetin, neomycin, or supplemental **potassium** may need extra cobalamin. Use of nicotine products or excessive alcohol can deplete B_{12}.

Resources

BOOKS

Bratman, Steven, and David Kroll. *Natural Health Bible*. CA: Prima Publishing, 1999.

Feinstein, Alice. *Prevention's Healing with Vitamins*. PA: Rodale Press, 1996.

Griffith, H. Winter. *Vitamins, Herbs, Minerals & Supplements: The Complete Guide*. AZ: Fisher Books, 1998.

Jellin, Jeff, Forrest Batz, and Kathy Hitchens. *Pharmacist's Letter/Prescriber's Letter Natural Medicines Comprehensive Database*. CA: Therapeutic Research Faculty, 1999.

Pressman, Alan H. and Sheila Buff. *The Complete Idiot's Guide to Vitamins and Minerals*. New York: Alpha Books, 1997.

Judith Turner

Vitamin B complex

Description

The vitamin B complex consists of 12 related water-soluble substances. Eight are considered essential vitamins because they need to be included in the diet. Four are not essential because the body can synthesize them. Although these vitamins are chemically distinct, they are grouped together because they are found with one another in the same foods. Since they are water-soluble, most are not stored for any length of time, and must be replenished daily. The eight vitamins have both names and corresponding numbers. They are:

- B_1 (thiamin)
- B_2 (riboflavin)
- B_3 (niacin)
- B_5 (pantothenic acid)
- B_6 (pyridoxine)
- B_7 (biotin)
- B_9 (folic acid)
- B_{12} (cobalamin)

Biotin is not always included among B complex supplements. The numbers that appear to have been skipped were found to be duplicate substances or non-vitamins. The four unnumbered components of the B complex that can be synthesized by the body are choline, inositol, PABA, and lipoic acid.

As a group, the B vitamins have a broad range of functions, including the maintenance of myelin, which is the covering of nerve cells. A breakdown of myelin can cause a large and devastating variety of neurologic symptoms. B vitamins are also key to producing energy from nutrients that are consumed. Three members of this group—folic acid, pyridoxine, and cobalamin—work together to keep homocysteine levels low. This is quite important, since high homocysteine levels are associated with **heart disease**. Some B vitamins prevent certain birth defects (including cleft palate and neural tube defects), maintain healthy red blood cells, support immune function, regulate cell growth, aid in hormone production, and may have a role in preventing certain types of **cancer**. They also help maintain healthy skin, hair, and nails.

General use

There are many claims regarding the usefulness of various B vitamins. **Thiamine** is thought to be supportive for people with **Alzheimer's disease**, a disorder that is also associated with low levels of pyridoxine and cobalamin.

High doses of niacin lower **cholesterol**, and balance high-density (HDL) and low-density (LDL) lipoproteins. This should be done under medical supervision only. Some evidence shows that niacin may prevent juvenile diabetes (type 1, insulin dependent) in at-risk children. It may maintain pancreatic excretion of some insulin for a longer time than would occur normally. Niacin has also been used to relieve intermittent claudication and **osteoarthritis**, although the dose for the latter may lead to liver problems. The frequency of migraines may be significantly reduced, and the severity decreased, by the use of supplemental riboflavin. Pyridoxine is used therapeutically to lower the risk of heart disease, to relieve **nausea** associated with **morning sickness**, and to treat **premenstrual syndrome** (PMS). In conjunction with **magnesium**, pyridoxine may have some beneficial effects on the behavior of children with **autism**. Cobalamin supplementation has been shown to improve male fertility. **Depression, dementia**, and mental impairment are often associated with deficiencies of both cobalamin and folic acid. Folic acid may reduce the odds of cervical or colon cancer in certain risk groups.

Deficiency

Vitamin B complex is most often used to treat deficiencies that are caused by poor vitamin intake, difficulties with vitamin absorption, or conditions causing increased metabolism, such as **hyperthyroidism**, which deplete vitamin levels at a higher than normal rate.

Biotin and pantothenic acid are rarely deficient since they are broadly available in foods, but often persons lacking one type of B vitamin are lacking other B components as well. An individual who may have symptoms due to an inadequate level of one vitamin may suffer from an undetected underlying deficiency as well. One possibility of particular concern is that taking folic acid supplements can cover up the symptoms of cobalamin deficiency. This scenario could result in permanent neurologic damage if the cobalamin shortage remains untreated.

Some of the B vitamins have unique functions within the body that allow a particular deficiency to be readily identified. Often, however, they work in concert so symptoms due to various inadequate components may overlap. In general, poor B vitamin levels will cause profound **fatigue** and an assortment of neurologic manifestations, which may include weakness, poor balance, confusion, irritability, **memory loss**, nervousness, tingling of the limbs, and loss of coordination. Depression may be an early sign of significantly low levels of pyridoxine, as well as other B vitamins. Additional symptoms of vitamin B deficiency are sleep disturbances, nausea, poor appetite, frequent **infections**, and skin lesions.

A certain type of **anemia** (megaloblastic) is an effect of inadequate cobalamin. This anemia can also occur if a person stops secreting enough intrinsic factor in the stomach. Intrinsic factor is essential for the absorption of cobalamin. A lack of intrinsic factor also leads to pernicious anemia, so called because it persists despite **iron** supplementation. Neurologic symptoms often precede anemia when cobalamin is deficient.

A severe and prolonged lack of niacin causes a condition called pellagra. The classic signs of pellagra are **dermatitis**, dementia, and **diarrhea**. It is very rare now, except in alcoholics, strict vegans, and people in areas of the world with very poor **nutrition**.

Thiamine deficiency is similarly rare, except among the severely malnourished and alcoholics. A significant depletion causes a condition known as beriberi, which can cause weakness, leg spasms, poor appetite, and loss of coordination. Wernicke-Korsakoff syndrome is the most severe form of deficiency, and occurs in conjunction with **alcoholism**. Early stages of neurologic symptoms are reversible, but psychosis and death may occur if the course is not reversed.

Risk factors for deficiency

People are at higher risk for deficiency if they have poor nutritional sources of B vitamins, take medications, or have conditions that impair absorption, or are affected by circumstances causing them to require above-normal levels of vitamin B components. Since the B vitamins often work in harmony, a deficiency in one type may have broad implications. Poor intake of B vitamins is most often a problem in strict vegetarians and the elderly. People who frequently fast or diet may also benefit from B vitamin supplements. Vegans need to use **brewer's yeast** or other sources of supplemental cobalamin, since the only natural sources are meats.

Risk factors that may decrease absorption of some B vitamins include **smoking**; excessive use of alcohol; surgical removal of portions of the digestive tract; and advanced age. Absorption is also impaired by some medications. Some of the drugs that may cause decreased absorption are corticosteroids, colchicine, metformin, phenformin, omeprazol, colestipol, cholestyramine, methotrexate, 5-fluorouracil, tricyclic antidepressants, and slow-release **potassium**.

A person's requirement for vitamin B complex may be increased by such conditions as **pregnancy**, breast-feeding, emotional **stress**, and physical stress due to surgery or injury. People who are very physically active require extra riboflavin. Use of birth control pills also increases the need for certain B vitamins.

Recent research indicates that children with **sickle cell anemia** are at high risk for elevated homocysteine levels and pyridoxine deficiency.

Studies of folic acid deficiency caused by cancer chemotherapy indicate that some patients are at greater risk than others due to genetic variations in metabolism of the B vitamins. Further research is needed to determine the role of these genetic factors in vitamin deficiency states.

Preparations

Natural sources

Although they are prevalent in many foods, fresh meats and dairy products are the best sources for most of the B vitamins. Cobalamin is only found naturally in animal source foods. Freezing of food and exposing foods or supplements to light may destroy some of the vitamin content. Dark-green leafy vegetables are an excellent source of folic acid. To make the most of the B vitamins contained in foods, they should not be overcooked. It is best to steam vegetables, rather than boil or simmer them.

Supplemental sources

B vitamins are generally best taken in balanced complement, unless there is a specific deficiency or need for an individual vitamin. An excess of one component may lead to depletion of the others. Injectable and oral forms of supplements are available. The injectable types may be more useful for those with deficiencies due to problems with absorption. B complex products vary in terms of components and dose level contained within them.

Individual components are also available as supplements. These are best used with the advice of a health care professional. Some are valuable when addressing specific problems such as pernicious anemia. Strict vegetarians will need to incorporate a supplemental source of B_{12} in their **diets**.

Precautions

In many cases, large doses of water-soluble vitamins can be taken with no ill effects since excessive amounts are readily excreted. However, liver inflammation may occur when niacin is taken at daily doses of over 500 mg. This problem occurs more often at doses six times as high. It is generally reversible once the supplementation is stopped. Niacin may also cause difficulty in controlling blood sugar in diabetics. It can increase uric acid levels, which will aggravate **gout**. Those with ulcers could be adversely affected, as niacin increases the production of stomach acid. Niacin also lowers blood pressure due to its vasodilatory effect, so it should not be taken in conjunction with medications that treat high blood pressure. If a form of niacin known as inositol hexaniacinate is taken, the beneficial effects on choles-terol are maintained without incurring the problems of flushing, gout, and ulcers.

High doses of pyridoxine may cause liver inflammation or permanent nerve damage. Megadoses of this vitamin are not necessary or advisable.

Thoseon medications for seizures, high blood pressure, and **Parkinson's disease** are at increased risk for interactions. Persons who have chronic health conditions, or take other medications, should seek the advice of a health professional before beginning any program of supplementation.

Side effects

In large amounts, niacin commonly causes flushing and **headache**, although this can be avoided by taking it in the form of inositol hexaniacinate. Large doses of riboflavin result in very bright yellow urine.

Interactions

Some medications may be affected by B vitamin supplementation, including those prescribed for high blood pressure; Parkinson's disease (such as levodopa, which is inactivated by pantothenic acid); and epileptiform conditions. Folic acid interacts with Dilantin (a brand name for phenytoin **sodium**), as well as other anticonvulsants. Large amounts of **vitamin C** taken within an hour of vitamin B supplements will destroy the cobalamin component. Niacin may interfere with control of blood sugar in people on antidiabetic drugs. Isoniazid, a medication to treat **tuberculosis**, can impair the proper production and utilization of niacin. Antibiotics potentially decrease the level of some B vitamins by killing the digestive tract bacteria that produce them.

Resources

BOOKS

Bratman, Steven, and David Kroll. *Natural Health Bible.* CA: Prima Publishing, 1999.

Feinstein, Alice. *Prevention's Healing with Vitamins.* PA: Rodale Press, 1996.

Griffith, H. Winter. *Vitamins, Herbs, Minerals & Supplements: The Complete Guide.* AZ: Fisher Books, 1998.

Janson, Michael. *The Vitamin Revolution in Health Care.* Arcadia Press, 1996.

Jellin, Jeff, Forrest Batz, and Kathy Hitchens. *Pharmacist's letter/Prescriber's Letter Natural Medicines Comprehensive Database.* CA: Therapeutic Research Faculty, 1999.

Pressman, Alan H., and Sheila Buff. *The Complete Idiot's Guide to Vitamins and Minerals.* New York: Alpha Books, 1997.

PERIODICALS

Wolters M., A. Strohle, and A. Hahn. "Age-associated changes in the metabolism of vitamin B_{12} and folic acid: Preva-

KEY TERMS

Beriberi—A condition caused by a thiamine deficiency, with peripheral neurologic (nerve), cerebral (brain), and cardiovascular (heart and blood vessel) symptoms.

Cleft palate—A birth defect characterized by a deep split in the roof of the mouth, associated with folic acid deficiency.

Homocysteine—An amino acid produced from the metabolization of other amino acids. High levels are an independent risk factor for heart disease.

Intermittent claudication—Calf pain that occurs while walking and is relieved at rest, and related to restricted blood flow to the legs.

Macrocytic anemia—A condition caused by cobalamin deficiency, which is characterized by red blood cells that are too few, too fragile, and abnormally large.

Megaloblastic anemia—A form of anemia involving large, irregularly shaped red blood cells, called megaloblasts, and related to vitamin B_{12} and folic acid deficiency.

Neural tube defect—Incomplete development of the brain, spinal cord, or vertebrae of a fetus, which is sometimes caused by a folic acid deficiency.

Pellagra—A deficiency disease caused by a lack of niacin in the diet, characterized by skin rash, diarrhea, and mental symptoms.

Pernicious anemia—A type of anemia that occurs when the stomach does not secrete enough intrinsic factor, which is necessary for the absorption of vitamin B_{12}.

Vasodilatory—Causing the veins in the body to dilate, or enlarge.

Vegan—A person who doesn't eat any animal products, including dairy and eggs.

Wernecke-Korsakoff Syndrome—A condition caused by thiamine deficiency and usually related to alcoholism. Symptoms occur alternately in the central nervous system (brain and spinal cord) and peripheral nervous system (nerves in the remaining parts of the body). Alcohol interferes with the body's ability to metabolize thiamine.

lence, aetiopathogenesis and pathophysiological consequences." Z Gerontol Geriatr. 2004 Apr;37(2):109-35. (article in German, reviewed in abstract only

Balasa, W., K. A. Kalinyak, J. A. Bean, et al. "Hyperhomocysteinemia is Associated with Low Plasma Pyridoxine Levels in Children with Sickle Cell Disease." *Journal of Pediatric Hematology and Oncology* 24 (June-July 2002): 374-9.

Fairfield, K. M., and R. H. Fletcher. "Vitamins for Chronic Disease Prevention in Adults: Scientific Review." *Journal of the American Medical Association (JAMA)* 287 (June 19, 2002): 3116-26.

McCaddon, A., B. Regland, P. Hudson, and G. Davies. "Functional Vitamin B_{12} Deficiency and Alzheimer's Disease." *Neurology* 58 (May 14, 2002): 1395-9.

Miller, J. W., R. Green, D. M. Mungas, et al. "Homocysteine, Vitamin B_6, and Vascular Disease in AD Patients." *Neurology* 58 (May 28, 2002): 1449-50.

Morris, M. S. "Folate, Homocysteine, and Neurological Function." *Nutrition in Clinical Care* 5 (May-June 2002): 124-32.

Prescott, N. J., and S. Malcolm. "Folate and the Face: Evaluating the Evidence for the Influence of Folate Genes on Craniofacial Development." *The Cleft Palate-Craniofacial Journal* 39 (May 2002): 327-31.

Ulrich, C. M., K. Robien, and R. Sparks. "Pharmacogenetics and Folate Metabolism— A Promising Direction." *Pharmacogenomics* 3 (May 2002): 299-313.

ORGANIZATIONS

American Dietetic Association. 216 West Jackson Blvd., Chicago, IL 60606. (312) 899-0040. <www.eatright.org>.

Rebecca J. Frey, Ph.D.
Samuel Uretsky, Pharm.D.

Vitamin B_1 see **Thiamine**

Vitamin B_2 see **Riboflavin**

Vitamin B_3 see **Niacin**

Vitamin B_5 see **Pantothenic acid**

Vitamin B_6 see **Pyridoxine**

Vitamin B_7 see **Biotin**

Vitamin C

Description

Vitamin C, or ascorbic acid, is naturally produced in fruits and vegetables. The vitamin, which can be taken in dietary or supplementary form, is absorbed by the intestines.

That which the body cannot absorb is excreted in the urine. The body stores a small amount, but daily intake, preferably in dietary form, is recommended for optimum health.

Certain health conditions may cause vitamin C depletion, including diabetes and high blood pressure. People who smoke and women who take estrogen may also have lower vitamin C levels. In addition, men are more likely to be vitamin C depleted, as are the elderly. High **stress** levels have also been linked to vitamin C deficiency.

In addition, certain medical and surgical procedures may lower the levels of vitamin C in the body. It has been found that hemodialysis causes patients with kidney disease to lose as much as 66 mg per session. Similarly, patients who have had kidney transplants are at increased risk of vitamin C deficiency.

Severe vitamin C deficiency leads to scurvy, a disease common on ships prior to the eighteenth century, due to the lack of fresh fruits and other dietary vitamin C sources. Symptoms of scurvy include weakness, bleeding, tooth loss, bleeding gums, bruising, and joint **pain**. Less serious vitamin C depletion can have more subtle effects such as weight loss, **fatigue**, weakened immune system (as demonstrated by repeated **infections** and colds), **bruises** that occur with minor trauma and are slow to heal, and slow healing of other **wounds**.

Low vitamin C levels have also been associated with high blood pressure, increased **heart attack** risk, increased risk for developing **cataracts**, and a higher risk for certain types of **cancer** (i.e., prostate, stomach, colon, oral, and lung).

General use

Vitamin C is a critical component of both disease prevention and of basic body building processes. The therapeutic effects of vitamin C include:

• Allergy and **asthma** relief. Vitamin C is present in the lung's airway surfaces, and insufficient vitamin C levels have been associated with bronchial constriction and reduced lung function. Some studies have associated vitamin C supplementation with asthmatic symptom relief, but results have been inconclusive and further studies are needed.

• Cancer prevention. Vitamin C is a known antioxidant and has been associated with reduced risk of stomach, lung, colon, oral, and prostate cancer.

• Cataract prevention. Long-term studies on vitamin C supplementation and cataract development have shown that supplementation significantly reduces the risk of cataracts, particularly among women. One study published in 2002 found that adequate vitamin C intake in women under 60 years of age reduced their risk of developing cataracts by 57%.

• Collagen production. Vitamin C assists the body in the manufacture of collagen, a protein that binds cells together and is the building block of connective tissues throughout the body. Collagen is critical to the formation and ongoing health of the skin, cartilage, ligaments, corneas, and other bodily tissues and structures. Vitamin C is also thought to promote faster healing of wounds and injuries because of its role in collagen production.

• Diabetes control. Vitamin C supplementation may assist diabetics in controlling blood sugar levels and improving metabolism.

• Gallbladder disease prevention. A study of over 13,000 subjects published in the *Archives in Internal Medicine* found that women who took daily vitamin C supplements were 34% less likely to contract gallbladder disease and **gallstones**, and that women deficient in ascorbic acid had an increased prevalence of gallbladder disease.

• Immune system booster. Vitamin C increases white blood cell production and is important to immune system balance. Studies have related low vitamin C levels to increased risk for infection. Vitamin C is frequently prescribed for HIV-positive individuals to protect their immune system.

• Neurotransmitter and hormone building. Vitamin C is critical to the conversion of certain substances into neurotransmitters, brain chemicals that facilitate the transmission of nerve impulses across a synapse (the space between neurons, or nerve cells). Such neurotransmitters as serotonin, dopamine, and norepinephrine are responsible for the proper functioning of the central nervous system, and a deficiency of neurotransmitters can result in psychiatric illness. Vitamin C also helps the body manufacture adrenal hormones.

Other benefits of vitamin C are less clear cut and have been called into question with conflicting study results. These include vitamin C's role in treating the **common cold**, preventing **heart disease**, and treating cancer.

Respiratory health

Doses of vitamin C may reduce the duration and severity of cold symptoms, particularly in people who are vitamin C deficient. The effectiveness of vitamin C therapy on colds seems to be related to the person's dietary vitamin C intake and their general health and lifestyle. In addition, however, other researchers have found that vitamin C is associated with improved lung function and overall respiratory health.

VITAMIN C DOSES FOR COMMON ILLNESSES

Illness	Dose per 24 hours
Asthma	5–20 grams (g); 4–8 doses per 24 hours
Hay fever	5–20 grams (g); 4–8 doses per 24 hours
Common cold	30–60 g; 6–10 doses per 24 hours
Influenza	100–150 g; 8–15 doses per 24 hours
Viral pneumonia	50–200+; 12–18 doses per 24 hours

Heart disease prevention

Some studies have indicated that vitamin C may prevent heart disease by lowering total blood **cholesterol** and LDL cholesterol and raising HDL, or good cholesterol, levels. The antioxidant properties of vitamin C have also been associated with protection of the arterial lining in patients with coronary artery disease. A study published in 2002 reported that the protective effects of vitamin C on the lining of the arteries reduces the risk of heart disease in patients who have received heart transplants.

On the other hand, the results of a recent study conducted at the University of Southern California and released in early 2000 have cast doubt on the heart protective benefits of vitamin C. The study found that daily doses of 500 mg of vitamin C resulted in a thickening of the arteries in study subjects at a rate 2.5 times faster than normal. Thicker arterial walls can cause narrow blood vessels and actually increase the risk for heart disease. Study researchers have postulated that the collagen-producing effects of vitamin C could be the cause behind the arterial thickening. Further studies will be needed to determine the actual risks and benefits of vitamin C in relation to heart disease and to establish what a beneficial dosage might be, if one exists. For the time being, it is wise for most individuals, particularly those with a history of heart disease, to avoid megadoses over 200 mg because of the risk of arterial thickening.

Blood pressure control

A 1999 study found that daily doses of 500 mg of vitamin C reduced blood pressure in a group of 39 hypertensive individuals. Scientists have hypothesized that vitamin C may improve high blood pressure by aiding the function of nitric oxide, a **gas** produced by the body that allows blood vessels to dilate and facilitates blood flow. Again, recent findings that vitamin C may promote arterial wall thickening seem to contradict these findings, and further long-term studies are needed to assess the full benefits and risks of vitamin C in relation to blood pressure control.

Cancer treatment

Researchers disagree on the therapeutic use of vitamin C in cancer treatment. On one hand, studies have shown that tumors and cancer cells absorb vitamin C at a faster rate than normal cells because they have lost the ability to transport the vitamin. In addition, radiation and chemotherapy work in part by stimulating oxidation and the growth of free radicals in order to stop cancer cell growth. Because vitamin C is an antioxidant, which absorbs free radicals and counteracts the oxidation process, some scientists believe it could be counterproductive to cancer treatments. The exact impact vitamin C has on patients undergoing chemotherapy and other cancer treatments is not fully understood, and for this reason many scientists believe that vitamin C should be avoided by patients undergoing cancer treatment.

On the other side of the debate are researchers who believe that high doses of vitamin C can protect normal cells and inhibit the growth of cancerous ones. In lab-based, in vitro studies, cancer cells were killed and/or stopped growing when large doses of vitamin C were administered. Researchers postulate that unlike normal healthy cells, which will take what they need of a vitamin and then discard the rest, cancer cells continue to absorb antioxidant vitamins at excessive rates until the cell structure is effected, the cell is killed, or cell growth simply stops. However, it is important to note that there have been no in vivo controlled clinical studies to prove this theory.

Based on the currently available controlled clinical data, cancer patients should avoid taking vitamin C supplementation beyond their recommended daily allowance.

Preparations

The U.S. recommended dietary allowance (RDA) of vitamin C was changed in 2000 to reflect growing recognition of the importance of vitamin C in the diet as an antioxidant as well as a protection against deficiency. The new values are as follows:

- men: 90 mg
- women: 75 mg
- pregnant women: 80 mg
- lactating women: 95 mg
- smokers: should consume an additional 35 mg

The National Academy of Sciences also established for the first time an upper limit (UL), or maximum daily dose, of 2,000 mg. Daily values for the vitamin as recommended by the U.S. Food and Drug Administration, the values listed on food and beverage labeling, remain at 60 mg for both men and women age four and older.

Many fruits and vegetables, including citrus fruits and berries, are rich in vitamin C. Foods rich in vitamin C include raw red peppers (174 mg/cup), guava (165 mg/fruit), orange juice (124 mg/cup), and black currants (202 mg/cup). Rose hips, broccoli, tomatoes, strawberries, papaya, lemons, kiwis, and brussels sprouts are also good sources of vitamin C. Eating at least five to nine servings of fruits and vegetables daily should provide adequate vitamin C intake for most people. Fresh, raw fruits and vegetables contain the highest levels of the vitamin. Both heat and light can reduce vitamin C potency in fresh foods, so overcooking and improper storage should be avoided. Sliced and chopped foods have more of their surface exposed to light, so keeping vegetables and fruits whole may also help to maintain full vitamin potency.

Vitamin C supplements are another common source of the vitamin. Individuals at risk for vitamin C depletion such as smokers, women who take birth control pills, and those with unhealthy dietary habits may benefit from a daily supplement. Supplements are available in a variety of different forms including pills, capsules, powders, and liquids. Vitamin C formulas also vary. Common compounds include ascorbic acid, **calcium** ascorbate, **sodium** ascorbate, and C complex. The C complex compound contains a substance called **bioflavonoids**, which may enhance the benefits of vitamin C. Vitamin C is also available commercially as one ingredient of a multivitamin formula.

The recommended daily dosage of vitamin C varies by individual need, but an average daily dose might be 200 mg. Some healthcare providers recommend megadoses (up to 40 g) of vitamin C to combat infections. However, the efficacy of these megadoses has not been proven, and in fact, some studies have shown that doses above 200 mg are not absorbed by the body and are instead excreted.

Precautions

Overdoses of vitamin C can cause **nausea, diarrhea,** stomach cramps, skin **rashes,** and excessive urination.

Because of an increased risk of kidney damage, persons with a history of kidney disease or **kidney stones** should never take dosages above 200 mg daily, and should consult with their healthcare provider before starting vitamin C supplementation.

A 1998 study linked overdoses (above 500 mg) of vitamin C to cell and DNA damage. However, other studies have contradicted these findings, and further research is needed to establish whether high doses of vitamin C can cause cell damage.

Side effects

Vitamin C can cause diarrhea and nausea. In some cases, side effects may be decreased or eliminated by adjusting the dosage of vitamin C.

Interactions

Vitamin C increases **iron** absorption, and is frequently prescribed with or added to commercial iron supplements for this reason.

Individuals taking anticoagulant, or blood thinning, medications should speak with their doctor before taking vitamin C supplements, as large doses of vitamin C may impact their efficacy.

Large amounts of vitamin C may increase estrogen levels in women taking hormone supplements or birth control medications, especially if both the supplement and the medication are taken simultaneously. Women should speak with their doctor before taking vitamin C if they are taking estrogen-containing medications. Estrogen actually decreases absorption of vitamin C, so larger doses of vitamin C may be necessary. A healthcare provider can recommend proper dosages and the correct administration of medication and supplement.

Persons who take aspirin, antibiotics, and/or steroids should consult with their healthcare provider about adequate dosages of vitamin C. These medications can increase the need for higher vitamin C doses.

Large dosages of vitamin C can cause a false-positive result in tests for diabetes.

Resources

BOOKS

Reavley, Nocola. *The New Encyclopedia of Vitamins, Minerals, Supplements, and Herbs.* New York: M. Evans & Company, 1998.

PERIODICALS

du Plessis, A. S., H. Randall, E. Escreet, et al. "Nutritional Status of Renal Transplant Patients." *South African Medical Journal* 92 (January 2002): 68-74.

KEY TERMS

Adrenal hormone—The adrenocortical hormones are cortisol and cortisone. They are anti-inflammatory substances that aid in the function of a number of body systems, including the central nervous system, the cardiovascular system, the musculoskeletal system, and the gastrointestinal system.

Antioxidants—Enzymes that bind with free radicals to neutralize their harmful effects.

Ascorbic acid—Another name for vitamin C, derived from its ability to prevent scurvy.

Bioflavonoids—Plant-derived substances that help to maintain the small blood vessels of the circulatory system.

Free radicals—Reactive molecules created during cell metabolism that can cause tissue and cell damage like that which occurs in aging and with disease processes such as cancer.

In vitro testing—A test performed in a lab setting rather than in a human or animal organism. The test may involve living tissue or cells, but takes place out of the body.

In vivo testing—A test performed on a living organism, such as a controlled clinical study involving human test subjects. In vivo is Latin for "in the living body."

Fang, J. C., S. Kinlay, J. Beltrame, et al. "Effect of Vitamins C and E on Progression of Transplant-Associated Arteriosclerosis: A Randomised Trial." *Lancet* 359 (March 30, 2002): 1108-1113.

Henderson, C.W."Prevalence Lower in Women with Increased Vitamin C Levels." *Women's Health Weekly* (April 22, 2000): 7.

Jacob, R. A., and G. Sotoudeh. "Vitamin C Function and Status in Chronic Disease." *Nutrition in Clinical Care* 5 (March-April 2002): 66-74.

Leibman, Bonnie."Antioxidants." *Nutrition Action Health Letter* (June 2000):9.

Morena, M., J. P. Cristol, J. Y. Bosc, et al. "Convective and Diffusive Losses of Vitamin C During Haemodiafiltration Session: A Contributive Factor to Oxidative Stress in Haemodialysis Patients." *Nephrology Dialysis Transplantation* 17 (March 2002): 422-427.

"New Questions About the Safety of Vitamin C Pills." *Tufts University Health & Nutrition Letter* (April 2000): 1.

Schunemann, H. J., S. McCann, B. J. Grant, et al. "Lung Function in Relation to Intake of Carotenoids and Other Antioxidant Vitamins in a Population-Based Study." *American Journal of Epidemiology* 155 (March 1, 2002): 463-471.

Taylor, A., P. F. Jacques, L. T. Chylack, Jr., et al. "Long-Term Intake of Vitamins and Carotenoids and Odds of Early Age-Related Cortical and Posterior Subcapsular Lens Opacities." *American Journal of Clinical Nutrition* 75 (March 2002): 540-549.

Tsuchiya, M., A. Asada, E. Kasahara, et al. "Smoking a Single Cigarette Rapidly Reduces Combined Concentrations of Nitrate and Nitrite and Concentrations of Antioxidants in Plasma." *Circulation* 105 (March 12, 2002): 1155-1157.

ORGANIZATIONS

United States Department of Agriculture. Center for Nutrition Policy and Promotion. 1120 20th Street NW, Suite 200, North Lobby, Washington, D.C. 20036. (202)418–2312. http://www.usda.gov/cnpp/. john.webster@usda.gov.

Paula Ford-Martin
Rebecca J. Frey, PhD

Vitamin D

Description

Vitamin D, also known as calciferol, is essential for strong teeth and bones. There are two major forms of vitamin D: D_2 or ergocalciferol and D_3 or cholecarciferol. Vitamin D can be synthesized by the body in the presence of sunlight, as opposed to being required in the diet. It is the only vitamin whose biologically active formula is a hormone. It is fat-soluble, and regulates the body's absorption and use of the minerals **calcium** and **phosphorus**. Vitamin D is important not only to the maintenance of proper bone density, but to the many calcium-driven neurologic and cellular functions, as well as normal growth and development. It also assists the immune system by playing a part in the production of a type of white blood cell called the monocyte. White blood cells are infection fighters. There are many chemical forms of vitamin D, which have varying amounts of biological activity.

General use

The needed amount of vitamin D is expressed as an Adequate Intake (AI) rather than an Required Daily Amount (RDA). This is due to a difficulty in quantifying the amount of the vitamin that is produced by the body with exposure to sunlight. Instead, the AI estimates the amount needed to be eaten in order to maintain normal function. It is measured in International Units (IU) and there are 40 IU in a microgram (mcg). The AI for vitamin D in the form of cholecarciferol or ergocalciferol for everyone under 50 years of age, including pregnant and lactating women, is 200 IU. It goes up to 400 IU for people 51-70 years old, and to 600 IU for those over age 70. A slightly higher dose of vitamin D, even as little as a total of 700 IU for those over age 65, can significantly reduce age-related **fractures** when taken with 500 mg of calcium per day.

One of the major uses of vitamin D is to prevent and treat **osteoporosis**. This disease is essentially the result of depleted calcium, but calcium supplements alone will not prevent it since vitamin D is required to properly absorb and utilize calcium. Taking vitamin D without the calcium is also ineffective. Taking both together may actually increase bone density in postmenopausal women, who are most susceptible to bone loss and complications such as fractures.

Osteomalacia and rickets are also effectively prevented and treated through adequate vitamin D supplementation. Osteomalacia refers to the softening of the bones that occurs in adults that are vitamin D deficient. Rickets is the syndrome that affect deficient children, causing bowed legs, joint deformities, and poor growth and development.

Vitamin D also has a part in **cancer** prevention, at least for colon cancer. A deficiency increases the risk of this type of cancer, but there is no advantage to taking more than the AI level. There may also be a protective effect against breast and **prostate cancer**, but this is not as well established. Studies are in progress to see if it can help to treat **leukemia** and lymphoma. The action of at least one chemotherapeutic drug, tamoxifen, appears to be improved with small added doses of vitamin D. Tamoxifen is commonly used to treat ovarian, uterine, and breast cancers.

Many older adults are deficient in vitamin D. This can affect hearing by causing poor function of the small bones in the ear that transmit sound. If this is the cause of the **hearing loss**, it is possible that supplementation of vitamin D can act to reverse the situation.

Some metabolic diseases are responsive to treatment with specific doses and forms of vitamin D. These include Fanconi syndrome and familial hypophosphatemia, both of which result in low levels of phosphate. For these conditions, the vitamin is given in conjunction with a phosphate supplement to aid in absorption.

A topical form of vitamin D is available, and can be helpful in the treatment of plaque-type **psoriasis**. It may also be beneficial for those with vitiligo or scleroderma. This cream, in the form of calcitriol, is not thought to affect internal calcium and phosphorus levels. Oral supplements of vitamin D are not effective for psoriasis. The cream is obtainable by prescription only.

Evidence does not support the use of vitamin D to treat **alcoholism**, **acne**, arthritis, cystic fibrosis, or herpes.

Preparations

Natural sources

Exposure to sunlight is the primary method of obtaining vitamin D. In clear summer weather, approximately ten minutes per day in the sun will produce adequate amounts, even when only the face is exposed. In the winter, it may require as much as two hours. Many people don't get that amount of winter exposure, but are able to utilize the vitamin that was stored during extra time in the sun over the summer. Sunscreen blocks the ability of the sun to produce vitamin D, but should be applied as soon as the minimum exposure requirement has passed, in order to reduce the risk of **skin cancer**. The chemical 7-dehydrocholesterol in the skin is converted to vitamin D_3 by sunlight. Further processing by first the liver, and then the kidneys, makes D_3 more biologically active. Since it is fat-soluble, extra can be stored in the liver and fatty tissues for future use. Vitamin D is naturally found in fish liver oils, butter, eggs, and fortified milk and cereals in the form of vitamin D_2. Milk products are the main dietary source for most people. Other dairy products are not a good supply of vitamin D, as they are made from unfortified milk. Plant foods are also poor sources of vitamin D.

Supplemental sources

Most oral supplements of vitamin D are in the form of ergocalciferol. It is also available in topical (calcitriol or calcipotriene), intravenous (calcitriol), or intramuscular (ergocalciferol) formulations. Products designed to be given by other than oral routes are by prescription only. As with all supplements, vitamin D should be stored in a cool, dry place, away from direct light, and out of the reach of children.

Deficiency

In adults, a mild deficiency of vitamin D may be manifested as loss of appetite and weight, difficulty sleeping, and **diarrhea**. A more major deficiency causes osteomalacia and muscle spasm. The bones become soft, fragile, and painful as a result of the calcium depletion. This is due to an inability to properly absorb and utilize calcium in the absence of vitamin D. In children, a severe lack of vitamin D causes rickets.

Risk factors for deficiency

The most likely cause of vitamin D deficiency is inadequate exposure to sunlight. This can occur with people who don't go outside much, those in areas of the world where pollution blocks ultraviolet (UV) light or where the weather prohibits spending much time outdoors. Glass filters out the rays necessary for vitamin formation, as does sunscreen. Those with dark skin may also absorb smaller amounts of the UV light necessary to effect conversion of the vitamin. In climates far to the north, the angle of the sun in winter may not allow adequate UV penetration of the atmosphere to create D_3 Getting enough sun in the summer, and a good dietary source, should supply enough vitamin D to last through the winter. Vegans, or anyone who doesn't consume dairy products in combination with not getting much sun is also at higher risk, as are the elderly, who have a decreased ability to synthesize vitamin D.

Babies are usually born with about a nine-month supply of the vitamin, but breast milk is a poor source. Those born prematurely are at an increased risk for deficiency of vitamin D and calcium, and may be prone to tetany. Infants past around nine months old who are not getting vitamin D fortified milk or adequate sun exposure are at risk of deficiency.

People with certain intestinal, liver and kidney diseases may not be able to convert vitamin D_3 to active forms, and may need at activated type of supplemental vitamin D.

Those taking certain medications may require supplements, including anticonvulsants, corticosteroids, or the cholesterol-lowering medications cholestyramine or colestipol. This means that people who are on medication for arthritis, **asthma**, **allergies**, autoimmune conditions, high **cholesterol**, **epilepsy**, or other seizure problems should consult with a healthcare practitioner about the advisability of taking supplemental vitamin D. As with some other vitamins, the abuse of alcohol also has a negative effect. In the case of vitamin D, the ability to absorb and store it is diminished by chronic overuse of alcohol products.

Populations with poor nutritional status may tend to be low on vitamin D, as well as other vitamins. This can be an effect of poor sun exposure, poor intake, or poor absorption. A decreased ability to absorb oral forms of vitamin D may result from cystic fibrosis or removal of portions of the digestive tract. Other groups who may need higher than average amounts of vitamin D include those who have recently had surgery, major injuries, or **burns**. High levels of **stress** and chronic wasting illnesses also tend to increase vitamin requirements.

Precautions

The body will not make too much vitamin D from overexposure to sun, but since vitamin D is stored in fat, toxicity from supplemental overdose is a possibility.

Symptoms are largely those of hypercalemia, and may include high blood pressure, **headache**, weakness, **fatigue**, heart arrhythmia, loss of appetite, **nausea**, **vomiting**, diarrhea, **constipation**, **dizziness**, irritability, seizures, kidney damage, poor growth, premature hardening of the arteries, and **pain** in the abdomen, muscles, and bones. If the toxicity progresses, **itching** and symptoms referable to renal disease may develop, such as thirst, frequent urination, proteinuria, and inability to concentrate urine. Overdoses during **pregnancy** may cause fetal abnormalities. Problems in the infant can include tetany, seizures, heart valve malformation, retinal damage, growth suppression, and mental retardation. Pregnant women should not exceed the AI, and all others over one year of age should not exceed a daily dose of 2000 IU. Infants should not exceed 1000 IU. These upper level doses should not be used except under the advice and supervision of a healthcare provider due to the potential for toxicity.

Individuals with hypercalemia, sarcoidosis, or hypoparathyroidism should not use supplemental calciferol. Those with kidney disease, arteriosclerosis, or **heart disease** should use ergocalciferol only with extreme caution and medical guidance.

Side effects

Minor side effects may include poor appetite, constipation, **dry mouth**, increased thirst, metallic taste, or fatigue. Other reactions, which should prompt a call to a healthcare provider, can include headache, nausea, vomiting, diarrhea, or confusion.

Interactions

The absorption of vitamin D is improved by calcium, choline, fats, phosphorus, and vitamins A and C. Supplements should be taken with a meal to optimize absorption.

There are a number of medications that can interfere with vitamin D levels, absorption, and metabolism. Rifampin, H_2 blockers, barbiturates, heparin, isoniazid, colestipol, cholestyramine, carbamazepine, phenytoin, fosphenytoin, and phenobarbital reduce serum levels of vitamin D and increase metabolism of it. Anyone who is on medication for epilepsy or another seizure disorder should check with a healthcare provider to see whether it is advisable to take supplements of vitamin D. Overuse of mineral oil, Olestra, and stimulant laxatives may also deplete vitamin D. Osteoporosis and hypocalcemia can result from long-term use of corticosteroids. It may be necessary to take supplements of calcium and vitamin D together with this medication. The use of thiazide diuretics in conjunction with vitamin D can cause hypercal-

KEY TERMS

Osteomalacia—Literally soft bones, a condition seen in adults deficient in vitamin D. The bones are painful and fracture easily.

Scleroderma—A condition causing thickened, hardened skin.

Tetany—Painful muscles spasms and tremors caused by very low calcium levels.

Vegan—A person who doesn't eat any animal products, including dairy and eggs.

Vitiligo—Patchy loss of skin pigmentation, resulting in lighter areas of skin.

cemia in individuals with hypoparathyroidism. Concomitant use of digoxin or other cardiac glycosides with vitamin D supplements may lead to hypercalcemia and heart irregularities. The same caution should be used with herbs containing cardiac glycosides, including black hellebore, Canadian hemp, digitalis, hedge mustard, figwort, lily of the valley, **motherwort**, oleander, pheasant's eye, **pleurisy**, squill, and strophanthus.

Resources

BOOKS
Bratman, Steven, and David Kroll. *Natural Health Bible.* CA: Prima Publishing, 1999.

Feinstein, Alice. *Prevention's Healing with Vitamins.* PA: Rodale Press, 1996.

Griffith, H. Winter. *Vitamins, Herbs, Minerals & Supplements: The Complete Guide.* AZ: Fisher Books, 1998.

Jellin, Jeff, Forrest Batz, and Kathy Hitchens. *Pharmacist's letter/Prescriber's Letter Natural Medicines Comprehensive Database.* CA: Therapeutic Research Faculty, 1999.

Pressman, Alan H., and Sheila Buff. *The Complete Idiot's Guide to Vitamins and Minerals.* New York: Alpha Books, 1997.

Judith Turner

Vitamin E

Description

Vitamin E is an antioxidant responsible for proper functioning of the immune system and for maintaining healthy eyes and skin. It is actually a group of fat soluble compounds known as tocopherols (i.e., alpha tocopherol

and gamma tocopherol). Gamma tocopherol accounts for approximately 75% of dietary vitamin E. Vitamin E rich foods include nuts, cereals, beans, eggs, cold-pressed oils, and assorted fruits and vegetables. Because vitamin E is a fat soluble vitamin, it requires the presence of fat for proper absorption. Daily dietary intake of the recommended daily allowance (RDA) of vitamin E is recommended for optimum health.

Vitamin E is absorbed by the gastrointestinal system and stored in tissues and organs throughout the body. Certain health conditions may cause vitamin E depletion, including liver disease, **celiac disease**, and cystic fibrosis. Patients with end-stage renal disease (kidney failure) who are undergoing chronic dialysis treatment may be at risk for vitamin E deficiency. These patients frequently receive intravenous infusions of **iron** supplements, which can act against vitamin E.

Vitamin E deficiency can cause **fatigue**, concentration problems, weakened immune system, **anemia**, and low thyroid levels. It may also cause vision problems and irritability. Low serum (or blood) levels of vitamin E have also been linked to major **depression**.

General use

Vitamin E is necessary for optimal immune system functioning, healthy eyes, and cell protection throughout the body. It has also been linked to the prevention of a number of diseases. The therapeutic benefits of vitamin E include:

• **Cancer** prevention and treatment. Vitamin E is a known antioxidant, and has been associated with a reduced risk of gastrointestinal, cervical, prostate, lung, and possibly **breast cancer**. In addition to its role as a cancer preventive, vitamin E is being studied as a cancer treatment. It has been shown to inhibit the growth of prostate tumors and to induce apoptosis (cell self-destruction) in cancer cells. Vitamin E is also being investigated as an adjunctive treatment for cancer patients undergoing radiation therapy; it is thought that high doses of dietary **antioxidants** may increase the efficacy of the radiation treatment while protecting healthy cells against damage.

• Immune system protection. Various studies have shown that vitamin E supplementation, particularly in elderly patients, boosts immune system function. Older patients have demonstrated improved immune response, increased resistance to **infections**, and higher antibody production. Vitamin E has also been used with some success to slow disease progression in HIV-positive patients.

• Eye disease prevention. Clinical studies on vitamin E have shown that supplementation significantly reduces

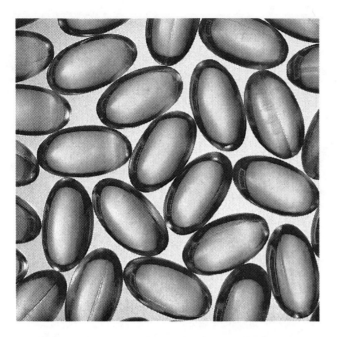

Vitamin E capsules, which are transparent yellow-orange.
(David Doody/FPG International Corp. Reproduced by permission.)

the risk for **cataracts** and for **macular degeneration**, particularly among women.

- Memory loss prevention. Vitamin E deficiency has been linked to poor performance on memory tests in some elderly individuals.

- Alzheimer's disease (AD) treatment. In a study performed at Columbia University, researchers found that Alzheimer's patients who took daily supplements of vitamin E maintained normal functioning longer than patients who took a placebo. In 2002, a group of Dutch epidemiologists reported on a much larger population-based study conducted in the Netherlands between 1990 and 1993, with follow-up examinations in 1994 and 1999. The study confirmed the findings of the Columbia researchers, that high dietary intake of vitamin E lowers the risk of developing AD.

- Liver disease treatment. Vitamin E may protect the liver against disease.

- Diabetes treatment. Vitamin E may help diabetic patients process insulin more effectively. It has also been found to be effective in the treatment of diabetic neuropathy, a family of nerve disorders caused by diabetes. Vitamin E appears to reduce the symptoms of diabetic neuropathy and to improve the speed of transmission of nerve impulses.

- **Pain** relief. Vitamin E acts as both an anti-inflammatory and analgesic (or pain reliever). Studies have indicated it may be useful for treatment of arthritis pain in some individuals.

- **Parkinson's disease** prevention. High doses of vitamin E intake was associated with a lowered risk of developing Parkinson's disease in one 1997 Dutch study.

- Tardive dyskinesia treatment. Individuals who take neuroleptic drugs for **schizophrenia** or other disorders may suffer from a side effect known as tardive dyskinesia, in which they experience involuntary muscle contractions or twitches. Vitamin E supplementation may lessen or eliminate this side effect in some individuals.

- Porphyria treatment. Vitamin E has been found to be beneficial in treating patients with porphyria, a group of disorders characterized by abnormalities in the metabolism of blood pigments, by lowering the level of excretion of these blood pigments in the urine.

Other benefits of vitamin E are less clear cut, and have been called into question with conflicting study results or because of a lack of controlled studies to support them. These include:

- **Heart disease** prevention. A number of epidemiological studies have indicated that vitamin E may prevent heart disease by lowering total blood **cholesterol** levels and preventing oxidation of LDL cholesterol. However, a large, controlled study known as the Heart Outcomes Prevention Evaluation (HOPE) published in early 2000 indicates that vitamin E does not have any preventative effects against heart disease. The study followed 9,500 individuals who were considered to be at a high risk for heart disease. Half the individuals were randomly chosen to receive vitamin E supplementation, and the other half of the study population received a placebo. After five years, there was no measurable difference in heart attacks and heart disease between the two patient populations. Still, vitamin E may still hold some hope for heart disease prevention. It is possible that a longer-term study beyond the five years of the HOPE study may demonstrate some heart protective benefits of vitamin E consumption. It is also possible that while the high-risk patient population that was used for the HOPE study did not benefit from vitamin E, an average-risk patient population might still benefit from supplementation. It is also possible that vitamin E needs the presence of another vitamin or nutrient substance to protect against heart disease. Further large, controlled, and long-term clinical studies are necessary to answer these questions.

- Skin care. Vitamin E is thought to increase an individual's tolerance to UV rays when taken as a supplement in conjunction with **vitamin C**. Vitamin E has also been touted as a treatment to promote faster healing of flesh **wounds**. While its anti-inflammatory and analgesic properties may have some benefits in reducing swelling and relieving discomfort in a wound, some dermatologists dispute the claims of faster healing, and there are no large controlled studies to support this claim.

- **Hot flashes.** In a small study conducted at the Mayo Clinic, researchers found that breast cancer survivors who suffered from hot flashes experienced a decrease in hot flashes after taking vitamin E supplementation.

- Muscle maintenance and repair. Recent research has demonstrated that the antioxidative properties of vitamin E may prevent damage to tissues caused by heavy endurance exercises. In addition, vitamin E supplementation given prior to surgical procedures on muscle and joint tissues has been shown to limit reperfusion injury (muscle damage that occurs when blood flow is stopped, and then started again to tissues or organs).

- Fertility. Vitamin E has been shown to improve sperm function in animal studies, and may have a similar effect in human males. Further studies are needed to establish the efficacy of vitamin E as a treatment for male **infertility**; as of 2002, its role in such treatment is still controversial.

Preparations

The U.S. recommended dietary allowance (RDA) of the alpha-tocopherol formulation of vitamin E is as follows:

- men: 10 mg or 15 IU

- women: 8 mg or 12 IU

- pregnant women: 10 mg or 15 IU

- lactating women: 12 mg or 18 IU

In April 2000, the National Academy of Sciences recommended changing the RDA for vitamin E to 22 international units (IUs), with an upper limit (UL), or maximum daily dose, of 1500 IUs. Daily values for the vitamin as recommended by the U.S. Food and Drug Administration, the values listed on food and beverage labeling, remain at 30 IUs for both men and women age four and older.

Many nuts, vegetable-based oils, fruits, and vegetables contain vitamin E. Foods rich in vitamin E include **wheat germ** oil (26.2 mg/tbsp), wheat germ cereal (19.5 mg/cup), peanuts (6.32 mg/half cup), soybeans (3.19 mg/cup), corn oil (2.87/tbsp), avocado (2.69 mg), and olive oil (1.68 mg/tbsp.). Grapes, peaches, broccoli, Brussels sprouts, eggs, tomatoes, and blackberries are also good sources of vitamin E. Fresh, raw foods contain the highest levels of the vitamin. Both heat and light can reduce vitamin and mineral potency in fresh foods, so overcooking and improper storage should be avoided. Sliced and chopped foods have more of their surface exposed to light, therefore keeping vegetables and fruits whole may also help to maintain full vitamin potency.

For individuals considered at risk for vitamin E deficiency, or those with an inadequate dietary intake, vitamin E supplements are available in a variety of different forms, including pills, capsules, powders, and liquids for oral ingestion. For topical use, vitamin E is available in ointments, creams, lotions, and oils. Vitamin E is also available commercially as one ingredient of a multivitamin formula.

The recommended daily dosage of vitamin E varies by individual need and by the amount of polyunsaturated fats an individual consumes. The more polyunsaturated fats in the diet, the higher the recommended dose of vitamin E, because vitamin E helps to prevent the oxidizing effects of these fats. Because vitamin E is fat soluble, supplements should always be taken with food.

Supplements are also available in either natural or synthetic formulations. Natural forms are extracted from wheat germ oil and other vitamin E food sources, and synthetic forms are extracted from petroleum oils. Natural formulas can be identified by a *d* prefix on the name of the vitamin (i.e., d-alpha-tocopherol).

Precautions

Overdoses of vitamin E (over 536 mg) can cause **nausea**, **diarrhea**, **headache**, abdominal pain, bleeding, high blood pressure, fatigue, and weakened immune system function.

Patients with rheumatic heart disease, iron deficiency anemia, **hypertension**, or thyroid dysfunction should consult their healthcare provider before starting vitamin E supplementation, as vitamin E may have a negative impact on these conditions.

Side effects

Vitamin E is well-tolerated, and side effects are rare. However, in some individuals who are **vitamin K** deficient, vitamin E may increase the risk for hemorrhage or bleeding. In some cases, side effects may be decreased or eliminated by adjusting the dosage of vitamin E and vitamin K.

Although the reasons are not yet clear, high intake of vitamin E has been associated with a statistically significant increased risk of breast cancer in men.

Vitamin E ointments, oils, or creams may trigger an allergic reaction known as **contact dermatitis**. Individuals who are considering using topical vitamin E preparations for the first time, or who are switching the type of vitamin E product they use, should perform a skin patch test to check for skin sensitivity to the substance. A small, dime sized drop of the product should be applied to a small patch of skin inside the elbow or wrist. The skin patch should be monitored for 24 hours to ensure no excessive redness, irritation, or rash occurs. If a reaction does occur, it may be in response to other ingredients in the topical preparation, and the test can be repeated with a different vitamin E formulation. Individuals who experience a severe reaction to a skin patch test of vitamin E are advised not to use the product topically. A dermatologist or other healthcare professional may be able to recommend a suitable alternative.

Interactions

Individuals who take anticoagulant (blood thinning) or anticonvulsant medications should consult their healthcare provider before starting vitamin E supplementation. Vitamin E can alter the efficacy of these drugs.

It is important for persons taking supplemental vitamin E to tell their surgeon if they are scheduled for an operation. Vitamin E may interact with some of the medications given prior to or during surgery; it has also been shown to increase bleeding time if the patient is taking such other herbal preparations as **feverfew** or gingko biloba.

Non-heme, inorganic iron supplements destroy vitamin E, so individuals taking iron supplements should space out their doses (e.g., iron in the morning and vitamin E in the evening).

Large doses of **vitamin A** can decrease the absorption of vitamin E, so dosage adjustments may be necessary in individuals supplementing with both vitamins.

Alcohol and mineral oil can also reduce vitamin E absorption, and these substances should be avoided if possible in vitamin E deficient individuals.

Resources

BOOKS

Reavley, Nocola. *The New Encyclopedia of Vitamins, Minerals, Supplements, and Herbs.* New York: M. Evans & Company, 1998.

PERIODICALS

Bolle, P., M. G. Evandri, and L. Saso. "The Controversial Efficacy of Vitamin E for Human Male Infertility." *Contraception* 65 (April 2002): 313-315.

Bonner, L. T., and E. R. Peskind. "Pharmacologic Treatments of Dementia." *Medical Clinics of North America* 86 (May 2002): 657-674.

Collins, S. C., and R. G. Dufresne Jr. "Dietary Supplements in the Setting of Mohs Surgery." *Dermatologic Surgery* 28 (June 2002): 447-452.

Engelhart, M. J., M. I. Geerlings, A. Ruitenberg, et al. "Dietary Intake of Antioxidants and Risk of Alzheimer's Disease."

KEY TERMS

Antioxidants—Enzymes that bind with free radicals to neutralize their harmful effects.

Apoptosis—A process of programmed cell death or cell self-destruction. Vitamin E is thought to induce apoptosis in cancer cells.

Contact dermatitis—Inflammation, redness, and irritation of the skin caused by an irritating substance.

Epidemiological study—A study that analyzes health events and trends in particular patient populations.

Free radicals—Reactive molecules created during cell metabolism that can cause tissue and cell damage like that occuring in aging and with disease processes such as cancer.

Macular degeneration—Degeneration, or breakdown, of the retina that can lead to partial or total blindness.

Non-heme iron—Dietary or supplemental iron that is less efficiently absorbed by the body than heme iron (ferrous iron).

Reperfusion—The reintroduction of blood flow to organs or tissues after blood flow has been stopped for surgical procedures.

Vitamin A—An essential vitamin found in liver, orange and yellow vegetables, milk, and eggs that is critical for proper growth and development.

Vitamin K—A fat-soluble vitamin responsible for blood clotting, bone metabolism, and proper kidney function.

Journal of the American Medical Association 287 (June 26, 2002): 3261-3263.

Johnson, K. C., S. Pan, and Y. Mao. "Risk Factors for Male Breast Cancer in Canada, 1994-1998." *European Journal of Cancer Prevention* 11 (June 2002): 253-263.

Pinelli, A., S. Trivulzio, L. Tomasoni, et al. "High-Dose Vitamin E Lowers Urine Porphyrin Levels in Patients Affected by Porphyria Cutanea Tarda." *Pharmacological Research* 45 (April 2002): 355-359.

Prasad, K. N., W. C. Cole, B. Kumar, and K. Che Prasad. "Pros and Cons of Antioxidant Use During Radiation Therapy." *Cancer Treatment Review* 28 (April 2002): 79-91.

Sytze Van Dam, P. "Oxidative Stress and Diabetic Neuropathy: Pathophysiological Mechanisms and Treatment Perspectives." *Diabetes/Metabolism Research and Reviews* 18 (May-June 2002): 176-184.

"Vitamin E: E for Exaggerated?" *Harvard Health Letter* 25, no. 5 (March 2000):6(3p).

Yu, A., P. Somasundar, A. Balsubramaniam, et al. "Vitamin E and the Y4 Agonist BA-129 Decrease Prostate Cancer Growth and Production of Vascular Endothelial Growth Factor." *Journal of Surgical Research* 105 (June 1, 2002): 65-68.

ORGANIZATIONS

American Dietetic Association. 216 West Jackson Blvd., Chicago, IL 60606. (312) 899-0040. <www.eatright.org>.

United States Department of Agriculture. Center for Nutrition Policy and Promotion. 1120 20th Street NW, Suite 200, North Lobby, Washington, D.C. 20036. (202) 418-2312. <www.usda.gov/cnpp>.

United States Food and Drug Administration (FDA). 5600 Fishers Lane, Rockville, MD 20857. (888) 463-6332. <www.fda.gov>.

Paula Ford-Martin
Rebecca J. Frey, PhD

Vitamin K

Description

Vitamin K originates from the German term *koajulation*. It is also known as antihemorrhagic factor, and is one of the four fat-soluble vitamins necessary for good health. The others are vitamins A, D, and E. The primary and best-known purpose of vitamin K is support of the process of blood clotting. Prothrombin and other clotting factors are dependent on vitamin K for production. It also plays a role in bone health, and may help to prevent **osteoporosis**. Appropriate growth and development are supported by adequate vitamin K.

There are several forms of the vitamin:

• K_1 or phylloquinone; also known as phytonadione

• K_2, a family of substances called menaquinones

• K_3 or menadione, a synthetic form of this vitamin

General use

The Required Daily Amount (RDA) of vitamin K is 5 micrograms (mcg) for infants less than six months old, 10 mcg for babies six months to one year old, 15 mcg for children aged one to three years, 20 mcg for those aged four to six years, and 30 mcg for those seven to ten years old. Males require 45 mcg from 11–14 years, 65 mcg from 15–18 years, 70 mcg from 19–24 years, and 80 mcg after the age of 24 years. Females need 45 mcg from 11–14 years, 55 mcg from 15–18 years, 60 mcg from 19–24 years, and 65 mcg after the age of 24, and for pregnant or lactating women. These values are based on an estimate of 1 mcg of vitamin K per kilogram of body weight.

The most common use of vitamin K is to supplement babies at birth, thus preventing hemorrhagic disease of the newborn. Routine administration of vitamin K to newborns is, however, being questioned by practitioners of evidence-based nursing. In 2003 the American Academy of Pediatrics (AAP) restated that prevention of bleeding from early vitamin K deficiency by administration of the vitamin is accepted practice. The AAP also noted that a possible link between supplemental vitamin K and early childhood **cancer** has not been proven as of 2003.

Others who may benefit from supplemental vitamin K include those taking medications that interact with it or deplete the supply. It also appears to have some effectiveness in preventing osteoporosis, but some studies done involved patients using a high dietary intake of the vitamin rather than supplements. In 2003, however, a group of Japanese researchers reported that supplemental doses of vitamin K_2 given together with vitamin D_3 appeared to reduce bone turnover and sustain bone density in postmenopausal women with mild osteoporosis.

People taking warfarin, a vitamin K antagonist, are able to use the vitamin as an antidote if the serum level of warfarin is too high, increasing the risk of hemorrhage. Vitamin K taken by mouth appears to be more effective than intramuscular injections of the vitamin when it is used to counteract the effects of warfarin.

Vitamin K is also used to treat bleeding from the esophagus and other complications of **cirrhosis**, a disease of the liver.

Some women find that supplemental vitamin K relieves the symptoms of **morning sickness** during **pregnancy**. This treatment is even more effective if vitamin K is taken together with **vitamin C**.

Topical formulations of vitamin K are sometimes touted as being able to reduce spider veins on the face and legs. The creams are quite expensive and the efficacy is questionable at best. However, recent clinical studies have shown that topical applications of vitamin K given to patients following laser treatments on the face are effective in minimizing bruising from the procedure.

More recently, researchers have been studying vitamin K intensively for its potential anticancer effects. Vitamin K_3 in particular may be useful as an adjuvant treatment for **ovarian cancer**.

Preparations

Natural sources

Dark green leafy vegetables are among the best food sources of vitamin K in the form of K_1. Seaweed is packed with it, and beef liver, cauliflower, eggs, and strawberries are rich sources as well. Vitamin K is fairly heat-stable, but gentle cooking preserves the content of other nutrients that are prone to breaking down when heated. Some of the supply for the body is synthesized as vitamin K_2 by the good bacteria in the intestines.

Supplemental sources

Vitamin K is not normally included in daily multivitamins, as deficiency is rare. Oral, topical, and injectable forms are available, but should not be used except under the supervision of a health care provider. Injectable forms are by prescription only. Supplements are generally given in the form of phytonadione since it is the most effective form and has a lower risk of toxicity than other types. Synthetic forms of vitamin K are also available for supplemental use.

Deficiency

Deficiency of vitamin K is uncommon in the general population but is of particular concern in neonates, who are born with low levels of vitamin K. Hemorrhagic disease of the newborn can affect infants who do not receive some form of vitamin K at birth. Affected babies tend to have prolonged and excessive bleeding following circumcision or blood draws. In the most serious cases, bleeding into the brain may occur. Most commonly an injection of vitamin K is given in the nursery following birth, but a series of oral doses is also occasionally used. The primary sign of a deficiency at any age is bleeding, and poor growth may also be observed in children.

Chronically low levels of vitamin K are correlated with higher risk of hip fracture in older men and women. A study done in 2003 reported that the current recommended dietary intake for vitamin K in adults may not be adequate for older women.

Risk factors for deficiency

Vitamin K deficiency is unusual, but may occur in certain populations, including those on the medications mentioned in interactions, alcoholics, and people with diseases of the gastrointestinal tract that impair absorption. Conditions that may be problematic include **Crohn's disease**, chronic **diarrhea**, sprue, and ulcerative colitis. Anything that impairs fat absorption also risks decreasing the absorption of the fat-soluble vitamins. Long term use of broad spectrum antibiotics destroys the bacteria in the intestinal tract that are necessary for the body's production of vitamin K.

Precautions

Allergic reactions to vitamin K supplements can occur, although they are rare. Symptoms may include flushed skin, **nausea**, rash, and **itching**. Medical attention should be sought if any of these symptoms occur. Infants receiving vitamin K injections occasionally suffer hemolytic **anemia** or high bilirubin levels, noticeable from the yellow cast of the skin. Emergency medical treatment is needed for these babies. Liver and brain impairment are possible in severe cases.

Certain types of liver problems necessitate very cautious use of some forms of vitamin K. Menadiol **sodium** diphosphate, a synthetic form also known as vitamin K_4, may cause problems in people with biliary fistula or obstructive **jaundice**. A particular metabolic disease called G6-PD deficiency also calls for careful use of vitamin K_4. The expertise of a health care professional is called for under these circumstances. Sheldon Saul Hendler, MD, PhD, advises there is no reason to supplement with more than 100 mcg daily except in cases of frank vitamin K deficiency.

Side effects

Oral forms of vitamin K_4 may occasionally irritate the gastrointestinal tract. High doses greater than 500 mcg daily have been reported to cause some allergic-type reactions, such as skin **rashes**, itching, and flushing.

Interactions

There are numerous medications that can interfere with the proper absorption or function of vitamin K. The long-term use of antacids may decrease the efficacy of the vitamin, as can certain anticoagulants. Warfarin is an anticoagulant that antagonizes vitamin K. Efficacy of the vitamin is also decreased by dactinomycin and sucralfate. Absorption is decreased by cholestyramine and colestipol, which are drugs used to lower blood **cholesterol** levels. Other drugs that may cause a deficiency include long-term use of mineral oil, quinidine, and sulfa drugs. Primaquine increases the risk of side effects from taking supplements.

Other types of prescription medications that may cause vitamin K depletion include anticonvulsants (drugs to prevent seizures), including valproic acid; macrolide, aminoglycoside, cephalosporin, and fluoroquinolone antibiotics; phenobarbital; and dapsone (used to treat leprosy and skin **infections**).

Resources

BOOKS

Bratman, Steven, and David Kroll. *Natural Health Bible.* Rocklin, CA: Prima Publishing, 1999.

Griffith, H. Winter. *Vitamins, Herbs, Minerals & Supplements: The Complete Guide.* AZ: Fisher Books, 1998.

Jellin, Jeff, Forrest Batz, and Kathy Hitchens. *Pharmacist's letter/Prescriber's Letter Natural Medicines Comprehensive Database.* CA: Therapeutic Research Faculty, 1999.

Pelletier, Kenneth R., MD. *The Best Alternative Medicine*, Part I: Food for Thought. New York: Simon & Schuster, 2002.

Pressman, Alan H., and Sheila Buff. *The Complete Idiot's Guide to Vitamins and Minerals*. New York: Alpha Books, 1997.

PERIODICALS

American Academy of Pediatrics Committee on Fetus and Newborn. "Controversies Concerning Vitamin K and the Newborn. American Academy of Pediatrics Committee on Fetus and Newborn." *Pediatrics* 112 (July 2003) (1 Pt 1): 191–192.

Booth, S. L., L. Martini, J. W. Peterson, et al. "Dietary Phylloquinone Depletion and Repletion in Older Women." *Journal of Nutrition* 133 (August 2003): 2565–2569.

Crowther, M. A., J. D. Douketis, T. Schnurr, et al. "Oral Vitamin K Lowers the International Normalized Ratio More Rapidly Than Subcutaneous Vitamin K in the Treatment of Warfarin-Associated Coagulopathy. A Randomized, Controlled Trial." *Annals of Internal Medicine* 137 (August 20, 2002): 251-254.

Iwamoto, J., T. Takeda, and S. Ichimura. "Treatment with Vitamin D_3 and/or Vitamin K_2 for Postmenopausal Osteoporosis." *Keio Journal of Medicine* 52 (September 2003): 147–150.

Lamson, D. W., and S. M. Plaza. "The Anticancer Effects of Vitamin K." *Alternative Medicine Review* 8 (August 2003): 303–318.

Libby, E. N., and D. A. Garcia. "A Survey of Oral Vitamin K Use by Anticoagulation Clinics." *Archives of Internal Medicine* 162 (September 9, 2002): 1893-1896.

Lucena, M. I., R. J. Andrade, G. Tognoni, et al. "Multicenter Hospital Study on Prescribing Patterns for Prophylaxis and Treatment of Complications of Cirrhosis." *European Journal of Clinical Pharmacology* 58 (September 2002): 435-440.

Medves, J. M. "Three Infant Care Interventions: Reconsidering the Evidence." *Journal of Obstetric, Gynecologic, and Neonatal Nursing* 31 (September-October 2002): 563-569.

Shah, N. S., M. C. Lazarus, R. Bugdodel, et al. "The Effects of Topical Vitamin K on Bruising After Laser Treatment." *Journal of the American Academy of Dermatology* 47 (August 2002): 241-244.

von Gruenigen, V. E., J. M. Jamison, J. Gilloteaux, et al. "The in vitro Antitumor Activity of Vitamins C and K_3 Against Ovarian Carcinoma." *Anticancer Research* 23 (July-August 2003): 3279–3287.

ORGANIZATIONS

American Academy of Pediatrics (AAP). 141 Northwest Point Boulevard, Elk Grove Village, IL 60007. (847) 434-4000. <http://www.aap.org>.

American Society for Clinical Nutrition. 9650 Rockville Pike, Bethesda, MD 20814. (301) 530-7110. <http://www.faseb.org/ascn>.

American Society of Hematology (ASH). 1900 M Street, NW, Suite 200, Washington, DC 20036. (202) 776-0544. <http://www.hematology.org>.

Judith Turner
Rebecca J. Frey, PhD

Vitex *see* **Chasteberry tree**

Vomiting

Definition

Vomiting is the forceful discharge of stomach contents through the mouth.

Description

Vomiting, also called emesis, is a symptomatic response to any number of harmful triggers. Vomiting is a forceful expulsion, and is different from regurgitation—the effortless return of stomach contents to the mouth. Although unpleasant, vomiting is an important function because it rids the body of harmful substances.

Vomiting is a complex process resulting from the coordinated interaction of nerve pathways, the brain, and muscles of the gastrointestinal system. The primary vomiting trigger point in the brain is called the area postrema. This structure is exposed to chemicals in the bloodstream and the cerebrospinal fluid (the fluid found in the brain and spinal cord). Scientific studies have shown that stimulation of the area postrema by a wide variety of drugs as well as bacterial toxins, radiation, and physiologic conditions, induces vomiting.

Certain nerve pathways (called afferent neural pathways) induce vomiting when triggered by motion, ear **infections** or tumors, **Ménière's disease** (a disease characterized by recurrent vertigo), odors, visual stimulation, **pain**, and bad tastes. Still other nerve pathways (peripheral afferent neural pathways) induce vomiting in response to stomach irritants, distension of the intestines and bile ducts, abdominal inflammation, and myocardial infarction (**heart attack**).

The physical act of vomiting is controlled by multiple sites of the brain stem. When activated, these structures send signals to the throat, diaphragm, and abdominal muscles. These signals result in the simultaneous contraction of these muscles, which brings the stomach contents up through the esophagus (the tube between the stomach and the throat) and out the mouth. During vomiting, breathing is inhibited, except for short breaths between discharges. Bradycardia (decrease in the heart rate) and changes in blood pressure may occur during retching and vomiting.

Causes & symptoms

Vomiting can be caused by many different things. Vomiting that lasts only one or two days is usually caused by infection, a reaction to medication, a toxin, uremia (accumulation of protein breakdown products in the bloodstream), and diabetic ketoacidosis (accumulation of toxins resulting from uncontrolled diabetes). Vomiting that lasts longer than one week can be caused by a long-term medical or psychiatric condition. Causes of vomiting include:

- Medications. Drugs are the most common cause of vomiting, especially during the first days of use. Drugs can induce vomiting by stimulation of the area postrema or by direct stimulation of peripheral nerve pathways. Medications that commonly cause vomiting include **cancer** drugs, pain relievers (especially opioids), heart medications, diuretics, hormones, antibiotics, antiasthmatics, gastrointestinal drugs, and medications that act on the brain.

- Infections. Infections of the gastrointestinal system or whole body can cause vomiting. Gastrointestinal infections are more common in infants, toddlers, and young adults (20–29 years old) who usually get 1.2 infections each year. Infections that can cause vomiting include bacterial, viral, and parasitic gastrointestinal infections, severe acute respiratory syndrome (SARS), otitis media

(**ear infection**), **meningitis** (infection of the membrane that surrounds the brain and spinal cord), and **hepatitis** (infection of the liver).

- Gastrointestinal and abdominal disorders. Disorders of the gastrointestinal system that can produce vomiting include blockage of the stomach or small intestine, motility disorders (muscles in the esophagus become discoordinated or weak, causing difficulty swallowing, regurgitation, and sometimes pain), **indigestion**, radiation therapy-induced changes, **Crohn's disease** (chronic recurrent inflammation of the intestines), peptic ulcer, worm infestations, or inflammation of the appendix, gall bladder, or pancreas.

- Nervous system disorders. Cancers, infarction (an area of dead tissue caused by an obstruction in the artery supplying the area), bleeding (hemorrhage), birth defects, ear disorders, **motion sickness**, weightlessness, ear tumors, Ménière's disease, unpleasant memories, psychogenic (caused by mental factors) issues, and bad tastes or smells can all cause vomiting.

- Hormones and physiological conditions. Hormonal and metabolic (physical and chemical processes of the body) conditions that can cause vomiting include: parathyroidism, diabetic ketoacidosis, **hyperthyroidism** (condition caused by excessive ingestion or production of thyroid hormone), Addison's disease, uremia, and **pregnancy**. Pregnancy is the most common cause of vomiting associated with the hormonal system. Vomiting associated with pregnancy is often called morning sickness.

- Postoperation. Anesthesia and pain medications can cause **nausea** and vomiting, which are complications associated with 17–39% of surgeries.

- Cyclic vomiting syndrome (CVS). This rare disorder occurs in children usually beginning at age five years, although it also occurs in adults. It is characterized by, on average, eight attacks of vomiting lasting for 20 hours each year. Although the exact cause is unknown, there seems to be a relationship between cyclic vomiting and migraine headaches.

- Poisons. Arsenic and other heavy metals, weed killers and household cleaning agents, and many other substances may cause vomiting if inhaled or swallowed.

- Miscellaneous causes. Excessive alcohol consumption causes vomiting by acting both on the gastrointestinal tract and the brain.

Nausea is often associated with vomiting. Vomiting may be preceded by retching, in which the muscles contract as for vomiting but without the discharge of stomach contents. The patient may hyperventilate (breathe rapidly and deeply) and salivate before vomiting begins.

Patients should consult a physician immediately if there is blood in the vomitus (expelled stomach contents).

Other symptoms associated with vomiting depend upon the cause. Gastrointestinal infection would also cause **fever**, muscle pain, and **diarrhea**. Patients with peptic ulcer, intestinal blockage, cholecystitis or **pancreatitis** (inflammation of the gall bladder or pancreas) would experience abdominal pain. Meningitis symptoms include neck stiffness, **headache**, vision changes, and changes in mental processes.

Diagnosis

Vomiting may be diagnosed by an internal medicine specialist or a gastroenterologist. A detailed medical history will be taken and will include specifics about the vomiting including frequency, a description of the vomitus, duration, how soon after meals vomiting occurs, and any other symptoms. The history alone can help the physician to narrow down the cause to a few choices. The patient's abdomen will be palpated (felt with the hands) to detect any abnormalities. Vital signs will be taken to identify any abnormalities in heart rate, blood pressure, or temperature.

Although the medical history and physical exam is usually sufficient to determine the cause of vomiting, certain laboratory tests may also be performed. Blood tests may be performed to check for dehydration (decreased water), **anemia** (decreased number of red blood cells or iron-poor blood), and electrolyte (blood chemicals) imbalances, as well as specific tests to confirm the suspected diagnosis.

In some cases, more advanced testing may be required. These include x rays, endoscopy (a thin, wand-like camera used to visualize internal organs), magnetic resonance imaging (MRI), ultrasound (using sound waves to visualize internal organs), and computed tomography (CT) scanning. In addition, there are tests that measure stomach emptying and the pressure and motility of the stomach and intestine.

Treatment

Alternative treatments can be effective in treating vomiting, but not the underlying cause. A physician should be consulted if vomiting is recurrent and/or lasts for more than a few days.

Dietary changes

The best dietary approach is to eat foods that can be quickly cleared from the stomach. Foods that are high in fat are slow to digest and place the patient at risk for additional vomiting. Ingestion of a low-fat, predominately liquid diet taken in frequent small meals can help relieve vomiting. Dry soda crackers are a good choice when nausea sets in. After vomiting, the patient should not eat for one hour, after which small servings of broth, bread, or flat soda may be taken. It is important to replenish the fluids lost by vomiting. Juice therapists recommend drinking a juice made from fresh **ginger**, apples, and carrots. Supplementation with vitamin B_6 was found to reduce the symptoms of **morning sickness** in pregnant women.

Herbals

The herbs that are effective in relieving nausea and vomiting include:

- apple tree (*Pyrus malus*) bark tea
- bergamot (*Monarda citriodora*) tea
- black **horehound** (*Ballota nigra*) infusion
- codonopsis (*Codonopsis pilosula*) decoction
- galangal (*Alpinia officinarum*) infusion
- ginger (*Zingiber officinale*) infusion or crystallized
- lemongrass (*Cymbogen citratus*) oil or tea
- nutmeg (*Myristica fragrans*) capsules
- turmeric (*Curcuma longa*) infusion

Chinese medicine

Practitioners of **traditional Chinese medicine** use **acupuncture**, ear acupuncture, herbals, and patent medicines in the treatment of vomiting. The following herbals may be made into soups, which are sipped frequently: Lu Gen (*Rhizoma phragmitis*); Zhu Ru (*Caulis bambusae in taeniis*), Bai Mao Gen (*Rhizoma imperatae*), and Pi Pa Ye (*Folium eriobotryae*); and Huo Xiang (*Herba agastachis*) and Pei Lan (*Herba eupatorii*). Placing a drop of Sheng Jiang (*Rhizoma zingiberis recens*) on the tongue can check vomiting. Patent medicines used to treat vomiting include: Huo Xiang Zheng Qi Wan (**Agastache** Pill to Rectify Qi), Yu Shu Dan (Jade Pivot Pill), Zuo Jin Wan (Left Metal Pill), and Bao He Wan (Preserve Harmony Pill).

Homeopathy

Homeopathic remedies are chosen based upon the specific set of symptoms displayed by the patient. **Ipecac** is chosen for strong nausea and vomiting. Bismuth or Phosphorous is indicated when vomiting is caused primarily by liquids. **Nux vomica** is recommended when vomiting is caused by emotional **stress** and for patients with **heartburn**, nausea, and retching. Tabacum is indicated for vomiting caused by motion. Veratrum album is indicated for the patient with nausea, vomiting, and diarrhea. Arsenicum is recommended for the patient with violent vomiting, diarrhea, abdominal pain, exhaustion, restlessness, and thirst. **Bryonia** is recommended for **gastroenteritis** (inflammation of the lining of the gastrointestinal system).

Ayurveda

Ayurvedic practitioners believe that vomiting is caused by high pitta in the stomach. Remedies for vomiting are:

- yogurt containing cardamon and honey
- warm milk containing cardamon and nutmeg
- tea prepared from cumin seeds and nutmeg
- fresh pineapple juice (1 cup with a pinch of ginger and black pepper and 0.5 tsp sugar) three times during a day of fasting
- water containing 10 drops lime juice, 0.5 tsp sugar, and 0.25 tsp baking soda
- cardamon seeds (chewed)
- ginger juice and onion juice (1 tsp each)
- water containing rose petal powder (0.5 tsp), sandalwood powder (0.25 tsp), rock candy powder (0.5 tsp), and lime juice (10 drops)

Other treatments

Various other treatments for vomiting include:

- Aromatherapy. The essential oil of **peppermint** is a traditional cure for vomiting.
- **Acupressure**. The acupressure points P5 and P6 located on the inner forearms are effective in treating vomiting. A wristband (Sea-Band) has been proven to be effective in reducing nausea and vomiting.
- Acupuncture. A National Institutes of Health consensus panel found that acupuncture is an effective treatment for chemotherapy and postoperative vomiting. A few people, however, experience nausea as a side effect of acupuncture.
- Behavioral interventions. Behavioral therapies such as desensitization, distraction, imagery, **relaxation**, and self-hypnosis have been shown to be effective in treating chemotherapy-induced vomiting.
- Hydrotherapy. Stomach upsets may be treated by drinking a glass of water containing **activated charcoal** powder.
- Reflexology. The reflex points solar plexus, chest, lung, diaphragm, esophagus, liver, stomach, gallbladder and thyroid, and pituitary and adrenal gland on the feet may help treat vomiting.

- Transcutaneous electrical nerve stimulation (TENS, which is a treatment where a mild electrical current is passed through electrodes on the skin to stimulate nerves and block pain signals). TENS can be effective in reducing postoperative vomiting.

Allopathic treatment

Treatment of vomiting depends upon the cause and severity but may include dietary changes, medications, and surgery. Replacement of lost fluids is an important component of treatment. Hospitalization may be required in some cases. Surgery may be needed to treat inflammatory conditions (such as cholecystitis) and physical abnormalities (such as blockage).

Medications used to treat vomiting are called antiemetics. Scopolamine, dimenhydrinate (Dramamine), and hyoscine are used to treat motion sickness; promethazine (Mepergan, Phenergan) is used to treat postoperative nausea; meclizine (Antivert, Bonine) is used to treat inner ear inflammation; and prochlorperazine (Compazine) is used for gastroenteritis, postoperative toxins, radiation, medications, and other causes of vomiting. Other medications that target the underlying cause of the vomiting may be used.

Newer drugs that have been developed to treat postoperative or postchemotherapy nausea and vomiting include ondansetron (Zofran) and granisetron (Kytril). Another treatment that has been found to lower the risk of nausea after surgery is intravenous administration of supplemental fluid before the operation.

Expected results

Most cases of vomiting resolve spontaneously. Complications of vomiting include dehydration, malnutrition, weight loss, and abnormalities of blood chemicals (including electrolytes, pH, and **potassium**). Vomiting by unconscious patients can lead to aspiration (inhalation of stomach contents), which can affect the lungs.

Prevention

Antiemetic drugs are effective at preventing vomiting. Some alternative treatments are effective at reducing nausea, which may prevent vomiting.

Resources

BOOKS

Cummings, Stephen and Dana Ullman. *Everybody's Guide to Homeopathic Medicines: Safe and Effective Remedies for You and Your Family.* 3rd. edition. New York, NY: Jeremy P. Tarcher/Putnam, 1997.
"Functional Vomiting." Section 3, Chapter 21 in *The Merck Manual of Diagnosis and Therapy*, edited by Mark H.

KEY TERMS

Area postrema—A structure of the brain stem that triggers vomiting in response to toxins in the bloodstream and cerebrospinal fluid.

Emesis—The medical term for vomiting.

Retching—The coordinated contraction of muscles as for vomiting but without the discharge of stomach contents.

Vomitus—The medical term for the contents of the stomach expelled during vomiting.

Beers, MD, and Robert Berkow, MD. Whitehouse Station, NJ: Merck Research Laboratories, 2002.

Hasler, William L. Approach to the Patient with Nausea and Vomiting. *Textbook of Gastroenterology.* 3rd edition, edited by Tadataka Yamada, et al. Philadelphia, PA: Lippincott Williams & Wilkins, 1999.

Reichenberg-Ullman, Judyth and Robert Ullman. *Homeopathic Self-Care: The Quick and Easy Guide for the Whole Family.* Rockland, CA: Prima Publishing, 1997.

Ying, Zhou Zhong and Jin Hui De. Vomiting. *Clinical Manual of Chinese Herbal Medicine and Acupuncture.* New York: Churchill Livingston, 1997.

PERIODICALS

Ali, S. Z., A. Taguchi, B. Holtmann, and A. Kurz. "Effect of Supplemental Pre-Operative Fluid on Postoperative Nausea and Vomiting." *Anaesthesia* 58 (August 2003): 780–784.

Cepeda, M. S., J. T. Farrar, M. Baumgarten, et al. "Side Effects of Opioids During Short-Term Administration: Effect of Age, Gender, and Race." *Clinical Pharmacology and Therapeutics* 74 (August 2003): 102–112.

Chung, A., L. Bui, and E. Mills. "Adverse Effects of Acupuncture. Which Are Clinically Significant?" *Canadian Family Physician* 49 (August 2003): 985–989.

O'Brien, C. M., G. Titley, and P. Whitehurst. "A Comparison of Cyclizine, Ondansetron and Placebo as Prophylaxis Against Postoperative Nausea and Vomiting in Children." *Anaesthesia* 58 (July 2003): 707–711.

Quinla, J. D., and D. A. Hill. "Nausea and Vomiting of Pregnancy." *American Family Physician* 68 (July 1, 2003): 121–128.

Ratnaike, R. N. "Acute and Chronic Arsenic Toxicity." *Postgraduate Medical Journal* 79 (July 2003): 391–396.

Tan, M. "Granisetron: New Insights Into Its Use for the Treatment of Chemotherapy-Induced Nausea and Vomiting." *Expert Opinion in Pharmacotherapy* 4 (September 2003): 1563–1571.

Tiwari, A., S. Chan, A. Wong, et al. "Severe Acute Respiratory Syndrome (SARS) in Hong Kong: Patients' Experiences." *Nursing Outlook* 51 (September-October 2003): 212–219.

Walling, Anne D. "Ginger Relieves Nausea and Vomiting During Pregnancy." *American Family Physician* 64 (November 15, 2001): 1745.

ORGANIZATIONS

American Gastroenterological Association (AGA). 7910 Woodmont Ave., 7th Floor, Bethesda, MD 20814. (310) 654-2055. http://www.gastro.org/index.html. aga001@aol.com.

Belinda Rowland
Rebecca J. Frey, PhD

Vulvovaginitis *see* **Vaginitis**

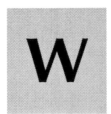

Warts

Definition

Warts, also called verrucae, are small benign growths usually caused by a viral infection of the skin or mucous membrane. The virus infects the surface layer of skin. The viruses that cause warts are members of the human papilloma virus (HPV) family, of which there are many different strains. Warts are not cancerous but some strains of HPV, usually not associated with warts, have been linked with **cancer** formation. Warts are contagious from person to person and from one area of the body to another on the same person.

Description

Particularly common among children, young adults, and women, warts are a problem for 7–10% of the population. There are close to 60 types of HPV that cause warts, each preferring a specific skin location. For instance, some types of HPV cause warts to grow on the skin, others cause them to grow inside the mouth, while still others cause them to grow on the genital and rectal areas. However, most can be active anywhere on the body. The virus enters through the skin and produces new warts after an incubation period of one to eight months. Warts are usually skin colored and feel rough to the touch, but they also can be dark, flat, and smooth.

Warts are passed from person to person, directly and indirectly. Some people are continually susceptible to warts, while others are more resistant to HPV and seldom get them. The virus takes hold more readily when the skin has been damaged in some way, which may explain why children who bite their nails tend to have warts located on their fingers. People who take a medication to suppress their immune system or are on long-term steroid use are also prone to a wart virus infection. The same is true for patients with **AIDS**.

The main categories of warts are common warts (face and hands), plantar warts (feet), and venereal warts.

Hand warts (verruca vulgaris) can grow anywhere on the hands, but usually occur where skin has been damaged in some way (e.g. picking or nail biting). This is a rough horny lesion varying in size from 1 mm–2cm in diameter.

Foot warts (verruca plantaris) known as plantar warts, are the most painful type of wart, due to the pressure exerted on them. They are most common in children and young adults, since they are often contracted in locker rooms and swimming pool areas. If left untreated, they can grow to an inch or more in circumference and spread into clusters. Those suffering from diabetes are more likely to suffer from plantar warts, and may also suffer complications due to the reduced potential for their bodies to heal themselves.

Flat warts tend to grow in great numbers and are smaller and smoother than other warts. They can erupt anywhere, appearing more frequently on the legs of women, the neck and dorsum of the hands, the faces of children, and on the areas of the face that are shaved by young adult males.

Genital warts, also called condylomata acuminata, moist warts, fig warts, or venereal warts, are one of the most common sexually transmitted diseases (STDs). Genital warts are more contagious than other types of warts. Approximately one million new cases of genital warts are diagnosed in the United States every year. It is estimated that two-thirds of persons coming into contact with genital warts will develop symptoms within three months.

Genital warts tend to be small flat bumps or they may be thin and pointed in shape. They are usually soft, moist, pink to red in color, occurring as a single lesion or in clusters that resemble a cauliflower, and not scaly like other warts. In women, genital warts appear on the external genitalia, within the vagina, on the cervix, and around the anus or within the rectum. In men, genital warts usually appear on the tip of the penis but may also be found on the scrotum or around the anus. Genital warts can also develop in the mouth of a person who has

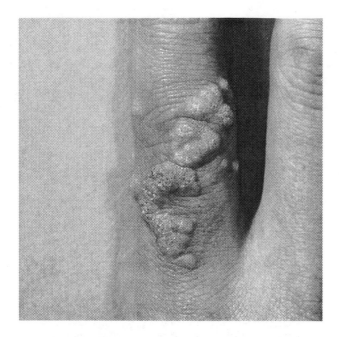

Cluster of warts on finger. *(Custom Medical Stock Photo. Reproduced by permission.)*

had oral sexual contact with an infected person. They may also appear, less often, between the toes.

Filiform wart is a long, horny, finger-like projection that is usually found in multiples. Seen most commonly in adult males, they occur in the bearded area of the face or on the eyelids and neck.

Causes & symptoms

Since warts are caused by a virus, they can only be caught by contact with a source of infection. This can be direct physical contact, or secondary contact with the shed skin of a wart (through a floor or a towel for example). As the incubation period for warts is quite long, it is often difficult to pinpoint sources of infection. Individuals whose immune systems are deficient most often contract warts. AIDS patients commonly suffer from warts, and it is not uncommon for warts to appear at the site of a trauma (**burns**, cuts or abrasions.)

Diagnosis

Common warts are rough, irregular, skin colored or brownish. Warts that are brownish in color, or that do not respond to treatment, should be checked by a physician to exclude the possibility that they may be malignant growths.

Treatment

Warts may need no treatment at all, since a large proportion of them (67% over a two-year period) disappear spontaneously. This is particularly so in the case of flat warts. However, a wart that appears unusual in any way should be checked by a physician, as a small proportion can become malignant. Generally, the main criterion for treatment of warts is a cosmetic one, if it is found to be embarrassing by the sufferer, or unpleasant to others.

Acupuncture

The aim with **acupuncture** will be to raise the general well-being of the patient, improve the functioning of the immune system, and free blockages of "chi" or life force. Warts and other health problems will be less likely to occur as general health and resistance are improved.

Aromatherapy

Since warts are caused by viral **infections**, the aim of an **aromatherapy** treatment would be to kill the virus with the application of an appropriate essential oil. There are many oils that have antiviral properties, so the therapist will also endeavor to choose oils that are appropriate for the patient. Onion and **garlic** oils both have powerful antiviral properties, but perhaps **tea tree oil**, which also possesses remarkable anti-viral properties, might be more acceptable as far as smell is concerned.

Colloidal silver

The use of **colloidal silver** against viruses of all kinds has proved very successful. It should be topically applied to the wart, but can be taken internally to promote functioning of the immune system, and thus prevent warts from occurring.

Herbal medicine

Herbal remedies for genital warts and other STDs have attracted considerable recent attention because of the epidemic spread of these diseases in developing countries where most people cannot afford allopathic treatments. One traditional herbal remedy from Colombia that is being studied is extracts of plants belonging to the Euphorbia family. These compounds have been used to treat ulcers, tumors, and warts for generations, and some of them appear to be effective in treating genital warts.

Before applying any herbal cure to a wart, as much of the wart as possible should be removed, in order to give the cure a head start.

Apple juice: Apply the juice of a sour apple. Action is due to the **magnesium** in the juice.

Banana skin: First the wart should be rubbed with an abrader, and a fresh banana skin (immediately after opening) should be applied and left overnight.

Cabbage: Apply fresh juice from a white cabbage.

Chickweed: Apply the juice to the wart.

Dandelion: The juice of the dandelion is a very old English cure for warts.

Garlic: Rub a raw clove on the wart every night until it disappears.

Green figs: The white milk from a green fig is excellent at removing warts.

House leek: This is a plant commonly found in rock gardens. It has thick fleshy leaves and its juice is rich in supermalate of **calcium**, which will destroy warts.

Pineapple: Cotton wool should be soaked in the fresh juice of a pineapple. The enzymes of the pineapple will dissolve the wart.

Rubber plant: If the stem of a leaf from a rubber plant is broken, white liquid will ooze out. If this is applied to the wart over a period of two to three days, the wart should disappear.

Naturopathy

Naturopathy, in common with many alternative therapies, works on the principle that given the right circumstances, such as pure air, pure water, and first class **nutrition**, the body will heal itself and become extremely resistant to illness. Naturopaths believe that such symptoms as warts are the result of toxins in the body, and an immune system that is not running efficiently. They may prescribe treatments such as **colonic irrigation**, alongside a program of healthy eating to raise the general level of health. A naturopath may suggest a paste made with **vitamin C**, applied to the wart daily for a period of a few weeks.

Visualization

This method, also known as creative imagery, has skeptically been described as "willing yourself well," but practically it has been found to be very effective for a range of conditions, both physical and emotional. The patient is required to sit in a relaxed state, breathing evenly, and visualize the self in the condition he or she would like to be. In this case, perhaps he or she visualizes the body overcoming the warts and absorbing them, leaving behind healthy skin. This method has been found particularly suitable for children, as it has no side effects and therapists claim it has a good success rate.

Folk remedies

There are many remedies for warts that have been handed down from generation to generation all over the world. The following remedies have excellent track records.

Thread: a length of thread should be tied around the wart, and tightened every day until the wart drops off.

Human saliva: the sufferer applies his or her saliva to the wart first thing every morning.

Allopathic treatment

Warts may be self-treated by a number of allopathic remedies, but care should be taken as they are fairly strong chemicals (usually salicylic acid). Those suffering from diabetes, **heart disease** or circulation problems, or any degree of **peripheral neuropathy**, should not attempt to treat themselves with any of these preparations, because of the risk of damage to tissue, and because of their increased susceptibility to infection.

In addition, the face and mucous membranes may scar, so it may be preferable to seek professional advice.

A physician may use cautery (use of heat) or cryosurgery (use of extreme cold, usually in the form of liquid nitrogen) to remove warts. These are processes that require precision, and therefore are highly skilled procedures. Another drawback is that they can be painful. Increasingly, laser treatments are also being used to treat warts, whereby the laser beam vaporizes the wart tissue. Pulsed laser treatments appear to be particularly effective in treating warts in the anogenital region of children.

A newer allopathic medication that shows promise in the treatment of resistant viral facial warts is diphencyprone (DPC), a drug that was developed to treat a type of **hair loss** known as alopecia areata. DPC has shown effectiveness in removing facial warts that were resistant to both cryosurgery and other topical drugs.

Expected results

Allopathic methods for the treatment of warts are generally successful, but they carry more risk of scarring than natural methods. More than one alternative method may have to be tried before success is achieved, but they carry the added bonus of adding to the well-being of the patient, and not harming the body. Allopathic treatments involve the use of strong chemicals, which carry risks and are not compatible with body chemistry. Usually, warts either disappear spontaneously or are treated successfully with no scarring or lasting effects. However, occasionally, what appears to be a wart is the beginning of a type of cancer, so those that are resistant to treatment should be seen by a physician.

Recurrent genital warts are a serious personal and public health concern. Even though genital warts may be removed, the virus itself continues to live. Certain types of HPV can cause tissue changes in the cervix of women with recurrent infection that may lead to cervical cancer. The general recommendation for women who have a history of genital warts is to see their doctors every six months for Pap smears to monitor any changes that may occur.

Prevention

To avoid foot warts, footwear should always be worn in public places and feet should be kept clean and dry. In general, warts should not be picked, to avoid cross infection, and any patch of damaged skin should be protected. Every effort should be made to keep the immune system in peak working condition.

Genital warts can be prevented by using condoms and avoiding unprotected sexual contact. Barrier protection will not, however, prevent the spread of wart-causing HPV to such uncovered areas as the pubis and upper thighs.

Although vaccines to prevent the spread of human papilloma virus are under investigation as of 2002, they will not be available for general use for at least several years.

Resources

BOOKS

Buchman, Dian Dincin. *Herbal Medicine.* London: Tiger Books International, 1991.

Kenton, Leslie. *The Joy of Beauty.* London: Century Publishing, 1993.

The Editors of Time-Life Books. *The Medical Advisor: The Complete Guide to Alternative and Conventional Treatments.* Alexandria, VA: Time-Life Books, 1997.

Renner, John H. *The Home Remedies Handbook.* Publications International, Ltd., 1994.

Stupik, Ramona. *AMA Complete Guide to Women's Health.* New York: Random House, 1996.

PERIODICALS

Betancur-Galvis, L. A., G. E. Morales, J. E. Forero, and J. Roldan. "Cytotoxic and Antiviral Activities of Colombian Medicinal Plant Extracts of the *Euphorbia* Genus." *Memorias do Instituto Oswaldo Cruz* 97 (June 2002): 541-546.

Brentjens, M. H., K. A. Yeung-Yue, P. C. Lee, and S. K. Tyring. "Human Papillomavirus: A Review." *Dermatologic Clinics* 20 (April 2002): 315-331.

Centers for Disease Control and Prevention. "Sexually Transmitted Diseases Treatment Guidelines 2002." *MMWR Recommendations and Reports* 51 (RR-6) (May 10, 2002): 1-78.

Garland, S. M. "Human Papillomavirus Update with a Particular Focus on Cervical Disease." *Pathology* 34 (June 2002): 213-224.

Pollock, B., and A. S. Highet. "An Interesting Response to Diphencyprone (DPC) Sensitization on Facial Warts: Review of DPC Treatment for Viral Warts." *Journal of Dermatological Treatment* 13 (June 2002): 47-50.

KEY TERMS

Condyloma acuminata (plural, condylomata)— The medical term for warts in the genital region or anus.

Cryotherapy—A technique of removing warts by freezing with liquid nitrogen.

Epidermis—The outer layer of human skin.

Human papilloma virus—A family of viruses that causes hand warts, foot warts, flat warts, and genital warts.

Salicylic acid—An agent prescribed in the treatment of hyperkeratotic skin conditions and fungal infections.

Verruca (plural, verrucae)—The medical term for warts.

Tuncel, A., M. Gorgu, M. Ayhan, et al. "Treatment of Anogenital Warts by Pulsed Dye Laser." *Dermatologic Surgery* 28 (April 2002): 350-352.

Vermani, K., and S. Garg. "Herbal Medicines for Sexually Transmitted Diseases and AIDS." *Journal of Ethnopharmacology* 80 (April 2002): 49-66.

ORGANIZATIONS

American Academy of Dermatology. P.O. Box 4014, 930 N. Meacham Rd., Schaumburg, IL 60168-5014. (847) 330-2300. Fax: (847)330-0050. <www.aad.org>.

American Academy of Family Physicians. 8880 Ward Parkway, Kansas City, MO 64114 (816) 333-9700. <www.aafp.org/health.info>.

American Podiatric Medical Association. 9312 Old Georgetown Rd, Bethesda, MD 20814–1698. (301) 571-9200. <www.apma.org>.

Centers for Disease Control and Prevention (CDC). 1600 Clifton Road, Atlanta, GA 30333. (404) 639-3311. <www.cdc.gov>.

OTHER

Medscape. http://www.medscape.com/micromedex/CareNotes/dermatology/ElectrocauteryWartRemoval.html.

Patricia Skinner
Rebecca J. Frey, PhD

Wasabi

Description

Wasabi (*Wasabia japonica*) is an edible plant member of the Cruciferae family, which includes cabbage, turnips, and mustard. Wasabi shares the anticancer benefits of this family. Native to Japan where it has been cultivated since the tenth century, it is still considered a staple condiment in that country. Traditional preparation involves using a sharkskin grater called an *oroshi*.

Wasabi's culinary popularity and chemical bioactivity make it valuable medicinally and industrially. Demand for wasabi has created a relatively short supply, higher prices, and new commercial opportunities. These new opportunities include research and development of cultivation technologies, particularly in Canada, and exportation from Japan of *seiyo wasabi*, or Western wasabi—imitations made of horseradish (*Cochlearia armoracia*). Western and Japanese wasabi are both highly prized.

Wasabi is a perennial, root-like rhizome that is cylindrical in shape. A brownish-green skin covers its pale green flesh. The plant grows to about 18 in (46 cm) in height and produces leaves on long stems from the crown of the plant. As the plant ages, the leaves fall off and a rhizome, or creeping underground stem, is formed, from which new buds arise as modified stems. The modified stem is the part of the plant that is used. The highest quality wasabi, whose translated name is mountain hollyhock (also known as *sawa wasabi*), thrives on cool water. It grows along the edges of cold mountain streams. When cultivated, rather than wild-crafted (harvested randomly from its natural growing places), it is grown on tree-shaded, terraced gravel beds covered by a thin layer of cool running mountain water or on artificially shaded gravel ridges formed in larger river beds. A lower quality wasabi (*oka wasabi*) is grown in fields. There are two varieties of wasabi, *Daruma*—considered to have a more attractive appearance—and *Mazuma*—considered to have more heat. Wasabi is described as being "hot and fiery without burning," which changes to a sweetness that lingers in the mouth.

General use

Historically, wasabi has been consumed as a condiment, used similarly to horseradish or mustard. Its pungent flavor and aroma may add a piquant flavor to sushi, marinades or sauces, and rice, noodle, and fish dishes. In Japanese restaurants across North America, sashimi and sushi may be served with a small mound of grated wasabi or wasabi paste. Nontraditional uses include adding wasabi to mashed potatoes, tuna sandwiches, or blending it with soy sauce. One source included it in a recipe for a unique Bloody Mary. Wasabi leaves marinated in sake, brine, or soy sauce, are eaten with a bowl of rice.

In addition to its flavor, wasabi has another benefit. Traditional Japanese cuisine includes raw fish, which is a potential source of parasites and bacteria. Wasabi's an-

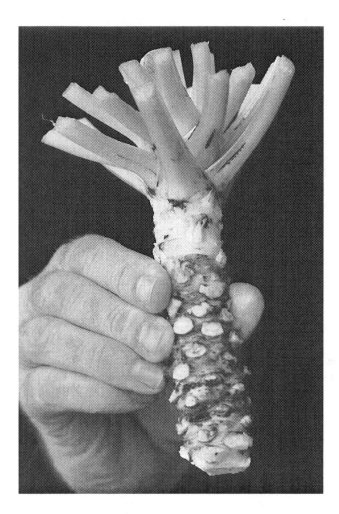

Wasabi root. (*Photograph by Don Ryan. AP Photos. Reproduced by permission.*)

tiparasitic, antimicrobial, and antibiotic abilities may be preventive against **food poisoning**. One source points specifically to wasabi's effectiveness against the Anisakis parasite. Another study, comparing the antibacterial activity of different foods against *Escherichia coli* (*E. coli*) and Staphylococcus bacteria, found that cruciferous plants possess antibacterial activity, with the highest activity found in wasabi (rhizome).

Other studies found that wasabi may be effective against the tooth-adhering ability of the bacteria *Streptococcus mutans*, thus inhibiting dental plaque and decay. Of special note are the numerous studies demonstrating wasabi's effectiveness against stomach **cancer** cells. One study found the induction of stomach cancer in rats was suppressed when they were given wasabi. The risk of hormone-related malignancies, such as breast and **prostate cancer**, may also be lowered. Some researchers believe that the cruciferous vegetables help the body eliminate excess endogenous (produced from within) and exogenous (produced from without but ingested or absorbed) hormones, such as estrogen. This action may be a result of wasabi's ability to stimulate the liver and gallbladder, aiding in the digestion of fatty foods and the processing of food nutrients.

Other medicinal benefits attributed to wasabi include its effectiveness against **diarrhea**, **blood clots**, inflammation, and **asthma**. Its pungent aroma may help relieve sinusitis and **bronchitis**. Although the amounts absorbed from culinary use may be negligible, wasabi reportedly also contains **potassium**, **calcium**, and **vitamin C**.

Industrial applications of wasabi under investigation include its usefulness in the development of other antibiotics, due to its own antibiotic qualities; its effectiveness as a fungicide against the blackleg fungus that threatens plants commercially valued for their oil, such as rapeseed and canola; and its possible use as an effective alternative to chemically toxic wood preservatives.

Preparations

Wasabi is most commonly found in powder or paste form. However, due to the scarcity and price of high quality wasabi, many of these preparations—including imports from Japan for retail sale and those served in Japanese restaurants—are imitations made of horseradish, mustard, a starchy binder, and coloring. Wasabi paste may be made from a powdered wasabi by adding water, and letting it stand 10 minutes to allow the flavor and heat to develop. One source noted that the powder may be safely stored in a cupboard, but recommended refrigerating the paste. A salad dressing may be made by combining 3 tablespoons of rice wine vinegar, 1 tablespoon honey, 1 teaspoon wasabi paste, 1 teaspoon soy sauce, and 1/2 teaspoon **sesame oil**.

Traditional wasabi is prepared freshly for each use, as its volatile oils are quickly dissipated. It is recommended that individuals select a fresh, cool, and succulent rhizome with nice color. It should be rinsed under cool water with a vegetable brush, cutting a fresh surface below or above the leaf node (a distinctive ridge as on bamboo stems). While maintaining a 90-degree angle to the grating surface, the wasabi should be grated in a circular motion against a traditional sharkskin, ceramic, or stainless steel grater. (It is not necessary to peel the wasabi rhizome before grating it.) Then it is gathered into a ball and allowed to sit momentarily at room temperature. It is best used within 15 to 20 minutes.

One source notes that wasabi products are often found in large grocery stores that sell Asian food products and ethnic condiments; Asian markets; fish markets; gourmet shops; and other alternative marketplaces. Prices are similar to other specialty condiments of equal quality.

Precautions

Wasabi should not come into contact with the eyes or nasal passages.

Due to its anti-inflammatory, antibiotic, antibacterial, antiparasitic, anticoagulant, and anti-asthmatic effects, the use of wasabi may magnify the effects of certain pharmaceutical drugs used for similar purposes. People with ulcers, esophageal reflux, kidney disorders, gastrointestinal disease, or those using hormone replacement therapy, are advised to consult with a healthcare professional before using wasabi.

Side effects

Due to its liver and gallbladder stimulating effects, eating wasabi may cause gastrointestinal disturbances, including diarrhea and **nausea**.

Interactions

One source notes that wasabi has possible interactions with anti-inflammatory analgesics, anesthetics, thyroid medications, corticosteroids, diuretics, and high blood pressure medications. This may be due in part to confusion with horseradish species. No other *Wasabia japonica*-drug interaction references are noted.

Resources

BOOKS
Black, Jacquelyn G. *Microbiology, Principles and Explorations,* 5th ed. Hoboken, NJ: John Wiley & Sons, 2002.

PERIODICALS
Cohen, S. "Wasabi May Make Sushi Safe." *Shape* (November 2002): 116.
Fuke, Y., Y. Ohishi, K. Iwashita, H. Ono, and K. Shinohara. "Growth Suppression of MKN-28 Human Stomach Cancer Cells by Wasabi (*Eutrema wasabi maxim*)." *Journal of the Japanese Society of Food Science & Technology* (1994): 709–11.
Fuke, Y., Y. Haga, H. Ono, T. Nomura, and K. Ryoyama. "Anticarcinogenic Activity of 6-methylsulfinylhexyl Isothiocyanate, an Active Anti-proliferative Principal of Wasabi (*Eutema wasabi maxim*)." *Cytotechnology* (1997): 197–203.
Hill, M., and G. Barclay. "Dig Up Great Taste." *The Herb Companion* (December 2003): 28–37.
Hodge, W. H. "Wasabi: Native Condiment Plant of Japan." *Economic Botany* (January 1974): 118–29.
Knittel, L. "10 Foods for a Healthy, Beautiful Smile." *Natural Health* (December 2002): 45–7.
Ono, H., S. Tesaki, S. Tanabe, and M. Watanabe. "6-Methlsulfinylhexyl Isothiocyanate and its Homologues as Food-oriented Compounds with Antibacterial Activity Against Escherichia coli and Staphylococcus aureus."

KEY TERMS

Crucifer—A type of vegetable that is now believed to guard against cancer, ulcers, and infections in the digestive tract. Examples of crucifers include wasabi, broccoli, cauliflower, mustard greens, and cabbage.

Rhizome—A subterranean plant stem that is distinguished from a true root by stem buds or nodes that develop into new shoots. A rhizome transports and stores water and nutrients. If a rhizome is cut, it does not die as would a root, but is capable of sprouting several new plants.

Sashimi—A traditional Japanese preparation of rice, fish, shell fish, mollusks, and other fish products, served with pickled vegetables.

Sushi—A traditional Japanese preparation of food wherein vinegared rice, vegetables, and fish or fish products, are wrapped in *nori* seaweed, cut, and served.

Bioscience, Biotechnology, and Biochemistry (February 1998): 363–5.

Tanida, N., A. Kawaura, A. Takahashi, K. Sawada, and T. Shimoyama. "Suppressive Effect of Wasabi (pungent Japanese spice) on Gastric Carcinogenesis Induced by MNNG in Rats." *Nutrition and Cancer* (1991): 53–8.

OTHER

American Chemical Society. *Wasabi! Sushi condiment may prevent cavities.* December 2000. <http://www.sciencedaily.com/>.

"Bamboo Select." *Botanical Features: Rhizomes.* [Cited May 22, 2004]. <http://www.bambooselect.com/UK/Botanical-features.htm>.

City Farmer, Canada's Office of Urban Agriculture. *Urban agricultural notes: Wasabia japonica.* <http://www.city-farmer.org/>.

Lerche-Davis, J. "Pull Out the Chop Sticks—Wasabi May Prevent Tooth Decay." *WebMD Medical News Archives* [cited June 14, 2004]. <http://www.mywedmd.com/>.

Mccauley, D. "Wasabi." *Canadian House & Home.* November 2000. [cited June 14, 2004]. <http://www. findarticles.com/>.

"Wasabi." *Wikipedia: The Free Encyclopedia* [cited June 14, 2004]. <http://en.wikipedia.org>.

Lee Ann Paradise
Katherine E. Nelson, N.D.

Water therapy *see* **Hydrotherapy**

Watsu *see* **Shiatsu**

Waxberry *see* **Bayberry**

Western cedar *see* **Red cedar**

Western herbalism *see* **Herbalism, Western**

Wheat germ

Description

Wheat germ is the embryo of the wheat kernel. It is separated from wheat being milled for flour. Wheat germ is **sodium** and **cholesterol** free, and dense in nutrients. It is rich in **vitamin E, magnesium, pantothenic acid, phosphorus**, thiamine, and **zinc**. It is also a source of coenzyme Q10 (ubiquinone) and PABA (para-aminobenzoic acid). Two tablespoons of wheat germ contains 65 calories, 6 grams protein, 2 grams of unsaturated fat, and 2 grams of fiber.

General use

Wheat germ is a food source, and is part of the breads and cereals food group. Its high vitamin and mineral content make it an extremely nutritious food. Wheat germ contains the following nutrients.

• Vitamin E. One cup of wheat germ contains 19.5 mg of vitamin E, and one tablespoon of wheat germ oil is packed with 26.2 mg of vitamin E. Vitamin E is an antioxidant, which is thought to protect the immune system.

• Magnesium. Magnesium assists the body in producing and transferring energy, and helps to maintain heart, bone, muscle, and circulatory system health.

• Pantothenic acid. The panthothenic acid in wheat germ helps the body process and use energy from food, and metabolizes cholesterol and fatty acids. There is approximately 1.24 mg of pantothenic acid, also called vitamin B_5, in 0.5 cup wheat germ. The U. S. recommended daily allowance (RDA) of pantothenic acid is 5 mg/day.

• Phosphorus. A quarter cup serving of wheat germ contains 232 mg of phosphorus. Phosphorus helps build bones and teeth and assists in metabolism. Adults should consume approximately 700 mg of the mineral daily.

• **Thiamine**. Thiamine, one of the B complex vitamins, is essential to normal growth, and to building healthy skin, muscle, bones, and hair. It also promotes normal functioning of the nervous system, and helps the body to metabolize alcohol. One cup of wheat germ contains

1.08 mg of thiamine, and the RDAs for men and women are 1.2 mg and 1.1 mg, respectively.

• Zinc. Wheat germ contains some zinc, a trace mineral and antioxidant essential for proper growth, immune system function, and hormone production.

• Coenzyme Q10. Coenzyme Q10, or ubiquinone, is an antioxidant that assists cells in transferring energy and oxygen.

• Para-aminobenzoic acid (PABA). PABA helps to maintain the balance of intestinal flora, or bacteria.

Wheat germ is also high in fiber, and contains approximately 1 gram of fiber per tablespoon. A diet high in fiber can be useful in regulating bowel function (i.e., reducing **constipation**), and may be recommended for patients at risk for colon disease, **heart disease**, and diabetes.

Preparations

Wheat germ is used extensively in animal feeds, but for human consumption, wheat germ cereals and wheat germ oil are the two most popular preparations of the grain. Both are available in most grocery and health food stores.

A jar of vacuum-packed wheat germ can be safely stored up to one year unopened. Opened jars should be refrigerated, where they can be stored up to nine months if stored properly and tightly sealed.

To increase fiber and nutrients in bread and cereal recipes, wheat germ may be used to replace 0.5–1 cup of regular flour.

Precautions

Because wheat germ contains fat, proper cold storage is necessary to prevent spoilage.

Side effects

There are no known side effects to wheat germ consumption at normal dietary levels.

Resources

BOOKS

Reavley, Nocola. *The New Encyclopedia of Vitamins, Minerals, Supplements, and Herbs.* New York: M. Evans & Company, 1998.

Paula Ford-Martin

Wheat grass therapy

Definition

Wheat grass, sometimes written as wheatgrass or wheat-grass, is a young green wheat plant (genus *Agropyron*) harvested before it develops grain kernels and turns the traditional yellow color associated with wheat stalks. Wheat grass is commonly prepared as a juice, and is consumed either alone, or as a mixture with other juices.

Wheat grass is a source of many nutrients. Differences between samples of wheat grass due to variable growing conditions, quality of seed, and other factors including dose amounts and form will produce variable amounts of nutrients in any single dose of wheat grass. The following is a partial list.

• biotin
• choline
• lutein
• lycopene
• betacarotene
• thiamine
• riboflavin
• niacin
• pantothenic acid
• pyridoxine
• folic acid
• vitamin C
• vitamin E
• vitamin K
• calcium
• cobalt
• copper
• alanine
• arginine

Although wheat grass contains a wide range of **amino acids** and other nutrients, the concentrations are

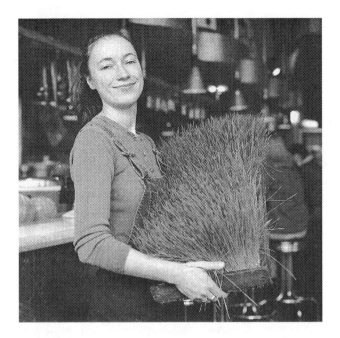

Woman carrying wheat grass, one of the ingredients to be made into a health drink. *(© Catherine Karnow/Corbis. Reproduced by permission.)*

low. Relatively large quantities of wheat grass may be required in order to provide significant nutritional benefits.

Origins

There is no well documented history of consumption of wheat grass. Wheat is one of the oldest crops known, and was cultivated as long as 9,000 years ago in the Euphrates Valley of the Middle East. At least one company has claimed that ingestion of wheat grass dates from the Essenes, a Jewish sect of about the first century A.D. Contemporary use seems to have originated with Ann Wigmore (1909–1994). Ms. Wigmore may be credited with many of the theories concerning enzymes, grasses, and living foods.

Benefits

Wheat grass, depending on the dose, is a dietary supplement, although the concentrations of some nutrients may be low. The sellers of wheat grass have made a large number of claims for the product. The following list is representative, but not complete.

• cure cancer

• cure chronic **fatigue** syndrome

• detoxify liver

• purify blood

• neutralize pollutants

• improve energy

• improve circulation

• slow aging

• increase immunity

• protect against biological warfare

Description

Wheat grass is usually grown indoors, either commercially or for personal use. The grass is harvested while still green, and before the wheat kernels have developed. The juice is extracted either with stone grinding, as with a mortar and pestle, or with a manual juicer. High-speed juicers are considered unsuitable, either because they will oxidize the chlorophyll or destroy the enzymes.

Wheat grass juice, according to Ann Wigmore, should be consumed within 30 minutes of juicing.

Wheat grass has a taste that has been described as pungent, however one manufacturer disputes these claims, and maintains that the product has a watermelon or **green tea** taste.

Preparations

Wheat grass may be purchased in a variety of ways. Kits are available, containing seed, soil, and pots, so that users may grow their own supplies. Alternately, the cut grass is available in packages of 8 or 16 ounces.

Powders and tablets made from dehydrated wheat grass are marketed.

Precautions

No special precautions are required. Because wheat grass juice does not contain gluten, the principle allergen in wheat, the juice may be expected to be safe even for people with wheat **allergies**.

Side effects

There are no established side effects of wheat grass.

Research & general acceptance

Wheat grass has not been accepted into conventional medicine at any level. The United States Food and Drug Administration (FDA) and the German Commission E have not reviewed the validity of wheat grass therapy claims. While some of the claims made for wheat grass are based on laboratory studies, there do not appear to be clinical studies or any form of confirmation from human studies of any form.

While wheat grass contains a large assortment of nutrients, the concentrations are low, and a large volume of juice or powder would be required in order to make a significant contribution to health. Arguments regarding the of benefits orally ingested enzymes have been generally rejected, because enzymes are destroyed during digestion.

Training & certification

There is no training required to prepare wheat grass, and no established rules for its use.

Resources

BOOKS

Blumenthal, M., et. al. *The Complete German Commission E Monographs—Therapeutic Guide to Herbal Medicine.* Austin, TX: American Botanical Council, 1998.

Meyerowitz, S., et. al. *Wheatgrass Nature's Finest Medicine: The Complete Guide to Using Grass Foods & Juices to Revitalize Your Health, 6th edition.* Great Barrington, MA: Sproutman Publications, 1999.

Wigmore, A. *The Wheatgrass Book.* Avery Penguin Putnam

PERIODICALS

Bauman, B. "The Benefits of Wheatgrass Fact or Fiction?" *Greater Baton Rouge Business Report*, August 29, 2000: 36.

Bradley, R. "You can reduce stress—lose weight—detoxify—stop smoking—increase energy with living foods." *Townsend Letter for Doctors and Patients* (April 2003): 86.

"11 Super Foods to Eat Right Now." *Vegetarian Times* (December 1998).

Gilbere, Gloria. "Nature's Immune Booster and pH Balancer." *Total Health* (August/September 2003): 40.

"Grass in a glass." *The University of California, Berkeley Wellness Letter* (November 1995): 4.

"Medicinal Antidotes from Dr. Chili: How to Protect Yourself Against the Effects of Chemical Weapons." *Earth First!* 21: 20

"Reports on the health aspects of wheat grass juice." *Environmental Nutrition* (May 2000): 7.

"Wheatgrass Therapy." *NCAHF Newsletter* (September-October 1994): 3.

Wigmore, A. "The wheatgrass way to super health and vitality: it's easy to grow your own!" *Health News & Review* (Spring 1992): B.

ORGANIZATIONS

American Botanical Council. 6200 Manor Rd, Austin, TX 78723. (512) 926-4900

Ann Wigmore Natural Health Institute, Inc. PO Box 429 Rincón, Puerto Rico 00677.

The National Council Against Health Fraud. 119 Foster Street Peabody, MA 01960.

Samuel Uretsky, Pharm.D.

Wheezing

Definition

Wheezing is a high-pitched whistling sound associated with labored breathing.

Description

Wheezing occurs when a person tries to breathe deeply through air passages (bronchia) that are narrowed because of muscle contractions or filled with mucus as a result of: allergy, infection, illness, or irritation. Wheezing is experienced by 10-15% of the population.

Wheezing most commonly occurs when a person is exhaling. It is sometimes accompanied by a mild sensation of tightness in the chest. **Anxiety** about not being able to breathe easily can cause muscle tension that makes the wheezing worse.

Causes & symptoms

Wheezing is the symptom most associated with **asthma**. It can be aggravated by dry air and high altitude. A 2001 study also found a connection between nighttime wheezing/asthma and gastroesophageal reflux, or the flow of stomach acid backward into the lower part of the esophagus. Wheezing can be caused by:

- exposure to allergens (food, pollen, and other substances that cause a person to have an allergic reaction)
- fumes
- ice-cold drinks, or very cold air
- medication
- strenuous exercise
- weather changes
- foreign objects trapped in the airway
- cystic fibrosis and other genetic disorders
- respiratory illnesses like **pneumonia**, **bronchitis**, congestive heart failure, and **emphysema**

The symptoms of wheezing are: labored breathing, whistling sound upon breathing, shortness of breath, and a tight or heavy feeling in the chest.

Medical emergencies

Breathing problems can be life-threatening. Immediate medical attention is required whenever a person:

- turns blue or gray and stops breathing
- becomes extremely short of breath, and is unable to speak
- coughs up bubbly pink or white phlegm
- seems to be suffocating
- develops a **fever** of 101°F (38.3°C) or higher
- wheezes most of the time, and coughs up gray or greenish phlegm

Diagnosis

A family physician, allergist, or pulmonary specialist takes a medical history that includes questions about **allergies**, or unexplained symptoms that may be the result of allergic reactions. If the pattern of the patient's symptoms suggests the existence of allergy, skin and blood tests are performed to identify the precise nature of the problem.

A pulmonary function test may be ordered to measure the amount of air moving through the patient's breathing passages. X rays are sometimes indicated for patients whose wheezing seems to be caused by chronic bronchitis or emphysema.

Treatment

Patients whose wheezing is related to asthma, chronic bronchitis, emphysema, or a severe allergic reaction may benefit from alternative medicine but they must continue to have their condition monitored by a conventional physician.

Mild wheezing may be relieved by drinking plenty of juice, water, weak tea, and broth. This helps to replace fluids lost because of rapid breathing and loosen mucus in the air passages. Ice-cold drinks should be avoided. A vaporizer can help clear air passages. A steam tent, created by lowering the face toward a sink filled with hot water, placing a towel over the head and sink, and inhaling the steam, can do likewise.

Herbal remedies

Several herbal remedies exist for the treatment of wheezing and asthma.

- Baical **skullcap** (*Scutellaria baicalensis*) decoction relieves wheezing.
- Coltsfoot tea may relieve wheezing.
- Cramp bark (*Viburnum opulus*) tincture eases breathing.

- Elecampane (*Inula helenium*) can help to clear mucus.
- Garlic (*Allium sativum*) can ease asthma symptoms.
- German **chamomile** (*Chamomilla recutita*) infusion can relieve wheezing.
- Ginkgo (*Ginkgo biloba*) eases asthma symptoms.
- Marsh mallow (*Althaea officinalis*) root eases asthma symptoms.
- Mullein (*Verbascum thapsus*) tea in a vaporizer relieves wheezing.
- Nettle (*Urtica dioca*) infusion relieves wheezing.
- Passionflower (*Passiflora incarnata*) relaxes muscle spasms leading to a reduction in wheezing.
- Thyme (*Thymus vulgaris*) infusion relieves wheezing.

Ayurvedic treatment

Wheezing can be alleviated by drinking **licorice** tea. The tea is prepared by steeping one teaspoon of licorice (*Yashti madbu*) root in one cup of water, adding 5-10 drops of mahanarayan oil just before drinking. The patient should take one sip every 5-10 minutes. A remedy for breathlessness is a mixture of onion juice (one quarter cup), black pepper (0.125 tsp), and honey (1 tsp).

Mustard seeds have bronchial system healing properties. Brown mustard oil may be massaged onto the chest. A mustard tea (one quarter teaspoon each ground mustard seed and pippali or black pepper) with honey may be drunk two or three times daily or sipped throughout the day. Another mustard remedy is taking brown mustard oil (1 tsp) with natural sugar (1 tsp) two or three times daily.

Homeopathy

Homeopathic remedies are chosen for each patient based on his or her pattern of symptoms. Arsenicum is indicated for patients who experience restlessness, fearfulness, wheezing, and shortness of breath between the hours of midnight and 3 A.M. Spongia is recommended for those who have dry wheezing, which may occur as the patient is falling asleep, a feeling of suffocation, and a dry **cough**. **Lobelia** is for patients with chest tightness and wheezing that is worsened in cold air. Sambucus is indicated for persons whose wheezing is worsened after midnight, but who don't experience the fear or restlessness experienced by an arsenicum patient. **Pulsatilla** is recommended for those who are affectionate, and feel stifled in warm rooms. **Ipecac** is for patients who have a lot of phlegm in the lungs (wheezing is accompanied by rattling sounds in the chest), coughing, and possibly **vomiting**. **Bryonia** is for patients with dry wheezing, who feel warm and thirsty, and whose symptoms are worsened by motion.

Other remedies

Other treatments for wheezing include:

• Aromatherapy. The **essential oils** of **lavender**, **eucalyptus**, and **rosemary** can relieve congestion. Adding German chamomile essential oil to a vaporizer can relieve wheezing.

• Diet. Eliminating red meat, and wheat and dairy products and following a **macrobiotic diet** of vegetarian foods may relieve asthma symptoms.

• Relaxation techniques. Because anxiety can worsen an asthma attack, and therefore wheezing, **meditation**, **biofeedback**, deep breathing, or other stress-reduction methods may help promote relaxation.

• Supplements. **Magnesium** may help to prevent bronchial spasms. The frequency of asthma attacks may be reduced by taking **vitamin C** and the B complex vitamins.

• Yoga. Certain yoga positions (Bridge, Cobra, Pigeon, and Sphinx) may relieve wheezing by improving breathing control and reducing stress.

Allopathic treatment

Bronchodilators (medications that help widen narrowed airways) may be prescribed for patients whose wheezing is the result of asthma. Antibiotics are generally used to cure acute bronchitis and other respiratory **infections**. Expectorants (cough-producing medications) or bronchodilators are prescribed to remove excess mucus from the breathing passages. If wheezing is caused by an allergic reaction, antihistamines will probably be prescribed to neutralize body chemicals that react to the allergen.

A new type of drug was being tested in late 2001 that blocks immunoglobulin E (IgE), an antibody produced in excessive levels in patients with **hay fever**. The drug also appears to prevent asthma in patients with chronic hay fever. The drug, called omalizumab, is the first in a new line of drugs expected to appear in the next few years.

If wheezing and asthma symptoms worsen in the nighttime, diagnosis and treatment of possible acid reflux in the stomach might ease symptoms.

Expected results

Mild wheezing caused by infection or acute illness usually disappears when the underlying cause is eliminated.

Some doctors believe that childhood respiratory infections may activate parts of the immune system that prevent asthma from developing.

Prevention

Stopping **smoking** can eliminate wheezing; so can reducing or preventing exposure to allergens or conditions that cause wheezing.

A person prone to wheezing should wear a scarf or surgical mask over the nose and mouth during physical exertion outdoors during cold weather. Likewise, wearing a surgical mask outdoors during the allergy season is helpful for persons whose wheezing is triggered by allergies.

Licorice root tea may prevent asthma (wheezing) attacks. Ayurvedic herbal remedies to prevent asthma symptoms include:

• cinnamon (1 tsp) and trikatu (0.25 tsp) tea with honey twice daily

• licorice and **ginger** (0.25 tsp each) tea

• bay leaf (0.5 tsp) and pippali (0.25 tsp) mixed in honey taken two or three times daily

• sitopaladi (0.5 tsp), punarnova (0.5 tsp), pippali (pinch), and abrak bhasma (pinch) mixed with honey taken once daily

• spinach juice (0.125 cup) and pippali (pinch) taken twice daily

Resources

BOOKS

Cummings, Stephen and Dana Ullman. *Everybody's Guide to Homeopathic Medicines: Safe and Effective Remedies for You and Your Family.* New York: Jeremy P. Tarcher/Putnam, 1997.

The Editors of Time-Life Books. *The Medical Advisor: The Complete Guide to Alternative and Conventional Therapies.* Alexandria, VA: Time-Life Books, 1996.

Lad, Vasant D. *The Compete Book of Ayurvedic Home Remedies.* New York: Harmony Books, 1998.

PERIODICALS

Avidan, B., et al. "Temporal Associations Between Coughing or Wheezing and Acid Reflux in Asthmatics." *Gut* (December 2001):767.

Blanc, Paul D., et al. "Alternative Therapies Among Adults with a Reported Diagnosis of Asthma or Rhinosinusitis: Data from a Population-Based Survey." *Chest* (November 2001): 1461.

Lanctot, Denise. "Case of the Out-Of-Control Wheeze." *Prevention* 48 (April 1996): 124+.

Langer, Stephen and Patricia Andersen-Parrado. "Stifling allergies." *Better Nutrition* 61(April 1999): 44+.

KEY TERMS

Allergen—A substance that causes an allergic reaction because of a hypersensitive immune system.

Bronchia—Air passages in the lungs. Wheezing occurs when bronchia become constricted (narrowed).

Plaut, Marshall. "Immune-Based, Tageted Therapy for Allergic Diseases." *JAMA, The Journal of the American Medical Association.* (December 19, 2001):3005.

ORGANIZATIONS

American Lung Association. 1740 Broadway, New York, NY 10019-4374. (800) 586-4872. http://www.lungusa.org.

Asthma and Allergy Foundation of America. (800) 7- ASTH-MA.

OTHER

"Kids in Daycare Three Times as Likely to Have Wheezing Illnesses." http://www.lungusa.org/footer.html (16 May 1998).

"Wheezing." http://www.mcare2.org/healthtips/homecare/wheezing.htm (16 May 1998).

"Wheezing." http://www.onhealth.com/bu/cond/ailments/htm/wheezing/htm (17 May 1998).

Belinda Rowland
Teresa Norris

White peony root

Description

Peonies are members of the same botanical family as the buttercup, Ranunculaceae, and belong to the genus *Paeonia*. They originated in Asia, and have been cultivated in both Japan and China for at least several centuries, perhaps even a millennium. Peonies are an early groundbreaker, producing reddish shoots as early as April in the Northern Hemisphere. They are a tall plant, ranging from 1–5 ft (30–150 cm) in height. Their branching stems produce glossy deep green leaves that taper to a point on each end, and grow up to 5 in (12.5 cm) in length. The peony root is brownish in color and tuberous.

The peony flowers are produced at the tips of the branching stems. Beginning as globular buds that produce a sweet, sticky exudate that attracts ants (that do no harm), these buds slowly open into large, showy flowers with diameters up to 10 in (20.5 cm) wide. The peony is an extremely long-lived plant, especially for a flowering one. It is not uncommon for peonies to live for a hundred years. They prefer moist, humus-rich loam and either full or partial sun. If peonies become overcrowded, the plants must be divided, and at the end of the growing season, it is best to cut the stems off at ground level and mulch for winter protection.

Though there are literally hundreds of hybrid varieties that have been developed over the centuries, most peonies share both a common origin and fairly similar characteristics. Many resemble a herbaceous shrub. Others that originated in western China have woody stems and are called tree peonies. Tree peonies do not die back completely in winter. In addition, tree peony root and red peony root are considered separate entities in **traditional Chinese medicine**.

Classification of these flowering plants is often based on when they bloom. The earliest produce blossoms in late April (in southern areas) or early May. Others flower in mid- or late May and into June. Another means of classifying peonies is based upon the shape of their flowers. Single peonies form a circle of five or more petals radiating symmetrically outward from a middle ring of yellow stamens, or male procreative structures. Japanese peonies have a similar appearance, but the stamens are both more narrow and more level and produce no pollen. Other varieties are either semi-double or double. Semi-double peonies have multiple rings of petals circling around visible stamens. Double peonies produce concentric rings of showy petals that hide the stamens.

Most of the varieties of peony admired in flower gardens today are hybrids of the two original species of this plant, *Paeonia officinalis* and *Paeonia lactiflora*, which differ slightly in appearance. *Paeonia officinalis* is the species most often seen in gardens and used as an ornamental flower. It reaches heights of 1.5-2 ft (45-60 cm) tall and its subspecies have a remarkable variation of colors. This species produces creeping roots that help to spread the plant.

Paeonia lactiflora, also called *Paeonia alba* or white peony, is the plant most often used in herbal medicine, particularly in Chinese herbal medicine. White peonies grow to 3 ft (1 m) tall, and are among the later-flowering peonies, coming into bloom in May and June in most climates. They have a sweeter scent than *Paeonia officinalis*. Despite the name of white peony, flowers can be several hues other than white depending upon the subspecies. There are rose-pink and scarlet varieties, as well as white peonies ornamented with other colors. White peonies can be either single, semi-double or fully double. *Paeonia rubra*, or red peony, is a separate herb.

General use

Under the name *bai shao*, white peony root is used in many diverse Chinese herbal formulas. It is considered a herb with strong blood-toning characteristics, used to treat the imbalance of blood in the body, cooling and providing nourishment to the blood and activating circulation. More specifically, red peony root is used to treat heat rash, to correct poor circulation and to stop hemorrhages. White peony root is used for irritability and muscle cramping, vaginal discharges, excessive menstrual bleeding, and excessive sweating. It is also given to treat a large variety of gynecological disorders and to avert miscarriage.

In the databases developed by the Agricultural Research Service of the United States Department of Agriculture, white peony root (from both *Paeonia albaflora* and subspecies *Paeonia albaflora trichocarpa*) has been shown to have chemical properties that restore the normal functioning of the digestive system; act as a laxative; relieve **pain**; reduce or stop spasms or seizures; lower blood pressure by dilating arteries; and improve the **nutrition** of blood. Peony root appears to have some positive effects in treating **anemia**, some types of **cancer**, convulsions, **gastritis**, **hypertension**, and some gynecological problems. It can also be used as an emmenagogue, which means that it can bring on a woman's menstrual period.

Preparations

Powdered peony root is used in combination with other herbs used in Chinese herbal medicine, including apricot seeds, bupleurum, inula, **cyperus**, clematis, **corydalis**, ginseng, **licorice**, pueraria, rehmannia, dogwood, and **gardenia**. The classic Chinese blood tonic is a mixture of rehmannia, *dang bui*, cnidium, and white peony. A Western herbalist suggests combining white peony with nettles and **yellow dock** for treating mild anemia or blood deficiency.

Precautions

Chinese herbalists advise against using white peony root when cold-deficiency **diarrhea** is present.

Western readers should remember that Chinese herbal medicine is based upon individual prescriptions developed for each patient and his or her unique symptoms. Chinese herbs should not be taken, either individually or in formulas, unless a practitioner of Chinese herbal medicine is first consulted.

Resources

BOOKS

Molony, David, and Ming Ming Pan Molony. *The American Association of Oriental Medicine's Complete Guide to*

Chinese Herbal Medicine. New York: Berkley Publishing, 1999.

Phillips, Ellen and C. Colston Burrell. *Rodale's Illustrated Encyclopedia of Perennials.* Emmaus, PA: Rodale Press, Inc., 1993.

Reid, Daniel. *A Handbook of Chinese Healing Herbs.* Boston: Shambhala Publications, Inc., 1995.

OTHER

Duke, James, MD. Dr. Duke's Phytochemical and Ethnobotanical Databases. http//www.ars-grin.gov/duke/ethnobot.htm.

Joan Schonbeck

White willow

Description

White willow (*Salix alba*) is a large tree that grows in Central and Southern Europe, Asia, and North America. Also known as European willow or baywillow, this tree prefers to root near streams and rivers and grows to a height of 35–75 ft (11–25 m). In the spring, the slender branches first sprout tiny, yellow flowers and then long, thin green leaves.

White willow belongs to the Salicaceae family. There are over 300 species of willow, but only several species are used medicinally: white willow (*S. alba*), purple willow (*S. purpurea*), violet willow (*S. daphnoides*), and crack willow (*S. fragilis*).

General use

White willow is the oldest recorded analgesic, or painkiller, in human history. Chinese physicians have used white willow since 500 B.C. to relieve **pain** and lower fevers. White willow was also used in ancient Assyrian, Egyptian, and Greek medicine as well. The Greek physicians Dioscorides, Hippocrates, and Galen recommended white willow to remedy fevers and pain. Native

American tribes, including the Cherokee, Blackfoot, Iroquois, and Eskimo peoples, created a tea from closely related species of the bark to relieve headaches, **fever**, sore muscles, **chills**, rheumatism, and general aches and pains. White willow was used in Europe to stop **vomiting**, remove **warts**, and suppress sexual desire in addition to treating fevers and pains.

In the mid-1700s, white willow was used in Britain as a remedy for **malaria** since the bark was similar to cinchona bark, a South American bark used to treat malaria. In 1828, European chemists extracted the constituent salicin from white willow bark and converted it to salicylic acid. At the end of the nineteenth century, acetylsalicylic acid was synthetically produced and aspirin was born. Due to the cheap and easy production of aspirin, white willow eventually lost its popularity as a pain and fever reliever.

In modern times, however, white willow is being recalled as nature's aspirin and gaining popularity around the world as an alternative treatment for fevers and inflammatory and painful conditions such as **bursitis, tendinitis**, headaches, **rheumatoid arthritis**, back pain, **osteoarthritis**, menstrual cramps, and muscle aches. White willow has been approved by the German Commission E for treating fevers, rheumatic ailments, and headaches. In France, white willow is used to remedy headaches, **toothache** pain, tendinitis, and muscle sprains. The British Herbal Compendium has administered white willow as a treatment for rheumatic and arthritic conditions, colds, and **influenza**.

How white willow works

The inner bark contains tannins, flavonoids, phenolic glycosides, and anti-inflammatory and fever-reducing salicylates. The high concentration of tannins may be responsible for relieving gastrointestinal disturbances and reducing tumors of the esophagus, stomach, colon, and rectum.

White willow's analgesic effect works to inhibit the production of prostaglandins, a hormone-like chemical that is produced by the body in response to injury and causes aches, pains, and inflammation. Thus, white willow is beneficial in treating acute and chronic pain and inflammation in conditions such as painful **menstruation**, arthritis, and **neuralgia**. White willow is best when used over long periods of time and can take days to improve conditions.

The active ingredient in white willow is salicin. Salicin is gradually converted along with other compounds in white willow into salicylic acid in the intestine and liver. Because of this conversion process, white willow generally takes longer to act than aspirin, but the effects may last for an extended period of time. As a result, white willow is mild on the stomach and usually does

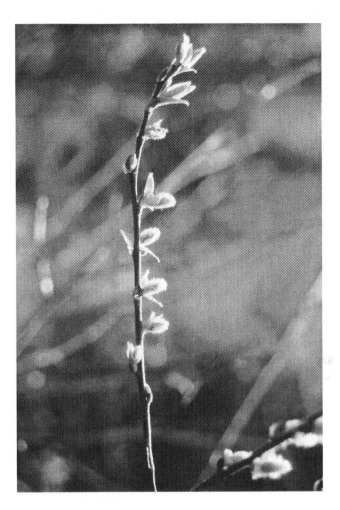

Willow branch (*Salix* sp.). *(Photo by Henriette Kress. Reproduced by permission.)*

not cause bleeding or other gastrointestinal discomfort that often occurs with aspirin usage.

White willow vs. aspirin

Herbalists claim that white willow can sometimes be used in the same conditions as aspirin. One benefit to white willow use is that the natural salicylic acid present in white willow reportedly produces fewer side effects than the synthetically produced acetylsalicylic acid of aspirin.

Aspirin has been recommended as a treatment to reduce the risk of heart attacks and **stroke** by lessening the chance of internal **blood clots**. Preventative benefits of white willow in these cases have not been determined, primarily because the salicin content of the bark varies. Herbal experts believe that most willow bark samples contain enough salicin to have a similar effect.

Preparations

The bark of young tree branches (two or three years old) is harvested during the early spring. The grayish bark is separated from the tree, then either dried or used fresh. White willow is commercially available in tincture, tablet, capsule, powder, or tea forms. When choosing a commercial preparation, it is recommended to use a standard product that contains 200–250 mg of white willow per dose.

The recommended daily dosage is 100–250 mg of white willow every four hours. To relieve arthritic, back, and muscle aches and pains, the recommended dosage is 225 mg of white willow bark four times daily.

A decoction made from willow bark is used both internally and externally. To make a decoction, combine 1 tsp chopped or powdered white willow bark with 8–10 oz of water. Bring to a boil, then simmer for five minutes. Drink three or four times daily. This mixture can also be gargled to help inflamed gums and tonsils. Cooled and applied externally, the decoction helps aid healing of sores, **burns**, or cuts.

Tincture dosage: 2 ml three times daily.

Precautions

Persons with **tinnitus** should not take white willow.

Pregnant or breastfeeding women should consult their healthcare practitioner before taking white willow.

Persons who are sensitive to aspirin should use caution when taking white willow as it may irritate their stomachs.

Administration of aspirin to children under the age of 16 to relieve symptoms of cold, flu, or **chickenpox** may cause a rare condition called Reye's syndrome. Reye's syndrome is characterized by vomiting, swelling of the brain, and liver damage; and may be fatal. *Reye's syndrome is a medical emergency and requires immediate treatment by qualified medical professionals.* The toll-free hot line number of the National Reye's Syndrome Foundation is listed below.

While white willow is metabolized differently from aspirin, there is still a similarity between the two, and it is recommended that white willow not be given in these situations.

Persons with a bleeding disorder, ulcer, colitis, **Crohn's disease**, kidney or liver disease, or diabetes should not take this herb.

Children over 12 and persons over 65 should take white willow in low initial doses. Children under the age of 12 should not use white willow at all.

Side effects

Excessive doses of white willow may cause stomach upset, **diarrhea**, **nausea**, or ringing in the ears. If this occurs, should be stopped white willow.

KEY TERMS

Analgesic—A medication or preparation given to relieve pain. White willow extract has analgesic effects.

Decoction—An herbal tea created by boiling herbs in water. Roots, bark, and seeds are used in decoctions; boiling the herbs brings out their medicinal properties.

Nonsteroidal anti-inflammatory drugs (NSAIDs)—A group of analgesic medications that also have anti-inflammatory effects when used over a period of time.

Reye's syndrome—A rare but potentially fatal disorder that is most likely to occur in children following a viral disease and associated with giving aspirin. The symptoms of Reye's syndrome include vomiting, liver damage, and swelling of the brain.

Salicin—A bitter-tasting water-soluble chemical found in willow bark that has analgesic properties.

Tinnitus—A condition that causes ringing in the ears.

Interactions

In general, persons considering taking white willow preparations should first consult a physician or registered pharmacist, as white willow interacts with a number of nonprescription as well as prescription medications.

Persons who are allergic to aspirin should not use white willow.

White willow should not be taken in combination with aspirin or such nonsteroidal anti-inflammatory drugs (NSAIDs) as ibuprofen or naproxen, alcohol, or blood-thinning medications.

White willow has been reported to have adverse interactions with bismuth subsalicylate (Pepto-Bismol), celecoxib (Celebrex), repaglinide (Prandin), and ticlopidine (Ticlid). It increases the action of metaclopramide (Reglan), but reduces the effectiveness of diclofenac (Voltaren, Cataflam), ketoprofen (Orudis), and nadolol (Corgard).

Resources

BOOKS

Pelletier, Kenneth R., MD. *The Best Alternative Medicine,* Chapter 6, "Western Herbal Medicine: Nature's Green Pharmacy." New York: Simon & Schuster, 2002.

Prevention. *The Complete Book of Natural and Medicinal Cures.* Rodale Press Inc., 1994.

PERIODICALS

Appelboom, T. "Arthropathy in Art and the History of Pain Management— Through the Centuries to Cyclooxygenase-2 Inhibitors." *Rheumatology (Oxford)* 41 (April 2002): Supplement 1, 28-34.

Brune, K. "Next Generation of Everyday Analgesics." *American Journal of Therapeutics* 9 (May-June 2002): 215-223.

Riddle, J. M. "History as a Tool in Identifying 'new' Old Drugs." *Advances in Experimental Medicine and Biology* 505 (2002): 89-94.

ORGANIZATIONS

American Herbalists Guild. 1931 Gaddis Road, Canton, GA 30115. (770) 751-6021. <www.americanherbalistsguild.com>.

National Reye's Syndrome Foundation. P. O. Box 829, Bryan, OH 43506. (800) 233-7393. lt;www.reyessyndrome.org>.

Jennifer Wurges
Rebecca J. Frey, PhD

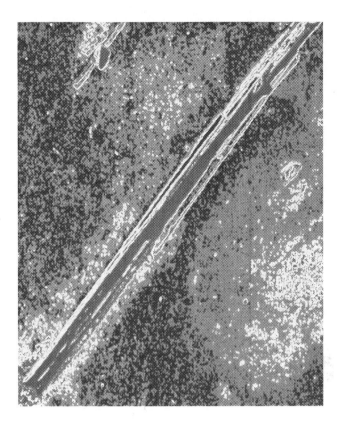

A magnified image of a pertussis toxin crystal that causes whooping cough. *(National Institutes of Health/Custom Medical Stock Photo. Reproduced by permission.)*

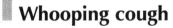

Whooping cough

Definition

Whooping cough, also known as pertussis, is a highly contagious disease that causes classic spasms (paroxysms) of uncontrollable coughing, followed by a sharp, high-pitched intake of air, which creates the characteristic whoop of the disease's name.

Description

Whooping cough is caused by a bacterium called *Bordetella pertussis*. *B. pertussis* causes its most severe symptoms by attaching itself to those cells in the respiratory tract that have cilia. Cilia are small, hair-like projections that beat continuously, and serve to constantly sweep the respiratory tract clean of such debris as mucus, bacteria, viruses, and dead cells. When *B. pertussis* interferes with this normal, janitorial function, mucus and cellular debris accumulate and cause constant irritation to the respiratory tract, triggering coughing and increasing further mucus production.

Whooping cough is a disease that exists throughout the world. While persons of any age can contract whooping cough, children under the age of two are at the highest risk for both the disease and for serious complications including death. Apparently, exposure to *B. pertussis* bacteria earlier in life gives a person some, but not complete, immunity against infection with it later on. Subsequent **infections** resemble the **common cold**.

It is estimated that as many as 120,000 persons in the United States get whooping cough each year. The number of cases has been increasing, with the largest increases found in older children and adults. Between 1993 and 1996, the number of cases increased by 40% in five-to nine-year-old children, 106% in 10–19 year olds, and 93% for persons aged 20 years and older.

Causes & symptoms

Whooping cough has four stages that partially overlap: incubation, catarrhal stage, paroxysmal stage, and convalescent stage.

A person usually acquires *B. pertussis* by inhaling droplets carrying the bacteria that were coughed into the air by someone already suffering with the infection. Incubation is the symptomless period of seven to 14 days after breathing in the *B. pertussis* bacteria, and during which the bacteria multiply and penetrate the lining tissues of the entire respiratory tract.

The catarrhal stage is often mistaken for an exceedingly heavy cold. The patient has teary eyes, **sneezing**, **fatigue**, poor appetite, and an extremely runny nose (rhinorrhea). This stage lasts about 10–14 days.

The paroxysmal stage, lasting two to four weeks, begins with the development of the characteristic whooping cough. Spasms of uncontrollable coughing, the whooping sound of the sharp inspiration of air, and **vomiting** are all hallmarks of this stage. The whoop is believed to occur due to inflammation and mucus that narrow the breathing tubes, causing the patient to struggle to get air into his/her lungs; the effort results in intense exhaustion. The paroxysms (spasms) can be induced by overactivity, feeding, crying, or even overhearing someone else cough.

The mucus that is produced during the paroxysmal stage is thicker and more difficult to clear than the more watery mucus of the catarrhal stage, and the patient becomes increasingly exhausted attempting to clear the respiratory tract through coughing. Severely ill children may have great difficult, maintaining the normal level of oxygen in their systems, and may appear somewhat blue after a paroxysm of coughing, due to the low oxygen content of their blood. Such children may also suffer from swelling and degeneration of the brain (encephalopathy), which is believed to be caused both by lack of oxygen to the brain during paroxysms, and also by bleeding into the brain caused by increased pressure during coughing. Seizures may result from decreased oxygen to the brain. Some children have such greatly increased abdominal pressure during coughing that hernias result (hernias are the abnormal protrusion of a loop of intestine through a weak area of muscle). Another complicating factor during this phase is the development of **pneumonia** from infection with another bacterial agent, which takes hold due to the patient's weakened condition.

If the patient survives the paroxysmal stage, recovery occurs gradually during the convalescent stage, usually taking about three to four weeks. However, spasms of coughing may continue to occur over a period of months, especially when a patient contracts a cold, or other respiratory infection.

Diagnosis

Diagnosis based only on the patient's symptoms is not particularly accurate, as the catarrhal stage may appear to be a heavy cold, a case of the flu, or a simple **bronchitis**. Other viruses and **tuberculosis** infections can cause symptoms similar to those found during the paroxysmal stage. The presence of a pertussis-like cough along with an increase of certain specific white blood cells (lymphocytes) is suggestive of pertussis (whooping cough). However, cough can occur from pertussis-like viruses. The most accurate method of diagnosis is to culture (grow in the laboratory) the organisms obtained from swabbing mucus out of the nasopharynx (the breathing tube continuous with the nose). *B. pertus-*

sis can then be identified by examining the culture under a microscope.

Researchers believe that as many as 90% of the cases are not diagnosed, mainly because of the nonspecific symptoms displayed by adults. An adult who has been coughing for months may have whooping cough.

Recent advances in the accuracy of diagnostic tests based on polymerase chain reactions (PCR) are now being applied to whooping cough. Researchers in Seattle are presently working on a PCR-based test for *Bordetella pertussis* that will improve the speed as well as the accuracy of diagnosing whooping cough.

Treatment

Whooping cough should always be treated with antibiotics and never with only alternative therapies. The following complementary therapies may reduce symptoms and speed recovery. Supportive treatment involves careful monitoring of fluids to prevent dehydration, rest in a quiet, dark room to decrease paroxysms, and suctioning of mucus. Sitting up during coughing attacks may help.

Herbals

The following herbal remedies may help to support antibiotic treatment of whooping cough:

- bryonia (*Bryonia alba*) tea: spasmodic coughing
- butterbur (*Pinguicula vulgaris*) infusion: infection and spasms
- evening primrose (*Oenothera biennis*) oil
- jamaican dogwood (*Piscidia erythrina*) root or bark: spasms
- lobelia (*Lobelia inflata*) tea or tincture: spasmodic coughing
- pansy (*Viola tricolor*) tea or tincture: spasms
- red clover (*Trifolium pratense*) tea
- santonica (*Artemisia cina*) powder, tablets, or lozenges
- sea holly (*Eryngium planum*) infusion: infection and spasms
- skunk cabbage (*Symplocarpus foetidus*) powder, extract, or tincture
- sundew (*Drosera rotundifolia*) infusion: infection and spasms
- thyme (*Thymus vulgaris*) infusion: infection and spasms
- wild cherry (*Prunus serotina*) bark infusion or syrup: infection, and spasmodic coughing

Homeopathy

Homeopathic remedies are chosen based upon the family of symptoms displayed by each patient. Remedies for symptom families include:

- Drosera: dry and tickly feeling in throat; violent coughing that induces vomiting; symptoms worse after midnight.
- *Kali carbonicum:* dry, hard, hacking cough at 3 A.M.; puffy eyelids; exhaustion; chilly feeling.
- Coccus: coughing worse when warm; drinking cold water brings relief; vomiting stringy, transparent mucus.
- Cuprum: coughing spasms cause breathlessness and exhaustion; blue lips; toe and finger cramping; drinking cold water brings relief.
- *Kali bichromicum:* coughing up yellow, stringy mucus.
- Belladonna: stomach **pain** before coughing; coughing worse at night; retching with coughing attacks; red face; puffy eyelids.
- Ipecac: sick feeling most of the time; paleness, rigidity, breathlessness, and then **relaxation** precede vomiting.

Chinese medicine

Traditional Chinese medicine (TCM) practitioners use a combination of herbals, **acupuncture**, and ear acupuncture to treat whooping cough during each stage. *Yi Zhi Huang Hua* (*Herba solidaginis*) decoction or a decoction of *Bai Mao Gen* (*Rhizoma imperatae*), *Lu Gen* (*Rhizoma phragmitis*), and *Si Gua Gen* (*Radix vascularis luffae*) may be taken for the early stage of whooping cough. Gasping cough can be treated with a mixture of *Wu Gong* (*Scolopendra*) and *Gan Cao* (*Radix glycyrrhizae*).

Other remedies

Other remedies may assist in the treatment of whooping cough.

- Dietary supplements include vitamins A and C, **beta carotene**, **acidophilus**, lung glandulars, **garlic**, and zinc.
- Dietary changes include drinking plenty of fluids, eating fruits, vegetables, brown rice, whole grain toast, vegetable broth, and potatoes, and avoiding dairy products.
- Juice therapists recommend orange and lemon juice or carrot and watercress juice.
- Hydrotherapy treatment consists of wet clothes or other material applied to the head or chest to relieve congestion.
- Aromatherapy uses **essential oils** of tea tree, **chamomile**, basil, camphor, **eucalyptus**, **lavender**, **peppermint**, or thyme.
- Osteopathic manipulation can reduce cough severity and make the patient feel more comfortable.

Allopathic treatment

Treatment with the antibiotic erythromycin is clearly helpful only in the very early stages of whooping cough, during incubation and early in the catarrhal stage. In general, however, physicians have used this antibiotic both for treatment of whooping cough itself and to prevent its spread to others in the patient's community. This type of preventive measure is known as prophylaxis.

Unfortunately, the benefits of antibiotic prophylaxis and treatment for whooping cough are limited because erythromycin-resistant strains of *B. pertussis* have spread throughout the United States since the first case of erythromycin resistance was identified in Arizona in 1994. Although erythromycin is still used as of 2003 for both treatment and prophylaxis of whooping cough, the Centers for Disease Control (CDC) is monitoring the five resistant strains of *B. pertussis* that have been identified so far.

Expected results

Just under 1% of all cases of whooping cough cause death; in 2000, only two deaths from whooping cough were reported in the United States. Children who die of whooping cough usually have one or more of the following three conditions:

- Severe pneumonia, perhaps with accompanying encephalopathy.
- Extreme weight loss, weakness, and metabolic abnormalities due to persistent vomiting during paroxysms of coughing.
- Other preexisting conditions, so that the patient is already in a relatively weak, vulnerable state (such conditions may include low-birth-weight babies, poor **nutrition**, infection with the **measles** virus, presence of other respiratory or gastrointestinal infections or diseases).

Prevention

The mainstay of prevention lies in the immunization program. In the United States, inoculations begin at two months of age. The pertussis vaccine, most often given as one immunization together with diphtheria and **tetanus** (called DTP), has greatly reduced the incidence of whooping cough. With one shot backed with a 70% immunization rate, two shots increase it to 75–80%, and three to only 85%, it is not a guarantee.

A new formulation of the pertussis vaccine is available. Unlike DTP, which is composed of dead bacterial cells, the newer acellular pertussis vaccine is made up of two to five chemical components of the *B. pertussis* bacteria. The acellular pertussis vaccine (called DTaP; when combined with diphtheria and tetanus vaccines) greatly reduces the risk of unpleasant reactions, including high **fever** and discomfort at the injection site.

Because adults are the primary source of infection for children, there has been some talk in the medical community about vaccinating or giving booster vaccinations to adults. A recent increase of pertussis cases among adults in France has led several French medical schools to recommend booster doses of vaccine for adults.

Resources

BOOKS

Fetrow, Charles W. *The Complete Guide to Herbal Medicines.* Springhouse, PA: Springhouse Corporation, 1999.

Lockie, Andrew and Nicola Geddes. *The Women's Guide to Homeopathy.* New York: St. Martin's Press, 1994.

Pertussis in Adults: Epidemiology, Signs, Symptoms, and Implications for Vaccination, edited by Sydney M. Finegold, et al. Chicago: The University of Chicago Press, 1999.

Ryan, Kenneth J., and Stanley Falkour. "Pertussis." In *Sherris Medical Microbiology: An Introduction to Infectious Diseases.* edited by Kenneth J. Ryan. Norwalk, CT: Appleton and Lange, 1994.

Stoffman, Phyllis. *The Family Guide to Preventing and Treating 100 Infectious Diseases.* New York: John Wiley and Sons, Inc., 1995.

Ying, Zhou Zhong and Jin Hui De. "Whooping Cough." In *Clinical Manual of Chinese Herbal Medicine and Acupuncture.* New York: Churchill Livingstone, 1997.

PERIODICALS

Decker, Michael D. and Kathryn M. Edwards. "Acellular Pertussis Vaccines." *Pediatric Clinics of North America* 47 (April 2000): 309-335.

Gilberg, S., E. Njamkepo, I. P. Du Chatelet, et al. "Evidence of *Bordetella pertussis* Infection in Adults Presenting with Persistent Cough in a French Area with Very High Whole-Cell Vaccine Coverage." *Journal of Infectious Diseases* 186 (August 2002): 415-418.

Henderson, C.W. "Disease Still Potentially Deadly." *World Disease Weekly* (11/29/99-12/6/99): 17+.

Jenkinson, Douglas. "Natural Course of 500 Consecutive Cases of Whooping Cough: A General Practice Population Study." *British Medical Journal* 310 (6975)(February 4, 1995): 299+.

Laliberte, Richard. "The Threat of Whooping Cough." *Parents* 74 (January 1999): 45+.

"Pertussis Deaths—United States, 2000." *Morbidity and Mortality Weekly Report* 51 (July 19, 2002): 616-618.

Qin, X., D. K. Turgeon, B. P. Ingersoll, et al. "*Bordetella pertussis* PCR: Simultaneous Targeting of Signature Se-

quences." *Diagnostic Microbiology and Infectious Disease* 43 (August 2002): 269-275.

Wilson, K. E., P. K. Cassiday, T. Popovic, and G. N. Sanden. "*Bordetella pertussis* Isolates with a Heterogeneous Phenotype for Erythromycin Resistance." *Journal of Clinical Microbiology* 40 (August 2002): 2942-2944.

ORGANIZATIONS

American Academy of Pediatrics. 141 Northwest Point Boulevard, Elk Grove Village, IL 60007. (847)434-4000. <www.aap.org>.

Centers for Disease Control and Prevention (CDC). 1600 Clifton Road, Atlanta, GA 30333. (404) 639-3311. <www.cdc.gov>.

Food and Drug Administration (FDA), Center for Biologics Evaluation and Research (CBER), 1401 Rockville Pike, Suite 200-N, Rockville, MD 20852. <www.fda.gov/cber>.

Belinda Rowland
Rebecca J. Frey, PhD

KEY TERMS

Catarrh—Inflammation of a mucous membrane, particularly in the respiratory system, that produces excessive secretions.

Cilia—Tiny hair-like projections from a cell. In the respiratory tract, cilia beat constantly in order to move mucus and debris up and out of the respiratory tree to protect the lung from foreign bodies.

Encephalopathy—Swelling and degeneration of the brain.

Paroxysm—A severe attack or a sudden increase in intensity of a disease.

Prophylaxis—The prevention of disease by protective measures.

Wigmore diet

Definition

The Wigmore diet is named for its creator, Ann Wigmore. She devised a nutritional system called the Living Foods Program, based on a combination of wheatgrass juice, live sprouts, and fresh raw foods. It is thought that this dietary regimen, which is sometimes called raw **nutrition**, detoxifies and rebuilds the body. Persons following the Wigmore diet also avoid using denatured processed commercial foods or anything containing chemicals, especially pesticides. Although the Wigmore diet is essentially a vegetarian diet, its distinctive feature is its emphasis on eating foods in their uncooked state.

Origins

The Wigmore diet was developed during the 1960s by Ann Wigmore, a woman who was born in Eastern Europe in 1909 and emigrated to the United States after World War I. She credited her grandmother with teaching her natural healing methods. She did not, however, use this folk wisdom immediately but returned to it after years of ill health that included colitis, headaches, and arthritis. When she finally learned that she had **cancer**, she returned to her grandmother's healing methods in order to regain her health.

After testing the results of a diet based on sprouts and wheat grass juice in her own life, she wanted others to benefit from what she had learned. Ann Wigmore founded the Hippocrates Health Institute in Boston in 1963, which still teaches her methods of self-healing through a live-foods diet. Although Ann Wigmore died in a fire in 1993, her diet still attracts new followers. In recent years, the Hippocrates Institute has opened branches in southern California and Florida.

Benefits

The Wigmore diet is based on the assumption that the high levels of living enzymes in fresh raw foods, particularly wheat grass juice and fresh sprouts, provide the body with substances needed to detoxify and regenerate it. In addition to increased vitality and a strengthened immune system, the Wigmore regimen is thought to help individuals overcome some serious diseases, including arthritis, digestive tract problems, **allergies,** and even **cancer**.

Description

Perhaps the essence of what she taught could best be described by Ann Wigmore herself: "Live foods **nutrition** is super nutrition because it recognizes and appreciates the differences between raw and cooked foods and between natural and synthetic nutrients. In the conventional nutrition-school curriculum there is little room for a discussion of either the value of enzymes and life forces in foods, or the merits of live (raw) versus cooked foods. Yet the difference, when translated into health terms, is the difference between being vitally healthy and alive, and just breathing."

The Wigmore diet classifies foods into four major groups: living foods, which include sprout mixtures, sunflower and buckwheat baby greens, living sauerkraut, and the fresh juices of wheat grass and barley; raw foods, which include fresh organic vegetables and ripe fruit, spices, herbs, and raw nuts; whole cooked foods, which include steamed or boiled vegetables, cooked whole grains, and baked root vegetables; and processed fast foods, which include all forms of "junk foods." People following the Wigmore diet believe that most human diseases are caused when a person's diet contains mostly foods in the last two groups.

Practitioners of the Wigmore diet encourage people to think of enzyme and oxygen levels as "bank accounts." The more oxygen and enzymes that can be stored in the cells, the healthier one feels. It has been shown that eating certain foods will maintain enzymes and oxygen at optimal preferred levels.

Other notable features of the Wigmore diet include its emphasis on wheat grass as a "living food medicine" and food combining as a key to good digestion. Wheat grass has been credited with more healings than any other factor in the program because it is supposed to be rich in over 90 enzymes and minerals that are needed to build up the blood and immune system. People following the Wigmore diet are encouraged to drink at least two 2-ounce servings of wheat grass juice every day. In addition, wheat grass enemas of 4–8 ounces can be taken "as often as possible" for best results during the **detoxification** process.

Food combining in the Wigmore diet is based on the assumption that certain food combinations cause stomach cramps, **indigestion**, **bad breath**, intestinal **gas**, or lowered energy levels. Foods are divided into nine groups: proteins (poultry, fish, dairy products, miso, and yeast); pre-digested proteins (nuts and seeds); starches; vegetables; acid fruits (citrus fruits and sour fruits); sub-acid fruits (apples, apricots, most berries, and peaches); sweet fruits (bananas, dates, and all dried fruits); melons; and neutral foods (avocados and lemons). Melons are to be eaten alone. While meals made up of foods from any one category are a good combination, for example, fruit and starch are a bad combination.

Another important point in the Wigmore diet is drinking water. Tap water is considered unsuitable, and some form of filter should be used. Distilled water or spring water are preferred.

Preparations

Preparations for the Wigmore diet include a gradual departure from less healthy foods; cleansing the digestive tract with **aloe** vera or similar products; and encouraging good digestion by eating food at room temperature as often as possible and eating raw or living foods before any cooked foods. It is thought that the cooked foods hold up the digestion of raw and living foods, causing intestinal gas. Ann Wigmore's *The Sprouting Book* discusses the proper preparation of the sprouts that play such a prominent role in her diet.

Precautions

Like all natural therapies, the Wigmore diet will be more effective if environmental as well as nutritional pollution of all types is avoided, and if a generally healthy lifestyle is followed. Such spiritual practices as **meditation**, visualization, and joining or starting a Living Foods support group are considered important features of a healthy lifestyle.

Side effects

Practitioners of the Wigmore diet warn people to expect certain side effects from detoxification, which is considered a key principle in the Living Foods lifestyle. The diet is believed to clear toxins from the body that have accumulated over years of poor nutritional habits. These toxins are released into the bloodstream and lymphatic system for eventual excretion. During the detoxification process, the dieter may feel less energetic and uncomfortable in their body. The program recommends daily non-strenuous **exercise**, high fiber intake to cleanse the colon, daily dry skin brushing over the entire body, and the use of **spirulina** (blue-green algae) products to ease the side effects of the detoxification process.

As the Wigmore diet is a purely organic regimen, and avoids the use of medications and all chemicals, the risk of other side effects is minimal. Nevertheless, some individuals will be unable to tolerate this diet, and others may be allergic to the foods that are prescribed.

Research & general acceptance

As with many holistic therapies, the Wigmore diet is met with skepticism from allopathic physicians. On the other hand, there are many clinical cases and testimonials consistent with Ann Wigmore's predicted benefits.

Training & certification

Anyone can follow the Wigmore regimen, as no special training or certification is required. Detailed information can be obtained from the organizations listed below, or from Ann Wigmore's books. Many holistic practitioners are familiar with Wigmore's works and can advise on the regimen.

Resources

ORGANIZATIONS

Ann Wigmore Foundation. PO Box 399, San Fidel, NM 87049-0399. (505) 552-0595. Fax: (505) 552-0596.

KEY TERMS

Detoxification—The process of purifying the body of poisons accumulated during years of poor eating habits.

Raw nutrition—A synonym for the Wigmore diet's emphasis on uncooked and living foods.

Spirulina—A genus of blue-green algae that is sometimes added to food to increase its nutrient value.

Wheat grass—Young green wheat sprouts, grown organically for juicing. Wheatgrass is a central element of the Wigmore diet.

Hippocrates Health Institute. Boston, MA. http://www.hippocratesinst.com.

Nature's First Law. P. O. Box 900202, San Diego, CA 91290. (619) 596-7979. (800) 205-2350. http://www.rawfood.com/wigmore.html.

Patricia Skinner

Wild endive *see* **Dandelion**

Wild thyme *see* **Thyme**

Wild oat

Description

Wild oat (*Avena sativa*) is a member of the grass family native to Scotland. There are approximately 25 varieties of the oat plants, and oat is now grown throughout the world. *Avena sativa* is the species that is used in herbal remedies. The mature seed of the oat plant is used as a cereal grain. However, much of the plant is used to maintain good health and to remedy disease conditions.

Before maturity oat seeds are in a liquid phase, and they are collected for use in tonics that treat nervous conditions. Wild oat is usually in this stage for two weeks during August.

The seeds mature in the late summer and early fall. If harvested then, the seeds are rolled or ground into oatmeal. If the seeds aren't harvested at that time, they are referred to as groats.

Once the seeds are harvested, the straw from the plant can be cut up and brewed as oatstraw tea. And the husks surrounding the seeds are used as oat bran.

The only part of this grain that is not used in alternative medicine is the root.

Wild oat is also known as oat, groats, oatstraw, and straw.

General use

Avena sativa is Latin for wild oat, a name that does not provide the complete picture of this grain's use in alternative and conventional medicine. The old saying "sowing your wild oats" is based on the observation that stallions given wild oat experienced greater sex drives. Wild oat was thought to have the same effect on men, although that has never been scientifically proven. Nevertheless, dietary supplements containing wild oats are still advertised and sold as boosting the male sex drive.

Wild oat may not be an aphrodisiac or a means of promoting fertility, but the grain has numerous other health benefits.

In the past, people recovering from illnesses ate oatmeal because it was easily digested. Doctors advised overworked people to drink a beverage consisting of wine and oats. The drink was said to restore nervous energy. Oatmeal also served as a treatment for skin conditions.

In contemporary times, oatmeal is acknowledged as a rich source of bran and fiber. The grain is associated with treating high **cholesterol** . Whole oat products with at least 0.02 oz (0.75 g) of soluble fiber in each serving can reduce the risk of **heart disease**. The U.S. Food and Drug Administration allowed manufacturers to make that statement, and add that the fiber product must be part of a diet that is low in **cholesterol** and saturated fat. A study published in the summer of 2002 reported that oat cereal is superior to wheat cereal in lowering LDL cholesterol levels in adult males.

A new use for the beta-glucans (complex carbohydrates) contained in oats is in the manufacture of functional foods for the management of Type 2 (adult-onset) diabetes. Functional foods are a relatively recent category of foods. They are not currently defined by any government regulatory body, but are commonly understood to be any potentially healthful food or food ingredient that may provide health benefits beyond the traditional nutrients it contains. Functional foods are sometimes called nutraceuticals.

Oat fiber is also used as a substrate, or growing medium, for *Lactobacillus* and other bacteria that are introduced into the digestive tract of patients suffering from severe **infections** of the pancreas. The "good" bacteria in the intestines help the body to fight off infections elsewhere in the digestive system. The oat fiber provides the bacteria with nourishment without causing any side effects to the patient.

Furthermore, pregnant women can benefit from the **calcium** and other trace nutrients found in oat straw.

Wild oat is recognized as a natural antidepressant and a mild sedative. It acts like a tonic to the nervous system, providing both nourishment and balance. Oat tea or an oat Bach flower remedy is used as a nervine (preparation given to calm the nerves).

In these capacities, wild oat can be used to treat conditions including headaches, **depression**, tension, **insomnia**, **anxiety**, and feelings of sadness. Wild oat is also a remedy for nerve **pain** and chronic **fatigue**.

Oatstraw can be used to ease emotional anxieties and to treat skin conditions such as **rashes**, **psoriasis**, **burns**, **eczema**, **warts**, and insect bites.

An oatmeal pack may be used to treat skin conditions. The oatmeal facial is a popular treatment for promoting smoother skin because the textured oat sloughs off dead skin when used as a mask or scrub. An oatstraw bath can provide more relief for skin conditions and **neuralgia**.

Wild oat is also believed to help with nicotine withdrawal, a remedy recommended by German doctors. The wild oat extract is said to be effective when used for this purpose, and oat cereal is also said to be helpful.

Preparations

Wild oat is available in various forms and is used in various alternative medicine traditions such as **homeopathy**. Commercial preparations include oatstraw tea, tincture, and the wild oat Bach flower remedy (a liquid concentrate called a stock). The packaged oatmeal sold in the grocery store can also be used for treatments.

Wild oat tea, which is also known as an infusion, is made by pouring 1 c (240 ml) of boiling water over 1–3 tsp (1.5–3 g) of the dried straw. The mixture is steeped for 10–15 minutes and then strained. Wild oat tea should be drunk three times a day.

When wild oat tincture is used, the dosage is 1 oz (1 mL) taken three times a day.

Wild oat can be combined with **skullcap** and **mugwort** to provide relief from depression and to improve sleep.

A flower remedy

Flower remedies are liquid concentrates made by soaking flowers in spring water. Also known as flower essences, 38 remedies were developed by homeopathic physician **Edward Bach** during the 1930s. Bach's wild oat remedy is taken to resolve conditions such as career anxiety and uneasiness about a lack of direction or commitment.

The daily dosage of the Bach wild oat flower remedy is 2–4 drops (1/8–1/4 ml) taken four times each day. The drops can be placed under the tongue or added to a glass of water. Another remedy is to add some stock to the bath water.

Oat baths

An oatstraw bath can provide relief for irritated skin and neuralgia. A bath is prepared by boiling 1 lb (500 g) of shredded oatstraw in 2 qt (0.95 L) of water. After boiling for 20 minutes, this mixture is strained and used in the bath. Another option is to place cooked rolled oats in a bag and the bag is put in the bath.

Precautions

Wild oat has not been associated with any health risks when taken in proper dosages, according to *Physician's Desk Reference for Herbal Medicines*, the 1998 book based on the findings of Germany's Commission E. The commission is the German counterpart of the U.S. Food and Drug Administration (FDA). The European group's findings about herbal remedies were published in a 1997 monograph.

However, people diagnosed with gluten sensitivity (**celiac disease**) should consult with a doctor or health practitioner to determine if they can safely take wild oat internally.

Side effects

There are no known side effects associated with designated dosages of wild oat.

Interactions

There are no known interactions associated with the use of wild oat and other medications or herbs.

Resources

BOOKS

Duke, James A. *The Green Pharmacy.* Emmaus, PA: Rodale Press, Inc., 1997.

Keville, Kathi. *Herbs for Health and Healing.* Emmaus, PA: Rodale Press, Inc., 1996.

PDR for Herbal Medicines. Montvale, NJ: Medical Economics Company, 1998.

Ritchason, Jack. *The Little Herb Encyclopedia.* Pleasant Grove, UT: Woodland Health Books, 1995.

Squier, Thomas Broken Bear with Lauren David Peden. *Herbal Folk Medicine.* New York: Henry Holt and Company, 1997.

Tyler, Varro and Steven Foster. *Tyler's Honest Herbal.* Binghamton, NY: The Haworth Herbal Press, 1999.

PERIODICALS

Davy, B. M., K. P. Davy, R. C. Ho, et al. "High-Fiber Oat Cereal Compared with Wheat Cereal Consumption Favorably

---

KEY TERMS

Aphrodisiac—A food or drug that stimulates or is thought to stimulate sexual desire.

Beta-glucans—Complex carbohydrates contained in oats and other cereal grains. They are thought to be useful in managing diabetes as well as lowering blood cholesterol levels.

Functional food—A food or food ingredient that is thought to confer health benefits in addition to the nutrients it contains.

Gluten—A grayish sticky compound found in oat flour and other grain flours, composed of two proteins, glutenin and gliadin.

Nervine—A type of medication or herbal preparation given to calm the nerves.

Nutraceutical—Another term for functional food.

Tincture—A method of preserving herbs with alcohol. Powdered herb is added to a 50 percent alcohol solution. The tincture steeps for two weeks and is shaken daily. It is strained and bottled.

Alters LDL-Cholesterol Subclass and Particle Numbers in Middle-Aged and Older Men." *American Journal of Clinical Nutrition* 76 (August 2002): 351-358.

Jenkins, A. L., D. J. Jenkins, U. Zdravkovic, et al. "Depression of the Glycemic Index by High Levels of Beta-Glucan Fiber in Two Functional Foods Tested in Type 2 Diabetes." *European Journal of Clinical Nutrition* 56 (July 2002): 622-628.

Olah, A., T. Belagyi, A. Issekutz, et al. "Randomized Clinical Trial of Specific *Lactobacillus* and Fibre Supplement to Early Enteral Nutrition in Patients with Acute Pancreatitis." *British Journal of Surgery* 89 (September 2002): 1103-1107.

ORGANIZATIONS

American Botanical Council. P.O. Box 201660, Austin, TX 78720. (512) 331-8868.

American Dietetic Association. 216 West Jackson Blvd., Chicago, IL 60606. (312) 899-0040. <www.eatright.org>.

Herb Research Foundation. 1007 Pearl St., Suite 200, Boulder, CO 80302. (303) 449-2265. <www.herbs.org>.

OTHER

Ask Dr. Weil. 2000. <www.askdrweil.com>.

MotherNature.com Health Encyclopedia. 2000. <www.mothernature.com/ency>.

Liz Swain
Rebecca J. Frey, PhD

Windflower *see* **Pulsatilla**

Wintergreen

Description

Though several different plants are called by this name, true wintergreen is *Gaultheria procumbens*, a low-growing species of shrub common in sandy coastal regions and woodlands of eastern North America from Georgia to New Foundland. It is a member of the heath, or Ericaceae, family. Other names by which wintergreen is known include aromatic wintergreen, boxberry, Canada tea, checkerberry, deerberry, ground berry, mountain tea, partidgeberry, spice berry, teaberry, and wax cluster.

Wintergreen plants have creeping underground stems from which small reddish stalks grow, normally less than 6 in (15 cm) high. Wintergreen leaves are spoon-shaped and less than 0.5 in (1 cm) in length. They are bright green, shiny, and have a leathery appearance. They are attached in tufts near the tip of a rigid, slender stalk. In June or July, wintergreen plants produce tiny wax-like, urn-shaped flowers, which are either white or pink in color. These unusual flowers are often difficult to find because the plant's leaves and other ground covers on the forest floor hide them so well. The fruit of the wintergreen, a startlingly brilliant red berry, appears in late autumn through the winter, and is much more visible than the wintergreen flower. Wintergreen is an evergreen plant, and even beneath deep snow it retains its shiny green leaves and scarlet berries.

Wintergreen leaves and berries are edible. In their natural state they have no particularly noticeable odor. The leaves have a tart, spicy, astringent taste, while the berries are sweet, with a unique, pleasant taste, which is often used in flavorings. Wintergreen leaves were formerly carried in the *United States Pharmacopoeia*, but now only the oil distilled from them is listed. But in many countries the whole plant is still used. When wintergreen leaves are distilled, they impart an oil, which is made up of 99% methyl salicylate, the chemical compound upon which all aspirin products are based. Before being distilled, wintergreen leaves have to be steeped in water for nearly a day before the oil will develop through fermentation. It is only after this fermentation and the chemical reaction of water and one component, gaultherin, that wintergreen emits its characteristic, pleasant aroma. Chemists have learned how to synthetically produce an oil with many of the same properties and a very similar product, also called oil of wintergreen, is extracted from the sweet birch tree, *Betula lenta*.

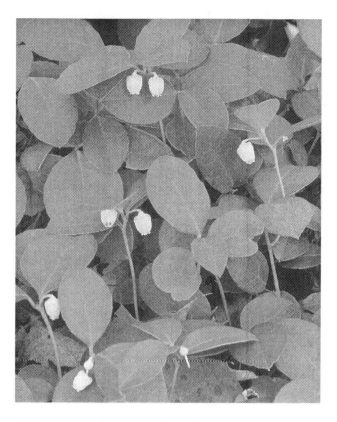

White wintergreen flowers. *(© Hal Horwitz/Corbis. Reproduced by permission.)*

The name wintergreen is also sometimes applied to two other members of the genus Gaultheria, as well as three other unrelated plants:

- *Gaultheria hispidula* is also called wintergreen. It is supposed to remove the predisposition to cancer from the body.

- *Gaultheria shallon*, sallol, is found in northwest America. Its berries are edible and quite tasty.

- *Pytola rotundiflora* is also known as false wintergreen or British wintergreen. It was formerly used as a vulnerary.

- *Chimophila umbellata* and *Maculata* are both called by a variety of names: bitter wintergreen, rheumatism weed, spotted wintergreen, or pipsissewa. North American natives used these two herbs for the treatment of **indigestion**, rheumatism, scrofula, and as a diuretic.

- *Trientalis europaea*, or **chickweed** wintergreen, is native to England and was used in the past externally in an ointment used in healing **wounds**, and internally as a tea to treat blood-poisoning and eczema.

General use

Wintergreen oil is used as flavoring for candies, chewing gum, and medicines. With **eucalyptus** or menthol, it is often used to flavor toothpaste and other dental products. The berry, often called checkerberry, is used for flavoring candies. It is sometimes used as a tea by itself, or combined with tea as a flavoring; hence its name teaberry.

Medicinally, wintergreen leaves are taken internally as a decoction to treat nephritis and bladder problems. It is used as a diuretic, for the treatment of **neuralgia**, as a systemic tonic, to stimulate menses, and to aid in bringing on lactation after **childbirth**. It has also been used to relieve children's headaches. Leaves have also been used for headaches and other pains, and as a gargle for a **sore throat** and mouth.

Externally, oil of wintergreen is widely used in liniments for the relief of muscular-skeletal **pain**, both from sports injuries and arthritis. Because of its aromatic and pain-relieving qualities, the oil is used in a number of products in aromatherapy, including stress-reducing pulse point creams, foot scrubs, and balms.

Preparations

Wintergreen leaves can actually be picked at any time of year, but summer is the most opportune time for gathering them. They must be dried in the shade to prevent loss of the volatile oil contained in the leaves, and should be stored in an airtight container in a dark, cool place. A decoction can be made by mixing 1 c (240 ml) of boiling water with 1 tsp (1.5 g) of the dried wintergreen leaves and allowing the mixture to steep for 15 minutes. This tea may be taken up to three times per day.

Oil of wintergreen, as noted previously, is made by first steeping wintergreen leaves in water for at least 24 hours, and then allowing this mixture to ferment and release its oil. Fermentation is known to have occurred when the characteristic wintergreen aroma is released. This oil is sometimes used externally in dilute solutions in combination with other products such as **aloe** and lanolin to produce ointments, but either the oil extracted from sweet birch or the synthetic version are more apt to be used.

Precautions

Oil of wintergreen should not be taken internally. In the past, it has been given in a capsule form to treat rheumatism, but excessive doses of it have actually caused death due to severe inflammation of the stomach and gastrointestinal hemorrhage.

Side effects

True oil of wintergreen, distilled from wintergreen leaves, is very rapidly absorbed by the skin and often causes severe skin irritation and painful, hive-like skin eruptions.

KEY TERMS

· ·

Eczema—General term for a group of acute or chronic inflammatory skin conditions characterized by redness, thickening, oozing, and the formation of papules, vesicles, and crusts.

Neuralgia—Severe pain caused by irritation of, or damage to, a nerve.

Papule—Superficial, solid elevation on the skin.

Rheumatism—A popular term for any disorder that causes pain and stiffness in muscles and joints and fibrous tissues, including minor aches and twinges, as well as disorders such as rheumatoid arthritis, osteoarthritis, and polymyalgia rheumatica.

Scrofula—Tuberculous inflammation of the lymph nodes of the neck in children, caused by bacteria in cattle; also called cervical adenitis.

Vesicle—Sac or hollow structure filled with fluid (i.e., a blister).

Vulnerary—An agent used for healing wounds.

Resources

BOOKS

Thayer, Henry. *Fluid and Solid Extracts.* Geo. C. Rand & Avery, 1866.

Grieve, M. and C. F. Leyel. *A Modern Herbal: The Medical, Culinary, Cosmetic and Economic Properties, Cultivation and Folklore of Herbs, Grasses, Fungi, Shrubs and Trees With All of Their Modern Scientific Uses.* Barnes and Noble Publishing, 1992.

Hoffman, David and Linda Quayle. *The Complete Illustrated Herbal: A Safe and Practical Guide to Making and Using Herbal Remedies.* Barnes and Noble Publishing, 1999.

Taber, Clarence Wilbur. *Taber's Cyclopedic Medical Dictionary.* F.A.Davis Co., 1997.

OTHER

Hobbs, Christopher. *Herbal Advisor.* http//www.AllHerb.com.

Joan Schonbeck

Witch hazel

Description

Witch hazel (*Hamamelis virginiana*) is a deciduous tree or shrub that is native to Atlantic North America,

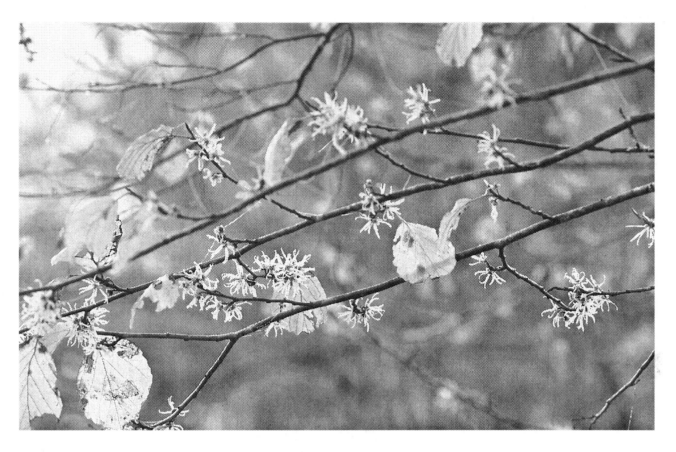

Witch hazel blooming in Great Smoky Mountains National Park. *(Photo Researchers, Inc. Reproduced by permission.)*

and it is now also cultivated in Europe and Asia. The shrub can reach a height of 15 ft (4.6 m). It flowers in the fall, producing vivid yellow flowers. Witch hazel is also known as hazel nut, snapping hazel, spotted alder, tobacco wood, winterbloom, and hamamelis water.

Native Americans used witch hazel leaves and bark as a poultice to reduce swelling and inflammation. Those are among the uses of this herb that has long been among the best known and widely used home remedies.

The word "witch" in the name of the herb is actually a derivative from the Anglo-Saxon word *wych* meaning flexible. The word described the flexibility of the branches that Native Americans used to make bows.

General use

Witch hazel is a very versatile remedy, with generally accepted uses ranging from facial care to soothing aching feet. It is also used for the treatment of **hemorrhoids**, inflammation of the mouth and throat, and other conditions, such as **varicose veins**, **wounds**, and **burns**.

Witch hazel has so many applications that **Andrew Weil**, M.D., called the decoction or tincture of the bark the "all–around astringent." Weil, who practices natural

and preventive medicine, recommended using witch hazel to ease the **pain** of **sunburn**, windburn, insect bites, poison ivy **blisters**, and sore and sprained muscles.

The medicinal element of witch hazel is the hamamelis water that is distilled, decocted, or tinctured from fresh and dried leaves, and fresh and dried bark and twigs. Tannins and volatile oils are the primary active ingredients of witch hazel that contribute to its astringent benefits. The tannin content of witch hazel leaves is 8%, and in witch hazel bark ranges from 1–3%, as the medicine derived from the bark will yield a higher tannin concentration than that from leaves. Recent research done in Asia indicates that it is the tannin content of witch hazel that is chiefly responsible for its strong antioxidant activity.

As with other herbal astringents, witch hazel reduces the irritation on the tissue surface through a form of numbing. Surface inflammation is reduced, and the astringent creates a partial barrier against infection. That barrier aids in the treatment of wounds and burns. The astringency helps to stop bleeding, so witch hazel is useful in treating **bruises**, cuts, and other skin abrasions.

In addition, a cold compress of witch hazel is said to ease a **headache**. Cosmetically, witch hazel is used as a facial skin freshener and astringent to reduce pore size, make-up remover, and to reduce bags under eyes. Products for men that contain witch hazel include herbal shaving cream and aftershave.

The above are among the mainstream applications of the herb that Native Americans regarded as a general tonic. They also brewed witch hazel as a tea for conditions including cuts, colds, heavy **menstruation**, tumors, and eye inflammation. Witch hazel was taken internally to stop bleeding from hemorrhage.

Some of those applications remain part of folk medicine. Other folk remedy applications of witch hazel include applications for backache, and internal use for **diarrhea**, nervousness, nosebleed, **vaginitis**, and venereal disease.

As of 2002, there has been relatively limited research on the uses of witch hazel in the United States. There is agreement among alternative health practitioners that external use of this herb is safe.

Research conducted in Europe provides more information about applications of witch hazel. There, witch hazel products were approved for skin injuries, inflammation of skin and mucous membranes, and varicose veins. Witch hazel and leaves were approved for the topical treatment of skin injuries, burns, varicose veins, and hemorrhoids. Recent studies carried out in Germany and the United Kingdom have established that witch hazel extract offers some protection against UV radiation prior to sun exposure as well as relieving the inflammation of sunburn.

In the United States, there is another controversy about the remedial benefit of witch hazel. Hamamelis water, when distilled, contains no tannin. Distilled witch hazel consists of a mixture of 14% alcohol in water with a trace of volatile oil. The astringent effect of witch hazel is due to an alcohol content similar to that of red wine. But the unstudied volatile oils exert some effects similar to topical tannin, and are also antimicrobial.

Preparations

Witch hazel is available in various forms. Commercial preparations include witch hazel water and gels, although much commercial witch hazel is not true distilled witch hazel water. Witch hazel is also an ingredient in products, such as face and body pads and hemorrhoid pads, including Preparation H ointment.

As a topical astringent, witch hazel water is applied directly to burns, bruises, insect bites, and aching muscles. It can also be used to clean oily skin, remove make-up, or mixed with water for a relaxing footbath. Uses for the gel include treating cuts, **diaper rash**, and **bedsores**.

An infusion of fresh or dried leaves has been "cautiously used" in the treatment of internal hemorrhaging or to reduce excessive menstrual flow.

Infusion is a process that preserves the astringent tannin in witch hazel, using the leaves. A decoction may be prepared by simmering, not boiling, the herb's bark. This is done by steeping 1 teaspoon of witch hazel powder or twigs in a cup of boiling water. The mixture is boiled and covered for 10 minutes, then strained. After it cools, it can be applied directly or mixed into an ointment base such as petroleum jelly.

Uses of witch hazel leaf include remedies for diarrhea and menstrual conditions. The bark is used for skin injuries, inflammation of the skin, locally inflamed swelling, hemorrhoids, and varicose veins.

Witch hazel dosages

Recommended dosages when using witch hazel are as follows:

- Witch hazel water (distillate) can be used as is or diluted at a 1:3 ratio with water.

- A poultice can be made by using 20–30% of witch hazel in semi-solid preparations.

- For an extract preparation, use a semi-solid and liquid preparation that corresponds to 5–10% of the drug.

- Decoctions of 5–10 grams of witch hazel extract per cup of water can be used for compresses and rinses.

- Ointment or gel is prepared by mixing 5 grams of witch hazel extract in 100 grams of an ointment base.

- The recommended dosage of suppositories is 0.1–1 gram of the drug. Suppositories in the rectum or vagina can be used from one to three times daily.

Applications

Witch hazel is a multi-faceted remedy that is administered in several ways. Applications of witch hazel include:

- Gargle with a decoction of 1 teaspoon of witch hazel bark that has been steeped 10 minutes in boiling water and then strained.

- For skin conditions, ointment or cream can be used twice a day or as needed.

- Tincture can be placed directly on affected areas.

- A poultice can be applied to wounds and sores.

- Witch hazel extracts can be applied in combination with warm, moist compresses in the morning or at bedtime.

- For bruises, a washcloth can be used for a witch hazel compress. An ice cube placed inside the cloth keeps the compress cold and diminishes swelling.

HEMORRHOID RELIEF. Witch hazel's applications include various methods for treating hemorrhoids:

- A hamamelis suppository can be inserted at bedtime to reduce inflammation of a swollen vein.
- For relief of hemorrhoids, Weil recommends moistening toilet paper with witch hazel. This compress is used to clean the anal area after bowel movements.

Combinations

Hemorrhoid treatment accounts for two remedies that combine witch hazel with another herb, such as pilewort. Pilewort is also known as celandine. Another hemorrhoid remedy combines witch hazel with **horse chestnut.**

Furthermore, witch hazel is combined with **aloe** vera in commercial products such as skin care treatments. Home recipes for facial cleanser and mask include witch hazel, **essential oils**, and other ingredients.

Precautions

When witch hazel is administered in designated therapeutic dosages, no health risks have been recorded. However, when witch hazel is taken internally, its tannin content can lead to digestive complaints. Furthermore, in rare cases, liver damage is conceivable following long term administration.

Witch hazel water is intended for external use and most sources cite recommended dosages are for adults. The amount should be adjusted for older people and the chronically ill. Individuals should check with their doctors about use of witch hazel.

External use of witch hazel may result in minor skin irritation for some people. When this occurs, the amount of witch hazel should be diluted.

While it is safe to use witch hazel for gargling, caution should be taken when using it internally. Witch hazel contains small amounts of safrole, a compound that the U. S. Food and Drug Administration (FDA) banned for use in food during the 1960s. That ban came after laboratory animals that ingested large amounts of the compound developed **cancer.** Witch hazel has not yet come under fire for safrole content. However, as of March 2000, there was little research information available. Additional study was needed on the safe use of this home remedy that was a staple for Native Americans.

Side effects

Opinion varies about the side effects caused when witch hazel is taken internally. The tannin content can cause stomach irritation or cramping. A dose of 1 gram of witch hazel will cause **nausea, vomiting,** or **constipation.**

The FDA has approved witch hazel distillate as safe for external use. Sources had reported no known side ef-

fects as of March of 2000. However, future studies may provide more information about the safety or side effects of witch hazel.

Interactions

The 1998 Commission E monograph reported no contraindications or interactions related to the use of witch hazel. However, there are well-known interactions between many drugs and high tannin herbs that are too numerous to list. Those on blood thinners for circulatory trouble should take internal witch hazel preparations with caution if at all. In addition, witch hazel should not be taken internally with medications containing alkaloids, as it interferes with their absorption. Alkaloid drugs include atropine and codeine.

Resources

BOOKS

Albright, Peter. *The Complete Book of Complementary Therapies.* Allentown, PA: People's Medical Society, 1997.

Castleman, Michael. *The Healing Herbs.* Emmaus, PA: Rodale Press, Inc., 1991.

Keville, Kathi. *Herbs for Health and Healing.* Emmaus, PA: Rodale Press, Inc., 1996.

Lockie, Andrew and Nicola Geddes. *The Complete Guide to Homeopathy.* New York: DK Publishing, 1995.

Medical Economics Company. *PDR for Herbal Medicines.* Montvale, N.J.: Medical Economics Co., 1998.

Ritchason, Jack. *The Little Herb Encyclopedia.* Pleasant Grove, UT: Woodland Health Books, 1995.

Squier, Thomas Broken Bear, with Lauren David Peden. *Herbal Folk Medicine.* New York: Henry Holt and Company, 1997.

Tyler, Varro and Steven Foster. *Tyler's Honest Herbal.* Binghampton, NY: The Haworth Herbal Press, 1999.

PERIODICALS

Choi, H. R., J. Choi, Y. N. Han, et al. "Peroxynitrite Scavenging Activity of Herb Extracts." *Phytotherapy Research* 16 (June 2002): 364-367.

Habtemariam, S. "Hamamelitannin from *Hamamelis virginiana* Inhibits the Tumour Necrosis Factor-Alpha (TNF)-Induced Endothelial Cell Death in Vitro." *Toxicon* 40 (January 2002): 83-88.

Hughes-Formella, B. J., A. Filbry, J. Gassmüller, and F. Rippke. "Anti-inflammatory Efficacy of Topical Preparations with 10% Hamamelis Distillate in a UV Erythema Test." *Skin Pharmacology and Applied Skin Physiology* 15 (March-April 2002): 125-132.

ORGANIZATIONS

American Botanical Council. P.O. Box 201660, Austin TX, 78720. (512) 331-8868. http://www.herbalgram.org.

Herb Research Foundation. 1007 Pearl St., Suite 200, Boulder, CO 80302. (303) 449-2265. http://www.herbs.org.

KEY TERMS

Antioxidant—An enzyme or other organic substance that is able to counteract the damaging effects of oxidation in living tissue. The hamamelitannin in witch hazel is a strong antioxidant.

Astringent—A substance that contracts body tissue and checks capillary bleeding. Witch hazel's astringent action is caused by tannins.

Decoction—System for releasing the herbal essence of bark or root bark. Those elements are simmered in a non–aluminum pan. Place 1 ounce of chopped bark or roots in 16 ounces or water. Bring to a boil, then simmer for 10 minutes. Strain, then squeeze out juices.

Pharynx—The cavity at the back of the throat that leads from the mouth and nasal passage to the larynx.

Poultice—A paste made of crushed herbs and a substance such as hot moist flour, corn meal, or bread and milk. The paste is placed on the skin.

Tannin—An astringent substance named for its uses in the tanning industry because it "fixes and preserves tissue," such as leather goods.

Tincture—A method of preserving herbs with alcohol. Powdered herb is added to a 50 percent alcohol solution. The tincture macerates for two weeks and is shaken daily. It is strained and bottled.

Topical—A type of medication that is applied to the external surface of the skin. Witch hazel is most commonly used in topical formulations.

OTHER

Ask Dr. Weil. http://www.askdrweil.com.
Holistic OnLine. http://www.holisticonline.com.

Liz Swain
Rebecca J. Frey, PhD

Worms

Definition

Worms are parasitic, soft-bodied organisms that can infect humans and animals. Parasitic worms fall into several different classes and include flukes, roundworm, and tapeworm.

Description

Worms are parasites that live within a host organism (human or animal) for the purpose of obtaining food. This relationship causes harm to the host, and, with severe cases of infection, can be fatal. The term worms commonly refers to intestinal worms, although worms can infect other organs and the bloodstream. Intestinal worms are helminths and fall into three classes: cestodes (tapeworms), nematodes (roundworms), and trematodes (flukes).

Cestodes

Tapeworms have a ribbon-like body composed of a scolex, which attaches the worm to the intestinal wall, and a long chain of progressively developing proglottids. Proglottids at the tail end of the worm contain eggs. Tapeworms can have 3–4,000 proglottids and be several meters long. Tapeworms that infect humans include *Taenia saginata*, *Taenia solium*, *Hymenolepis nana*, and *Diphyllobothrium latum*. Tapeworms live in the small intestine and absorb food from the intestinal contents.

The complex life cycles of cestodes differ with each genus and involve two or three different hosts. In general, one host (the intermediate host) ingests eggs that develop into a larval stage. A second host (the definitive host) ingests the larva, which develop into adult worms in the intestine. Humans can become infected with tapeworm by eating raw or inadequately cooked, contaminated fish, pork, or beef. Humans can serve as both intermediate and definitive hosts for certain cestodes. Although humans can experience severe disease when serving as an intermediate host, they may show few signs of disease when harboring adult tapeworms.

Nematodes

Intestinal nematodes, or roundworms, are the most worm-like of all the helminths and resemble the earthworm. Nematodes have a mouth with either three lips or teeth (hookworms), a complete digestive tract, and separate sexes. Nematodes can range from a few millimeters to over one meter long. Roundworms that can infect humans include *Trichuris trichiura* (whipworm), *Enterobius vermicularis* (pinworm), *Capillaria philippinensis*, *Trichostrongylus* species, *Ascaris lumbricoides*, *Ancylostoma duodenale* (hookworm), *Necator americanus* (hookworm), and *Strongyloides stercoralis*. Infection occurs following contact (ingestion or skin) with contaminated soil. Pinworms are not uncommon in children and are easily spread to other family members.

There are five stages (four larval and one adult) in the life cycle of the roundworm. Each genus has a unique life cycle that can be classified into one of three patterns. A person becomes infected by ingesting eggs or larva or through skin penetration by larva. Once ingested, depending upon the genus, eggs may either develop into adult worms in the intestines, or a larval stage may gain access to the bloodstream, enter the lungs, be swallowed, and then develop into adult worms in the intestines. For certain genera, larva penetrate the skin, arrive at the lungs via the bloodstream, are swallowed, and become mature worms in the intestines. Eggs are passed out in the stool, or with pinworms, the female lays eggs on the skin surrounding the anal opening.

Trematodes

Trematodes, or flukes, are flat, leaf-shaped, and range in length from a few millimeters to 75 millimeters. Intestinal flukes are primarily found in the Asian continent. Intestinal flukes that can infect humans are *Fasciolopsis buski*, *Heterophyes heterophyes*, *Metagonimus yokogawai*, *Echinostoma* species, and *Nanophyetus salmincola*.

The life cycles of all flukes involve freshwater snails as an intermediate host. Flukes are contracted by ingestion of eggs or encysted (encased) larva from contaminated water, raw water plants (water chestnuts, water bamboo shoots, etc.), or raw or inadequately cooked fish or snails. The eggs or larva mature into adult worms in the intestines.

Causes & symptoms

Infection by worms is caused by the ingestion of or skin contact with helminth eggs or larva, as described above.

Symptoms of helminth **infections** vary depending upon the genera and number of worms involved. Infection with adult tapeworms often causes no symptoms, however, some patients may experience **diarrhea**, abdominal **pain**, **anemia**, and/or **vitamin B_{12}** deficiency. Roundworm infection often causes no symptoms but some patients may experience abdominal pain, diarrhea, growth retardation, anemia, and bloody, mucusy stools. Pinworms cause irritated, itchy skin surrounding the anal opening. **Itching** may be more severe at night and interfere with sleep. Mild infection with flukes may cause no symptoms, but heavy infections can cause diarrhea, abdominal pain, and profuse stools containing undigested food.

One side effect of worm infestation that is presently being studied for potential applications in treating atopy (a type of inherited allergic response) is the release of certain anti-inflammatory chemicals in the body. These chemicals, called cytokines, may prove to be useful in preventing atopy.

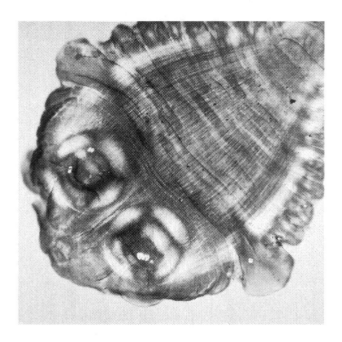

The head of an adult beef tapeworm. *(Custom Medical Stock Photo. Reproduced by permission.)*

Diagnosis

The patient will be questioned about travel and ingestion of high-risk foods. Worms are diagnosed by microscopic examination of stool samples to identify eggs and adult worms. Three samples may be taken: two from normal bowel movements and one following the use of a laxative. Pinworms are diagnosed using the "Scotch tape" method in which a piece of tape is applied to the skin surrounding the anal opening. Pinworm eggs, and occasionally an adult worm, adhere to the tape and are identified by microscopic examination.

Treatment

Although alternative remedies may help treat worms, the patient should consult a physician to obtain an accurate diagnosis and appropriate antihelmintic medication.

Dietary modifications help to rid a person of worm infection. Processed foods and foods that contain sugar, white flour, and milk products should be avoided. The diet should be comprised of 25% fat, 25% protein, and 50% complex carbohydrates. At least two tablespoons of unprocessed sesame, safflower, canola, or flax oil should be taken daily.

Herbals

Herbals that may kill and expel worms include:

• aloe (*Aloe vera*)

- ash (*Fraxinus americana*) bark ashes
- bayberry (*Myrica cerifera*) bark tea
- black walnut bark
- *Brassica oleracea* decoction
- butternut root bark
- citrin (*Garcinia cambogia*) extract
- clove (*Eugenia caryophyllus*)
- cranberry powder
- erba ruggine (*Ceterach officinarum*)
- fennel (*Foeniculum officinale*)
- garlic (*Allium sativum*)
- *Chenopodium ambrosioides*
- ginger (*Zingiber officinale*)
- goldenseal (*Hydrastis canadensis*)
- lemon (*Citrus limon*)
- male fern
- orange (*Citrus sinensis*) peel
- onion (*Allium cepa*)
- palmarosa (*Cymbopogon martinii*)
- pinkroot (*Spigelia*)
- pumpkin (*Cucurbita pepo*) seeds
- *Punica granatum* bark infusion
- sage (*Salvia officinalis*)
- tansy
- wood betony (*Stachys officinalis*) tea
- wormwood (*Artemisia absinthium*) tincture

Chinese herbal medicines

Roundworms are treated with the herbs Chuan Lian Gen Pi (*Cortex meliae radicis*) and Bing Lang (*Semen arecae*) and the patent medicines Wu Mei Wan (Mume Pill) and Qu Hui Wan (Dispel Roundworms Pill). Pinworms are treated with the herbs Ku Lian Gen Pi (*Cortex meliae radicis*) and Shi Jun Zi (*Fructus quisqualis*). Flukes are treated with the herbs Bing Lang (*Semen arecae*) and a mixture of Bing Lang (*Semen arecae*), Da Huang (*Radix et rhizoma rhei*), and Qian Niu Zi (*Semen pharbitidis*). Hookworm is treated with the herbs Lei Wan (*Sclerotium omphaliae*) and a combination of Guan Zhong (*Rhizoma dryopteris crassirhizomae*), Ku Lian Gen Pi (*Cortex meliae radicis*), Tu Jing Jie (*Herba chenopodii ambrosioidis*), and Zi Su Ye (*Folium perillae*).

Other alternative remedies

Other remedies for intestinal worms include:

- **Acupuncture.** Acupuncture may be used as an adjunct to other treatments to relieve pain and regulate the Spleen and Stomach.
- Ayurveda. Ayurvedic remedies for pinworms include eating one-quarter teaspoon twice daily with water of the herbal mixture: vidanga (5 parts), shardunika (2 parts), and trikatu (one eighth part). Also, the patient may take one-half teaspoon **triphala** in warm water each night.
- Homeopathy. The most common remedy for pinworms is wormseed (*Cina*). Pinworms associated with other conditions are treated with stinging **nettle** (*Urtica urens*) for **hives**, Mexican grass (*Sabadilla*) for **hay fever**, cat **thyme** (*Teucrium*) for polyps, pinkroot (*Spigelia*) for heart palpitations or facial pain, and krameria (*Ratanhia*) for rectal fissures.

Allopathic treatment

Intestinal worm infection is treated with medications, many of which are effective with one oral dose. Helminth infections are treated with albendazole (Albenza), levamisole (Ergamisol), mebendazole (Vermox), praziquantel (Biltricide), pyrantel (Antiminth, Ascarel, Pin-X), or thiabendazole (Mintezol).

In treating tapeworm infestations, it is important to completely eliminate the head and neck regions of the tapeworm, as the entire worm can regenerate from these parts.

Expected results

Medications are very effective in eliminating helminth infections; however, reinfection is always a possibility. Some types of worms appear to trigger changes in the human immune system that make reinfection easier. Patients should be retested following treatment to ensure that the infection has been eliminated. Complications of severe untreated infections include anemia, growth retardation, malnourishment, intestinal blockage, rectal prolapse (when the rectum extrudes out of the anal opening), and death.

Prevention

Most intestinal worm infections may be prevented by properly washing the hands after using the bathroom, washing skin after contact with soil, wearing shoes outside, and eating thoroughly cooked fish, meats (including meat from wild game), and freshwater plants. A number of cases of worm infections caused by eating raw salmon and crayfish were reported in North America in 2003; in addition, there was an outbreak of trichinellosis in Saskatchewan in 2000 that was traced to infected bear meat.

Skin penetration by larva may be reduced by eating foods rich in **vitamin A** including squash, carrots, sweet potatoes, yams, and greens.

People who live on farms, or have dogs or cats as house pets, should have their animals checked by a veterinarian on a regular basis and have them dewormed if necessary.

The Centers for Disease Control and Prevention (CDC) recommends that people traveling abroad should wash their hands with soap and water before handling food; should wash and peel all raw vegetables and fruits before eating; and should drink only bottled or boiled water, or carbonated drinks in cans or bottles.

As of late 2003, researchers in developing countries are working on a vaccine for pigs to help control worms transmitted by pigs to humans; however, the vaccine is not likely to be available for several years.

Resources

BOOKS

"Cestodes (Tapeworms)." Section 13, Chapter 161 in *The Merck Manual of Diagnosis and Therapy*, edited by Mark H. Beers, MD, and Robert Berkow, MD. Whitehouse Station, NJ: Merck Research Laboratories, 2002.

Garcia, Lynne S. and David A. Bruckner. *Diagnostic Medical Parasitology.* Washington, DC: American Society for Microbiology, 1997.

Markell, Edward K., David T. John, and Wojciech A. Krotoski. *Markell and Voge's Medical Parasitology.* 8th edition. Philadelphia: W.B. Saunders Company, 1999.

"Nematode (Roundworm) Infections." Section 13, Chapter 161 in *The Merck Manual of Diagnosis and Therapy*, edited by Mark H. Beers, MD, and Robert Berkow, MD. Whitehouse Station, NJ: Merck Research Laboratories, 2002.

Pearson, Richard D. *Parasitic Diseases: Helminths.* Textbook of Gastroenterology, 3rd edition. Edited by Tadataka Yamada et al. Philadelphia: Lippincott Williams & Wilkins, 1999.

Ying, Zhou Zhong and Jin Hui De. "Common Parasitoses." In *Clinical Manual of Chinese Herbal Medicine and Acupuncture.* New York: Churchill Livingston, 1997.

PERIODICALS

Albonico, Marco, D.W.T. Crompton, and L. Savioli. "Control Strategies for Human Intestinal Nematode Infections." *Advances in Parasitology* (1999): 277-341.

Castilla, E. A., R. Jessen, D. N. Sheck, and G. W. Procop. "Cavitary Mass Lesion and Recurrent Pneumothoraces Due to *Paragonimus kellicotti* Infection: North American Paragonimiasis." *American Journal of Surgical Pathology* 27 (August 2003): 1157–1160.

Couture, C., L. Measures, J. Gagnon, and C. Desbiens. "Human Intestinal Anisakiosis Due to Consumption of Raw Salmon." *American Journal of Surgical Pathology* 27 (August 2003): 1167–1172.

Ferreira, M. B., S. L. da Silva, and A. G. Carlos. "Atopy and Helminths." *Allergy and Immunology (Paris)* 34 (January 2002): 10-12.

Gittleman, Ann Louise. "Parasites." *Total Health* (May/June 1997): 47+.

Guarrera, Paolo Maria. "Traditional Antihelmintic, Antiparasitic and Repellent Uses of Plants in Central Italy." *Journal of Ethnopharmacology* (1999): 183-192.

Jenson, J. S., R. O'Connor, J. Osborne, and E. Devaney. "Infection with Brugia Microfilariae Induces Apoptosis of CD4(+) T Lymphocytes: A Mechanism of Immune Unresponsiveness in Filariasis." *European Journal of Immunology* 32 (March 2002): 858-867.

Kumaran, A. M., P. D'Souza, A. Agarwal, et al. "Geraniol, the Putative Anthelmintic Principle of *Cymbopogon martinii*." *Phytotherapy Research* 17 (September 2003): 957.

Roy, S. L., A. S. Lopez, and P. M. Schantz. "Trichinellosis Surveillance—United States, 1997–2001." *Morbidity and Mortality Weekly Report Surveillance Summaries* 52 (July 25, 2003): 1–8.

Schellenberg, R. S., B. J. Tan, J. D. Irvine, et al. "An Outbreak of Trichinellosis Due to Consumption of Bear Meat Infected with *Trichinella nativa*, in 2 Northern Saskatchewan Communities." *Journal of Infectious Diseases* 188 (September 15, 2003): 835–843.

ORGANIZATIONS

American Veterinary Medical Association (AVMA). 1931 North Meacham Road, Suite 100, Schaumburg, IL 60173-4360. <http://www.avma.org>.

Centers for Disease Control and Prevention. 1600 Clifton Rd., NE, Atlanta, GA 30333. (800) 311-3435, (404) 639-3311. <http://www.cdc.gov>.

Belinda Rowland
Rebecca J. Frey, PhD

Wormwood

Description

Wormwood (*Artemisia absinthium*) is a perennial that is native to Europe and parts of Africa and Asia but now grows wild in the United States. It is extensively cultivated. Also called shrub wormwood, *Artemisia absinthium* is a member of the daisy or Asteraceae family. The species name, *absinthium*, means "without sweetness." Many species of the genus *Artemisia* have medicinal properties.

Wormwood grows alongside roads or paths. This shrubby plant is 1-3 ft (0.3-0.9 m) tall and has gray-green or white stems covered with fine hairs. The yellowish-green leaves are hairy and silky and have glands that contain resinous particles where the natural insecticide is stored. Wormwood releases an aromatic odor and has a spicy, bitter taste.

Constituents and bioactivities

Wormwood contains a wide variety of biologically active compounds that contribute to its medicinal value. The constituents of wormwood include:

- acetylenes (trans-dehydromatricaria ester, C13 and C14 trans-spiroketalenol ethers and others)
- ascorbic acid (vitamin C)
- azulenes (chamazulene, dihydrochamazulenes, bisabolene, camphene, cadinene, sabinene, trans-sabinylacetate, phellandrene, pinene, and others)
- carotenoids
- flavonoids (quercitin 3-glucoside, quercitin 3-rhamnoglucoside, spinacetin 3-glucoside, spinacetin 3-rhamnoglucoside, and others)
- lignins (diayangambin and epiyangambin)
- phenolic acids (p-hydroxyphenylacetic, p-coumaric, chlorogenic, protocatechuic, vanillic, syringic, and others)
- tannins
- thujone and isothujone
- sesquiterpene lactones (absinthin, artabsin, anabsinthin, artemetin, artemisinin, arabsin, artabin, artabsinolides, artemolin, matricin, isoabsinthin, and others)

Wormwood is a strong bitter that affects the bitter-sensing taste buds on the tongue that send signals to the brain to stimulate the entire digestive system (salivation, stomach acid production, intestinal tract movement, etc.). This bitter taste also stimulates the production of bile by the liver and storage of bile in the gall bladder. The azulenes in wormwood have anti-inflammatory activity. The sesquiterpene lactones are insecticidal and have anti-tumor activity. The toxin thujone is a brain stimulant. Wormwood also has anti-inflammatory, anti-depressant, carminative (relieves intestinal **gas**), tonic (restores tone to tissues), antibacterial, antifungal, anti-amoebic, antifertility, hepatoprotective (prevents and cures liver damage), febrifugal (reduces **fever**), and vermifugal (expels intestinal **worms**) activities.

General use

Wormwood has been used in European traditional medicine as a restorative of impaired cognitive functions (thinking, remembering, and perception).

Wormwood is often used as a digestive stimulant. It is helpful in treating **indigestion**, **heartburn**, **irritable bowel syndrome**, stomach **pain**, gas, and bloating. By increasing the production of stomach acids and bile, wormwood can be useful to persons with poor digestion. It helps persons recover after a long illness and improves the uptake of nutrients.

As the name suggests, wormwood is used to eliminate intestinal worms, especially pinworms and roundworms. It is also used as an insect repellent and insecticide.

More recently, one of the sesquiterpene lactones, artemisinin, has shown promise as a treatment for **breast cancer**. Artemisinin was extracted from wormwood by the Chinese thousands of years ago to cure **malaria**, and is presently used in Asia and parts of Africa for that purpose. Recent experiments have shown that artemisinin is effective against the malaria parasite because it reacts with the high levels of **iron** in the parasite to produce free radicals. The free radicals then destroy the cell walls of the malaria parasite. **Cancer** researchers then applied the same principle to target cancer cells, which have a higher concentration of iron than normal cells. The researchers tested samples of breast cancer cells and normal breast cells that had first been treated to maximize their iron content and then treated with a water-soluble form of artemisinin. The normal cells showed little change, but within 16 hours, almost all of the cancer cells were dead.

Wormwood is also helpful in treating gall bladder inflammation, **hepatitis**, **jaundice**, fever, **infections**, and mild **depression**. Wormwood may also protect the liver from harmful chemicals and stimulate **menstruation** or miscarriage. It has been used to treat the pains associated with **childbirth**, cancers, muscle aches, arthritic joints, sprains, dislocated joints, and broken bones.

Wormwood has a historical dark side: absinthe. This clear green alcoholic beverage, which contains essential oil of wormwood and other plant extracts, is highly toxic and presently banned in many countries. A favorite liqueur in nineteenth-century France, absinthe was addictive and associated with a collection of serious side effects known as absinthism (irreversible damage to the central nervous system). The toxic component of wormwood that causes absinthism is thujone. Wormwood may contain as much as 0.6% thujone. On the other hand, wormwood soaked in white wine is used to produce the liqueur called vermouth (derived from the German word for wormwood, *Wermuth*), which contains very little thujone.

Preparations

Wormwood is harvested immediately prior to or during flowering in the late summer. All the aerial portions (stem, leaves, and flowers) have medicinal uses. Wormwood is used either fresh or dried.

Wormwood may be taken as an infusion (a tea), as a tincture (an alcohol solution), or in pill form. Wormwood should be taken only under the supervision of a professional. It should be taken in small doses as directed, and for no longer than four to five weeks at a time.

The infusion is prepared by steeping 0.5-2 tsp of wormwood in 1 cup of boiling-hot water for 10-15 minutes. The usual dosage is 3 cups daily, for a period not to exceed four weeks.

Wormwood tincture can be prepared by adding 1.5 cups of fresh, finely chopped wormwood or 8 tbsp of powdered wormwood to 2 cups of whiskey. The herb and alcohol mixture is shaken daily and allowed to steep for 11 days. The solids are strained out and the tincture is stored in a tightly capped bottle in a cool place. This tincture may be used externally (to relieve pain) or internally. Ten to twenty drops of tincture are added to water, which is taken 10–15 minutes before each meal. As with the infusion, wormwood tincture should not be taken for longer than four weeks.

Wormwood preparations are usually sipped because the strong bitter taste is an important component of its therapeutic effect on stomach ailments. The bitter taste of wormwood infusion or tincture may be masked with honey or molasses when the bitter action is not necessary, as in the treatment of worms, fever, or liver ailments.

Powdered wormwood is available in a pill form that can be used in the treatment of intestinal worms. An essential oil of wormwood is available for use in **aromatherapy**; it is toxic if used excessively.

Insect repellent can be made from wormwood by mixing thoroughly crushed fresh wormwood leaves with apple cider vinegar. This mixture is put into a small piece of gauze or cheesecloth. The ends are folded up and tied to make a little bag, and the bag is rubbed over the skin of humans or pets to repel mosquitoes, gnats, and horseflies.

Precautions

Excessive use of wormwood leads to toxic levels of thujone in the body. The long-term use of wormwood oil containing thujone, or alcoholic drinks containing thujone oil (e.g., absinthe) can be addictive and cause seizures, brain damage, temporary kidney failure, and possibly death. Using wormwood for longer than four weeks or at higher than recommended doses may lead to **nausea**, **vomiting**, restlessness, **insomnia**, vertigo, **tremors**, and seizures. Women who are pregnant or lactating (breast-feeding) should not use wormwood.

Side effects

Significant side effects are not encountered when wormwood is taken in small doses for only two to four weeks. One report stated, however, that using as much as 1 mL of wormwood tincture three times a day for up to nine months caused no side effects.

The U.S. Food and Drug Administration (FDA) states that wormwood may cause neurological symptoms, including delirium, paralysis, loss of intellect, and numbness of the legs and arms. The side effects associated with absinthism include auditory (hearing) and visual (seeing) hallucinations; tremors and convulsions; sleeplessness; paralysis; stomach problems; brain damage; and an increased risk of psychological disorders and suicide.

Interactions

As of mid-2000, there are no identified interactions between wormwood and any other drug or herbal medicine.

Resources

BOOKS

Chevallier, Andrew. *The Encyclopedia of Medicinal Plants.* New York: DK Publishing, 1996.

Heinerman, John. *Heinerman's Encyclopedia of Healing Herbs and Spices.* Englewood Cliffs, NJ: Parker Publishing Company, 1996.

PERIODICALS

"Ancient Chinese Folk Remedy May Hold Key to Nontoxic Cancer Treatment." *Health & Medicine Week* (December 17, 2001): 6.

Belinda Rowland
Rebecca J. Frey, PhD

Wounds

Definition

A wound occurs when the integrity of any tissue is compromised, for example, when skin breaks, muscle tears, **burns**, or bone **fractures**. A wound may be caused by an act, such as a gunshot, fall, or surgical procedure; by an infectious disease; or by an underlying condition.

Description

Types and causes of wounds are wide ranging, and health care professionals have several different ways of classifying them. They may be chronic, such as the skin ulcers caused by **diabetes mellitus**, or acute, such as a gunshot wound or animal bite. Wounds may also be referred to as open, in which the skin has been compromised and underlying tissues are exposed, or closed, in which the skin has not been compromised, but trauma to underlying structures has occurred, such as a bruised rib or cerebral contusion. Emergency personnel and first-aid workers generally place acute wounds in one of eight categories:

• Abrasions. Also called scrapes, they occur when the skin is rubbed away by friction against another rough surface (e.g. rope burns and skinned knees).

• Avulsions. These occur when an entire structure or part of it is forcibly pulled away, such as the loss of a permanent tooth or an ear lobe. Explosions, gunshots, and animal bites may cause avulsions.

• Contusions. Also called **bruises**, these result from forceful trauma that injures an internal structure without breaking the skin. Blows to the chest, abdomen, or head with a blunt instrument (e.g. a football or a fist) can cause contusions.

• Crush wounds occur when a heavy object falls onto a person, splitting the skin and shattering or tearing underlying structures.

• Cuts are slicing wounds made with a sharp instrument, leaving even edges. They may be as minimal as a paper cut or as significant as a surgical incision.

• Lacerations. Also called tears, these are separating wounds that produce ragged edges. They are produced by a tremendous force against the body, either from an internal source as in **childbirth**, or from an external source like a punch.

• Missile wounds. Also called velocity wounds, they are caused by an object entering the body at a high speed, typically a bullet.

• Punctures are deep, narrow wounds produced by sharp objects such as nails, knives, and broken glass.

Causes & symptoms

Acute wounds have a wide range of causes. Often, they are the unintentional results of motor vehicle accidents, falls, mishandling of sharp objects, or sports-related injury. Wounds may also be the intentional result of violence involving assault with weapons, including fists, knives, or guns.

The general symptoms of a wound are localized **pain** and bleeding. Specific symptoms include:

• An abrasion usually appears as lines of scraped skin with tiny spots of bleeding.

• An avulsion has heavy, rapid bleeding and a noticeable absence of tissue.

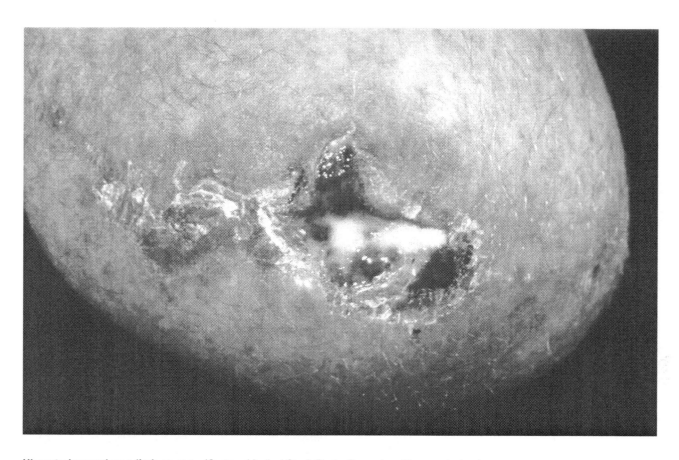

Ulcerated wound on a limb stump. *(Custom Medical Stock Photo. Reproduced by permission.)*

- A contusion may appear as a bruise beneath the skin or may appear only on imaging tests; an internal wound may also generate symptoms such as weakness, perspiration, and pain.

- A crush wound may have irregular margins like a laceration; however, the wound will be deeper and trauma to muscle and bone may be apparent.

- A cut may have little or profuse bleeding depending on its depth and length; its even edges readily line up.

- A laceration too may have little or profuse bleeding; the tissue damage is generally greater and the wound's ragged edges do not readily line up.

- A missile entry wound may be accompanied by an exit wound, and bleeding may be profuse, depending on the nature of the injury.

- A puncture wound will be greater than its length, therefore there is usually little bleeding around the outside of the wound and more bleeding inside, causing discoloration.

Diagnosis

A diagnosis is made by visual examination and may be confirmed by a report of the causal events. Medical personnel will also assess the extent of the wound and what effect it has had on the patient's well-being (e.g. profound blood loss, damage to the nervous system or skeletal system). In cases of severe injury, or when a physician suspects possible internal injury, tests might be made to determine the extent of a wound. In late 2001, a new ultrasound (imaging inside the body via sound waves) technique was introduced that might help doctors diagnose internal bleeding, a serious complication of some injuries. The technique could help prevent invasive surgery for diagnosis.

Treatment

Treatment of wounds involves stopping any bleeding, then cleaning and dressing the wound to prevent infection. Additional medical attention may be required if the effects of the wound have compromised the body's ability to function effectively.

Stopping the bleeding

Most bleeding may be stopped by direct pressure. Direct pressure is applied by placing a clean cloth or dressing over the wound and pressing the palm of the hand over the entire area. This limits local bleeding without disrupting a significant portion of the circulation. The cloth absorbs blood and allows clot formation; the clot should not be disturbed, so if blood soaks through the cloth, another cloth should be placed directly on top rather than replacing the original cloth.

If the wound is on an arm or leg that does not appear to have a broken bone, the wound should be elevated to a height above the person's heart while direct pressure is applied. Elevating the wound allows gravity to slow down the flow of blood to that area.

If severe bleeding cannot be stopped by direct pressure or with elevation, the next step is to apply pressure to the major artery supplying blood to the area of the wound. In the arm, pressure would be applied to the brachial artery by pressing the inside of the upper arm against the bone. In the leg, pressure would be applied to the femoral artery by pressing on the inner crease of the groin against the pelvic bone.

If the bleeding from an arm or leg is so extreme as to be life-threatening and if it cannot be stopped by any other means, a tourniquet—a device used to check or prevent bleeding or blood flow—may be required. However, in the process of limiting further blood loss, the tourniquet also drastically deprives the limb tissues of oxygen. As a result, the patient may live but the limb may die.

Dressing the wound

Once the bleeding has been stopped, cleaning and dressing the wound is important for preventing infection. Although the flowing blood flushes debris from the wound, running water should also be used to rinse away dirt. Embedded particles such as wood slivers and glass splinters, if not too deep, may be removed with a needle or pair of tweezers that has been sterilized in rubbing alcohol or in the heat of a flame. Once the wound has been cleared of foreign material and washed, it should be gently blotted dry, with care not to disturb the blood clot. An antibiotic ointment may be applied. The wound should then be covered with a clean dressing and bandaged to hold the dressing in place.

Homeopathic remedies

In addition to the conventional treatments described above, there are alternative therapies that may help support the injured person. **Homeopathy** can be very effective in acute wound situations. **Ledum** (*Ledum palustre*) is recommended for puncture wounds (taken internally). **Calendula** (*Calendula officinalis*) is the primary homeopathic remedy for wounds.

Other effective treatments

A naturally occurring antiseptic is **tea tree oil** (*Melaleuca* spp.), which can be mixed with water for cleaning wounds. **Aloe** (*Aloe barbadensis*) can be applied topically to soothe skin during healing. When wounds affect the nerves, especially in the arms and legs, **St. John's wort** (*Hypericum perforatum*) can be helpful when taken internally or applied topically. Also, an important Chinese herb preparation called Yunnan Bai Yao, which includes the main herbal ingredient san chi, is used very effectively to stop bleeding, and promote healing for all sorts of wounds. Other herbal remedies include Hypericum for nerve pain, and **arnica** for soft tissue damage. **Acupuncture** can help support the healing process by restoring the energy flow in the meridians that have been affected by the wound. In some cases, **vitamin E** taken orally or applied topically can speed healing and lessen scarring.

Allopathic treatment

A person who has become impaled on a fixed object, such as a fence post or a stake in the ground, should only be moved by emergency medical personnel. Foreign objects embedded in the eye should only be removed by a doctor. Larger penetrating objects, such as a fishhook or an arrow, should only be removed by a doctor to prevent further damage as they exit.

Additional medical attention is necessary in several instances. Wounds that penetrate the muscle beneath the skin should be cleaned and treated by a doctor. Such a wound may require stitches to keep it closed during healing. Some deep wounds, which do not extend to the underlying muscle may only require butterfly bandages to keep them closed during healing. Wounds to the face and neck, even small ones, should always be examined and treated by a doctor to preserve sensory function and minimize scarring. Deep wounds to the hands and wrists should be examined for nerve and tendon damage. Puncture wounds may require a **tetanus** shot to prevent serious infection. Animal bites should always be examined and the possibility of **rabies** infection determined.

Infection

Wounds that develop signs of infection should also be brought to a doctor's attention. Signs of infection are swelling, redness, tenderness, throbbing pain, localized warmth, **fever**, swollen lymph glands, the presence of pus either in the wound or draining from it, and red streaks spreading away from the wound.

Emergency treatment

With even as little as one quart of blood lost, a person may lose consciousness and go into traumatic shock. Because this is life-threatening, emergency

KEY TERMS

Abrasion—Also called a scrape. The rubbing away of the skin surface by friction against another rough surface.

Avulsion—The forcible separation of a piece from the entire structure.

Butterfly bandage—A narrow strip of adhesive with wider flaring ends (shaped like butterfly wings) used to hold the edges of a wound together while it heals.

Cut—Separation of skin or other tissue made by a sharp edge, producing regular edges.

Laceration—Also called a tear. Separation of skin or other tissue by a tremendous force, producing irregular edges.

Plasma—The straw-colored fluid component of blood, without the other blood cells.

Puncture—An injury caused by a sharp, narrow object deeply penetrating the skin.

Tourniquet—A device used to control bleeding, consisting of a constricting band applied tightly around a limb above the wound. It should only be used if the bleeding is life-threatening and cannot be controlled by other means.

Traumatic shock—A condition of depressed body functions as a reaction to injury with loss of body fluids or lack of oxygen. Signs of traumatic shock include weak and rapid pulse, shallow and rapid breathing, and pale, cool, clammy skin.

Whole blood—Blood that contains red blood cells, white blood cells, and platelets in plasma.

medical assistance should be called immediately. If the person stops breathing, artificial respiration (also called mouth-to-mouth resuscitation or rescue breathing) should be administered. In the absence of a pulse, cardiopulmonary resuscitation (CPR) must be performed. Once the person is breathing unassisted, the bleeding may be attended to.

In cases of severe blood loss, medical treatment may include the intravenous replacement of body fluids. This may be infusion with saline or plasma, or a transfusion of whole blood.

Expected results

Without the complication of infection, most wounds heal well with time. Depending on the depth and size of the wound, it may or may not leave a visible scar.

Prevention

Most actions that result in wounds are preventable. Injuries from motor vehicle accidents may be reduced by wearing seat belts and placing children in size-appropriate car seats in the back seat. Sharp, jagged, or pointed objects or machinery parts should be used according to the manufacturer's instructions and only for their intended purpose, as well as educating children on the proper way to hold and handle them, or keeping them out from their reach. Firearms and explosives should be used only by adults with explicit training; they should also be kept locked and away from children. Persons engaging in sports, games, and recreational activities should wear all proper protective equipment and follow safety rules.

Resources

BOOKS

American Red Cross Staff. *Standard First Aid.* St. Louis: Mosby Yearbook, 1992.

The Editors of Time-Life Books. *The Medical Advisor: The Complete Guide to Alternative and Conventional Treatments.* Alexandria, VA: Time-Life Books, 1996.

PERIODICALS

"Sound Waves Beat the Knife." *The Economist* (December 8, 2001).

ORGANIZATIONS

American Red Cross. P.O. Box 37243, Washington, D.C. 20013. http://www.redcross.org.

Kathleen Wright
Teresa G. Odle

Writing therapy *see* **Journal therapy**

Wu bing shao *see* **Pinellia**

Wu wei zi *see* **Schisandra**

Xin yi hua *see* **Magnolia**

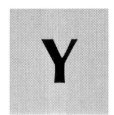

Yarrow

Description

Yarrow (*Achillea millefolium*) is an aromatic member of the Asteraceae (Compositae) family. This perennial European native with lovely, fern-like foliage is also named millefoil, or thousand leaves, because of its finely-divided leaves. There are many species and subspecies of yarrow, including a similar native American variety known as *A. Millefolium var. lanulosa*. Yarrow is naturalized throughout North America and can be found growing wild in meadows, fields, and along roadsides. Introduced to North America by early colonists, yarrow soon became a valued remedy used by many tribes of indigenous people. American Shakers gathered yarrow for use in numerous medicinal preparations. The plant was listed in the official *U.S. Pharmacopoeia* from the mid- to late nineteenth century.

Yarrow's hardy rhizome, or underground stem, develops from underground runners as the extensive root system spreads. The lacy, finely-divided leaves are multi-pinnate, and grow alternately, clasping at the base along the simple, erect and angular stem. The feather-like leaves may reach 6 in (15.2 cm) in length. They mound near the ground in early growth; then the slightly hairy stems reach upwards to 3 ft (0.91 m) in height during flowering. The tiny blossoms may be rose or lilac colored, or a creamy white; they flower from June until October. Yarrow blossoms grow in flat-topped composite clusters at the top of the stems.

Human relationships with this healing plant reach back to ancient times. The fossilized pollen of yarrow has been found in Neanderthal burial caves from as far back as 60,000 years. Yarrow has long been associated with magic and divination, and is considered by some folk herbalists as a sacred plant with special spiritual powers to offer protection. Yarrow stalks are traditionally used to cast the *I Ching*, the Chinese book of prophecy. The herb was also believed to be useful in love charms and in conjuring. One folk name for yarrow is devil's

nettle. Other names include bloodwort, carpenter's weed, sanguinary, staunchweed, dog daisy, old man's pepper, field **hops**, nosebleed, knight's milfoil, soldier's woundwort, and military herb. Yarrow accompanied soldiers into battle and was relied upon for its hemostatic action to treat **wounds**. This use may have been the source of yarrow's generic name, taken from the legend of Achilles. The Greek hero is said to have used yarrow in the Trojan War to staunch the blood flowing from the wounds of fallen comrades. Yarrow was used in battlefield first aid as recently as World War I (1914–1918).

General use

Scientists have identified over one hundred active chemical compounds in yarrow, including the intensely blue-colored azulene derivatives found in the essential oil of yarrow and at least two species of **chamomile** (*Chamaemelum nobile (L.)* and *Matricaria recutita*). Other chemical constituents in yarrow include lactones, flavonoids, tannins, coumarins, saponins, sterols, sugars, a bitter glyco-alkaloid, and **amino acids**. The aerial parts of yarrow, particularly the wild white-flowered variety, are most often used in medicinal remedies.

External uses

Yarrow is well known for its wound healing capabilities, particularly in staunching the flow of blood. The herb is considered a vulnerary and hemostatic with antiseptic and antibacterial properties. The astringent action of the leaf, when inserted into a nostril, may stop a nosebleed. An infusion of the leaf, stems, and flowers will speed the healing of **rashes**, **hemorrhoids**, and skin ulcers. Dried and powdered yarrow sprinkled on cuts and abrasions may also facilitate healing. Native Americans used yarrow in poultice form to treat skin problems. Infusions of yarrow have been used as a hair rinse in attempts to prevent baldness.

Internal uses

In folk medicine, freshly gathered yarrow root mashed in whiskey was used as a primitive anesthetic.

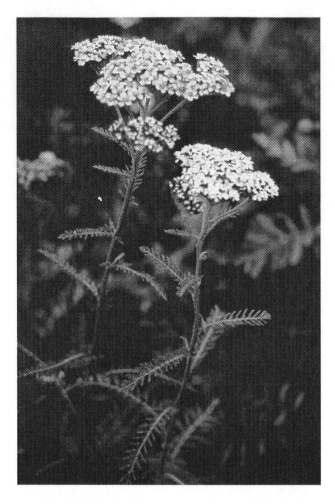

Yarrow (*Achillea millefolium*). *(Photo by Henriette Kress. Reproduced by permission.)*

Yarrow has also been used to stop internal bleeding, and as a bitter digestive tonic. Its emmenagogic action promotes the flow of bile. Yarrow tea taken warm acts as a diaphoretic, or medication given to induce sweating. It is particularly beneficial in the treatment of **fever**, colds, and **influenza**, as well as the early stages of **measles** and **chickenpox**. The essential oil, extracted by steam distillation of the flowers, is dark blue in color and has anti-inflammatory, anti-allergenic, and antispasmodic properties. Fresh yarrow leaf chewed slowly is said to relieve **toothache**. The herb has also been used to induce nosebleed in an attempt to relieve migraine **headache**. Yarrow appears to be beneficial in reducing high blood pressure. Flavonoids in the herb act to dilate the peripheral arteries and help to clear **blood clots**.

Preparations

Yarrow should be harvested while the herb is in flower, on a dry day after the morning dew has evaporated. The leaves, stems, and blossoms are all used medicinally. The leaves should be cut from the stems and spread out on a paper-lined tray to dry in a bright, airy room, out of direct sunlight. Blossoms may be left on the stems and hung in small bunches upside-down in a very warm room. Dried flowers should be stored separately, and dry stems cut into small segments before storage in an airtight, dark glass container, clearly labeled to indicate the contents and the date and place of harvest.

Leaf infusion: Place 2 oz of fresh yarrow leaf, less if dried, in a warmed glass container. Bring 2.5 cups of fresh, nonchlorinated water to the boiling point and add it to the yarrow. Cover. Steep the tea for 10 to 15 minutes, then strain. Drink warm or cold throughout the day, up to three cups per day. The prepared tea can be stored for about two days in the refrigerator.

Tincture: Combine 4 oz of fresh yarrow leaf and stalks cut fine (or 2 oz dry powdered herb) with 1 pint of brandy, gin, or vodka in a glass container. The alcohol should be enough to cover the plant parts and have a 50/50 ratio of alcohol to water. Cover and store the mixture away from the light for about two weeks, shaking several times each day. Strain and store in a tightly capped, clearly labeled dark glass bottle. A standard dose is 10 to 15 drops of the tincture in water, up to three times a day.

Precautions

Yarrow may have a cumulative medicinal effect on the system. Patients should avoid the frequent use of yarrow in large doses for long periods of time. Yarrow is a uterine stimulant; pregnant or lactating women should therefore not use the herb internally.

Side effects

People with **allergies** to ragweed, another member of the Asteraceae family of plants, may also want to avoid taking yarrow internally. In some cases yarrow may cause skin rashes or photosensitivity after ingestion.

Interactions

No interactions between yarrow and standard pharmaceutical preparations have been reported.

Resources

BOOKS

Coon, Nelson. *An American Herbal: Using Plants For Healing.* Emmaus, PA: Rodale Press, 1979.

Foster, Steven, and James A. Duke. *Peterson Field Guide to Eastern/Central Medicinal Plants.* New York: Houghton Mifflin Company, 1990.

Hutchens, Alma R. *A Handbook of Native American Herbs.* Boston: Shambhala, 1992.

KEY TERMS

Astringent—A substance that causes soft tissue to contract or constrict. Yarrow has some astringent properties.

Diaphoretic—A substance or medication given to induce or promote sweating.

Hemostatic—A substance used to stop bleeding or hemorrhaging. Yarrow has hemostatic properties.

Infusion—The most potent type of extraction of a herb into water. Infusions are steeped for a longer period of time than teas.

Pinnate—Having leaflets arranged on each side of a common stalk. Yarrow has a multi-pinnate leaf.

Tincture—The extraction of a herb into an alcohol solution for either internal or external use.

Vulnerary—A substance or medication used to speed the healing of external wounds. Yarrow was traditionally used as a vulnerary.

McIntyre, Anne. *The Medicinal Garden.* New York: Henry Holt and Company, 1997.

Ody, Penelope. *The Complete Medicinal Herbal.* New York: Dorling Kindersley, 1993.

PDR for Herbal Medicines. Montvale, NJ: Medical Economics Company, 1998.

Tyler, Varro E., Ph.D. *The Honest Herbal.* New York: Pharmaceutical Products Press, 1993.

OTHER

Alternative Herbal Index. http://www.onhealth.com.

Clare Hanrahan

Yeast infection

Definition

Yeast infection is most often caused by a species of the yeast *Candida*, most commonly *Candida albicans*, thus it is often referred to as candidiasis. *Candida* is a common cause of vaginal **infections** in women, and *Candida* may cause mouth infections in people with reduced immune function, or in patients taking certain antibiotics. *Candida* can be found in virtually all normal people, but causes problems in only a fraction. In recent years, however, several serious categories of candidiasis have become more common, due to the increased use of antibiotics, the rise of **AIDS**, the increase in the number of organ transplantations, and the use of invasive devices (catheters, artificial joints and valves)—all of which increase a patient's susceptibility to infection.

Description

Vaginal candidiasis

Over one million women in the United States develop vaginal yeast infections each year. It is not life-threatening, but it can be uncomfortable and frustrating.

Oral candidiasis

This disorder, also known as thrush, causes white, curd-like patches in the mouth or throat.

Deep organ candidiasis

Also known as invasive candidiasis, deep organ candidiasis is a serious systemic infection that can affect the esophagus, heart, blood, liver, spleen, kidneys, eyes, and skin. Like vaginal and oral candidiasis, it is an opportunistic disease that strikes when a person's resistance is lowered, often due to another illness. There are many diagnostic categories of deep organ candidiasis, depending on the tissues involved.

Causes & symptoms

Vaginal candidiasis

Most women with vaginal candidiasis experience severe vaginal **itching**. They also have a discharge that often looks like cottage cheese and has a sweet or bread-like odor. The vulva and vagina can be red, swollen, and painful. Sexual intercourse may also be painful.

Oral candidiasis

Whitish patches can appear on the tongue, inside of the cheeks, or the palate. Oral candidiasis typically occurs in people with abnormal immune systems. These can include people undergoing chemotherapy for **cancer,** people taking immunosuppressive drugs to protect transplanted organs, or people with HIV infection.

Deep organ candidiasis

Anything that weakens the body's natural barrier against colonizing organisms, including stomach surgery, **burns**, nasogastric tubes, and catheters, can predispose a person for deep organ candidiasis. Rising numbers of AIDS patients, organ transplant recipients, and other individuals whose immune systems are compro-

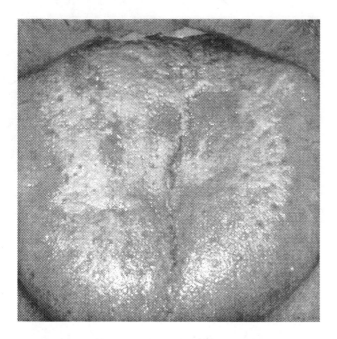

This patient's tongue is infected with candidiasis. *(Photograph by Edward H. Gill, Custom Medical Stock Photo. Reproduced by permission.)*

mised help account for the dramatic increase in deep organ candidiasis in recent years. Patients with granulocytopenia (deficiency of white blood cells) are particularly at risk for deep organ candidiasis.

Diagnosis

Often clinical appearance gives a strong suggestion about the diagnosis. Generally, a clinician will take a sample of the vaginal discharge or swab an area of oral plaque, and then inspect this material under a microscope. Under the microscope, it is possible to see characteristic forms of yeasts at various stages in the life cycle.

Fungal blood cultures should be taken for patients suspected of having deep organ candidiasis. Tissue biopsy may be required for a definitive diagnosis.

Treatment

Home remedies for vaginal candidiasis include vinegar douches or insertion of a paste made from *Lactobacillus acidophilus* powder into the vagina. In theory, these remedies will make the vagina more acidic, and therefore, less hospitable to the growth of *Candida*. Also effective for treatment is the dietary addition of berberis, **thyme**, **grapefruit seed extract**, and tea tree. Fresh **garlic** (*Allium sativum*) is believed to have antifungal action, so incorporating it into the diet or inserting a peeled garlic clove wrapped in gauze into the vagina may be helpful. The insert should be changed twice daily. Some

women report success with these remedies; they should try a conventional treatment if an alternative remedy is not effective, or seek the advice from a licensed naturopathic physician.

Some prescription drugs, particularly antibiotics, may disrupt the bacteria normally present in the intestine and vagina, causing the unpleasant symptoms of **constipation**, **diarrhea**, or **vaginitis**. Because *Lactobacillus acidophilus* is one such regular inhabitant that can prevent bacterial or yeast overgrowth, consumption of yogurt or *L. bacillus* capsules or tablets has been found to be effective in decreasing the incidence of candidiasis.

Allopathic treatment

Vaginal candidiasis

In most cases, vaginal candidiasis can be treated successfully with a variety of over-the-counter antifungal creams or suppositories. These include Monistat, Gyne-Lotrimin, and Mycelex. However, infections often recur. If a women has frequent recurrences, she should consult her doctor about prescription drugs such as Vagistat-1, Diflucan, and others.

Oral candidiasis

This is usually treated with prescription lozenges or mouthwashes. Some of the commonly used prescriptions are nystatin mouthwashes (Nilstat or Nitrostat) and clotrimazole lozenges.

Deep organ candidiasis

The recent increase in deep organ candidiasis has led to the creation of treatment guidelines. Patients who have been diagnosed with deep organ candidiasis should have catheters removed, and antifungal chemotherapy should be started to prevent the spread of the disease. Drugs should be prescribed based on a patient's specific history and defense status.

Expected results

Vaginal candidiasis

Although most cases of vaginal candidiasis are cured reliably, these infections can recur. To limit recurrences, women may need to take a prescription antifungal drug such as terconazole (sold as Terazol), or take other antifungal drugs on a preventive basis.

Oral candidiasis

These infections can also recur, sometimes because the infecting Candida develops resistance to one drug. Therefore, a physician may need to prescribe a different drug.

KEY TERMS

Biopsy—The removal and examination of tissue from a live body.

Colonize—To become established in a host.

Granulocytopenia—A condition characterized by a deficiency of white blood cells.

Nasogastric—Tube inserted through the nasal passages into the stomach.

Opportunistic—Infection caused by microorganisms that are usually harmless, but which can cause disease when a host's resistance is lowered.

Systemic—Afflicting an entire body system or the body in general.

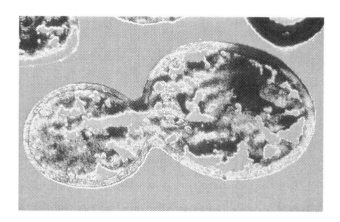

A transmission electron microscopy (TEM) of *Candida albicans.* (Custom Medical Stock Photo. Reproduced by permission.)

Deep organ candidiasis

The prognosis depends on the category of disease, as well as the condition of the patient when the infection strikes. Patients who are already suffering from a serious underlying disease are more susceptible to deep organ candidiasis that spreads throughout the body.

Prevention

Because *Candida* is part of the normal group of microorganisms that co-exist with all people, it is impossible to avoid contact with it. Good vaginal hygiene and good oral hygiene might reduce problems, but they are not guarantees against candidiasis. Other risk factors include low protein or vegetarian **diets**, a diet high in sugar, and use of antibiotics. There are also a number of ways vaginal candidiasis may be avoided:

• Frequent douching and use of feminine sprays and bath products should be avoided, as these products may disturb the normal vaginal pH balance.

• Drying the outside vaginal area thoroughly, and avoiding prolonged wear of a wet bathing suit, or damp undergarments.

• Wiping from the front to the rear, away from the vagina, after a bowel movement or urination.

• Avoiding sexual intercourse during treatment.

• Using unscented sanitary pads during menstruation.

• The use of cotton underpants, and the avoidance of tight fitting clothing.

Because hospital-acquired (nosocomial) deep organ candidiasis is on the rise, people need to be made aware of it. Patients should be sure that catheters are properly maintained and used for the shortest possible time. The frequency, length, and scope of courses of antibiotic treatment should also be cut back.

Resources

BOOKS

Carlson, K.J., S.A. Eisenstat, and T. Ziporyn. *The Harvard Guide to Women's Health.* Harvard University Press, 1996.

PERIODICALS

Greenspan, Deborah, and John S. Greenspan. "HIV-related oral disease." *The Lancet* 348 (September 14, 1996):729-734.

Tobin, Marla J. "Vulvovaginal candidiasis: topical vs. oral therapy." *American Family Physician* 51 (May 15, 1995): 1715-1723.

OTHER

Monistat.com: Yeast Infection Resource Center. http://www. monistat.com.

Kathleen D. Wright

Yellow dock

Description

Yellow dock (*Rumex crispus*) is a small, leafy plant that grows wild throughout the world. It belongs to the buckwheat or Polygonaceae family. It has yellowish-brown roots, which accounts for its common name. The roots are 8-12 in (20-30 cm) long, about 0.5 in (1.27 cm) thick, fleshy, and usually not forked. The stem is 1-3 ft (0.3-0.9 m) high and branched. Yellow dock is also known as curly or curled dock because of its long lance shaped leaves that are slightly ruffled along its edges. The leaves are 6-10 in (15-25 cm) long. Its leaves are used for food while both roots and leaves are used as herbal remedies. Yellow dock is closely related to rhubarb and sorrel.

In terms of chemical analysis, yellow dock contains anthraquinone glycosides, tannins, rumicin, and oxalates, including **potassium** oxalate.

General use

Yellow dock is primarily used in the treatment of digestive problems, liver diseases, and skin disorders. It has been described as an alterative, astringent, cholagogue, hepatic, laxative, and nutritive.

Yellow dock contains relatively small amounts of anthraquinone glycosides, which are strong laxatives in larger doses. Since yellow dock contains only small amounts of these chemicals, however, it is used as a mild laxative. Yellow dock is also used to help support and restore liver function, which is why it is called a hepatic.

Applied externally as an antiseptic and an astringent, yellow dock has been used to treat skin cuts, swelling, **rashes, boils, burns**, bleeding **hemorrhoids**, dog and insect bites, and **wounds**. An ancient British charm that was chanted when dock is applied to skin irritations caused by stinging **nettle** illustrates the use of yellow dock as a skin treatment: "Nettle out, dock in, dock remove the nettle sting."

Yellow dock is also taken internally as a treatment for such skin conditions as **psoriasis, eczema, acne**, poison ivy, and other rashes, often in combination with such other herbs as **red clover** (*Trifolium pratense*), **dandelion** root (*Taraxacum officinalis*), cleavers (*Galium aparine*), and burdock (*Arctium lappa*).

Yellow dock also has been used in the treatment of liver and gallbladder disorders. It is called a cholagogue because it is thought to stimulate the production of bile and digestive fluids.

Yellow dock is nutritious, as it contains **vitamin C, iron, calcium**, and **phosphorus**. It even contains enough tannin to use in tanning leather.

Other uses of yellow dock by traditional herbalists have included the treatment of:

• vaginitis

• fibroids

• anemia

• swollen glands

Preparations

Both the roots and leaves of yellow dock are used in remedies. Due to the mild and general nature of its actions, yellow dock is rarely used alone, but in combination with other herbal remedies. The roots are dug in late summer and autumn between the months of August and October. They are cleaned well and split lengthwise before drying. The roots are ground or crushed and then are used in preparing ointments, tinctures, decoctions, or teas. The ground root is kept cool and dry but not frozen.

Tea is prepared by boiling 1-2 tsp (5-10 g) of yellow dock root in 500 mL (2 cups) water for 10 minutes. Syrup is made by boiling 0.5 lb of crushed root in a pint of syrup. Dried extracts of yellow dock are also prepared as pills or capsules, and are available commercially. These commercial preparations are often a mixture of several different types of herbs. The directions on the label of the commercial product should be followed for recommended dosages.

For external applications, both roots and leaves are used. The root may be pounded and applied as a poultice. Fresh or boiled leaves and stems are directly placed on skin irritations. An ointment is made by boiling the root in vinegar until the fiber is softened. The pulp is then mixed with a solid grease such as petroleum jelly, animal fat, or vegetable shortening.

The young leaves of yellow dock may be eaten cooked as greens, but should not be eaten raw. If the plant is too bitter, it may be parboiled, washed, added to clear water, and cooked until tender. Since the leaves contain oxalic acid (similar to spinach), they should not be eaten frequently in large amounts as the oxalic acid can prevent the absorption of calcium. The seeds of yellow dock have been ground and used as flour.

Precautions

Since no safe dosage has been established, pregnant or breastfeeding women and infants and children under the age of six should avoid the use of yellow dock. Persons with any chronic diseases of the gastrointestinal tract, such as duodenal ulcers, esophageal reflux, spastic colitis, diverticulosis, or **diverticulitis**, should not take yellow dock.

A person with a history of **kidney stones** should not use yellow dock, since the oxalates and tannins present in yellow dock may aggravate that condition.

When used as a laxative, yellow dock should not be used for more than a week, unless a doctor has ordered otherwise. Overuse of a laxative may lead to dependence. Any sudden changes in bowel habits or function that last longer than two weeks should be checked by a doctor be-

KEY TERMS

Alterative—A herb that changes one's physical condition, especially a blood cleanser.

Astringent—A substance that constricts or binds skin cells.

Cholagogue—A substance that stimulates the flow of bile.

Hepatic—A herb that acts as a liver tonic.

Infusion—The most potent form of extraction of a herb into water. Infusions are steeped for a longer period of time than teas.

Oxalic acid—A white crystalline water-soluble acid, found in yellow dock, sorrel, and spinach. In its pure form it is used as a cleanser and bleaching agent.

fore using a laxative. Children up to six years of age should not take a laxative unless prescribed by a doctor.

Side effects

The side effects, especially if larger doses of yellow dock are taken, include **diarrhea**, skin eruptions, **nausea**, and **vomiting**. Kidney damage, characterized by blood in urine, decreased urine flow, and swelling of hands and feet may also occur.

Interactions

To enhance the activity of yellow dock, it should be used in combination with such other herbs as red clover (*Trifolium pratense*), dandelion root (*Taraxacum officinalis*), cleavers (*Galium aparine*), and burdock (*Arctium lappa*).

Resources

BOOKS

Heatherly, Ana Nez. *Healing Plants: A Medicinal Guide to Native North American Plants and Herbs.* New York: The Lyons Press, 1998.

Judith Sims

Yerba santa

Description

Yerba santa (*Eriodictyon glutinosum* and *Eriodictyon californicum*) is a short evergreen shrub that grows in dry,

hilly areas of California and Northern Mexico. The plant, part of the Hydrophyllaceae family, grows in clusters and is approximately 3 ft (1 m) in height. The smooth stem and thick yellow leaves are covered with a resin, and the plant has blue flowers that cluster together in groups of six to 10. The leaves are 2–5 in (5–12 cm) long. The plant contains chrysocriol, eridonel, eriodictyol, formic acid, glucose, glycerides of fatty acids, homoeriodictyol, resin, tannic acids, tannins, volatile oil, and zanthoeridol. The leaves should be gathered in the spring and early summer.

General use

Yerba santa, which literally means sacred herb in Spanish, has been used for centuries for a variety of illnesses, such as **bronchitis**, colds, coughs, **diarrhea**, and **stomach aches**. The Spanish came to know of its medicinal value through Native Americans, who either smoked or made infusions of yerba santa. The herb, also known as bear's weed, consumptive's weed, gum bush, and mountain balm, is still primarily used for respiratory congestion, either from acute **asthma**, colds, or coughs. Yerba santa has also been found effective for a number of symptoms, including gastrointestinal disorders and **fatigue**. When used externally for **bruises**, mosquito bites, or sprains, yerba santa can be applied as a poultice. The herb also used as a tonic to cleanse the blood, tone the nervous system, stimulate the mind, and control the appetite. It is also believed to enhance the action of other herbs when used in combination. It has a sweet, slightly bitter taste.

Respiratory conditions

Yerba santa is best known for its use in respiratory conditions, especially when there is a lot of mucus stuck in the body. It is considered one of the best decongestants, working as an expectorant by breaking up thick mucus and facilitating its expulsion from the body. For acute colds and coughs with upper respiratory and sinus congestion, yerba santa is extremely helpful. As a muscle relaxant, yerba santa works well for asthmatics as it dilates the bronchial tubes and allows air to flow more easily into the lungs. For asthma, yerba santa is often smoked in a pipe, for instance.

Acute illnesses

At the onset of a cold, especially when there is a **cough** or bronchial irritation, yerba santa can eradicate or at least alleviate the symptoms.

Digestive aid

As a sialagogue, a substance that promotes salivation, yerba santa helps digestion. The excess saliva pro-

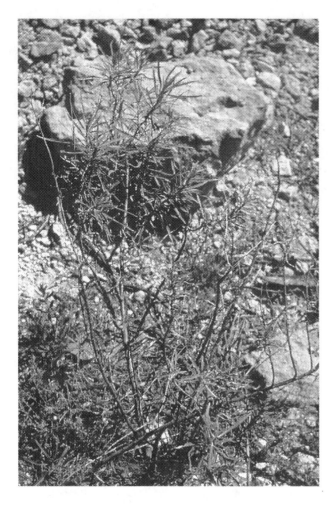

Yerba santa plant (*Eriodictyon* sp.). *(Photo by Henriette Kress. Reproduced by permission.)*

duction helps the digestive process and can alleviate digestive problems.

Fatigue

Because yerba santa is a stimulant, it reduces **fatigue** and curbs the appetite.

Skin conditions

A poultice of yerba santa should be applied to **bruises**, insect bites, sprains, and **wounds**.

Preparations

For a yerba santa infusion, take 1 tbsp of the fresh or dried leaves to 1 c of boiling water and let it steep for 10 minutes. If a tincture is taken, then one dose should be from 10–30 drops, taken four times a day. If dried leaves are used, then the tincture is best with an alcohol base.

Precautions

Yerba santa should not be taken by women who are pregnant or nursing. It is also an herb that should not be used by people who are suffering from chronic gastrointestinal disorders. As a stimulant, it should also be used sparingly by those who have **sleep disorders** or bouts of **insomnia**.

Side effects

As a stimulant, yerba santa may cause sleeplessness and contribute to a lack of appetite.

Interactions

When it is taken internally, as an infusion, tincture, or in capsule form, be aware that yerba santa can affect how **iron** and other minerals are absorbed into the body. Those who tend to be iron deficient may want to supplement their **diets** with iron while taking yerba santa. It is best to consult with a physician or other health practitioner before attempting to self-medicate.

Resources

BOOKS
Ritchason, Jack. *The Little Herb Encyclopedia.* Woodland Health Books, 1995.
Tierra, Michael. *The Way of Herbs.* Pocket Books, 1980.

OTHER
Grieve, Mrs. M. *A Modern Herbal.* http://www.botanical.com.
Herbal Dave Homepage. http://www.herbaldave.com.
InfoStructure. http://www.mind.net.
Thrive Online. http://www.thriveonline.com.

Katherine Y. Kim

Yoga

Definition

The term *yoga* comes from a Sanskrit word that means yoke or union. Traditionally, yoga is a method joining the individual self with the Divine, Universal Spirit, or Cosmic Consciousness. Physical and mental

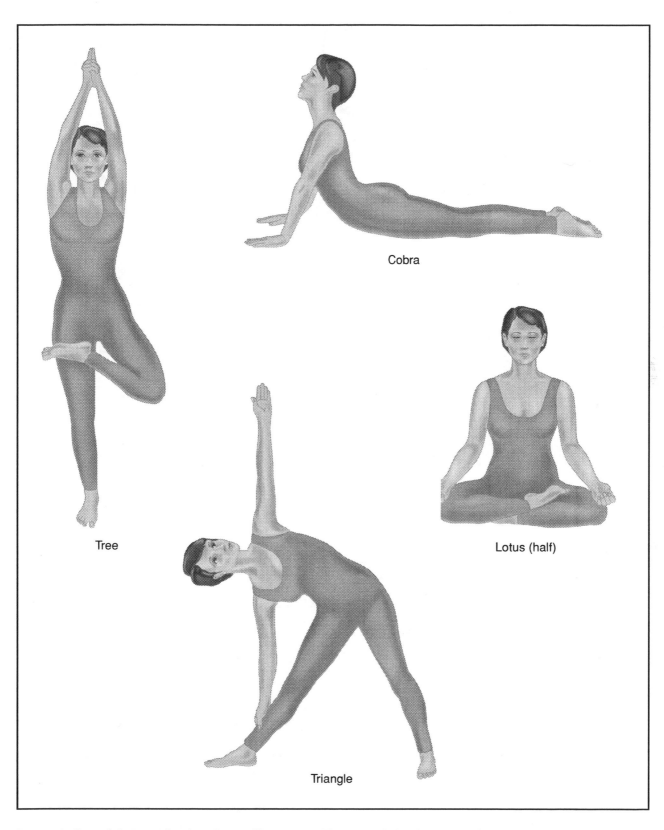

Tree

Cobra

Lotus (half)

Triangle

Demonstrations of the tree, triangle, cobra, and lotus poses. The tree and triangle are good for balance and coordination. Cobra stretches the pelvic and strengthens the back. Lotus is a meditative pose. (Illustration by Electronic Illustrators Group. The Gale Group.)

YOGA POSITIONS

Name	Description
Abdominal massage	Kneel with arms folded. Bend torso toward ground and lower forehead to the floor. Slowly raise up, switch arms, and repeat.
Boat	Lying on stomach, raise head, torso, arms, and legs off the ground and stretch. Arms should be outstretched and pointing towards feet.
Bow	Lying on stomach, hold ankles from behind and slowly raise head, torso, and thighs off floor.
Bridge	Lying on back with knees bent and feet flat on floor, raise pelvis off floor and arch back. Arms should be stretched out on floor with hands grasped.
C	On hands and knees, move head and buttocks as far left as possible. Inhale as you return center and repeat on the right side.
Camel	While kneeling, arch back and bend head back toward feet. Hold heels with hands and exhale while in movement.
Cat	On hands and knees, arch back and exhale while in movement, rounding shoulders and back.
Child	Kneeling with arms to the side, roll torso to floor and rest forehead on the ground.
Cobra	Stretched out on floor with stomach down, place elbows parallel to shoulders and raise torso up. Arms should straighten with hands flat on floor.
Corpse	Lie on back with feet and arms outstretched. Breathe deeply.
Dog	On hands and knees, dip back and lift head and buttocks up. Exhale.
Downward Dog	On hands and knees form an inverted V by pushing pelvis up and pressing hands and heels to floor. Exhale while in movement.
Half Cobra	Stretched out on floor with stomach down, place elbows parallel to shoulders and raise torso up. Keep arms bent and only raise torso off the ground as far as the navel.
Half Locust	Lying on stomach with hands beneath the body, raise legs one at a time while tensing buttocks. Repeat with other leg.
Half Lotus	Sit with legs crossed (only one leg should be over the other) and knees touching the floor.
Half-Moon	Standing with feet together, hold hands above the head with arms outstretched. Exhale and stretch to the left. Inhale and return to center. Repeat on other side.
Hand and thumb squeeze	Make a fist around thumb and squeeze. Release slowly and repeat on other hand.
Head to knee	Sitting with right leg outstretched and the left leg bent toward the body with the left foot touching the right leg, stretch head to right knee. Repeat on other side.
Hero	On hands and knees, cross left knee in front of right knee while sitting back between the heels. Hold heels with hands.
Knee down twist	Lying on back with arms outstretched, place right foot on left knee and swivel right knee to the left side of floor. While in movement, turn head to left side. Repeat on opposite side.

exercises are designed to help achieve this goal, also called self-transcendence or enlightenment. On the physical level, yoga postures, called *asanas*, are designed to tone, strengthen, and align the body. These postures are performed to make the spine supple and healthy and to promote blood flow to all the organs, glands, and tissues, keeping all the bodily systems healthy. On the mental level, yoga uses breathing techniques (*pranayama*) and **meditation** (*dyana*) to quiet, clarify, and discipline the mind. However, experts are quick to point out that yoga is not a religion, but a way of living with health and peace of mind as its aims.

Origins

Yoga originated in ancient India and is one of the longest surviving philosophical systems in the world. Some scholars have estimated that yoga is as old as

YOGA POSITIONS (CONTD.)

Locust	Lying on stomach with hands under the body, squeeze buttocks and lift legs up and outward. Keep legs straight.
Mountain	Standing with feet together, inhale while raising arms straight above the head and clasp hands together. Exhale while lowering arms.
Pigeon	Kneeling, slide the left leg straight out from behind and inhale, stretching torso up. Release and repeat on other side.
Plow	Lying on back, inhale and raise legs over head while keeping hands flat on floor for support.
Posterior stretch	Sitting with legs outstretched and feet together, stretch head to toes.
Rag Doll	While standing, exhale and bend over toward toes, cupping elbows with hands. Breathe deeply.
Seated angle	Sitting with legs outstretched in a V shape, stretch arms to toes and head to floor.
Shoulder crunch	With back straight, slowly lift shoulder to ear and lower. Repeat on other side.
Shoulder stand	Lying on back, lift legs up and support back with hands. Slowly angle legs over head and then extend upward.
Sphinx	Lying on stomach with elbows parallel to shoulders and palms on the ground, push torso up and look upward.
Spider	Press fingertips together and move palms in and out.
Spinal twist	Sit with right foot crossed over left leg and right leg held with left arm. Twist while supporting body with right hand on the floor. Repeat on other side.
Standing angle	Inhale and step into V position, stretching arms out and then down toward floor.
Standing yoga mudra	Standing with arms at sides, inhale and raise arms in front. Exhale and swing arms to back.
Tree	While standing, place one foot on the opposite thigh and outstretch arms above the head. Hold hands above with index fingers straight and the remaining fingers clasped.
Triangle	With arms parallel to floor and legs outstretched, turn one foot out and stretch to that side, keeping arms straight. Repeat on other side.
Upward Dog	Lying on stomach with hands down near the chest, lift torso off the floor while raising on toes. Hands should raise, but remain palms down. Arch back slightly.
Warrior I	Raise arms over head with palms together and lunge forward with one foot, keeping thigh parallel to the ground.
Warrior II	With arms straight out and parallel to the ground and legs in V, turn one foot out and lunge to the side, keeping hips straight.
Yoga Mudra	Sitting on heels, round torso to the ground with forehead to the floor while stretching arms overhead. Inhale while in movement and exhale while lowering arms.

5,000 years; artifacts detailing yoga postures have been found in India from over 3000 B.C. Yoga masters (*yogis*) claim that it is a highly developed science of healthy living that has been tested and perfected for all these years. Yoga was first brought to America in the late 1800s when Swami Vivekananda, an Indian teacher and yogi, presented a lecture on meditation in Chicago. Yoga slowly began gaining followers, and flourished during the 1960s when there was a surge of interest in Eastern phi-losophy. There has since been a vast exchange of yoga knowledge in America, with many students going to India to study and many Indian experts coming here to teach, resulting in the establishment of a wide variety of schools. Today, yoga is thriving, and it has become easy to find teachers and practitioners throughout America. A recent Roper poll, commissioned by *Yoga Journal*, found that 11 million Americans do yoga at least occasionally and six million perform it regularly. Yoga stretches are

PATANJALI
(C. 2ND CENTURY B.C.)

There is little historical information available on Patanjali, who is credited with developing yoga, one of the six systems of Hindu philosophy. Several scholars suggest several persons may have developed yoga under the pseudonym of Patanjali. In any case, Patanjali existed around 150 B.C. in India. He developed yoga based on a loose set of doctrines and practices from the Upanishads, themselves a set of mystical writings. The Upanishads are part of the Aranyakas, philosophical concepts that are part of the Veda, the most ancient body of literature of Hinduism. Patanjali gave these combined philosophical and esoteric writings a common foundation in his *Yoga Sutra*, a set of 196 concise aphorisms (wise sayings) that form the principles of yoga. He also drew upon Samkhya, the oldest classic system of Hindu philosophy. Patanjali's yoga accepted Samkhya metaphysics and the concept of a supreme soul. He established an eight-stage discipline of self-control and meditation. The individual sutras (verses) lay out the entire tradition of meditation. They also describe the moral and physical disciplines needed for the soul to attain absolute freedom from the body and self.

Ken R. Wells

used by physical therapists and professional sports teams, and the benefits of yoga are being touted by movie stars and Fortune 500 executives. Many prestigious schools of medicine have studied and introduced yoga techniques as proven therapies for illness and **stress**. Some medical schools, like UCLA, even offer yoga classes as part of their physician training program.

Benefits

Yoga has been used to alleviate problems associated with high blood pressure, high **cholesterol**, migraine headaches, **asthma**, shallow breathing, backaches, **constipation**, diabetes, **menopause**, **multiple sclerosis**, **varicose veins**, and many chronic illnesses. It also has been studied and approved for its ability to promote **relaxation** and reduce stress. On the other hand, some researchers are now questioning claims that yoga is beneficial for such conditions as **carpal tunnel syndrome**.

As of late 2002, yoga is increasingly recommended for **dysmenorrhea**, **premenstrual syndrome**, and other disorders in premenopausal women, in Europe as well as in the United States.

Yoga can also provide the same benefits as any well-designed **exercise** program, increasing general health and stamina, reducing stress, and improving those conditions brought about by sedentary lifestyles. Yoga has the added advantage of being a low-impact activity that uses only gravity as resistance, which makes it an excellent physical therapy routine; certain yoga postures can be safely used to strengthen and balance all parts of the body. A study published in late 2002 summarized recent findings about the benefits of yoga for the cardiovascular and musculoskeletal systems. The review noted that yoga is still viewed as a "trendy" form of exercise rather than one with documented medical benefits.

Meditation has been much studied and approved for its benefits in reducing stress-related conditions. The landmark book, *The Relaxation Response*, by Harvard cardiologist Herbert Benson, showed that meditation and breathing techniques for relaxation could have the opposite effect of stress, reducing blood pressure and other indicators. Since then, much research has reiterated the benefits of meditation for stress reduction and general health. Currently, the American Medical Association recommends meditation techniques as a first step before medication for borderline **hypertension** cases. Some 2002 studies indicate that yogic meditation by itself is effective in lowering serum cholesterol as well as blood pressure.

Modern psychological studies have shown that even slight facial expressions can cause changes in the involuntary nervous system; yoga utilizes the mind/body connection. That is, yoga practice contains the central ideas that physical posture and alignment can influence a person's mood and self-esteem, and also that the mind can be used to shape and heal the body. Yoga practitioners claim that the strengthening of mind/body awareness can bring eventual improvements in all facets of a person's life.

Description

Classical yoga is separated into eight limbs, each a part of the complete system for mental, physical, and spiritual well-being. Four of the limbs deal with mental and physical exercises designed to bring the mind in tune with the body. The other four deal with different stages of meditation. There are six major types of yoga, all with the same goals of health and harmony but with varying techniques: hatha, raja, karma, bhakti, jnana, and tantra yoga. **Hatha yoga** is the most commonly practiced branch of yoga in America, and it is a highly developed system of nearly 200 physical postures, movements, and breathing techniques designed to tune the body to its optimal health. The yoga philosophy believes the breath to be the most important facet of health, as the breath is the largest source of *prana*, or life force, and hatha yoga utilizes *pranayama*, which literally means the science or control of breathing. Hatha yoga was originally developed as a system to make the body strong and healthy enough to enable mental awareness and spiritual enlightenment.

There are several different schools of hatha yoga in America; the two most prevalent ones are Iyengar and ashtanga yoga. Iyengar yoga was founded by B.K.S. Iyengar, who is widely considered as one of the great living innovators of yoga. Iyengar yoga puts strict emphasis on form and alignment, and uses traditional hatha yoga techniques in new manners and sequences. Iyengar yoga can be good for physical therapy because it allows the use of props like straps and blocks to make it easier for some people to get into the yoga postures. Ashtanga yoga can be a more vigorous routine, using a flowing and dance-like sequence of hatha postures to generate body heat, which purifies the body through sweating and deep breathing.

The other types of yoga show some of the remaining ideas that permeate yoga. Raja yoga strives to bring about mental clarity and discipline through meditation, simplicity, and non-attachment to worldly things and desires. Karma yoga emphasizes charity, service to others, non-aggression and non-harming as means to awareness and peace. **Bhakti yoga** is the path of devotion and love of God, or Universal Spirit. Jnana yoga is the practice and development of knowledge and wisdom. Finally, tantra yoga is the path of self-awareness through religious rituals, including awareness of sexuality as sacred and vital.

A typical hatha yoga routine consists of a sequence of physical poses, or asanas, and the sequence is designed to work all parts of the body, with particular emphasis on making the spine supple and healthy and increasing circulation. Hatha yoga asanas utilize three basic movements: forward bends, backward bends, and twisting motions. Each asana is named for a common thing it resembles, like the sun salutation, cobra, locust, plough, bow, eagle, and tree, to name a few. Each pose has steps for entering and exiting it, and each posture requires proper form and alignment. A pose is held for some time, depending on its level of difficulty and one's strength and stamina, and the practitioner is also usually aware of when to inhale and exhale at certain points in each posture, as breathing properly is another fundamental aspect of yoga. Breathing should be deep and through the nose. Mental concentration in each position is also very important, which improves awareness, poise, and posture. During a yoga routine there is often a position in which to perform meditation, if deep relaxation is one of the goals of the sequence.

Yoga routines can take anywhere from 20 minutes to two or more hours, with one hour being a good time investment to perform a sequence of postures and a medi-

tation. Some yoga routines, depending on the teacher and school, can be as strenuous as the most difficult workout, and some routines merely stretch and align the body while the breath and heart rate are kept slow and steady. Yoga achieves its best results when it is practiced as a daily discipline, and yoga can be a life-long exercise routine, offering deeper and more challenging positions as a practitioner becomes more adept. The basic positions can increase a person's strength, flexibility, and sense of well-being almost immediately, but it can take years to perfect and deepen them, which is an appealing and stimulating aspect of yoga for many.

Yoga is usually best learned from a yoga teacher or physical therapist, but yoga is simple enough that one can learn the basics from good books on the subject, which are plentiful. Yoga classes are generally inexpensive, averaging around 10 dollars per class, and students can learn basic postures in just a few classes. Many YMCAs, colleges, and community health organizations offer beginning yoga classes as well, often for nominal fees. If yoga is part of a physical therapy program, its cost can be reimbursed by insurance.

Preparations

Yoga can be performed by those of any age and condition, although not all poses should be attempted by everyone. Yoga is also a very accessible form of exercise; all that is needed is a flat floor surface large enough to stretch out on, a mat or towel, and enough overhead space to fully raise the arms. It is a good activity for those who cannot go to gyms, who do not like other forms of exercise, or have very busy schedules. Yoga should be done on an empty stomach, and teachers recommend waiting three or more hours after meals. Loose and comfortable clothing should be worn.

Precautions

People with injuries, medical conditions, or spinal problems should consult a doctor before beginning yoga. Those with medical conditions should find a yoga teacher who is familiar with their type of problem and who is willing to give them individual attention. Pregnant women can benefit from yoga, but should always be guided by an experienced teacher. Certain yoga positions should not be performed with a **fever**, or during **menstruation**.

Beginners should exercise care and concentration when performing yoga postures, and not try to stretch too much too quickly, as injury could result. Some advanced yoga postures, like the headstand and full lotus position, can be difficult and require strength, flexibility, and gradual preparation, so beginners should get the help of a teacher before attempting them.

Yoga is not a competitive sport; it does not matter how a person does in comparison with others, but how aware and disciplined one becomes with one's own body and limitations. Proper form and alignment should always be maintained during a stretch or posture, and the stretch or posture should be stopped when there is **pain**, **dizziness**, or **fatigue**. The mental component of yoga is just as important as the physical postures. Concentration and awareness of breath should not be neglected. Yoga should be done with an open, gentle, and non-critical mind; when one stretches into a yoga position, it can be thought of as accepting and working on one's limits. Impatience, self-criticism, and comparing oneself to others will not help in this process of self-knowledge. While performing the yoga of breathing (pranayama) and meditation (dyana), it is best to have an experienced teacher, as these powerful techniques can cause dizziness and discomfort when done improperly.

Side effects

Some people have reported injuries by performing yoga postures without proper form or concentration, or by attempting difficult positions without working up to them gradually or having appropriate supervision. Beginners sometimes report muscle soreness and fatigue after performing yoga, but these side effects diminish with practice.

Research & general acceptance

Although yoga originated in a culture very different from modern America, it has been accepted and its practice has spread relatively quickly. Many yogis are amazed at how rapidly yoga's popularity has spread in America, considering the legend that it was passed down secretly by handfuls of followers for many centuries.

There can still be found some resistance to yoga, for active and busy Americans sometimes find it hard to believe that an exercise program that requires them to slow down, concentrate, and breathe deeply can be more effective than lifting weights or running. However, ongoing research in top medical schools is showing yoga's effectiveness for overall health and for specific problems, making it an increasingly acceptable health practice.

Training & certification

Many different schools of yoga have developed in America, and beginners should experiment with them to find the best-suited routine. Hatha yoga schools emphasize classical yoga postures, and raja yoga schools concentrate on mental discipline and meditation techniques. In America, there are no generally accepted standards for the certification of yoga teachers. Some schools certify teachers in a few intensive days and some require years of study before certifying teachers. Beginners should search for teachers who show respect and are careful in their teaching, and should beware of instructors who push them into poses before they are ready.

Resources

BOOKS

Ansari, Mark, and Liz Lark. *Yoga for Beginners*. New York: Harper, 1999.

Bodian, Stephan, and Georg Feuerstein. *Living Yoga*. New York: Putnam, 1993.

Carrico, Mara. *Yoga Journal's Yoga Basics*. New York: Henry Holt, 1997.

Iyengar, B.K.S. *Light on Yoga*. New York: Schocken, 1975.

Pelletier, Kenneth R., MD. *The Best Alternative Medicine*, Chapter 10, "Ayurvedic Medicine and Yoga: From Buddha to the Millennium." New York: Simon & Schuster, 2002.

PERIODICALS

Engebretson, J. "Culture and Complementary Therapies." *Complementary Therapies in Nursing and Midwifery* 8 (November 2002): 177–184.

Gerritsen, A. A., M. C. de Krom, M. A. Struijs, et al. "Conservative Treatment Options for Carpal Tunnel Syndrome: A Systematic Review of Randomized Controlled Trials." *Journal of Neurology* 249 (March 2002): 272–280.

Kronenberg, F., and A. Fugh-Berman. "Complementary and Alternative Medicine for Menopausal Symptoms: A Review of Randomized, Controlled Trials." *Annals of Internal Medicine* 137 (November 19, 2002): 805–813.

Manocha, R., G. B. Marks, P. Kenchington, et al. "Sahaja Yoga in the Management of Moderate to Severe Asthma: A Randomized Controlled Trial." *Thorax* 57 (February 2002): 110–115.

Raub, J. A. "Psychophysiologic Effects of Hatha Yoga on Musculoskeletal and Cardiopulmonary Function: A Literature Review." *Journal of Alternative and Complementary Medicine* 8 (December 2002): 797–812.

Tonini, G. "Dysmenorrhea, Endometriosis and Premenstrual Syndrome." [in Italian] *Minerva Pediatrica* 54 (December 2002): 525–538.

Vyas, R., and N. Dikshit. "Effect of Meditation on Respiratory System, Cardiovascular System and Lipid Profile." *Indian Journal of Physiology and Pharmacology* 46 (October 2002): 487–491.

Yoga International Magazine. R.R. 1 Box 407, Honesdale, PA 18431. <http://www.yimag.com>.

Yoga Journal. P.O. Box 469088, Escondido, CA 92046. <http://www.yogajournal.com>.

ORGANIZATIONS

American Yoga Association. <www.americanyogaassociation.org.>.

International Association of Yoga Therapists (IAYT). 4150 Tivoli Ave., Los Angeles, CA 90066.

Yoga Research and Education Center (YREC). 2400A County Center Drive, Santa Rosa, CA 95403. (707) 566-0000. <www.yrec.org.>.

OTHER

Yoga Directory. <http://www.yogadirectory.com>.

Yoga Finder Online. <http://www.yogafinder.com>.

Douglas Dupler
Rebecca J. Frey, PhD

Yohimbe

Description

Yohimbe (*Corynanthe yohimbe*) is an herb derived from the bark of the yohimbe tree found primarily in the West African nations of Cameroon, Gabon, and Zaire. The major active constituent of the bark is yohimbine. In prescription doses, the active ingredient is yohimbine hydrochloride.

General use

Yohimbe has been used for centuries in African folk medicine to treat fevers, leprosy, coughs, and as a local anesthetic. But its most popular use has been as an aphrodisiac and a mild hallucinogen. It has been widely used in Europe for about 75 years to treat male erectile dysfunction, formerly called **impotence**. The U. S. Food and Drug Administration (FDA) approved yohimbe as a treatment for impotence in the late 1980s. It is sold as an over-the-counter dietary supplement and as a prescription drug under brand names such as Yocon, Aphrodyne, Erex, Yohimex, Testomar, Yohimbe, and Yovital.

There is no clear medical research that indicates exactly how or why yohimbe works in treating impotence.

It is generally believed that yohimbe dilates blood vessels and stimulates blood flow to the penis, causing an erection. It also prevents blood from flowing out of the penis during an erection. It may also act on the central nervous system, specifically the lower spinal cord area where sexual signals are transmitted. Studies show it is effective in 30-40% of men with impotence. It is primarily effective in men with impotence caused by vascular, psychogenic, or diabetic problems. It usually does not work in men whose impotence is caused by organic nerve damage. In men without erectile dysfunction, yohimbe in some cases appears to increase sexual stamina and prolong erections.

Yohimbe is also used for weight loss, although not to the extent it is used for treating impotence. Some alternative health practitioners believe it is more effective and safer than the stimulant **ephedra** (also known as *ma huang*) in achieving weight loss. Yohimbe is often prescribed for weight loss by natural health practitioners at Bastyr University in Kenmore, Washington. "It's my number one choice for weight loss," Lise Alschuler, medical director of the school's natural health clinic, said in a January 1998 article in *Vegetarian Times*. "I prescribe it in very small doses and slowly increase intake while monitoring patients' tolerance levels." Dosing starts at 1 mg of yohimbine three times a day.

A 1994 study by the Eastern Virginia Medical School also found yohimbine may be effective in treating **narcolepsy**. While the study involved only eight people with the sleep disorder, seven of them given yohimbine were able to stay awake for an eight-hour work day. The researchers believe yohimbine works by counteracting the brain chemistry that causes narcolepsy, and remains effective even after a few weeks of regular use.

Preparations

The usual dosage of yohimbine extract to treat erectile dysfunction is 5.4 milligrams (mg) three times a day. It may take three to six weeks for it to take effect. In the event of side effects, dosage is usually reduced to one-half a tablet three times a day, then gradually increased to one tablet three times a day. Prescription yohimbe containing yohimbine is standardized at 5.4 mg per tablet. The retail price for a name brand yohimbe is generally $18-36 for 30 tablets. A generic prescription for yohimbine is about $6-12 for 30 tablets. Most yohimbe sold over the counter is in tablet or capsule form and contains 500-1,000 mg of yohimbe bark, and contains only a small percentage of the active ingredient yohimbine. The strength of yohimbe bark extract sold over the counter varies greatly and may not be a reliable source of yohimbine. A 1995 study by the FDA looked at 26 over-the-counter yohimbe products and did not find any that had enough yohimbine to effectively treat erectile dysfunction. Yohimbe bark extract is also sold over the counter in combination with other herbs and dietary supplements. The best way to ensure that a patient is getting enough active ingredient to treat erectile dysfunction is to ask a physician for a prescription yohimbe product.

Precautions

Since yohimbe can cause confusion, **dizziness**, and disorientation, it should not be taken while operating machinery, driving, or performing hazardous activities. It should not be taken by people with chronic health problems, such as heart, liver, or kidney disease, diabetes, **glaucoma**, **hypertension** (high blood pressure), or mental illness. Children, women, or men with prostate problems should not use yohimbe. Persons should consult their physician or health care practitioner before they start taking yohimbe.

Side effects

There can be several serious side effects associated with yohimbe. An allergic reaction is possible with symptoms such as difficulty breathing, throat constriction, **hives**, and swelling of the face, lips, or tongue. It can also cause an irregular or rapid heartbeat, and disorientation. Minor side effects can include dizziness, **anxiety**, shaking, headaches, skin flushing, and irritability.

Yohimbe is also reported to have produced hallucinogenic properties in some people. The effects have been compared to the drug LSD and can last from two to four hours. These effects include audio and visual hallucinations, and feelings of euphoria. They usually occur when yohimbe is taken in higher than recommended doses.

Interactions

Yohimbe should not be used by people who are taking tranquilizers, antidepressants, sedatives, antihistamines, amphetamines or other stimulants, including **caffeine**. Since yohimbe is a short-term monoamine oxidase (MAO) inhibitor, it should not be taken with hypertension medication. It should not be taken with food or drink that contains high amounts of tyramine, such as wine, beer, cheese, cured meats, dried fish, bananas, red plumbs, oranges, dried fruit, avocado, tomato, eggplant, and soy sauce. Doing so can cause a rise in blood pressure. Yohimbe should not be used with other prescription erectile dysfunction drugs, such as Viagra.

Resources

BOOKS

Foster, Steven and Varro E. Tyler. *Tyler's Honest Herbal: A Sensible Guide to the Use of Herbs and Related Remedies.* Binghamton, NY: The Haworth Press, Inc. 1999.

> ## KEY TERMS
>
> **Aphrodisiac**—Any substance, aroma, or image that arouses sexual desire.
>
> **Erectile dysfunction**—Formerly called impotence, the inability of a male to have or maintain an erection.
>
> **Glaucoma**—A disease of the eye marked by increased pressure within the eyeball that can cause damage and lead to a gradual loss of vision.
>
> **Hypertension**—Abnormally high arterial blood pressure, which if left untreated can lead to heart disease and stroke.
>
> **Leprosy**—A chronic disease characterized by lesions on the body, especially the face, that enlarge and spread if left untreated, leading to paralysis, muscle wasting, and deformities.
>
> **Monoamine oxidase inhibitor**—A class of antidepressant drugs.
>
> **Narcolepsy**—A condition characterized by brief attacks of deep sleep outside of the normal sleep cycle.
>
> **Tyramine**—A compound derived from tyrosine, an amino acid that is a precursor to various alkaloids, and found in various types of food.

Miller, Lucinda G. and Wallace J. Murray (Editors). *Herbal Medicinals: A Clinician's Guide.* Binghamton, NY: The Haworth Press, Inc. 1999.

Poche, Henry Z. *Medical Biology of Yohimbine & Its Easy Use in Male Sex Erectile Dysfunction.* Washington, DC: ABBE Publishers Association of Washington, DC. 1997.

Robbers, James E. and Varro E. Tyler. *Tyler's Herbs of Choice: The Therapeutic Use of Phytomedicinals.* Binghamton, NY: The Haworth Press, Inc. 1998.

Tenny, Deanne. *Yohimbe (The Woodland Health Series.)* Pleasant Grove, UT: Woodland Publishing. 1997.

PERIODICALS

Berger, Laurie. "The Lowdown on natural Fat Fighters." *Vegetarian Times* (January 1998): 82-84.

Campbell, Adam. "Soft Science: The Exclusive World on Which Sex Supplements may Help and Which Won't." *Men's Health* (May 2002): 100.

Castleman, Michael. "Recipes for Lust." *Psychology Today* (July/August 1997): 50-58.

Millman, Christian. "Natural Disasters." *Men's Health* (April 1999): 90.

Puotinen, C. J. "Herbs for Virility: Natural Ways to Spruce Up Your Sex Appeal." *Vegetarian Times* (May 1997): 80-82.

"Yohimbe Tree Bark: Herbal Viagra Better Gotten by Rx." *Environmental Nutrition* (February 1999): 8.

ORGANIZATIONS

American Herbalist Guild. P.O. Box 70, Roosevelt, UT 84066. (435) 722-8434. <http://www.healthy.net:80/pan/pa/herbalmedicine/ahg.htm>.

OTHER

Natural Health Encyclopedia . "Yohimbe." Personal Health Zone. 2000. <http://www.personalhealthzone.com/pg000251.html>.

"Yohimbe (*Pausinystalia yohimbe*)." MotherNature.com. <http://www.mothernature.com/ency/herb/yohimbe.asp>.

"Yohimbine." drkoop.com. http://www.drkoop.com/hcr/drugstory/pharmacy/leaflets/english/d01386a1.asp.

Ken R. Wells
Teresa G. Odle

Yucca

Description

The yucca plant is native to the high deserts of the southwestern United States and Mexico. It is also found less commonly in parts of the eastern United States and West Indies. Extracts from the plant's root are used in alternative medicine as a soap and as an herbal dietary supplement. The yucca has at least 40 species, including *Yucca filamentosa*, the most common type, *Yucca brevifolia* (Joshua tree), *Yucca aloifolia* (Spanish bayonet), and *Yucca gloriosa* (Spanish dagger). Two other species, *Yucca baccata* and *Yucca glauca*, are called soap plant because their roots are especially good for making soap.

Yucca plants are tree-like succulents of the lily family (Liliaceae) with stemless stiff, pointed leaves that end in a sharp needle. The Joshua tree, the namesake of Joshua Tree National Park near Palm Springs, California, is believed to have been named by Mormon settlers because the plant's angular branches resembled the outstretched arms of Joshua leading them out of the desert. The yucca flower is a series of white or purple blossoms on a long stalk.

General use

Native American tribes in the southwestern United States and Northern Mexico found numerous uses for the yucca, dating back hundreds of years. Several tribes, including the Western Apaches on the Fort Apache Reservation in Arizona, use the plant today. The most common use seems to be for hygiene. Roots of the yucca baccata are pounded to remove extracts that are made into shampoo and soap. The Apaches also use yucca leaf fibers to make dental floss and rope. Historically, Western Apaches mixed ground **juniper** berries with yucca fruit to make a gravy. They also made a fermented drink from juniper berries and yucca fruit pounded to a pulp and soaked in water. Other Native American groups used yucca soap to treat **dandruff** and **hair loss**.

Native Americans also used yucca plants for a variety of other non-medical purposes, including making sandals, belts, cloth, baskets, cords, and mats. Such uses can still be found today among Hopi, Papago, and Ute Indians. The Zuni used a mixture of soap made from yucca sap and ground aster to wash newborn babies to stimulate hair growth. Navajos would tie a bunch of yucca fibers together and use it as a brush for cleaning metates.

The primary medical use of yucca is to treat arthritis and joint **pain** and inflammation. Native Americans used sap from the leaves in poultices or baths to treat skin lesions, sprains, inflammation, and bleeding. Teas made from yucca mixed together with other herbs are still brewed by folk healers in northern New Mexico to treat **asthma** and headaches. Constituents of the yucca are used today to treat people with **osteoarthritis** and **rheumatoid arthritis**. The plant's medical properties are found in saponins, precursors of cortisone, which prevent the release of toxins from the intestines that restrict normal cartilage formation. Saponins are produced naturally in the body by the adrenal glands. It is believed yucca works best for arthritis when taken over an extended period of time.

Yucca extract is used to treat a variety of other conditions, including migraine headaches, colitis, ulcers, **wounds, gout, bursitis, hypertension** (high blood pressure), and high LDL **cholesterol** (also called bad cholesterol). Liver, kidney, and gallbladder disorders are also treated with yucca extract. More recently, researchers have found that resveratrol, a compound found in yucca extract as well as in red wine, inhibits the aggregation or clumping of blood platelets. This finding suggests that yucca extract may be useful in preventing **blood clots**.

A number of commercial uses for yucca extract have been found, including adding it to root beer, alcoholic beer, and cocktail mixers as a foaming agent. The bittersweet dark brown extract is also used as an additive in ice cream and other foods.

The extract of the *Yucca schidigera* (Mojave or Mohave yucca) is also used as an additive in natural pet foods. It is reported to speed up bowel elimination, reduce fecal and urine odor, and improve digestion in dogs and cats. It can also be added to pet food as a spray or drops. Several studies also show that when added to animal feed, *Yucca schidigera* extract can reduce noxious ammonia

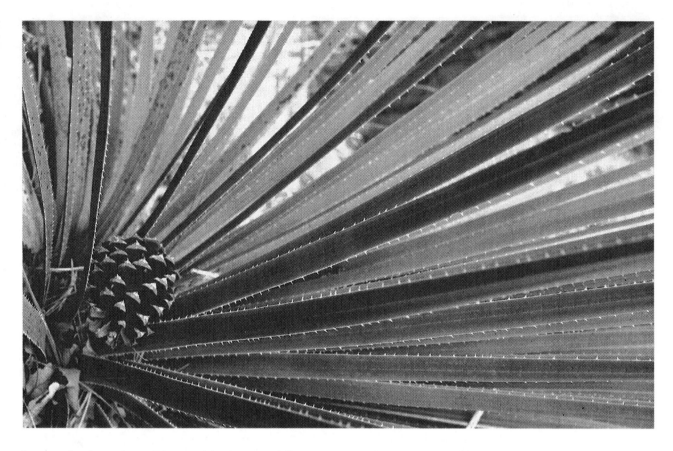

Leaves of a yucca plant. *(Photograph by Robert J. Huffman. Field Mark Publications. Reproduced by permission.)*

gas in the waste products of poultry, pigs, cows, and horses. A decrease in ammonia levels can increase egg production in chickens and milk production in dairy cattle.

Preparations

The standard dosage of concentrated yucca saponins is two to four tablets or capsules a day. Yucca concentrate is also available as a tea, with the usual dosage being 3–5 cups a day. Capsules and tablets are commonly sold in doses of 500 milligrams. A bottle of 30, 60, 90, or 100 units costs $6–10 and can usually be found in health food stores.

Precautions

Since yucca has rarely been studied in a scientific setting, it is not known whether it is safe in children, pregnant or lactating women, or people with a history of severe kidney or liver diseases, **heart disease**, or **cancer**. It appears to be nontoxic to other mammals, including such household pets as cats and dogs.

Side effects

Saponins extracted from yucca plants are generally considered safe when used in traditional doses and forms based on several hundred years of use by Native Americans, both as food and medicine. In recent years, the only reported minor problems are rare cases of **diarrhea** and **nausea**. Some people who are sensitive to plant allergens may develop a mild skin rash from contact with yucca sap.

Interactions

Long-term internal use of yucca extract may interfere with the absorption of such fat-soluble vitamins as A, D, E, and K. As of 2002, however, no interactions between yucca and standard prescription medications have been reported.

Resources

BOOKS

Foster, Steven and Varro E. Tyler. *Tyler's Honest Herbal: A Sensible Guide to the Use of Herbs and Related Remedies.* Binghamton, NY: The Haworth Press, Inc. 1999.

Heinerman, John. *Aloe Vera, Jojoba, and Yucca.* Chicago, IL: Keats Publishing, 1990.

Kavasch, E. Barrie, and Karen Baar. *American Indian Healing Arts: Herbs, Rituals, and Remedies for Every Season of Life.* New York: Bantam Books, 1999.

KEY TERMS

. . . .

Adrenal glands—A pair of endocrine organs near the kidneys that produce steroids such as sex hormones, hormones associated with metabolic functions, and epinephrine.

Bursitis—An inflammation of a sac between a tendon and bone, usually in the shoulder or elbow.

Cholesterol—A fatty substance manufactured in the liver and carried throughout the body in the bloodstream.

Colitis—An inflammation of the colon.

Cortisone—A drug used in the treatment of rheumatoid arthritis.

LDL cholesterol—Low density lipid cholesterol, which causes fatty buildup in blood vessels and can lead to heart disease.

Metates—Stone slabs used by Native Americans to grind corn and other grains.

Poultice—Medicinal herbs or remedies held together by a piece of cloth tied together at its corners, heated, and applied to sores or lesions to promote healing.

Saponins—A group of glucosides that occur in plants and produce a soapy lather.

Miller, Lucinda G., and Wallace J. Murray, eds. *Herbal Medicinals: A Clinician's Guide.* Binghamton, NY: The Haworth Press, Inc. 1999.

Null, Gary. *Secrets of the Sacred White Buffalo.* Paramus, NJ: Prentice Hall. 1998.

Robbers, James E. and Varro E. Tyler. *Tyler's Herbs of Choice: The Therapeutic Use of Phytomedicinals.* Binghamton, NY: The Haworth Press, Inc. 1998.

PERIODICALS

Miyakoshi, M., et al. "Antiyeast Steroidal Saponins from *Yucca Schidigera* (Mohave Yucca), a New Anti-Food-Deteriorating Agent." *Journal of Natural Products* (March 2000): 332-338.

Nyerges, Christopher. "Naturally Clean: How to Find and Use Some of Nature's Most Common Soaps." *Mother Earth News* (August-September 1997): 18-19.

Olas, B., B. Wachowicz, A. Stochmal, and W. Oleszek. "Anti-Platelet Effects of Different Phenolic Compounds from *Yucca schidigera Roezl.* Bark." *Platelets* 13 (May 2002): 167-173.

Vanderjagt, T. J., R. Ghattas, D. J. Vanderjagt, et al. "Comparison of the Total Antioxidant Content of 30 Widely Used Medicinal Plants of New Mexico." *Life Sciences* 70 (January 18, 2002): 1035-1040.

Wang, Y., et al. "Effect of Steroidal Saponin from *Yucca Schidigera* Extract on Ruminal Microbes." *Journal of Applied Microbiology* (May 2000): 887-896.

ORGANIZATIONS

American Association of Naturopathic Physicians (AANP). 3201 New Mexico Avenue, NW, Suite 350, Washington, DC 20016. (202) 895-1392. <www.naturopathic.org>.

Southwest School of Botanical Medicine. P. O. Box 4565, Bisbee, AZ 85603. (520) 432-5855. <www.swsbm.com>.

OTHER

"Yucca." MotherNature.com. <www.mothernature.com/ency/herb/yucca.asp>.

Ken R. Wells
Rebecca J. Frey, PhD

Z

Zhi zi *see* **Gardenia**

Zinc

Description

Zinc is a mineral that is essential for a healthy immune system, production of certain hormones, wound healing, bone formation, and clear skin. It is required in very small amounts, and is thus known as a trace mineral. Despite the low requirement, zinc is found in nearly every cell of the body and is a key to the proper function of more than 300 enzymes, including superoxide dismutase. Normal growth and development cannot occur without it.

General use

The U.S. Recommended Dietary Allowance (RDA) for zinc is 5 milligrams (mg) for children under one year of age, 10 mg for children aged one to 10 years old, 15 mg for males 11 years or older, 12 mg for females 11 years or older, 15 mg for women who are pregnant, and 16-19 mg for women who are lactating.

Zinc has become a popular remedy for the **common cold**. Evidence shows that it is unlikely to prevent upper respiratory **infections**, but beginning a supplement promptly when symptoms occur can significantly shorten the duration of the illness. The only form of zinc proven effective for this purpose is the zinc gluconate or zinc acetate lozenge. Formulations of 13-23 mg or more appear to be most effective, and need to be dissolved in the mouth in order to exert antiviral properties. Swallowing or sucking on oral zinc tablets will not work. The lozenges can be used every two hours for up to a week or two at most.

People who are deficient in zinc are prone to getting more frequent and longer lasting infections of various types. Zinc acts as an immune booster, in part due to stimulation of the thymus gland. This gland tends to shrink with age, and consequently produces less of the hormones that boost the production of infection-fighting white blood cells. Supplemental zinc, at one to two times RDA amounts, can reverse this tendency and improve immune function.

In another immune stimulant capacity, zinc can offer some relief from chronic infections with *Candida albicans*, or yeast. Most women will experience a vaginal **yeast infection** at some time, and are particularly prone to them during the childbearing years. Some individuals appear to be more susceptible than others. One study showed yeast-fighting benefits for zinc even for those who were not deficient in the mineral to begin with. Other supplements that will complement zinc in combating yeast problems are **vitamin A**, **vitamin C**, and **vitamin E**. Another measure that can help to limit problems with *Candida* is eating yogurt, which is an excellent source of *Lactobacillus*, a friendly bacteria that competes with yeast. Limiting sweets in the diet and eating **garlic** or odor-free garlic supplements may also prove helpful.

People who are going to have surgery are well advised to make sure they are getting the RDA of zinc, vitamin A, and vitamin C in order to optimize wound healing. A deficiency of any of these nutrients can significantly lengthen the time it takes to heal. Adequate levels of these vitamins and minerals for at least a few weeks before and after surgery can speed healing. The same nutrients are important to minimize the healing time of **bedsores**, **burns**, and other skin lesions.

There are two male health problems that can potentially benefit from zinc supplementation. Testosterone is one of the hormones that requires zinc for production. Men with **infertility** as a result of low testosterone levels may experience improvement from taking a zinc supplement. Another common condition that zinc can be helpful for is benign prostatic hypertrophy, a common cause of abnormally frequent urination in older men. Taking an extra 50 mg a day for three to six months offers symptomatic relief for some men.

Teenagers are often low in zinc, and also tend to experience more **acne** than the general population. The doses used in studies have been in the high range, requiring medical supervision, but increasing dietary zinc or taking a modest supplement in order to get the RDA amount is low risk and may prove helpful for those suffering from acne. People should consult a knowledgeable health care provider before taking large doses of any supplement.

There is some evidence that zinc supplementation may slightly relieve the symptoms of **rheumatoid arthritis**, but the studies are not yet conclusive. It's possible that those who initially had low zinc levels benefited the most.

In 2002, new research showed certain concentrations of zinc improved the effect of a therapy called interferon for some patients with chronic **hepatitis** C. Although the trial was preliminary, it showed promise for further research into zinc's effects in enhancing interferon therapy.

Zinc is sometimes promoted as an aid for memory. This may be true to the extent that vitamin B_6 and neurotransmitters are not properly utilized without it. However, in the case of people with **Alzheimer's disease**, zinc can cause more harm than good. Some experiments indicate that zinc actually decreases intellectual function of people with this disease. Under these circumstances, it is probably best to stick to the RDA of 15 mg as a maximum daily amount of zinc.

The frequency of sickle-cell crisis in patients with sickle-cell **anemia** may be decreased by zinc supplementation. The decrease was significant in one study, although the severity of the attacks that occurred was not affected. Use of zinc supplementation or other treatment for sickle-cell anemia, a serious condition, should not be undertaken without the supervision of a health care provider.

Both the retina of the eye, and the cochlea in the inner ear contain large amounts of zinc, which they appear to need in order to function properly. Dr. George E. Shambaugh, Jr., M.D., is a professor emeritus of otolaryngology and head and neck surgery at Northwestern University Medical School in Chicago. In *Prevention's Healing with Vitamins*, he "estimates that about 25% of the people he sees with severe **tinnitus** are zinc-deficient." He adds that they sometimes have other symptoms of zinc deficiency. Large doses may be used in order to provide relief for this problem. Medical supervision and monitoring are necessary to undertake this course of treatment.

Topical zinc can be useful for some conditions, including cold sores. It is also available in a combination formula with the antibiotic erythromycin for the treatment of acne. Zinc oxide is a commonly used ingredient in the strongest sun block preparations and some creams for the treatment of **diaper rash** and superficial skin injuries. Men can use topical zinc oxide to speed the healing of **genital herpes** lesions, but it is too drying for women to use in the vaginal area.

There is still not enough information on some of the claims that are made for zinc. A few that may have merit are the prevention or slowing of **macular degeneration**, and relieving **psoriasis**. One should consult a health care provider for these uses.

Deficiency

It is not uncommon to have mild to moderately low levels of zinc, although serious deficiency is rare. Symptoms can include an increased susceptibility to infection, **rashes**, **hair loss**, poor growth in children, delayed healing of **wounds**, rashes, acne, male infertility, poor appetite, decreased sense of taste and smell, and possible swelling of the mouth, tongue, and eyelids.

A more serious, chronic deficiency can cause severe growth problems, including dwarfism and poor bone maturation. The spleen and liver may become enlarged. Testicular size and function both tend to decrease. **Cataracts** may form in the eyes, the optic nerve can become swollen, and color vision is sometimes affected by a profound lack of zinc. Hearing is sometimes affected as well.

Since meats are the best sources of zinc, strict vegetarians and vegans are among the groups more likely to be deficient. The absorption of zinc is inhibited by high fiber foods, so people who have **diets** that are very high in whole grain and fiber need to take supplements separately from the fiber. Zinc is needed in larger amounts for women who are pregnant or breastfeeding. Deficiency during **pregnancy** may lower fetal birthweight, as well as increase maternal risk of toxemia. A good prenatal vitamin is likely to contain an adequate amount. People over age 50 don't absorb zinc as well, nor do they generally have adequate intake, and may require a supplement. Alcoholics generally have poor nutritional status to begin with, and alcohol also depletes stored zinc.

There is an increased need for most vitamins and minerals for people who are chronically under high **stress**. Those who have had surgery, severe burns, wasting illnesses, or poor **nutrition** may require larger amounts of zinc than average.

Some diseases increase the risk of zinc deficiency. Sickle-cell anemia, diabetes, and kidney disease can all affect zinc metabolism. People with **Crohn's disease**, sprue, chronic **diarrhea**, or babies with acrodermatitis enteropathica also have an increased need for zinc. Consult a health care provider for appropriate supplementation instructions.

Preparations

Natural sources

Oysters are tremendously high in zinc. Some sources, such as whole grains, beans, and nuts, have good zinc content but the fiber in these foods prevents it from being absorbed well. Foods with better utilized zinc include beef, chicken, turkey, milk, cheese, and yogurt. Pure maple syrup also is a good source of zinc.

Supplemental sources

Zinc supplements are available as oral tablets in various forms, as well as lozenges. Zinc gluconate is the type most commonly used in lozenge form to kill upper respiratory viruses. One should select brands that do not use citric acid or tartaric acid for flavoring, as these appear to impair the effectiveness. The best-absorbed oral types of zinc may include zinc citrate, zinc acetate, or zinc picolinate. Zinc sulfate is the most likely to cause stomach irritation. Topical formulations are used for acne and skin injuries. Oral zinc should not be taken with foods that will reduce its absorption, such as coffee, bran, protein, phytates, **calcium**, or **phosphorus**. Supplements should be stored in a cool, dry location, away from direct light, and out of the reach of children.

Precautions

Toxicity can occur with excessively large doses of zinc supplements, and produce symptoms, including **fever**, **cough**, abdominal **pain**, **nausea**, **vomiting**, diarrhea, drowsiness, restlessness, and gait abnormalities. If doses greater than 100 mg per day are taken chronically, it can result in anemia, immune insufficiency, heart problems, and **copper** deficiency. High doses of zinc can also cause a decrease in high density lipoprotein (HDL), or good, **cholesterol**.

People who have hemochromatosis, are allergic to zinc, or are infected with HIV should not take supplemental zinc. Ulcers in the stomach or duodenum may be aggravated by supplements as well. Those with **glaucoma** should use caution if using eye drops containing zinc. Overuse of supplemental zinc during pregnancy can increase the risk of premature birth and stillbirth, particularly if the supplement is taken in the third trimester. This increase in adverse outcomes has been documented with zinc dosages of 100 mg taken three times daily.

KEY TERMS

Acrodermatitis enteropathica—Hereditary metabolic problem characterized by dermatitis, diarrhea, and poor immune status. Oral treatment with zinc is curative.

Benign prostatic hypertrophy—Enlargement of the prostate gland, which surrounds the male urethra, causing frequent urination. This condition is very common in older men.

Hemochromatosis—A hereditary condition, which results in excessive storage of iron in various tissues of the body.

Macular degeneration—Deterioration of part of the retina, causing progressive loss of vision. This is the most common cause of blindness in the elderly.

Sickle-cell anemia—A genetic malformation of red blood cells that can cause periodic crises in sufferers.

Tinnitus—Perceived ringing, buzzing, whistling, or other noise heard in one or both ears that has no external source. There are a number of conditions that may cause this.

Side effects

Zinc may cause irritation of the stomach, and is best taken with food in order to avoid nausea. The lozenge form used to treat colds has a strong taste, and can alter the sense of taste and smell for up to a few days.

Interactions

The absorption of vitamin A is improved by zinc supplements, but they may interfere with the absorption of other minerals taken at the same time, including calcium, **magnesium**, **iron**, and copper. Supplements of calcium, magnesium, and copper should be taken at different times than the zinc. Iron should only be taken if a known deficiency exists. Thiazide and loop diuretic medications, sometimes used for people with high blood pressure, congestive heart failure, or liver disease, increase the loss of zinc. Levels are also lowered by oral contraceptives. Zinc can decrease the absorption of tetracycline and quinolone class antibiotics, antacids, soy, or **manganese**, and should not be taken at the same time of day. Drinking coffee at the same time as taking zinc can reduce the absorption by as much as half. Even moderate amounts of alcohol impair zinc metabolism and increase its excretion. Chelation with EDTA can deplete zinc, so patients undergoing chelation need to supplement with zinc, according to the instructions of the health care provider.

Resources

BOOKS

Bratman, Steven and David Kroll. *Natural Health Bible.* California: Prima Publishing, 1999.

Feinstein, Alice. *Prevention's Healing with Vitamins.* Pennsylvania: Rodale Press, 1996.

Griffith, H. Winter. *Vitamins, Herbs, Minerals & supplements: the complete guide.* Arizona: Fisher Books, 1998.

Jellin, Jeff, Forrest Batz, and Kathy Hitchens. *Pharmacist's letter/Prescriber's Letter Natural Medicines Comprehensive Database.* California: Therapeutic Research Faculty, 1999.

Pressman, Alan H. and Sheila Buff. *The Complete Idiot's Guide to Vitamins and Minerals.* New York: alpha books, 1997.

PERIODICALS

Vernarec, Emil. "Zinc May Enhance the Efficacy of Interferon." *RN* (May 2002): 28.

Judith Turner
Teresa G. Odle

The Zone diet

Definition

The Zone Diet program is a food management system that claims to promote optimal metabolic efficiency in the body by balancing the hormones insulin and glucagon. Insulin is responsible for converting, in the blood, incoming nutrients into cells. Glucagon regulates glucose in the liver. The Zone's food plan consists of a dietary intake of 40% carbohydrates, 30% protein, and 30% fat.

Origins

In 1995, Dr. Barry Sears, Ph.D., a former biotechnology researcher for the Massachusetts Institute of Technology, authored *The Zone*. Since that time, the book has sold over one million copies. One of the more popular carbohydrate-restrictive **diets**, the Zone's success has recently spawned several Zone "knock-off" diets. The Zone Diet is based on a program Dr. Sears developed almost twenty years earlier to treat **heart disease** in Type 2 diabetics. One of his key inspirations for developing this program was his own genetic history, which demonstrated an inclination for premature **heart attack**.

In a web interview for WebMD Health, *Spending a Week in the Zone with Barry Sears, Ph.D.,* Dr. Sears ex-plained that he believed that the primary cause of heart disease was not high **cholesterol** but high levels of insulin; and that the Zone Diet is designed to control insulin levels and thus promote better health. Dr. Sears continues to promote his diet through speeches and his web site, http://www.drsears.com/.

Benefits

The name of Dr. Sears' diet refers to an expression used by athletes to describe a euphoric state of optimal physical and mental efficiency. At its heart, the Zone Diet strives to control two metabolic hormones, insulin and glucagons, as well as properly balance eicosanoid metabolism. Eicosanoids, found in fatty acids, are important in the regulation of inflammatory, immunological and hemostatic (arresting hemorrhage) processes. Metabolism is the chemical process in living cells that provides the body with energy and new material to repair waste. In addition to permanent weight loss, this hormonal balance is said to increase longevity and blood flow, improve the immune system, and promote a sense of general well being. Furthermore, the Zone Diet is thought to assist in the prevention of chronic ailments such as diabetes, heart disease, and high blood pressure.

Description

The diet asserts that by controlling the glucagons-insulin ratio in the body, it promotes long-term weight loss as the body burns excess fat. In addition, it is claimed that balancing levels of eicosanoids further increases mental and physical performance and reduces inflammation and hunger. This state of hormonal balance, also referred to as "the Zone," is achieved, according to the diet, by maintaining a dietary ratio of 40% carbohydrates, 30% fat, and 30% protein. It is this dietary ratio that has led people to call the Zone a "40/30/30 diet."

The Zone diet requires eating five times a day—three full meals as well as a mid-afternoon and pre-bedtime snack. The dieter is told that he/she should eat at least once every five hours to maintain proper insulin levels. There are two distinct methods used when preparing a Zone meal: the Eyeball Method and the Block Method. Following either method should provide a daily caloric intake of roughly 1,200 calories for women and 1,500 calories for men.

With the Eyeball Method, the dieter's hand is used to judge portion sizes. For low fat proteins (chicken and fish), the portion should be approximately the size and thickness of the dieter's palm. This equals roughly three ounces of protein for women and four ounces for men. Then carbohydrates are added to the meal. For "favorable" carbohydrates, such as most fruits and vegetables,

DR. BARRY SEARS 1940–

Dr. Barry Sears grew up in Long Beach, California, where he exhibited both an athletic and scientific bent. After graduating from Palisades High School at the age of 17, Sears went to Occidental College to major in chemistry. He played both basketball and volleyball in college, and even after he earned his Ph.D. in biochemistry from Indiana University in 1969, he continued to play volleyball at the national level. Sears became keenly interested in understanding heart disease when his father died of a massive heart attack at the age of 53. Within several years, his father's three brothers all also died of heart attacks. This left Sears with a goal to find some way to combat heart disease. He came upon a study published by two researchers at a San Francisco hospital that claimed that arteriosclerosis, or hardening of the arteries, had been cured in rabbits by the injection of naturally occurring fats called phospholipids. Seizing on this one study, he started his own company in 1976, Lipid Specialties, Inc. The aim of Lipid Specialties was to come up with a phospholipid that could be created in the laboratory, and was thus patentable. Sears came up with several "new" phospholipids, and collaborated on animal studies of their effects with the drug manufacturer Upjohn.

After running out of private funding, Sears shifted his study of the effects of phospholipids on heart disease to a new venture: using phospholipid technology to deliver cancer-fighting drugs. Some drugs that were highly effective at shrinking tumors were nevertheless too toxic to help cancer patients unless they could be modified to go directly to the tumor sites. Sears' phospholipids could safely carry new cancer drugs in the bloodstream. He took out several patents for drug-delivery systems using phospholipids.

But Sears' interest veered again with the awarding of the Nobel Prize for Physiology and Medicine in 1982 to three researchers who had uncovered the functioning of a class of hormones known as eicosanoids. Eicosanoids control a variety of systems within the body, including the cardiovascular system, the immune system, and the body's system for regulating fat storage. The fatty acids Sears had been studying for years in his lipids work were also the building blocks of the eicosanoids. At this point Sears made a leap from biochemical research to nutritional science. He deduced that many diseases could be traced to an imbalance of eicosanoids. The best way to regulate eicosanoids, he theorized, was through food. In the early 1980s, Sears elaborated a theory of nutritional control of eicosanoids that evolved into the Zone diet.

two loose, fist-sized portions may be added. For "unfavorable" carbohydrates, such as pasta and grains, only one tight, fist-sized portion may be added. Finally, a "dash" of dietary fat is added, which can consist of a few nuts, olives, or guacamole.

The second, and more precise, method for the Zone diet is the Block Method. In this method, each "Zone Food Block" consists of three "mini-blocks," which each represent one portion each of low-fat protein, favorable carbohydrates, and dietary fat. These mini-blocks contain a precise measurement of these macronutrients, specifically seven grams of protein, nine grams of carbohydrates, and 1.5 grams of fat. Each of the three daily meals and snacks consists of a set number of blocks. Women should consume three blocks per meal and one block for each snack, totaling eleven blocks each day. Men should consume four blocks per meal and one block for each snack, totaling 14 blocks each day. These are considered the minimum daily nutritional requirements for an adult. Different factors, such as increased muscle mass and **pregnancy**, may increase the daily food block requirements.

The Zone diet is only one of four key elements in the entire nutritional program proposed by Dr. Sears. The other three elements are the use of monounsaturated fats, dietary supplementation of Omega-3 fish oils, and **exercise**. These other elements, it is asserted, will help control metabolic function, produce "good" eicosanoids, and lower insulin levels. These four elements combined should produce a positive hormonal balance and thus increased health and permanent weight loss.

Preparations

There are few preparations required for going on the Zone diet. However, as with going on any diet, it is wise to consult with a physician beforehand. A physical examination and blood work are suggested, particularly to determine levels of cholesterol, glucose, insulin, and triglycerides (fatty acids). Dieters should also prepare their kitchens by purchasing proper measuring tools and a food scale. In addition, they should empty their cupboards of all foods with high-density carbohydrates. Zone "quick start" kits are also available from various retailers and on-line stores.

Precautions

As every individual possesses a unique biochemistry, achieving "the Zone," the state of optimal mental and physical efficiency, can be very subjective. This subjectivity can lead to confusion and frustration as individuals attempt to find their perfect metabolic balance using the 40/30/30 diet plan. Some critics believe the Zone diet is too strict, making it too difficult to maintain over a long period of time.

Due to its high protein ration (30%), the Zone diet is not recommended for people with impaired liver or kidney function. Protein metabolizes in the liver and is then excreted by the kidneys. The added strain of a high protein diet can cause long-term damage to these organs, as well as cause **kidney stones** and bone loss. Some experts further believe that these high protein requirements also contra-indicate the Zone diet for people with or at risk of heart disease, due to the higher level of saturated fat and cholesterol in many high protein foods. Clinical studies have shown that high fat/high protein/low carbohydrate diets can also increase the risk of serious diseases such as high blood pressure, **stroke**, and adult-onset diabetes.

Despite Dr. Sears' claims to the contrary, many scientific studies show that the Zone diet may actually impair physical performance rather than enhance it. **Fatigue** experienced by athletes during exercise may be due to the diet's low proportions of dietary intake of carbohydrates (as stated above) as well as inadequate caloric intake. Additionally, the suggested benefits of risk reduction and increased health may be overstated.

Side effects

Dr. Sears states there are few or no side effects associated with his diet. However, many nutritional experts disagree. The Zone diet requires an intake of carbohydrates below the minimum nutritional daily requirements (100–120 g) agreed upon by most health experts. This deficiency can lead to several health risks such as cardiac problems, ketosis, and orthostatic hypotension (temporarily lowered blood pressure, usually from standing up quickly, causing temporary blood flow reduction and lack of oxygen to the brain, then lightheadedness and sometimes loss of consciousness). Mineral and vitamin deficiencies caused by low carbohydrate consumption may increase the risk of numerous diseases. The diet's high protein intake places added **stress** on kidney functions, increasing the risk of **gout**, **osteoporosis**, kidney stones, and kidney damage. One researcher, Sachiko St. Jeor, and colleagues concluded that dieters following diets like the Zone are potentially at risk for vitamin and mineral deficiencies.

Research & general acceptance

Although the Zone diet is not as strongly criticized as most high protein/low carbohydrate diets, few health organizations and nutritionists endorse it. Indeed, organizations such as the American College of Sports Medicine and the American Dietetic Association have publicly disagreed with the 40/30/30 plan. Most experts note the Zone diet's lack of scientific credibility, either claiming that the majority of Dr. Sears' observations and findings are supported by poorly controlled studies, unproven theories, non-validated results, and half-truths, or that the majority of published scientific research points to the detrimental effects of the Zone rather than to its health benefits. The long-term effects of the Zone diet have not been fully researched; therefore, the diet's long-term health benefits and risks are still undefined.

Training & certification

There is no formal training or certification required for the Zone diet. As Dr. Sears stated, "All you need [to start on the diet] is one hand and one eye."

Resources

BOOKS

Sears, Barry. *The Zone*. New York: Harper-Collins, 1995.
Sears, Barry. *Mastering the Zone*. New York: Regan Books, 1997.

PERIODICALS

Cheuvront, Samuel. "The Zone Diet and Athletic Performance." *Sports Medicine* (April 2000): 289–294.
Cheuvront, Samuel. "The Zone Diet Phenomenon: A Closer Look at the Science behind the Claims." *Journal of the American College of Nutrition* (February, 2003): 9–17.
Coleman, Ellen. "The BioZone Nutrition System: A Dietary Panacea?" *International Journal of Sports Nutrition* (March, 1996): 19–21.
Jarvis, Mark, Alan Seddon, Lars McNaughton, and Dylan Thompson. "The Acute 1-Week Effects of the Zone Diet on Body Composition, Blood Lipid Levels, and Performance in Recreational Endurance Athletes." *The Journal of Strength and Conditioning Research*. (February 2002):50–57.
Kendall, Pat. "Zoning in on the Zone." *Nutrition News* (September 1997).
St. Jeor, Sachiko, Barbara Howard, Elaine Prewitt, Vicki Bovee, Terry Bazzarre, and Robert Eckel. "Dietary Protein and Weight Reduction." *Circulation* (October 2001): 1869–1874.

OTHER

Babal, Ken. "The Zone: Sound Advice or Just Another Diet?" [cited June 13, 2004]. <http://www.healthwell.com/hn-breakthroughs/feb98/thezonediet.cfm>.
"Introduction to the Zone." Zone Perfect [cited June 13, 2004]. <http://www.zoneperfect.com>.
McDougall, John. "The Great Debate: High vs. Low Protein Diets" [cited June 13, 2004]. <http://www.drmcdougall.com/debate.html>.
Sears, Barry. "Zone Diet." DrSears.com [cited June 13, 2004]. <http://www.drsears.com>.

KEY TERMS

Carbohydrates—Neutral compounds of carbon, hydrogen, and oxygen found in sugar, starches, and cellulose.

Eicosanoids—Local, short–lived fatty acid substances with hormone-like properties, derived from arachidonic acid, that have strong physiological effects, even in very low concentrations. They influence several vital functions, such as the regulation of inflammatory, immunological and hemostatic processes.

Glucagon—A hormone from the pancreas that is responsible for releasing glucose stored in the liver.

Insulin—The hormone responsible for conveying incoming blood nutrients into cells.

Ketogenic diet—A diet that results in energy produced through the metabolism of fatty acids, usually from stored fat. By eating a very high amount of fat (80 percent) and low amounts of carbohydrates and protein, the body burns stored fat. Close medical supervision is necessary because of serious possible side effects, including ketosis.

Ketosis—An abnormal accumulation of ketones in the body, usually found in people who have diabetes mellitus or who are fasting, pregnant, starving, or on a high fat diet. Ketosis can cause serious side effects, including dehydration, kidney stones, gall stones, inflammation of the pancreas, decreased bone density, vitamin deficiency, eye problems.

Orthostatic hypotension—A drop in systolic blood pressure, which can result in dizziness or loss of consciousness.

Triglycerides—A blood fat lipid that increases the risk for heart disease.

"Spending a Week in the Zone with Barry Sears, Ph.D." WebMD Health [cited June 13, 2004]. <http://my.webmd.com/content/article/1/1700_50101>.

"The Zone Diet." Healthwell.com [cited June 13, 2004]. <http://www.healthwell.com/healthnotes.cfm?ContentID=1069001>.

"The Zone Diet." Weight-loss Institute [cited June 13, 2004]. <http://www.weight-loss-institute.com/zone_diet.htm>.

Lee Ann Paradise

Zone therapy *see* **Reflexology**

Zoster *see* **Shingles**

ORGANIZATIONS

The list of organizations is arranged in alphabetical order. Although the list is comprehensive, it is by no means exhaustive. It is a starting point for further information that can be used in conjunction with the Resources section of each main body entry, as well as other online and print sources. E-mail addresses and urls listed were provided by the associations; Thomson Gale is not responsible for the accuracy of the addresses or the contents of the websites.

A

Academy of Dermatology
930 N. Meacham Road
PO Box 4014
Schaumberg, IL 60168-4014
Phone: (708) 330-0230
Website: http://www.aad.org/zoster. html

Academy for Guided Imagery
PO Box 2070
Mill Valley, CA 94942
Phone: (800) 726-2070
Website: http://www.academyforguided
    imagery.com/

Academy of General Dentistry
Suite 1200, 211 East Chicago Avenue
Chicago, IL 60611
Phone: (312) 440-4300
Website: http://www.agd.org

Academy of General Dentistry
Suite 1200, 211 East Chicago Avenue
Chicago, IL 60611
Phone: (312) 440-4300
Email: agdjournal@agd.org
Website: http://www.agd.org

Academy of Psychosomatic Medicine
5824 N. Magnolia
Chicago, IL 60660
Phone: (773) 784-2025
Website: http://www.amp.org

Acupressure Institute
1533 Shattuck Avenue
Berkeley, CA 94709
Phone: (510) 845-1059.
Email: info@acupressure.com
Website: http://www.acupressure.com

**Aerobic and Fitness Association of
    America**
15250 Ventura Blvd., Suite 200
Sherman Oaks, CA 91403
Phone: (877) 968-2639
Website: http://www.afaa.com

**Agency for Toxic Substances and
    Disease**
Registry Public Information Office
1600 Clifton Road, NE
Atlanta, GA 30333
Phone: (404) 639-0501
Email: ATSDRIC@cdc.gov
Website: http://www.atsdr.cdc.gov

**Agoraphobics Building Independent
    Lives**
400 West 32nd Street
Richmond, VA 23225
Phone: (804) 353-3964
Email: answers@anxietysupport.org
Website: http://www.anxietysupport.
    org/

Agoraphobics In Motion
1719 Crooks
Royal Oak, MI 48067
Phone: (248) 547-0400
Email: anny@ameritech.net
Website: http://www.aim-hq.org/

AIDS Treatment Data Network
The NETWORK
611 Broadway, Suite 613,
New York, NY 10012
Phone: (212) 260-8868 or (800)734-
    7104
Fax: (212) 260-8869
Email: network@atdn.org
Website: http://www.atdn.org

Al-Anon, Alanon Family Group, Ínc
PO Box 862
Midtown Station
New York, NY 10018-0862
Phone: (800) 356-9996
Website: http://www.recovery.org/aa

Alcoholics Anonymous
World Service Organization
PO Box 459
New York, NY 10163
Phone: (212) 870-3400
Website: http://www.aa.org

**Alexander Graham Bell Association
    for the Deaf**
3417 Volta Place NW
Washington, DC 20007-2778
Phone: (202) 337-5220
Website: http://www.agbell.org

Alexander Technique International
1692 Massachusetts Ave., 3rd Floor,
Cambridge, MA 02138
Phone: (888) 321-0856
Fax: (617) 497-2615
Email: ati@ati-net.com
Website: http://www.ati-net.com

Alliance for Alternative Medicine
PO Box 59
Liberty Lake, WA 99019
Website: http://www.naam-cancer.lle.
    org/

Alliances, Inc
2121 Eisenhower Avenue, Suite 603
Alexandria, VA 22314
Phone: (800) 463-6482
Website: http://www.medsource.com

Aloha International
PO Box 665

Kilauea, HI 96754
Phone: (808) 828-0302
Website: http://www.huna.org/

ALS Association
21021 Ventura Blvd., Suite #321
Woodland Hills, CA 91364
Phone: (818) 340-7500
Website: http://www.alsa.org/

ALS Therapy Development Foundation
215 First Street
Cambridge, MA 02142
Website: http://www.als.net/

Alternative Medicine Foundation, Inc
5411 W. Cedar Lane, Suite 205-A
Bethesda, MD 20814
Phone: (301) 581-0116
Website: http://www.amfoundation.org/

Alzheimer's Disease Education & Referral (ADEAR) Center
The National Institute of Aging (NIA)
PO Box 8250
Silver Spring, MD 20907-8250
Phone: (800) 438-4380
Website: http://www.alzheimers.org

Alzheimer's Association
919 North Michigan Ave., Suite 1000
Chicago, IL 60611
Phone: (800) 272-3900 or (312) 335-8882
Website: http://www.alz.org/

American Academy of Alternative Medicine (AAAM)
16126 E. Warren
Box 24224
Detroit, MI 48224-0224
Phone: (313) 882-0641
Fax: (313) 882-0972

American Academy of Audiology
11730 Plaza America Drive, Suite 300,
Reston, VA 20190
Phone: (703) 790-8466
Website: http://www.audiology.org

American Academy of Child and Adolescent Psychiatry
3615 Wisconsin Avenue, NW
Washington, DC 20016-3007
Phone: (202) 966-7300
Fax: (202) 966-2891
Website: http://www.aacap.org

American Academy of Clinical Sexologists
1929 18th Street NW, Suite 1166
Washington, DC 20009
Phone: (202) 462-2122

American Academy of Clinical Toxicology
777 East Park Drive

PO Box 8820
Harrisburg, PA 17105
Phone: (717) 558-7750
Website: www.clintox.org

American Academy of Dermatology (AAD)
PO Box 4014
Schaumburg, IL 60168-4014
Phone: (847) 330-0230 or (888) 462-DERM
Fax: (847) 330-0050
Website: http://www.aad.org

American Academy of Environmental Medicine
East Kellogg, Suite 625
Wichita, KS 67207
Phone: (316) 684-5500
Website: http://www.aaem.com

American Academy of Family Physicians
11400 Tomahawk Creek Parkway,
Leawood, KS 66211
Phone: (913) 906-6000 or (800) 24-2247
Email: fp@aafp.org
Website: http://www.aafp.org

American Academy of Medical Acupuncture (AAMA)
4929 Wilshire Blvd., Suite 428
Los Angeles, CA 90010
Phone: (323) 937-5514
Email: JDWODEN@prodigy.net
Website: http://www.medicalacupuncture.org

American Academy of Neural Therapy
410 East Denny Way, Suite 18
Seattle, WA 98122
Phone: (206) 749-9967
Website: http://www.Neuraltherapy.com

American Academy of Neurology
1080 Montreal Ave.
St. Paul, MN 55116
Phone: (612) 695-1940
Website: http://www.aan.com

American Academy of Ophthalmology (National Eyecare Project)
PO Box 429098
San Francisco, CA 94142-9098
Phone: (800) 222-EYES
Website: http://www.eyenet.org

American Academy of Orthopaedic Surgeons (AAOS)
6300 North River Road
Rosemont, IL 60018
Phone: (847) 823-7186 or (800) 346-AAOS
Website: http://www.aaos.org

American Academy of Otolaryngology, Head and Neck Surgery, Inc
One Prince Street
Alexandria, VA 22314-3357
Phone: (703) 836-4444
Website: http://www.entnet.org

American Academy of Pain Management
13947 Mono Way #A
Sonora, CA 95370
Phone: (209) 533-9744
Website: http://www.aapainmanage.org

American Academy of Pain Medicine
4700 W. Lake
Glenview, IL 60025
Phone: (847) 375-4731
Website: http://www.painmed.org

American Academy of Pediatrics (AAP)
141 Northwest Point Boulevard, Elk
Grove Village, IL 60007
Phone: (847) 434-4000
Email: kidsdocs@aap.org
Website: http://www.aap.org

American Academy of Sleep Medicine (AASM)
One Westbrook Corporate Center, Suite 920
Westchester, IL 60154
Phone: (708) 492-0930
Website: http://www.aasmnet.org

American Alliance of Aromatherapy
PO Box 750428
Petaluma, California 94975

American Anorexia/Bulimia Association, Inc
293 Central Park West
New York, NY 10024
Phone: (212) 501-8351
Fax: (212) 501-0342

American Apitherapy Society (AAS)
1209 Post Road
Scardsale, NY 10583
Phone: (914) 725-7944
Fax: (914) 23-0920
Email: info@apitherapy.org
Website: http://www.apitherapy.org

American Art Therapy Association
1202 Allanson Rd.
Mundelein, IL 60060-3808
Phone: (888) 290-0878 or (847) 949-6064
Fax: 847-566-4580. arttherapy@ntr.net
Website: http://www.arttherapy.org

American Association for Chronic Fatigue Syndrome
7 Van Buren Street
Albany, NY 12206

Phone: (518) 435-1765
Website: http://weber.u.washington.
edu/~dedra/aacfs1.html

American Association for Marriage and Family Therapy
1100 17th Street NW,
10th Floor, Washington, DC 20036-4601
Phone: (202) 452-0109

American Association For Pediatric Ophthalmology and Strabismus c/o Denise De Losada Wilson
PO Box 193832
San Francisco, CA 94119-3832
Phone: (415) 561-8505
Email: aapos@aao.org
Website: http://med-aapos.bu.edu

American Association for Therapeutic Humor
222 S. Meramec, Suite 303
St. Louis, MO 63105
Phone: (314) 863-6232
Website: http://www.aath.org

American Association of Acupuncture and Oriental Medicine
433 Front St.
Catasaugua, PA 18032
Phone: (610) 266-1433

American Association of Clinical Endocrinologists (AACE)
1000 Riverside Avenue, Suite 205
Jacksonville, FL 32204
Phone: (904) 353-7878
Fax: (904) 353-8185
Website: http://www.aace.com/

American Association of Colleges of Osteopathic Medicine
5550 Friendship Blvd., Suite 310
Chevy Chase, MD 20815-7231
Phone: (301) 968-4100
Website: http://www.aacom.org

American Association of Naturopathic Physicians (AANP)
3201 New Mexico Avenue NW, Suite 350
Washington, DC 20016
Phone: (202) 895-1392 or (866) 538-2267
Fax: (202) 274-1992
Email: member.services@Naturopathic.org
Website: http://www.naturopathic.org

American Association of Neurological Surgeons (AANS)
5550 Meadowbrook Drive
Rolling Meadows, IL 60008
Phone: (888) 566-AANS or (847) 378-0500
Fax: (847) 378-0600
Website: http://www.aans.org

American Association of Nutritional Consultants
400 Oak Hill Drive
Winona Lake, IN 46590
Phone: (888) 828-2262
Fax: (574) 269-4060
Email: registrar@aanc.net
Website: http://www.aanc.net

American Association of Oriental Medicine (AAOM)
433 Front Street
Catasauqua, PA 18032
Phone: (610) 266-1433
Fax: (610) 264-2768
Email: AAOMI@aol.com
Website: http://www.aaom.org

American Association of Orthopedic Medicine
PO Box 29551
Buena Vista, CO 81211
Phone: (800) 992-2062
Fax: (719) 395-5615
Email: Aaom@aaomed.org
Website: http://www.aaomed.org

American Association of Pastoral Counselors
9504-A Lee Highway
Fairfax, VA 22031
Phone: (703) 385-6967
Email: info@aapc.org
Website: http://www.aapc.org

American Association of Poison Control Centers
3201 New Mexico Avenue, Suite 310
Washington, DC 20016
Phone: (800) 222-1222
Website: http://www.aapcc.org

American Association of Sex Educators
Counselors & Therapists
PO Box 238
Mt Vernon, IA 52314
Website: http://www.aasect.org

American Board of Hypnotherapy
16842 Von Karman Avenue, Suite 476
Irvine, CA 92714
Website: http://www.hypnosis.com/

American Botanical Council
6200 Manor Rd.
Austin, TX 78714
Phone: (12) 926-4900
Fax: (512) 926-2345
Email: abc@herbalgram.org
Website: http://www.herbalgram.org

American Cancer Society (National Headquarters)
1599 Clifton Road, N.E.
Atlanta, GA 30329
Phone: (800) ACS-2345
Website: http://www.cancer.org

American Chiropractic Association
1701 Clarendon Blvd.
Arlington, VA 22209
Phone: (800)986-4636
Website: http://www.amerchiro.org/

American Chronic Pain Association
PO Box 850
Rocklin, CA 95677-0850
Phone: (916) 632-0922
Website: http://members.tripod.com/
~widdy/ACPA.html

American College for Advancement in Medicine
23121 Verdugo Drive, Suite 204
Laguna Hills, CA 92653
Website: http://www.acam.org

American College of Acupuncture and Oriental Medicine
9100 Park West Drive
Houston, TX 77063
Phone: (800) 729-4456
Website: http://www.acaom.edu

American College of Allergy, Asthma, and Immunology
85 West Algonquin Road, Suite 550
Arlington Heights, IL 60005
Phone: (847) 427-1200
Website: http://www.acaai.org

American College of Chiropractic Consultants (ACCC)
28 E. Jackson Bldg., 10th Fl., Suite 1020
Chicago, IL 60604
Website: http://www.accc-chiro.com

American College of Gastroenterology
4900-B South Thirty-First Street
Arlington, VA 22206-1656
Phone: (703) 820-7400
Website: http://www.acg.cgi.gi.org/acg
home/html

American College of Obstetricians and Gynecologists (ACOG)
409 12th St., SW.
PO Box 96920
Washington, DC 20090-6920
Website: http://www.acog.org

American College of Occupational and Environmental Medicine (ACOEM)
1114 North Arlington Heights Road
Arlington Heights, IL 60004
Phone: (847) 818-1800
Website: http://www.acoem.org

American College of Rheumatology
1800 Century Place, Suite 250
Atlanta, GA 30345
Phone: (404) 633-3777
Email: acr@rheumatology.org
Website: http://www.rheumatology.org

American College of Sports Medicine
401 W. Michigan St.
Indianapolis, IN 46202-3233
Phone: (317) 637-9200
Fax: (317) 634-7817
Email: publicinfo@acsm.org
Website: http://www.acsm.org

American College of Traditional Chinese Medicine
455 Arkansas Street
San Francisco, CA 94107
Phone: (415) 282-7600
Website: http://www.actcm.edu

American Council for Headache Education
Phone: (ACHE)
19 Mantua Road
Mt. Royal, NJ 08061
Phone: (609) 423-0043 or (800) 255-2243
Website: http://www.achenet.org/

American Council on Exercise
5820 Oberlin Dr., Suite 102
San Diego, CA 92121-0378
Phone: (858) 535-8227
Website: http://www.acefitness.org

American Dance Therapy Association
Phone: (410) 997-4040. info@adta.org
Website: http://www.adta.org

American Dental Association
211 E Chicago Ave.
Chicago, IL 60611
Phone: (312) 440-2500
Website: http://www.ada.org

American Diabetes Association
1701 North Beauregard Street
Alexandria, VA 22311
Phone: (800) DIABETES
Email: AskADA@diabetes.org
Website: http://www.diabetes.org

American Dietetic Association
Phone: (ADA) 120 South Riverside Plaza, Suite 2000
Chicago, IL 60606
Phone: (800) 877-1600
Website: http://www.eatright.org

American Epilepsy Society
638 Prospect Avenue
Hartford, CT 06105-4298
Phone: (205) 232-4825

American Foundation for AIDS Research
120 Wall Street 13th Floor
New York, NY 10005
Phone: (212) 806-1600 or 800-39-am fAR
Fax: (212) 806-1601
Website: http://www.amfar.org/

American Foundation for Homeopathy
1508 S. Garfield
Alhambra, CA 91801

American Foundation for the Prevention of Venereal Disease, Inc
799 Broadway, Suite 638
New York, NY 10003
Phone: (212) 759-2069

American Foundation for Urologic Disease, Inc
1000 Corporate Boulevard, Suite 410
Linthicum, MD 21090
Phone: (800) 828-7866
Phone: (410) 689-3990
Email: memberservices@nafc.org
Website: http://www.afud.org

American Foundation of Traditional Chinese Medicine (AFTCM)
505 Beach Street
San Francisco, CA 94133
Phone: (415) 776-0502
Fax: (415) 392-7003
Email: aftcm@earthlink.net

American Gastroenterological Association (AGA)
7910 Woodmont Ave., 7th Floor
Bethesda, MD 20814
Phone: (310) 654-2055
Email: aga001@aol.com
Website: http://www.gastro.org/index.html

American Heart Association National Center
7272 Greenville Avenue
Dallas, TX 75231
Phone: (800) 242-8721
Website: http://www.americanheart.org

American Herbal Products Association
8484 Georgia Ave., Suite 370
Silver Spring, MD 20910
Phone: (301) 588-1174
Website: http://www.ahpa.org

American Herbalist Guild
PO Box 70
Roosevelt, UT 84066
Phone: (435) 722-8434
Website: http://www.healthy.net:80/pan/pa/herbalmedicine/ahg.htm

American Herbalists Guild
1931 Gaddis Road
Canton, GA 30115
Phone: (770) 751-6021
Fax: (770) 751-7472
Email: ahgoffice@earthlink.net
Website: http://www.americanherbalistsguild.com

American Holistic Health Association
Dept. R, PO Box 17400
Anaheim, CA 92817
Phone: (714) 779-6152
Email: ahha@healthy.net
Website: http://www.healthy.net/pan/chg/ahha/rosen.html

American Holistic Medical Association (AHMA)
12101 Menaul Blvd. NE, Suite C
Albuquerque, NM 87112
Phone: (505) 292-7788
Fax: (505) 293-7582
Email: info@holisticmedicine.org
Website: http://www.holisticmedicine.org

American Indian Science and Engineering Society (AISES)
5661 Airport Blvd.
Boulder, CO 80301-2339
Phone: (303) 939-0023
Fax: (303) 939-8150
Email: aisehq@spot.colorado.edu
Website: http://www.colorado.edu/aises

American Industrial Hygiene Association
2700 Prosperity Avenue, Suite 250
Fairfax, VA 22031
Phone: (703) 849-8888
Website: http://www.aiha.org

American Institute of Homeopathy
1585 Glencoe
Denver, CO 80220
Phone: (303) 898-5477
Website: http://www.homeopathyusa.org/

American Institute of Stress
124 Park Avenue
Yonkers, NY 10703
Phone: (914) 963-1200
Fax: (914) 965-6267
Website: http://www.stress.org

American Institute of Vedic Studies
PO Box 8357
Santa Fe, NM 87504
Phone: (505) 983-9385
Fax: (502) 982-5807
Website: http://www.vedanet.com

American Legion. Gulf War Veteran Issues. 1608 K Street, N.W
Washington, D.C. 20006
Phone: (202) /861-2700
Website: http://www.legion.org/veterans/vt_gulfvet_info.htm

American Liver Foundation
1425 Pompton Ave.
Cedar Grove, NJ 07009
Phone: (800) 465-4837
Website: http://www.liverfoundation.org

American Lung Association
61 Broadway, 6th Floor
New York, NY 10006
Phone: (800) 586-4872 or (212) 315-8700
Website: http://www.lungusa.org

American Macular Degeneration Foundation
PO Box 515
Northampton, MA 01061
Phone: (888) MACULAR or (413) 268-7660
Email: amdf@macular.org
Website: http://www.macular.org

American Massage Therapy Association
820 Davis St., Suite 100
Evanston, IL 60201
Phone: (847) 864-0123
Fax: (847) 864-1178
Email: info@inet.amtamassage.org
Website: http://wwww.amtamassage.org

American Medical Association
515 N. State Street
Chicago, IL 60612
Phone: (312) 464-5000
Website: http://www.ama-assn.org

American Menopause Foundation
350 Fifth Ave., Ste. 2822
New York, NY 10118
Phone: (212) 714-2398
Website: http://www.americanmenopause.org

American Music Therapy Association, Inc
8455 Colesville Road, Suite 1000
Silver Spring, MD 20910
Phone: (301) 589-3300
Website: http://www.musictherapy.org

American Natural Hygiene Society
PO Box 30630
Tampa, FL 33630
Phone: (813) 855-6607
Email: anhs@anhs.org
Website: http://www.anhs.org/index.html

American Obesity Association (AOA)
1250 24th Street NW, Suite 300
Washington, DC 20037
Phone: (202) 776-7711 or (800) 98-OBESE
Website: http://www.obesity.org

American Optometric Association
243 N Lindbergh Blvd.
St. Louis, MO 63141
Phone: (314) 991-4100
Website: http://www.aoanet.org

American Oriental Bodywork Therapy Association (AOBTA)
50 Maple Place
Manhassett, NY 11030
Phone: (856) 782-1616

American Orthopedic Foot and Ankle Society
222 South Prospect
Park Ridge, IL 60068

American Osteopathic Association (AOA)
142 East Ontario Street
Chicago, IL 60611
Phone: (800) 621-1773
Email: info@aoa-net.org
Website: http://www.aoa-net.org

American Osteopathic Board of Neuromusculoskeletal Medicine
3500 DePauw Boulevard, Suite 1080
Indianapolis, IN 46268

American Pain Society
4700 W. Lake Ave.
Glenview, IL 60025
Phone: (847) 375-4715
Website: http://www.ampainsoc.org/

American Parkinson Disease Association, Inc
1250 Hylan Blvd., Suite 4B
Staten Island, NY 10305
Phone: (800) 223-2732
Email: apda@apdaparkinson.org
Website: http://www.apdaparkinson.com

American Physical Therapy Association (APTA)
1111 North Fairfax Street
Alexandria, VA 22314
Phone: (703) 684-APTA or (800) 999-2782
Website: http://www.apta.org

American Podiatric Medical Association
9312 Old Georgetown Rd
Bethesda, MD 20814
Phone: (301) 571-9200
Website: http://www.apma.org

American Polarity Therapy Association
PO Box 19858
Boulder, CO 80308
Phone: (303) 545-2080
Fax: (303) 545-2161
Email: HQ@polaritytherapy.org
Website: http://www.polaritytherapy.org

American Psychiatric Association (APA)
1000 Wilson Boulevard, Suite 1825
Arlington, VA 22209
Phone: (703) 907-7300

Email: apa@psych.org
Website: http://www.psych.org

American Psychological Association (APA)
Office of Public Affairs
750 First St. NE
Washington, DC 20002
Phone: (202) 336-5700 or (800) 374-2721
Website: http://www.apa.org/

American Psychosomatic Society
6728 Old McLean Village Drive
McLean, VA 22101
Phone: (703) 556-9222
Website: http://www.psychosomatic.org

American Psychotherapy & Medical Hypnosis Association
210 S Sierra
Reno, NV 89501
Website: http://members.xoom.com/Hypnosis/

American Red Cross
2025 E Street, NW
Washington, DC 20006
Phone: (202) 303-4498
Website: http://www.redcross.org

American Rose Society
8877 Jefferson Paige Rd.
Shreveport, LA 71119
Phone: (318) 938-5402
Email: ars@ars-hq.org
Website: http://www.ars.org

American School of Ayurvedic Sciences
2115 112th Avenue NE
Bellevue, WA 98004
Phone: (425) 453-8002

American Skin Association, Inc
150 E. 58th Street, 3rd floor
New York, NY 10155-0002
Phone: (212) 688-6547

American Sleep Apnea Association
1424 K Street NW, Suite 302
Washington, DC 20005
Phone: (202) 293-3650
Fax: (202) 293-3656
Website: http://www.sleepapnea.org

American Sleep Disorders Association
1610 14th Street NW, Suite 300
Rochester, MN 55901
Phone: (507) 287-6006

American Social Health Association
PO Box 13827
Research Triangle Park, NC 27709
Phone: (919) 361-8400
Fax: (919) 361-8425
Website: http://www.ashastd.org

American Society for Bariatric Surgery
7328 West University Avenue, Suite F
Gainesville, FL 32607
Phone: (352) 331-4900
Website: http://www.asbs.org

American Society for Clinical Nutrition
9650 Rockville Pike
Bethesda, MD 20814
Phone: (301) 530-7110
Website: http://www.faseb.org/ascn

American Society for Reproductive Medicine
1209 Montgomery Highway
Birmingham, AL 35216-2809
Phone: (205) 978-5000
Website: http://www.asrm.com

American Society for the Alexander Technique
401 East Market Street
PO Box 835
Charlottesville, VA 22902
Phone: (800) 473-0620 or (804) 295-2840
Fax: 804-295-3947
Email: alexandertec@earthlink.net
Website: http://www.alexandertech.org

American Society of Bariatric Physicians
5453 East Evans Place
Denver, CO 80222-5234
Phone: (303) 770-2526
Website: http://www.asbp.org

American Society of Clinical Hypnosis
140 N Bloomingdale Rd.
Bloomingdale, IL 60108
Phone: (630) 980-4740
Fax: (630) 351-8490
Email: info@asch.net
Website: http://www.asch.net/

American Society of Dowsers
PO Box 24
Danville, Vermont 05828
Phone: (802) 684-3417
Website: http://www.dowsers.org/

American Society of Exercise Physiologists
Department of Exercise Physiology
The College of St. Scholastica
1200 Kenwood Ave.
Duluth, MN 55811
Phone: (218) 723-6297
Website: http://www.css.edu/asep

American Society of Hematology (ASH)
1900 M Street, NW, Suite 200
Washington, DC 20036
Phone: (202) 776-0544

Website: http://www.hematology.org

American Thyroid Association
Montefiore Medical Center
111 E. 210th St.
Bronx, NY 10467
Website: http://www.thyroid.org

American Tinnitus Association
PO Box 5
Portland, Oregon 97207
Phone: (800) 634-8978 or (503) 248-9985
Website: http://www.ata.org

American Urological Association (AUA)
1120 North Charles Street
Baltimore, MD 21201
Phone: (410) 727-1100
Website: http://www.auanet.org

American Veterinary Medical Association (AVMA)
1931 North Meacham Road, Suite 100
Schaumburg, IL 60173-4360
Website: http://www.avma.org

American Yoga Association
PO Box 19986
Sarasota, FL 34276
Phone: (941) 927-4977
Fax: (941) 921-9844
Email: patricia.rockwood@american yogaassociation.org
Website: http://www.americanyoga association.org

Anglo-European College of Chiropractic (AECC)
13-15 Parkwood Rd.
Bournemouth BH5 2DF, United Kingdom
Phone :44 1202 436200
Fax: 44 1202 436312
Email: aecc@aecc.ac.uk
Website: http://www.aecc.ac.uk

Ann Wigmore Foundation
PO Box 399
San Fidel, NM 87049-0399
Phone: (505) 552-0595
Fax: (505) 552-0596
Email: livingfood@wigmore.org
Website: http://www.wigmore.org/

Ann Wigmore Natural Health Institute, Inc
PO Box 429
Rincón, Puerto Rico 00677
Email: wigmore@coqui.net
Website: http://www.annwigmore.org/

Anorexia Nervosa and Related Eating Disorders, Inc
PO Box 5102
Eugene, OR 97405
Phone: (541) 344-1144

Anthroposophic Press
PO Box 960
Herndon, VA 20172
Phone: (703) 661-1594 or (800) 856-8664
Fax: (703) 661-1501
Email: service@steinerbooks.org
Website: http://www.steinerbooks.org

Anti-Aging Institute
843 William Hilton Parkway
Hilton Head, SC 29928
Phone: (912) 238-3383
Website: http://www.anti-aging.org

Anxiety Disorders Association of America
8730 Georgia Avenue, Suite 600
Silver Spring, MD 20910
Phone: (240) 485-1001
Fax: (240) 485-1035
Website: http://www.adaa.org

Anxiety Network Homepage
Website: http://www.anxietynetwork. com

Aromatherapy Organisation Council
PO Box 6522
Desborough
Kettering NN14 2YX, United Kingdom
Phone: 44 870 7743477
Fax: 44 870 7743477
info@aocuk.net
Website: http://www.aocuk.net

Art Through Touch
41 Westbury Ct.
Nightingale Ln.
London SW4 9AB, United Kingdom
Phone: 44 20 86735389
Website: http://members.aol.com/AT Touch/

Artemesia. The Association for Anthroposophical Renewal of Healing
1923 Geddes Avenue
Ann Arbor, MI 48104
Phone: (734) 930-9462

Arthritis Foundation
PO Box 7669
Atlanta, GA 30357
Phone: (800) 283-7800
Website: http://www.arthritis.org

Ashtanga Yoga Center—Moscow, St. Petersburg
Metro station Novokuznetskaya or m. Tretyakovskaya 7,
Stary Tolmachevsky pereulok
Moscow, Russia
Phone: +7 (095) 953-69-57
Email: yoga108@mail.ru
Website: http://www.yoga108.com/

Asia-Pacific Association of Psychotherapists (APAP)
4/4 Charles St.
Petersham, NSW 2049, Australia
Phone: 61 2 85851085
Fax: 61 2 85851010

Association for Applied Psychophysiology and Biofeedback (AAPB)
10200 W. 44th Avenue, Suite 304
Wheat Ridge, CO 80033
Phone: (303) 422-8436
Website: http://www.aapb.org

Association of Aromatherapists Southern Africa (AOASA)
PO Box 23924
Claremont 7735, Republic of South Africa
Phone: 27 21 5317314

Association for NLP
PO Box 78
Stourbridge, UK DY8 2YP

Association for Past Life Research and Therapies, Inc
PO Box 20151
Riverside, CA 92516
Website: http://www.pastlifehealing.com/

Association for Psychosomatic Medicine
4560 Delafield Ave.
Bronx, NY 10471-3905
Website: http://www.theamp.org

Association of Reflexologists
27 Old Gloucester St.
London WC1N 3XX, United Kingdom
Phone: 44 870 5673320
Fax: 44 1823 336646
Email: info@aor.org.uk
Website: http://www.aor.org.uk

Association for Repetitive Motion Syndromes
PO Box 471973
Aurora, CO 80047
Phone: (303) 369-0803
Website: http://www.certifiedpst.com/arms/index.html

Association of Labor Assistants and Childbirth Educators (ALACE)
PO Box 390436
Cambridge, MA 02139
Phone: (617) 441-2500 or (888) 222-5223
Fax: (617) 441-3167
Email: info@alace.org
Website: http://www.alace.org

Association of Oncology Social Work
1211 Locust Street
Philadelphia, PA 19107

Phone: (215) 599-6093
Website: http://www.aosw.org

Association for Research and Enlightenment, Inc.
215 67th St., Virginia Beach, VA 23451
Phone: (757) 428-3588 or
Phone: (800) 333-4499. are@edgar cayce.org
Website: http://www.are-cayce.com/index.htm

Asthma and Allergy Foundation of America
1233 20th Street, NW, Suite 402
Washington, D.C. 20036
Phone: (202) 466-7643 or (800) 7-ASTHMA
Fax: (202)466.8940
Email: info@aafa.org
Website: http://www.aafa.org/

Aston Training Center
PO Box 3568
Incline Village, NV 89450
Phone: (775) 831-8228
Website: http://www.aston-patterning.com

Australian Association of Massage Therapists (AAMT)
85 Queen St., Level 2
Melbourne, VIC 3000, Australia
Phone: 61 3 96708878
Fax: 61 3 96422466
Email: info@aamt.com.au
Website: http://www.amta. asn.au

Australian Association of Professional Hypnotherapists and NLP Practitioners, Inc
PO Box 1526
Southport, Gold Coast
Queensland 4215 Australia
Website: http://www.members.tripod.com/~aaphan/index.html

Australian Hypnotherapists' Association
5/5 Karrabee Ave.
Tarban, NSW 2111, Australia

Australian Music Therapy Association (AMTA)
PO Box 79
Turramurra, NSW 2074, Australia
Phone: 61 2 94495279
Fax: 61 2 99883856
Email: info@austmta.org.au
Website: http://www.austmta.org.au

Australian Society of Teachers of the Alexander Technique AUSTAT Inc
PO BOX 716
Darlinghurst, NSW 2010
Email: info@alexandertechnique.org.au
Website: http://www.alexander technique.org.au/

Australian Traditional-Medicine Society (ATMS)
PO Box 1027
Meadowbank, NSW 2114, Australia
Phone: 61 2 98096800
Fax: 61 2 98097570
Email: info@atms.com.au
Website: http://www.atms.com.au

Austrian Society for Acupuncture (ASA)
Kaiserin-Elisabeth Hospital
Huglgasse 1-3
A-1150 Vienna, Austria
Phone: 43 1 981045758
Fax: 43 1 981045759
Email: aku@kes.magwien.gv.at
Website: http://www.akupunktur.at

Ayurveda Holistic Center
Bayville
Long Island, NY
Phone: (516)759-7731
Email: mail@Ayurvedahc.com
Website: http://www.Ayurvedahc.com

Ayurvedic and Naturopathic Medical Clinic
2115 112th Ave NE
Bellevue, WA 98004
Phone: (425) 453-8022
Fax: (425) 451-2670
Website: http://www.ayurvedicscience.com/

Ayurvedic Institute of Albuquerque
PO Box 23445
Albuquerque, NM 87192
Phone: (505) 291-9698

B

Bach Centre
Mount. Vernon, Bakers Lane
Sotwell, Oxon, OX10 OPX UK
Email: centre@bachcentre.com
Website: http://www.bachcentre.com

Baltimore Academy of Behavioral Optometry
16 Greenmeadow Drive, Suite 103
Timonium, MD 21093
Phone: (800) 447-0370

Bastyr University of Natural Health Sciences
14500 Juanita Dr. NE
Kenmore, WA 98028
Phone: (425) 823-1300
Fax: (425) 823-6222
Website: http://www.bastyr.edu/

Better Hearing Institute
515 King Street, Suite 420

Alexandria, VA 22314
Phone: (703) 684-3391
Email: mail@betterhearing.org
Website: http://www.betterhearing.org/

Biofeedback Certification Institute of America
10200 W. 44th Avenue, Suite 310
Wheat Ridge, CO 80033
Phone: (303) 420-2902
Email: bcia@resourcenter.com
Website: http://www.bcia.org

Boiron Research Foundation
1208 Amosland Road
Norwood, PA 19074

Bonnie Prudden Pain Erasure Clinic and School for Physical Fitness and Myotherapy
PO Box 65240
Tucson, AZ 85728
Phone: (520) 529-3979
Fax: (520) 529-6679
Website: http://www.bonnieprudden.com

Brazilian Association of Homeopathic Medicine Associacao Medica Homeopatica Brasileira
SEPS 714/914 Ed. Santa Maria, Sala 312
70390-145 Brasilia, Federal District, Brazil
Phone: 55 61 3456077
Fax: 55 61 3456077
Email: amhb@amhb.org.br
Website: http://www.amhb.org.br

The Breema Center
6076 Claremont Ave.
Oakland, CA 94618
Phone: (510) 428-0937.
Fax: (510) 428-9235
Website: http://www.breema.com

Barbara Brennan School of Healing
500 NE Spanish River Blvd., Suite 108
Boca Raton, FL 33431-4559
Phone: (561) 620-8767 or (800) 924-2564
Fax: (561) 620-9028
Website: http://www.barbarabrennan.com/main.html

Brentforton Scientific and Medical Trust
Brentforton Hall
Vale of Evesharm, Worcs., WR11 5JH England
Phone: (01)386-830537

British Acupuncture Association and Register (BAAR)
34 Aldernay St.
London SW1V 4EU, United Kingdom
Phone: 44 171 8346229

British Acupuncture Council
63 Jeddo Rd.
London W12 9HQ, United Kingdom
Phone: 44 208 7350400
Fax: 44 208 7350404
Email: info@acupuncture.org.uk
Website: http://www.acupuncture.org.uk

British Chiropractic Association
Blagrave House
17 Blagrave St.
Reading RG1 1QB, United Kingdom
Phone: 44 118 9505950
Fax: 44 118 9588946
Email: enquiries@chiropractic-uk.co.uk
Website: http://www.chiropractic-uk.co.uk

British Holistic Medical Association
59 Landsdowne Place
East Sussex
Hove BN3 1FL, United Kingdom
Phone: 44 1273 725951
Fax: 44 1273 725951
Email: bhma@bhma.org
Website: http://www.bhma.org

British Homeopathic Association
15 Clerkenwell Close
London EC1R 0AA, United Kingdom
Phone: 44 207 5667800
Fax: 44 207 5667815
Email: info@trusthomeopathy.org

British Institute of Homeopathy Canada
1445 St. Joseph Blvd.
Gloucester, ON K1C 7K9 Canada
Phone: (613) 830-4759
Website: http://www.homeopathy.com

British Massage Therapy Council
17 Rymers Lane, Oxford OX4 3JU.
01865-774123
Website: http:\\www.bmtc.co.uk

British Natural Hygiene Society
Shalimar, 3 Harold Grove
Frinton on Sea, Essex England, CO13 9BD
Phone: 011-44-1255 672823
Website: http://members.rotfl.com/bnhs

British Osteopathic Association
Langham House West
Mill St.
Luton LU1 2NA, United Kingdom
Phone: 44 158 2488455
Fax: 44 158 2481533
Email: enquiries@osteopathy.org
Website: http://www.osteopathy.org

British Society of Dowsers
Sycamore Cottage, Tamley Lane
Hastingleigh, Ashford,
Kent TN26 5HW, United Kingdom

Buddhist Association of the United States (BAUS)
1384 Broadway, 19th Floor
New York, NY 10018
Phone: (212) 398-8886
Website: http://www.baus.org

Buffalo Trust
PO Box 89
Jemez Springs, NM 87025-0089
Phone: (505) 829-3635
Fax: (505) 829-3450
Website: natachee@aol.com

C

Cèdres Recyclés
60 Adrien Robert
Hull, Quebec, Canada J8Y 3S2
Phone: (819) 771-3446
Fax: (819) 771-0067
Website: http://cedarleaf.org

California Colon Hygienist Society
333 Miller Ave., Suite 1
Mill Valley, CA 94941
Phone: (415) 383-7224

Cambridge Institute for Better Vision
65 Wenham Rd.
Topsfield, MA 01983
Phone: (978) 887-3883 or (800) 372-3937
Fax: 978-887-3885
Email: info@bettervision.com
Website: http://www.bettervision.com/msbio.html

Canada Academy and Association of Chinese Acupuncture
c/o Dr. Peter Yea, Ch. Off.
3852 Finch Ave. E, No. 407
Toronto, ON, Canada M1T 3T6
Phone: (416) 298-3070

Canadian Association of Rubenfeld Synergists
112 Lund St.
Richmond Hill, ON, Canada L4C 5V9
Phone: (905) 883-3158
Website: http://www.rubenfeldsynergy.com/

Canadian Centre for Occupational Health and Safety
135 Hunter Street
East Hamilton, ON Canada L8N 1M5
Phone: (800) 668-4284
Fax: 905) 572-2206
Email: clientservices@ccohs.ca
Website: http://www.ccohs.ca

Canadian Chiropractic Association (CCPA)
L'Association de Protection Chiropratique Canadienne
1396 Eglinton Ave. W
Toronto, ON, Canada M6C 2E4
Phone: (416) 781-5656
Fax: (416) 781-0923 or (800) 668-2076
Email: ccachiro@ccachiro.org
Website: http://www.ccachiro.org

Canadian College of Massage & Hydrotherapy
Calgary Campus
4104 MacLeod Trail SW
Calgary, Alberta
Phone: (403) 875-4585

Canadian College of Naturopathic Medicine (CCNM)
1255 Sheppard Ave. E
Toronto, ON, Canada M2K 1E2
Phone: (416) 498-1255
Fax: (416) 498-1576 or (866) 241-2266
Email: info@ccnm.edu
Website: http://www.ccnm.edu

Canadian Coordinating Office for Health Technology Assessment
Website: www.ccohta.ca/pubs/english/ sleep/treatmnt

Canadian Federation of Aromatherapists (CFA)
456136 45th Line, RR No. 5
Embro, ON, Canada N0J 1J0
Phone: (519) 475-9038
Fax: (519) 475-9078 or (888) 340-4445
Email: manager@cfacanada.com
Website: http://www.cfacanada.com/

Canadian Institute of Traditional Chinese Medicine
136 17th Ave NE
Calgary, AB T2E 1L6 Canada
Phone: (403) 520-5258 or (888) 859-8686
Fax: (403) 520-5286

Canadian Naturopathic Association/Association canadienne de naturopathie
1255 Sheppard Avenue
East at Leslie, North York, ON M2K 1E2
Phone: (800) 551-4381 or (416) 496-8633
Website: http://www.naturopathicassoc.ca

Canadian Neuro-Optic Research Institute
PO Box 29053
4324 Dewdney Ave.
Regina, Saskatchewan S4T 7X3.
Canada
Phone: (306) 359-7694

Fax: (306) 525-2659
Email: cnricontacts@cnri.edu
Website: http://www.cnri.edu/

Canadian Osteopathic Aid Society (COAS)
Societe Canadienne d'Assistance Osteopathique (SCAO)
PO Box 24081
London, ON, Canada N6H 5C4
Phone: (519) 681-1500
Fax: (519) 681-1500
Email: coas@rogers.com

Canadian Reiki Association (CRA)
PO Box 74072, Hillcrest RPO
Vancouver, BC, Canada V5V 5C8
Phone: (604) 699-9049
Fax: (604) 521-9557 or (800) 835-7525
Email: reiki@reiki.ca
Website: http://www.reiki.ca/

Canadian Taijiquan Federation
PO Box 421
Milton, Ontario Canada L9T 4Z1
Website: http://www.canadiantaijiquan federation.ca

Cancer Care, Inc
275 7th Ave.
New York, NY, 10001
Phone: (800) 813-HOPE
Email: info@cancercare.org
Website: http://www.cancercareinc.org

Cancer Prevention Coalition
c/o University of Illinois School of Public Health
2121 West Taylor Street
Chicago, IL 60612
Phone: (312) 996-2297
Email: epstein@uic.edu
Website: http://www.preventcancer.com

Cancer Research Institute (National Headquarters)
681 Fifth Avenue
New York, NY 10022
Phone: (800) 992-2623
Website: http://www.cancerresearch.org

CancerNet
Phone: (800) 4-CANCER
Website: http://wwwicic.nci.nih.gov

Celiac Disease Foundation
13251 Ventura Blvd., Suite 1
Studio City, CA 91604-1838
Phone: (818) 990-2354
Website: http://www.cdf@celiac.org

Celiac Sprue Association/United States of America (CSA/USA)
PO Box 31700
Omaha, NE 68131
Phone: (877) CSA-4CSA.
Fax: 402-558-1347
Email: celiacs@csaceliacs.org

Website: http://www.csaceliacs.org/

Center for Attitudinal Healing
33 Buchanan Drive
Sausalito, California 94965
Phone: (415) 331-616
Fax: (415) 331-4545
Website: http://www.localcommunities. org/servlet/lc_ProcServ/dbpage= page&mode=display&gid=0100401 1550947263615155189

Center for Biologics Evaluation and Research (CBER)
U. S. Food and Drug Administration (FDA)
1401 Rockville Pike
Rockville, MD 20852-1448
Phone: (800) 835-4709 or (301) 827-1800
Website: http://www.fda.gov/cber

Center for Cell and Gene Therapy. Baylor College of Medicine
1102 Bates St, Suite 1100
Houston, TX 77030-2399
Phone: (713) 770-4663
Website: http://www.bcm.tmc.edu/gene therapy

Center for Classical Homeopathy Similia
105005, 10 Ladojskaja str.,
Moscow, Russia
Phone: (095) 265 5064, 5026762, 473 5552 (inf)
Email: similial@aha.ru
Website: http://similia.rusmedserv.com/

Center for Complementary and Alternative Medicine Research in Asthma, Allergy, and Immunology
University of California at Davis
3150B Meyer Hall
Davis, CA 95616
Phone: (916) 752-6575
Website: http://www-camra.ucdavis.edu

Center for Food Safety and Applied Nutrition, U.S. Department of Health and Human Services
5100 Paint Branch Parkway
College Park, MD 20740
Phone: (888) SAFEFOOD
Website: http://www.cfsan.fda.gov

Center for Food Safety and Applied Nutrition. Food and Drug Administration
(CFSAN/FDA)
5100 Pain Branch Pkwy
College Park MD 20740
Website: http://www.cfsan.fda.gov/list. html

Center for Journal Therapy
12477 W. Cedar Drive, #102
Lakewood, CO 80228

Website: http://www.journaltherapy.com

Center for Mind/Body Medicine
PO Box 1048
La Jolla, CA 92038
Phone: (619)794-2425

Center for Mind-Body Medicine
5225 Connecticut Ave. NW, Suite 414
Washington, DC 20015
Phone: (202) 966-7338

Center for Mindfulness in Medicine, Health Care and Society
Stress Reduction Clinic
University of Massachusetts Memorial
Health Care
55 Lake Avenue North
Worcester, MA 01655
Phone: (508) 856-2656
Fax: (508) 856-1977
Email: jon.kabat-zinn@banyan@um
med.edu
Website: http://www.umassmed.edu/cfm

Center for Occupational and Environmental Medicine
7510 Northforest Drive
North Charleston, SC 29420
Phone: (843) 572-1600
Email: allanl@coem.com
Website: http://www.coem.com

Center for Science in the Public Interest
1875 Connecticut Avenue NW, Suite 300
Washington, DC, 20009. 202-332-9110
Website: http://www.cspinet.org

Center for the Study of Anorexia and Bulimia
1 W. 91st St.
New York, NY 10024
Phone: (212) 595-3449

Centers for Disease Control and Prevention (CDC) Cancer Prevention and Control Program
4770 Buford Highway NE, MS K64
Atlanta, GA 30341
Phone: (888) 842-6355
Fax: (770) 488-4760
Email: cancerinfo@cdc.gov
Website: http://www.cdc.gov/cancer/
comments.htm

Centers for Disease Control and Prevention (CDC)
1600 Clifton Rd
Atlanta, GA 30333
Phone: (404) 639-3311 or (800) 311-3435
Website: http://www.cdc.gov/

Centers for Disease Control and Prevention (CDC). International Traveler's Hotline
Phone: (404) 332-4559
Website: http://www.cdc.gov/travel/

Centers for Disease Control and Prevention. National Center for Infectious Diseases
Division of Parasitic Diseases
1600 Clifton Road
Atlanta, GA 30333
(404) 639-3534
(800) 311-3435
Website: http://www.cdc.gov/ncidod/
dpd/parasites/lice/default.htm

Centers for Disease Control and Prevention. National Immunization Hotline
1600 Clifton Rd. NE
Atlanta, GA 30333
Phone: (800) 232- 2522 (English) or
(800) 232-0233 (Spanish)
Website: http://www.cdc.gov

Centers for Disease Control and Prevention. National Institute for Occupational Safety and Health (NIOSH)
Phone: (800) 35-NIOSH
Fax: (513) 533-8573
Website: http://www.cdc.gov/niosh

Centers for Disease Control Malaria Hotline
Phone: (770) 332-4555

Centers for Disease Control Travelers Hotline
Phone: (770) 332-4559

Central Institute of Medical Medicinal and Aromatic Plants (CIMAP)
c/o Dr. Ashok Sharma, Coord.
Kukrail Picnic Spot Rd.
PO Box CIMAP
Lucknow 226 015, Uttar Pradesh, India
Phone: 91 522 2357133
Fax: 91 522 344159
Email: ashoksharma@cimap.org
Website: http://www.cimap.org

Centre for Economic Botany
Royal Botanic Gardens, Kew
Richmond, Surrey TW9 3AE United
Kingdom
Phone: +44 (0)20 8332 5768
Website: http://www.rbgkew.org.uk

Centre for International Ethnomedicinal Education and Research (CIEER)
Email: info@cieer.org
Website: http://www.cieer.org

Chalice of Repose Project at St. Patrick Hospital
312 East Pine Street
Missoula, MT 59802
Phone: (406) 329-2810
Fax: (406) 329-5614
Website: http://www.saintpatrick.org/
chalice/

Chelation Therapy
Dr. Fabio Solano, M.D.
Calle 24-28 Avenida Primera
San JosÈ, Costa Rica
Phone: (506) 221-81-20
Fax: (506)257-04-39
Email: elpaso@sol.racsa.co.cr
Website: http://www.edenia.com/
medical/solano.htm

China Academy of Traditional Chinese Medicine
18 Beixincang, Dongzhimennai
Beijing 100900, People's Republic of
China
Phone: 86 10 446661 NATIONAL

China Spiritual Therapy Study Association
5 Alley 11, Lane 131, Olung St.
Taipei, Taiwan

Chinese Association of Urine Therapy
72 Wu Kon Lio Road
Wuku Industrial Park
Taipei Hsien, Taiwan, Republic of
China
Phone: 886-2-22988446
Website: http://www.everlifepharm.
com/urine/

Chinese Kung-Fu Wu-Su Association
28 West 27th Street
New York, NY 10001
Phone: (212) 725-0535
Email: questions@kungfuwusu.com
Website: http://www.kungfu-wusu.com/

Chiropractic Association of South Africa (CASA)
Chiropraktiese Vereniging van Suid-
Afrika
PO Box 706
Bethlehem 9700, Republic of South
Africa
Phone: 27 58 3034571
Fax: 27 58 3034571
Email: drreg@mweb.co.za
Website: http://www.chiropractic.co.za

Chiropractic Doctors' Association of Hong Kong (CDAHK)
Hong Kong, People's Republic of
China
Phone: 852 81085688
Email: chairman@cda.org.hk
Website: http://www.cda.org.hk

**Chiropractors' Association of
Australia (CAA)**
148 Station St., Ste. 4
PO Box 6246
South Penrith, NSW 2750, Australia
Phone: 61 2 47318011
Fax: 61 2 47318088
Email: nhq@caa.asn.au
Website: http://www.chiropractors.asn.
au

Chuang Yen Monastery
2020, Route 301
Carmel, NY 10512
Phone: (845) 225-1819 or (845) 228-
4288

Church of Christ, Scientist
Email: heal@ChristianScience.org
Website: http://www.ChristianScience.
org

Civil Aerospace Medical Institute
PO Box 20582
Oklahoma City, OK 73125
Phone: (202) 366-4000
Website: http://www.cami.jccbi.gov

**College of Maharishi Ayur-Ved,
Maharishi International University**
1000 4th Street
Fairfield, IA 52557
Phone: (515) 472-7000

**College of Optometrics in Vision
Development**
PO Box 285
Chula Vista, CA 91912
Phone: (619) 425-6191
Fax: (619) 425-0733

College of Syntomic Optometry
Phone: (717) 387-0900
Website: http:\\www.syntonicphoto
therapy.com

Continence Restored, Inc.
407 Strawberry Hill Avenue
Stanford, CT 06902
Phone: (914) 493-1470

Cosmetic Ingredient Review (CIR)
1101 17th Street NW, Suite 310
Washington, DC 20036
Phone: (202) 331-0651
Fax: (202) 331-0088
Website: http://www.cir-safety.org

**Council for Homeopathic
Certification**
PO Box 157
Corte Madera, CA 94976
Website: http://www.homeopathic
directory.com/

**Craniosacral Therapy Association of
North America (CSTNA)**
12 Sato St.

Whitby, ON, Canada L1R 2E6
Phone: (905) 666-0681
Email: info@craniosacraltherapy.org
Website: http://www.craniosacral
therapy.org

**Crohn's & Colitis Foundation of
America, Inc.**
386 Park Avenue South, 17th Floor
New York, NY 10016-8804
Phone: (800) 932-2423
Email: Info@cfa.org
Website: http://www.ccfa.org/

Cultural Survival
96 Mount Auburn St.
Cambridge, MA 02138
Phone: (617) 441-5400.
Fax: (617) 441-5417
Email: csinc@cs.org
Website: http://www.cs.org

Cystic Fibrosis Foundation
6931 Arlington Road
Bethesda MD 20814
Phone: (301) 951-4422 or (800) FIGHT
CF (344-4823)
Fax: (301) 951-6378
Email: info@cff.org
Website: http://www.cff.org

D

Day-Break Geriatric Massage Project
PO Box 1815
Sebastopol, CA 95473

Delta Society
875 124th Ave NE, Ste 101
Bellevue, WA 98005
Phone: (425) 226-735
Fax: (425) 235-1076
Email: info@deltasociety.org
Website: http://www.deltasociety.org/

Depression After Delivery (D.A.D.)
PO Box 1282
Morrisville, PA 19067
Phone: (800) 944-4773
Website: http://www.depressionafter
delivery.com

**Dietitians of Canada/Les diététistes
du Canada**
480 University Avenue, Suite 604
Toronto, ON M5G IV2
Phone: (416) 596-0857
Website: http://www.dietitians.ca/

**Digestive Disease National Coalition
(DDNC)**
711 Second Street NE, Suite 200
Washington, DC 20002
Phone: (202) 544-7497

Website: http://www.ddnc.org

Digestive Health Initiative
7910 Woodmont Avenue, #914
Bethesda, MD 20814
Phone: (800) 668-5237
Website: http://www.gastro.org./dhi.html

**Dine College, Office of Continuing
Education**
PO Box 731
Tuba City, AZ 86045
Phone: (520) 283-6321
Fax: (520) 283-4590
Email: nccce@crystal.ncc.cc.nm.us
Website: http://www.dinecollege.edu/
dcce/index.php

E

Edward Bach Centre
Mount Vernon
Bakers Lane
Sotwell, Oxon United Kingdom OX10
0PZ
Phone: +44 (0) 1491-834-678
Fax: +44 (0) 1491-825-022
Website: http://www.bachcentre.com

**Eating Disorder Awareness &
Prevention, Inc**
603 Stewart St., Suite 803
Seattle, WA 98101
Phone: (206) 382-3587
Email: info@NationalEatingDisorders.
org
Website: http://www.edap.org

Endocrine Society
8401 Connecticut Avenue, Suite 900
Chevy Chase, MD 20815
Phone: (301) 941-0200
Website: http://www.endo-society.org/

**Endometriosis Association
International Headquarters**
8585 North 76th Place
Milwaukee,WI 53223
Phone: (800) 992-3636
Website: http://EndometriosisAssn.org

**Environmental Health Center, a
Division of the National Safety
Council**
1025 Connecticut
Avenue, NW, Suite 1200
Washington, DC 20036
Phone: (202) 293-2270
Website: http://www.nsc.org

Environmental Protection Agency
Ariel Rios Building
1200 Pennsylvania Avenue, NW
Washington, DC 20460

Phone: (202) 272-0167
Website: http://www.epa.gov/

Epilepsy Concern International Service Group
1282 Wynnewood Drive
West Palm Beach,FL 33417
Phone: (407) 683-0044

Epilepsy Foundation of America
4251 Garden City Drive
Landover, MD 20875-2267
Phone: (301) 459-3700 or (800) 532-1000
Fax: (301) 577-2684

Epilepsy Information Service
Phone: (800) 642-0500

European Herbal Infusions Association (EHIA)
Gotenstrasse 21
D-20097 Hamburg, Germany
Phone: 49 40 23601614
Fax: 49 40 23601610
Email: ehia@wga-hh.de
Website: http://www.ehia-online.org

European Herbal Practitioners Association (EHPA)
45A Corsica St.
London N5 1JT, United Kingdom
Phone: 44 20 73545067
Fax: 44 20 73543605
Email: info@euroherb.com
Website: http://www.euroherb.com

European Liaison Committee for Osteopaths (ELCO)
Comite de Liaison Europeen des Osteopathes (CLEO)
116 Av. des Champs Elysee's
F-75008 Paris, France
Phone: 33 1 44218075

European Institute of Vedic Studies
B.P. 4
30170 Monoblet, France
TÈl : 0033 (0)4 66 53 76 87
Fax: 0033 (0)4 66 53 76 88
Email: info@atreya.com
Website: http://www.atreya.com/

F

Faculty of Homeopathy
Hahnemann House
29 Park St. W
Luton LU1 3BE, United Kingdom
Phone: 44 870 4443955
Fax: 44 870 4443960
Email: info@trusthomeopathy.org
Website: http://www.trusthomeopathy.org

Fasting Center International
32 West Anapurna St., #360
Santa Barbara, CA 93101
Website: http://www.fasting.com

Federation of Feminist Women's Health Centers
633 East 11th Ave.
Eugene, OR 97401
Phone: (503) 344-0966

Feldenkrais Guild of North America
3611 SW Hood Avenue, Suite 100
Portland, OR 97201
Phone: (800) 775-2118 or (503) 221-6612
Fax: (503) 221-6616
Website: http://www.feldenkrais.com

Feminist Women's Health Center
106 East E Street
Yakima, WA 98901
Phone: (509) 575-6473
Email: Info@fwhc.org
Website: http://www.fwhc.org

Florida Institute of Psychophysical Integration: Quantum Balance
3301 Bayshore Blvd., Ste 1502
Tampa, FL 33629
Phone: (813) 902-9092
Fax: (813) 902-1902
Email: Dr.Joy@JohnsonMail.com
Website: http://www.quantumbalance.com/home.htm

Florida Institute of Traditional Chinese Medicine
5335 66 St. N
St. Peterbsburg, FL 33709
Phone: (727) 546-6565 or (800) 565-1246
Email: fitcm@gte.net

Flower Essence Society
PO Box 459
Nevada City, CA 95959
Phone: (800) 736-9222
Email: mail@flowersociety.org
Website: http://www.flowersociety.org

Food and Drug Administration (FDA)
5600 Fishers Lane
Rockville, MD 20857
Phone: (888) 463-6332
Website: http://www.fda.gov

Food and Drug Administration (FDA), Center for Biologics Evaluation and Research (CBER)
1401 Rockville Pike, Suite 200-N
Rockville, MD 20852
Website: http://www.fda.gov/cber

Foundation Fighting Blindness
Executive Plaza I, Suite 800
11350 McCormick Rd.,

Hunt Valley, MD 21031-1014
Phone: (888) 394-3937
Website: http://www.blindness.org

Foundation for Homeopathic Education and Research
21 Kittredge St.
Berkeley, CA 94704
Phone: (510) 649-8930

Freedom From Fear
308 Seaview Ave.
Staten Island, NY 10305
Phone: (718) 351-1717
Website: http://www.freedomfromfear.com

G

Gay Men's Health Crisis, Inc.
The Tisch Building
119 West 24 Street
New York, NY 10011
Phone: (212) 367-1000
Website: http://www.gmhc.org/

General Council and Register of Naturopaths
Goswell House
2 Goswell St.
Somerset BA16 0JG, United Kingdom
Phone: 44 870 7456984
Fax: 44 870 7456985
Email: admin@naturopathy.org.uk
Website: http://www.naturopathy.org.uk

Geomancy, the Feng Shui Education Association
2939 Ulloa Street
San Francisco, CA 94116
Phone: (415) 753-6408
Website: http://www.geofengshui.com

George Ohsawa Macrobiotic Foundation
PO Box 3998
Chico, CA 95927
Phone: (800) 232-2372
Website: http://www.gomf.macrobiotic.net

German Group Psychotherapeutic Society (GGPS)
Deutsche Gruppenpsychotherapeutische Gesellschaft (DGG)
Kantstrabe 120-121
D-10625 Berlin, Germany
Phone: 49 30 3132698
Fax: 49 30 3136959
Email: dgg@dynpsych.de

Gerson Institute
PO Box 430
Bonita, CA 91908-0440

Phone: (888) 4GERSON
Website: http://www.gerson.org

Gilpen Street Holistic Center
Dr. Philip Incao, M.D.
1624 Gilpen Street
Denver, CO 80218
Phone: (303) 321-2100

Gluten Intolerance Group
15110 10th Ave SW, Suite A
Seattle, WA 98166
Phone: (206) 246-6652
Fax: (206) 246-6531
Email:info@gluten.net
Website: http://www.gluten.net

Grand Forks Human Nutrition Research Center
2420 2nd Ave North
Grand Forks, ND 58202
Website: http://www.gfhnrc.ars.usda.gov

Guild for Structural Integration
209 Canyon Blvd
PO Box 1868
Boulder, CO 80306-1868
Phone: (303) 449-5903 or (800) 530-8875
Website: http://www.rolfguild.org

H

Hawaiian Lomilomi Association
456 Palo Alto Avenue
Mountain View, CA 94041
Phone: (650) 938-8615
Email:HLA@HaleOle.com
Website: http://www.HaleOle.com/HLA

Healing Light Center Church
261 E. Alegria Ave. #12
Sierra Madre, CA 91024
Phone: (626) 306-2170
Fax: (626) 355-0996

Health and Rejuvenation Research Center. A division of the Association for Research and Enlightenment, Inc
215 67th Street
Virginia Beach, VA 23451-2061
Phone: (757) 428-3588 ext. 7340
Email: hrrc@are-cayce.com

Healthy Mothers, Healthy Babies National Coalition
409 12th St.
Washington, DC 20024
Phone: (202) 638-5577

Hellerwork
406 Berry St.
Mt. Shasta, CA 96067

Phone: (530) 926-2500
Website: http://www.hellerwork.com

Hepatitis Foundation International
30 Sunrise Terrace
Cedar Grove, NJ 07009-1423
Phone: (800)891-0707
Fax: (973)857-5044
Website: http://www.hepfi.org/

Herb Research Foundation
1007 Pearl St., Suite 200
Boulder, CO 80302
Phone: (303) 449-2265
Email:Info@herbs.org
Website: http://www.herbs.org

Herbal Advisor
Website: http//www.AllHerb.com

Herbal Association of South Africa (HAOSA)
PO Box 1831, Escourt
Kwazulu 3310, Republic of South Africa
Phone: 27 33 2631227
Fax: 27 33 2631227

Hippocrates Health Institute
Boston, MA
Website: http://www.hippocratesinst.com

Holistic Dental Association
PO Box 5007
Durango, Colorado 81301
Website: http://www.holisticdental.org

Homeopathic Educational Services
2124 Kittredge Street
Berkeley, CA 94704
Phone: (510) 649-0294 or (800) 359-9051
Fax: (510) 649-1955
Website: http://www.homeopathic.com/

Homeopathic Pharmacopoeia of the United States
PO Box 2221
Southeastern, PA 19399-2221
Phone: (610) 783-5124
Fax: (610) 783-5180

Huna Research, Inc
1760 Anna Street
Cape Girardeau, MO 63701-4504
Phone: (573) 334-3478
Email: hunahq@compuserve.com

Hypnotherapy Practitioners Association
Wellbeing House,
262 Spendmore Lane,
Chorley, Lancashire, PR7 5DE
Phone: 01257 795627
Email: johndove@hypnosis.fsworld.co.uk
Website: http://www.hypnotherapy practitioners.com

Hypoglycemia Association, Inc
18008 New Hampshire Ave.
PO Box 165
Ashton, MD 20861-0165

I

Impotence Institute of America, Impotents Anonymous
10400 Little Patuxent Parkway,Suite 485
Columbia, MD 21044-3502
Phone: (800) 669-1603

Indigenous Traditional Healing Council
PO Box 646
Tempe, AZ 85280
Phone: (602) 209-4759
Website: http://www.azitlan.org/sweat lodge/council/htm

Insight Meditation Society
1230 Pleasant
St. Barre, MA 01005
Phone: (978) 355-4378
Fax: (978) 355-6398
Website: http://www.dharma.org

Institut Pasteur
25-28, rue du Dr. Roux
75015 Paris, France
Phone: +33 (0) 1 45 68 80 00
Website: http://www.pasteur.fr/haut_ext.html

Institute for Frontier Science
6114 LaSalle Ave
Oakland, CA 94611
Phone: (510) 531-5767
E-mail: brubik@compuserve.com
Website: http://www.healthy.net/frontierscience/

Institute of Chinese Materia Medica
China Academy of Traditional Chinese Medicine
Beijing, 100700

Institute of Traditional Medicine
2017 SE Hawthorne Blvd
Portland, OR 97214
Phone: (503) 233-4907
Website: http://www.itmonline.org

International Academy of Osteopathy
Schipholpoort 100
NL-2034 MC Haarlem, Netherlands
Phone: 31 23 5300485
Fax: 31 23 5300437
Website: http://www.iao.be

International Acupuncture Institute
301 Nathan Rd., Rm. 1304
Hong Kong, People's Republic of China
Phone: 852 27711066
Fax: 852 23888836

International Alliance of Healthcare Educators (IAHE)
11211 Prosperity Farms Road, D-325
Palm Beach Gardens, FL 34410
Phone: (561) 622-4334 or (800) 311-9204
Website: http://www.iahe.com

International Aromatherapy and Herb Association
3541 West Acapulco Lane
Phoenix, AZ 85053-4625
Phone: (602) 938-4439
Website: http://www.aztec.asu.edu./iaha/

International Acupuncture Institute
301 Nathan Rd., Rm. 1304
Hong Kong, People's Republic of China
Phone:852 27711066
Fax: 852 23888836

International Association of Crystal Healing Therapists
PO Box 344
Manchester, M60 2EZ, United Kingdom.
Phone: (UK) 01200-426061
Fax: (UK) 01200-444776
Email: info@iacht.co.uk
Website: http://www.iacht.co.uk/

International Association of Enterstomal Therapy
27241 La Paz Road, Suite 121
Laguna Niguel, CA 92656

International Association of Infant Massage
PO Box 1045
Oak View, CA 93022
Website: http://www.iaim.net/

International Association of Reiki Professionals
PO Box 481
Winchester, MA 01890
Website: http://www.iarp.org

International Association for the Study of Traditional Asian Medicine (IASTAM)
Euston House,
24 Eversholt Street
LONDON NW1
Email: e.ford@ucl.ac.uk
Website: http://www.iastam.org/

International Association of Yoga Therapists (IAYT)
4150 Tivoli Ave
Los Angeles, CA 90066

International Bio-Oxidative Medicine Foundation (IBOMF)
PO Box 891954
Oklahoma City, OK 73109
Phone: (405) 634-7855
Fax: (405) 634-7320

International Center for Health & Humor
2930 Hidden Valley Road
Edmond, OK 73013
Phone: (405) 341-8115
Website: http://www.humorandhealth.com

International Center for Infertility Information Dissemination
PO Box 6836
Arlington, VA 22206
Phone: (703) 379-9178
Website: http://www.inciid.org

International Chi Kung/Qi Gong Directory
2730 29th Street
Boulder, CO 80301
Phone: (303) 442-3131

International Childbirth Education Association (ICEA)
PO Box 20048
Minneapolis, MN 55420-0048
Phone: (612) 854-8660
Website: http://www.icea.org

International College of Applied Kinesiology
6405 Metcalf Ave., Suite 503
Shawnee Mission, KS 66202
Phone: (913) 384-5336
Website: http://www.icakusa.com and http://www.icak.com

International Committee of Homeopathic Pharmacists
Comite International des Pharmaciens Homeopathiques (CIPH)
Laboratories Boiron
Avenida Valdelaparra 27
Alcobendas
E-28108 Madrid, Spain
Phone: 34 91 4840438

International Council of Reflexologists (ICR)
PO Box 78060, Westcliffe Postal Outlet
Hamilton, ON, Canada L9C 7N5
Phone:(905) 387-8449
Fax: (905) 387-6199
Email: icr@mountaincable.net
Website: http://www.icr-reflexology.org/

International Council for Control of Iodine deficiency Disorders (ICCIDD)
Prof. Jack Ling. Director, ICEC
1501 Canal Street, Suite 1304
New Orleans, LA 70112

Phone: (504) 584-3542
Fax: (504) 585-4090
Email: ICEC@mailhost.tcs.tulane.edu
Website: http://www.people.virginia.edu/~jtd/iccidd/

International Council for Medical and Clinical Therapists
7361 McWhorter Place, Suite 300
Annandale, VA 22003-5469
Website: http://www.ultradepth.com/ICMCT.htm

International Federation of Aromatherapists (Australian Branch)
PO Box 786
Templestowe, VIC 3106, Australia
Phone: 61 3 98509254
Fax: 61 3 98505730
info@ifa.org.au
Website: http://www.ifa.org.au/

International Federation of Reflexologists
76-78 Edridge Rd.
Croydon CRO 1EF, United Kingdom
Phone: 44 208 6459134
Fax: 44 208 6499291
Email: ifr44@aol.com
Website: http://www.reflexology-ifr.com

International Food Information Council
1100 Connecticut Avenue, NW, Suite 430
Washington, DC, 20036
Phone: (202) 296-6540
Website: http://www.ific.org

International Foundation for Functional Gastrointestinal Disorders
PO Box 17864
Milwaukee, WI 53217
Phone: (888) 964-2001
Website: http://www.execpc.com/iffgd

International Foundation for Homeopathy
PO Box 7
Edmonds, WA 98020
Phone: (206) 776-4147
Fax: (206) 776-1499
Email: ifh@hwlink.com

International Foundation for the Promotion of Homeopathy
2366 Eastlake Avenue East,Suite 301
Seattle, WA 98102
Phone: (206) 324-8230

International Institute of Infant Massage
605 Bledsoe Rd. NW
Albuquerque, NM 87107
Phone: (505) 341-9381

Fax: (505) 341-9386
Website: http://www.infantmassage.com

International Institute of Islamic Medicine & The Islamic Medical Association of North America
Website: http://www.iiim.org/

International Institute of Reflexology
5650 First Avenue North
PO Box 12642
St Petersburg, FL 33733
Phone: (727) 343-4811
Fax: (727) 381-2807
Email: iir@tampabay.rr.com
Website: http://www.reflexology-usa.net/

International Iridology Research Association
PO Box 1442
Solano Beach, CA 92075-2208
Phone: (888) 682-2208
Email: IIRAOffice@aol.com
Website: http://www.iridologyassn.org/

International Medical and Dental Hypnotherapy Association
4110 Edgeland, Suite 800
Royal Oak, MI 48073-2285
Website: http://www.infinityinst.com

International Meditation Centre
54 Cessnock Road
Sunshine, NSW 2264, Australia
Tel: +61 2 49 705 433
Fax: +61 2 49 705 749
Website: http://www.imcnsw.com/

International Meditation Centre
Lot 78, Jacoby Street
Mahogany Creek WA 6072, Australia
Tel: +61 89 295 2644
Fax: +61 89 295 3435
Website: http://members.iinet.net.au/ ~imcperth/

International Meditation Centre
A-9064 St. Michael/Gurk 6, Austria
Tel: +43 4224 2820
Fax: +43 4224 2820 14
Website: http://www.imc-austria.com/

International Meditation Centre— Canada
336 Sandowne Drive, Waterloo, Ontario, N2K 1V8, Canada
Tel: (519) 747-4762

International Meditation Centre— Germany
Sayagyi U Ba Khin Gesellschaft
In Der Wann 39,
65037 Marburg, Germany
Tel: +49 6421 34 660
Website: http://www.subk-vipassana.de/

International Meditation Centre— Japan
Sayagyi U Ba Khin Memorial Trust
Komatsuri-Cho 861,
Kisshiwada-Shi, Osaka-Prefecture 596-0821, Japan,
Tel: +81 724 45 0057
Fax: +81 72445 0057 or +81 722 97 3201

International Meditation Centre— Switzerland
Sayagyi U Ba Khin Gesellschaft
Chutzenstrasse 67,
3007 Bern, Switzerland
Phone/Fax: +41 31 372 9844
Website: http://www.ubakhin.ch/

International NLP Trainers Association, Ltd
Coombe House, Mill Road
Fareham, Hampshire UK PO16 0TN
Phone: (044) 01489 571171

International Ozone Association, Ind. Pan American Group
31 Strawberry Hill Ave
Stamford, CT 06902
Phone: (203) 348-3542
Fax: (203) 967-4845

International School of Shiatsu
10 South Clinton Street
Doylestown, PA 18901
Phone: (215) 340-9918
Fax: (215) 340-9181
Email: info@shiatsubo.com
Website: http://www.shiatsubo.com/

International Sivananda Yoga Vedanta Center (ISYVC)
673 8th Ave.
Val Morin, QC, Canada J0T 2R0
Phone: (819) 322-3226
Fax: (819) 322-5876 or (800) 263-9642
Email: hq@sivananda.org
Website: http://www.sivananda.org

International Society for the Study of Subtle Energies and Energy Medicine (ISSSEEM)
356 Goldco Circle
Golden, CO 80401
Phone: (303) 278-2228
Website: http://www.vitalenergy.com/ ISSSEEM

International Society for Traumatic Stress Studies
60 Revere Dr., Ste. 500
Northbrook, IL 60062
Phone: (847) 480-9028
Website: http://www.istss.org

International Tremor Foundation
7046 West 105th Street
Overland Park, KS 66212
Phone: (913) 341-3880

International Trepanation Advocacy Group (ITAG), Inc
PO Box 65
Wernersville, PA 19565
Phone: (610) 693-6869
Fax: (610) 693-3261
Website: http://www.trepan.com

International Vegetarian Union (IVU)—Africa
PO Box 2178,
Gaborone, Botswana
Phone: +267 3552136
Fax: +267 356591 (Attn: Dr. Jain)
Email: africa@ivu.org (English, Hindi)
Website: http://www.ivu.org/

International Vegetarian Union (IVU)—Asia
114-A, Mittal Court
Nariman Point, Mumbai 400 021, India
Phone: +91 22 285 5755/56 or 285 3592/93
Fax: +91 22 284 5040
Email: asia@ivu.org
Website: http://www.ivu.org/

International Vegetarian Union (IVU)—Australasia
2 Hull Street
Dianella WA 6059, Australia
Phone: +61 (08) 9275 5682
Email: australasia@ivu.org (English)
Website: http://www.ivu.org/

International Vegetarian Union (IVU)—Latin America
Servid„o do Nilton, 412
Praia de CacupÈ
88050-170 FlorianÛpolis SC Brazil
Phone: 0055 48 2351609
Email: latinam@ivu.org (English, Spanish, Portuguese)
Website: http://www.ivu.org/

International Yoga Teachers' Association (IYTA)
PO Box 31
Thornleigh, NSW 2120, Australia
Phone:61 2 9489848
Fax: 61 2 94849848
Email: info@iyta.org.au
Website: http://www.iyta.org.au/

Intestinal Health Institute
4427 East Fifth St
Tucson, AZ 85711
Phone: (520) 325-9686
Email: info@sheilas.com
Website: http://www.sheilas.com

Irish Society of Homeopaths (ISHom)
Ruxton Ct.
35-37 Dominick St.
Galway, Ireland
Phone: 353 91 565040

Fax: 353 91 565040
Email: ishom@eircom.net
Website: http://www.irishsocietyof
homeopaths.com/

Italian Society of Therapeutic Psychosynthesis
Societa Italiana Psicosintesi
Terapeutica (SIPT)
Via S Domenico, 16
I-50133 Florence, Italy
Phone: 39 055570140
Fax: 39 055570140
Email: istituto@psicosintesi.it

ITL Cancer Clinic (Bahamas) Ltd
PO Box F-42689
Freeport, Grand Bahama, Bahamas
Phone: (877) 785-7460
Email: info@immunemedicine.com
Website: http://www.iatclinic.com

J

Japan Society for Oriental Medicine
Nihonbashi Nakadori Building 4F 2-2-20
Nihonbashi,Chuo-ku, Tokyo 103-0027
Phone: 81-3-3274-5060

Japanese Chiropractic Association (JCA)
IK Bldg.
6-20-11 Shinbashi
Minato-ku
Tokyo 105-0004, Japan
Phone: 81 3 54010961
Fax: 81 3 54010956
Website: http://www.chiro.co.jp/jca/
ejca/htm

Jiva Ayurveda
6/103, Kaushalya Park, Hauz Khas
New Delhi-16, India
Tel/Fax: +91-11-51655846
Email: yuvraj@jiva.org
info@ayurvedic.org

Juvenile Diabetes Foundation International
120 Wall Street
New York, NY 10005-4001
Phone: (212) 785-9595
Phone: (800) JDF-CURE
Fax: (212) 785-9595
Email: info@jdrf.org
Website: http://www.jdf.org/

K

KidsHealth/Nemours Foundation
4600 Touchton Road East
Building 200, Suite 500
Jacksonville, FL 32246
Website: http://www.kidshealth.org

Kneipp Corporation of America
105-107 Stonehurst Court
Northvale, NJ 07647
Phone: (201) 750-0600 or (800) 937-4372
Website: http://www.kniepp.com

Korean Academy of Psychotherapists (KAP)
178-23 Song-buk dong
Song-buk-ku
Seoul 136-020, Republic of Korea
Phone:82 2 7648432
Fax: 82 2 7659776
Email: bjlee@medigate.net
Website: http://www.daopsychotherapy.
org

Kushi Institute
PO Box 7
Becket, MA 01223
Phone: (800) 975-8744 or (413) 623-5741
Email: kushi@macrobiotics.org
Website: http://www.macrobiotics.org

L

Labyrinth Enterprises
128 Slocum Avenue
St. Louis, MO 63119
Phone: (800) 873-9873 or (314) 968-5557
Fax: (314) 968-5539
Website: http://www.labyrinth-enter
prises.com

The Labyrinth Society (TLS)
PO Box 144
New Canaan, CT 06840
Phone: (877) 446-4520
Website: http://www.labyrinthsociety.
org

LaLeche League
1400 N. Meacham Rd.
Schaumburg, IL 60173-4048
Phone: (847) 519-7730
Website: http://www.lalecheleague.org

LaStone Therapy
2919 E. Broadway Blvd., Suite 224
Tucson, AZ 85716
Phone: (520) 319-6414

Website: http://www.lastonetherapy.com

Learning Disabilities Association of America
4156 Library Road
Pittsburgh, PA 15234-1349
Phone: (412) 341-1515
Website: http://www.ldanatl.org

Leukemia and Lymphoma Society
600 Third Avenue
New York, NY 10016
Phone: (800) 955-4572
Website: http://www.leukemia.org

Life Extension Foundation
995 SW 24th Street
Fort Lauderdale, FL 33315
Phone: (954) 766-8433 or (877) 900-9073
Website: http://www.lef.org

Light on Yoga Italia (LYI)
Via San Gervasio 18
I-50131 Florence, Italy
Phone: 39 55 576182
Fax: 39 55 576182
Email: info@iyengaryoga.it
Website: http://www.iyengaryoga.it

The Lighthouse
111 East 59th Street
New York, NY 10022
Phone: (800) 334-5497
Website: http://www.lighthouse.org

Linus Pauling Institute
Oregon State University
571 Weniger Hall
Corvalis, OR 97331
Phone: (541) 737-5075
Email: Lpi@orst.edu
Website: http://osu.orst.edu/dept/lpi/
resagenda/timeline.html

Livingston Foundation Medical Center
3232 Duke St.
San Diego, CA 92110
Phone: (619)224-3515
Phone: (888) 777-7321
Website: http://www.livingstonmed
centr.com

Lonjer Oncology Hospital
No. 232 Renmin Road, Anqiu,
Shandong Province, P.R.China.
262100
Phone: 86536-4262226
Fax: 86536-4220109
Email: doctor@orient-hospital.com
Email: manager@orient-hospital.com
Website: http://www.orient-hospital.
com/

Lupus Foundation of America, Inc
1300 Piccard Dr., Suite 200
Rockville, MD 20850

Phone: (800) 558-0121
Website: http://www.lupus.org

Lyme Disease Foundation, Inc
One Financial Plaza
Hartford, CT 06103
Phone: (800) 886-LYME
Website: http://www.lyme.org

Lyme Disease Network of NJ, Inc
43 Winton Road
East Brunswick, NJ 08816
Website: http://www.lymenet.org

Lymphedema and Wound Care Clinic of Austin
5750 Balcones Dr., Ste. 110
Austin, TX 78731
Phone: (512) 453-1930
Website: http://www.lymphedema.com

Lymphoma Research Foundation of America, Inc
8800 Venice Boulevard, Suite 207
Los Angeles, CA 90034
Phone: (310) 204-7040
Website: http://www.lymphoma.org

M

Macular Degeneration Foundation
PO Box 531313
Henderson, NV 89053
Phone: (888) 633-3937
Website: http://www.eyesight.org

Macular Degeneration Partnership
8733 Beverly Boulevard, Suite 201
Los Angeles, CA 90048-1844
Phone: (888) 430-9898 or (310) 423-6455
Website: http://www.amd.org

March of Dimes Resource Center
1275 Mamaroneck Avenue
White Plains, NY 10605
Phone: (888) 663-4637
Website: http://www.modimes.org

Massage Therapy Association
PO Box 53320
Kenilworth 7745, Republic of South Africa
Phone: 27 21 6715313
Email: aoasa@global.co.za

Max Gerson Memorial Cancer Center
Phone: (800) 759-2966
Email: 75141.2044@compuserve.com
Website: http://www.1999.com/gerson

Mayo Clinic
Website: http://www.mayoclinic.com

McDougall Wellness Center
PO Box 14039
Santa Rosa, CA 95402
Phone: (707) 576-1654
Website: http://www.crmcdougall.com

Memorial Sloan-Kettering Cancer Center
1275 York Ave. 68th St.
New York, NY 10021
Phone: (212) 639-2000
Website: http://www.mskcc.org

Meningitis Foundation of America
7155 Shadeland Station, Suite 190
Indianapolis, IN 46256-3922
Phone: (800) 668-1129
Website: http://www.musa.org/welcome.htm

Meridian Institute
1853 Old Donation Parkway, Suite 1
Virginia Beach, VA 23454
Phone: (757) 496-6009
Email: meridian@meridianinstitute.com
Website: http://www.meridianinstitute.com

Michael J. Fox Foundation for Parkinson's Research
Grand Central Station
PO Box 4777
New York, NY 10163
Phone: (800) 708-7644
Website: http://www.michaeljfox.org

Milne Institute Inc
PO Box 2716
Monterey, CA 93942-2716
Phone: (831) 649-1825
Fax: (831) 649-1826
Email: milneinst@aol.com
Website: http://www.milneinstitute.com

Mind-Body Medical Institute
Beth Israel Deaconess Medical Center
One Deaconess Road,
Boston, MA 02215
Phone: (617) 632-9525
Website: http://www.mbmi.org

Mozart Center (Tomatis method)
PO Box 76
Jenner, CA 95450
Phone: (707) 632-6976
Website: http://www.mozartcenter.com

Multiple Sclerosis Association of America (MSAA)
706 Haddonfield Road
Cherry Hill, NJ 08002-2652
Phone: (800) LEARN-MS (532-7667)
Fax: (609) 661-9797
Website: http://www.msaa.com

Multiple Sclerosis Foundation, Inc (MSF)
6350 North Andrews Ave
Fort Lauderdale, FL 33309
Phone: (954) 776-6805 or (800) 225-6495
Fax: (954) 351-0630
Email: support@msfocus.org
Website: http://www.msfocus.org

Muscular Dystrophy Association
3300 East Sunrise Drive
Tucson, AZ 85718
Phone: (520) 529-2000 or (800) 572-1717
Website: http://www.mdausa.org

Mushroom Council
11875 Dublin Boulevard, Suite D-262
Dublin, CA 94568
Phone: (925) 556-5970
Website: http://www.mushroomcouncil.com

Myopia International Research Foundation
1265 Broadway, Room 608
New York, NY 10001
Phone: (212) 684-2777

N

Narcolepsy Network
10921 Reed Hartman Highway
Cincinnati, OH 45242
Phone: (513) 891-3522
Website: http://www.websciences.org/narnet/

National Academy of Sciences
500 Fifth Street, NW
Washington, DC 20001
Website: http://www4.national academies.org/nas/nashome.nsf

National Aeronautics and Space Administration
Office of Biological and Physical Research
Website: http://www.spaceresearch.nasa.gov

National AIDS Hot Line
Phone: (800) 342-AIDS (English)
Phone: (800) 344-SIDA (Spanish)
Phone: (800) AIDS-TTY (hearing-impaired)

National Alliance for the Mentally Ill (NAMI)
Colonial Place Three
2107 Wilson Blvd., Suite 300
Arlington, VA 22201

Phone: (703) 524-7600 or (800) 950-NAMI
Fax: (703) 524-9094
Email: campaign@nami.org
Website: http://www.nami.org

National Alliance of Breast Cancer Organizations
9 East 37th St., 10th floor
New York,NY 10016
Phone: (888) 80-NABCO
Website: http://www.nabco.org

National Alliance on Alcoholism and Drug Dependence, Inc
12 West 21st St.
New York, NY 10010
Phone: (212) 206-6770

National Anxiety Foundation
3135 Custer Dr.
Lexington, KY 40517
Phone: (606) 272-7166
Website: http://www.lexington-on-line.com/naf.html

National Arthritis and Musculoskeletal and Skin Diseases Information Clearinghouse
National Institutes of Health
1 AMS Circle
Bethesda, MD 20892
Phone: (301) 495-4484
Website: http://www.nih.gov/niams

National Association of Cognitive-Behavioral Therapists
PO Box 2195
Weirton, WV 26062
Phone: (800) 853-1135
Website: http://www.nacbt.org/

National Association for Continence
PO Box 1019
Charleston, SC 29402
Phone: (800) BLADDER (252-3337) or (843) 377-0900
Fax: (843) 377-0905
Email: memberservices@nafc.org
Website: http://www.nafc.org

National Association for Parents of the Visually Impaired, Inc
PO Box 317
Watertown, MA 02471
Phone: (800) 562-6265
Fax: (617) 972-7444
Website: http://www.spedex.com/napvi

National Association of Alternative Medicines (NAAM)
PO Box 35189
Chicago, IL 60707-0189
Phone: (708) 453-0080
Fax: (708) 453-0083

National Association of Anorexia Nervosa and Associated Disorders
Box 7
Highland Park, IL 60035
Phone: (708) 831-3438
Email: anad20@aol.com

National Association of Holistic Aromatherapy
836 Hanley Industrial Court
St. Louis, MO 63144
Phone: (888) ASK-NAHA
Website: http://www.naha.org

National Association of Jewish Chaplains
901 Route 10
Whippany, NJ 07981-1156
Phone: (973) 736-9193
Website: http://www.najc.org

National Association of Karate and Martial Arts Schools
Rosecraig
Bullockstone Rd.
Herne Bay CT6 7NL, United Kingdom
Phone: 44 1227 370055
Email: nakmas@aol.com
Website: http://www.nakmas.org.uk

National Association of Nurse Massage Therapists
1710 East Linden St.
Tucson, AZ 85719

National Association of Pregnancy Massage Therapy
Phone: (888) 451-4945

National Association of Rubenfeld Synergists
1000 River Road, Suite 8H
Belmar, NJ 07719
Phone: (800) 484-3250 code 8516
Website: http://www.rubenfeldsynergy.com

National Association of the Deaf
814 Thayer Ave
Silver Spring, MD 20910-4500
Phone: (301) 587-1788
Website: http://www.nad.org

National Board for Hypnotherapy and Hypnotic Anaesthesiology
7841 West Ludlow Drive, Suite A
Peoria, AZ 85381
Website: http://www.nbha-medicine.com/index.html

National Cancer Institute (National Institutes of Health)
6116 Executive Boulevard, Room 3036A
Bethesda, MD 20892
Phone: (800) 4-CANCER (422-6237)
Website: http://www.nci.nih.gov/

National Cancer Institute. Cancer Information Service (CIS)
6116 Executive Boulevard, Room 3036A. Bethesda, MD 20892
Phone: (800) 4-CANCER (422-6237)
Website: http://cancernet.nci.nih.gov

National Center for Complementary and Alternative Medicine (NCCAM)Clearinghouse
PO Box 7923
Gaithersburg, MD 20898
Phone: (888) 644-6226
Fax: (866) 464-3616
Email: info@nccam.nih.gov
Website: http://nccam.nih.gov/health/clearinghouse/

National Center for Environmental Health. Centers for Disease Control and Prevention
Mail Stop F-29
4770 Buford Highway NE
Atlanta, GA 30341-3724
Phone: (888) 232-6789
Website: http://www.cdc.gov/nceh/ncehhome.htm

National Center for Homeopathy (NCH)
801 North Fairfax Street, Suite 306
Alexandria, VA 22314
Phone: (703) 548-7790 or (877) 624-0613
Fax: (703) 548-7792
Email: info@homeopathic.org
Website: http://www.homeopathic.org/index.html

National Center for Learning Disabilities (NCLD)
381 Park Avenue South, Suite 1401
New York, NY 10016
Phone: (410) 296-0232
Website: http://www.ncld.org

National Center for the Preservation of Medicinal Herbs
3350 Beech Grove Road
Rutland, OH 45775
Phone: (740) 742- 4401
Fax: (740) 742-8303
Website: http://home.frognet.net/~rural8/

National Certification Board for Therapeutic Massage and Bodywork
8201 Greensboro Drive, Suite 300
McLean, VA 22102
Phone: (703) 610-9015 or (800) 296-0664
Fax: (703) 610-9005
Email: info@ncbtmb.com
Website: http://www.ncbtmb.com/

National Cholesterol Education Program. NHLBI Information Center
PO Box 30105
Bethesda, MD 20824-0105
Website: http://www.nhlbi.nih.gov

National Chronic Pain Outreach
PO Box 274
Millboro, VA 24460
Phone: (540) 997-5004
Website: http://www.chronicpain.org/

National Clearinghouse for Alcohol and Drug Information
Website: http://www.health.org

National Commission for Certification of Acupuncturists
1424 16th St. NW, Suite 501
Washington, DC 20036
Phone: (202) 232-1404

National Council Against Health Fraud
119 Foster Street
Peabody, MA 01960.
Phone: (978) 532-9383
Website: http://www.ncahf.org/

National Council of Strength & Fitness
PO Box 557486
Miami, FL 33255
Phone: (800) 772-6273
Website: http://www.ncsf.org

National Depressive and Manic Depressive Association(NDMDA)
730 Franklin Street, Suite 501
Chicago, IL 60610
Phone: (800) 826-3632
Fax: (312) 642-7243
Website: http://www.ndmda.org

National Diabetes Information Clearinghouse
1 Information Way
Bethesda, MD 20892-3560
Phone: (301) 654-3327
Fax: 301-907-8906
Website: http://www.niddk.nih.gov/

National Digestive Diseases Information Clearinghouse
2 Information Way
Bethesda, MD 20892
Phone: (800) 891-5389 or (301) 654-3810
Email: nddic@info.niddk.nih.gov
Website: http://digestive.niddk.nih.gov/

National Eating Disorders Association
603 Stewart Street, Suite 803
Seattle, WA 98101
Phone: (800) 931-2237

Website: http://www.nationaleating disorders.org

National Emphysema Foundation
15 Belden Avenue
Norwalk, CT 06850
Phone: (203) 849 9000
Fax: (203) 286 1105
Website: http://emphysemafoundation. org/

National Eye Institute
2020 Vision Place
Bethesda, MD 20892
Phone: (301) 496-5248
Website: http://www.nei.nih.gov

National Guild of Hypnotists
PO Box 308
Merrimack, NH
Phone: (603) 429-9438
Email: ngh@ngh.net
Website: http://www.ngh.net

National Headache Foundation
428 West St. James Place
Chicago, IL 60614
Phone: (773) 388-6399 or (800) 843-2256
Website: http://www.headaches.org

National Heart, Lung, and Blood Institute (NHLBI)
PO Box 30105
Bethesda, MD 20824-0105
Phone: (301) 592-8573
Email: nhlbiinfo@nhlbi.nih.gov
Website: http://www.nhlbi.nih.gov

National Heartburn Alliance
303 East Wacker Drive, Suite 440
Chicago, IL 60601
Phone: (877) 471-2081
Email: nhbainformation@heartburn alliance.org
Website: http://www.heartburnalliance. org/

National Hypoglycemia Association, Inc
PO Box 120
Ridgewood, NJ 07451
Phone: (201) 670-1189

National Institute for Occupational Safety and Health, US Department of Health and Human Services
4676 Columbia Parkway
(Mail Drop R2)
Cincinnati, OH 45226
Website: http://www.cdc.gov/niosh/home page.html

National Institute of Aging, Alzheimer's Education, and Referral Center
Phone: (800) 438-4380

National Institute of Allergy and Infectious Diseases
6610 Rockledge Drive, MSC 6612,
Bethesda, MD 20892
Website: http://www.niaid.nih.gov/

National Institute of Arthritis and Musculoskeletal and Skin Diseases (NIAMS). National Institutes of Health (NIH)
1 AMS Circle
Bethesda, Maryland 20892-3675
Phone: (301) 495-4484 or (877) 22-NIAMS
Fax: (301) 718-6366
Email: niamsinfo@mail.nih.gov
Website: http://www.niams.nih.gov/

National Institute of Ayurvedic Medicine
584 Milltown Road
Brewster, NY 10509
Phone: (845) 278-8700
Fax: 845-278-8215
Email: drgerson@erols.com
Website: http://www.niam.com

National Institute of Child Health and Human Development
PO Box 3006
Rockville, MD 20847
Phone: (800) 370-2943
Fax: (301) 496-7101
Email: NICHDInformationResource Center@mail.nih.gov

Website: http://www.nichd.nih.gov/
National Institute of Dental and Craniofacial Research (NIDCR). National Institutes of Health
Bethesda, MD 20892
Phone: (301) 496-4261
Email: nidcrinfo@mail.nih.gov
Website: http://www.nidr.nih.gov

National Institute of Diabetes and Digestive and Kidney Disorders. National Institutes of Health
Building 31, room 9A04
Center Drive, MSC 2560
Bethesda, MD 20892B
Website: http://www.niddk.nih/gov/

National Institute of Mental Health (NIMH)
6001 Executive Boulevard
Room 8184, MSC 9663
Bethesda, MD 20892-9663
Phone: (866) 615-NIMH or (301) 443-4513
Email: nimhinfo@nih.gov
Website: http://www.nimh.nih.gov

National Institute of Mental Health Eating Disorders Program
Building 10, Room 3S231
9000 Rockville Pike

Bethesda, MD 20892
Phone: (301) 496-1891

National Institute of Mental Health Anxiety Disorders Education Program
6001 Executive Blvd
Room 8184, MSC 9663
Bethesda, MD 20892
Phone: (800) 64-PANIC
Website: http://www.nimh.nih.gov/

National Institute of Neurological Disorders and Stroke
PO Box 5801
Bethesda, MD 20824
Phone: (800) 352-9424 or (301) 496-5751
Website: http://www.ninds.nih.gov/index.htm

National Institute on Aging
Building 31, Room 5C27
31 Center Drive, MSC 2292
Bethesda, MD 20892
Phone: (301) 496-1752
Website: http://www.nia.nih.gov/

National Institute on Deafness and Other Communication Disorders
(NIDCD). National Institutes of Health
31 Center Drive
MSC 2320
Bethesda, MD 20892-2320
Phone: (800) 241-1044 or TTY (800) 241-1055
Fax: (301) 402-0018
Email: lel@ms.nidcd.nih.gov
Website: http://www.nidcd.nih.gov

National Institutes of Health. Office of Research on Women's Health
Email: chunkom@od.nih.gov
Website: www4.od.nih.gov/orwh

National Jewish Center for Immunology and Respiratory Medicine
1400 Jackson Street
Denver, CO 80206

National Kidney and Urologic Diseases Information Clearinghouse
3 Information Way
Bethesda, MD 20892
Phone: (800) 891-5390
Website: http://www.kidney.niddk.nih.gov/

National Kidney Foundation
30 East 33rd St
New York, NY 10016
Phone: (800) 622-9010 or (212) 889-2210
Fax: (212) 689-9261

National Lead Information Center
801 Roeder Road, Suite 600

Silver Spring, MD 20910
Phone: (800) 424-LEAD (5323)
Website: http://www.epa.gov/lead/nlic.htm

National Lead Information Center, National Safety Council
1025 Connecticut Ave. NW, Suite 1200
Washington, DC 20036
Phone: (800) LEAD-FYI or (800) 424-LEAD
Website: http://www.nsc.org/ehc/lead.htm

National Lymphedema Network
Latham Square
1611 Telegraph Ave, Suite 1111
Oakland, CA 94612
Phone: (800) 541-3259 or (510) 208-3200
Fax: (510) 208-3110.
Website: http://www.lymphnet.org/

National Mental Health Association
2001 N. Beauregard St
12th floor
Alexandria, VA 22311
Phone: (800) 969-NMHA
Website: http://www.nmha.org

National Multiple Sclerosis Society (NMSS)
733 3rd Avenue
New York, NY 10017-3288
Phone: (800) 344-4867 or (212) 986-3240
Website: http://www.nmss.org

National Organization for Rare Disorders (NORD)
55 Kenosia Ave
PO Box 1968
Danbury, CT 06813
Phone: (203) 744-0100 or (800) 999-6673
Fax: (203) 798-2291
Email: orphan@rarediseases.org
Website: http://www.rarediseases.org/

National Oriental Medicine Accreditation Agency (NOMAA)
3445 Pacific Coast Highway, Suite 300
Torrance, CA 90505
Phone: (213) 820-2045
Website: http://www.nomaaa.org

National Osteoporosis Foundation
1232 22nd Street NW, Washington, DC 20037
Phone: (202) 223-2226
Website: http://www.nof.org

National Parkinson Foundation, Inc
1501 NW Ninth Ave./Bob Hope Road
Miami, FL 33136
Phone: (305) 243-6666 or (800) 327-4545
Fax: (305) 243-5595

Email: contact@parkinson.org
Website: http://www.parkinson.org

National Pediculosis Association (NPA), Inc
50 Kearney Road
Needham, MA 02494
Phone: (781) 449-NITS
Email: npa@headlice.org
Website: http://www.headlice.org

National Prostate Cancer Coalition
1154 15th St., NW
Washington, DC 20005
Phone: (202) 463-9455 or (888) 245-9455
Fax: (202) 463-9456
Email: info@pcacoalition.org
Website: http://www.4npcc.org/

National Psoriasis Foundation
6600 S.W. 92nd Avenue, Suite 300
Portland, OR 97223
Phone: (800) 723-9166
Website: http://www.psoriasis.org

National Reye's Syndrome Foundation
PO Box 829
Bryan, OH 43506
Phone: (800) 233-7393
Website: http://www.reyessyndrome.org

National Rosacea Society
800 S. Northwest Highway, Suite 200
Barrington, IL 60010
Phone: (888) 662-5874
Website: http://www.rosacea.org

National Scoliosis Foundation
5 Cabot Place
Stoughton, MA 02072
Phone: (800) 673-6922
Email: NSF@scoliosis.org
Website: http://www.scoliosis.org

National Sleep Foundation
1522 K Street, NW, Suite 500
Washington, DC 20005
Phone: (202) 347-3471
Fax: (202) 347-3472
Email: nsf@sleepfoundation.org
Website: http://www.sleepfoundation.org./

National Stroke Association
9707 E Easter Lane
Englewood, CO. 80112
Phone: (800) STROKES or (303) 649-9299
Fax: (303) 649-1328
Website: http://www.stroke.org

National Toxicology Program (NTP)
Liaison and Scientific Review Office
PO Box 12233
MD A3-01
Research Triangle Park, NC 27709

Phone: (919) 541-0530
Website: http://ntp-server.niehs.nih.gov

National Vaginitis Association
117 South Cook Street, Suite 315
Barrington, IL 60010
Phone: (800) 909-8745
Email: VagAssoc@aol.com
Website: http://www.vaginalinfection.com

National Women's Health Information Center
8550 Arlington Blvd., Suite 300
Fairfax, VA 22031
Phone: (800) 994-9662
Website: http://www.4woman.gov

National Women's Health Network
514 10th Street NW, Suite 400
Washington DC 20004
Phone: (202) 347-1140
Fax: (202) 347-1168
Email: nwhn@nwhn.org
Website: http://www.nwhn.org/

Natural Woman Foundation
8539 Sunset Blvd, No. 135
Los Angeles, CA 90069
Phone: (888) 489-6626
Email: Chriscoprd@aol.com
Website: http://www.naturalwoman.org

Naturopathic Physicians Licensing Examination Board (NPLEX)
PO Box 69657
Portland, OR 97201
Phone: (503) 250-9141
Website: http://www.nabne.org/html/index2.html

Nelson Bach USA, Ltd
100 Research Drive
Wilmington, MA 01887
Phone: (800) 319-9151 or (978) 988-3833
Fax: (978) 988-0233
Website: http://www.nelsonbach.com/usa.html

New York Botanical Garden
Bronx River Parkway at Fordham Road
Bronx, NY 10458
Phone: (718) 817-8700
Website: http://www.nybg.org

New York Ginseng Association
PO Box 127
Roxbury, NY 12474
Phone: (607) 326-3005

New Zealand Society for Music Therapy (NZSMT)
47 The Crows Nest
Whitby Porirua 6006 New Zealand
Phone: 64 4 2347192
Fax: 64 4 2347191
Email: lewishome@xtra.co.nz

New Zealand Vegetarian Society
PO Box 26664
Epsom
Auckland, New Zealand
Phone: 64 9 5234686
Fax: 64 9 5234686
Email: nzvs@ivu.org .
Website: http://www.ivu.org/nzvs

North American Association for the Study of Obesity
8630 Fenton St., Suite 412
Silver Spring, MD, 20910
Phone: (301) 563-6526
Website: http://www.naaso.org

North American Menopause Society
PO Box 94527
Cleveland, OH 44101
Phone: (440) 442-7550 or (800) 774-5342
Fax: (440) 442-2660
Email: info@menopause.org
Website: http://www.menopause.org

North American Riding for the Handicapped Association (NARHA)
PO Box 33150
Denver, CO 80233
Phone: (303) 452-1212 or (800) 369-RIDE
Website: http://www.narha.org

North American Society of Homeopaths
10700 Old County Rd. 15, #350
Minneapolis, MN 55441
Phone: (612) 593-9458
Website: http://www.homeopathy.org/

North American Vegetarian Society (NAVS)
PO Box 72
Dolgeville, NY 13329
Phone: (518) 568-7970
Email: navs@telenet.net
Website: http://www.navs-online.org/

Northeast Center for Environmental Medicine
PO Box 2716
Syracuse, NY 13220
Phone: (800) 846-ONUS

Northwest Academy of Preventative Medicine
15615 Bellevue-Redmond Road
Bellevue, WA 98008
Phone: (206) 881-9660

Northwest Center for Environmental Medicine
177 NE 102nd St.
Portland, OR 97220
Phone: (503) 561-0966

Norwegian Acupuncture Association (NFKA)
Norsk Forening for Klassisk Akupunktur
St. Olavsgt. 12
N-0165 Oslo, Norway
Phone: 47 22 988144
Fax: 47 22 361853
Email: nfka@akupunktur.no
Website: http://www.akupunktur.no

Novato Institute for Research & Training
1516 W. Grant Avenue, Suite 212
Novato, CA 94945
Phone: (415) 897-0336
Website: http://www.somatics.com/

Nurse Healers Professional Associates International(NH-PAI), the Official Organization of Therapeutic Touch
3760 S. Highland Drive
Salt Lake City, UT 84106
Phone: (801) 273-3399
Email: nhpai@therapeutic-touch.org
Website: www.therapeutic-touch.org

Nutrition Health Review
171 Madison Avenue
New York, NY 10016

Nutrition Science News
1401 Pearl Street
Boulder, CO 80302
Phone: (303) 939-8440

O

Office of Dietary Supplements (ODS). National Institutes of Health
6100 Executive Boulevard
Room 3B01, MSC 7517
Bethesda, MD 20892
Email: ods@nih.gov
Website: http://ods.od.nih.gov

Office of the Special Assistant for Gulf War Illnesses
5111 Leesburg Pike, Suite 901
Falls Church, VA 22041
Phone: (703) 578-8518
Email: brostker@gwillness.osd.mil
Website: http://www.gulflink.osd.mil

Office of Water Resources Center, Environmental Protection Agency
Mail Code (4100), Room 2615
East Tower Basement
401 M St. SW
Washington, DC 20460
Phone: (800) 426-4791

Website: http://www.epa.gov/ow/

Oldways Preservation and Exchange Trust
266 Beacon Street
Boston, MA 02116
Phone: (617) 421-5500
Fax: (617) 421-5511
Email: oldways@oldwayspt.org
Website: http://www.oldwayspt.org/

Omega Nutrition
6515 Aldrich Rd
Bellingham, WA 98226
Phone: (360) 384-1238
Fax: (360) 384-0700
Email: info@omeganutrition.com
Website: http://www.flaxseedoil.com/

Oncolink. Abramson Cancer Center of the University of Pennsylvania
3400 Spruce Street-2 Donner
Philadelphia, PA 19104
Fax: 215-349-5445
Website: http://cancer.med.upenn.edu

Ontario College of Naturopathic Medicine
60 Berl Avenue
Toronto, Ontario M8Y3C7

Open International University for Alternative Medicines
Indian Board Of Alternative Medicines
80,Chowringhee Road, Calcutta - 700 020, India
Phone: 0091-33-2247 0157/2476 9361
Fax: 0091-33-2485 3845
Email: info@altmeduniversity.com
Website:
    http://www.altmeduniversity.com/

Optometric Extension Program Foundation
2912 South Daimler Street, Suite 100
Santa Ana, CA 92705
Phone: (949) 250-8070

Osteoporosis and Related Bone Diseases. National Resource Center
2 AMS Circle
Bethesda, MD 20892
Phone: (800) 624-BONE or (202) 223-0344
Fax: (202) 293-2356
Email: OsteoInfo@osteo.org
Website: http://www.osteo.org/

Osterreichischer Judo Verband (OJV)
Wassergasse 26
A-1030 Vienna, Austria
Phone: 43 1 7147331
Fax: 43 1 7147333133
E-Mail: office@oejv.com

Overeaters Anonymous World Service Office
PO Box 44020
Rio Rancho, NM 87174
Phone: (505) 891-2664
Fax: (505) 891-4320
Website: http://www.overeaters anonymous.org/

P

Parkinson Alliance
PO Box 308
Kingston, NJ 08528-0308
Phone: (800) 579-8440
Email: admin@parkinsonalliance.org
Website: http://www.parkinsonalliance. net

Parkinson's Action Network
1000 Vermont Ave. NW
Washington, DC 20005
Phone: (800) 850-4725 or (202) 842-4101
Email: info@parkinsonsaction.org
Website: http://parkinsonsaction.org

Parkinson's Disease Foundation
710 West 168th Street
New York, NY 10032
Phone: (800) 457-6676 or (212) 923-4778
Email: info@pdf.org
Website: http://www.parkinsons-foundation.org

Patience T'ai Chi Association
2620 East 18th Street
Brooklyn, NY 11235
Phone: (718) 332-3477
Website: http://www.patiencetaichi.com

People Against Cancer
604 East Street
PO Box 10
Otho, IA 50569
Phone: (515) 972-4444
Fax: (515) 972-4415
Email: info@PeopleAgainstCancer.net
Website: http://www.peopleagainst cancer.net

PhysicalMind Institute
1807 Second Street, Suite 15/16
Santa Fe, New Mexico 87505
Phone: (505) 988-1990 or (800) 505-1990
Fax: (505) 988-2837
Email: themethod@trail.com
Website: http:\\www.the-method.com

Physicians Association for Anthroposophical Medicine (PAAM)
1923 Geddes Avenue
Ann Arbor, MI 48104
Phone: (734) 930-9462
Fax: (734) 662-1727
Email: paam@anthroposophy.org
Website: http://www.paam.net

Pittsburgh School of Pain Management
1312 E. Carson Street
Pittsburgh, PA 15203
Phone: (412) 481-2553
Website: http://www.painschool.com

Plants For a Future
The Field, Penpol
Lostwithiel, Cornwall PL22 0NG England
Phone: (+44 1208) 872963
Website: http://www.scs.leeds.ac.uk/pfaf/

Polycystic Ovarian Syndrome Association
PO Box 80517
Portland, OR 97280
Phone: (877) 775-PCOS
Website: http://www.pcosupport.org

Postpartum Support International
927 North Kellog Avenue
Santa Barbara, CA 93111
Phone: (805) 967-7636
Website: http://www.postpartum.net

Prevent Blindness America (Diabetes and Eyesight)
500 East Remington Rd.
Schaumburg, IL 60173
Phone: (800) 331-2020
Website: http://www.diabetes-sight.org

Preventive Medicine Research Institute
900 Bridgeway, Suite 200
Sausalito, CA 94965.
Phone: (415) 332-2525
Fax: (415) 332-5730
Website: http://www.pmri.org/

Professional Association of German Yoga Instructors
Berufsverband der Yogalehrenden in Deutschland e.V.
Judenstr. 37
D-37073 Gottingen, Germany
Phone: 49 551 4883808
Fax: 49 551 4883860
Email: info@yoga.de
Website: http://www.yoga.de

Prostate Health Council. American Foundation for Urologic Disease
1000 Corporate Boulevard, Suite 410
Linthicum, Maryland 21090

Phone: (410) 689-3990 or (800) 828-7866
Website: http://www.afud.org/education/prostate/prostatecancer.asp

Q

Qigong Human Life Research Foundation
PO Box 5327
Cleveland, OH 44101
Phone: (216) 475-4712

R

The Radionics Association
Baerlein House, Goose Green
Deddington, Oxon. OX15 0SZ United Kingdom
Phone: (01869) 338852
Website: http://www.interlog.com/~radionic/#institute

Radionics Institute
411 W 75 Eastdale
Toronto, Canada M4C 5N3
Website: http://www.mystical-www.co.uk/dowsing.html

Reflexology Association of America
4012 Rainbow St
KPMB#585
Las Vegas, NV 89103-2059
Website: http://www.reflexology-usa.org/

Reflexology Association of Australia (RAA)
PO Box 366
Cammeray, NSW 2062, Australia
Phone: 61 3 98994760

RESOLVE
1310 Broadway
Somerville, MA 02144-1779
Phone: (617) 623-1156
Website: http://www.resolve.org

Restless Legs Syndrome Foundation
1904 Banbury Road
Raleigh, NC 27608-4428
Phone: (919) 781-4428
Website: http://www.rls.org

Rocky Mountain Herbal Institute
PO Box 579
Hot Springs, MT 59845
Phone: (406) 741-3811
Website: http://www.rmhiherbal.org

Rocky Mountain Institute of Yoga and Ayurveda
PO Box 1091
Boulder, CO 80306
Phone: (303) 443-6923
Website: http://www.rmiya.org/

Rosenthal Center for Complementary and Alternative Medicine Research in Aging and Women's Health
Columbia University, College of Physicians and Surgeons
630 W. 168th St.,
New York, NY 10032
Website: http://www.rosenthal.hs.columbia.edu

Rubenfeld Synergy Center
45 West 60th Street, Apt. 11A
New York, NY 10023
Phone: (212) 315-3533
Website: http://members.aol.com/rubenfeld/synergy

Russian Chiropractic Association (RCA)
2 Leontivski Pereolo, 3rd entrance
Moscow, Russia
Phone: 7 503 2349656
Fax: 7 95 9520983
Email: spine@redline.ru
Website: http://www.sport-dc.com/rca.html

S

The Scoliosis Association
PO Box 811705
Boca Raton, FL 33481-1705
Phone: (407) 368-8518
Email: normlipin@aol.com
Website: http://www.scoliosis-assoc.org

Scoliosis Research Society
611 East Wells Street
Milwaukee, WI 53202
Phone: (414) 289-9107
Email: Tjackson@execinc.com
Website: http://www.srs.org

Scottish Institute of Reflexology (SIR)
110 Easterhouse Rd., Flat 1/2
Glasgow G34 9RG, United Kingdom
Phone: 44 141 7730018
Email: mmreflex@aol.com
Website: http://www.scottishreflexology.org

Self Help for Hard of Hearing People, Inc
7910 Woodmont Avenue, Suite 1200
Bethesda, MD 20814

Phone: (301) 657-2248
Website: http://www.shhh.org

Sensory Integration International/The Ayres Clinic
1514 Cabrillo Avenue
Torrance, CA 90501-2817
Website: http://www.sensoryint.com

Serafin AG, Naturopathic Clinic
Kronenstrasse 745
CH-9427 Wolfhalden
Switzerland
Phone: + 41 (0) 71 891 32 40
Fax: + 41 (0)71 891 32 47
Email: cheitz@serafin.ch
Website: http://www.serafin.ch/

Shalem Institute for Spiritual Formation
Mount Saint Alban
Washington, DC 20016
Website: http://www.shalem.org

Shiatsu Therapists Alliance (STA)
1054 Centre St., Ste. 431
Thornhill, ON, Canada L4J 8E5
Phone: (416) 579-5373
Email: shiatsutherapistsalliance@yahoo.ca

Shintaido of America
PO Box 38-1672
Cambridge, MA 02238
Website: http://www.shintaido.org

Shriners Hospitals for Children
2900 Rocky Point Drive
Tampa, FL 33607-1435
Website: http://www.shrinershq.org/hospitals/index.html

Sickle Cell Disease Association of America
200 Corporate Point, Suite 495
Culver City, CA 90230-7633
Phone: (310) 216-6363 or (800) 421-8453
Website: http://sicklecelldisease.org/

Sickle Cell Disease Program, Division of Blood Diseases and Resources. National Heart, Lung, and Blood Institute
II Rockledge Centre
6701 Rockledge Dr
MSC 7950
Bethesda, MD 20892-7950
Phone: (301) 435-0055

Smoking, Tobacco, and Health Information Line. Centers for Disease Control and Prevention
Mailstop K-50
4770 Buford Highway NE
Atlanta, GA 30341-3724
Phone: (800) 232-1311
Website: http://www.cdc.gov/tobacco

Society for Clinical and Experimental Hypnosis
6728 Old McLean Village Drive
McLean, VA 22101
Website: http://ijceh.educ.wsu.edu/sceh/scehframe.htm

Society for Light Treatment and Biological Rhythms
824 Howard Ave
New Haven, CT 06519
Fax: (203) 764-4324
Email: sltbr@yale.edu
Website: http://www.sltbr.org

Society for Ortho-Bionomy International
5875 North Lincoln Avenue, Suite 225
Chicago, IL 60659
Phone: (800) 743-4890
Website: http://www.ortho-bionomy.org

Society of Cosmetic Chemists (SCC)
120 Wall Street, Suite 2400
New York, NY 10005-4088
Phone: (212) 668-1500
Fax: (202) 668-1504
Website: http://www.scconline.org

Society of Neuro-Lingustic Programming
PO Box 424
Hopatcong, NJ 07843
Phone: (201) 770-3600

Society of Teachers of the Alexander Technique
Website: www.stat.org.uk

Sound Healers Association
PO Box 2240
Boulder CO, 80306
Phone: (303) 443-8181
Website: http://www.healingsounds.com

Southwest School of Botanical Medicine
PO Box 4565
Bisbee, AZ 85603
Phone: (520) 432-5855
Website: http://www.swsbm.com

Spiritualist Yoga Fellowship (SYF)
PO Box 1445 Sta. H
Montreal, QC, Canada H3G 2N3
Phone:(514) 937-8359
Fax: (514) 937-5380
Email: mrossner@iiihs.com

Stanford Center for Narcolepsy
Stanford University School of Medicine
701-B Welch Road, Room 146
Palo Alto, CA 94304
Phone: (650) 725-6517
Website: http://www-med.stanford.edu/school/Psychiatry/narcolepsy

StoneCircle Services
893 Noe Street
San Francisco, CA 94114
Phone: (415) 826-0904
Fax: (415) 826-1893
Email: info@stonecircledesign.com
Website: http://www.stonecircledesign.com

Stress and Anxiety Research Society (STAR)
Website: http://www.star-society.org

Supreme Master Ching Hai International Association
PO Box 730247
San Jose, CA 95173-0247
Website: http://www.godsdirectcontact.org

Swedish Psychoanalytical Society

Svenska Psykoanalytiska Foreningen
Vasterlanggatan 60
S-111 29 Stockholm, Sweden
Phone :46 8 108095
Fax: 46 8 108095
Email: spaf@spaf.a.se
Website: http://www.spaf.a.se

Swedish Vegan Federation

Svenska Veganforeningen
Klovervagen 6
S-647 30 Mariefred, Sweden
Phone: 46 159 34404
Website: http://www.vegan.org.se

Swedish Vegetarian Federation
Svenska Vegetariska Foreningen
Sagargat 4 bu
S-11636 Stockholm, Sweden
Phone: 46 8 7021116
Fax: 46 8 7021117
Email: svf@vegetarian.se
Website: http://www.vegetarian.se

T

Telesound LTD
31 Hall Green
Malvern, Worcestershire UK WR14 3QY
Phone: (0) 1684 572506
Email: sales@telesound.co.uk
Website: http://www.telesound.co.uk

Texas Heart Institute Heart Information Service
PO Box 20345
Houston, TX 77225-0345
Phone: (800) 292-2221
Website: http://www.tmc.edu/thi/his.html

Thyroid Foundation of America, Inc
Ruth Sleeper Hall, RSL 350
Boston, MA 02114-2968
Phone: (800) 832-8321 or (617) 726-8500
Website: http://www.clark.net/pub/tfa

Thyroid Society for Education and Research
7515 S. Main St., Suite 545
Houston, TX 77030
Phone: (800) THYROID or (713) 799-9909

TMJ Association, Ltd
PO Box 26770
Milwaukee, WI 53226-0770
Phone: (414) 259-3223
Fax: (414) 259-8112
Website: www.tmj.org

Tomatis Method
Website: http://www.tomatis.com

Touch for Health Kinesiology Association
11262 Washington Blvd
Culver City, CA 90230-4616
Phone: (310) 313-5580 or (800) 466-8342
Website: http://www.tfh.org

Tourette Syndrome Association, Inc.
42-40 Bell Boulevard
Bayside, NY 11361-2820
Phone: (718) 224-2999
Fax: (718) 279-9596
Email: ts@tsa-usa.org
Website: http://www.tsa-usa.org

Trager Institute
21 Locust Ave
Mill Valley, CA 94941-2806
Phone: (415) 388-2688
Fax: (415) 399-2710
Email: admin@trager.com
Website: http://www.trager.com

Trans-Hyperboreau Institute of Science
PO Box 2344
Sausalito, CA 94966
Phone: (415) 331-0230 or (800) 485-8095
Fax: (415) 331-0231

Trigeminal Neuralgia/Tic Douloureux Association
PO Box 340
Barnegat Light, NJ 08006
Phone: (609) 361-1014

TTEAM/Ttouch in Canada
Rochdell Road, Vernon, BC V1B 3E8
Phone: (250) 545-2336
Website: www.tellingtontouch.com

TTEAM/Ttouch in USA
PO Box 3793
Santa Fe, NM 87506
Phone: (800) 854-8326
Website: http://www.tellingtontouch.com

U

Union of French Physiotherapy Masseurs
70 rue Aqueduc
F-75010 Paris, France
Phone: 33 1 42059032
rdefrance00@cegetel.rss.fr

U.S. Department of Agriculture and U.S. Department of Health and Human Services
Phone: (888) 878-3256
Website: http://www.usda.gov/Food AndNutrition

U.S. Food and Drug Administration (FDA)
5600 Fishers Lane
Rockville, MD 20857-0001
Website: http://www.fda.gov

U.S. Food and Drug Administration Office of In Vitro Diagnostic Device Evaluation and Safety
HFZ-440 2098 Gaither Road
Rockville, MD 20850
Phone: (301) 594-3084
Website: http://www.fda.gov/cdrh/oivd

U.S. Food and Drug Administration
HFI-40 2098 Gaither Road
Rockville, MD 20850
Phone: (888) 463-6332
Email: webmail@oc.fda.gov
Website: http://www.fda.gov/bbs/to pics/ANSWERS/ANS00309.htm

U.S. Food and Drug Administration
Office of Consumer Affairs
FDA (HFE-88)
5600 Fishers Lane
Rockville, MD 20857
Phone: (301) 827-5006
Website: http://www.fda.gov
To report adverse effects of a cosmetic product, call:
Phone: (800) 270-8869

U.S. Fund for UNICEF
333 East 38th Street
New York, NY 10016
Email: webmaster@unicefusa.org
Website: http://www.unicefusa.org/ issues99/sep99/learn.html

Unani Tibbi Herbal Healing
311 North Robertson Blvd

PMB 396
Beverly Hills, CA 90211
Phone: (310) 308-9881 or (310) 284-3626
Fax: (561)325-6252
Email: Consult-free@unanitibb.com
Website: http://unanitibb.com/

United Network for Organ Sharing
1100 Boulders Parkway, Suite 500
PO Box 13770,
Richmond, VA 23225-8770
Phone: (804) 330-8500
Website: http://www.unos.org

United Plant Savers
PO Box 98
East Barre, VT 05649
Phone: (802)479-9825
Fax: (802)-476-3722
Website: http://www.plantsavers.org

United States Department of Agriculture (USDA)
Agricultural Research Service (ARS)
5601 Sunnyside Avenue, Beltsville, MD 20705
Phone: (301) 504-1651
Website: http://www.ars.usda.gov

United States Department of Agriculture
Center for Nutrition Policy and Promotion
1120 20th Street NW, Suite 200
North Lobby, Washington, DC 20036
Phone: (202) 418-2312
Website: http://www.usda.gov/cnpp

United States Food and Drug Administration (FDA)
5600 Fishers Lane
Rockville, MD 20857
Phone: (888) 463-6332
Website: http://www.fda.gov

United States Food and Drug Administration (FDA)
Center for Food Safety and Applied Nutrition
5100 Paint Branch Parkway
College Park, MD 20740
Phone: (888) SAFEFOOD
Website: http://www.cfsan.fda.gov

United States Pharmacopoeia (USP)
12601 Twinbrook Parkway
Rockville, MD 20852
Phone: (800) 822-8772
Website: www.usp.org

Upledger Institute
11211 Prosperity Farms Road
Palm Beach Gardens, FL 33410
Phone: (800) 233-5880
Fax: (561) 622-4771
Website: http://www.upledger.com

USA Karate Federation
1300 Kenmore Boulevard
Akron, OH 44314
Phone: (330) 753-3114
Website: http://www.usakarate.org/

Uruguayan Association of the Analytical Psychotherapy
Asociacion Uruguaya de Psicoterapia Psicoanalitica (AUDEPP)
Canelones 2208
11200 Montevideo, Uruguay
Phone: 598 2 4084985
Fax: 598 2 4022066
Email: contacto@audepp.org
Website: http://www.audepp.org/

V

Vaidya M. P. Nanal Ayurvedic Foundation
c/o Vaidya Vilas M. Nanal
606, Sadashiv Peth, Kunte Chowk, Laxmi Road,
Vaidya Nanal Niwas,
Pune - 411030
MS (India)
Phone: +91 - 020 - 445 2950
Fax: +91 - 020 - 422 2312
Email: nanalvm@giaspn01.vsnl.net.in
Website: http://www.nanalfoundation. org/

Valley Cedar Leaf Oil
RR #5
Eganville, Ontario, Canada K0J 1T0
Phone: (613) 628-2892
Website: http://www.valleycedarleafoil. com

Vegan Outreach
211 Indian Drive
Pittsburgh, PA 15238
Phone: (412) 968-0268
Website: http://www.veganoutreach.org/about /about.html

Vegan Society—England (VS)
7 Battle Rd.
St. Leonards-on-Sea TN37 7AA, United Kingdom
Phone: 44 1424 427393
Fax: 44 1424 717064
Email: info@vegansociety.com
Website: http://www.vegansociety.com

Vegan Society of Australia
PO Box 85
Seaford, VIC 3198, Australia
Phone: 61 3 97764425
Email: info@veganaustralia.org
Website: http://www.veganaustralia.org

Vegan Society of Finland
Vegaaniliitto
PO Box 320
FIN-00151 Helsinki, Finland
Phone: 358 50 3449524
Fax: 358 9 7732328
Email: info@vegaaniliitto.fi
Website: http://www.vegaaniliitto.fi

Vegetarian Resource Group
PO Box 1463
Baltimore, MD 21203
Phone: (410) 366-8343
Website: http://www.vrg.org/

Vegetarian Society of Ireland
PO Box 3010
Ballsbridge 4, Dublin Ireland
Phone: 353 1 8730451
Email: vegsoc@ireland.com
Website: http://www.vegetarian.ie

Vegetarian Society of the United Kingdom
Parkdale
Dunham Rd.
Altrincham WA14 4QG, United Kingdom
Phone: 44 161 9252000
Fax: 44 161 9269182
Email: info@vegsoc.org
Website: http://www.vegsoc.org

Vestibular Disorders Association
PO Box 4467
Portland, OR 97208-4467
Phone: (800) 837-8428
Website: http://www.vestibular.org

Veterans Administration
Persian Gulf Medical Information Helpline
400 South 18th Street
St. Louis, Missouri 63103-2271
Phone: (800) 749-8387
Website: http://www.va.gov

Veterans Administration
Persian Gulf Registry
Phone: (800) PGW-VETS (800) 749-8387
Website: http://www.va.gov

Vivaholistic Institute for Natural Health
Beatrice Missbauer
Residencial Park
IBIZA Baleares, Balearic Island 07800
Phone: 0034971312733
Fax: 0034971312 852
Website: http://www.vivaholistic.com

W

Weight-control Information Network (WIN)
1 WIN Way, Bethesda, MD 20892-3665
Phone: (202) 828-1025 or (877) 946-4627

Women's Association for Natural Medicinal Therapy
Private Mail Bag
Suva, Fiji
Phone: 679 315021
Fax: 679 315021
Email: wainimate@is.com.fj

Women's Cancer Resource Center
3023 Shattuck Ave
Berkeley, CA 94705
Phone: (510) 548-9272

World Federation of Acupuncture-Moxibustion Societies (WFAS)
18 Beixincang
Beijing 100700, People's Republic of China
Phone: 86 10 64063648
Fax: 86 10 64013968
Website: http://wfas.acutimes.com

World Health Organization (WHO)
CH-1211 Geneva 27, Switzerland.
Phone: +41 22 791 2111.
Fax: +41 22 791 0746
Telex: 45 415416.
Email: postmaster@who.ch.
Website: http://www.who.ch

World Federation of Acupuncture-Moxibustion Societies (WFAS)
18 Beixincang
Beijing 100700, People's Republic of China
Phone: 86 10 64063648
Fax: 86 10 64013968
Website: http://wfas.acutimes.com

World Hypnosis Organization, Inc
2521 W. Montrose Avenue
Chicago, IL 60618
Website: http://www.worldhypnosis.org/about.html

World Karate Federation
Federation Mondiale de Karate
c/o Hellenic Karate Federation
149 Vizantiou Str.
GR-14235 Athens, Greece
Phone: 30 210 2717564
Fax: 30 210 2717563
Email: secretariat@wkf.net
Website: http://www.wkf.net

World Taekwondo Federation (WTF)
5th Fl., Shinmunne Bldg.
238 Shinmunno 1st-ga

Jongro-gu
Seoul 110-061, Republic of Korea
Phone: 82 2 5662505
Fax: 82 2 5334728
Email: wtf@unitel.co.kr
Website: http://www.wtf.org

XYZ

Yasodhara Ashram Society (YAS)
Box 9
Kootenay Bay, BC, Canada V0B 1X0
Phone: (250) 227-9224 or (800) 661-8711
Fax: (250) 227-9494
Email: yashram@netidea.com
Website: Website: http://www.yasodhara.org

Yoga Alliance
122 West Lancaster Avenue, Suite 204
Reading, PA 19607-1874
Phone: (610) 777-7793
Fax: (610) 777-0556
Website: http://www.yogaalliance.org

Yoga Research and Education Center (YREC)
2400A County Center Drive
Santa Rosa, CA 95403
Phone: (707) 566-0000
Website: http://www.yrec.org

Yoga Research and Education Center (YREC)
PO Box 426
Manton, CA 96059
Phone: (530) 474-5700
Website: http://www.yrec.org

Yoga Research and Education Center
PO Box 1386
Lower Lake, CA 95457
Phone: (707) 928-9898
Website: http://www.yrec.com

Zimbabwe National Traditional Healers Association (ZINATHA)
PO Box 116
Reliance House
Corner of Takcawira and Speke Ave.
Harare, Zimbabwe
Phone: 263 4 751902

GLOSSARY

A

ABLATION To remove or destroy tissue or a body part, such as by burning or cutting.

ABORTIFACIENT An agent that induces abortion.

ABRASION Also called a scrape. The rubbing away of the skin surface by friction against another rough surface.

ABSCESS A localized collection of pus in the skin or other body tissue caused by infection.

ABSORPTION SPECTROMETRY A scientific procedure to determine the chemical composition of an unknown substance.

ABSTINENCE The act of doing without something, such as sex, voluntarily.

ACANTHOSIS NIGRICANS A skin condition characterized by darkly pigmented areas of velvety wart-like growths. Acanthosis nigricans usually affects the skin of the armpits, neck, and groin.

ACCOMMODATION The ability of the lens to change its focus from distant to near objects and vice versa. It is achieved through the action of the ciliary muscles that change the shape of the lens.

ACETALDEHYDE An intermediate product in the breakdown pathway of ethanol. Acetaldehyde is believed to cause hangover.

ACETYLCHOLINE The ability of the lens to change its focus from distant to near objects and vice versa. It is achieved through the action of the ciliary muscles that change the shape of the lens.

ACHENE Any small, dry, hard seed case or fruit that does not split open at maturity to discharge the seed. Dandelion seeds are held inside achenes.

ACONITINE A toxic alkaloid contained in aconite. As little as 2 mg taken internally may be fatal.

ACOUSTIC NEUROMA A benign tumor that grows on the nerve leading from the inner ear to the brain. As the tumor grows, it exerts pressure on the inner ear and causes severe vertigo.

ACRODERMATITIS ENTEROPATHICA Hereditary metabolic problem characterized by dermatitis, diarrhea, and poor immune status. Oral treatment with zinc is curative.

ACTIN A protein that functions in muscular contraction by combining with myosin.

ACUPOINT A point or site on the body where qi tends to accumulate. Acupoints are pressed or manipulated in Chinese massage in order to activate or redirect the patient's qi.

ACUPRESSURE An ancient form of Asian healing massage that involves applying pressure to special points or areas on the body in order to maintain good health, cure disease, and restore vitality.

ACUPUNCTURE Healing technique in traditional Chinese medicine utilizing the insertion of thin needles and other methods.

ACUTE PRESCRIBING Homeopathic treatment for self-limiting illnesses with abrupt onset.

ACUTE RETROVIRAL SYNDROME A group of symptoms resembling mononucleosis that often are the first sign of HIV infection.

ACUTE Refers to a disease or symptom that has a sudden onset and lasts a relatively short period of time.

ACYCLOVIR An antiviral drug that is available under the trade name Zovirax, in oral, intravenous, and topical forms. The drug prevents the varicella zoster virus from replicating.

ADAMS TEST A screening test in which a child being examined for scoliosis is asked to bend forward with the feet together and the knees straight.

ADAPTOGEN A substance that improves the body's ability to adapt to stress.

ADDICTION The state of being both physically and psychologically dependent on a substance.

ADENOCARCINOMA A cancerous tumor derived from epithelial (surface) cells or a gland-like tumor.

ADENOID A collection of lymph tissue located in the nasopharynx.

ADENOVIRUS A type of virus that can cause upper respiratory tract infections.

ADHESIONS Web-like scar tissue that may develop as a result of endometriosis and bind organs to one another.

ADHESIVE CAPSULITIS Adhesions and inflammation in the shoulder capsule that restrict movement.

ADIPOSE TISSUE Fat tissue.

ADJUNCTIVE Refers to a form of treatment that is not strictly necessary to a therapy regimen but is helpful. Music therapy is an example of an adjunctive form of treatment.

ADJUSTMENT DISORDER A psychiatric disorder marked by inappropriate or inadequate responses to a change in life circumstances.

ADJUSTMENT In chiropractic treatment, a very specific type of manipulation of the spine designed to return it to proper structural and functional form.

ADJUVANT THERAPY Treatment involving radiation, chemotherapy (drug treatment), or hormone therapy, or a combination of all three.

ADJUVANT Auxiliary or supplementary. An adjuvant treatment is one given to aid or assist the effects of other forms of therapy.

ADRENAL GLANDS A pair of endocrine organs near the kidneys that produce steroids such as sex hormones, hormones associated with metabolic functions, and epinephrine.

ADRENAL HORMONE The adrenocortical hormones are cortisol and cortisone. They are anti-inflammatory substances that aid in the function of a number of body systems, including the central nervous system, the cardiovascular system, the musculoskeletal system, and the gastrointestinal system.

ADRENALINE Also known as the **EMERGENCY HORMONE**, adrenaline is produced by the body during times of stress. Excess adrenaline levels can increase blood pressure and heart rate, leading to heart disease.

ADSORPTION A process in which an extremely thin layer of one substance (liquid, gas, or solid) forms on the surface of another substance. French green clay works as a cosmetic treatment by adsorbing toxic substances from the skin.

ADULTERANT A substance that makes something impure or inferior.

AEROBIC EXERCISE Exercise training that is geared to provide a sufficient cardiovascular overload to stimulate increases in cardiac output.

AEROBICS Any of various forms of sustained vigorous exercise, such as jogging, calisthenics, or jazz dancing, intended to stimulate and strengthen the heart and respiratory system.

AESCINATE A chemical found in horse chestnut that is effective in relieving the tissue swelling associated with varicose veins.

AFFECTIVE DISORDER An emotional disorder involving abnormal highs and/or lows in mood. Now termed mood disorder.

AFFECTIVE FLATTENING A loss or lack of emotional expressiveness. It is sometimes called blunted or restricted affect.

AFFERENT Sensory signals that go from the sensory cells at the periphery of the body back to the brain and spinal cord.

AGE-RELATED MACULAR DEGENERATION (AMD, ARMD) Macular degeneration that accompanies aging. The most common form of MD.

AGGRAVATION In homeopathy, a temporary worsening or intensification of the patient's symptoms prior to improvement and healing.

AGNI Ayurvedic term for strength of digestion.

AGNUSIDE The active ingredient in chasteberry.

AGONIST A drug or other chemical that produces a predictable response by means of a specific cellular affinity.

AGORAPHOBIA Abnormal anxiety regarding public places or situations from which the person may wish to flee or in which he or she would be helpless in the event of a panic attack.

AIDS DEMENTIA COMPLEX A type of brain dysfunction caused by HIV infection that causes difficulty thinking, confusion, and loss of muscular coordination.

AIDS Acquired Immune Deficiency Syndrome; a disease in which the immune response is impaired. The disease is caused by the Human Immunodeficiency Virus (HIV) which is spread by direct contact with infted body fluids such as blood and semen.

AIKIDO A Japanese martial art developed during the early twentieth century by Morihei Ueshiba. Literally translated, aikido means "the way of harmony with universal energy" or "the way of a loving spirit."

AKA In Huna (an esoteric Polynesian psychology), the shadow body of the low self. The aka forms threads or cords between the low self and other persons, objects, or the High Self. These aka threads serve as energy channels.

AKATHISIA Agitated or restless movement, usually affecting the legs and accompanied by a sense of discomfort. It is a common side effect of neuroleptic medications.

AKINESIA (an esoteric Polynesian psychology)

ALBUMINURIA The presence of high levels of the protein albumin in the urine.

ALDOSTERONE A hormone produced by the adrenal gland, instrumental in the regulation of sodium and potassium resorption by the kidney.

ALENDRONATE A nonhormonal drug used to treat osteoporosis in postmenopausal women.

ALEXANDER TECHNIQUE A technique developed by Frederick Alexander that focuses on the variations in body posture, muscles, and breathing. Defects in these functions can lead to stress, nervous tension, or possible loss of function.

ALGAE A group of primarily aquatic plants that have chlororphyll or other pigments and carry on photosynthesis. They range from single-cell to large multicellular organisms.

ALKALOID A type of chemical commonly found in plants and often having medicinal properties.

ALLERGEN A substance that provokes an allergic response.

ALLERGIC REACTION An immune system reaction to a substance in the environment; symptoms include rash, inflammation, sneezing, itchy watery eyes, and runny nose.

ALLERGIC RHINITIS Inflammation of the mucous membranes of the nose and eyes in response to an allergen.

ALLOPATHIC An immune system reaction to a substance in the environment; symptoms include rash, inflammation, sneezing, itchy watery eyes, and runny nose.

ALLOPATHY Conventional medical treatment of disease symptoms that uses substances or techniques to oppose or suppress the symptoms.

ALLOPURINOL A drug that corrects hyperuricemia by inhibiting urate production.

ALOE CONCENTRATE Aloe gel from which the water has been removed.

ALOE GEL Thick, undiluted substance from the central portion of the aloe leaf.

ALOE JUICE A product for oral use, which is composed of at least 50% aloe gel.

ALOE LATEX Bitter yellow sap from the middle leaf layer of the aloe plant.

ALPHA-$_2$ AGONIST A class of drugs that bind to and stimulate alpha-$_2$-adrenergic receptors, causing responses similar to those of adrenaline and noradrenaline, by inhibiting aqueous humor production.

ALPHA-FETOPROTEIN A substance produced by a fetus' liver that can be found in the amniotic fluid and in the mother's blood. Abnormally high levels of this substance suggest there may be defects in the fetal neural tube, a structure that will include the brain and spinal cord when completely developed. Abnormally low levels suggest the possibility of Down's syndrome.

ALPHA-TOCOPHEROL An antioxidant derivative of vitamin E that stabilizes cell membranes.

ALTERATIVE A medicinal substance that acts gradually to nourish and improve the system.

ALVEOLI The tiny air sacs clustered at the ends of the bronchioles in the lungs in which oxygen-carbon dioxide exchange takes place.

ALZHEIMER'S DISEASE A degenerative brain disease caused by physiological changes inside the brain. As a result, there is impaired memory and thought processes.

AMARGOGENTIN An extremely bitter substance found in gentian that makes it an effective digestive stimulant.

AMBIENT Surrounding.

AMEBIASIS An infection caused by an amoeba, which is a type of protozoan, especially by *Entamoeba histolytica*.

AMENORRHEA The absence or abnormal stoppage of menstrual periods.

AMINO ACID DECARBOXYLATE (AADC) INHIBITORS Drugs, such as carbidopa and benserazide, that block the enzyme AADC, which breaks down levodopa in the blood.

AMINO ACID An organic compound composed of both an amino group and an acidic carboxyl group. Amino acids are the basic building blocks of proteins. There are 20 types of amino acids (eight are essential amino acids which the body cannot make and must therefore be obtained from food).

AMPHETAMINES A group of drugs that stimulate the central nervous system. They are used medically to counteract depression, but are often used illegally as stimulants.

AMPULLA OF VATER The widened portion of the duct through which the bile and pancreatic juices enter the intestine. *Ampulla* is a Latin word describing a bottle with a narrow neck that opens into a wide body.

AMPUTATION The surgical removal of a part of the body.

AMSLER GRID A checkerboard pattern with a dot in the center that is used to diagnose MD.

AN MO A form of Chinese massage that treats the whole body and emphasizes balancing yin and yang techniques in the treatment. Its name means "press and stroke" in Chinese.

ANABOLIC STEROIDS A group of mostly synthetic hormones sometimes taken by athletes to temporarily increase muscle size.

ANAEROBIC An organism that grows and thrives in an oxygen-free environment.

ANALGESIC A pain-relieving substance.

ANAPHRODISIAC A substance or medication that suppresses sexual desire.

ANAPHYLACTIC SHOCK A severe allergic reaction that causes blood pressure drop, racing heart, swelling of the airway, rash, and possibly convulsions.

ANAPHYLAXIS Also called anaphylactic shock; a severe allergic reaction characterized by airway constriction, tissue swelling, and lowered blood pressure.

ANDROGENS Hormones (specifically testosterone) responsible for male sex characteristics.

ANDROPAUSE Midlife hormonal changes in men.

ANEMIA A condition in which the level of hemoglobin falls below normal values due to a shortage of mature red blood cells. Common symptoms include paleness, fatigue, and shortness of breath.

ANESTHESIA reatment with medicine that causes a loss of feeling, especially pain. Local anesthesia numbs only part of the body; general anesthesia causes loss of consciousness.

ANEURYSM A weakened area in the wall of a blood vessel which causes an outpouching or bulge. Aneurysms may be fatal if these weak areas burst, resulting in uncontrollable bleeding.

ANGINA Angina pectoris, or chest pain, caused by an insufficient supply of oxygen and decreased blood flow to the heart muscle. Angina is frequently the first sign of coronary artery disease.

ANGIOEDEMA Patches of circumscribed swelling involving the skin and its subcutaneous layers, the mucous membranes, and sometimes the organs frequently caused by an allergic reaction to drugs or food. Also called angioneurotic edema, giant urticaria, Quincke's disease, or Quincke's edema.

ANGIOGENESIS Patches of circumscribed swelling involving the skin and its subcutaneous layers, the mucous membranes, and sometimes the organs frequently caused by an allergic reaction to drugs or food. Also called angioneurotic edema, giant urticaria, Quincke's disease, or Quincke's edema.

ANGIOGRAPHY The procedure that enables blood vessels to be seen on film after the vessels have been filled with a contrast medium (a substance that shows up opaque on x rays).

ANGIOPLASTY Surgery to dilate the narrowed or blocked part of a blood vessel.

ANISOMETROPIA An eye condition in which there is an inequality of vision between the two eyes. There may be unequal amounts of nearsightedness, farsightedness, or astigmatism, so that one eye will be in focus while the other will not.

ANKYLOSING SPONDYLITIS A type of arthritis that causes gradual loss of flexibility in the spinal column. It occurs most commonly in males between the ages of 16 and 35, and may be initiated by a food allergy component, such as an allergy to wheat.

ANKYLOSING Refers to fusion, stiffness, or rigidity of a joint.

ANNUAL A plant that grows every year.

ANNULUS FIBROSIS The peripheral ring of fibrous tissue in an intervertebral disk.

ANODYNE A medicinal herb that relieves distress or soothes pain.

ANOREXIA NERVOSA An eating disorder marked by an unrealistic fear of weight gain, self-starvation, and distortion of body image. It most commonly occurs in adolescent females.

ANOREXIA Lack or loss of appetite.

ANTACID Common medication that neutralizes stomach acid for the short-term treatment of heartburn.

ANTHELMINTIC A medication that destroys or expels parasitic worms from the digestive tract.

ANTHOCYANOSIDES Flavonoid antioxidants from plant pigments that are particularly active in the eye.

ANTHRAQUINONES A group of chemicals contained in the latex of the Aloe plant and having strong laxative properties.

ANTHRAX A bacterial infection, primarily of livestock, that can be spread to humans. In humans it affects the skin, intestines, or lungs.

ANTHROPOLOGY The study of the origin and physical, social, and cultural development and behavior of groups of people.

ANTI-ANDROGEN DRUGS Drugs that block the activity of the male hormone.

ANTIANDROGEN A substance that blocks the action of androgens, the hormones responsible for male characteristics.

ANTIBIOTIC An agent able to kill or interfere with the development of bacteria and other micro-organisms.

ANTIBODY A bacterial infection, primarily of livestock, that can be spread to humans. In humans it affects the skin, intestines, or lungs.

ANTICHOLINERGIC A medication or other substance that blocks the action of the neurotransmitter acetylcholine. They are used to lessen muscle spasms in the intestines, lungs, bladder, and eye muscles.

ANTICOAGULANT A medication used to prevent clot formation or to prevent a clot that has formed from enlarging. Anticoagulant drugs inhibit clot formation by blocking the action of clotting factors or platelets. They fall into three groups: inhibitors of clotting factor synthesis, inhibitors of thrombin, and antiplatelet drugs.

ANTICONVULSANT A medication used to prevent convulsions or seizures. They often are prescribed in the treatment of epilepsy.

ANTIDEPRESSANT A type of medication that is used to treat depression; it is also sometimes used to treat autism.

ANTIDIURETIC A substance that diminishes the formation of urine.

ANTIDOTE A remedy to counteract a poison or injury. Also refers to a substance which cancels the effect of homeopathic remedies.

ANTIEMETIC A medication that helps control nausea; also called an antinausea drug.

ANTIFUNGAL A drug or compound effective in treating fungal infections.

ANTIGEN A substance (usually a protein) identified as foreign by the body's immune system, triggering the release of antibodies as part of the body's immune response.

ANTIHYPERTENSIVE A medication given to lower blood pressure.

ANTI-INFLAMMATORY A medication or substance that reduces the symptoms of fever and inflammation.

ANTIMALARIAL Any substance that reduces the effects of the tropical disease malaria.

ANTIMICROBIAL A substance that acts to inhibit the growth of harmful microorganisms, or acts to destroy them.

ANTI-MOTILITY MEDICATIONS Medications such as loperamide (Imodium), diphenoxylate (Lomotil), or medications containing codeine or narcotics that decrease the ability of the intestine to contract. These can worsen the condition of a patient with dysentery or colitis.

ANTIOXIDANT An enzyme or other organic substance that is able to counteract the damaging effects of oxidation in living tissue.

ANTIPRURITIC A type of medication applied to the skin to stop itching.

ANTIPSORIC A homeopathic remedy that is an effective constitutional treatment for the psoric miasm.

CALCAREA CARBONICA is one of three major antipsoric remedies.

ANTIPSYCHOTIC DRUG A class of drugs used to control psychotic symptoms in patients with psychotic disorders such as schizophrenia and delusional disorder. Antipsychotics include risperidone (Risperdal), haloperidol (Haldol), and chlorpromazine (Thorazine).

ANTIPYRETIC A substance or medication that combats fever with cooling properties.

ANTISCORBUTIC An agent that is effective against scurvy, like the vitamin C found in cramp bark.

ANTISEPTIC A substance that checks the growth or action of microorganisms especially in or on living tissue.

ANTISPASMODIC A substance that relieves muscle spasms or cramping.

ANTITOXIN An antibody against an exotoxin, usually derived from horse serum.

ANTITUSSIVE A drug used to suppress coughing.

ANTIVENIN An antitoxin to a specific animal venom. Antivenin is extracted from the blood serum of horses (or other animals) that have been immunized against the toxin.

ANUS The opening at the lower end of the rectum. The anus and rectum are both part of the large intestine, a digestive system organ.

ANXIETY DISORDER A mental disorder characterized by prolonged, excessive worry about circumstances in one's life. Anxiety disorders include agoraphobia and other phobias, obsessive-compulsive disorder, post-traumatic stress disorder, and panic disorder.

ANXIOGENIC Tending to produce anxiety.

ANXIOLYTIC A medication that alleviates anxiety.

APANA Life-sustaining energy centered in the larger intestine; the fifth of the five airs of Ayurvedic philosophy; the life force governing expulsion activity.

APHRODISIAC Any substance that excites sexual desire.

APIGENIN A bioflavonoid contained in chamomile that appears to inhibit *H. pylori*.

APITHERAPY A form of alternative therapy based on the use of honey and other bee products.

APLASTIC Exhibiting incomplete or faulty development.

APNEA The temporary absence of breathing.

APOCRINE A type of glandular secretion in which the top portion of the secreting cells is released along with the secreted substances.

APOPTOSIS Cell death.

APPETITE SUPPRESSANT A drug that decreases feelings of hunger. Most work by increasing levels of serotonin or catecholamine, chemicals in the brain that control appetite.

AQUEOUS HUMOR A transparent liquid, contained within the eye, that is composed of water, sugars, vitamins, proteins, and other nutrients.

AREA POSTREMA A structure of the brain stem that triggers vomiting in response to toxins in the bloodstream and cerebrospinal fluid.

AROMATHERAPY The therapeutic use of plant-derived, aromatic essential oils to promote physical and psychological well-being.

ARRHYTHMIA An abnormal rate or rhythm of the heartbeat.

ART THERAPY The use of art media to assess and treat an individual's development, abilities, personality, interests, concerns, or conflicts.

ARTEMINISININS A family of antimalarial products derived from an ancient Chinese herbal remedy. Two of the most popular varieties are artemether and artesunate, used mainly in southeast Asia in combination with mefloquine.

ARTEMISININ An antimalarial agent derived from an ancient Chinese herbal remedy. Two of the most popular varieties are artemether and artesunate, used mainly in Southeast Asia in combination with mefloquine.

ARTERIES Blood vessels that carry blood to organs and other tissues of the body.

ARTERIOLE The tiny extensions of arteries that lead into the capillaries.

ARTERIOSCLEROSIS A disease characterized by build-up on the artery walls that can lead to the obstruction of blood flow.

ARTHRALGIA Joint pain.

ARTHRITIS Inflammation of a joint that may lead to changes in the joint's structure. It causes pain and swelling. Rheumatoid arthritis is a chronic disease that leads to crippling deformities.

ARTHROGRAPHY An imaging technique that is sometimes used to evaluate TMJ associated with internal derangement.

ARTICULAR BONES Two or more bones which are connected with each other via a joint.

ASANA A position or stance in yoga.

ASANAS Physical postures associated with the practice of hatha yoga.

ASCENDING INFECTION Infection which begins in the urinary bladder and travels through the ureters up to the kidneys.

ASCOMYCETE Any class of higher fungi with septate hyphae and spores formed in the asci.

ASCORBIC ACID Another name for vitamin C, a nutrient found in fresh fruits and vegetables. Good sources of vitamin C in the diet are citrus fruits like oranges, lemons, limes, and grapefruits, berries, tomatoes, green peppers, cabbage, broccoli, and spinach.

ASCOSPORES Any spores contained in the ascus, which is the oval or tubular spore case of an ascomycete.

ASPERGER SYNDROME Children who have autistic behavior but no problems with language.

ASPIRATION BIOPSY The removal of cells in fluid or tissue from a mass or cyst using a needle for microscopic examination and diagnosis.

ASPIRATION Inhalation of food or saliva.

ASTHMA A disease in which the air passages of the lungs become inflamed and narrowed, causing wheezing, coughing, and shortness of breath.

ASTIGMATISM An eye condition in which the cornea doesn't focus light properly on the retina, resulting in a blurred image.

ASTRAL Of or from the stars.

ASTRINGENT A substance or compound that causes contraction or constriction of soft tissue.

ATAXIA A substance or compound that causes contraction or constriction of soft tissue.

ATHEROSCLEROSIS A process in which the walls of the arteries thicken due to the accumulation of plaque in the blood vessels. Atherosclerosis is the cause of most coronary artery disease.

ATHETOID The type of cerebral palsy that is marked by slow, writhing, involuntary muscle movements.

ATHLETE'S FOOT A fungal infection between the toes, officially known as tinea pedis.

ATOPIC DERMATITIS An intensely itchy inflammation often found on the face of people prone to allergies. In infants and early childhood, it's called infantile eczema.

ATOPIC ECZEMA Inflammation of the skin caused by allergic reaction.

ATOPY An inherited type of allergic hypersensitivity associated with IgE antibodies. Studies of the effects of worm infestation on the human immune system are providing new clues to the prevention of atopy.

ATRIAL TACHYCARDIA A heart rate of more than 100 beats per minute in the small antechambers of the heart.

ATRIOVENTRICULAR BLOCK A blockage of the electrical signal between the heart's chambers and its ventricles; the severity of the block varies.

ATROPHIC VAGINITIS An inflammation of the vagina that develops when the estrogen levels in the body drop. It is usually associated with normal menopause or with surgical removal of the ovaries, but can occur with breast-feeding or premature menopause.

ATROPHIC Characterized by a wasting away of a part of the body.

ATROPHY A progressive wasting and loss of function of any part of the body.

ATTENTION DEFICIT DISORDER (ADD) Disorder characterized by a short attention span, impulsivity, and in some cases hyperactivity.

ATTUNEMENT Life energy teaching given by a Reiki master to a student.

AUDIOLOGIST A health care professional who performs diagnostic testing of impaired hearing.

AUGMENTATIVE COMMUNICATION DEVICES Computers, picture boards, and other devices that increase the ability to communicate, either with or without speech.

AURA A light or radiance that is claimed to emanate from the body and to be visible to certain persons with psychic or spiritual powers.

AURICULAR ACUPUNCTURE Acupuncture using only points found on the ears.

AUTHENTIC MOVEMENT A type of movement that is influenced heavily by Jungian analysis, and works by analyzing the internal images of the patient. Patients are also urged to dance only when they feel the **IMPULSE** to move.

AUTISM A developmental disability that appears early in life, in which normal brain development is disrupted and social and communication skills are retarded, sometimes severely.

AUTODIGESTION A process in which pancreatic enzymes are activated prematurely and begin to digest the pancreas itself.

AUTOGENIC TRAINING A form of self-hypnosis developed in Germany that appears to be beneficial to migraine sufferers.

AUTOGENOUS VACCINE A vaccine made of dead bacteria from a patient's own body.

AUTOHEMOTHERAPY A form of ozone therapy in which a small quantity of the patient's blood is withdrawn, treated with a mixture of ozone and oxygen, and reinfused into the patient.

AUTOIMMUNE DISORDER One of a group of disorders, like rheumatoid arthritis and systemic lupus erythematosus, in which the immune system is overactive and has lost the ability to distinguish between self and nonself. The body's immune cells turn on the body, attacking various tissues and organs.

AUTOIMMUNE Pertaining to an immune response by the body against one of its own tissues or types of cells.

AUTOIMMUNITY A condition in which the body's immune system produces antibodies in response to its own tissues or blood components instead of to foreign particles or microorganisms.

AUTOINTOXICATION Self-poisoning by toxic products formed within the body during intestinal digestion. This term was coined around 1885 as part of a theory that regarded intestinal function as a central aspect of health.

AUTONOMIC NERVOUS SYSTEM (ANS) The part of the nervous system that supplies nerve endings in the blood vessels, heart, intestines, glands, and smooth muscles; it also governs their involuntary functioning. The autonomic nervous system is responsible for the biochemical changes involved in experiences of anxiety.

AVALOKITESVARA The Sanskrit name of Quan yin.

AVULSION FRACTURE A fracture caused by the tearing away of a fragment of bone where a strong ligament or tendon attachment forcibly pulls the fragment away from the bone tissue.

AXON A process of a neuron that conducts impulses away from the cell body. Axons are usually long and straight.

AYURVEDA In Sanskrit, *Ayur,* means life, and *veda* means knowledge. Ayurveda is a system of holistic medicine from India that aims to bring the individual into harmony with nature. It provides guidance regarding food and lifestyle, so that healthy people can stay healthy and people with health challenges can improve their health.

AYURVEDIC MEDICINE A system of holistic medicine from India that aims to bring the individual into harmony with nature. It provides guidance regarding food and lifestyle, so that healthy people can stay healthy and people with health challenges can improve their health.

AZOLE Any member of a group of chemical compounds with five-membered rings containing one or more nitrogen atoms. Several azoles are used as antifungal medications.

B

BABESIOSIS A disease caused by protozoa of the genus *Babesia* characterized by a malaria-like fever, anemia, vomiting, muscle pain, and enlargement of the spleen. Babesiosis, like Lyme disease, is carried by a tick.

BACILLUS CALMETTE-GUÉRIN (BCG) A vaccine made from a damaged bacillus similar to the tubercle bacillus, which may help prevent serious pulmonary TB and its complications.

BACOSIDES The name of two chemicals found in brahmi that appear to aid memory by improving the efficiency of nerve impulse transmission.

BACTEREMIA Bacterial infection of the blood.

BACTERICIDAL An agent that destroys bacteria (e.g., *Staphylococci aureus, Streptococci pneumoniae, Escherichia coli, Salmonella enteritidis*).

BACTERICIDE A substance that kills bacteria.

BACTERIURIA The presence of bacteria in the urine.

BAICALEIN A compound found in skullcap that appears to be a cancer chemopreventive.

BARBITURATE One of a group of medicines (including Seconal and Nembutal) that act as sedatives. They slow breathing and lower the body temperature and blood pressure. Since they can be habit forming, they are now used chiefly for anesthesia.

BARIATRICS The branch of medicine that deals with the prevention and treatment of obesity and related disorders.

BARRETT'S ESOPHAGUS OR BARRETT'S SYNDROME Changes in the type of cells lining the esophagus. Sometimes associated with the development of esophageal cancer.

BASAL GANGLIA (SINGULAR, GANGLION) Masses of gray matter in the cerebral hemispheres of the brain that are involved in the regulation of voluntary movements. Tourette syndrome has been linked to these areas of the brain.

BEHAVIOR MODIFICATION A form of therapy that uses rewards to reinforce desired behavior. An example would be to give a child a piece of chocolate for grooming appropriately.

BEHAVIORAL MEDICINE The branch of medicine that studies mind/body relationships.

BEHAVIORAL THERAPY A form of therapy that uses rewards to reinforce desired behavior. An example would be to give a child a piece of chocolate for grooming appropriately.

BELLERGAL A potent combination of ergotamine tartrate (a blood vessel constricting substance often used for migraines), belladona alkaloids (a potentially poisonous substance with sedative and anti-spasmodic effects), and phenobarbitol (an hypnotic, long acting sedative and anticonvulsant). Bellergal is one of the early synthetic patented formulations prescribed for relief of hot flashes due to its actions on the central nervous system, but now avoided due to its addictive capacity.

BELL'S PALSY Facial paralysis or weakness with a sudden onset, caused by swelling or inflammation of the seventh cranial nerve, which controls the facial muscles. Disseminated Lyme disease sometimes causes Bell's palsy.

BENIGN PROSTATIC HYPERPLASIA (BPH) A noncancerous condition of the prostate that causes growth of the prostate tissue, thus enlarging the prostate and obstructing urination.

BENIGN Not malignant, noncancerous.

BENTONITE CLAY A green clay of aluminum silicate containing magnesium and trace minerals. The clay can draw out agents of infection.

BENZODIAZEPINE A class of drugs that have a hypnotic and sedative action, used mainly as tranquilizers to control symptoms of anxiety.

BERBERINE A white or yellow water-soluble alkaloid with antibacterial properties. Coptis, goldenseal, and barberry are all plants that contain berberine.

BERIBERI A serious disease caused by a deficiency in vitamin B_1 and characterized by a slow degeneration of the nerves of the digestive system and heart.

BEST-CASE SERIES A preliminary study that relies on assumptions about patient outcomes without a specific treatment, compared with similar patients receiving the best available conventional treatments. There are no control cases.

BETA AGONIST Class of substances that relieve bronchoconstriction, among other effects.

BETA-AMYRIN PALMITATE A compound found in lobelia that has antidepressant properties.

BETA-BLOCKER A class of drugs that bind beta-adrenergic receptors and thereby decrease the ability of the body's own natural epinephrine to bind to those receptors, leading to the reduction of aqueous humor secretion.

BETA-GLUCANS Complex carbohydrates contained in oats and other cereal grains. They are thought to be useful in managing diabetes as well as lowering blood cholesterol levels.

BETA-SITOSTEROL A plant lipid with considerable biological activity; even in very amounts it is found to be anti-inflammatory and to have positive effects in treating BPH.

BIENNIAL A plant that requires two years to complete the cycle from seed to maturity and death.

BILE A serious disease caused by a deficiency in vitamin B_1 and characterized by a slow degeneration of the nerves of the digestive system and heart.

BILIARY DUCT DISEASE Disease of the anatomic duct from the liver, which joins the duct from the gall bladder to form the common bile duct before entering the small intestine.

BILIARY SYSTEM The gallbladder and the system of tubes that carry bile from the liver into the intestines.

BILIRUBIN When gathered in large amounts, this water-insoluble pigment occurs in bile and blood.

BINGE EATING A pattern of eating marked by episodes of rapid consumption of large amounts of food, usually food that is high in calories.

BINGE To consume large amounts of food uncontrollably within a short time period.

BIOACCUMULATION The process in which toxic chemicals collect in the tissues of humans and other animals toward the top of the food chain.

BIOAVAILABILITY The amount of a substance that can enter the bloodstream and be utilized effectively by the body.

BIOCIDE Any chemical that works to kill microorganisms and other forms of life by poisoning. Hospital disinfectants are examples of biocides.

BIODEGRADABLE Capable of being broken down by the actions of living organisms. Inulin from chicory roots can be used to produce biodegradable substances used in industry.

BIOENERGETICS A system of therapy that combines breathing and body exercises, psychological therapy, and the free expression of emotions to release blocked physical and psychic energy.

BIOFEEDBACK The process in which toxic chemicals collect in the tissues of humans and other animals toward the top of the food chain.

BIOFIELD THERAPIES A subgroup of energy therapies that make use of energy fields (biofields) thought to exist within or emanate from the human body. Biofield therapies include such approaches as aura therapy, Reiki, therapeutic touch, qigong, and polarity balancing.

BIOFLAVONOID A large group of phytochemicals with antioxidant and immune-boosting properties.

BIOIDENTICAL Molecules that are identical in chemical formulae and similar or identical in chemical structures, actions, and effects to naturally occurring biological molecules.

BIOPSY The surgical removal and microscopic examination of living tissue for diagnostic purposes.

BIOTERRORISM The use of biological agents, including plant-derived toxic materials like ricin, to frighten and intimidate large populations.

BIOTIN A B complex vitamin, found naturally in yeast, liver, and egg yolks.

BIPHOSPHONATES Compounds (like alendronate) that slow bone loss and increase bone density.

BISMUTH A substance used in medications to treat diarrhea, nausea, and indigestion.

BITTER A substance that reduces toxins, fights infection and fever, and acts as a mild tonic.

BLACKHEAD A plug of fatty cells capped with a blackened mass.

BLADDER NECK The place where the urethra and bladder join.

BLADDER SPHINCTER The outlet that releases urine into the urethra.

BLASTOCYST A cluster of cells representing multiple cell divisions that have occurred in the fallopian tube after successful fertilization of an ovum by a sperm. This is the developmental form that must enter the uterus and implant to achieve pregnancy.

BLEPHARITIS An inflammation of the eyelid.

BLOCKING PROTEIN FACTOR (BPF) A serum component that may prevent the immune system from recognizing cancer cells.

BLOOD CHEMISTRY PANEL A general set of tests measuring substances in the blood that may indicate common diseases.

BLOOD CULTURE A procedure where blood is collected from a vein and is placed in a small bottle that contains a special liquid; the liquid will make any organisms that are present in the blood sample grow. These organisms can then be grown and identified in the laboratory so that the proper antibiotic can be given to the patient.

BLOOD PRESSURE The pressure of the blood in the arteries measured in millimeters of mercury by a sphygmomanometer or by an electronic device.

BLOOD In TCM, it is the fluid that transports physical and emotional nourishment.

BLOOD-BRAIN BARRIER An arrangement of cells within the blood vessels of the brain that prevents the passage of toxic substances, including infectious agents, from the blood and into the brain. It also makes it difficult for certain medications to pass into brain tissue.

BODHISATTVA A Buddhist holy person who has attained enlightenment, but postpones nirvana in order to help others become enlightened.

BODY DYSMORPHIC DISORDER A psychiatric disorder marked by preoccupation with an imagined physical defect.

BODYWORK A term that covers a variety of therapies that include massage, realignment of the body, and similar techniques to treat deeply ingrained stresses and traumas carried in the tissues of the body.

BONE MARROW SUPPRESSION Decrease in production of blood components, including red blood cells, white blood cells, and platelets. This can result in anemia, increased susceptibility to infections, and excessive bleeding.

BONE MARROW TRANSPLANTATION A medical procedure in which normal bone marrow is transferred from a healthy donor to an ailing recipient. An illness that prevents production of normal blood cells—such as sickle cell anemia—may be treated with a bone marrow transplant.

BONE MARROW A spongy tissue located in the hollow centers of certain bones, such as the skull and hip bones. Bone marrow is the site of blood cell generation.

BONE SCAN An x-ray study in which patients are given an intravenous injection of a small amount of a radioactive material that travels in the blood. When it reaches the bones, it can be detected by x ray to produce an image of their internal structure.

BOUCHARD'S NODES Swelling of the middle joint of the finger.

BOWEL ASTRINGENT A substance that causes bowel tissue to dry and shrink by reducing its ability to absorb water.

BOWEL OBSTRUCTION A blockage in the intestine that prevents the normal flow of waste down the length of the intestine.

BRADYKINESIA Slow movement.

BRAHMI A herb used in Ayurvedic and Japanese medicine that appears to improve a person's ability to remember new information. Brahmi is also called bacopa.

BRAXTON HICKS CONTRACTIONS Short, fairly painless uterine contractions during pregnancy that may be mistaken for labor pains. They allow the uterus to grow and help circulate blood through the uterine blood vessels.

BROMHIDROSIS A medical condition in which a person's sweat always smells unpleasant.

BRONCHI Singular, bronchus; the large tubular passages that carry air to the lung and allow air to be expelled from the lungs.

BRONCHIAL TUBES The major airways from the back of the throat to the lungs and their main branches.

BRONCHIOLES Small tubes in the lungs leading to the alveoli, where gas exchange occurs.

BRONCHITIS Inflammation of the air passages of the lungs.

BRONCHODILATORS Inflammation of the air passages of the lungs.

BRONCHOSCOPE A lighted instrument that is inserted into the windpipe to view the bronchi and bronchioles, to remove obstructions, or to withdraw specimens for testing.

BRONCHOSCOPY An examination of the lungs and airway passages using a flexible fiberoptic instrument.

BRUXISM Habitual clenching and grinding of the teeth as a result of stress. The behavior usually occurs during sleep.

BUDDHISM A philosophy founded in India in the sixth century B.C. *AND BASED ON THE TEACHINGS OF THE HISTORICAL BUDDHA, BORN SIDDARTHA GAUTAMA.*

BULBAR MUSCLES Muscles of the mouth and throat responsible for speech and swallowing.

BULIMIA NERVOSA An eating disorder characterized by episodic binge eating followed by self-induced vomiting or laxative abuse.

BUPLEURUM An Asian plant used in traditional Chinese and Japanese medicines to treat infected or inflamed skin.

BURNOUT An emotional condition, marked by tiredness, loss of interest, or frustration, that interferes with job performance. Burnout is usually regarded as the result of prolonged stress.

BURSA A closed sac lined with a synovial membrane and filled with fluid, usually found in areas subject to friction, such as where a tendon passes over a bone.

BURSITIS Inflammation of a bursa, a fluid-filled cavity or sac. In the body, bursae are located at places where friction might otherwise develop.

BUTTERFLY BANDAGE A narrow strip of adhesive with wider flaring ends (shaped like butterfly wings) used to hold the edges of a wound together while it heals.

C

CACHEXIA General physical wasting and malnutrition, usually associated with such chronic diseases as cancer and AIDS.

CADMIUM A heavy metal.

CADUCEUS The ancient and universal symbol of medicine consisting of the winged staff of Mercury and two intertwining serpents.

CALCITONIN A naturally occurring hormone made by the thyroid gland that can be used as a drug to treat osteoporosis and Paget's disease of the bone.

CALCIUM CARBONATE A salt that is used in many antacids.

CALCIUM CITRATE A form of calcium containing citric acid.

CALCIUM A silvery-yellow metal that is the basic element of lime and makes up about 3% of the earth's crust. It is the most abundant mineral in the human body. Calcium and phosphorous combine as calcium phosphate, the hard material of bones and teeth.

CALCIUM-CHANNEL BLOCKER A drug that blocks the entry of calcium into the muscle cells of small blood vessels (arterioles) and keeps them from narrowing.

CALCULUS Plural, calculi. Any type of hard concretion (stone) in the body, but usually found in the gallbladder, pancreas, and kidneys. They are formed by the accumulation of excess mineral salts and other organic material such as blood or mucous. Calculi (pl.) can cause problems by lodging in and obstructing the proper flow of fluids, such as bile to the intestines or urine to the bladder. In dentistry, calculus refers to a hardened yellow or brown mineral deposit from unremoved plaque, also called tartar.

CALORIC TESTING Flushing warm and cold water into the ear stimulates the labyrinth and causes vertigo and nystagmus (involuntary movement of the eyes in a horizontal direction) if all the nerve pathways are intact.

CAMPYLOBACTER A bacterium that can invade the lining of the intestine.

CANCER A disease caused by uncontrolled abnormal cell growth.

CANDIDIASIS A common fungal infection caused by yeast that thrives in moist, warm areas of the body.

CANTHARIDIN The irritating poison produced by Spanish fly that serves as the active ingredient in cantharis. Because of cantharidin, high doses of cantharis are highly toxic.

CAPACITOR PLATES An apparatus that can carry electricity and stores an electrical charge.

CAPSAICIN A colorless, bitter compound that is present in cayenne and gives it its heat.

CARBOHYDRATES Neutral compounds of carbon, hydrogen, and oxygen found in sugar, starches, and cellulose.

CARBUNCLE A Staphylococcal skin infection that affects the hair follicles. The term may also be used to refer to a group of boils.

CARCINOGENS Substances in the environment that cause cancer, presumably by inducing mutations, with prolonged exposure.

CARDIAC ARRYTHMIA The irregular beating of the heart.

CARDIAC CATHETERIZATION A treatment using a narrow tube to clear out a blocked blood vessel.

CARDIAC GLYCOSIDES Drugs that block the enzyme that regulates the electrical activity of the heart

CARDIAC TONIC Any of a diverse group of remedies intended to relieve heart symptoms. Most tonics contain herbal extracts, vitamins, and minerals.

CARDIOMYOPATHY A condition of damaged, diseased, thickened, or stretched heart muscle, resulting in weakness of the heart. Cardiomyopathy often occurs following heart attacks due to scarring, but may also have an infectious or nutritional origin.

CARDIOVASCULAR Related to the heart and lungs.

CARIES Cavities in the teeth.

CARMINATIVE Any medication or preparation given to expel gas from the digestive tract.

CARNOSOL An antioxidant compound found in rosemary that appears to have anticancer properties.

CAROTENOID A large class of red and yellow pigments found in some plants and in animal fat.

CAROTENOSIS (CAROTENODERMIA, CAROTENEMIA) A yellowish pigmentation of the skin caused by high levels of carotene in the blood.

CARPAL TUNNEL SYNDROME A condition caused by compression of the median nerve in the carpal tunnel of the hand, characterized by pain.

CARPAL TUNNEL A passageway in the wrist, created by the bones and ligaments of the wrist, through which the median nerve passes.

CARRIER OIL An oil used to dilute essential oils for use in massage and other skin care applications.

CARTILAGE A tough, elastic connective tissue found in the joints, outer ear, nose, larynx, and other parts of the body.

CARVONE The chemical compound that gives spearmint its characteristic flavor. Carvone is a pale yellow or colorless liquid when extracted from the plant.

CATACHIN A flavonoid found in fo ti that has antioxidant and tumor-inhibiting qualities.

CATALYST A substance that changes the rate of a chemical reaction, but is not physically changed by the process.

CATAPLEXY A symptom of narcolepsy in which there is a sudden episode of muscle weakness triggered by emotions. The muscle weakness may cause the person's knees to buckle, or the head to drop. In severe cases, the patient may become paralyzed for a few seconds to minutes.

CATARACTS A condition in which the lens of the eye becomes cloudy.

CATARRH Inflammation of a mucous membrane, especially of the nose and air passages.

CATECHIN A yellow, slightly bitter antioxidant found in evening primrose oil. Catechin appears to slow tumor growth and to protect against heart disease.

CATECHOL-O-METHYLTRANSFERASE (COMT) INHIBITORS Drugs, such as entacapone and tolcapone, that block COMT, an enzyme that breaks down levodopa in the blood.

CATHARSIS Therapeutic discharge of emotional tension by recalling past events.

CATHETER A rubber or plastic tube placed through the urethra into the bladder to remove excess urine when the flow of urine is cut off, or to prevent urinary infection.

CAUDA EQUINA The roots nerves of the final portion of the spine, controlling movement and sensation in the legs. These nerve roots resemble a horse's tail.

CAULOSAPONIN The chemical compound found in blue cohosh that is used to stimulate uterine contractions during labor. It can have toxic side effects in humans.

CAUTERIZATION Sealing tissue or blood vessels by burning with a heat source or electrical current.

CAUTERIZE To seal tissue or blood vessels using a heat or electrical source.

CAUTERY INSTRUMENT A device that uses heat applied to the tissues to destroy damaged or diseased areas.

CAVITY A hole or weak spot in the tooth surface caused by decay.

CD4 A type of protein molecule in human blood, sometimes called the T4 antigen, that is present on the surface of 65% of immune cells. The HIV virus infects cells with CD4 surface proteins, and as a result, depletes the number of T cells, B cells, natural killer cells, and monocytes in the patient's blood. Most of the damage to an AIDS patient's immune system is done by the virus' destruction of CD4+ lymphocytes.

CELIAC DISEASE An intestinal disorder characterized by intolerance of gluten, a protein present in the grains of wheat, rye, oats, and barley.

CELLULOSE The primary substance composing the cell walls or fibers of all plant tissues.

CENTRAL NERVOUS SYSTEM (CNS) The brain, spinal cord, and nerves throughout the body.

CENTRIFUGE A machine that rotates rapidly and uses centrifugal force to separate substances of different densities.

CEPHAELINE A chemical compound found in ipecac that irritates the stomach lining and triggers the vomiting reflex.

CEPHALALGIA The medical term for headache.

CEREBROSPINAL FLUID (CSF) Fluid made in chambers within the brain which then flows over the surface of the brain and spinal cord. CSF provides nutrition to cells of the nervous system, as well as providing a cushion for the nervous system structures. It may accumulate abnormally in some disease processes, causing pressure on and damage to brain structures.

CERVICAL Relating to the top part of the spine that is composed of the seven vertebrae of the neck and the disks that separate them.

CERVIX A small, cylindrical structure about an inch or so long and less than an inch around that makes up the lower part and neck of the uterus. The cervix separates the body and cavity of the uterus from the vagina.

CESTODES Tapeworms, which are long, flat, segmented parasitic intestinal worms.

CHAKRA One of seven major energy centers in the body, as defined by Hindu and yoga philosophy.

CHALAZION A small cyst on the eyelid that develops because the Meibomian gland becomes plugged.

CHANCRE The initial skin ulcer of primary syphilis, consisting of an open sore with a firm or hard base.

CHARANTIN A compound with hypoglycemic effects that can be extracted from bitter melon with alcohol.

CHARCOT-MARIE-TOOTH SYNDROME (CMT) The most common form of inherited peripheral neuropathy.

CHELATE A chemical that binds to heavy metals in the blood, thereby helping the body to excrete them in urine.

CHELATION THERAPY A treatment using chelating agents, compounds that surround and bind to target substances allowing them to be excreted from the body.

CHELATION The process by which a molecule encircles and binds to a metal and removes it from tissue.

CHEMOPREVENTATIVE A chemical or drug that is thought to prevent a disease.

CHEMOTHERAPEUTIC AGENT A medication used to treat cancer.

CHEMOTHERAPY Any treatment of an illness with chemical agents. The term is usually used to describe the treatment of cancer with drugs that inhibit cancer growth or destroy cancer cells.

CHI Universal life energy as defined by traditional Chinese medicine. Also known as qi.

CHILBLAIN Redness and swelling of the skin often accompanied by burning, itching, and blisters. A condition caused by excessive exposure to the cold.

CHIROPRACTIC A method of treatment based on adjustment or manipulation of the segments of the spinal column.

CHITIN A transparent horny substance found in the outer coverings of shellfish. Chitin is used to make commercial preparations of glucosamine.

CHLAMYDIA A common sexually transmitted disease in the United States that often accompanies gonorrhea. It is caused by a rickettsia called *Chlamydia trachomatis*.

CHLOASMA A skin discoloration common during pregnancy, also known as the "mask of pregnancy" or melasma, which blotches of pale brown skin appear on the face. The blotches may appear in the forehead, cheeks, and nose, and may merge into one dark mask. It usually fades gradually after pregnancy, but it may become permanent or recur with subsequent pregnancies.

CHLOROPHYLL A green plant pigment found in plants, algae, and some bacteria. Chlorophyll is responsible for capturing the light energy needed for photosynthesis.

CHLOROQUINE An antimalarial drug that was first used in the 1940s, until the first evidence of quinine resistance appeared in the 1960s. It is now ineffective against falciparum malaria almost everywhere. However, because it is inexpensive, it is still the antimalarial drug most widely used in Africa. Native individuals with partial immunity may have better results with chloroquine than a traveler with no previous exposure.

CHOLAGOGUE Stimulates the flow of bile from the liver to the intestines.

CHOLECYSTECTOMY Surgical removal of the gallbladder.

CHOLESTEROL ABSORPTION INHIBITOR A substance that decreases the absorption of cholesterol in the intestines.

CHOLESTEROL A steroid fat found in animal foods that is also produced in the body from saturated fat for several important functions. Excess cholesterol intake is linked to many diseases.

CHOLINE AND INOSITOL Two of the vitamins in the B vitamin complex.

CHONDROITIN A complex carbohydrate found in human and animal cartilage that is used to treat several physical disorders, most importantly arthritis.

CHOREA A nervous system disorder that causes involuntary jerking or spasms. Also known as St. Vitus dance.

CHOROID The middle vascular layer of the eyeball, behind the retina.

CHOROIDAL NEOVASCULARIZATION (CNV) The proliferation of new, fragile blood vessels in the choroid layer. Leakage from these vessels causes wet AMD.

CHRONIC BRONCHITIS A smoking-related respiratory illness in which the membranes that line the bronchi, or the lung's air passages, narrow over time. Symptoms include a morning cough that brings up phlegm, breathlessness, and wheezing.

CHRONIC NEPHROTIC SYNDROME Chronic nephrotic syndrome is long-term inflammation of the kidney.

CHRONIC Refers to a disease or condition that progresses slowly but persists or recurs over time.

CHVOSTEK'S SIGN A facial spasm caused when the doctor taps lightly on the patient's facial nerve. A positive Chvostek's sign may indicate that the patient has hypomagnesemia.

CILIA Tiny, hair-like projections from a cell. Within the respiratory tract, the cilia act to move mucus along, in an effort to continually flush out and clean the respiratory tract.

CIRCADIAN RHYTHM Any body rhythm that recurs in 24-hour cycles such as the sleep-wake cycle.

CIRCADIAN Events that occur on a 24 hour rhythmic cycle; a biological clock.

CIRRHOSIS The end result of many forms of liver disease, the condition of the liver when its cells have been damaged or destroyed and are replaced by scar tissue.

CITRAL A pale yellow liquid drived from lemongrass used in making perfumes and to flavor food.

CLAIRVOYANT A person who has the power to see within their mind a future event or an event or thing out of their visual range.

CLEFT PALATE Refers to a disease or condition that progresses slowly but persists or recurs over time.

CLINDAMYCIN An antibiotic that can be used instead of penicillin to treat certain infections.

CLINICAL NUTRITION The use of diet and nutritional supplements as a way to enhance health and prevent disease.

CLOSE WORK Tasks which cause the eyes to focus on something close at hand, such as reading, writing, computer work, and sewing.

CLOSTRIDIUM A genus of deadly bacteria that are responsible for tetanus and other serious diseases, including botulism and gangrene from war wounds. It thrives without oxygen.

COBB ANGLE A measure of the curvature of scoliosis, determined by measurements made on x rays.

COCHLEA The hearing part of the inner ear. This snail-shaped structure contains fluid and thousands of microscopic hair cells tuned to various frequencies, in addition to the organ of Corti (the receptor for hearing).

COENZYME Q$_{10}$ A substance used by cells in the human body to produce energy for cell maintenance and growth. It is being studied as a possible preventive for migraine headaches.

COENZYME A non-protein organic compound that plays an essential role in the action of particular enzymes.

COGNITIVE BEHAVIORAL THERAPY A therapy that focuses on changing negative behavior in order to alter the attitudes or harmful thinking patterns that cause the behavior.

COGNITIVE RESTRUCTURING The process of replacing maladaptive thought patterns with constructive thoughts and beliefs.

COLCHICINE A drug used to treat painful flare-ups of gout.

COLD In Chinese pathology, the term defines a condition that has insufficient warmth, either objective (hypothermia) or subjective (feeling cold).

COLD-DEFICIENCY DIARRHEA In Chinese herbal medicine, this condition is described as cold settling in the abdomen when resistance is low, causing cramping, gas, and loose stools.

COLITIS An inflammation of the colon.

COLLAGEN Collagen is a white, fibrous protein that is found in skin, bones, ligaments, tendons, cartilage and all other connective tissue.

COLLARETTE The slightly raised area of scaly skin that forms at the borders of the herald patch and later lesions of pityriasis rosea.

COLON The part of the large intestine that lies between the cecum and the rectum, and is divided by name into three parts, the ascending, transverse and descending colon. In a healthy person, the ascending colon rises upward intra-abdominally from above the right leg toward the right hip, the transverse colon crosses over to the left hip, and the descending colon segment joins the rectum intra-abdominally, near the top of the left leg. An unhealthy colon may droop, drape or twist, and be enlarged or otherwise irregularly shaped.

COLONIZE To become established in a host.

COLONOSCOPY Examination of an area of the gastrointestinal tract by putting a lighted scope, usually bearing a fiber-optic camera, into the rectum, and passing it through the intestine.

COLOSTOMY A surgical procedure in which an opening is made in the wall of the abdomen to allow a part of the large intestine (the colon) to empty outside the body. Colostomies are usually required because portions of the intestine have been removed or an intestinal obstruction exists.

COLTSFOOT A common weed, *Russilago farfara*, used to treat chest complaints.

COMEDO A hard plug composed of sebum and dead skin cells, also called a blackhead. The mildest type of acne.

COMMENSAL BACTERIA Bacteria that live in or on the human body and are in an often beneficial relationship with the human host. For example, some bacteria in the digestive tract produce needed B vitamins.

COMMON BILE DUCT A hard plug composed of sebum and dead skin cells, also called a blackhead. The mildest type of acne.

COMMON COLD A mild illness caused by upper respiratory viruses. Usual symptoms include nasal congestion, coughing, sneezing, throat irritation, and a low-grade fever.

COMPLEMENT One of several proteins in the blood that acts with other proteins to assist in killing bacteria.

COMPLETE PROTEIN A protein food that has all the essential amino acids the body requires to digest it.

COMPLEX CARBOHYDRATES One of several proteins in the blood that acts with other proteins to assist in killing bacteria.

COMPLEX SUGARS A category of carbohydrate compounds within plants, found to have antiviral and anti-inflammatory effects; they have a more complex structure than the sweet, simple dietary sugars.

COMPOUNDING PHARMACY A pharmacy that uses bulk materials to fill prescriptions according to a physician's formulation; a formulating pharmacy.

COMPRESS A cloth used to apply heat, cold, or medications to the skin.

COMPULSION A repetitive or ritualistic behavior that a person performs to reduce anxiety. Compulsions often develop as a way of controlling or **UNDOING** obsessive thoughts.

COMPUTED TOMOGRAPHY (CT) SCAN An imaging technique in which cross-sectional x rays of the body are compiled to create a three-dimensional image of the body's internal structures.

CONDUCT DISORDER A behavioral and emotional disorder of childhood and adolescence. Children with a conduct disorder act inappropriately, infringe on the rights of others, and violate societal norms.

CONDUCTIVE HEARING LOSS Hearing loss caused by loss of function in the external or middle ear.

CONDYLOMA ACUMINATA (PLURAL, CONDYLO-MATA) The medical term for warts in the genital region or anus.

CONDYLOMATA LATA Highly infectious patches of weepy pink or gray skin that appear in the moist areas of the body during secondary syphilis.

CONES Receptor cells, located in the retina of the eye, that allow the perception of colors.

CONGENITAL Existing at or before birth; a condition that developed while the fetus was in utero or as a consequence of the birth process.

CONIFER Any of several families of trees and shrubs, mostly evergreen, belonging to the order Coniferales, distinguished by bearing seeds and pollen in the form of dry scales arranged in a cone.

CONIZATION Surgical removal of a cone-shaped piece of tissue from the cervix.

CONJUNCTIVITIS An inflammation of the mucous membranes that cover the outer eyeball and line the eyelids. The eye appears red or pink and is itchy or sore.

CONNECTIVE TISSUE Tissue that supports and binds other body tissue and parts.

CONSOLIDATION A condition in which lung tissue becomes firm and solid rather than elastic and air-filled because it has accumulated fluids and tissue debris.

CONSTIPATION Difficulty passing stools, infrequent stools, or insufficient stools.

CONSTITUTIONAL PRESCRIBING Homeopathic treatment based on a total assessment of the person's life history, heredity, lifestyle, and present environment, as distinct from prescribing based on immediate acute symptoms.

CONSTITUTIONAL REMEDY A homeopathic medicine prescribed according to each person's character and temperament as well as symptoms.

CONSTITUTIONAL Involving the whole body. A constitutional symptom, for example, is one that is not focused entirely in the diseased organ system, but affects the whole system (such as fever).

CONTACT DERMATITIS Inflammation of the skin as a result of contact with a substance.

CONTAMINATED Becoming unclean or infected by contact with or addition of something.

CONTINUOUS POSITIVE AIRWAY PRESSURE (CPAP) A ventilation system that blows a gentle stream of air into the nose to keep the airway open.

CONTRACT To squeeze down, become smaller.

CONTRACTURE A tightening or shortening of muscles that prevents normal movement of the associated limb or other body part.

COPROLALIA The involuntary use of vulgar or obscene language.

CORNEA The clear, dome-shaped outer covering of the eye that lies in front of the iris and pupil. The cornea lets light into the eye.

CORONARY ARTERIES The two arteries that provide blood to the heart. The coronary arteries surround the heart like a crown, coming out of the aorta, arching down over the top of the heart, and dividing into two branches. These are the arteries where coronary artery disease occurs.

CORONARY ARTERY DISEASE A narrowing or blockage, due to atherosclerosis, of the arteries that provide oxygen and nutrients to the heart. When blood flow is cut off, the result is a heart attack.

CORONAVIRUS One of a family of RNA-containing viruses known to cause severe respiratory illnesses. In March 2003, a previously unknown coronavirus was identified as the causative agent of severe acute respiratory syndrome, or SARS.

CORPUS CAVERNOSUM Plural, corpora cavernosa. Rods of spongy tissue in the penis that become engorged with blood in order to produce an erection.

CORPUS STRIATUM Regions on each side of the brain that transmit signals for movement in response to dopamine from the substantia nigra.

CORTICAL Regarding the cortex, or the outer layer of the brain, as distinguished from the inner portion.

CORTICOSTEROIDS A group of hormones produced naturally by the adrenal gland or manufactured synthetically. They are often used to treat inflammation. Examples include cortisone and prednisone.

CORTISOL A steroid hormone released by the cortex (outer portion) of the adrenal gland when a person is under stress.

CORTISONE A drug used in the treatment of rheumatoid arthritis.

CORYDALINE An alkaloid derived from corydalis that has some effectiveness as a pain reliever.

COSMIC RADIATION Radiation of high penetrating power originating in outer space. It consists partly of high-energy atomic nuclei.

COTYLEDON A seed leaf, from the embryo of a seed plant.

COUMARIN A chemical compound found in plants that breaks down red blood cells.

CRABS An informal term for pubic lice.

C-REACTIVE PROTEIN (CRP) A protein present in blood serum in various abnormal states, like inflammation.

CREATININE The metabolized by-product of creatine, an organic acid that assists the body in producing muscle contractions. Creatinine is found in the bloodstream and in muscle tissue. It is removed from the blood by the kidneys and excreted in the urine. Higher than normal levels of this substance may indicate kidney disease.

CREEPING ERUPTION Itchy irregular, wandering red lines on the skin made by burrowing larvae of the hookworm family and some roundworms. Also called cutaneous larva migrans.

CRETINISM Severe hypothyroidism that is present at birth.

CRIGLER-NAJJAR SYNDROME A moderate to severe form of hereditary jaundice.

CROCETIN A reddish-yellow plant pigment found in saffron that is being studied for its anticancer effectiveness.

CROHN'S DISEASE A disease characterized by inflammation of the intestines. Its early symptoms may resemble those of IBS.

CROSS LATERALIZATION A term used to describe what was believed to be a difference in the way the mind works in persons with and without dyslexia. It was believed that functions processed in the right half of the brain by a person without dyslexia were processed in the left half by a person with dyslexia.

CROWN The part of a tooth that is covered by enamel.

CRUCIFER A type of vegetable that is now believed to guard against cancer, ulcers, and infections in the digestive tract. Examples of crucifers include wasabi, broccoli, cauliflower, mustard greens, and cabbage.

CRYOGENICS A science examining the freezing of living tissue for preservation and use at a later time.

CRYOSURGERY Freezing and destroying abnormal cells.

CRYOTHERAPY A technique of removing warts by freezing with liquid nitrogen.

CT (COMPUTER TOMOGRAPHY) SCAN The diagnostic technique in which the combined use of a computer and x rays passed through the body at different angles produces clear, cross-sectional images *(slices)* of the tissue being examined.

CUCURMIN (SOMETIMES SPELLED CURCUMIN) A yellow material that gives turmeric root its characteristic color.

CULTURE TEST A laboratory test to grow samples of an infecting organism from discharge or samples of affected tissue.

CULTURING To grow cells in a special substance, or media, in the laboratory.

CUMULATIVE Increasing in effects or quantity by successive additions.

CUPPING A type of percussion stroke in which the massage therapist strikes or thumps the muscles with cupped hands.

CURETTAGE The removal of tissue or growths by scraping with a curette.

CUSHING'S SYNDROME A hormonal disorder caused by an abnormally high level of cortisol, a corticosteroid hormone that is produced by the adrenal glands. It is most commonly caused by taking medications containing the hormone over a long period of time or more rarely by a pituitary or adrenal gland tumor that stimulates the body to produce excessive amounts of cortisol.

CUT A slicing wound made with a sharp instrument, leaving even edges.

CYANOSIS A bluish tinge to the skin that can occur when the blood oxygen level drops too low.

CYCLOSPORIN A drug that suppresses the immune system and has been used to treat severe psoriasis. Recent research indicates that cyclosporin increases the risk of skin cancer for psoriasis patients.

CYME A flower cluster whose main branch ends in a flower that blooms before the others at its side or base.

CYSTIC FIBROSIS (CF) A disorder of the exocrine glands that affects many organs of the body, especially the sweat glands and glands in the lungs and pancreas.

CYSTINURIA Excess cystine, lysine, arginine, and ornithine in urine due to defective transport system of these acids in kidney and intestines.

CYSTITIS An inflammation or irritation of the bladder and uterus.

CYSTOSCOPE An instrument used to view and introduce treatments into the urinary tract.

CYTOCHROME A substance that contains iron and acts as a hydrogen carrier for the eventual release of energy in aerobic respiration.

CYTOKINES Chemicals made by T cells that act on other cells to stimulate or inhibit their function.

CYTOSTATIC Suppressing the growth and multiplication of cells.

CYTOTOXIC An agent that destroys the cells of a specific organ. Anticancer agents are cytotoxic.

D

DAIDZEIN A soy isoflavone used to produce ipriflavone.

DAILY VALUE (DV) The percentage of the RDA of a nutrient that is present in a food or supplement.

DAOISM Also called Taoism, Dao means **THE WAY**. Daoism is a holistic spiritual philosophy of the universe that is based on the idea that all elements in the universe are interactive and interdependent with each other and that the universe and natural world are in a constant state of change, or flux.

DARKFIELD A technique of microscopic examination in which light is directed at an oblique angle through the slide so that organisms look bright against a dark background.

DAWN SIMULATION A form of light therapy in which the patient is exposed while asleep to gradually brightening white light over a period of an hour and a half.

DE-BLOCKING PROTEIN FACTOR (DPF) A serum component used in IAT that is claimed to inactivate or remove BPF.

DEBRIDE To surgically remove dead tissue.

DEBRIDEMENT The surgical removal of dead tissue.

DECIBEL A unit of the intensity of sound or a measure of loudness. Normal speech is typically spoken in the range of about 20-50 decibels.

DECIDUOUS A tree or bush that sheds its leaves seasonally.

DECILITER (DL) A fluid measurement that is equal to one-tenth of a liter, or 100 cubic centimeters (27 fluid drams or teaspoonfuls).

DECOCTION A liquid extract of a herb, made by simmering or boiling the herb in water, then straining out the plant parts.

DEFECATE Pass feces through the anus for elimination.

DEFECATION Passage of feces through the anus.

DEFINITIVE HOST The host organism for the final (adult) stage in the life cycle of a parasite.

DEGAS To release and vent gases. New building materials often give off gases and odors and the air should be well circulated to remove them.

DEGENERATIVE DISORDER A disorder by which the body or a part of the body gradually loses its ability to fucntion.

DEHYDRATION A condition in which the body lacks the normal level of fluids, potentially impairing normal body functions.

DEHYDROEPIANDROSTERONE (DHEA) A hormone precursor to testosterone, estrogen, and other hormones.

DELIRIUM TREMENS A complication that may accompany alcohol withdrawal. The symptoms include body shaking (tremulousness), insomnia, agitation, confusion, hearing voices or seeing images that are not really there (hallucinations), seizures, rapid heart beat, profuse sweating, high blood pressure, and fever.

DEMENTIA Loss of memory and other higher functions, such as thinking or speech, lasting six months or more.

DEMINERALIZATION A loss or decrease of minerals in the bones.

DEMULCENT A gelatinous or oily substance that has a protective or soothing influence on irritated mucous membranes.

DENATURED Food which has been processed and is no longer of benefit to the body.

DENDRITES Branching projections that grow out of a nerve cell.

DENTAL CARIES A disease of the teeth in which microorganisms convert sugar in the mouth to acid, which then erodes the tooth.

DENTINE The hard major portion of a tooth below the enamel.

DEPENDENCE A state in which a person requires a steady concentration of a particular substance in order to avoid experiencing withdrawal symptoms.

DEPRESSION A psychological condition, with feelings of sadness, sleep disturbance, fatigue, and inability to concentrate.

DERMATITIS HERPETIFORMIS A chronic, very itchy skin disease with groups of red lesions that leave spots behind when they heal. It is sometimes associated with cancer of an internal organ.

DERMATITIS Inflammation of the skin.

DERMATOLOGIST A physician specializing in the branch of medicine concerned with skin.

DERMATOPHYTE A type of fungus that is parasitic on skin and causes a skin disease.

DERMOID TUMOR A skin-like benign growth that may appear on the ovary and resemble a cyst.

DERVISH A member of the Sufi order. Their practice of meditation involves whirling ecstatic dance.

DESENSITIZATION A treatment for phobias which involves exposing the phobic person to the feared situation. It is often used in conjunction with relaxation techniques. Also used to describe a technique of pain reduction in which the painful area is stimulated with whatever is causing the pain.

DETOXIFICATION The process of purifying the body of poisons accumulated during years of poor eating habits.

DEVIATED SEPTUM A hole or perforation in the septum, the wall that divides the two nasal cavities.

DHEA Dehydroepiandrosterone, a hormone produced by the adrenal glands, that is important in making other hormones, especially estrogen and testosterone.

DIABETES MELLITUS A degenerative disease characterized by inadequate production or absorption of insulin, excessive urine production, and excessive amounts of sugar in the blood and urine.

DIABETES TYPE 2 A form of diabetes mellitus that usually occurs in adults. The pancreas produces insulin, but the muscle cells are resistant to the effects of the insulin. This was formerly called maturity (or adult) onset diabetes.

DIABETIC COMA A life-threatening, reduced level of consciousness that occurs in persons with uncontrolled diabetes mellitus.

DIABETIC KETOACIDOSIS A potentially serious condition in which ketones become present in the blood stream because of the metabolism of fats *burned* in lieu of carbohydrates that would normally be used. This occurs because there is insufficient insulin available to cause carbohydrates to be used as fuel.

DIABETIC PERIPHERAL NEUROPATHY The sensitivity of nerves to pain, temperature, and pressure is dulled particularly in the legs and feet.

DIABETIC RETINOPATHY A condition seen most frequently in individuals with poorly controlled diabetes mellitus where the tiny blood vessels to the retina, the tissues that sense light at the back of the eye, are damaged. This damage causes blurred vision, sudden blindness, or black spots, lines, or flashing light in the field of vision.

DIADZIN An isoflavone contained in kudzu that appears to be useful in treating alcoholism.

DIAGENESIS Recombination or rearrangement of a substance resulting in a new compound.

DIAGNOSIS The art or act of identifying a disease from its signs and symptoms.

DIAN XUE The Chinese name for acupressure. This form of massage can be done at home as well as by a trained therapist.

DIAPHORETIC A substance that induces sweating.

DIAPHRAGM BREATHING Method of deep breathing using the entire lungs.

DIASTOLIC BLOOD PRESSURE Blood pressure when the heart is resting between beats.

DIAZINON A member of the organophosphate family of pesticides. This chemical causes nerve and reproductive damage.

DIETARY SUPPLEMENT According to the United States Food and Drug Administration (FDA), any product intended for ingestion as a supplement to the diet.

DIGESTIVE ENZYMES Proteins that catalyze the breakdown of large molecules (usually food) into smaller molecules.

DIGESTIVE TRACT The long tubular structure that handles all digestion, and the structures that connect to it, including the mouth, esophagus, stomach, and intestines.

DIGITALIS A naturally occuring compound used in the preparation of the medication, digoxin, prescribed to increase the heart rate and strengthen the force of the heart's contractions.

DIHYDROTESTOSTERONE (DHT) A testosterone metabolite implicated in the increase in size and number of prostatic cells.

DILATE To expand in diameter and size.

DIMER A molecule consisting of two identical simpler molecules.

DIMERCAPROL (BAL) A chemical agent used to remove excess lead from the body.

DIOPTER (D) A unit of measure for describing the refractive power of a lens.

DIOSGENIN A phytohormone extracted from Mexican yams that is used to make natural and synthetic progesterone.

DIOXIN A toxic chemical used in the manufacture of some pesticides and herbicides.

DIPLEGIA Paralysis affecting like parts on both sides the body, such as both arms or both legs.

DIRECT FLUORESCENT ANTIBODY TEST (DFA TEST) A test in which a fluorescent dye is linked to an antibody for diagnostic purposes.

DIRECTION In the Alexander technique, direction involves bringing about the free balance of the head on the spine and the resulting release of the erector muscles of the back and legs to establish improved coordination.

DIRTY BOMB A bomb made with conventional explosives that also contains radioactive isotopes. When the bomb explodes, the radioactive material spreads contamination over a wide area.

DISK Dense tissue between the vertebrae that acts as a shock absorber and prevents damage to nerves and blood vessels along the spine.

DISSEMINATED Spread to other tissues.

DISSOCIATION A reaction to trauma in which the mind splits off certain aspects of the traumatic event from conscious awareness. Dissociation can affect the patient's memory, sense of reality, and sense of identity.

DISSOCIATIVE AMNESIA A dissociative disorder characterized by loss of memory for a period or periods of time in the patient's life.

DISTILLATE When a substance is distilled (vaporized and condensed to separate out different compounds), the material that is obtained through that process is called the distillate.

DISULFIRAM-LIKE POISON Disulfiram is a chemical compound that causes a severe physiological reaction to alcohol. This poison behaves like disulfiram.

DISUSE ATROPHY Condition of muscles that have lost size, strength, and function due to lack of mobility.

DIURETIC A substance that promotes urination.

DIURNAL Events that happen in the daytime, daily; associated with circadian rhythms.

DIVINING The act of locating an object using a special sense or instinct.

DNA Deoxyribonucleic acid; the genetic material in cells that holds the inherited instructions for growth, development, and cellular functioning.

DOJO A martial arts school.

DONEPEZIL A drug, sold under the trade name Aricept, commonly prescribed for Alzheimer's disease that provides temporary improvement in cognitive functions for some patients with mild-to-moderate forms of the disease.

DOPAMINE AGONIST (DA) A drug that binds to dopamine receptors on cell surfaces and mimics the effects of dopamine.

DOPAMINE RECEPTOR ANTAGONISTS (DAS) The older class of antipsychotic medications, also called neuroleptics. These primarily block the site on nerve cells that normally receives the brain chemical dopamine.

DOPAMINE A neurotransmitter made in the brain that is involved in many brain activities, including movement and emotion.

DORSAL RHIZOTOMY A surgical procedure that cuts nerve roots to reduce spasticity in affected muscles.

DORSAL ROOT ENTRY ZONE (DREZ) A type of nerve surgery for postherpetic neuralgia that is occasionally used when the patient can get no other pain relief. The surgery destroys the area where damaged nerves join the central nervous system, thereby interfering with inappropriate pain messages from nerves to the brain.

DOSHA One of three constitutional types, either vata, pitta, or kapha, found in Ayurvedic medicine.

DOUBLE BLIND PLACEBO CONTROLLED STUDY A study in which neither the patient nor the drug administrator knows who is receiving the trial drug and who the placebo.

DOUBLE-BLIND RANDOMIZED CONTROLLED TRIAL A scientific, or clinical, study which uses two groups of subjects. One group receives the treatment being tested, while the other group (the control group) receives a placebo. Double-blind means that neither the subjects nor the researchers know which subjects are in which group.

DOULA A doula is someone who undergoes special training to enable them to support women during childbirth and into the postpartum period.

DOWN SYNDROME A genetic disorder caused by an extra human chromosome 21 (trisomy 21), characterized by mental retardation, muscular weakness, and folds over the patient's eyelids. Patients with Down's syndrome often begin to lose their memory in midlife.

DRUG TOLERANCE A phenomenon whereby a drug user becomes physically accustomed to a particular dose of a substance, and requires ever-increasing dosages in order to obtain the same effects.

DRUSEN Yellowish-white fatty deposits on the retina, including the macula.

DSM-IV Diagnostic and Statistical Manual of Mental Disorders, Fourth Edition (DSM-IV). This reference book, published by the American Psychiatric Association, is the diagnostic standard for most mental health professionals in the United States.

DTAP Diphtheria and tetanus toxoids and accellular Pertussis combination vaccine.

DTP Diphtheria, tetanus, and whole-cell pertussis vaccine.

DUODENUM The first of the three segments of the small intestine. The duodenum is about 10 in (25 cm) long and connects the stomach and the jejunum.

DYANA The yoga term for meditation.

DYSBIOSIS The condition that results when the natural flora of the gut are thrown out of balance, such as when antibiotics are taken.

DYSKINESIA An abnormal involuntary movement or tic.

DYSLEXIA A term applied to a kind of learning disability particularly noted for reversals and spatial shifts, making reading, writing, spelling and math very difficult.

DYSMENORRHEA Painful menstruation.

DYSMOTILITY Abnormally slow or fast rhythmic movement of the stomach or intestine.

DYSPEPSIA Recurrent or persistent pain in the upper abdomen.

DYSPLASIA Abnormal changes in cells.

DYSPNEA Difficulty in breathing, usually associated with heart or lung diseases.

DYSSOMNIA A primary sleep disorder in which the patient suffers from changes in the quantity, quality, or timing of sleep.

DYSTONIA Painful involuntary muscle cramps or spasms.

DYSTONIC Dystonic refers to a condition called dystonia, in which fine motor control is confused.

DYSURIA Painful or difficult urination.

E

ECCHYMOSIS The medical term for a bruise, or skin discoloration caused by blood seeping from broken capillaries under the skin.

ECCRINE A type of gland that produces a clear watery secretion without releasing cells or cell contents into the secretion.

ECHINACEA A popular herbal remedy used to treat colds, the flu, and urinary tract infections.

ECLECTICS Nineteenth century herbal scientists in the United States who founded the Reformed Medical School. Their outlook was based on herbal medicines of Europe, Asia, and Indian.

ECT Electroconvulsive therapy sometimes is used to treat depression or mania when pharmaceutical treatment fails.

ECTOPIC PREGNANCY A pregnancy that develops outside of the mother's uterus, such as in the fallopian tube. Ectopic pregnancies often cause severe pain in the lower abdomen and are potentially life-threatening because of the massive blood loss that may occur as the developing embryo/fetus ruptures and damages the tissues in which it has implanted.

ECTOPIC Out of place or located away from the normal position.

ECZEMA A superficial type of inflammation of the skin that may be very itchy and weeping in the early stages; later, the affected skin becomes crusted, scaly, and thick. There is no known cause.

EDEMA The presence of abnormally large amounts of fluid in the intercellular tissue spaces of the body.

EDETATE CALCIUM DISODIUM (EDTA CALCIUM) A chemical agent used to remove excess lead from the body.

EFFERENT Motor signals that go from brain and spinal cord out to the muscles of the body.

EFFICACY The power to bring about intended results.

EFFLEURAGE A massage technique that involves light stroking with the palms or thumbs.

EFFUSION A collection of fluid that has leaked out into some body cavity or tissue.

EICOSANOIDS Local, short–lived fatty acid substances with hormone-like properties, derived from arachidonic acid, that have strong physiological effects, even in very low concentrations. They influence several vital functions, such as the regulation of inflammatory, immunological and hemostatic processes.

EICOSAPENIAENOIC ACID A type of acid derived from gamma-linoleic acid.

EJACULATORY INCOMPETENCE Inability to ejaculate inside the vagina.

ELASTIN A yellow fibrous protein that is the basic component of elastic connective tissue.

ELECAMPANE A perennial herb with large yellow flowers used primarily as a digestive stimulant.

ELECTRICAL IMPEDANCE This technique uses a small electrical current passing through the body. Fat impedes or slows down electrical current. The faster the current runs through the body, the less fat there is.

ELECTROCARDIOGRAPHY A test that uses electrodes attached to the chest with an adhesive gel to transmit the electrical impulses of the heart muscle to a recording device.

ELECTROCAUTERY A procedure that to remove small growths on the skin using an instrument that generates heat from an electric current.

ELECTRODESICCATION To make dry, dull, or lifeless with the use of electrical current.

ELECTROLYTES Substances in the blood, such as sodium and potassium, that help to regulate fluid balance in the body.

ELECTROMAGNETIC ENERGY Energy created by electromagnetism, the forces of electricity and magnetism.

ELECTROMYOGRAPHIC BIOFEEDBACK A method for relieving jaw tightness by monitoring the patient's attempts to relax the muscle while the patient watches a gauge. The patient gradually learns to control the degree of muscle relaxation.

ELECTROMYOGRAPHY (EMG) A diagnostic test that records the electrical activity of muscles. In the test, small electrodes are placed on or in the skin; the patterns of electrical activity are projected on a screen or over a loudspeaker. This procedure is used to test for muscle disorders, including muscular dystrophy.

ELECTRONYSTAGMOGRAPHY A method for measuring the electricity generated by eye movements. Electrodes are placed on the skin around the eye and the individual is subjected to a variety of stimuli so that the quality of eye movements can be assessed.

ELECTRORETINOGRAM An instrument for measuring electrical signals from a point in the macula.

ELEUTHEROSIDE The active chemical found in Siberian ginseng.

ELIXIR Similar to a liquid extract, sweetened, and with added aromatic principals, said to be one of the most common forms of liquid herbal medicines for oral consumption.

ELLAGIC ACID A yellow crystalline compound derived from tannins and used to prevent bleeding. It is found in raspberries and is thought to help prevent cancer.

EMBOLI, EMBOLUS Emboli is the plural form of embolus. Embolus refers to any mass of air, blood clot, or foreign body that travels through the bloodstream and is capable of lodging in smaller blood vessels where it can obstruct the blood flow to that vessel.

EMBOLISM A blood clot, air bubble, or mass of foreign material that travels and blocks the flow of blood in an artery. When blood supply to a tissue or organ is blocked by an embolism, infarction, or death of the tissue the artery feeds, occurs. Without immediate and appropriate treatment, an embolism can be fatal.

EMBOLIZATION A technique to stop or prevent hemorrhage by introducing a foreign mass, such as an air-filled membrane (balloon), into a blood vessel to block the flow of blood. This term also refers to an alternative to splenectomy that involves injecting silicone or a similar substances into the splenic artery to shrink the size of the spleen.

EMBOLUS Plural, emboli. An embolus is something that blocks the blood flow in a blood vessel. It may be a gas bubble, a blood clot, a fat globule, a mass of bacteria, or other foreign body that forms somewhere else and travels through the circulatory system until it gets stuck.

EMBRYO In humans, the developing individual from the time of implantation to about the end of the second month after conception. From the third month to the point of delivery, the individual is called a fetus.

EMESIS An act or episode of vomiting.

EMETIC A medication intended to cause vomiting. Emetics are sometimes used in aversion therapy in place of electric shock. Their most common use in mainstream medicine is in treating accidental poisoning.

EMMENAGOGUE A type of medication that brings on or increases a woman's menstrual flow.

EMOLLIENT A substance that softens and smoothes the skin.

EMPHYSEMA A type of medication that brings on or increases a woman's menstrual flow.

EMPYEMA An infection that causes pus to accumulate in the pleural space which may cause a tear in the pleural membrane and allow the infection to spread to other areas in the body.

ENAMEL The hard outermost surface of a tooth.

ENCEPHALITIS Inflammation of the brain, usually caused by a viral infection.

ENCEPHALOPATHY Any abnormality in the structure or function of brain tissues.

ENDARTERECTOMY A procedure in which the diseased inner portions of an artery, including any deposits, are removed.

ENDEMIC Natural to or characteristic of a particular place, population, or climate.

ENDOCARDITIS Inflammation of the inner membrane lining heart and/or of the heart valves caused by infection.

ENDOCRINE GLAND A ductless gland, such as the pituitary, thyroid, or adrenal gland, that secretes its products directly into the blood or lymph.

ENDOCRINE SYSTEM The network of glands that produces hormones and releases them into the bloodstream. The thyroid gland is part of the endocrine system.

ENDODONTIST A dentist who specializes in diagnosing and treating diseases of the pulp and other inner parts of the tooth.

ENDOGENOUS OPIOID A natural pain reliever produced by the body that is also associated with the sensation of itching.

ENDOMETRIAL IMPLANTS Growths of endometrial tissue that attach to organs, primarily in the pelvic cavity.

ENDOMETRIAL Pertaining to the endometrium, a mucous membrane lining the uterus.

ENDOMETRIOSIS A condition in which the tissue that normally lines the uterus (endometrium) grows in other areas of the body, causing pain, irregular bleeding, and frequently, infertility.

ENDOMETRIUM The mucosal layer lining the inner cavity of the uterus. The endometrium's structure changes with age and with the menstrual cycle.

ENDORPHINS A group of chemicals resembling opiates that are released in the body in response to trauma or stress. Endorphins react with opiate receptors in the brain to reduce pain sensations.

ENDOSCOPE A medical instrument that can be passed into an area of the body (the bladder or intestine, for example) to allow visual examination of that area. The endoscope usually has a fiber-optic camera that allows a greatly magnified image to be shown on a television screen viewed by the operator. Many endoscopes also allow the operator to retrieve a small sample (biopsy) of the area being examined, to more closely view the tissue under a microscope.

ENDOSCOPY Visual examination of an organ or body cavity using an endoscope, a thin, tubular instrument containing a camera and light source. Many endoscopes also allow the retrieval of a small sample (biopsy) of the area being examined, in order to more closely view the tissue under a microscope.

ENDOTHELIUM A thin layer of smooth tissue that lines the inside of blood vessels, the heart and abdomen, and other body cavities.

ENDURANCE The time limit of a person's ability to maintain either a specific force or power involving muscular contractions.

ENERGY Includes nonmaterial (eg, Qi) as well as material (eg, blood) vital forces that create and sustain life.

ENGRAM A permanent trace left in nerve tissue by a stimulus; in psychology, a latent memory picture or lasting trace left in the psyche by any experience.

ENTERITIS Inflammation of the mucosal lining of the small intestine.

ENTEROPATHY A disease of the intestinal tract.

ENTRAINMENT The patterning of body processes and movements to the rhythm of music.

ENZYME THERAPY An alternative approach to the treatment of digestive disorders and other illnesses related to nutritional problems. Enzyme therapy emphasizes the use of animal- or plant-derived digestive enzymes as dietary supplements.

ENZYME Any of a group of complex proteins that originate in living cells and help to break down organic compounds into simpler molecules.

EOSINOPHILIA MYALGIA SYNDROME (EMS) A chronic, painful disease of the immune system that causes joint pain, fatigue, shortness of breath, and swelling of the arms and legs. EMS can be fatal.

EPICONDYLE A projection on the surface of a bone; often an area for muscle and tendon attachment.

EPICONDYLITIS A painful and sometimes disabling inflammation of the muscle and surrounding tissues of the elbow caused by repeated stress and strain on the forearm near the lateral epicondyle of the humerous (arm bone).

EPIDEMIC PAROTITIS The medical name for mumps.

EPIDEMIC A widespread regional disease outbreak.

EPIDEMIOLOGICAL STUDY Medical research that deals with the incidence, distribution, and control of disease in a population; the sum of factors controlling the presence or absence of a disease, or pathogens.

EPIDERMIS The outermost layer of skin cells.

EPIDURAL SPACE The space immediately surrounding the outer most membrane of the spinal cord.

EPIGLOTTITIS A serious bacterial infection that can develop rapidly and lead to airway obstruction.

EPILEPSY A neurological disorder characterized by recurrent seizures with or without a loss of consciousness.

EPILEPTOLOGIST A physician who specializes in the treatment of epilepsy.

EPINEPHRINE Also called adrenalin, a secretion of the adrenal glands (along with norepinephrine) that helps the liver release glucose and limits the release of insulin. Norepinephrine is both a hormone and a neurotransmitter, a substance that transmits nerve signals.

EPISIOTOMY A surgical incision of the vaginal opening made during childbirth to avoid tearing during delivery.

EPITHELIUM The layer of tissue that covers body surfaces or lines the inner surfaces of body cavities and hollow organs.

EPSOM SALTS A preparation of magnesium sulfate, used internally as a laxative or externally in compresses or warm baths to reduce swelling, inflammation, and itching from minor skin problems.

EPSTEIN-BARR VIRUS (EBV) A virus in the herpes family that causes mononucleosis.

EQUINE-FACILITATED THERAPY Another term for therapeutic riding.

EQUINOVARUS A condition in which the foot is commonly pulled inward.

EQUINUS The most common postural deformity, the foot is extended by the strong pull of the rear calf muscles, causing the toes to point.

ERECTILE DYSFUNCTION Impotence; the inability of a man to achieve and/or maintain an erection of sufficient quality for sexual intercourse.

ERGONOMICS A branch of applied science that coordinates the physical design and arrangement of furniture, machines, and other features of a living or working environment with the needs and requirements of the individuals in that environment.

ERGOT PREPARATIONS A classification of drugs made from a fungus, used primarily for the treatment of migraines.

ERUPTION Emergence of teeth through the gums.

ERYTHEMA MIGRANS (EM) A red skin rash that is one of the first signs of Lyme disease in about 75% of patients.

ERYTHEMA A diffuse red and inflamed area of the skin.

ERYTHROBLASTOSIS FETALIS A type of hemolytic anemia of newborn infants caused by incompatibility (involving either the Rh factor and/or the ABO blood groups) between a mother's blood and her unborn baby's blood. As a result of this incompatibility, the baby's red blood cells are destroyed by antibodies that have crossed the placenta from the mother's blood.

ERYTHROCYTE SEDIMENTATION RATE (ESR) The rate at which red blood cells settle out in a tube of unclotted blood, expressed in millimeters per hour; elevated sedimentation rates indicate the presence of inflammation.

ERYTHROCYTES Known as red blood cells, erythrocytes carry oxygen to every part of the body.

ERYTHROGENIC TOXIN A toxin or agent produced by the scarlet fever-causing bacteria that causes the skin to turn red.

ERYTHROMYCIN An antibiotic that can be used instead of penicillin.

ESOPHAGITIS Inflammation of the esophagus.

ESOPHAGUS Muscular tube, about 10 in (25 cm) long, connecting the throat to the stomach.

ESSENCE The constituent of a plant that determines its characteristics.

ESSENTIAL AMINO ACID An amino acid that the body requires but cannot make.

ESSENTIAL FATTY ACID (EFA) A fatty acid that the body cannot make but must obtain from the diet. EFAs include omega-6 fatty acids found in primrose and safflower oils, and omega-3 fatty acids oils found in fatty fish and flaxseed, canola, soybean, and walnuts.

ESSENTIAL OIL A concentrated oil that has been distilled from a plant.

ESSENTIAL TREMOR An uncontrollable (involuntary) shaking of the hands, head, and face. Also called familial tremor because it is a sometimes inherited, it can begin in the teens or in middle age. The exact cause is not known.

ESTROGEN Female hormone produced by the ovaries and released by the follicles as they mature. After menopause, the production of the hormone gradually stops.

ESTROGENIC Having properties that mimic the functions of the female hormone, estrogen.

ESTROGEN-RECEPTOR ASSAY A test to see if a breast cancer needs estrogen to grow.

ETHANOL The chemical name for beverage alcohol. It is also sometimes called ethyl alcohol or grain alcohol to distinguish it from isopropyl or rubbing alcohol.

ETHEREAL Something that is of or from the heavens, usually used in a metaphysical sense.

ETHNOBOTANY The study of the plant lore and agricultural practices of a people or culture.

ETHNOMEDICINE Medicine pertaining to a particular ethnic group.

EUSTACHIAN TUBE A thin tube between the middle ear and the pharynx. Its purpose is to equalize pressure on either side of the ear drum.

EXACERBATIONS Increase in severity of a disease or condition.

EXANTHEM A skin eruption or rash. The term is also used for diseases that have skin rashes as a prominent feature (e.g., measles). Pityriasis rosea is an example of an exanthem.

EXCISION Surgical removal of tissue.

EXFOLIATE To shed skin. In skin care, the term exfoliate describes the process of removing dead skin cells.

EXOCRINE Refers to a system of organs that produces chemicals that go through a duct (or tube) to reach other organs or body surfaces whose functioning they affect.

EXPECTORANT A substance or medication given to bring up phlegm or mucus from the respiratory tract.

EXTENSOR MUSCLES A group of muscles in the forearm that serve to lift or extend the wrist and hand. Tennis elbow results from overuse and inflammation of the tendons that attach these muscles to the outside of the elbow.

EXTRACT A concentrated form of the herb made by pressing the herb with a hydraulic press, soaking it in water or alcohol, then letting the excess water or alcohol evaporate.

EXTRAPYRAMIDAL SYMPTOMS (EPS) A group of side effects associated with antipsychotic medications. EPS include parkinsonism, akathisia, dystonia, and tardive dyskinesia.

EXUVIUM A cast-off shell of an insect or crustacean. Cicada in traditional Chinese medicine is made from the molted shell of a cicada.

F

FALLOPIAN TUBE The tube leading from the ovary into the uterus.

FALSE-NEGATIVE A laboratory result that does not detect the presence of a disease that is actually present.

FAMCICLOVIR An oral antiviral drug that is available under the trade name Famvir. The drug prevents the varicella zoster virus from replicating.

FARSIGHTEDNESS Being able to see more clearly those objects far away as opposed to those that are near. Also called hyperopic.

FASCIA The sheet of connective tissue that covers the body under the skin and envelops every muscle, bone, nerve, gland, organ, and blood vessel. Fascia helps the body to retain its basic shape.

FASCICULATION Small involuntary muscle contractions visible under the skin.

FASTING Avoiding food for a period of time.

FAT One of the nutrients that supplies calories to the body.

FEBRIFUGE A substance or medication that lowers or dispels fevers.

FEBRILE SEIZURE Convulsions brought on by fever.

FEBRILE Characteristic of fever.

FECES Undigested food and other waste that is eliminated through the anus. Feces are also called fecal matter or stools.

FEEDBACK RESPONSE A response to information carried back to the brain, or to other areas or glands from target tissues that generates a follow up response.

FELDENKRAIS An educational method dedicated to improved movement and enhanced functioning originated by Moshe Feldenkrais (1904-1984), an engineer, physicist and Judo expert.

FEMUR The main bone in the human thigh and the strongest bone in the body.

FERRITIN An iron storage protein found in the blood. High levels of serum ferritin may indicate iron overload.

FETUS An unborn child from the end of the eighth week after fertilization until birth.

FIBRINOGEN A protein that is important in blood clotting.

FIBRINOLYSIS The breakdown of fibrin, an insoluble protein that is the end product of blood clotting. Fibrinolysis results in the dissolution of small clots.

FIBROBLASTS Found in connective tissue, these fat, oval cells help build fibrous tissue.

FIBROCARTILAGE Cartilage that consists of dense fibers.

FIBROCYSTIC DISEASE A common condition in middle aged women, characterized by the growth of one or more cysts in the breasts. Cysts are small inclusions filled with fluid. These are harmless, but may cause pain and tenderness.

FIBROIDS Fibrous non-cancerous growths on the uterus or surrounding tissue.

FIBROMYALGIA A chronic syndrome characterized by fatigue, widespread muscular pain, and pain at specific points on the body.

FIBROSIS The formation of fibrous, or scar, tissue which may follow inflammation and destruction of normal tissue.

FIGHT-OR-FLIGHT RESPONSE The body's reaction to stress or threats.

FIRE An extremely high internal heat condition characterized by severe dehydration, red eyes, red face, constipation, insomnia, and agitation. Fire often affects Lungs, Liver, and Stomach.

FISTULA An abnormal channel that creates an open passageway between two structures that do not normally connect.

FIVE ELEMENTS The five basic substances (water, wood, fire, earth, and metal) that symbolize the fundamental qualities of the universe. In Chinese food cures, the five elements are correlated with the internal organs of the body and with the five basic food tastes.

FIVE SUBSTANCES The basic entities in the human body that serve its development and maintenance. They include chi (qi), vital essence, spirit, blood, and fluids.

FLAKE A small, thin skin mass.

FLAVONE A colorless crystalline compound found in skullcap and other plants that is the parent substance of a group of yellow plant pigments.

FLAVONOID Any of a group of water-soluble plant pigments that are thought to have antioxidative, anti-inflammatory, and antiviral properties.

FLUID EXTRACT Made by simmering a plant and reducing the water until the mixture is thickened. This resulting liquid has a concentrated form of the active constituents of a plant. Alcohol, glycerin, or tincture of Benzoin may be added as a preservative.

FLUORESCEIN ANGIOGRAPHY A method that uses a fluorescent dye for photographing blood vessels of the retina.

FLUORIDE A chemical compound containing fluorine that is used to treat water or applied directly to teeth to prevent decay.

FLUOROQUINOLONES A group of newer antibiotics that are used to treat penicillin-resistant staphylococcal infections.

FLUOROURACIL An anticancer drug.

FLUOUROQUINOLONES A group of medications used to treat bacterial infections in many different parts of the body. They are often used to treat bacteria that have become resistant to penicillin and other antibiotics.

FOLLICLE-STIMULATING HORMONE (FSH) A pituitary hormone that in females stimulates the ovary to mature egg capsules (follicles) and in males stimulates sperm production.

FOMITE An inanimate object that can transmit infectious organisms.

FONTANELLE A membrane-covered soft spot in an infant's skull where the bone has not yet completely formed.

FORENSIC Pertaining to courtroom procedure or evidence used in courts of law.

FORMALDEHYDE A chemical preservative used in many building materials such as adhesives, furnishings, and manufactured woods (plywood and particle board). It can cause eye, nose, and throat irritation and it has been listed as a cancer-causing agent.

FORSKOLIN Chemical compound extracted from coleus root that appears to be effective in treating asthma, eczema, colic, and other conditions.

FRAGILE X SYNDROME A genetic condition related to the X chromosome that affects mental, physical, and sensory development.

FREE OXYGEN RADICALS Also called free radicals, these are by-products of oxygen that cause oxidative damage to the body's cells.

FREE RADICAL An unstable molecule that causes oxidative damage by stealing electrons from surrounding molecules, thereby disrupting activity in the body's cells.

FREUDIAN ANALYSIS A type of psychological treatment where the therapist seeks to help the patient resolve conflicts and traumas buried in the subconscious.

FRIEDREICH'S ATAXIA An inherited disease that usually manifests in childhood or adolescence, characterized by loss of muscular coordination (ataxia), curvature of the spine, impaired speech, and cardiomyopathy.

FRUCTOSE A type of natural sugar found in many fruits, vegetables, and in honey.

FUNCTIONAL CYST A benign cyst that forms on the ovary and resolves on its own without treatment.

FUNCTIONAL FOOD A food or food ingredient that is thought to confer health benefits in addition to the nutrients it contains.

FUNDOPLICATION Surgical procedure that increases pressure on the LES (lower esophageal sphincter), reducing reflux.

FUNGICIDE A substance that kills fungi.

FUNGUS A member of a group of simple organisms that are related to yeast and molds.

FURANOSESQUITERPENES A sub-class of compounds known as terpenes in the oils of plants and foods that do not contain an alcohol portion. These compounds tend to be found in volatile oils, and are related to the aroma of volatile and essential oils.

FUROCOUMARIN A toxic compound found in ruta that can cause nausea, vomiting, and convulsions in humans.

FURUNCLE The medical name for a boil.

G

GALACTOGOGUE A substance or medication that increases the flow of breast milk in nursing mothers.

GAMMA LINOLENIC ACID (GLA) An essential fatty acid that is found in borage seed oil.

GAMMA RADIATION High energy electromagnetic waves emitted in some nuclear reactions.

GANGRENE Decay or death of body tissue because the blood supply is cut off. Tissues that have died in this way must be surgically removed.

GASTRIC ACID Also, stomach acid. Helps break up fats and proteins for further digestion, aids in the absorption of nutrients through the walls of the intestines into the blood, and helps protect the gastrointestinal tract from harmful bacteria.

GASTRITIS Inflammation of the stomach, particularly of its mucous membrane.

GASTROESOPHAGEAL REFLUX DISEASE (GERD) A disorder of the lower end of the esophagus in which the lower esophageal sphincter does not open and close normally. As a result the acidic contents of the stomach can flow backward into the esophagus and irritate the tissues.

GASTROESOPHAGEAL REFLUX Upward flow of stomach contents into the esophagus, causing heartburn.

GASTROINTESTINAL TRACT The entire length of the digestive system, running from the stomach, through the small intestine, large intestine, and out the rectum and anus.

GASTROINTESTINAL Pertaining to the stomach and intestine.

GAUCHER'S DISEASE A rare genetic disease caused by a deficiency of enzymes needed for the processing of fatty acids.

GEL ELECTROPHORESIS A laboratory test that separates molecules based on their size, shape, or electrical charge.

GENE THERAPY A method of treating a disorder by replacing damaged or abnormal genes with normal ones. Some researchers think that gene therapy may offer a new way to treat impotence.

GENERAL PARESIS A form of neurosyphilis in which the patient's personality, as well as his or her control of movement, is affected. The patient may develop convulsions or partial paralysis.

GENIOPLASTY An operation performed to reshape the chin. Genioplasties are often done to treat OSA because the procedure changes the structure of the patient's upper airway.

GENISTEIN A plant isoflavone, found as genistin in soy, that is used to produce ipriflavone.

GENOTYPE The genetic makeup of an organism or group of organisms with respect to a biological trait or set of traits.

GENU VALGUS Deformity in which the legs are curved inward so that the knees are close together, nearly or actually knocking as a person walks with ankles widely apart.

GENUS With regard to botany, genus refers to a plant's classification. Plants within the same genus have one or more common characteristics.

GEOPATHIC STRESS Any variation in normal energy patterns which some believe can cause illness.

GERMAN COMMISSION E The world standard to regulate herbal products.

GERMANDER A plant, *Teucrium chamaedrys*, that belongs to the mint family and may have been used to adulterate skullcap products reported to cause liver damage.

GERMICIDAL Known to kill germs.

GESTALT THERAPY A humanistic therapy technique that focuses on gaining an awareness of emotions and behaviors in the present rather than in the past. It stresses the interconnectedness of self-awareness, behavior, and experience.

GESTATION The period from conception to birth, during which the developing fetus is carried in the uterus.

GESUNDHEIT A German expression wishing good health, usually used when a person sneezes.

GHEE Butter heated to removed the fat, used in Ayurvedic foods and remedies.

GHRELIN A recently discovered peptide hormone secreted by cells in the lining of the stomach. Ghrelin is important in appetite regulation and maintaining the body's energy balance.

GILBERT'S SYNDROME A mild hereditary form of jaundice.

GINGIVITIS Inflammation of the gums.

GINGKO BILOBA A shade tree native to China that has fan-shaped leaves and fleshy seeds. Gingko extract is being studied as a sunburn remedy and preventative.

GINKGO EXTRACT Made from the leaves of the *Ginkgo biloba* tree, this extract, used in other countries to treat circulatory problems, may improve the symptoms of patients with dementia.

GINSENG INTOXICATION Possible side effects of taking *Panax ginseng* products.

GINSENOCIDE Active substances found in ginseng.

GLANDS Collections of tissue that produce chemicals needed for chemical reactions elsewhere in the body.

GLAUCOMA A common eye disease characterized by increased fluid pressure in the eye that damages the optic nerve, which carries visual impulses to the brain. Glaucoma can be caused by another eye disorder, such as a tumor or congenital malformation, or can appear without obvious cause, but if untreated it generally leads to blindness.

GLOBIN One of the component protein molecules found in hemoglobin. Normal adult hemoglobin has a pair each of alpha-globin and beta-globin molecules.

GLOBUS PALLIDUS Areas on each side of the brain that transmit signals controlling movement.

GLOMERULONEPHRITIS An inflammation of the filtering units of the kidney (glomeruli). The condition hinders removal of waste products, salt, and water from the bloodstream, leading to serious complications. It is the most common cause of renal failure.

GLOSSOPHARYNGEAL NEURALGIA Sharp recurrent pain deep in the throat that extends to the area around the tonsils and possibly the ear. It is triggered by swallowing or chewing.

GLOTTIS The opening between the vocal cords at the upper part of the larynx.

GLUCAGON A hormone produced in the pancreas that raises the level of glucose in the blood. An injectable form of glucagon, which can be bought in a drug store, is sometimes used to treat insulin shock.

GLUCAN A complex sugar molecule consisting of smaller units of glucose.

GLUCOCORTICOIDS A general class of adrenal cortical hormones that are mainly active in protecting against stress and in protein and carbohydrate metabolism. They are widely used in medicine anti-inflammatories and immunosuppresives.

GLUCOSAMINE A complex carbohydrate composed of glucose and an amino acid called glutamine. It is an important building block of cartilage and is often taken together with chondroitin as a treatment for osteoarthritis.

GLUCOSE A sugar that serves as the body's primary source of fuel.

GLUCOSE-6-PHOSPHATE DEHYDROGENASE (G6PD) DEFICIENCY A hereditary disorder that can lead to episodes of hemolytic anemia in combination with certain medications.

GLUTATHIONE PEROXIDASE An enzyme that functions as an antioxidant, in the activation of other enzymes, and in the transport of minerals and amino acids. Human glutathione is dependent on selenium.

GLUTATHIONE A water-soluble peptide composed of cysteine, glycine, and glutamic acid. It functions as an antioxidant. The body uses ademetionine to form glutathione.

GLUTEN A protein found in wheat, rye, barley, and oats.

GLYCEMIC INDEX (GI) A numeric scale for measuring the level and speed of blood glucose increase that carbohydrate-containing food creates upon consumption.

GLYCEMIC The presence of glucose in the blood.

GLYCOPROTEINS Complex proteins that protect immune factors and growth factors from being broken down by stomach acids. Glycoproteins are also called protease inhibitors.

GLYCOSIDE An herbal carbohydrate that exerts powerful effect on hormone-producing tissues. The glycoside breaks down into a sugar and a non-sugar component.

GLYCYRRHIZIN A sweet-tasting compound in licorice root that has a number of beneficial effects on the cardiovascular and digestive systems.

GNRH ANTAGONISTS A group of medications that affect the reproductive hormones. These medications are used to treat fibroids, endometriosis, and infertility.

GOBO A variety of burdock that can be used as a vegetable for soups and salads. It is sometimes known as Japanese burdock.

GOITER Chronic enlargement of the thyroid gland.

GONADS Organs that produce gametes (eggs or sperm), i.e. the ovaries and testes.

GONIOSCOPE An instrument used to examine the anterior chamber of the eye. It consists of a magnifier and a lens equipped with mirrors, which sits on the patient's cornea during the examination.

GONOCOCCUS The bacterium *Neisseria gonorrheae*. The gonococcus causes gonorrhea, a sexually transmitted infection of the genitals and urinary tract that may occasionally affect the eye, causing blindness if not treated.

GOSSYPOL A chemical found in cotton seed oil that is thought to immobilize sperm.

GOUT A metabolic disorder characterized by sudden recurring attacks of arthritis caused by deposits of crystals that build up in the joints due to abnormally high uric acid blood levels. In gout, uric acid may be overproduced, underexcreted, or both.

GRAM-POSITIVE/NEGATIVE A classification system that differentiates bacteria into two classes based upon staining characteristics determined by the composition of the cell wall. Usnea are effective against gram-positive bacteria.

GRAM-POSITIVE Refers to a bacteria that takes on a purplish color when exposed to the Gram stain. Common examples of gram-positive bacteria include several species of streptococci, staphylococci, and clostridia.

GRANULATION TISSUE A kind of tissue formed during wound healing. It has a rough or irregular surface and a rich supply of blood capillaries.

GRANULES Small packets of reactive chemicals stored within cells.

GRANULOCYTOPENIA A condition characterized by a deficiency of white blood cells.

GUIDED IMAGERY The use of relaxation and mental visualization to improve mood and/or physical well-being.

GUILLAIN-BARRÉ SYNDROME Also called acute idiopathic polyneuritis, this condition is a neurologic syndrome that can cause numbness in the limbs and muscle weakness following certain viral infections.

GUMMA A symptom that is sometimes seen in tertiary syphilis, characterized by a rubbery swelling or tumor that heals slowly and leaves a scar.

GYNECOLOGIST A physician with specialized training in diseases and conditions of the female reproductive system.

H

H₂ ANTAGONIST A type of drug that relieves indigestion by reducing the production of stomach acid.

HABIT Referring to the particular set of physical and mental tensions present in any individual.

HACHIMIJIOGAN A Chinese herbal formula that is thought to protect the eyes against cataracts by increasing the glutathione content of the lens.

HAIR FOLLICLES Tiny organs in the skin, each one of which grows a single hair.

HAIRY LEUKOPLAKIA OF THE TONGUE A white area of diseased tissue on the tongue that may be flat or slightly raised. It is caused by the Epstein-Barr virus and is an important diagnostic sign of AIDS.

HALLUCINOGEN A drug that distorts sensory perceptions and disturbs emotion, judgment, and memory.

HASHIMOTO'S DISEASE Disease in which the body makes antibodies to destroy the thyroid. Tendency toward this disease is thought to be inherited.

HATHA YOGA A form of yoga using postures, breathing methods, and meditation.

HDL CHOLESTEROL High-density lipoprotein cholesterol is a component of cholesterol that helps protect against heart disease. HDL is nicknamed good cholesterol.

HEALING CRISIS In homeopathy, the healing crisis is a temporary worsening of the patient's symptoms during successive stages of treatment. In the more general context of alternative medicine, a healing crisis occurs when the cells release toxins into the bloodstream simultaneously, throwing the body into a state of toxic overload until the **BACKLOG** is cleared. During the healing crisis unpleasant sensations, such as headache or nausea, may be experienced.

HEARTBURN A popular term for an uncomfortable burning sensation in the stomach and lower esophagus, sometimes caused by the reflux of small amounts of stomach acid.

HEAT CONDITION A disease whose symptoms include fever, rashes, redness, dehydration, and inflammation.

HEAT In Chinese pathology, the term defines a condition that has excessive heat, either objective (fever, infection) or subjective (feeling hot).

HEAVY METAL POISON A metal with a specific gravity greater than about 5.0, especially one that is poisonous, such as lead or mercury.

HEAVY METAL One of 23 chemical elements that has a specific gravity (a measure of density) at least five times that of water.

HEBERDEN'S NODES Swelling or deformation of the finger joints closest to the fingertips.

HELICOBACTER PYLORI The bacterium that is implicated in most cases of nonerosive gastritis.

HELMINTH A type of parasitic worm, including flukes, tapeworms, and roundworms.

HEMATOLOGIST A medical specialist who specializes diseases and disorders of the blood and blood-forming organs.

HEMATURIA The presence of blood in the urine.

HEME The iron-containing molecule in hemoglobin that serves as the site for oxygen binding.

HEMIPLEGIA Paralysis of one side of the body.

HEMOCHROMATOSIS A hereditary condition which results in excessive storage of iron in various tissues of the body.

HEMODIALYSIS The blood processing procedure used when kidney function is lost. Blood is removed from a vein, processed through a dialysis machine (artificial kidney), and put back into a vein.

HEMOGLOBIN An iron-containing pigment of red blood cells composed of four amino acid chains (alpha, beta, gamma, delta) that delivers oxygen from the lungs to the tissues of the body.

HEMOGLOBIN A Normal adult hemoglobin which contains a heme molecule, two alpha-globin molecules, and two beta-globin molecules.

HEMOGLOBIN S Hemoglobin that is produced in association with the sickle cell trait; the beta-globin molecules of hemoglobin S are defective.

HEMOLYSIS The process of breaking down of red blood cells. As the cells are destroyed, hemoglobin, the component of red blood cells which carries the oxygen, is liberated.

HEMOLYTIC ANEMIA A blood disorder characterized by destruction of red blood cells.

HEMOLYTIC Able to break down or dissolve red blood cells.

HEMOPHILIA Any of several hereditary blood coagulation disorders occurring almost exclusively in males. Because blood does not clot properly, even minor injuries can cause significant blood loss that may require a blood transfusion, with its associated minor risk of infection.

HEMORRHAGE Severe, massive bleeding that is difficult to control. The bleeding may be internal or external.

HEMORRHAGING Heavy or uncontrollable bleeding.

HEMORRHOID An area around the anus or in the rectum where veins become dilated and the tissue swells, causing itching and pain.

HEMOSTATIC A substance used to stop bleeding or hemorrhaging. Yarrow has hemostatic properties.

HEPATIC ENCEPHALOPATHY Brain and nervous system damage that occurs as a complication of liver disorders.

HEPATIC Promotes the well being of the liver.

HEPATITIS An inflammation of the liver, with accompanying liver cell damage or cell death, caused most frequently by viral infection, but also by certain drugs, chemicals, or poisons. May be either acute (of limited duration) or chronic (continuing). Symptoms include jaundice, nausea, vomiting, loss of appetite, tenderness in the right upper abdomen, aching muscles, and joint pain. In severe cases, liver failure may result.

HEPATOTOXIC Poisonous to the liver.

HERALD PATCH The initial skin eruption of pityriasis rosea, usually on the back or chest, that occurs a week or two before the main outbreak. It is sometimes called the mother patch.

HERB In naturopathy, a plant or plant derivative or extract prescribed for health or healing.

HERNIATED Characterized by an abnormal protrusion of a body part. In a herniated disk, the disk protrudes into the spinal canal between the vertebrae.

HERNIORRHAPHY Surgical repair of a hernia.

HERPES SIMPLEX VIRUS A virus that can cause fever and blistering on the skin, mucous membranes, or genitalia.

HERPES ZOSTER VIRUS Acute inflammatory virus attacking the nerve cells on the root of each spinal nerve with skin eruptions along a sensory nerve ending.

HIATAL HERNIA Protrusion of part of the stomach through the diaphragm to a position next to the esophagus.

HIATUS Opening in the diaphragm through which the stomach connects to the esophagus.

HIGH SELF The Huna term for the level of the personality that functions as a guardian spirit and forms the person's connection with God.

HIGH SPOT An area of a tooth or restoration that feels abnormal or uncomfortable because it hits its opposing tooth before other teeth meet.

HIPPOCAMPUS A horseshoe-shaped ridge in the brain that is part of the limbic system. The hippocampus is associated with the formation of short-term memory and with the sense of spatial orientation.

HIRSUITISM An abnormal growth of hair on the face and other parts of the body caused by an excess of androgens. Also known as hypertrichosis.

HISTAMINE RECEPTOR 2 (H2) BLOCKER Heartburn medication that reduces the production of stomach acid.

HISTAMINE A substance released by immune system cells in response to the presence of an allergen. It stimulates widening of blood vessels and increased porousness of blood vessel walls so that fluid and protein leak out from the blood into the surrounding tissue, causing localised inflammation of the tissue.

HLA-B27 An antigen or protein marker on cells that may indicate ankylosing spondylitis.

HMG-COA REDUCTASE Hepetic hydroxy-methyl-glutaryl coenzyme A is an enzyme created in the liver that promotes the production of cholesterol.

HODGKIN'S DISEASE One of two general types of lymphoma (cancers that arise in the the lymphatic system and can invade other organs), Hodgkin's disease is characterized by lymph node enlargement and the presence of a large polyploid cells called Reed-Sternberg cells.

HOLISTIC A practice of medicine that focuses on the whole patient, and addresses the social, emotional, and spiritual needs of a patient as well as their physical treatment.

HOMEOPATH A homeopathic physician.

HOMEOPATHIC Healthcare practice that uses remedies and treatments that cause similar effects to the symptoms they are intended to treat in an effort to stimulate the natural immune response of the body.

HOMEOPATHIC REMEDY A substance used to treat illnesses that manifest symptoms similar to those that the remedy itself causes, but administered in extremely diluted doses to prevent any toxic effects.

HOMEOPATHY A holistic system of treatment developed in the eighteenth century. It is based on the idea that substances that produce symptoms of sickness in healthy people will have a curative effect when given in very dilute quantities to sick people who exhibit those same symptoms. Homeopathic remedies are believed to stimulate the body's own healing processes.

HOMEOSTASIS The statch the body has reached its optimal level of internal balance and stability.

HOMOCYSTEINE An sulfur-containing amino acid.

HONOKIOL A compound derived from magnolia that is used in some Japanese herbal preparations as a mild tranquilizer. Honokiol may also be useful in treating lung cancer.

HOOK-UP A state of effortless connection with a life-enhancing force. Trager practitioners enter a state of hook-up before working with clients in order to focus on their needs. Trager himself described hook-up as a meditative process of "becoming one with the energy force that surrounds all living things."

HORDEOLUM The medical term for stye; an infection or small abscess formation in the hair follicle glands of the eyelids.

HORMONE REPLACEMENT THERAPY (HRT) Also called estrogen replacement therapy, this controversial treatment is used to relieve the discomforts of menopause. Estrogen and another female hormone, progesterone, are usually taken together to replace the estrogen no longer made by the body. It has the added effect of stopping bone loss that occurs at menopause.

HORMONE THERAPY Treatment for prostate and breast cancer, that involves reducing the levels of the male hormone testosterone, so that the growth of the prostate cancer cells is inhibited.

HORMONE A chemical messenger secreted by a gland and released into the blood, where it travels to distant cells to exert an effect.

HOT FLASH A temporary sensation of warmth that starts in the chest and radiates into the neck and face, usually associated with the menopause in women. It is sometimes called a hot flush.

HUBBARD TANK A large water tank or tub used for underwater exercises.

HUMAN CHORIONIC GONADOTROPIN (HCG) A hormone produced by the placenta during pregnancy.

HUMAN IMMUNODEFICIENCY VIRUS (HIV) A transmissible retrovirus that causes AIDS in humans. Two forms of HIV are now recognized: HIV-1, which causes most cases of AIDS in Europe, North and South America, and most parts of Africa; and HIV-2, which is chiefly found in West African patients.

HUMAN PAPILLOMAVIRUS (HPV) A virus that causes common warts of the hands and feet, as well as lesions in the genital and vaginal area. More than 50 types of HPV have been identified, some of which are linked to cancerous and precancerous conditions, including cancer of the cervix.

HUNTINGTON'S CHOREA A hereditary disease that typically appears in midlife, marked by gradual loss of brain function and voluntary movement. Some of its symptoms resemble those of schizophrenia.

HUNTINGTON'S DISEASE A rare hereditary disease that causes progressive chorea (jerky muscle movements) and mental deterioration that ends in dementia. Huntington's symptoms usually appear in patients in their 40s. Also called Huntington's chorea.

HYDROGEN PEROXIDE A colorless, unstable compound of hydrogen and oxygen (H_2O_2). An aqueous solution of hydrogen peroxide is used as an antiseptic and bleaching agent.

HYDROGENATED FAT An unsaturated fat, commonly vegetable oil, that is processed with high heat and hydrogen to make it solid at room temperature. Margarine is a common hydrogenated fat.

HYDROTHERAPY A family of therapies that treat illness by using water either externally or internally.

HYPERALIMENTATION A method of refeeding anorexics by infusing liquid nutrients and electrolytes directly into central veins through a catheter.

HYPERAROUSAL A state or condition of muscular and emotional tension produced by hormones released during the fight-or-flight reaction.

HYPERBARIC OXYGEN THERAPY (HBO) A form of oxygen therapy in which the patient breathes oxygen in a pressurized chamber.

HYPEREMESIS Severe vomiting during pregnancy. Hyperemesis appears to increase a woman's risk of postpartum depression.

HYPERGLYCEMIA A condition characterized by excessively high levels of glucose in the blood. It occurs when the body does not have enough insulin or cannot use the insulin it does have to turn glucose into energy.

HYPERHIDROSIS Excessive sweating. Hyperhidrosis can be caused by heat, overactive thyroid glands, strong emotion, menopause, or infection.

HYPERKALEMIA An abnormally high level of potassium in the blood.

HYPERLIPIDEMIA A condition characterized by abnormally high levels of lipids in blood plasma.

HYPERMAGNESEMIA A condition in which the levels of magnesium in body fluids are too high. It is almost always caused by a combination of low calcium levels and taking too much magnesium as a dietary supplement. Patients with hypermagnesemia may have central nervous system depression, muscle weakness, fatigue, or sleepiness.

HYPERMETABOLIC Conditions that increase the rate of metabolism, such as fever and hyperthyroidism.

HYPERPLASIA A condition where cells, such as those making up the prostate gland, rapidly divide abnormally and cause the organ to become enlarged.

HYPERPLASTIC OBESITY Excessive weight gain in childhood, characterized by an increase in the number of new fat cells.

HYPERREFLEXIA Reflexes that are abnormally brisk.

HYPERSENSITIVITY The state where even a tiny amount of allergen can cause severe allergic reactions.

HYPERSOMNIA An abnormal increase of 25% or more in time spent sleeping. Individuals with hypersomnia usually have excessive daytime sleepiness.

HYPERTENSION Abnormally high arterial blood pressure, which if left untreated can lead to heart disease and stroke.

HYPERTHYROIDISM A condition characterized by abnormal over-functioning of the thyroid glands. Patients are hypermetabolic, lose weight, are nervous, have muscular weakness and fatigue, sweat more, and have increased urination and bowel movements. Also called thyrotoxicosis.

HYPERTROPHIC OBESITY Excessive weight gain in adulthood, characterized by expansion of already existing fat cells.

HYPERTROPHY A technical term for enlargement, as in BPH (benign prostatic hypertrophy).

HYPERURICEMIA High levels of uric acid in the bloodstream.

HYPNAGOGIC HALLUCINATION A vivid, dream-like hallucination, such as the sensation of falling, that occurs at the onset of sleep.

HYPNOSIS A sleeplike condition that can be artificially induced in people, in which they are susceptible to suggestions from the hypnotist.

HYPOCALCEMIA Calcium deficiency in the blood.

HYPOCRETINS Chemicals secreted in the hypothalamus that regulate the sleep/wake cycle.

HYPOGLYCEMIA A condition characterized by abnormally low levels of glucose in the blood.

HYPOKALEMIA An abnormally low level of potassium in the bloodstream.

HYPOMAGNESEMIA A condition characterized by an abnormally low concentration of magnesium in the blood.

HYPOMANIA A milder form of mania that is characteristic of bipolar II disorder.

HYPONATREMIA A condition characterized by an abnormally low concentration of sodium in the blood.

HYPOPNEA Shallow or excessively slow breathing usually caused by partial closure of the upper airway during sleep.

HYPOTHALAMUS The part of the brain that controls the endocrine system.

HYPOTHYROIDISM A condition that is characterized by decreased activity of the thyroid gland (a hormone-producing gland at the front of the neck) that often results in weight gain, tiredness, dry skin, and other symptoms.

HYPOTONIC Hypotonic refers to a condition called hypotonia, in which fine motor control is floppy, without tone.

HYSTERECTOMY Surgical removal of the uterus.

I

ICTERUS Another name for jaundice.

IDEAL WEIGHT Weight corresponding to the lowest death rate for individuals of a specific height, gender, and age.

IDIOPATHIC Of unknown origin.

IEP Individualized Education Plan. Under federal law governing special education, every child in public schools who is determined through assessment to have special mental disability needs has an IEP. An IEP is typically developed by a team of professionals that may include special education teachers, physical, occupational and speech therapists, psychologists, parents or guardians, and others who may be called on to provide expertise. The team meets at least once a year to set goals for the next school year and to assess progress on already established goals. Parents who are not satisfied with school-based assessments have the right to ask for independent assessments that must be paid for by the school system.

ILLITE A family of hydrous potassium aluminosilicate clays, characterized by a three-layer structure and a gray, light green, or yellow-brown color. The name is derived from Illinois, where these clays were first classified in 1937. French green clay belongs to this group of clays.

IMMUNE FUNCTION The body's defense system against bacteria, viruses and fungi, and any malfunction of the organism.

IMMUNE RESPONSE The protective reaction by the immune system against foreign antigens (substances that the body perceives as potentially dangerous). The immune system combats disease by neutralizing or destroying antigens.

IMMUNE SUPPRESSING Anything that reduces the activity of the immune system.

IMMUNE SYSTEM The system of specialized organs, lymph nodes, and blood cells throughout the body that work together to defend the body against foreign invaders (bacteria, viruses, fungi, etc.).

IMMUNOCOMPROMISED Having a damaged immune system.

IMMUNODEFICIENCY A condition in which the body's immune response is damaged, weakened, or is not functioning properly.

IMMUNOFLUORESCENT ASSAY A laboratory technique using a fluorescent dye and a special microscope to identify the cause of an infection.

IMMUNOGLOBULIN G (IGG) Immunoglobulin type gamma, the most common type found in the blood and tissue fluids.

IMMUNOGLOBULIN Any of several classes of proteins in the blood that function as antibodies.

IMMUNOGLOBULINS A group of globulin proteins that function as antibodies.

IMMUNOSUPPRESSIVE Anything that acts to suppress or weaken the body's immune system, thus making it more susceptible to disease.

IMMUNOTHERAPY Treatment of cancer by stimulating the body's immune defense system.

IMPACTED TOOTH Any tooth that is prevented from reaching its normal position in the mouth by another tooth, bone, or soft tissue.

IMPETIGO A bacterial infection of the skin characterized by skin blistering.

IMPOTENCT Unable to achieve or maintain an erection of the penis.

IN VITRO TESTING A test performed in a lab setting rather than in a human or animal organism. The test may involve living tissue or cells, but takes place out of the body.

IN VITRO An artificial environment; not in a living organism.

INCARCERATED HERNIA A hernia of the bowel that can not return to its normal place without manipulation or surgery.

INCONTINENCE A hernia of the bowel that can not return to its normal place without manipulation or surgery.

INCONTINENTIA PIGMENTI SYNDROME (IPS) An inherited skin disorder characterized by blistered lesions in infancy, which heal but leave uneven pigmentation of the skin.

INCUBATION PERIOD The time period between exposure to an infectious agent, such as a virus or bacteria, and the appearance of symptoms of illness. Also called the latent period.

INDEX CASE The first case of a contagious disease in a group or population that serves to call attention to the presence of the disease.

INDOCYANIN GREEN ANGIOGRAPHY A sensitive method for examining retinal blood vessels.

INFERTILITY Inability to have children, which may occur as a result of pelvic infections.

INFEST To be parasitic in a host.

INFLAMMATION A localized reaction to tissue injury or damage, usually characterized by pain, swelling, and redness.

INFLUENZA An infectious disease caused by a virus that affects the respiratory system, causing fever, congestion, muscle aches, and headaches.

INFUSION A medicine or herbal preparation made by steeping plant parts or other substances in water to extract their medicinal principles.

INHIBITION Restraint of or interference with a biological process, such as the clumping of blood cells. In the Alexander technique, inhibition refers to the moment in an Alexander lesson when the student refrains from beginning a movement in order to avoid tensing the muscles.

INK BAG The part of a cuttlefish that contains their dye, also known as sepia.

INNERVATE To supply a part of the body with nerves. For example, the vagus nerve supplies nerve function to the eardrum; therefore, we say that the eardrum is innervated by the vagus nerve.

INSECTICIDE Any substance used to kill insects.

INSOMNIA A sleep disorder characterized by inability either to fall asleep or to stay asleep.

INSULIN RESISTANCE Also called metabolic syndrome, a condition in which the body fails to properly respond to the insulin it produces.

INSULIN A hormone or chemical produced by the pancreas that is needed by cells of the body in order to use glucose (sugar), a major source of energy for the human body.

INSULIN A hormone produced by the pancreas that is needed by cells of the body to use glucose (sugar), the body's main source of energy.

INTERFERON A substance proved to be necessary in the body to help fight cancer cells.

INTERMEDIATE HOST The host organism for an intermediate (larval) stage in the life cycle of a parasite.

INTERMITTENT CLAUDICATION Cramp-like leg pain and weakness caused by poor circulation of blood to leg muscles and brought on by walking.

INTERNAL DERANGEMENT A condition in which the cartilage disc in the temporomandibular joint lies in front of its proper position.

INTERNATIONAL UNIT (IU) A measurement of biological activity in which one IU is equal to one mg (milligram).

INTERSTITIAL CYSTITIS A chronic inflammatory condition of the bladder involving symptoms of bladder pain, frequent urination, and burning during urination. Diagnosis is confirmed by cystoscopy with the bladder distended by fluid.

INTERSTITIAL SPACES Areas of the body occurring outside the vessels or organs, between the cells.

INTESTINAL DYSBIOSIS An imbalance among the various microorganisms that live in the digestive tract.

INTESTINAL FLORA The beneficial bacteria that live in the digestive tract and aid digestion of food.

INTESTINAL MICROFLORA The bacteria and other microorganisms that live in the human gastrointestinal tract.

INTESTINES Also called the bowels and divided into the large and small intestine, they extend from the stomach to the anus, where waste products exit the body. The small intestine is about 20 ft (6.1 m) long and the large intestine, about 5 ft (1.5 m) long.

INTRACELLULAR Inside the cells.

INTRAVENOUS (IV) THERAPY Administration of fluids through the veins.

INTRAVENOUS FLUIDS Nutrients and medicines that can be fed quickly and directly into the veins.

INTRAVENOUS Into a vein; a needle is inserted into a vein in the back of the hand, inside the elbow, or some other location on the body.

INTUBATION A procedure in which a tube is inserted through the mouth and into the trachea to keep the airway open and to help a patient breathe.

INULIN A starchlike complex sugar obtained from chicory roots that is used to improve the texture of processed foods.

IQ Intelligence quotient; a measure of intellectual functioning determined by performance on standardized intelligence tests.

IRIS The circular membrane that forms the colored portion of the eye and expands or contracts around the pupil.

IRRADIATION The act of exposing something to ultraviolet rays or x rays.

IRRITABLE BOWEL SYNDROME (IBS) A condition affecting the small and large intestine, usually associated with emotional stress. There may be complaints of diarrhea and pain the lower abdomen.

ISCHEMIC Refers to ischemia, a decrease in the blood supply to an area of the body caused by obstruction or constriction of blood vessels.

ISLES OF LANGERHANS Cellular masses of tissue in a space within the pancreas that secrete insulin.

ISOFLAVONE A phytoestrogen found in soybeans and other plants that sometimes is used as an estrogen supplement.

ISOMERS Two chemicals identical in chemical composition (contain the same atoms in the same amounts) that have differing structures. The normal prion protein and the infectious prion protein are conformational isomers of one another. They have the same chemical structures, but for some reason, assume different shapes.

ISOTOPE Any of two or more species of atoms of a chemical element with the same atomic number and nearly identical chemical behavior but with differing atomic mass and physical properties.

ISOTRETINOIN A drug that decreases sebum production and dries up acne pimples.

ITAI-ITAI DISEASE The first reported cases of cadmium poisoning in the world, seen in Japan circa 1950. The name means **OUCH-OUCH** and represents the sufferers' screams of pain. The disease caused bone and kidney defects. It was caused by cadmium pollution from mines.

J

JACUZZI A trademark name for a whirlpool bath.

JARISCH-HERXHEIMER REACTION A temporary reaction to penicillin treatment for syphilis that includes fever, chills, and worsening of the skin rash or chancre.

JAUNDICE A condition characterized by higher-than-normal levels of bilirubin in the bloodstream and an accompanying yellowing of the skin and eyes.

JOINT A structure that holds two or more bones together.

JUNGIAN ANALYSIS A method of psychological treatment where the patient strives to understand the internal, often mythic images in his or her thoughts and dreams.

K

KAHUNA A native Hawaiian priest or healer.

KAMPO Traditional Japanese system of herbal medicine.

KAPOSI'S SARCOMA A cancer of the skin, mucous membranes, and blood vessels that begins as soft brown or purplish red lesions on the skin. It occurs most often in men with AIDS.

KARATE A native Okinawan fighting style brought to Japan in the early twentieth century.

KAVALACTONES Medically active compounds in kava root that act as local anesthetics in the mouth and as minor tranquilizers

KELOID An overgrowth of scar tissue that does not resolve.

KERATOCONUS An eye condition in which the central part of the cornea bulges outward, interfering with normal vision. Usually both eyes are affected.

KESHAN DISEASE A form of heart disease in children, first discovered in the Keshan region of China. It may represent a selenium deficiency syndrome.

KETOACIDOSIS A condition due to starvation or uncontrolled Type I diabetes. Ketones are acid compounds that form in the blood when the body breaks down fats and proteins. Symptoms include abdominal pain, vomiting, rapid breathing, extreme tiredness, and drowsiness.

KETOCONAZOLE An antifungal medication.

KETOGENIC DIET A diet that supplies an abnormally high amount of fat, and small amounts of carbohydrates and protein.

KETONES Poisonous acidic chemicals produced by the body when fat instead of glucose is burned for energy. Breakdown of fat occurs when not enough insulin is present to channel glucose into body cells.

KETOSIS An abnormal accumulation of ketones in the body, usually found in people who have diabetes mellitus or who are fasting, pregnant, starving, or on a high fat diet. Ketosis can cause serious side effects, including dehydration, kidney stones, gall stones, inflammation of the pancreas, decreased bone density, vitamin deficiency, eye problems.

KIDNEY DIALYSIS A process by which blood is filtered through a dialysis machine to remove waste products that would normally be removed by the kidneys. The filtered blood is then circulated back into the patient. This process is also called renal dialysis.

KIDNEY STONE A hard mass that occurs in the kidney, a kidney stone can cause pain, bleeding, obstruction, or infection. Stones are primarily made up of calcium. Also called a renal calculus or nephrolith.

KINESIOLOGY The study of the anatomy and physiology of body movement, particularly in relation to therapy.

KNEE AND ANKLE JERK REFLEXES Normal reflexes elicited usually by testing with a reflex hammer and demonstrating, by being present, a healthy and intact nervous system.

KOOSH BALL A lightweight, **FURRY** ball of rubber band material used in Davis technique exercises for retraining neuropathways in the brain of a person with dyslexia.

KOPLIK'S SPOTS Tiny spots occurring inside the mouth, especially on the inside of the cheek. These spots consist of minuscule white dots (like grains of salt or sand) set onto a reddened bump. Unique to measles.

KUNDALINI YOGA A type of yoga that focuses on the body's innate psychospiritual energy (*kundalini shakti* or "serpent power" in Sanskrit) through breathing exercises, meditation, yoga postures, and chanting. Its goal is to empower the individual's consciousness to merge with universal consciousness.

KUNDALINI In Indian yoga, a vital force or energy at the base of the spine that is activated or released by certain yoga postures or breathing techniques. This release is called the **AWAKENING** term: of the kundalini. Some Westerners have had kundalini experiences that were diagnosed as psychotic episodes or symptoms of schizophrenia.

KUNG FU Another name for qigong; today it more commonly means a Chinese martial arts practice.

L

LACERATION Also called a tear. Separation of skin or other tissue by a tremendous force, producing irregular edges.

LACTIC ACID A by-product of muscular work out; slow clearance of lactic acid from tissues is associated with muscular fatigue.

LACTOBACILLUS The healthy bacteria found in the intestine.

LACTOFERRIN A protein found in colostrum that carries iron to red blood cells and appears to have anti-cancer activity.

LACTO-OVO VEGETARIAN People who do not eat meat, but do include dairy products and eggs in their diets.

LACTOSE INTOLERANCE An inability to properly digest milk and dairy products.

LACTOSE A sugar found in milk and milk products. Some people are lactose intolerant, meaning they have trouble digesting lactose. Lactose intolerance can produce symptoms resembling those of IBS.

LAETRILE The chemical amygdalin, obtained from apricots, peaches, and bitter almonds.

LAMINITIS A veterinary term for inflammation in the foot of a horse.

LANCEOLATE A narrow, leaf shape that is longer than it is wide, and pointed at the end.

LANUGO A soft, downy body hair that develops on the chest and arms of anorexic women.

LAPACHOL The name given to the active ingredient in pau d'arco, which appears to have some anti-cancer properties.

LAPAROSCOPE An optical or fiberoptic instrument that is inserted by incision in the abdominal wall and is used to view the interior of the peritoneal cavity.

LAPAROSCOPY An examination of the interior of the abdomen with a lighted tube called a laparoscope.

LAPAROTOMY A surgical procedure in which the abdominal cavity is opened up.

LARYNX Also known as the voice box, the larynx is the part of the airway that lies between the pharynx and the trachea. It is composed of cartilage that contains the apparatus for voice production—the vocal cords and the muscles and ligaments that move the cords.

LASER-ASSISTED IN-SITU KERATOMILEUSIS (LASIK) A procedure that uses a cutting tool and a laser to modify the cornea and correct moderate to high levels of myopia (nearsightedness).

LATCHING A term used to describe a baby's mouth hold on his or her mother's nipple.

LATENT PERIOD Also called incubation period, the time between infection with a disease-causing agent and the development of disease.

LATENT A nonactive virus in a dormant state within a cell. Herpes virus is latent in the nervous system.

LATERAL NAIL FOLD The fold of skin along the side of the nail.

LAW OF SIMILARS The basic principle of homeopathic medicine that governs the selection of a specific remedy. It holds that a substance of natural origin that produces certain symptoms in a healthy person will cure those same symptoms in a sick person.

LAWS OF CURE A set of three rules used by homeopaths to assess the progress of a patient's recovery.

LAXATIVE Substance or medication that encourages a bowel movement.

LAZY BOWEL SYNDROME An inability to have a bowel movement without the aid of chemical laxatives.

LDL CHOLESTEROL Low-density lipoprotein cholesterol is the primary cholesterol molecule. High levels of LDL increase the risk of coronary heart disease. LDL is nicknamed bad cholesterol.

LEFT BRAIN The left cerebral hemisphere, which controls activity on the right side of the body in humans. The left brain is thought to be specialized for language use and mathematical calculation; it is also associated with logical analysis, fact-based decisions, and planning or organization. A maze is considered a left-brain puzzle.

LEGUMES A family of plants, including beans, peas, and lentils, that bear edible seeds in pods. These seeds are high in protein, fiber, and other nutrients.

LEIOMYOMA A benign tumor composed of muscle tissue. Leiomyomas in the uterus are sometimes called fibroids.

LEISHMANIASIS A disease of the tropics transmitted by sandflies.

LEMON BALM A herb with antiviral properties that is also used to alleviate anxiety or insomnia. The botanical name for lemon balm is *Melissa officinalis*.

LENS The transparent, elastic, curved structure behind the iris (colored part of the eye) that helps focus light on the retina. Also refers to any device that bends light waves.

LENTINAN A compound found in shiitake mushrooms that helps to boost the immune system.

LEPROSY A chronic, contagious skin and nervous system disease that leads, in the more serious form, to numbness, muscle weakness, and paralysis. Leprosy is sometimes referred to as Hansen's disease.

LEPTIN A protein hormone that affects feeding behavior and hunger in humans. At present it is thought that obesity in humans may result in part from insensitivity to leptin.

LESION A disruption of the normal structure and function of a tissue by an injury or disease process. Wounds, sores, rashes, and boils are all lesions.

LEUCINE An amino acid produced by the hydrolysis of proteins by pancreatic enzymes during digestion, and by putrefaction of nitrogenous organic matter.

LEUKOCYTES Also called white blood cells, leukocytes fight infection and boost the immune system.

LEUKORRHEA White discharge from the vagina, normally occurring during the menstrual cycle, pregnancy, lactation, and menopause. A change in color, amount, or odor is a symptom of a reproductive tract disorder.

LEUKOTRIENES Substances that are produced by white blood cells in response to antigens and contribute to inflammatory and asthmatic reactions.

LEVODOPA A naturally occurring amino acid that is converted to dopamine in the brain; the primary treatment for Parkinson's disease.

LICHEN PLANUS A noncancerous, chronic, itchy skin disease that causes small, flat purple plaques on wrists, forearm, and ankles.

LICHEN A fungus that grows a symbiotic relationship with algae.

LICORICE ROOT An herb believed to be helpful in treating ulcers, respiratory problems, and a variety of other conditions.

LIGAMENT A type of tough, fibrous tissue that connects bones or cartilage and provides support and strength to joints.

LIGASE CHAIN REACTION A laboratory technique for detecting sexually transmitted disease organisms in urine by rapidly copying and recopying the organism's DNA, thus making the presence of infection easier to detect.

LIGATION Tying off a blood vessels or other tube with wire or suture, usually during surgery.

LIGNANS Chemicals found in plants that have estrogen-like, liver-protective, and anti-inflammatory activities.

LIMBIC SYSTEM A group of structures in the brain that includes the hypothalamus, amygdala, and hippocampus. The limbic system plays an important part in regulation of human moods and emotions.

LINDANE An organic chloride, neurotoxic insecticide that kills lice.

LINOLEIC ACID An essential fatty acid that is found in sesame oil.

LIPIDS A group of organic compounds consisting of fats, oils, and related substances that, along with proteins and carbohydrates, are the structural components of living cells.

LIPOPOLYSACCHARIDE A complex carbohydrate with lipids (organic fats and waxes) attached to its molecule.

LIPOPROTEIN(A) A type of bad cholesterol that increases the risk of heart attack or stroke.

LIPOSUCTION The surgical removal of fatty tissue underneath the skin through a small incision in the skin.

LIPOTROPIC Substances that help prevent or correct excessive fat deposits in liver.

LITHOTRIPSY A nonsurgical technique for removing gallstones by breaking them apart with high-frequency sound waves.

LIVER ENCEPHALOPATHY A condition in which the brain is affected by a buildup of toxic substances that would normally be removed by the liver. The condition occurs when the liver is too severely damaged to cleanse the blood effectively.

LOBECTOMY Surgical removal of an entire lobe of the lung.

LOBELINE An alkaloid compound found in lobelia that resembles nicotine in its pharmacological effects. It has been studied by researchers in the field of tobacco addiction and drug abuse.

LOCKJAW Refers to a common name given to the disease taken from its most pervasive symptom.

LODESTONE A variety of magnetite that possesses magnetic polarity.

LOTUS SUTRA One of the most sacred texts of Buddhism, regarded as a summary of the supreme Buddhist teaching that leads one directly to enlightenment.

LOW SELF The Huna term for the subconscious mind. The word "low" does not mean inferior in value, but refers only to what is below the level of consciousness.

LOW-DENSITY LIPOPROTEIN LDL, the so-called bad cholesterol.

LOWER BURNER A TCM term for the kidneys.

LOWER ESOPHAGEAL SPHINCTER (LES) Muscle at the base of the esophagus that opens to allow food to enter the stomach and closes to prevent reflux back into the esophagus.

LOZENGE A medicated candy intended to be dissolved slowly in the mouth to soothe irritated tissues of the throat.

LUES MALIGNA A skin disorder of secondary syphilis in which areas of ulcerated and dying tissue are formed. It occurs most frequently in HIV-positive patients.

LUMBAGO Lower back pain caused by rheumatoid arthritis, muscle strain, osteoarthritis, or a ruptured spinal disk.

LUMBAR PUNCTURE (LP) A procedure in which the doctor inserts a small needle into the spinal cavity in the lower back to withdraw spinal fluid for testing. Also known as a spinal tap.

LUMBAR SPINE The segment of the human spine above the pelvis that is involved in low back pain. There are five vertebrae, or bones, in the lumbar spine.

LUMBAR VERTEBRAE Five bones in the lower spine.

LUMBOSACRAL Referring to the lower part of the backbone or spine.

LUMPECTOMY Surgical procedure in which only the cancerous tumor is removed, together with a rim of normal tissue.

LUNGS In TCM, the parts of the body associated with breathing, such as the lungs and the skin. It also regulates the movement of water and qi through the body channels.

LUPUS ERYTHEMATOSUS An autoimmune disease that can damage skin, joints, kidneys, and other organs.

LUPUS NEPHRITIS Kidney damage associated with Systemic lupus erythematosis, an autoimmune disease. The kidney damage is gradual, but leads to complete kidney failure.

LUTEIN An antioxidant carotenoid found in large quantities in dark-green, leafy vegetables such as spinach and kale. Lutein is deposited on the lens and macula of the eye where it protects cells from damage caused by ultraviolet and blue light.

LUX The International System unit for measuring illumination, equal to one lumen per square meter.

LYME BORRELIOSIS Another name for Lyme disease.

LYME DISEASE An acute recurrent inflammatory disease involving one or a few joints, believed to be transmitted by a tickborne virus. The condition was originally described in the community of Lyme, Connecticut, but has also been reported in other parts of the United States and other countries. Knees and other large joints are most commonly involved with local inflammation and swelling.

LYMPH NODES Small, bean–shaped masses of tissue scattered along the lymphatic system that act as filters: removing fluids, bacteria, or cancer cells that travel through the lymph system. Breast cancer cells in the lymph nodes under the arm or in the chest are a sign that the cancer has spread, and that it might recur.

LYMPH An alkaline fluid found in the lymphatic vessels that is usually clear, transparent fluid, unless it is draining from the intestines when it then appears milky.

LYMPHATIC SYSTEM The vessels, nodes, and organs that carry the clear lymph fluid, containing lymphocytes and other white blood cells, throughout the body and that filter the blood to remove dead cells and other debris.

LYMPHOCYTE A type of white blood cell that is important in the formation of antibodies and that can be used to monitor the health of AIDS patients.

LYMPHOMA A diverse group of cancers of the lymphatic system characterized by abnormal growth of lymphatic cells. Two general types are commonly recognized—Hodgkin's disease and non-Hodgkin's lymphoma.

M

MACROBIOTICS A diet emphasizing grains, certain vegetables, legumes, and fish.

MACROCYTIC ANEMIA A condition caused by cobalamin deficiency, which is characterized by red blood cells that are too few, too fragile, and abnormally large.

MACROPHAGE A large white blood cell that engulfs and digests foreign invaders, such as bacteria and viruses, in an attempt to stop them from causing disease within the body.

MACULA The central part of the retina where the rods and cones are densest.

MACULAR DEGENERATION Deterioration of part of the retina, causing progressive loss of vision. This is the most common cause of blindness in the elderly.

MAGNETIC RESONANCE IMAGING (MRI) An imaging technique that uses a large circular magnet and radio waves to generate signals from atoms in the body. These signals are used to construct images of internal structures.

MAGNETISM (Animal magnetism) A discredited theory put forth by Viennese physician Franz Anton Mesmer stating that all persons possess magnetic forces that can be used to influence magnetic fluid in other people and therefore effect healing. Mesmer opened a clinic in Paris in 1878, and appeared to cure people apparently suffering from hysterical conditions, such as emotionally caused paralysis.

MAJOR MINERAL One of three important nonorganic elements in human nutrition, distinguished from trace elements (minor minerals) and electrolytes. Magnesium is a major mineral, along with calcium and phosphorus.

MALABSORPTION The inability of the digestive tract to absorb all the nutrients from food due to some malfunction or disability.

MALADAPTIVE Unsuitable; maladaptive behavior is behavior that is inappropriate to a given situation.

MALATHION An organic phosphate, neurotoxic insecticide that kills lice.

MALIGNANT HYPERTHERMIA A rare, inherited condition in which a person develops a very high fever when given certain anesthetics or muscle relaxants in preparation for surgery.

MALIGNANT MELANOMA The most serious of the three types of skin cancer, malignant melanoma arises from the melanocytes, the skin cells that produce the pigment melanin.

MALIGNANT Cancerous.

MALNUTRITION Any disorder of nutrition caused by insufficient or unbalanced diet that can result in impaired absorption or use of foods.

MALOCCLUSION The misalignment of opposing teeth in the upper and lower jaws.

MAMMOGRAPHY X–ray imaging of the breast that can often detect lesions in the tissue too small or too deep to be felt.

MANA The Hawaiian word for life energy. According to Huna, mana can be transferred from the conscious mind into parts of the body needing healing or into talismans or crystals to charge them with energy.

MANDALA A design, usually circular, that appears in religion and art. In Buddhism and Hinduism, the mandala has religious ritual purposes and serves as a yantra (a geometric emblem or instrument of contemplation).

MANDIBLE The medical name for the lower jaw.

MANIA Hyperelevated, or excessively excited mood.

MANOMETRY A technique for measuring changes in pressure.

MANTRA A sacred word or formula that is repeated as an incantation to focus the mind and spirit, or to induce a mystical state.

MARTIAL ARTS Group of diverse activities originating from the ancient fighting techniques of the Orient.

MASSAGE A rubbing or kneading with hands or other parts of the body to stimulate circulation, make joints more supple, and relieve tension.

MAST CELLS A type of immune system cell that is found in the lining of the nasal passages and eyelids and participates in the allergic response by releasing histamine.

MASTITIS Inflammation of the breast.

MASTOID PROCESS The protrusions of bone behind the ears at the base of the skull.

MATERIA MEDICA A Latin phrase that means "the materials of medicine." In homeopathy, a *materia medica* is a book that lists the various homeopathic remedies together with the symptoms that they treat.

MATURATION The process by which stem cells transform from immature cells without a specific function into a particular type of blood cell with defined functions.

MAZE A network of paths or passages intended to confuse, with numerous choices at different points. Unlike a labyrinth, a maze often has high walls intended to block the visitor's line of sight.

MCCUNE-ALBRIGHT SYNDROME (MCAS) A genetic disorder that includes bone, endocrine, and skin abnormalities. Some individuals with this syndrome show the effects of excessive secretion of pituitary growth hormone.

MEDIAN NERVE A nerve which runs through the wrist and into the hand. It provides sensation and some movement to the hand, the thumb, the index finger, the middle finger, and half of the ring finger.

MEDICINE BUNDLE A leather bag or animal skin in which a Native American healer carries herbs, stones, and various ritual objects as a sign of his or her healing powers.

MEDITATION A practice of concentrated focus upon a sound, object, visualization, the breath, movement, or attention itself in order to increase awareness of the present moment, reduce stress, promote relaxation, and enhance personal and spiritual growth.

MEDITERRANEAN DIET A low-cholesterol diet that emphasizes vegetables and fish, and limits consumption of red meat and eggs.

MEFLOQUINE An antimalarial drug that was developed by the United States Army in the early 1980s. Today, malaria resistance to this drug has become a problem in some parts of Asia (especially Thailand and Cambodia).

MEGA-DOSES Very high doses of vitamins intended to treat a variety of ailments, as recommended by ortho-molecular practitioners.

MEGALOBLAST A large erythroblast (a red marrow cell that synthesizes hemoglobin).

MEGALOBLASTIC ANEMIA A form of anemia involving large, irregularly shaped red blood cells, called megaloblasts, and related to vitamin B_{12} and folic acid deficiency.

MELANIN A pigment that creates hair, skin, and eye color. Melanin also protects the body by absorbing ultraviolet light.

MELANOMA A highly malignant form of skin cancer associated with overexposure to ultraviolet radiation from sunlight.

MELATONIN A naturally occurring hormone involved in regulating the body's internal clock.

MENARCHE The first menstrual period or the establishment of the menstrual function.

MÉNIÈRE'S DISEASE A disease of the labyrinth in the ear, characterized by dizziness, hearing loss, ringing in the ears, and nausea.

MENINGES The three-layer membranous covering of the brain and spinal cord, composed of the dura, arachnoid, and pia. It provides protection for the brain and spinal cord, as well as housing many blood vessels and participating in the appropriate flow of CSF.

MENINGITIS An infection or inflammation of the membranes that cover the brain and spinal cord. It is usually caused by bacteria or a virus.

MENISCOCYTOSIS Another word for sickle cell disease.

MENISCUS A wedge of cartilage that separates the articulating bones in certain joints.

MENOPAUSE The permanent cessation of menstruation; also called the change of life or climacteric.

MENORRHAGIA Heavy and painful periods.

MENSTRUATION A monthly occurrence of blood and uterine material discharge from a woman's vagina while she is in her reproductive years.

MENTASTICS The active phase of Trager therapy. Mentastics are a form of movement reeducation in which clients learn to reexperience movement as pleasurable and positive.

MERCURY A metallic element that is a silvery liquid at ordinary temperatures.

MERIDIAN In traditional Chinese medicine, the channels which run beneath the skin through which the body's energy (chi) flows. Also refers to a section of a sphere, such as the line connecting the North and South Poles on the face of the Earth.

MESOTHELIOMA A tumor consisting of spindle cells or fibrous tissue, usually in the lining of the lung.

META-ANALYSIS An analysis of previous medical studies.

METABOLIC Refers to the chemical reactions in living organisms.

METABOLISM The physical and chemical changes that allow the body to grow, function, and to convert food into energy.

METABOLITE A by-product of the physical and chemical change process known as metabolism.

METABOLIZE For food and nutritional components, to convert food into energy and then break it down into simpler substances for excretion.

METASTASIS The spreading of cancer from the original site to other parts of the body.

METATES Stone slabs used by Native Americans to grind corn and other grains.

METFORMIN An anti-diabetic drug of the biguanide class. This drug increases the sensitivity of cells to insulin, but is capable of causing very severe adverse reactions, including lactic acidosis and anemia.

METHAMPHETAMINE A form of amphetamine that is a potent stimulant of the central nervous system and is highly addictive. Slang terms for methamphetamine include "meth," "ice," "speed," and "chalk."

METHANOL A liquid alcohol, used as a solvent or denaturant for ethanol.

METHIONINE An essential sulfur-containing amino acid, found in protein foods.

METRONIDAZOLE An anti-infective agent regarded as the best available drug for treating trichomoniasis. It is sold under the trade names Flagyl and MetroGel.

MIASM In homeopathic theory, a general weakness or predisposition to chronic disease that is transmitted down the generational chain.

MICROANGIOPATHIC Pertaining to disorders of the small blood vessels.

MICROFLORA The bacterial population in the intestine.

MICRONIZED A crystal that is ground to a very fine powder.

MICRONUTRIENT An element essential to health that is required only in very small amounts. Micronutrients are sometimes called trace elements.

MIDDLE EAR The inner portion of the ear made up of an air-filled chamber, which is separated from the outer ear by the tympanic membrane.

MIDDLE SELF The Huna term for the conscious mind, including the ability to reason. The middle self is what others recognize as an individual's personality.

MIGRAINE A very severe headache, often accompanied by nausea and vomiting. It is usually experienced on one side of the head, and may be preceded by visual symptoms.

MILIARY TUBERCULOSIS A form of TB in which the bacillus spreads through all body tissues and organs, producing many thousands of tiny tubercular lesions. Miliary TB is often fatal unless promptly treated.

MILK ALKALI SYNDROME A disorder of the kidneys caused by long-term treatment of ulcers with antacids, particularly alkaline compounds such as sodium bicarbonate, and large amounts of calcium.

MIND'S EYE A term referring to an imaginary point from which the mind views what the eyes look at or what the imagination presents. In dyslexia, the mind's eye is unanchored to one location, and sends many signals to the brain about what it sees, which causes disabling confusion.

MINERALS Inorganic chemical elements that are found in plants and animals and are essential for life. There are two types of minerals: major minerals, which the body requires in large amounts, and trace elements, which the body needs only in minute amounts.

MINI-MENTAL STATUS EXAMINATION (MMSE) A brief test of memory and cognitive function that is used to evaluate the presence and extent of memory loss, and to monitor the effects of treatment for memory loss.

MIOTIC A drug that causes pupils to contract.

MISCARRIAGE Case when a fetus is prematurely ejected from the uterus during pregnancy.

MISO A fermented paste made from soybeans, salt, and rice or barley, used to flavor soups and sauces in Oriental cooking.

MITE An insect parasite belonging to the order Acarina. The organism that causes scabies is a mite.

MITTELSCHMERZ A German word for the pain that some women experience at ovulation.

MIXED HEMISPHERIC DOMINANCE A term later used to describe what was believed to be a difference in the way the mind works in persons with and without dyslexia. It was believed that functions processed in the right half of the brain by a person without dyslexia were sometimes processed in the left half by a person with dyslexia.

MIXED MANIA/MIXED STATE A mental state in which symptoms of both depression and mania occur simultaneously.

MODALITY A factor or circumstance that makes a patient's symptoms better or worse. Modalities include such factors as time of day, room temperature, the patient's level of activity, sleep patterns, etc.

MONACOLIN An HMG-CoA reductase inhibitor, which assists in the lowering of cholesterol levels.

MONOAMINE OXIDASE (MAO) INHIBITORS A group of anti-depressant drugs.

MONOCLONAL ANTIBODY A protein substance that is produced in the laboratory from a single clone of a B-cell, the type of cell of the immune system that makes antibodies. Monoclonal antibodies are used in cancer treatment.

MONOCYTE A large white blood cell that is formed in the bone marrow and spleen.

MONOMER A molecule that can combine with others to form a dimmer or a polymer.

MONONUCLEOSIS A flu-like illness caused by the Epstein-Barr virus.

MOOD DISORDER A group of mental disorders involving a disturbance of mood, along with either a full or partial excessively happy (manic) or extremely sad (depressive) syndrome not caused by any other physical or mental disorder. Mood refers to a prolonged emotion.

MOTHER TINCTURE The first stage in the preparation of a homeopathic remedy, made by soaking a plant, animal, or mineral product in a solution of alcohol.

MOTILITY The movement or capacity for movement of an organism or body organ. Indigestion is sometimes caused by abnormal patterns in the motility of the stomach.

MOTOR NEURON A nerve cell that specifically controls and stimulates voluntary muscles.

MOXIBUSTION A treatment where crushed leaves of the mugwort, or moxa, plant (*Artemisia vulgaris*) are shaped into a cigar-like form that is lit and held directly over the skin of the area being treated.

MRI (MAGNETIC RESONANCE IMAGING) The diagnostic technique which provides high quality cross-sectional images of organs or structures within the body through the use of a high-speed magnetic imaging device.

MUCILAGE A gelatin-like plant substance found in leaves and stems. Any substance that resembles mucilage in having a thick or sticky texture is said to be mucilaginous.

MUCILAGINOUS Having a moist, soft, and sticky quality. The inner rind of slippery elm bark is an example of a mucilaginous plant product.

MUCOPOLYSACCHARIDE An older term for a class of large sugar molecules that are found in cartilage and other forms of connective tissue. Mucopolysaccharides are now called glycosaminoglycans.

MUCOUS MEMBRANES The thin skin layers that line, lubricate and protect body passages and cavities such as the nose.

MUCOUS MEMBRANES Thin sheets of tissue that cover and protect body passages that open to the outside. These membranes secrete mucus and absorb water and various salts.

MUCUS The slippery secretion of the mucous membranes of the respiratory tract.

MUGWORT-SPICE SYNDROME A type of food allergy that occurs in people who are sensitized to mugwort, celery, carrots, and other spices. It often takes the form of a skin rash.

MULLEIN A plant related to the figwort, used by Native Americans to treat inflammations. It is still recommended by naturopaths to reduce the discomfort of swimmer's ear.

MULTIPLE CHEMICAL SENSITIVITY A condition characterized by severe and crippling allergic reactions to commonly used substances, particularly chemicals. Also called environmental illness.

MULTIPLE ENDOCRINE NEOPLASIA Tumor formation characterized by a progressive, abnormal multiplication of cells that are not necessarily malignant in any of the glands that secrete chemicals directly into the blood stream, such as the thyroid gland, adrenal glands, or ovaries.

MULTIPLE SCLEROSIS (MS) A progressive, autoimmune disease of the central nervous system characterized by damage to the myelin sheath that covers nerves. The disease, which causes progressive paralysis, is marked by periods of exacerbation and remission.

MUSCLE BALANCE AND FUNCTION DEVELOPMENT (MBF) A movement therapy that strives to realign body posture through a series of exercises.

MUTATION A change in a gene's DNA. Whether a mutation is harmful is determined by the effect on the product for which the gene codes.

MYALGIA Muscle pain.

MYASTHENIA GRAVIS A muscle weakness that occurs because the body makes antibodies to the natural chemical that facilitates transmission of impulses between the nerve and the muscle.

MYCELIUM Fine thread-like tendrils sent out by a fungus to seek nutrition, capable of invading body organs.

MYCOBACTERIA A group of bacteria that includes *Mycobacterium tuberculosis*, the bacterium that causes tuberculosis, and other forms that cause related illnesses.

MYCOBACTERIUM AVIUM (MAC) INFECTION A type of opportunistic infection that occurs in about 40% of AIDS patients and is regarded as an AIDS-defining disease.

MYELIN A fatty sheath surrounding nerves throughout the body that helps them conduct impulses more quickly.

MYELOGRAPHY A medical test in which a special dye is injected into a nerve to make it visible on an x ray.

MYELOPATHY Any disease of the spinal cord or bone marrow.

MYOCARDIAL INFARCTION Heart attack. Sudden death of part of the heart muscle characterized in most cases by severe, unremitting chest pain.

MYOCARDIUM The thick middle layer of the heart that forms the bulk of the heart wall and contracts as the organ beats.

MYOPATHY Any abnormal condition or disease of muscle tissue, characterized by muscle weakness and wasting.

MYOSIN A protein found in muscle tissue that interacts with another protein called actin during muscle contraction.

MYOSITIS Inflammation of the muscle.

MYOTHERAPY A form of trigger point therapy that relies on deep massage of the trigger points rather than injections to relieve pain.

MYOTONIA The inability to normally relax a muscle after contracting or tightening it.

MYRCENE A compound found in the essential oil of lemongrass that has pain-relieving properties.

MYRINGOTOMY A surgical procedure performed to drain an infected middle ear. A newer type of myringotomy uses a laser instead of a scalpel.

MYXEDEMA A condition that can result from a thyroid gland that produces too little of its hormone. In addition to a decreased metabolic rate, symptoms may include anemia, slow speech, an enlarged tongue, puffiness of the face and hands, loss of hair, coarse and thickened skin, and sensitivity to cold.

N

N.D. OR DOCTOR OF NATUROPATHIC MEDICINE In some states, Naturopathic doctors, medically trained in diagnostics and natural and alternative therapies, are licensed as Naturopathic physicians. In other states, they may be licensed or registered as Naturopathic doctors. They are distinct from other naturopathic doctors, who may be correspondence school trained in traditional alternatives, by being medically trained graduates of accredited programs in naturopathic medicine, and board certified by a state's Department of Health. Information on finding a naturopathic physician may be found at www.naturopathic.org.

N-ACETYLCYSTEINE (NAC) A compound amino acid and antioxidant that protects the liver, supports the immune system, and helps break up mucous.

NAIL PLATE The horny plate covering the tips of the fingers and toes. Commonly called the nail.

NARCOLEPSY A lifelong sleep disorder marked by four symptoms: sudden brief sleep attacks, cataplexy, temporary paralysis, and hallucinations.

NASOGASTRIC INTUBATION Insertion of a tube through the nose and mouth for delivery of food and oxygen.

NASOGASTRIC Tube inserted through the nasal passages into the stomach.

NASOPHARYNX The part of the airway leading into the nose.

NATURAL KILLER (NK) CELL A lymphocyte that acts as a primary immune defense against infection.

NATURALIZED Plants which are introduced in the wild.

NATUROPATHY A type of alternative medicine that does not use surgery or synthetic drugs to treat disease but relies on fasting and special diets to assist the body's healing processes.

NEARSIGHTEDNESS Being able to see more clearly those objects that are near as opposed to those in the distance. Also called myopia.

NECROSIS The death of tissue in response to injury or disease.

NEMATODES Roundworms, which are parasitic intestinal worms resembling earthworms.

NEPHRECTOMY Surgical removal of a kidney.

NEPHRITIS An inflammation or irritation of the kidneys.

NEPHRITIS An inflammation or irritation of the kidney.

NERVE Fibers that carry sensory information, movement stimuli, or both from the brain and spinal cord to other parts of the body and back again. Some nerves, including the vagus nerve, innervate distantly separated parts of the body.

NERVINE A type of medication or herbal preparation given to calm the nerves.

NERVOUS TIC A repetitive, involuntary action, such as the twitching of a muscle or repeated blinking.

NEURAL TUBE DEFECTS (NTDS) A group of birth defects caused by failure of the neural tube to close completely during the formation of the baby's central nervous system. Recent research indicates that methionine deficiency in pregnant women increases the risk of NTDs in their newborns.

NEURALGIA Severe nerve pain.

NEURALLY MEDIATED HYPOTENSION A rapid fall in blood pressure that causes dizziness, blurred vision, and fainting, and is often followed by prolonged fatigue.

NEURASTHENIA Nervous exhaustion. A disorder with symptoms of irritability and weakness, commonly diagnosed in the late 1800s.

NEURASTHENIA Nervous exhaustion; a disorder with symptoms of irritability and weakness, commonly diagnosed in the late 1800s.

NEURODERMATITIS An itchy skin disease (also called lichen simplex chronicus) found in nervous, anxious people.

NEUROFIBRILLARY TANGLE Twisted masses of protein inside nerve cells that develop in the brains of people with AD.

NEUROIMAGING The use of x ray studies and magnetic resonance imaging (MRIs) to detect abnormalities or trace pathways of nerve activity in the central nervous system.

NEUROLEPTIC Another name for the older type of antipsychotic medications given to schizophrenic patients.

NEUROLOGICAL SYSTEM The system that initiates and transmits nerve impulses including the brain, spinal cord, and nerves.

NEUROMUSCULAR The body system of nerves and muscles as they function together.

NEURON A nerve cell.

NEUROPATHY Abnormality of the nerves which may be manifested as numbness, tingling, or weakness of the affected area.

NEUROSIS A term commonly used to describe a range of relatively mild psychiatric disorders in which the sufferer remains in touch with reality. Neurotic disorders include mild depression, anxiety disorders (including phobias and obsessive compulsive disorders), somatization disorders, dissociative disorders, and psychosexual disorders.

NEUROTOXIN A chemical compound that is toxic to the central nervous system.

NEUROTRANSMISSION When a neurotransmitter, or chemical agent released by a particular brain cell, travels across the synapse to act on the target cell to either inhibit or excite it.

NEUROTRANSMITTER A chemical in the brain that transmits messages between neurons, or nerve cells.

NICOTINE REPLACEMENT THERAPY (NRT) A method of weaning a smoker away from both nicotine and the oral fixation that accompanies a smoking habit by giving the smoker smaller and smaller doses of nicotine in the form of a patch or gum.

NICOTINE The addictive ingredient of tobacco, it acts on the nervous system and is both stimulating and calming.

NIGHT GUARD A removable custom-fitted plastic appliance that fits between the upper and lower teeth to prevent them from grinding against each other.

NIRVANA In Buddhism, release from the cycle of reincarnation through conquering one's hatreds, passions, and delusions.

NIT The egg sac laid by adult female lice.

NOCICEPTOR A specialized type of nerve cell that senses pain.

NOCTURIA Excessive need to urinate at night. Nocturia is a symptom of OSA and often increases the patient's daytime sleepiness.

NOCTURNAL MYOCLONUS A disorder in which the patient is awakened repeatedly during the night by cramps or twitches in the calf muscles. Also called periodic limb movement disorder (PLMD).

NODULOCYSTIC ACNE A disorder of the sebaceous (oil-secreting) glands in which deep, and sometimes painful, cysts and pustules are formed.

NOH THEATRE A Japanese theatrical form developed in the fourteenth century, featuring masks, extravagant costumes, bare stages, and restrained movements.

NONCOMEDOGENIC A substance that contains nothing that would cause blackheads or pimples to form on the skin. Jojoba oil is noncomedogenic.

NON-ESSENTIAL AMINO ACIDS The remaining amino acids that are produced in the human body.

NONGONOCOCCAL URETHRITIS (NGU) A sexually transmitted urethral infection that is not gonorrhea.

NON-HEME IRON Dietary or supplemental iron that is less efficiently absorbed by the body than heme iron (ferrous iron).

NON-SMALL CELL LUNG CANCER A group of lung cancers: squamous cell carcinoma, adenocarcinoma, and large cell carcinoma.

NONSTEROIDAL ANTI-INFLAMMATORY DRUGS (NSAIDS) A term used for a group of pain-relieving medications that also reduce inflammation when used over a period of time. NSAIDs are often given to patients with osteoarthritis.

NOSOCOMIAL Contracted in a hospital. Staph infections are the most common type of nosocomial infections.

NOSODE A homeopathic medicine made from disease material. Nosodes are given in order to prevent infectious diseases.

NOURISH YIN In TCM, to cool the body and replenish its fluids.

NUCLEIC ACID A type of chemical that is used as a component for building DNA. The nucleic acids found in DNA are adenine, thymine, guanine, and cytosine.

NUCLEOSIDES Any of various compounds consisting of a sugar and a purine or pyrimidine base, especially a compound obtained by hydrolysis of a nucleic acid

NUCLEUS PULPOSUS The center portion of the intervertebral disk that is made up of a gelatinous substance.

NUMMULAR DERMATITIS A skin infection in which the areas of irritated skin are coin-shaped.

NUTRACEUTICAL Any food or food ingredient that is thought to provide health benefits, including the prevention and treatment of disease. Flaxseed is considered a nutraceutical.

NYSTAGMUS An involuntary, rapid movement of the eyeball, usually from side to side.

O

OBSESSION A recurring, distressing idea, thought, or impulse that feels "foreign" or alien to the individual.

OBSESSIVE-COMPULSIVE DISORDER (OCD) A disorder that may accompany bulimia, characterized by the tendency to perform repetitive acts or rituals in order to relieve anxiety.

OBSTRUCTION A blockage.

OBSTRUCTIVE SLEEP APNEA (OSA) A potentially life-threatening condition characterized by episodes of breathing cessation during sleep alternating with snoring or disordered breathing. The low levels of oxygen in the blood of patients with OSA may eventually cause heart problems or stroke.

OCCIPITAL NEURALGIA Pain on one side of the back of the head caused by entrapment or pinching of an occipital nerve.

OCCLUSION The way upper and lower teeth fit together during biting and chewing.

OCCLUSIVE Closing off. One of the newest treatments for stress urinary incontinence in women is an external occlusive single-use cap that covers the urethral opening.

OFFAL Waste parts of an animal that are usually discarded.

OFFICINALIS Denoting that the substance is available without prescription.

OLEIC ACID Oily acid found in most vegetable and animal oils and fats. Used to make ointments.

OLIGOMENORRHEA Scanty or infrequent menstrual periods.

OLIGOMERIC PROANTHOCYANIDINS (OPCS) Part of a large group of phytochemicals called bioflavonoids.

OLIGURIA A condition in which the kidneys produce small amounts of urine.

OMEGA-3 FATTY ACIDS. Fatty acids from fish and vegetable oils that appear to protect against blood clots.

OMEGA-6 FATTY ACIDS A group of essential fatty acids that the humans body cannot produce on its own and must be obtained through diet..

ONCOLOGIST A doctor who specializes in treating cancer.

ONYCHOCRYPTOSIS The medical term for ingrown nail.

OPHTHALMOLOGIST A physician who specializes in treating diseases and disorders of the eye.

OPHTHALMOSCOPE An instrument, with special lighting, designed to view structures in the eye.

OPPORTUNISTIC INFECTION A type of infection caused only under certain circumstances, as when a person's immune system is impaired.

OPTIC NERVE A bundle of nerve fibers that carries visual messages from the retina in the form of electrical signals to the brain.

OPTICAL COHERENCE TOMOGRAPHY (OCT) A diagnostic method for imaging eye tissue.

OPTOKINETIC A reflex that causes a person's eyes to move when their field of vision moves.

OPTOMETRIST A health care professional who examines and tests the eyes for disease and treats visual disorders by prescribing corrective lenses and/or vision therapy. In many states, optometrists are licensed to use diagnostic and therapeutic drugs to treat certain ocular diseases.

ORCHITIS Inflammation of one or both testes, accompanied by swelling, pain, fever, and a sensation of heaviness in the affected area.

OREXIN Another name for hypocretin, a chemical secreted in the hypothalmus that regulates the sleep/wake cycle. Narcolepsy is sometimes described as an orexin deficiency syndrome.

ORGAN OF CORTI A spiral structure inside the cochlea that converts vibration to signals that are passed to the brain.

ORGANIC FOOD Food grown without the use of synthetic pesticides and fertilizers.

ORGANIC ILLNESS A physically, biologically based illness.

ORGASMIC DISORDER Impairment of the ability to reach sexual climax.

ORTHOKERATOLOGY A method of reshaping the cornea using a contact lens. It is not considered a permanent method to reduce myopia.

ORTHOPEDICS A medical specialty concerned with treating diseases, injuries, and malformations of the bones and supporting structures, such as tendons, ligaments, and muscles.

ORTHOPEDIST A specialist who is concerned with the bones, muscles, and joints and their points of interaction.

ORTHOSTATIC HYPOTENSION A drop in systolic blood pressure, which can result in dizziness or loss of consciousness.

ORTHOSTATIC Related to or caused by an upright position.

ORTHOTIC A device or brace used to control, correct, or compensate for a bone deformity.

OSSICLES A group of tiny bones in the middle ear that conduct sound through vibration. The bones are the malleus (or anvil), incus (or hammer), and stapes (or stirrup).

OSTEOARTHRITIS A degenerative disease of the joints, characterized by pain and stiffness related to loss or destruction of the cartilage in the joints.

OSTEOARTHRITIS A type of arthritis marked by chronic degeneration of the cartilage of the joints, leading to pain and sometimes loss of function.

OSTEOBLASTS Cells in the body that build new bone tissue.

OSTEOCLASTS Cells that break down and remove old bone tissue.

OSTEOMALACIA Softening, weakening, and removal of the minerals from bone in adults caused by vitamin D deficiency.

OSTEOPATHIC MANIPULATIVE TREATMENT (OMT) A collective term that refers to the variety of hands-on manipulative techniques practiced by osteopaths to diagnose and prevent disorders as well as to treat them.

OSTEOPATHY System of health care that emphasizes the musculoskeletal system.

OSTEOPENIA A disease of the bone, characterized by reduced bone mass leading to increased susceptibility to fractures. It is common among teenaged girls, and is often responsible for fractures of the lower arm.

OSTEOPOROSIS A disease in which the bones become extremely porous, are subject to fracture, and heal slowly.

OTITIS EXTERNA Inflammation of the outer ear. Otitis externa is the medical term for swimmer's ear.

OTOSCLEROSIS A disease that scars and limits the motion of the small conducting bones in the middle ear.

OTOSCOPE A lighted medical instrument that can be used to visualize the ear canal and the tympanic membrane.

OTOTOXIC Damaging to the nerves controlling the senses of hearing and balance.

OVARY The female organ in which eggs (ova) are stored and mature.

OVULATION The monthly release of an egg from an ovary.

OVUM The reproductive cell of the female that contains genetic information and participates in the act of fertilization. Also popularly called the egg.

OXALIC ACID A white crystalline water-soluble acid, found in yellow dock, sorrel, and spinach. In its pure form it is used as a cleanser and bleaching agent.

OXIDATION The loss of electrons from a molecule by their bonding to an oxygen molecule, rendering the donor molecule positive in charge and the recipient oxygen negative in charge (free radical).

OXIDIZE When oxygen reacts with a substance, it causes a decomposition of its living elements.

OXIDIZED METABOLITE The result of a process in which one molecule or substance is utilized by the body by first adding oxygen.

OZONE A form of oxygen with three atoms in its molecule (O_3), produced by an electric spark or ultraviolet light passing through air or oxygen. A layer of ozone about 15 mi (24 km) above Earth's surface helps protect living things from the damaging effects of the sun's ultraviolet rays. Ozone is used therapeutically as a disinfectant and oxidative agent.\

P

PACEMAKER Device that is surgically implanted in those suffering from heart disease or disorders, that regulates the beating of the heart.

PACLITAXEL A drug derived from the common yew tree (*Taxus baccata*) that is the mainstay of chemotherapy for ovarian cancer.

PAGET'S DISEASE A common disease of the bone of unknown cause usually affecting middle-aged and elderly people, characterized by excessive bone destruction and unorganized bone repair.

PALLIDOTOMY Surgery that destroys a small amount of tissue in the globus pallidus, which is over-stimulated by the corpus striatum in PD. The surgery can improve tremors, rigidity, and bradykinesia.

PALMATE A type of leaf that has lobes or leaflets radiating from a central point.

PALPATE Feel.

PALPATION A diagnostic technique in which the examiner gently presses, or palpates, a specific area of the patient's body. Palpation is used in the diagnosis of varicose veins.

PALPITATION Rapid, forceful, throbbing, or fluttering heartbeat.

PANAX GINSENG A popular longevity herb cultivated in Asia, Russia, and the United States. Described by some herbalists as an adaptogen, it is purported to strengthen the immune system and have a number of other beneficial effects.

PANCARDITIS Inflammation the lining of the heart, the sac around the heart, and the muscle of the heart.

PANCHAKARMA Intensive Ayurvedic cleansing and detoxification program.

PANCREAS The organ beneath the stomach that produces digestive juices, insulin, and other hormones.

PANDEMIC Worldwide outbreak of an infection, afflicting millions of victims.

PANTETHEINE A growth factor substance essential in humans, and a constituent of coenzyme A.

PAPANICOLAU (PAP) SMEAR A diagnostic test using a sampling of tissue from the cervix.

PAPILLOMA A benign growth on the skin or mucous membrane.

PAPULE A small, hard bump on the skin.

PARADIGM SHIFT A philosophical or spiritual change in the pattern or model by which one lives and views the world.

PARADIGM A pattern or model.

PARAMYXOVIRUS A genus of viruses that includes the causative agent of mumps.

PARASITE An organism that lives on or within a host organism for the purpose of obtaining food.

PARASITIC Behaving like a parasite; an organism that lives on, with, or in another organism. It draws its energy from the host, without providing any benefit to the host.

PARASITICIDE A substance destructive to parasites.

PARASOMNIA A primary sleep disorder in which the person's physiology or behaviors are affected by sleep, the sleep stage, or the transition from sleeping to waking.

PARASYMPATHETIC NERVOUS SYSTEM A part of the autonomic nervous system that is concerned with conserving and restoring energy. It is the part of the nervous system that predominates in a state of relaxation.

PARASYMPATHETIC RESPONSE A state of deep relaxation and the mechanism by which the body naturally regenerates itself and maintains chemical and metabolic balance.

PARENCHYMA A term used to describe the supportive tissue surrounding a particular structure. An example is that tissue that surrounds and supports the actually functional lung tissue.

PARESTHESIA The sensation of pins and needles or tingling that is often the result of nerve compression.

PARKINSONISM A set of symptoms originally associated with Parkinson's disease that can occur as side effects of neuroleptic medications. The symptoms include trembling of the fingers or hands, a shuffling gait, and tight or rigid muscles.

PARKINSON'S DISEASE A progressive disease caused by degeneration of the basal ganglia of the brain. Its most common symptoms are tremors and muscular rigidity.

PAROTITIS Inflammation and swelling of one or both of the parotid salivary glands.

PAROXYSM A severe attack or a sudden increase in intensity of a disease.

PARTHENOLIDE A sesquiterpene lactone isolated from feverfew that is thought to be responsible for most of its medical effectiveness.

PARTURITION Childbirth.

PASSIVE DIFFUSION A process whereby a liquid will migrate from a solution of lower concentration to a solution of higher concentration, making the latter more dilute.

PASSIVE SMOKING A term that refers to a person's having to breathe in smoke from someone else's cigarette or pipe. Other terms for passive smoking are exposure to secondhand smoke or exposure to environmental tobacco smoke (ETS).

PASTIA'S LINES Red lines in the folds of the skin, especially in the armpit and groin, that are characteristic of scarlet fever.

PATCH TEST A skin test that is done to identify allergens. A suspected substance is applied to the skin. After 24–48 hours, if the area is red and swollen, the test is positive for that substance.

PATENT FORMULAS Chinese herbal formulas that were patented centuries ago and are believed to be proven over centuries of use and study.

PATHOGENIC BACTERIA Bacteria that produce illness.

PATHOGENS Micro-organisms capable of causing disease.

PATHOLOGICAL, OR, NON-PATHOLOGICAL Terms indicating whether a condition is considered a disease state.

PATHOLOGIST A physician specializing in the study of disease, particularly as is involves cellular changes in the body and laboratory tests and methods.

PEDICULICIDE Any substance that kills lice.

PEDICULOSIS (PLURAL, PEDICULOSES) A lice infestation.

PELLAGRA A condition caused by a dietary deficiency of niacin, one of the B vitamins. The patient will have dementia, diarrhea and dermatitis.

PELVIC INFLAMMATORY DISEASE (PID) An infection of the upper genital tract.

PELVIC LYMPHADENECTOMY Surgical removal of the lymph nodes and passageways within the pelvis.

PEMPHIGUS VULGARIS An autoimmune skin disorder that causes blistering of the skin and mucous membrane.

PENICILLAMINE (CUPRIMINE, DEPEN) A drug used to treat medical problems (such as excess copper in the body and rheumatoid arthritis) and to prevent kidney stones. It is also sometimes prescribed to remove excess lead from the body.

PENICILLIN An antibiotic that is used to treat bacterial infections.

PENILE IMPLANT An artificial device inserted by surgery in the penis to produce an erection. Implantation of rigid or semi-rigid bars produces a permanent erection; use of an inflatable device allows the man to produce an erection at will.

PEPTIC ULCER DISEASE (PUD) A stomach disorder marked by corrosion of the stomach lining due to the acid in the digestive juices.

PERCUTANEOUS ABSORPTION The process by which certain strong medications, such as selenium compounds, can enter the body through the skin.

PERCUTANEOUS Medical procedure that is performed through the skin using a needle. Abscess drainage and urinary stones may be treated percutaneously.

PERENNIAL A plant that lives for many years; comes back yearly without replanting.

PERFORATION A hole that develops in a body tissue. In otitis media, the eardrum sometimes perforates because of the pressure of fluid behind it.

PERIMENOPAUSE The time span just before a woman reaches menopause. It usually begins when a woman is in her 40s and may produce many of the symptoms associated with menopause.

PERINATAL ASPHYXIA Asphyxia, or lack of oxygen, that occurs during birth.

PERINEAL AREA The genital area between the vulva and anus in a woman, and between the scrotum and anus in a man.

PERINEOMETER A device for measuring PC-muscle contraction.

PERIODIC LIMB MOVEMENTS IN SLEEP (PLMS) Random movements of the arms or legs that occur at regular intervals of time during sleep.

PERIODONTAL DISEASE Disease of the gums and teeth. Symptoms include bleeding and receding gums, gingivitis, abscesses, and loose teeth.

PERIODONTITIS A gum disease that destroys the structures supporting the teeth, including bone.

PERIOSTEUM The specialized layer of connective tissue that covers all bones in the body.

PERIOSTITIS Inflammation of the tissue covering the bone.

PERIPHERAL NEUROPATHY Damage to the nerve endings of the hands and feet, often as a result of diabetes.

PERIPHERAL VISION The ability to see objects that are not located directly in front of the eye. Peripheral vision allows people to see objects located on the side or edge of their field of vision.

PERISTALSIS The smooth muscle contractions that move food, bile, and urine through their respective passageways.

PERMETHRIN A synthetic pyrethroid for killing lice.

PERNICIOUS ANEMIA A type of anemia that occurs when the stomach does not secrete enough intrinsic factor, which is necessary for the absorption of vitamin B_{12}.

PERSISTENT GENERALIZED LYMPHADENOPATHY (PGL) A condition in which HIV continues to produce chronic painless swellings in the lymph nodes during the latency period.

PERSONALITY DISORDER A group of conditions characterized by a general failure to learn from experience or adapt appropriately to changes, resulting in personal distress and impairment of social functioning.

PESTICIDES Chemicals used to kill insects and weeds.

PETIT MAL SEIZURES A less severe form of epileptic seizure.

PETRISSAGE A massage technique in which the therapist kneads or squeezes the muscles with both hands.

PETROLEUM JELLY OR OINTMENT Petrolatum, a gelatinous substance obtained from oil that is used as a protective dressing.

PEYOTE One of the dried tops of the mescal cactus. Peyote contains mescaline, a hallucinogen that is sometimes used in Native American healing ceremonies.

PEYRONIE'S DISEASE A disease resulting from scarring of the corpus cavernosa, which causes painful erections.

PH A measurement of the acidity or alkalinity (basicity) of a solution. A low pH indicates an acid solution; a high pH indicates a base, or alkaline, solution. The normal vaginal pH is 4-4.5.

PHARMACODYNAMICS The study of the relationships and interactions of herbs.

PHARMACOGNOSIST A person involved in pharmacognosy, the science concerned with the medical products of plants in their natural state.

PHARMACOPOEIA A reference book containing a list of medicinal substances used by a particular medical stream or area.

PHARYNX The part of the throat that lies between the mouth and the larynx or voice box.

PHENACETIN A compound formerly used to ease pain or fever, but withdrawn because of its serious side effects.

PHENOTHIAZINES A parent compound for the synthesis of some antipsychotic compounds.

PHENYLALANINE An essential amino acid that cannot be consumed by people with a metabolic disease known as phenylketonuria (PKU).

PHENYLKETONURIA (PKU) An enzyme deficiency present at birth that disrupts metabolism and causes brain damage. This rare inherited defect may be linked to the development of autism.

PHEOCHROMOCYTOMA A tumor of the sympathoadrenal system that produces hypertension resulting in excessive headaches, sweating, and palpitation, apprehension, flushing of the face, nausea, and vomiting.

PHEROMONE HORMONES Substances secreted in order to bring out a response from other members of the same species, particularly in regard to sexual arousal.

PHLEBITIS Inflammation of a vein, often accompanied by swelling and the formation of blood clots.

PHLEGM A thick secretion of mucus produced in response to irritation that may clog the airway passages.

PHOBIA In psychoanalytic theory, a psychological defense against anxiety in which the patient displaces anxious feelings onto an external object, activity, or situation.

PHONICS A system to teach reading by teaching the speech sounds associated with single letters, letter combinations, and syllables.

PHOSPHOROUS Referring to a chemical element occurring in all living cells.

PHOTODYNAMIC THERAPY (PDT) A therapy that uses light-activated drugs to destroy rapidly-dividing cells or new blood vessels in the eye.

PHOTORECEPTORS Specialized nerve cells (rods and cones) in the retina that are responsible for vision.

PHOTOREFRACTIVE KERATECTOMY (PRK) A procedure that uses an excimer laser to reshape the cornea and permanently correct nearsightedness (myopia).

PHOTOSENSITIVITY An abnormal reaction to light exposure caused by a disorder or resulting from the use of certain drugs.

PHOTOTOXIC Causes a harmful skin reaction when exposed to sunlight.

PHYCOCYANIN A protein found in spirulina that gives the alga its blue color. Phycocyanin has anti-inflammatory effects.

PHYLLOQUINONE An alternate name for vitamin K_1.

PHYSICAL MANIPULATION The use of deep massage, spinal alignment, and joint manipulation to stimulate tissues.

PHYSIOLOGIC Refers to physiology, particularly normal, healthy, physical functioning.

PHYTO-, AS IN PHYTOCHEMICAL, PHYTOMEDICINAL, AND PHYTOTHERAPY Meaning, or pertaining to, a plant or plants.

PHYTOALEXIN A type of compound formed in a plant at the site of invasion by microorganisms that helps the plant resist disease. A phytoalexin called resveratrol appears to be useful in treating boils.

PHYTOCHEMICAL A naturally occurring chemical substance in a plant.

PHYTOESTROGENS Compounds found in plants that can mimic the effects of estrogen in the body.

PHYTOHORMONES Steroid hormones found in plants, including phytoestrogens and phytoandrogens.

PHYTOMEDICINALS Medicinal substances derived from plants.

PHYTONADIONE Another name for vitamin K_1. It is the form of vitamin K most often used to treat patients on anticoagulant therapy.

PHYTOPLANKTON Very small free-floating aquatic plants found in plankton.

PHYTOSTEROLS Plant-based oils that appear to have a cholesterol-lowering effect.

PHYTOTHERAPY A form of treatment that uses plants or plant extracts either externally or internally.

PICA An abnormal appetite or craving for non-food items, often such substances as chalk, clay, dirt, laundry starch, or charcoal.

PIGMENTED RETINAL EPITHELIUM The dark-colored cell layer that supports the retina. It may thin or become detached with MD.

PINEAL GLAND A gland about the size of a pea at the base of the brain that is part of the endocrine system.

PINNATE Having leaflets arranged on each side of a common stalk. Parsley has a tripinnate leaf.

PIOGLITAZONE An anti-diabetic drug of the thiazolidinedione class. This drug increases the sensitivity of the cells to insulin, but is capable of causing severe adverse reactions, including congestive heart failure.

PIPERONYL BUTOXIDE A liquid organic compound that enhances the activity of insecticides.

PIRIFORMIS A muscle in the pelvic girdle, or hip bones, that is closely associated with the sciatic nerve.

PITTING EDEMA A swelling in the tissue under the skin, resulting from fluid accumulation, that is measured by the depth of indentation made by finger pressure over a boney prominence.

PITUITARY GLAND The **MASTER GLAND** at the base of the brain that secretes a number of hormones responsible for growth, reproduction, and other activities. Pituitary hormones stimulate the ovaries to release estrogen and progesterone.

PLACEBO EFFECT The tendency of an ineffective therapy to benefit a patient who believes in the healing ability of the therapy.

PLACEBO An inactive substance with no pharmacological action that is administered to some patients in clinical trials to determine the relative effectiveness of another drug administered to a second group of patients.

PLACENTA The organ that develops in the uterus during pregnancy that links the blood supplies of the mother and baby.

PLANKTON A mass of tiny animals and plants floating in the sea or in lakes, usually near the surface.

PLANTAR FASCIA A tough fibrous band of tissue surrounding the muscles of the sole of the foot.

PLANTAR FASCITIS Inflammation of the plantar fascia.

PLANTAR WARTS Warts located on the sole of the foot.

PLASMA A clear yellowish fluid that is a component of blood.

PLATELET AGGREGATION The clumping together of blood cells, possibly forming a clot.

PLATELET The smallest kind of blood cell, usually found in large quantities, that plays an important part in blood clotting. Also called thrombocytes.

PLEURISY Inflammation of the pleura (lining of the chest cavity) usually caused by a lung infection.

PLEXOPATHY Compression of a nerve where it is part of a bundle of nerves called a plexus.

PNEUMOCYSTIS CARINII PNEUMONIA (PCP) An opportunistic infection caused by a fungus that is a major cause of death in patients with late-stage AIDS.

PNEUMONECTOMY Surgical removal of an entire lung.

PNEUMONIA A condition caused by bacterial or viral infection that is characterized by inflammation of the lungs and fluid within the air passages.

PNEUMONITIS Inflammation of lung tissue.

PNEUMOTHORAX Air inside the chest cavity, which may cause the lung to collapse. Pneumothorax is both a complication of pulmonary tuberculosis and a means of treatment designed to allow an infected lung to rest and heal.

PODIATRY A medical specialty concerned with treating diseases, injuries, and malformations of the feet.

POINT OF VIEW In a person with dyslexia, this term is used to describe the angle from which their mind's eye views an object. This point of view may be unanchored and moving about, as if several different people were telling what they see all at the same time.

POLLEN COUNT The amount of pollen in the air; often broadcast on the daily news during allergy season. It tends to be lower after a heavy rain that washes the pollen out of the air and higher on warm, dry, windy days.

POLYCHREST A homeopathic remedy that is used in the treatment of many ailments.

POLYCYSTIC OVARIAN SYNDROME (PCOS) A condition in which the eggs are not released from the ovaries and instead form multiple cysts.

POLYCYSTIC OVARIAN SYNDROME PCOS, a hormonal condition in women that if untreated can lead to the inability to have children.

POLYP A benign, tumor-like outgrowth.

POLYPHENOL Acid compound in plants.

POLYPHENOLS Phytochemicals that act as an antioxidant, protecting cells against damaging free radicals.

POLYSOMNOGRAPHY A group of tests administered to analyze heart, blood, and breathing patterns during sleep.

POLYUNSATURATED A group of fats that are less likely to be converted into cholesterol in the body than other fats.

POSITIVE IONS Ion particles having a positive electrical charge.

POST-HERPETIC NEURALGIA (PHN) The term used to describe the pain after the rash associated with herpes zoster is gone.

POSTHERPETIC NEURALGIA Persistent pain that occurs as a complication of a herpes zoster infection. Although the pain can be treated, the response is variable.

POSTPARTUM Following childbirth.

POSTPRANDIAL After eating or after a meal.

POTENCY The number of times that a homeopathic remedy has been diluted and succussed (shaken). In centesimal potencies, one part of the medicinal substance has been diluted with 99 parts of water or alcohol; in decimal potencies, the ratio is 1:9.

POTENTIATE To intensify the effects of another herb or prescription medication.

POTENTIATION A type of drug interaction in which one drug or herbal preparation intensifies or increases the effects of another.

POTENTIZATION The process of increasing the power of homeopathic preparations by successive dilutions and succussions of a mother tincture.

POTENTIZE To trigger effectiveness of a substance.

POULTICE A soft cloth filled with a warm moist mass of grains, herbs, or other medications applied to sores or injured parts of the body.

PRAKRITI An individual's unique dosha pattern.

PRANA Yoga term for life-enhancing nutrient found in air, food and water; an Hindu word that refers to the spiritual energy or vital force within a person.

PRANAYAMA The yogic discipline of controlling the breath. It is sometimes used to refer to a form of yoga that emphasizes breathing exercises.

PREBIOTIC A type of nondigestible substance found in chicory and some other plants that supports the growth and activity of beneficial bacteria in the colon.

PREDNISONE A steroid, immune suppressing, anti-inflammatory medication used to treat the symptoms of rheumatoid arthritis, auto-immune, and many inflammatory conditions.

PREECLAMPSIA A toxemia of pregnancy that causes increasing hypertension, headaches, and swelling of the lower extremities.

PREGNENOLONE A steroid ketone formed by the oxidation of other steroids, such as cholesterol, and is a precursor to the hormone progesterone.

PREMATURE EJACULATION Rapid ejaculation before the person wishes it, usually in less than one to two minutes after beginning intercourse.

PREMENSTRUAL SYNDROME (PMS) A group of symptoms that occur several days prior to the beginning of menstruation, including irritability, emotional tension, anxiety, and mood changes such as depression, headache, breast tenderness with or without swelling, and water retention. Symptoms usually subside shortly after the onset of the flow.

PRESSURE POINTS Specific locations on the feet and hands that correspond to nerve endings that connect to the organs and glands of the human body via the spinal cord.

PRIMARY ENERGY PATTERN a spiral motion that radiates from the umbilicus; the energy pattern associated with a child in the womb.

PRIMARY HEADACHE A headache that is not caused by another disease or medical condition.

PROANTHOCYANIDINS Bioflavenoids found in cranberries, responsible for the fruit's effectiveness in preventing urinary tract infections.

PROBIOTIC Favoring the support of life; related to promoting life and life conditions.

PROBIOTICS The use of beneficial microbes to treat various diseases, including diarrhea.

PROCAINE PENICILLIN An injectable form of penicillin that contains an anesthetic to reduce the pain of the injection.

PRODROMAL Referring to warning symptoms that occur before the onset of a disease or disorder.

PRODROME Symptoms that warn of the beginning of disease. The herpes prodrome consists of pain, burning, tingling, or itching at a site before blisters are visible.

PROGESTERONE Female hormone that prepares the uterus for the fertilized egg. Progesterone is normally produced in the ovaries, except when a woman is pregnant, then it is produced in the placenta. The adrenal glands also produce small amounts of progesterone.

PROGESTIN A type of hormone used to treat some types of breast cancer.

PROGNOSIS Referring to the expected outcome of a disease and its treatment.

PROGRESSIVE MULTIFOCAL LEUKOENCEPHALOPATHY (PML) A disease caused by a virus that destroys white matter in localized areas of the brain. It is regarded as an AIDS-defining illness.

PROKINETIC A drug that works to speed up the emptying of the stomach and the motility of the intestines.

PROLACTIN A hormone found in lactating women, and in men. Levels are increased by drinking beer.

PROLAPSED An organ fallen down from its normal body position.

PROLINE-RICH POLYPEPTIDE (PRP) A hormone found in colostrum that regulates the thymus gland and the immune system. It helps to make colostrum an effective treatment for autoimmune disorders and possibly heart disease. Proline is an amino acid.

PRONATION The lowering or descending of the inner edge of the foot while walking.

PROPHYLACTIC A preventative treatment.

PROPHYLAXIS The prevention of disease by protective measures.

PROPOLIS A sticky resin made by honeybees to seal the holes in their hives.

PROPRIOCEPTIVE Pertaining to proprioception, or the awareness of posture, movement, and changes in equilibrium and the knowledge of position, weight, and resistance of objects as they relate to the body.

PROSTAGLANDINS Unsaturated fatty acids that are associated with the contraction of smooth muscle, control of inflammation, and regulation of body temperature. Researchers think that prostaglandins may hold a clue to the cause of Raynaud's.

PROSTASIN A blood protein that appears to be a reliable early indicator of ovarian cancer.

PROSTATE A gland in males that secretes a fluid into the semen that improves the movement and viability of sperm.

PROSTATECTOMY The surgical removal of the prostate gland.

PROSTATIC SECRETIONS Normal secretions of the prostate gland intended to nourish and protect sperm, improving fertility.

PROSTATITIS An inflammation or irritation of the prostate.

PROTEASE ENZYME Any of a group of enzymes that help to break down proteins into smaller amino acid compounds. Bromelain belongs to this enzyme group.

PROTEASE The enzyme that digests proteins.

PROTEIN Complex groups of substances (including nitrogen, carbon, oxygen, iron, and hydrogen) that contain amino acids. Protein is vital to all animals because it makes up the hormones and enzymes controlling the body's actions.

PROTHROMBIN One protein component of the cascade reaction which results in clot formation.

PROTON PUMP INHIBITOR (PPI) Medication that inhibits stomach acid production in severe heartburn.

PROTOZOA Single-celled microorganisms belonging to the subkingdom Protozoa that are more complex than bacteria. About 30 protozoa cause diseases in humans.

PROTOZOAN A single-celled, usually microscopic organism that has a nucleus and is, therefore different from bacteria.

PROVING Case study of the effect of a homeopathic medicine.

PROVITAMIN A A carotenoid, such as beta carotene, that can be converted into vitamin A in the liver.

PRURITUS The medical term for itching. Pruritus is a common symptom of pityriasis rosea.

PSA TEST A blood test to determine prostate specific antigen levels in men, which can help determine the risk for prostate cancer.

PSA Prostatic Specific Antigen, elevated levels of which are a precondition to the development of cancer of the prostate gland.

PSEUDOCYST A fluid-filled space that may arise in the setting of pancreatitis.

PSEUDOMEMBRANOUS COLITIS A potentially life-threatening inflammation of the colon, caused by a toxin released by the Clostridium difficile bacterium that multiplies rapidly following antibiotic treatment.

PSORA According to Hahnemann, the oldest and most universal miasm, responsible for human vulnerability to the majority of non-venereal chronic diseases.

PSORIASIS A common chronic skin disorder that causes red patches anywhere on the body.

PSYCHOANALYSIS A psychological theory and therapeutic method based on the idea that the mind works on conscious and unconscious levels and that childhood events have a psychological influence on people throughout their lives.

PSYCHODYAMIC The scientific study of mental or conditional forces developing especially in early childhood and their effect on behavior and mental states.

PSYCHODYNAMIC THERAPY A therapeutic approach that assumes improper or unwanted behavior is caused by unconscious, internal conflicts and focuses on gaining insight into these motivations.

PSYCHOMOTOR AGITATION Disturbed physical and mental processes (e.g., fidgeting, wringing of hands, racing thoughts); a symptom of major depressive disorder.

PSYCHOMOTOR RETARDATION Slowed physical and mental processes (e.g., slowed thinking, movement, and talking); a symptom of major depressive disorder.

PSYCHONEUROIMMUNOLOGY The study of the relationships among mind, nervous system, and immune response.

PSYCHOSIS A severe mental disorder characterized by delusions, hallucinations, and other evidence of loss of contact with reality. Some psychiatrists regard shamanic experiences as evidence of psychosis.

PSYCHOSOCIAL Relating to both the psychological and the social aspects of a person.

PSYCHOSOMATIC ILLNESS A condition in which unresolved emotional distress manifests as physical symptoms of illness.

PSYCHOTHERAPY A medical treatment that seeks to resolve psychological traumas and conflicts, often by discussing them and emotionally reliving difficult events in the past.

PTYALISM Excess salivation.

PUBERTY The period of life in which boys' and girls' sexual organs begin to reach maturity and the ability to reproduce begins.

PUBOCOCCYGEAL (PC) MUSCLES The muscles of the lower pelvic girdle, or pelvic floor, which support the bladder, urethra, and urethral sphincter; the muscle group at the neck of the bladder that acts as a spigot for controlling urine flow into the urethra, vagina, uterus, and rectum.

PULEGONE The toxic chemical found in pennyroyal oil.

PULP The soft innermost part of a tooth, containing blood vessels and nerves.

PULPITIS Inflammation of the pulp of a tooth that involves the blood vessels and nerves.

PUMICE STONE A volcanic rock that can be used to remove overgrowths and smooth the skin.

PUNCTURE An injury caused by a sharp, narrow object deeply penetrating the skin.

PUPIL The black hole in the center of the iris through which light enters on the way to the lens and retina.

PUPILLARY REACTION The normal change in the size of the pupil due to the amount of ambient light. Under normal circumstances, both pupils respond simultaneously and equally.

PURGATIVE A substance that encourages bowel movements.

PURGE To rid the body of food and calories, commonly by vomiting or using laxatives.

PURGING The use of vomiting, diuretics, or laxatives to clear the stomach and intestines after a binge.

PURIFIED PROTEIN DERIVATIVE (PPD) An extract of tubercle bacilli that is injected into the skin to find out whether a person presently has or has ever had tuberculosis.

PURINE A substance found in foods that is broken down into urate and may contribute to hyperuricemia and gout.

PURPURA A group of disorders characterized by purple, red, or brown areas of discoloration visible through the skin.

PUS A fluid formed in infected tissue, consisting of while blood cells and cellular debris.

PUSTULAR Resembling a blister and usually containing pus.

PUSTULE A small, pus-filled bump on the skin.

PYELONEPHRITIS Infection and inflammation of the kidney.

PYOGENIC Capable of generating pus. Streptococci, staphylococci, and bowel bacteria are the primary pyogenic organisms.

PYRETHRIN, PYRETHROID Naturally-occurring insecticide extracted from chrysanthemum flowers. It paralyzes lice so that they cannot feed.

PYRIDOXINE Another name for vitamin B_6.

PYROGEN A chemical circulating in the blood that causes a rise in body temperature.

Q

QI The Chinese term for life force or vital energy. It is sometimes spelled *chi* or *ki*.

QIGONG An exercise practice derived from traditional Chinese medicine that is designed to facilitate energy flow throughout the body.

QUADRIPLEGIA Paralysis of all four limbs.

QUERCETIN A flavonoid (chemical compound/biological response modifier) found in onions and garlic that may be a useful dietary supplement for asthma patients.

QUININE One of the first treatments for malaria, quinine is a natural product made from the bark of the Cinchona tree. It was popular until being superseded by the development of chloroquine in the 1940s. In the wake of widespread chloroquine resistance, however, it has become popular again. Quinine, or its close relative quinidine, can be given intravenously to treat severe *Falciparum* malaria.

QUINOLONES A group of antibiotics, often used to treat bacterial infections, that sometimes cause tendinitis.

QUINSY Acute inflammation of the tonsils and throat area that often results in abscesses.

QV Quantum vacuum, a theory coined by physicists, which defines the interactions of energy that combine to form reality.

R

RADIAL KERATOTOMY (RK) A surgical procedure involving the use of a diamond-tipped blade to make several spoke-like slits in the peripheral (non-viewing) portion of the cornea to improve the focus of the eye and correct myopia by flattening the cornea.

RADIATION THERAPY Treatment using high energy radiation from x-ray machines, cobalt, radium, or other sources.

RADICULAR Pain that is caused by compression or impingement at the root of a nerve.

RADICULOPATHY Compression of a nerve root at the point where it exits the spinal cord.

RADIODERMATITIS Red, irritated, and inflamed skin caused by x rays, radiation treatment, or other type of radiation exposure.

RADIOISOTOPE A chemical tagged with radioactive compounds that is injected during a nuclear medicine procedure to highlight organs or tissue.

RANSON'S SIGNS A set of 11 signs used to evaluate the severity of a case of pancreatitis.

RAPID EYE MOVEMENT SLEEP A stage of sleep during which dreams occur. This stage usually alternates with a heavier, more restful stage of sleep.

RASH A spotted, pink or red skin eruption that may be accompanied by itching and is caused by disease, contact with an allergen, food ingestion, or drug reaction.

RATES The subtle emanations of energy which may be detected with radionic equipment.

RAW NUTRITION A synonym for the Wigmore diet's emphasis on uncooked and living foods.

RAYNAUD'S DISEASE A vascular disorder in which the patient's fingers ache and tingle after exposure to cold or emotional stress, with characteristic color changes from white to blue to red. Raynaud's phenomenon may be seen in scleroderma and systemic lupus erythematosus.

RECEPTOR A cell-surface molecule that binds a specific hormone to produce a specific biological effect.

RECOMMENDED DAILY ALLOWANCE (RDA) Guidelines for the amounts of vitamins and minerals necessary for proper health and nutrition. The RDA was established by the National Academy of Sciences in 1989.

RECOMMENDED DIETARY ALLOWANCE (RDA) The average daily dietary intake of a nutrient that is sufficient to meet the nutritional requirements of 97–98% of healthy individuals of a given age and gender.

RECTAL PROLAPSE A condition where the lining of the rectum, the last part of the large intestine, protrudes through the anus.

RECTUM The last 5–6 in (13-16 cm) of the intestine that leads to the anus.

RECURRENCE The return of an active infection following a period of latency.

RED BLOOD CELL Hemoglobin-containing blood cells that transport oxygen from the lungs to tissues. In the tissues, the red blood cells exchange their oxygen for carbon dioxide, which is brought back to the lungs to be exhaled.

REDUCIBLE HERNIA A hernia that can be gently pushed back into place or that disappears when the person lies down.

REFERRED PAIN Pain that is experienced in one part of the body but originates in another organ or area. The pain is referred because the nerves that supply the damaged organ enter the spine in the same segment as the nerves that supply the area where the pain is felt.

REFLEXOLOGY Belief that reflex areas in the feet correspond to every part of the body, including organs and glands, and that stimulating the correct reflex area can affect the body part.

REFLUX The backward flow of a body fluid or secretion. Indigestion is sometimes caused by the reflux of stomach acid into the esophagus.

REFRACTION The turning or bending of light waves as the light passes from one medium or layer to another. In the eye it means the ability of the eye to bend light so that an image is focused onto the retina.

REFRACTIVE EYE SURGERY A general term for surgical procedures that can improve or correct refractive errors of the eye by permanently changing the shape of the cornea.

REFRACTIVE POWER The degree of refraction of an eye.

REFRACTIVE SURGERY Eye surgery to correct a defect in the eye's ability to focus accurately on an image.

REGRESSION THERAPY Traveling back and reliving emotions experience through prior lives while meditating.

REIKI Form of therapeutic bodywork that strives to heal the body's energy field.

REISHI MUSHROOM Another name for ganoderma.

RELAPSE A return to a disease state after recovery appeared to be occurring. In alcoholism, relapse refers to a patient beginning to drink alcohol again after a period of avoiding it.

RELAXATION RESPONSE The body's response to relaxation techniques,during which metabolism and stress levels decrease and immune response increases.

REMEDY ANTIDOTE Certain foods, beverages, prescription medications, aromatic compounds, and other environmental elements that counteract the efficacy of homeopathic remedies.

REMISSION Disappearance of a disease as a result of treatment. Complete remission means that all disease is gone. Partial remission means that the disease is significantly improved by treatment, but residual traces of the disease are still present.

RENAL ARTERY STENOSIS Disorder in which the arteries that supply blood to the kidneys constrict.

RENAL FAILURE A state when the kidneys are so extensively damaged that they can no longer function.

REPERFUSION The reintroduction of blood flow to organs or tissues after blood flow has been stopped for surgical procedures.

REPERTORIES Homeopathic reference books consisting of descriptions of symptoms. The process of selecting a homeopathic remedy from the patient's symptom profile is called repertorizing.

REPERTORY Reference manual of homeopathic remedies.

REPETITIVE STRAIN INJURY Injury resulting from a repeated movement such as typing or throwing a ball.

RESIDUAL VOLUME The amount of air trapped inside the lungs as a result of incompletely exhaling.

RESIN A sticky substance used for medicinal purposes and in the manufacture of varnishes, obtained from the bark of certain trees.

RESORPTION The breakdown or dissolving of bone tissue by biochemical processes in the body.

RESTLESS LEGS SYNDROME (RLS) A disorder in which the patient experiences crawling, aching, or other disagreeable sensations in the calves that can be relieved by movement.

RESVERATROL An enzyme that promotes health and is found in 72 varieties of plants.

RETCHING The coordinated contraction of muscles as for vomiting but without the discharge of stomach contents.

RETINA The inner, light-sensitive layer of the eye that transforms images into electrical messages which are sent to the brain.

RETINITIS PIGMENTOSA A group of inherited degenerative eye disorders characterized by deterioration of the retina. This deterioration of the retina causes vision impairment and ultimately blindness, usually by the time the individual reaches middle age.

RETINOIDS Any of the group of substances which comprise active vitamin A, including retinaldehyde, retinol, and retinoic acid.

RETINOL EQUIVALENT (RE) 1 ¶g of all-*trans* retinol (vitamin A), 6 ¶g of all-*trans* beta carotene.

RETROGRADE EJACULATION A condition in which the semen spurts backward into the bladder.

RETROGRADE MENSTRUATION Menstrual flow that travels into the body cavity rather than out through the vagina.

RETROVIRUS A virus that contains a unique enzyme called reverse transcriptase that allows it to replicate within new host cells.

RETT SYNDROME An X-linked disorder of the nervous system found almost exclusively in girls. Children with Rett's syndrome often develop bruxism, for reasons as yet unknown.

REYE'S SYNDROME A rare but potentially fatal disorder that is most likely to occur in children following a viral disease and associated with giving aspirin. The symptoms of Reye's syndrome include vomiting, liver damage, and swelling of the brain.

RHABDOMYOLYSIS The necrosis or disintegration of skeletal muscle.

RHABDOVIRUS A type of virus named for its rod- or bullet-like shape.

RHEUMATIC FEVER A heart disease that is a complication of a strep infection.

RHEUMATIC Refers to any of a variety of disorders marked by inflammation, deterioration, or metabolic damage of the body's connective tissues, especially the joints.

RHEUMATISM A popular term for any disorder that causes pain and stiffness in muscles and joints and fibrous tissues, including minor aches and twinges, as well as disorders such as rheumatoid arthritis, osteoarthritis, and polymyalgia rheumatica.

RHEUMATOID ARTHRITIS A chronic autoimmune disorder marked by inflammation and deformity of the affected joints.

RHEUMATOLOGY The branch of medicine that specializes in the treatment of arthritis and related conditions, including Raynaud's disease.

RHINOPHYMA Long-term swelling and overgrowth in skin tissue of the nose that leaves it with a knobby, bulb-like look.

RHINOVIRUS A virus that infects the upper respiratory system and causes the common cold.

RHIZOME A fleshy plant stem that grows horizontally under or along the ground; roots are sent out below this stem and leaves or shoots are sent out above it.

RHODOPSIN The light-sensitive photopigment contained in rods which discriminates between different levels of light intensity.

RHOMBOHEDRAL A parallelogram with four equal sides, sometimes with no right angles.

RHYTHM METHOD The oldest method of contraception with a very high failure rate, in which partners periodically refrain from having sex during ovulation. Ovulation is predicted on the basis of a woman's previous menstrual cycle.

RICIN An extremely poisonous protein derived from castor beans.

RICKETS A condition caused by the deficiency of vitamin D, calcium, and usually phosphorus, seen primarily in infancy and childhood, and characterized by abnormal bone formation.

RIGHT BRAIN The right cerebral hemisphere, which controls activity on the left side of the body in humans. It is associated with spatial and nonverbal concepts, intuition, emotions, and creativity. Labyrinth walking is thought to stimulate the right brain.

RINGWORM A fungal skin infection that predominantly affects children. The condition is characterized by reddish, scaly rings on the skin.

RODS Photoreceptors, located in the retina of the eye, that are highly sensitive to low levels of light.

ROLFING A deep-tissue therapy that involves manipulating the body's fascia to realign and balance the body's structure.

ROUGHAGE Another name for dietary fiber.

ROYAL JELLY Special substance secreted by bees to feed the young queen bees.

RUBELLA Also known as German measles. When a woman contracts rubella during pregnancy, her developing infant may be damaged. One of the problems that may result is autism.

RUMINANT Any of various hoofed, even-toed, usually horned mammals of the suborder Ruminantia, such as cattle, sheep, goats, deer, and giraffes.

RUSSELL'S SIGN Scraped or raw areas on the patient's knuckles, caused by self-induced vomiting.

RUTIN A bright greenish-yellow flavonoid (plant pigment) found in ruta that has been credited with antioxidant properties.

S

SACRAL NERVES The five pairs of nerves that arise from the lowermost segments of the spinal cord and control bladder, bowel, and pelvic functions. Stimulation of the sacral nerves by an implanted device is a newer treatment for urinary incontinence.

SACRO-ILIAC The joint at which the upper hip bone joins the backbone to the pelvis.

SAIKOSAPONINS Chemical compounds found in bupleurum that have anti-inflammatory effects.

SALICIN A bitter-tasting water-soluble chemical found in willow bark that has analgesic properties.

SALICYLIC ACID An agent prescribed in the treatment of hyperkeratotic skin conditions and fungal infections.

SALIVARY DUCT Tube through which saliva is carried from the salivary gland to the mouth.

SALIVARY GLAND Gland in which saliva is formed.

SALVE Topical ointment or paste made by blending it with olive oil, then mixing it with melted beeswax.

SAMANA life sustaining energy of the smaller intestine; the fourth of the five airs of Ayurvedic philosophy; the life force governing side-to-side motion.

SAME An active compound made from methionine and adenosine triphosphate (ATP), an enzyme found in muscle tissue.

SANSKRIT The classical literary language of India. It is considered the oldest living language of the Indo-Aryan family.

SAPONINS A group of glucosides that occur in plants and produce a soapy lather.

SARCOIDOSIS A rare disease of currently unknown cause that occurs mostly in young adults. Inflammation occurs in the lymph nodes and other tissues throughout the body, usually including the lungs, liver, skin, and eyes.

SARCOMA A malignant growth in the connective tissue, bone, cartilage or muscle; usually the most lethal form of cancer.

SASHIMI A traditional Japanese preparation of rice, fish, shell fish, mollusks, and other fish products, served with pickled vegetables.

SATURATED FAT Fat that is usually solid at room temperature, found mainly in meat and dairy products but also in vegetable sources such as some nuts, seeds, and avocados.

SCABIES A contagious rash caused by the *Sarcoptes scabiei* mite, which burrows into the upper layer of the skin in order to lay eggs. Scabies is characterized by intense itching.

SCALE Any thin, flaky, plate-like piece of dry skin.

SCARLET FEVER A childhood disease characterized by a red skin rash appearing on the chest, neck, elbows, and thighs. Scarlet fever, which may also be accompanied by sore throat and fever, is caused by the bacterium *Streptococcus pyogenes*.

SCHEMAS Fundamental core beliefs or assumptions that are part of the perceptual filter people view the world through. Cognitive-behavioral therapy seeks to change maladaptive schemas.

SCHISTOSOMIASIS Also called bilharziasis, this is a disease caused by bodily infestation of blood flukes.

SCHIZOPHRENIA Schizophrenia is a psychotic disorder that causes distortions in perception (delusions and hallucinations), inappropriate moods and behaviors, and disorganized or incoherent speech and behavior.

SCIATICA Pain along the course of the sciatic nerve, running from pelvis down the back of leg to the foot caused by a compression or irritation of the fifth lumbar spinal root.

SCLERA A dense white fibrous membrane that, together with the cornea, forms the outer covering of the eyeball.

SCLERODERMA A chronic autoimmune disorder in which connective tissue anywhere in the body becomes hard and rigid.

SCOLIOMETER A tool for measuring trunk asymmetry; it includes a bubble level and angle measure.

SCOLIOSIS A lateral curvature of the spine.

SCROFULA Tuberculous inflammation of the lymph nodes of the neck in children, caused by bacteria in cattle; also called cervical adenitis.

SCROFULODERMA Abscesses on the skin that are a symptom of the lung disease tuberculosis.

SCRUPULOSITY A spiritual disorder characterized by perfectionism and obsessive fears of God's punishment. Some patients with OCD also develop religious scrupulosity.

SCURVY A disease caused by the absence of vitamin C in the diet.

SEASONAL AFFECTIVE DISORDER (SAD) Depression caused by decreased daylight during the winter months.

SEBACEOUS GLANDS The oil- or grease-producing glands of the body.

SEBORRHEIC DERMATITIS An inflammatory condition of the skin of the scalp, with yellowish greasy scaling of the skin and itching. Other areas of the body may also be affected. Mild seborrheic condition is called dandruff.

SEBUM An oily skin moisturizer produced by sebaceous glands.

SECONDARY HEADACHE A headache that is caused by another disease or disorder.

SECONDARY INFECTION An infection by a microbe that occurs during an infection by a different kind of microbe.

SEDATIVE A substance given to calm or soothe.

SEDIMENTARY Formed by deposits of sediment, or material that settles on the bottom in a liquid.

SELECTIVE ESTROGEN RECEPTOR MODULATOR A hormonal preparation that offers the beneficial effects of hormone replacement therapy (HRT) without the increased risk of breast and uterine cancer associated with HRT.

SELECTIVE SEROTONIN REUPTAKE INHIBITORS (SSRIS) A class of antidepressants that work by blocking the reabsorption of serotonin in brain cells, raising the level of the chemical in the brain. SSRIs include Prozac, Zoloft, Luvex, and Paxil.

SELENIUM A mineral supplement with antioxidant properties that may be useful for reducing breast pain and tenderness associated with fibrocystic breast disease. The recommended daily allowance of selenium is 70 mcg for men and 55 mcg for women.

SELF-BREEMA A personalized form of Breema bodywork that the individual performs on his or her own body, without an instructor as partner. It is intended to supplement Breema bodywork treatment sessions with an instructor.

SEMEN A whitish, opaque fluid containing sperm released at ejaculation.

SEMINAL VESICLES The pouches above the prostate that store semen.

SENESCENCE Aging.

SENILE PLAQUE Structures composed of parts of neurons surrounding brain proteins called beta-amyloid deposits and found in the brains of people with AD.

SENSITIZATION The process of becoming sensitive or hypersensitive.

SENSORINEURAL HEARING LOSS Hearing loss caused by damage to the nerves or parts of the inner ear that control the sense of hearing.

SENSORY AWARENESS Bringing attention to the sensations of tension and/or release in the muscles.

SENSORY ROOT GANGLION A bundle of nerves that help conduct physical sensations.

SEPSIS A bacterial infection of the bloodstream or tissues of the body.

SEQUELA (PLURAL, SEQUELAE) An abnormal condition resulting from a previous disease or disorder.

SERIAL CASTING A series of casts designed to gradually move a limb into a more functional position, as opposed to doing it all at once with one cast, as would be done in setting a broken bone.

SEROTONIN DOPAMINE ANTAGONISTS (SDAS) The newer second-generation antipsychotic drugs, also called atypical antipsychotics. SDAs include clozapine (Clozaril), risperidone (Risperdal), and olanzapine (Zyprexa).

SEROTONIN SYNDROME A potentially life-threatening reaction to increased levels of the neurotransmitter serotonin in the central nervous system, most often as a result of drug interactions. St. John's wort has been implicated in several cases of serotonin syndrome.

SEROTONIN One of three major types of neurotransmitters found in the brain that is linked to emotions.

SERUM, PL. SERA The clear liquid that remains after cellular components are removed from blood by clotting; a blood derivative containing an antitoxin for diagnostic or therapeutic use.

SESSILE A botanical term to describe a leaf that emerges from the plant stem without a stalk.

SEXUAL AROUSAL DISORDER The inhibition of the general arousal aspect of sexual response.

SEXUALLY TRANSMITTED DISEASES (STDS) A group of diseases that are transmitted by sexual contact. In addition to gonorrhea, this group generally includes chlamydia, HIV (AIDS), genital herpes, syphilis, and genital warts.

SHAMAN Among certain tribal peoples, a man or woman who is thought to be an intermediary between natural and supernatural forces, and to have unusual abilities to heal illness or foretell the future.

SHEEP BLOOD AGAR PLATE A petri dish filled with a nutrient gel containing red blood cells that is used to detect the presence of streptococcal bacteria in a throat culture. Streptococcal bacteria will break down the red blood cells, leaving a clear spot around the bacterial colony.

SHEN NONG A legendary emperor, he was called the "Divine Farmer" of China. Shen Nong made many discoveries concerning herbal medicine and cataloged 365 species of medicinal plants. An early herbal text, written around 400 A.D., *WAS NAMED AFTER HIM.*

SHEN One of the five body energies. It influences mental, spiritual, and creative energy. Shen tonics address deficiencies in this type of energy.

SHIATSU Japanese form of acupressure massage.

SHINGLES An disease caused by an infection with the *Herpes zoster* virus, the same virus that causes chickenpox. Symptoms of shingles include pain and blisters along one nerve, usually on the face, chest, stomach, or back.

SHOCK WAVE THERAPY A method of treating tennis elbow and other musculoskeletal injuries that involves directing bursts of high-pressure sound waves at the affected area.

SHOCK An abnormal condition resulting from low blood volume. Signs of shock include rapid pulse and breathing; cool, moist, pale skin; and bluish lips and fingernails.

SIALAGOGUE An agent that increases salivation.

SICK BUILDING SYNDROME An illness related to multiple chemical sensitivity in which a person develops symptoms in response to chronic exposure to airborne environmental chemicals found in a tightly sealed building.

SICKLE CELL DISEASE A hereditary defect in hemoglobin synthesis that changes the shape of red cells and makes them more fragile.

SIDESTREAM SMOKE The smoke that is emitted from the burning end of a cigarette or cigar, or that comes from the end of a pipe. Along with exhaled smoke, it is a constituent of second-hand smoke.

SIGMOID COLON The final portion of the large intestine which empties into the rectum.

SILICOSIS A serious lung disease caused by prolonged inhaling of dust from stone or sand that contains silicon dioxide. It is also called grinder's disease.

SIMPLE A type of leaf that is not divided into parts.

SINUS TRACT A channel connecting a body part with the skin outside.

SINUSITIS An infection of the sinus cavities characterized by pain in the eyes and cheeks, fever, and difficulty breathing through the nose.

SITZ BATH A hydrotherapy treatment for soaking the pelvic or genital areas.

SJÖGREN'S SYNDROME An autoimmune disorder in which the body's white cells attack the glands that produce saliva and tears. Dry mouth is a core symptom of Sjögren's syndrome.

SKIN GRAFT Surgery used to cover burned or injured areas of the body with new skin.

SKIN LESION BIOPSY A procedure in which a sliver of tissue from the skin is removed in order to examine it and establish a diagnosis.

SLEEP APNEA A condition in which a person stops breathing while asleep. These periods can last up to a minute or more, and can occur many times each hour. In order to start breathing again, the person must become semi-awake. The episodes are not remembered, but the following day the client feels tired and sleepy. If severe, sleep apnea can cause other medical problems.

SLEEP DISORDER Any condition that interferes with sleep. At least 84 have been identified, according to the American Sleep Disorders Association.

SLEEP LATENCY The amount of time that it takes a person to fall asleep.

SLEEP PARALYSIS An abnormal episode of sleep in which the patient cannot move for a few minutes, usually occurring on falling asleep or waking up. Often found in patients with narcolepsy.

SLIT LAMP A special viewing device used by eye specialists to examine the eye for cataracts.

SOFT PALATE The structure at the roof of the mouth that separates the mouth and the pharynx.

SOYBEAN The seed of the plant *Glycine max.*

SPASM Involuntary contraction of a muscle.

SPASMOLYTIC A substance or medication that relieves cramping.

SPASTIC Spastic refers to a condition in which the muscles are rigid, posture may be abnormal, and fine motor control is impaired.

SPAWN Grain, often rye or millet, that has been inoculated with mushroom spores and is used to grow mushrooms commercially.

SPECIFIC PHOBIA An intense but irrational fear of a specific place, object, or animal. Common specific phobias include fear of spiders, snakes, or dogs; fear of flying or highway driving; fear of blood; and fear of elevators and other closed spaces.

SPERM The reproductive cell of the male that contains genetic information and participates in the act of fertilization of an ovum.

SPERMATOGENESIS The process by which sperm develop to become mature sperm, capable of fertilizing an ovum.

SPERMATORRHEA A term describing the involuntary discharge of semen without an orgasm occurring; sperm leakage.

SPHYGMOMANOMETER An instrument used to measure blood pressure.

SPINA BIFIDA A congenital defect in which part of the vertebrae fail to develop completely, leaving a portion of the spinal cord exposed.

SPINAL STENOSIS Usually the result of arthritis of the spine, causing narrowing of the spinal canal in the lumbar vertebrae. The narrowing puts pressure on the roots of the sciatic nerve. It may cause sciatica, but not necessarily.

SPINES These sharp needle-like protrusions serve the plant in three important ways. Not only do they conduct water and reduce water loss, but they also protect the plant from herbivores.

SPIROCHETE A spiral-shaped bacterium. The bacteria that cause Lyme disease and syphilis, for example, are spirochetes.

SPIRULINA A nutritionally valuable organism that is rich in vitamins, minerals, essential fatty acids, and antioxidants.

SPLEEN In TCM, the system of organs that includes the pancreas, large muscles, the lips, the eyelids, the lymph system, and the spleen. It also includes the functions that extract nourishment and convert it into qi and Blood.

SPLENECTOMY Surgical removal of the spleen.

SPONDYLITIS An inflammation of the spine.

SPONDYLOSIS Arthritis of the spine.

SPORE The asexual reproductive body of a mushroom or other nonflowering plant.

SPRUE A disorder in which the absorption of nutrients from the diet by the small intestine (malabsorption) is impaired resulting in malnutrition. Two forms of sprue exist: tropical sprue, which occurs mainly in tropical regions; and celiac sprue, which occurs more widely and is due to sensitivity to the wheat protein gluten.

SPUTUM Secretions produced in a patient's infected lung and coughed up. Sputum is routinely used as a specimen for culturing the tubercle bacillus in the laboratory.

STAGE A term used to describe the size and extent of cancer.

STAGING Using various methods of diagnosis to determine the extent of disease present in an individual. Staging is important as a way of determining the appropriate type of treatment for a particular disease, as well as helping to predict an individual's chance for cure from a particular disease.

STAMEN The male fertilizing organ of flowering plants, bearing pollen.

STANDARDIZED HERBAL EXTRACT An herbal product created by using water or alcohol to dissolve and concentrate the active ingredients, which are then quantified for medicinal pharmacological effect.

STANDARDIZED To cause to conform to a standard. In medicine and pharmacy, this means that a given weight of an herb will contain a standardized percentage or weight of the active principle.

STAPHYLOCOCCUS A genus of bacteria that resembles a cluster of grapes, that can infect various body systems.

STARCH Complex carbohydrates.

STASIS Stagnation in the flow of blood or any body fluid.

STATIN An HMG-CoA reductase inhibitor, which assists in the lowering of cholesterol levels.

STATINS A class of drugs used primarily, but not exclusively, to treat high cholesterol.

STEAM DISTILLATION A process of extracting essential oils from plant products through a heating and evaporation process.

STENT A small springlike device made of stainless steel or a biodegradable plastic that can be inserted into the urethra to widen it during voiding.

STIGMA The thread-like filament found in the center of a flower where pollen collects.

STIGMASTEROL A plant steroid that is extracted from soybeans and used to produce natural human hormones.

STIMULANT LAXATIVES Powerful laxatives that increase the frequency of bowel movements by stimulating muscle contractions that accelerate the passage of stool.

STIMULUS Anything capable of eliciting a response in an organism or a part of that organism.

STOMACHIC A medication or herbal preparation given to improve the functioning of the digestive system.

STRABISMUS Failure of the two eyes to direct their gaze at the same object simultaneously due to muscle imbalance.

STRANGULATED HERNIA A hernia that is so tightly incarcerated outside the abdominal wall that the intestine is blocked and the blood supply to that part of the intestine is cut off.

STRAWBERRY TONGUE A sign of scarlet fever in which the tongue appears to have a red coating with large raised bumps.

STREET DRUG A substance purchased from a drug dealer. It may be a legal substance, sold illicitly (without a prescription, and not for medical use), or it may be a substance which is illegal to possess.

STRESS HARDINESS A personality characteristic that enables persons to stay healthy in stressful circumstances. It includes belief in one's ability to influence the situation; being committed to or fully engaged in one's activities; and having a positive view of change.

STRESS MANAGEMENT A category of popularized programs and techniques intended to help people deal more effectively with stress.

STRESS URINARY INCONTINENCE (SUI). Urine leakage upon straining, coughing, laughing, or sneezing.

STRESSOR A stimulus or event that provokes a stress response in an organism. Stressors can be categorized as acute or chronic, and as external or internal to the organism.

STRIDOR A noisy wheezing sound during breathing that may indicate an airway obstruction.

STROKE A condition caused by the blockage of blood flow and oxygen to the brain. Paralysis, coma, and death may result.

STRUCTURAL INTEGRATION The term used to describe the method and philosophy of life associated with Rolfing. Its fundamental concept is the vertical line.

STRYCHNINE A colorless, crystalline poison obtained from the seeds of nux vomica.

SUBCHONDRAL CYSTS Fluid-filled sacs that form inside the marrow at the ends of bones as part of the development of OA.

SUBCUTANEOUS Beneath the skin.

SUBDURAL HEMATOMA Bleeding into the space between the outermost and middle membranes covering the brain.

SUBLINGUAL Taken underneath the tongue.

SUBLUXATION A partial or incomplete dislocation of the bones that form a joint.

SUBSTANTIA NIGRA Movement control centers of the brain containing dopamine-producing cells.

SUCCIMER (CHEMET) OR DMSA A drug used to remove excess lead from the body.

SUCCUSSION A process integral to the creation of a homeopathic remedy in which a solution is repeatedly struck against a firm surface. This is performed to thoroughly mix the substance and magnify its healing properties.

SUET Refers to the hard fat found around cattle and sheep kidneys and loins; it is used in cooking.

SULFADOXONE/PYRIMETHAMINE (FANSIDAR) An antimalarial drug developed in the 1960s. It is the first drug tried in some parts of the world where chloroquine resistance is widespread. It has been associated with severe allergic reactions due to its sulfa component.

SUNSCREEN Products that block the damaging rays of the sun. Good sunscreens contain either para-aminobenzoic acid (PABA) or benzophenone, or both. Sunscreen protection factors range from 2-45.

SUPERANTIGEN A type of bacterial toxin that triggers abnormal activation of T-cells, which regulate the body's response to infected or malignant cells. *Streptococcus pyogenes* is responsible for the production of a number of different superantigens.

SUPERIOR MESENTERIC ARTERY SYNDROME A condition in which a person vomits after meals due to blockage of the blood supply to the intestine.

SUPPOSITORY A herbal treatment prepared to be inserted into the vagina or the rectum.

SUSHI A traditional Japanese preparation of food wherein vinegared rice, vegetables, and fish or fish products, are wrapped in *nori* seaweed, cut, and served.

SWIMMER'S EAR An inflammation or infection of the ear canal due to overexposure to water.

SWIMMER'S ITCH An allergic skin inflammation caused by a sensitivity to flatworms that die under the skin, causing an itchy rash.

SYMBIOTIC The living together of two different organisms. Symbiotic relationships can be mutually beneficial, beneficial to one partner and not harmful to the other partner, or beneficial to one partner and harmful to the other partner.

SYMPTOM In homeopathy, a positive sign of the body's self-defense and self-healing that assists the practitioner to choose the correct remedy. Symptoms include the patient's emotional state and psychological characteristics as well as physical symptoms in the narrow sense.

SYNCOPE Dizziness or brief loss of consciousness resulting from an inadequate flow of oxygenated blood to the brain.

SYNDROME A collection of abnormalities that occur together often enough to suggest that they have a common cause.

SYNERGISTIC EFFECT. A compounding effect greater than the effect otherwise expected from adding the involved components.

SYNERGISTIC Describes an association which improves the effectiveness of members of the association.

SYNERGY Combined action or effects. Some researchers think that the side effects and interactions reported for kava kava are related to synergy among the various compounds in the herb.

SYNOVIA A clear, somewhat sticky lubricating fluid secreted by membranes that surround the joints.

SYNOVIAL FLUID Fluid surrounding the joints which acts as a lubricant, reducing the friction between the joints.

SYNOVIAL JOINT A type of joint that allows articular bones to move.

SYNOVIAL MEMBRANE The membrane that lines the inside of the articular capsule of a joint and produces a lubricating fluid called synovial fluid.

SYRUP An herbal preparation that is made generally by boiling the herb with water, adding sugar as a preservative, and boiling until it thickens. The syrup may be stored.

SYSTEMIC LUPUS ERYTHEMATOSUS A chronic, inflammatory, autoimmune disorder in which the individual's immune system attacks, injures, and destroys the body's own organs and tissues. It may affect many organ systems including the skin, joints, lungs, heart, and kidneys.

SYSTEMIC Involving the whole body; the opposite of localized.

SYSTOLIC BLOOD PRESSURE Blood pressure when the heart contracts (beats).

T

TABES DORSALIS A progressive deterioration of the spinal cord and spinal nerves associated with tertiary syphilis.

TABLEWORK The passive phase of Trager therapy, in which the practitioner uses gentle and noninvasive movements to allow the client to relax deeply and experience physical movement as free and effortless.

TACRINE A drug commonly prescribed for Alzheimer's disease that provides temporary improvement in cognitive functions for some patients with mild-to-moderate forms of the disease.

TACTILE SENSE Receiving information about the body and the environment via contact with the skin. When this is lost through illness, a person may receive injuries without being aware of it.

TACTILE The perception of touch.

T'AI CHI A Chinese system of meditative physical exercise, characterized by slow methodical circular and stretching movements.

TAMOXIFEN A drug used to treat cancer.

TANNINS These astringent plant chemicals are the medicinal constituent of an herb that enables it to facilitate healing of wounds.

TAOISM A Chinese religion and philosophy based on the doctrines of Laotse which advocates simplicity and selflessness.

TAOISM The system of thought that shaped the view of creation underlying traditional Chinese medicine.

TAPOTEMENT A group of massage techniques in which the therapist strikes the soft tissues with the sides of the hands or with loose fists. It is intended to invigorate and tone the body.

TARGET TISSUES Tissues specifically receptive to a given hormone.

TARTAR A hard, yellowish-brown gritty deposit that collects on the teeth. It is also called dental calculus.

T-CELL A type of lymphocyte that develops in the thymus gland, circulates in the blood and lymph, and regulates the body's immune response to infected or malignant cells.

TD The abbreviation for tetanus and diptheria vaccine.

TELANGIECTASIA Small blood veins visible at the surface of the skin of the nose and cheeks.

TELLINGTON TOUCH (TTOUCH) A form of energy therapy that combines aspects of the Feldenkrais method of bodywork with aura therapy.

TEMPEH A dense high-fiber food product made from fermented soybeans.

TEMPORAL BONES The compound bones that form the left and right sides of the skull.

TEMPOROMANDIBULAR JOINT (TMJ) The joint responsible for movement of the jawbone.

TEMPOROMANDIBULAR JOINT DISORDER Inflammation, irritation, and pain of the jaw caused by improper opening and closing of the temporomandibular joint. Other symptoms include clicking of the jaw and a limited range of motion.

TENDINITIS Inflammation of tissues that connect muscles to bones. Tendinitis is usually caused by strain or an injury.

TENDON A band or cord of thick white fibrous tissue that connects a muscle to bone.

TENDONS Refers to the tough, fibrous connective tissue that connects muscles to bones.

TENOTOMY Surgical procedure that cuts the tendon of a contractured muscle to allow lengthening.

TERPENES Hydrocarbons found especially in essential oil.

TEST ANXIETY A name for the stress and anxiousness that commonly occur in students before they take exams.

TESTICLES Two egg-shaped glands that produce sperm and sex hormones.

TESTOSTERONE A male hormone produced in the testes or made synthetically that is responsible for male secondary sex characteristics.

TETANUS A potentially fatal infection of the central nervous system, found in wounds.

TETANY A disorder of the nervous system characterized by muscle cramps, spasms of the arms and legs, and numbness of the extremities. It is a symptom of an abnormality in calcium metabolism.

THALAMOTOMY Surgery that destroys a small amount of tissue in the thalamus to control PD tremors.

THALAMUS An important relay center for sensory signals in the cerebral cortex of the brain.

THALASSEMIA A group of several genetic blood diseases characterized by absent or decreased production of normal hemoglobin. Individuals who have thalassemia have to undergo frequent blood transfusions, and are at risk for iron overload.

THEOBROMINE A stimulant that occurs naturally in chocolate as well as in kola nut. Foods and drinks containing theobromine are poisonous to domestic pets.

THERAPEUTIC TOUCH (TT) An American form of energy therapy based on the ancient tradition of the laying-on of hands. TT is thought to work by removing energy blockages or disturbances from the patient's aura.

THERMAL BURN Tissue injury caused by extreme heat.

THERMOGENESIS The production of heat, especially within the body.

THIAZOLADINEDIONES A class of drugs typically used to treat diabetes and insulin resistance.

THIRD EYE A term used to refer to the inner eye or eye of the mind. Opening the third eye refers to admission to a new level of consciousness.

THORACIC OUTLET SYNDROME Spasticity of the muscles of the upper back, neck, and/or shoulders.

THROMBOCYTES Thrombocytes, also called platelets, help the blood to clot so that wounds can heal.

THROMBOPHLEBITIS Inflammation of a vein together with clot formation.

THROMBOTIC Pertaining to a blood clot formed within an intact blood vessel as opposed to a clot formed to seal the wall of a blood vessel after an injury.

THROMBUS A blood clot that forms within a blood vessel or the heart.

THRUSH A yeast infection of the mouth characterized by white patches on the inside of the mouth and cheeks.

THUJONE A natural chemical compound found in sage as well as in wormwood and certain other spices. Thujone in large quantities can cause hallucinations and convulsions.

THYROIDECTOMY Removal of the thyroid gland.

THYROID-STIMULATING HORMONE (TSH) A hormone secreted by the pituitary gland that controls the release of T_4 by the thyroid gland.

THYROTOXICOSIS An excess of thyroid hormones in the blood causing a variety of symptoms that include rapid heart beat, sweating, anxiety, and tremor.

THYROXINE (T_4) A thyroid hormone that regulates many essential body processes.

TIA (TRANSIENT ISCHEMIC ATTACK) Occlusion of smaller blood vessels to the brain which can produce stroke-like symptoms for anywhere from a few minutes to 24 hours, but leaves no permanent damage.

TIBB NABAWI Prophetic medicine (another name for unani-tibbi).

TIBIA One of the long bone of the lower leg.

TIC An involuntary, sudden, spasmodic muscle contraction.

TINCTURE A liquid extract of an herb prepared by steeping the herb in an alcohol and water mixture. Tinctures can also be prepared using vinegar or glycerin, instead of alcohol.

TINEA CRURIS The medical term for jock itch.

TINEA A term that refers to any of several fungal infections of the skin, especially ringworm.

TINNITUS Ringing or other noises in the ears, sometimes caused by skeletal misalignment.

TISANE A decoction of herbs, usually drunk for medicinal purposes.

TITRATION Gradually adjusting dosage of a supplement until the desired result is obtained, but no unwanted side effects appear.

TOFU A high-protein curd made from soybeans, used in meat and dairy replacement products.

TONIC PUPIL A pupil that is slow to change.

TONIC A preparation or medicine that invigorates, strengthens, or restores tone to body tissues.

TONIFICATION Acupuncture technique for strengthening the body.

TONSILS Oval-shaped masses of glandular tissue located on both sides at the back of the throat. Tonsils act like filters to trap bacteria and viruses.

TOPHUS (PLURAL, TOPHI) A chalky deposit of a uric acid compound found in gout. Tophi occur most frequently around joints and in the external ear.

TOPICAL Applied to the skin or external surface of the body.

TORSION The accidental twisting of tissues in the body that may decrease the blood and oxygen supply to the affected area.

TOTAL PELVIC EXENTERATION Surgical procedure involving removal of the rectum, lower portion of the large intestine, the urinary bladder, the pelvic reproductive organs, lymph nodes, pelvic muscles, and perineum. Both urinary and fecal diversions are required for this surgery.

TOURNIQUET A device used to control bleeding, consisting of a constricting band applied tightly around a limb above the wound. It should only be used if the bleeding in life-threatening and cannot be controlled by other means.

TOXEMIA Poisoning of the blood.

TOXIC SHOCK SYNDROME (TSS) A potentially serious bacterial infection associated with the use of tampons to absorb menstrual flow.

TOXICOLOGY The branch of medical pharmacology dealing with the detection, effects, and antidotes of poisons.

TOXIFICATION When the body is unable to eliminate poisonous substances, they remain clogged in the system and eventually cause a breakdown of normal function.

TOXIN A substance that has poisonous effects on the body.

TRACE ELEMENT An element that is required in only minute quantities for the maintenance of good health. Trace elements are also called micronutrients.

TRACHEA A cartilage tube in the area of the throat that carries air to the lungs.

TRACHEOTOMY A surgical procedure in which a small hole is cut into the trachea, or windpipe, below the level of the vocal cords.

TRADITIONAL CHINESE MEDICINE Ancient Chinese healing system involving acupuncture, herbal remedies, dietary therapies, and other healing techniques.

TRANSCENDENTAL MEDITATION (TM) A meditation technique based on Hindu practices that involves the repetition of a mantra.

TRANSCRANIAL MAGNETIC STIMULATION A procedure used to treat patients with depression.

TRANSCUTANEOUS ELECTRICAL NERVE STIMULATION (TENS) A treatment for chronic pain that involves the use of a self-operated portable device. The device sends electrical impulses through electrodes placed over the painful area.

TRANSENDENTAL MEDITATION A focusing of the mind based in part on Hindu meditation techniques in which each person is given a word or phrase to meditate upon.

TRANS-FATTY ACID A toxic type of fat created by hydrogenating oils and by deep frying foods.

TRANSIENT Of short duration.

TRANS-RECTAL ULTRASOUND A procedure where a probe is placed in the rectum. High-frequency sound waves that cannot be heard by humans are sent out from the probe and reflected by the prostate. These sound waves produce a pattern of echoes which are then used by the computer to create sonograms, or pictures of areas inside the body.

TRANSVAGINAL ULTRASOUND A technique for imaging the ovaries using sound waves generated by a probe inserted into the vagina. This diagnostic imaging procedure serves as the baseline for a hysterosonographic examination.

TRAUMATIC SHOCK A condition of depressed body functions as a reaction to injury with loss of body fluids or lack of oxygen. Signs of traumatic shock include weak and rapid pulse, shallow and rapid breathing, and pale, cool, clammy skin.

TRAVELER'S DIARRHEA Diarrhea caused by ingesting local bacteria to which one's digestive system has not yet adapted.

TREMATODES Flukes, which are flat, leaf-shaped parasitic worms.

TREPHINE A saw- or drill-like instrument used to remove a circular piece of bone from the skull. It is also called a trepan.

TRICHINELLOSIS A parasitic disease caused by tissue-dwelling roundworms of the species *Trichinella spiralis*, usually acquired by eating infected meat.

TRICYCLIC ANTIDEPRESSANT (TCA) A group of antidepressant drugs that all have three rings in their chemical structure. Their mechanism of action is not fully understood, but they appear to extend the duration of action of some neurohormones, including serotonin and norepinephrine. They have also been used to treat some forms of chronic pain. Common brand names are Aventyl, Elavil, Surmontil, and Vivactil.

TRICYCLICS A type of antidepressant; Elavil, for example.

TRIDOSHA the combination of three basic principles of energy, or biological humor, that comprise life, according to Ayurvedic philosophy.

TRIGEMINAL NEURALGIA OR TIC DOULOUREUX An affliction of the trigeminal or fifth cranial nerve. The condition is characterized by attacks of shooting, stabbing pain on one side of the face. These episodes are triggered by touching the affected area.

TRIGGER POINTS Hypersensitive muscle locations that cause pain in response to undue stress.

TRIGLYCERIDE A fat that comes from food or is made from other energy sources in the body. Elevated triglyceride levels contribute to the development of atherosclerosis.

TRIGONELLINE An alkaloid compound found in fenugreek.

TRIIODOTHYRONINE (T_3) A thyroid hormone similar to thyroxine but more powerful. Preparations of triiodothyronine are used in treating hypothyroidism.

TRIMESTER One-third or 13 weeks of pregnancy.

TRIMYRISTIN A chemical found in nutmeg that causes anxiety.

TRIPLE BURNER The pathways and relationships between the Spleen, the Lungs and the Kidney.

TRITURATION A method of preparing a homeopathic remedy from an insoluble substance by grinding or pounding it into a fine powder. *Calcarea carbonica* is prepared from shells by trituration.

TUBAL PREGNANCY A pregnancy that implants in the fallopian tube instead of inside the uterus. This often occurs as a result of sexually transmitted infections such as chlamydia. It is also known as ectopic pregnancy

TUBER The thick, fleshy, underground stem of a plant.

TUBERCLES Small, pea-sized tubers that grow on *Dioscorea* plants in the angles between the leaves and the stem. They are used in the cultivation of Chinese yam.

TUBEROUS SCLEROSIS A genetic disease that causes skin problems, seizures, and mental retardation. It may be confused with autism.

TUI NA A form of Chinese massage in which the therapist vigorously pushes and kneads the soft tissues of the patient's body. Its name means "push and grasp."

TUMOR ANTIBODY FACTOR (TAF) A component of IAT sera, possibly tumor necrosis factor (TNF), that may induce antibodies that destroy tumors.

TUMOR COMPLEMENT FACTOR (TCF) A component of IAT sera that stimulates antibody production.

TUMOR An uncontrolled growth of tissue, which may be cancerous.

TUMOR-INDUCING FACTOR (TIF). A blood component that can initiate tumor growth.

TYRAMINE A compound derived from tyrosine, an amino acid that is a precursor to various alkaloids, and found in various types of food.

TZANCK PREPARATION A procedure in which skin cells from a blister are stained and examined under the microscope. The presence of large skin cells with many cell centers or nuclei points to a diagnosis of herpes zoster when combined with results from a physical examination.

TZANCK TEST A laboratory test using a microscope to examine tissue samples that have been stained with certain dyes.

U

UDANA life sustaining energy of the diaphragm, the third of the five airs of Ayurvedic philosophy, the life force governing upward motion.

ULCER A site of damage to the skin or mucous membranes characterized by the formation of pus and the death of tissue. It is frequently accompanied by inflammation.

ULCER An open sore on the skin, resulting from tissue destruction, that is usually accompanied by redness, pain, or infection.

ULCERATION A pitted area or break in the continuity of a surface, such as the skin or mucous membrane.

ULCERATIVE COLITIS An inflammation in the walls of the bowel that causes internal sores, called ulcers, on the lining of the bowel.

ULTRASOUND This medical device uses sound waves bouncing off body organs or tissues, which are reflected back as images on the screen. Ultrasound can show shape, size, and certain characteristics of the tissues.

ULTRAVIOLET RADIATION (UV) Electromagnetic radiation that is shorter than visible light rays but longer than x rays. UV is thought to be responsible for sunburns, skin cancers, and cataract formation.

UNAPPROVED DRUG The FDA is responsible for ensuring that biological products are safe and effective and in compliance with the law and FDA regulations. Biological products are licensed under the provisions of Section 351 of the Public Health Service Act (42USC)(PHS Act).

UNICURSAL A curve or series of curves that forms one path, without branching or splitting. A true labyrinth is unicursal in design.

UNSATURATED FAT A type of fat found in plant foods that is typically liquid (oil) at room temperature. Unsaturated fats are the most commonly recommended dietary fats.

UNSATURATED FAT Fat found in plant foods that is typically liquid (oil) at room temperature. They can be monounsaturated or polyunsaturated, depending on the chemical structure. Unsaturated fats are the most recommended dietary fats.

UREA A colorless compound that is the primary component of urine in mammals and that results from the oxidation of proteins.

URETERS The tubes that carry urine from the kidney into the bladder for storage.

URETHERA The tube that drains the bladder.

URETHRA The canal that carries urine from the bladder.

URETHRAL SPHINCTER Circular muscle that controls the movement of urine from the bladder to the urethra.

URETHRITIS Inflammation of the urethra.

URIC ACID A compound that can form deposits in joints and tissues. This disease is known as gout or hyperuricemia.

URINARY RETENTION The result of progressive obstruction of the urethra by an enlarging prostate, causing urine to remain in the bladder even after urination.

UROLOGIST A physician who specializes in treating problems of the urinary tract.

URTICARIA Itchy pustules that may be caused by a hypersensitivity to food, drugs, or other substances.

USP The *U.S. Pharmacopoeia.* Nationally and internationally recognized drug standards published by the United States Pharmacopeia Convention, Inc. and used as a standard by FDA and other federal regulatory agencies.

UTERUS Female reproductive organ that contains the developing fetus during pregnancy.

UTERUS The organ that carries and provides nutrition to a developing baby. Also called the womb.

UVEITIS Inflammation of the uvea, which is a continuous layer of tissue consisting of the iris, the ciliary body, and the choroid. The uvea lies between the retina and sclera.

UVULOPALATOPHARYNGOPLASTY (UPPP) An operation to remove excess tissue at the back of the throat to prevent it from closing off the airway during sleep.

V

VACCINE A substance prepared from a weakened or killed virus which, when injected, helps the body to form antibodies that will attack an invading virus and may prevent infection altogether.

VAGINAL CONE A weighted cone held in the vagina for Kegel excercising.

VAGINISMUS A condition in which muscles around the outer third of the vagina have involuntary spasms in response to attempts at vaginal penetration, thus making penetration impossible or difficult.

VAGINITIS An inflammation of the mucous membrane that lines the interior of the vagina. It often results from a *Candida* or other fungal infection, and is accompanied by pain, itching, and discharge.

VAGINOSIS Bacterial infection of the vagina, caused by an overgrowth of bacteria that normally live in the vagina.

VALACYCLOVIR An oral antiviral drug that is available under the trade name Valtrex. The drug prevents the varicella zoster virus from replicating.

VARICELLA-ZOSTER IMMUNE GLOBULIN (VZIG) A substance that can reduce the severity of chickenpox symptoms.

VARICELLA-ZOSTER VIRUS The virus that causes chicken pox and shingles.

VARICOSE VEINS Swollen veins that can no longer maintain proper blood pressure.

VARIVAX A vaccine for the prevention of chicken pox.

VAS DEFERENS The duct that stores sperm and carries it from the testicles to the urethra.

VASODILATATION A widening of the blood vessels.

VASODILATOR Any drug that relaxes blood vessel walls.

VASODILATORY Having the effect of relaxing or widening the blood vessels.

VATA One of the three main constitutional types found under Ayurvedic principles. Keeping one's particular constitution in balance is considered important in maintaining health.

VECTOR An animal carrier that transfers an infectious organism from one host to another. The vector that transmits Lyme disease from wildlife to humans is the deer tick or black-legged tick.

VECTOR An animal or insect that carries a disease-producing organism.

VEGAN DIET A vegetarian diet that excludes meat and dairy products.

VEGAN A person who doesn't eat any animal products, including dairy and eggs.

VEGETARIANISM The theory or practice of living only on vegetables and fruits.

VENTRICLE One of the two lower chambers of the heart.

VENTRICULAR TACHYCARDIA A heart rate of more than 100 beats per minute in the large chambers of the heart.

VENTRICULAR Pertaining to the two lower chambers of the heart.

VERMIFUGE A medication or preparation given to expel worms and other intestinal parasites.

VERRUCA (PLURAL, VERRUCAE) The medical term for warts.

VERTEBRAE The component bones of the spine.

VERTIGINOUS ATTACKS Attacks of vertigo or dizziness.

VERTIGO A feeling of dizziness together with a sensation of movement and a feeling of rotating in space.

VESICLE Sac or hollow structure filled with fluid (i.e., a blister).

VESTIBULAR SYSTEM The brain and parts of the inner ear that work together to detect movement and position.

VESTIBULAR Pertaining to the vestibule; regarding the vestibular nerve of the ear which is linked to the ability to hear sounds.

VIAGRA Trade name of an orally administered drug for erectile failure first cleared for marketing in the United States in March 1998. Its generic name is sildenafil citrate.

VIGILANCE Attentiveness or alertness.

VILLI Tiny, finger-like projections that enable the small intestine to absorb nutrients from food.

VIPASSANA A Buddhist meditative practice that emphasizes deep attentiveness to the present moment.

VIREMIA The measurable presence of virus in the bloodstream that is a characteristic of acute retroviral syndrome.

VIRILIZATION The development of male characteristics in women.

VIRUS A tiny particle that can cause infections by duplicating itself inside a cell using the cell's own machinery.

VISUAL ACUITY Visual sharpness and resolving ability, usually measured by the ability to read numbers and letters.

VISUALIZATION TECHNIQUES A form of meditation, contemplation, and imagination that seeks to alter physical processes and directions of behavior or outcomes by focused mental awareness on specific images.

VITAL FORCE Innate wisdom and energy of the body.

VITAMIN A (RETINOL). An essential nutrient for vision that is obtained from animal products or made in the liver from carotenoids such as beta carotene.

VITAMIN K A fat-soluble vitamin responsible for blood clotting, bone metabolism, and proper kidney function.

VITAMINS Any of various organic carbon-containing substances that are essential in minute amounts for normal growth and activity of the body, and are obtained naturally from plant and animal foods.

VITILIGO Patchy loss of skin pigmentation, resulting in lighter areas of skin.

VOLATILE OR ESSENTIAL OILS Simple molecules that give the plant its scent. When applied to the skin, volatile oil extracts are absorbed into the bloodstream through the fatty layer of the skin.

VOLATILE ORGANIC COMPOUNDS Compounds from common sources such as cleaning materials and furnishings that vaporize, or become a gas, at room temperature.

VOLATILE Something that vaporizes or evaporates quickly when exposed to air.

VOLUNTARY MUSCLE A muscle under conscious control; contrasted with smooth muscle and heart muscle.

VOMITUS The medical term for the contents of the stomach expelled during vomiting.

VULNERARY An agent used for healing wounds.

VULVA The external genital organs of a woman, including the outer and inner lips, clitoris, and opening of the vagina.

VULVAR VESTIBULITIS Inflammation of the vestibule of the vulva or vagina.

VULVOVAGINAL CANDIDIASIS A yeast-like fungal infection of the vulva and vagina, which can be related to regular consumption of cranberry.

VYANA life sustaining energy of the heart and lungs; the second of the five airs of Ayurvedic philosophy; the life force governing circular motion.

W

WARFARIN A blood-thinning drug, known by the brand name Coumadin.

WART A small, fleshy skin growth caused by a virus.

WASTING SYNDROME A progressive loss of weight and muscle tissue caused by the AIDS virus.

WATER-SOLUBLE VITAMINS Vitamins that are not stored in the body and are easily excreted. These vitamins must be consumed regularly as foods or supplements to maintain health.

WEDGE RESECTION Removal of only a small portion of a cancerous lung.

WERNECKE-KORSAKOFF SYNDROME A condition caused by thiamine deficiency and usually related to alcoholism. Symptoms occur alternately in the central nervous

system (brain and spinal cord) and peripheral nervous system (nerves in the remaining parts of the body). Alcohol interferes with the body's ability to metabolize thiamine.

WERNICKE-KORSAKOFF SYNDROME A disorder of the central nervous system resulting from long-term thiamine deficiency. It is characterized by amnesia, confusion, visual problems, and unsteady gait; and is most commonly seen in alcoholics.

WHEAL A smooth, slightly elevated area on the body surface, which is redder or paler than the surrounding skin.

WHEATGRASS Young green wheat sprouts, grown organically for juicing. Wheatgrass is a central element of the Wigmore diet.

WHEY PROTEIN The protein found in cow's milk after the casein, the most common milk protein (curds), has been removed.

WHOLE BLOOD Blood that contains red blood cells, white blood cells, and platelets in plasma.

WILDCRAFTING The art of gathering or harvesting herbs or other plants from their native wild environment for human use.

WILSON'S DISEASE An inborn defect of copper metabolism in which free copper may be deposited in a variety of areas of the body. Deposits in the brain can cause tremor and other symptoms of Parkinson's disease.

WINDOW A perspective adopted to assess the property of a given plant.

WITHDRAWAL SYMPTOMS A group of physical or mental symptoms that may occur when a person suddenly stops using a drug or substance to which he or she has become dependent.

X

XEROSTOMIA The medical term for dry mouth.

Y

YAG Yttrium aluminum garnet, a type of laser used to perform surgery on secondary cataracts.

YANG ASPECTS In traditional Chinese medicine, yang aspects are qualities of nature such as warmth, activity, light, and dryness.

YIN AND YANG In Taoist thought, the two primordial opposing yet interdependent cosmic forces.

YIN ASPECTS Yin aspects are the opposite of yang aspects and are represented by qualities such as cold, stillness, darkness, and passiveness.

YOGA A system of physical, mental, and breathing exercises developed in India.

YOGI (FEMININE, YOGINI) A trained yoga expert.

Z

ZEAXANTHIN An antioxidant carotenoid that is the mirror image of lutein.

ZEN A form of meditation that emphasizes direct experience.

ZOLLINGER-ELLISON SYNDROME A disorder characterized by the presence of tumors (gastrinomas) that secrete a hormone (gastrin), which stimulates the production of digestive juices.

ZONE THERAPY Also called zone analgesia, a method of relieving pain by applying pressure to specific points on the body. It was developed in the early twentieth century by Dr. William Fitzgerald.

ZOONOSIS (PLURAL, ZOONOSES) Any disease of animals that can be transmitted to humans under natural conditions. Lyme disease and rabies are examples of zoonoses.

ZYGOTE The result of the sperm successfully fertilizing the ovum. The zygote is a single cell that contains the genetic material of both the mother and the father.

INDEX

References to individual volumes are listed in **boldface**; numbers following a colon refer to page numbers. **Boldface** page ranges indicate main topical essays. Illustrations are highlighted with an *italicized* page number; tables are also indicated with *italics* followed by a lowercase "t."

A

A-200 pediculicides, **3**:1213
AA (Alcoholics Anonymous), **1**:46
AAAAI (American Academy of Allergy, Asthma and Immunology), **4**:1883
AAAOM (American Association of Acupuncture and Oriental Medicine), **1**:20, 169
AAMA (American Academy of Medical Acupuncture), **1**:20, 169
AANP (American Association of Naturopathic Physicians), **1**:445, **3**:1433
AAPC (American Association of Pastoral Counselors), **3**:1627
AAPM (American Academy of Pain Management), **4**:2049
AASECT (American Association of Sexual Educators, Counselors and Therapists), **4**:1833
AAT (Animal assisted therapy). *See* Pet therapy
AATA (American Art Therapy Association), **1**:133, **2**:1127
Abana, for ischemia, **2**:1109
ABCT (American Board of Chelation Therapy), **1**:419
Abdominal pain
    from appendicitis, **1**:111
    corydalis for, **1**:552
    evodia fruit for, **2**:721
    magnolia for, **3**:1274
    See also Stomachaches
ABHM (American Board of Holistic Medicine), **2**:978
Abnormal uterine bleeding, defined, **3**:1337, 1339
Abortifacients
    bayberry, **1**:188, 189
    blue cohosh, **1**:268

cotton root bark, **1**:553
    pennyroyal, **3**:1567
Abraham, Irwin, **3**:1652
Abrak bhasma, for wheezing, **4**:2142
Abrams, Albert, **3**:1698, 1699
Abrasions, **4**:2166
Abscess, **1**:1–3
    Crohn's disease and, **1**:568, 570
    diverticulitis and, **2**:637, 638
    drainage of, **1**:2
    from epididymitis, **2**:699
    fritillaria for, **2**:789
    with gum diseases, **2**:887
    hepar sulphuris for, **2**:940
    from staphylococcal infections, **4**:1922
    usnea for, **4**:2072
Absence seizures, **2**:704, 705
Absinthe, **4**:2165
Absorption (Physiology)
    chelated minerals and, **1**:417
    Crohn's disease and, **1**:568
ABT Global Pharmaceutical, **3**:1367
Abumrad, Naji N., **1**:213
Academic disorders. *See* Learning disorders
Academy for Guided Imagery, **3**:1365
Academy of Lymphatic Studies, **3**:1257
ACAM (American College of Advancement in Medicine), **1**:419–420
Acamprosate, for alcoholism, **1**:46
Acanthosis nigricans, insulin resistance and, **2**:1087
Accidental poisoning. *See* Acute poisoning
Accumulation (Biological). *See* Bioaccumulation
Accutane. *See* Isotretinoin
ACD (Allergic contact dermatitis), **1**:538–539
Acemannan, aloe vera and, **1**:61
Acetaldehyde, hangovers and, **2**:894

Acetaminophen
    for chills, **1**:447
    for cuts and scratches, **1**:582
    for dysmenorrhea, **2**:655
    for fever, **1**:430, 447
    for migraine, **3**:1356
    for mononucleosis, **3**:1371
    See also Analgesics
Acetaminophen overdose
    methionine for, **3**:1350, 1351
    milk thistle for, **3**:1359
Acetazolamide, for glaucoma, **2**:847–848
Acetylated mannose. *See* Acemannan
Acetylcysteine. *See* N-acetyl cysteine
Acetyl-L-carnitine
    for chronic fatigue syndrome, **1**:481
    for memory loss, **3**:1320
    See also Carnitine
ACHE (American Council for Headache Education), **2**:906
Aches and pains. *See* Pain
Achillea millefolium. See Yarrow
Acid indigestion. *See* Heartburn; Indigestion
Acid reflux. *See* Gastroesophageal reflux
Acidophilus, **1**:3–4, **3**:1645–1646, 1647
    for acne, **1**:6
    for chlamydia, **1**:464
    for chronic fatigue syndrome, **1**:481
    for colic, **1**:512
    detoxification and, **2**:612
    for diarrhea, **2**:629–630
    for food poisoning, **2**:778
    for fungal infections, **2**:794
    for gastroenteritis, **2**:821
    for gonorrhea, **2**:860
    for heavy metal poisoning, **2**:931
    for Lyme disease, **3**:1254
    for vaginitis, **4**:2085
    for whooping cough, **4**:2149
    for yeast infections, **4**:2174
Acidosis, methionine and, **3**:1351

Index

Affinity of herbs, in traditional Chinese medicine, **2**:947

Aframomum melegueta roscoe. See Grains-of-paradise fruit

African medicine. *See* Traditional African medicine

African pygeum, **1**:25–27
 for hair loss, **2**:892
 for male infertility, **2**:1071
 in traditional African medicine, **4**:2032, 2033

Agalsidase alfa, **2**:694

Agastache, **1**:27–28

Agastache and Pig's Bladder Pill, for rhinitis, **3**:1743

Agastache to Rectify Qi. *See* Huo Xiang Zheng Qi

Agatston, Arthur, **4**:1902–1903, 1904

Agave, for stomachaches, **4**:1928

Age spots, hydroxy acids for, **1**:209

Ageless Body, Timeless Mind (Chopra), **1**:176

Age-Related Eye Disease Study, **1**:206

Age-related macular degeneration. *See* Macular degeneration

Aging, **1**:28–32, *29, 176*
 astragalus and, **1**:147
 atherosclerosis and, **1**:149
 bee pollen and, **1**:195
 cataracts and, **1**:373
 chills and, **1**:446
 Chinese foxglove root and, **1**:448
 DHEA for, **2**:615
 fo ti for, **2**:772–773
 grape seed extract for, **2**:872
 hearing loss and, **2**:912
 heart attacks and, **2**:915
 heart disease and, **2**:920
 infertility and, **2**:1068
 ledum for, **3**:1199
 melatonin for, **1**:30, **3**:1316
 memory loss and, **3**:1318, 1320
 natural hormone replacement therapy and, **3**:1424
 nummular dermatitis, **2**:608
 osteoarthritis, **3**:1502
 pine bark extract for, **3**:1593
 royal jelly for, **3**:1763
 stroke risk and, **4**:1939–1940
 t'ai chi for, **2**:724
 See also Elderly

Agoraphobia, **1**:199, **3**:1581,1582,1583

Agriculture, biodynamic, **1**:98

Agrimony, **2**:768*t*, 770
 for rashes, **3**:1701
 for urinary incontinence, **4**:2067

Agropyron species. *See* Wheat grass therapy

Ague tree. *See* Sassafras

Ague-weed. *See* Boneset

AHAs. *See* Alpha hydroxy acids

Ahimsa, **4**:2095

AHMA (American Holistic Medical Association), **2**:687, 979

AHPA (American Herbal Products Association), **2**:1144

AI (Adequate Intake). *See* Estimated Safe and Adequate Dietary Intake

Ai ye. *See* Mugwort

AIDS, **1**:32–41, *33, 34, 35t*
 apitherapy for, **4**:2103
 astragalus for, **1**:147
 cat's claw for, **1**:379
 chills in, **1**:446, 447
 coenzyme Q10 for, **1**:37
 common cold and, **1**:529
 DHEA for, **2**:615
 essiac tea for, **2**:713
 glutamine for, **2**:851
 glutathione for, **2**:853
 hyperthermia for, **2**:1029
 Kaposi's sarcoma and, **1**:*34*, 35–36, **2**:*1142*, 1142–1143
 Korean ginseng for, **2**:842
 maitake for, **3**:1276–1277
 marijuana for, **3**:1290
 medium-chain triglycerides for, **3**:1314
 melatonin for, **3**:1316
 mesoglycan for, **3**:1347
 methionine for, **3**:1350
 mistletoe for, **3**:1366, 1367
 neurolinguistic programming for, **3**:1452
 omega-3 fatty acids for, **3**:1485
 shingles and, **4**:1846
 Siberian ginseng for, **2**:845
 stages, **1**:34–36
 traditional African medicine for, **4**:2032
 traditional Chinese medicine for, **2**:948
 transmission, **1**:32–34
 treatment, **1**:36–38
 See also HIV

AIDS dementia complex, **1**:35

Aikido, **1**:105, **3**:1295–1296

Aikido Association of America, **3**:1296, **3**:1296–1297

Air pollution
 lung cancer and, **3**:1239
 poisoning and, **1**:422

Air quality, indoor. *See* Indoor air quality

Airborne allergens, **1**:53, 55

Airport malaria, **3**:1278, 1281

Airsickness. *See* Motion sickness

AIT. *See* Auditory integration training

Ajna, **1**:408

Ajuga. *See* Bugle weed

Ajwan, for stomachaches, **4**:1929

Al Anon, **1**:46

Al Razi, **4**:2064

Al Zahrawi, **4**:2064

ALA. *See* Alpha-linolenic acid

Alanine, for gout, **2**:866

Alanylglutamine supplements, **2**:851

Albuterol, for asthma, **1**:141

Alchemilla vulgaris. See Lady's mantle

Alcohol abuse. *See* Alcoholism

Alcoholic beverages
 cancer and, **1**:346
 cluster headaches and, **2**:907
 elimination diet and, **2**:677
 frostbite and, **2**:791, 793
 gingko and, **2**:836
 hangovers, **2**:893–895
 heart disease and, **2**:918–919, 924
 ischemia and, **2**:1110
 lead poisoning and, **3**:1191
 lemon balm in, **3**:1200
 mistletoe in, **3**:1367
 mushroom poisoning and, **2**:778
 osteoporosis and, **3**:1513
 for tremor, **4**:2042

Alcoholics Anonymous, **1**:46

Alcohol-induced disorders, **1**:44

Alcoholism, **1**:41–47, *42t*
 acupuncture for, **1**:16, 45
 cirrhosis and, **1**:43, 494, 495, 497
 Gulf War syndrome and, **2**:883
 kudzu for, **2**:1170–1171
 linoleic acid and, **3**:1221
 lobelia for, **3**:1224
 nux vomica for, **3**:1469
 pancreatitis and, **3**:1535
 potassium for, **3**:1619
 thiamine deficiency and, **4**:2009
 See also Substance abuse and dependence

Alder buckthorn/dogwood. *See* Buckthorn

Alder, Janet, **2**:589

Aldosterone, glycyrrhizin and, **2**:596

Alefacept, for psoriasis, **3**:1663

Alendronate, for osteoporosis, **3**:1512

Aletrius farinosa. See True unicorn root

Alexander, Charles, **3**:1309

Alexander, Frederick Matthias, **1**:47–49

Alexander technique, **1**:47–50, **3**:1380
 during pregnancy, **3**:1632
 Rubenfeld synergy method and, **3**:1767

Alexander Technique International, **1**:49

Alexander's archangel. *See* Angelica

Alfalfa, **1**:50–52, *51*
 for angina, **1**:88
 for atherosclerosis, **1**:150
 for osteoporosis, **3**:1511
 for PMS, **3**:1637

Algae
 chlorella, **1**:466–468, **2**:931
 Dunaliella, **1**:204
 for genital herpes, **2**:825
 usnea and, **4**:2071–2072
 See also Spirulina

Algin, in kelp, **2**:1152

Alisma, **1**:52–53

Allergens
 asthma and, **1**:136–137, 137*t*

American Vegan Society, **4**:2094
American Veterinary Medical Association, **3**:1690
American water plantain. *See* Alisma
American white oak. *See* Oak
American Yoga Association, **1**:215
Amino acids, **1**:71–74, **3**:1463–1464
   ademetionine and, **1**:20
   for ADHD, **1**:159
   as antioxidant, **1**:102
   for cataracts, **1**:374
   for gastritis, **2**:816
   for gout, **2**:866
   for juvenile rheumatoid arthritis, **2**:1136
   for lead poisoning, **3**:1193
   for Lou Gehrig's disease, **3**:1232
   for Parkinson's disease, **3**:1550
   for retinopathy, **3**:1734
   See also specific amino acids, e.g., Arginine
Amino sugars, **2**:848
Amla powder, for gum diseases, **2**:886
Ammi visnaga, for allergies, **1**:56
Amoebic abscess, **1**:2
Amoracia rusticana. See Horseradish
Amoxicillin
   with acidophilus, **1**:4
   for Lyme disease, **3**:1254
Amphetamine substance abuse, **4**:1944
Ampicillin, with acidophilus, **1**:4
Ampligen, for chronic fatigue syndrome, **1**:482
Amputation, for gangrene, **2**:804
AmSAT. *See* American Society for the Alexander Technique
Amsler grid, for macular degeneration detection, **3**:1265
Amygdalin, **1**:117–118
Amylases, **2**:693
Amyloid precursor protein, **1**:66
Amyotrophic lateral sclerosis. *See* Lou Gehrig's disease
An mo massage, **1**:450
ANA. *See* American Naturopathic Association
Anacardium, for contact dermatitis, **1**:539
Anal itching, **2**:1112
Analgesic abuse headaches. *See* Rebound headaches
Analgesics, **3**:1529–1530
   ademetionine, **1**:21
   arnica, **1**:121
   Balm of Gilead, **1**:181
   black cumin, **1**:246
   cayenne, **1**:384
   for childbirth, **1**:438
   eucalyptus, **2**:717
   evodia fruit, **2**:721–722
   for fibrocystic breast disease, **2**:757
   for fractures, **2**:785
   gastrodia, **2**:818
   grape seed extract, **2**:872

   for headaches, **2**:909
   for herniated disks, **2**:956
   for influenza, **2**:1078
   kava kava, **2**:1144
   lemongrass, **3**:1202
   for low back pain, **3**:1237
   marijuana, **3**:1290
   MSM, **3**:1386
   for osteoarthritis, **3**:1504
   for otitis media, **2**:662
   for sciatica, **4**:1804
   sesame oil, **4**:1829
   shiatsu massage, **4**:1840
   for shin splints, **4**:1848
   for sprains and strains, **4**:1917
   for teething, **4**:1991
   for toothache, **4**:2025
   white willow, **4**:2144–2145
   See also Pain management
Anaphylaxis
   from allergies, **1**:55–56
   bee venom for, **4**:2104
   treatment of, **1**:57
Anas barbariae hepatis, for common cold, **1**:531
Anatomy of an Illness (Cousins), **2**:1009
Anatomy of the Spirit (Myss), **2**:687
Ancient Greece
   herbal medicine and, **2**:949–950
   labyrinths and, **3**:1173
   mint and, **4**:1907
Ancient Rome, labyrinths and, **3**:1173
Ancylostoma duodenale. See Hookworm
Androgen replacement (Natural hormone replacement therapy), **3**:1424, 1425, 1426–1427, 1428
Androgenetic alopecia, **2**:891
Andrographis, **1**:74–75, **4**:1861
Andropause, natural hormone replacement therapy and, **3**:1424, 1426–1427
Androstenedione, **1**:75–77, **3**:1427
Anemarrhena, **1**:77–79
Anemia, **1**:79–84, *80*
   anise for, **1**:90
   chills from, **1**:446
   codonopsis for, **1**:500
   dandelion for, **2**:592
   dong quai for, **2**:645
   ferrum phosphoricum for, **2**:747
   gymnema for, **2**:888
   homeopathy for, **2**:1101
   iron phosphate for, **2**:1101
   veganism and, **4**:2095
   white peony for, **4**:2144
Anesthetics
   acupuncture as, **1**:11, **1**:16
   for canker sores, **1**:357
   electroacupuncture, **2**:676
   for epididymitis, **2**:700
   hypnotherapy and, **2**:1033, 1034
   local, **3**:1449, **3**:1451
   neural therapy and, **3**:1450–1451

Anethole, in anise, **1**:89–90
Aneurysm, **4**:1939, 1940
Angelica, **1**:84–86, *85*
   for digestive disorders, **2**:646
   for irritable bowel syndrome, **2**:1105
   for PMS, **3**:1637
   for stomachaches, **4**:1928
   in Sun's soup, **4**:1956
Angelica archangelica. See Angelica
Angelica atropurpurea (American angelica), **2**:646
Angelica sinensis. See Dong quai
Angina, **1**:86–89
   bromelain for, **1**:302
   carnitine for, **1**:360
   fish oil for, **2**:760
   hawthorn for, **1**:88, **2**:900, 901
   heart disease and, **2**:920, 921, 922
   vs. heartburn, **2**:927
   ischemia and, **2**:1107, 1108
   kudzu for, **2**:1169, 1171
   magnesium for, **3**:1269
   marijuana for, **3**:1290
Angioedema, defined, **2**:968
   See also Hives
Angiogenesis theory, **1**:368
Angiography
   for angina, **1**:87
   for atherosclerosis, **1**:149
   for diverticulitis, **2**:637–638
   for heart disease, **2**:921–922
   for ischemia, **2**:1108
Angioplasty
   for angina, **1**:88
   for cerebral vascular insufficiency, **1**:403
   See also Balloon angioplasty
Angostura bitters, **1**:238
Animal bites. *See* Bites and stings
Animal enzymes, **2**:693
Animal-assisted therapy. *See* Pet therapy
Animals. *See* Veterinary medicine
Anise, **1**:89–92, *90*
   for anemia, **1**:82
   for bronchitis, **1**:304
   for common cold, **1**:530
   for cough, **1**:555
   for digestion, **2**:635
   for heartburn, **2**:927
   for influenza, **2**:1078
   for irritable bowel syndrome, **2**:1105
   for laryngitis, **3**:1183
   for lice infestation, **3**:1212
   for nausea, **3**:1437
   for stomachaches, **4**:1928
Anise hyssop. *See* Agastache
Aniseed. *See* Anise
Anisocoria. *See* Adie's pupil
Anisometropia, lazy eye from, **3**:1187–1188

Bandler, Richard, **3**:1451
Bangkok massage. *See* Thai massage
Bao He Wan, for vomiting, **4**:2127
Baptisia tinctoria. See Wild indigo
Barberry, **1**:*181–183*, *182*
   for hangovers, **2**:895
   for irritable bowel syndrome,
     2:1105
   for psoriasis, **3**:1661
   for UTIs, **1**:256, 257
   for yeast infections, **4**:2174
Barbiturates
   for anxiety, **1**:106
   for Ménière's disease, **3**:1324
Barium enema, for IBD, **2**:1074
Barium swallow. *See* Upper GI x-ray
   series
Barley grass, **1**:183–185
Barney de Cruz, Margarita, **3**:1641
Barosma betulina. See Buchu
Barré, Jean-Alexandre, **1**:23
Barrett's esophagus, **2**:925, 926, 928
Barrier contraception methods, **1**:438
Bartenieff fundamentals, **3**:1379
Bartenieff, Irmgard, **3**:1379
Barton, Benjamin Smith, **2**:857
Basal cell carcinoma, **4**:1864–1865,
   1866
   See also Skin cancer
Base chakra, **1**:408
Base oils. *See* Carrier oils (Aromather-
   apy)
Basil, **2**:974, 1161
Bastard ginseng. *See* Codonopsis
Bastard saffron. *See* Safflower flower
Bastyr University of Natural Health
   Sciences (Seattle)
    homeopathy and, **2**:984, 987, 992
    naturopathic medicine and, **3**:1434
    panchakarma and, **3**:1534
    yohimbe and, **4**:2185
Bates Association for Vision Education,
   1:187
Bates method, **1**:185–188
   for astigmatism, **1**:143
   for hyperopia, **2**:1020
   for myopia, **3**:1409
Bates, William H., **1**:185–186, 196
Bathing. *See* Hydrotherapy; Hygiene;
   Therapeutic baths
Battle fatigue. *See* Post-traumatic stress
   disorder
Battle's sign, **1**:307
Bay laurel
   in aromatherapy, **1**:123*t*
   for stomachaches, **4**:1929
   for wheezing, **4**:2142
Bayberry, **1**:188–190, *189*
   for common cold, **1**:530
   for worms, **4**:2162
Baylor College of Medicine (Texas),
   3:1272
Baylor University, **3**:1525
Baywillow. *See* White willow

BCG. *See* Bacille Calmette-Guérin
Beano, for gas, **2**:814
Bearberry. *See* Uva ursi
Beard, John, **2**:1149
Beard moss. *See* Usnea
Bear's grape. *See* Uva ursi
Bear's weed. *See* Yerba santa
Beating percussion, **3**:*1298*
Beaver tree. *See* Magnolia
Becker, Robert O., **1**:14
Bedsores, **1**:190–192, *191*
Bedwetting, **1**:192–194
   cornsilk for, **1**:548, 549
   cornus for, **1**:550
   lycopodium for, **3**:1250
   sepia for, **4**:1828
   uva ursi for, **4**:2079
Bee bread. *See* Red clover
Bee pollen, **1**:194–196, *195*, **2**:903
Bee sting therapy. *See* Apitherapy
Bee stings. *See* Bites and stings
Bee venom. *See* Apis
Bee venom therapy. *See* Apitherapy
Beebread. *See* Borage oil
Beech, **2**:768*t*, 770, **3**:1701
Beechdrops. *See* Blue cohosh
Beer industry. *See* Breweries
Bee's milk. *See* Royal jelly
Beggarweed. *See* Cuscuta
Behavioral homework, **1**:198
Behavioral medicine. *See* Mind/body
   medicine
Behavioral optometry, **1**:196–197
Behavioral therapy, **1**:197–200, **3**:1670,
   1671–1672
   for ADHD, **1**:158
   for alcoholism, **1**:45
   for autism, **1**:172
   for bedwetting, **1**:193
   for binge eating disorder, **1**:218
   for bulimia nervosa, **1**:317
   for depression, **2**:602
   for hyperopia, **2**:1020
   for insomnia, **2**:1084
   for irritable bowel syndrome,
     2:1106
   for obesity, **3**:1476
   for schizophrenia, **4**:1801
   for sexual dysfunction, **4**:1833
   for stress, **4**:1937
   for Tourette syndrome, **4**:2028
   for trichotillomania, **2**:892
   for urinary incontinence, **4**:2067
   for vomiting, **4**:2128
   See also Cognitive-behavioral therapy
Belladonna, **1**:*201*, 201–204
   for abscess, **1**:2
   for boils, **1**:272
   for breast cancer effects, **1**:291
   for bursitis, **1**:326
   for chickenpox, **1**:430
   for conjunctivitis, **1**:533
   for earaches, **2**:658

   for endometriosis, **2**:685
   for fever, **4**:1794
   for headaches, **2**:909
   for irritable bowel syndrome,
     2:1105
   for knee pain, **2**:1161
   for measles, **3**:1305
   for mumps, **3**:1400
   for otitis media, **2**:661
   for pelvic inflammatory disease,
     3:1565
   for rubella, **3**:1766
   for sore throat, **4**:1897
   for strep throat, **4**:1934
   for tonsillitis, **4**:2023
   for whooping cough, **4**:2149
Bellanti, Joseph A., **1**:110
Bellergal, for hot flashes, **2**:1007
Bellis perennis, for low back pain,
   3:1236
Bell's palsy, apitherapy for, **4**:2103
Belshaw, Chris, **3**:1508
Ben Cao Gang Mu-Dan Shi Bu Yi (Chinese pharmacopeia), **3**:1711
Bencao gangmu (Shiz-Hen), **3**:1679
Benign prostatic hypertrophy. *See*
   Prostate enlargement
Benign tumors. *See* Tumors
Benne. *See* Sesame oil
Benor, Daniel, **2**:687, 688–689
Benson, Herbert
   breath therapy, **1**:297
   meditation, **3**:1309, 1625, 1626,
    4:2182
   relaxation therapy, **3**:1362, **3**:1723,
    1724
Bentonite clay
   for abscess, **1**:2
   for contact dermatitis, **2**:607
   for fungal infections, **2**:794
Benzodiazepines
   abuse of, **4**:1943, 1944
   for anxiety, **1**:106
   for bipolar disorder, **1**:231
   for headaches, **2**:909
   for insomnia, **2**:1085
   for panic disorder, **3**:1542
Benzoin
   for bronchitis, **1**:304
   for cuts and scratches, **1**:581
   for juvenile rheumatoid arthritis,
    2:1135
   for laryngitis, **3**:1183
Ber, Abram, **3**:1658
Berard, Guy, **1**:162, **4**:1899
Berard method. *See* Auditory integration training
Berberine compounds
   from coptis, **1**:544
   for diabetes, **2**:948
   for parasitic infections, **3**:1547
Berberis species. *See* Barberry
Bergamot
   for boils, **1**:272

devil's claw for, **2:**614
diathermy for, **2:**631
glucosamine for, **2:**849
knee pain and, **2:**1160
Russian massage for, **3:**1768
vitamin B12 for, **4:**2108
Burton, Lawrence, **2:**1050–1051, 1053
Burzynski, Stanislaw, **1:**350, **3:**1517
Butcher's broom, **1:327–329,** *328,*
2:938, **3:**1580
Buteyko, **1:329–331**
Buteyko, Konstantin, **1:**329
Butin abscess, **1:**1
Butterbur. *See* Coltsfoot
Butterflyweed, **2:**903, **3:**1603–1604
Butternut. *See* Black walnut
BVT. *See* Apitherapy
Byakujutsu. *See* Atractylodes
Byers, Dwight, **3:**1714
Bypass surgery. *See* Coronary artery
bypass surgery

C

Cabbage
hypothyroidism and, **2:**851
for itching, **2:**1113
for peptic ulcers, **4:**2061
for warts, **4:**2133
Cactus
for insulin resistance, **2:**1088
for ischemia, **2:**1109
prickly pear, **3:**1640–1644
Cadmium poisoning, **1:333–334,**
2:930, 931
Caesarean section, **1:**435
Caffeine, **1:334–337,** 335*t*
for asthma, **1:**140
bedwetting and, **1:**194
dry mouth and, **2:**648
ephedra and, **2:**696
epididymitis and, **2:**700
fatigue and, **2:**736, 737
in green tea, **2:**878
in kola nuts, **2:**1165, 1166
McDougall diet and, **3:**1303
senior nutrition and, **4:**1819
CAG Functional Foods, **3:**1647
Caisse, Rene, **2:**713–714
Calamine lotion, **1:**430, 539
Calamus, for diverticulitis, **2:**638
Calcarea carbonica, **1:337–339, 2:**927,
3:1512
Calcarea fluor. See Calcium fluoride
Calcarea phos. See Calcium phosphate
Calcarea sulph. See Calcium sulfate
Calciferol. *See* Vitamin D
Calcitonin, for osteoporosis, **3:**1512
Calcium, **1:339–343,** 416
for ADHD, **1:**159
for adolescents, **4:**1986
in bonemeal, **1:**273, 274

boron and, **1:**281
for chickenpox, **1:**429
for children, **1:**441
for constipation, **1:**536, 537
for coronary heart disease, **2:**917
for dysmenorrhea, **2:**654
for endometriosis, **2:**685
for fatigue, **2:**735
fractures and, **2:**785–786
gallstones and, **2:**797
for gum diseases, **2:**887
for heart disease, **2:**922
for heavy metal poisoning, **2:**931
ipriflavone and, **2:**1096
for kidney stones, **2:**643
kidney stones and, **2:**1156
for knee pain, **2:**1162
lead contamination of, **1:**416,
2:643–644
for lead poisoning, **3:**1193
for leukemia, **3:**1207
for lung cancer, **3:**1241
for Lyme disease, **3:**1254
lysine and, **3:**1259
magnesium and, **3:**1269–1270
for menopause, **3:**1333
for menstruation disorders, **3:**1339
for mononucleosis, **3:**1370
for muscle cramps, **3:**1404
for osteoporosis, **1:**542, **3:**1512
for Parkinson's disease, **3:**1550
phosphorus and, **3:**1585
for PMS, **3:**1637
potassium and, **3:**1621
senior nutrition and, **4:**1819
for shingles, **4:**1845
for sleep disorders, **4:**1877
for temporomandibular joint syndrome, **4:**1993
for tinnitus, **4:**2021
Calcium fluoride, **1:**387, 388, **2:**937
Calcium phosphate, **1:**319, 387
Calcium sulfate, **1:**387
Calcium sulfide. *See Hepar sulphuris*
Calendula, **1:343–345,** *344*
for abscess, **1:**2
for allergies, **1:**56
for athlete's foot, **1:**152
for bedsores, **1:**191
with bitters, **1:**240
for blisters, **1:**260
for burns, **1:**323, 324
for canker sores, **1:**357
for chickenpox, **1:**430
for contact dermatitis, **1:**539
for corns and calluses, **1:**547
for cradle cap, **1:**557
for cuts and scratches, **1:**580, 581
for dermatitis, **2:**607
for diaper rash, **2:**627
for earaches, **2:**657
for eczema, **2:**669
for fractures, **2:**785
for fungal infections, **2:**794

for gonorrhea, **2:**860
for ingrown nails, **2:**1081
for itching, **2:**1113
for mumps, **3:**1400
for pelvic inflammatory disease,
3:1565
for peptic ulcers, **4:**2061
for radiation injuries, **3:**1695
for rashes, **3:**1701
for retinopathy, **3:**1735
for shingles, **4:**1845
for sore throat, **4:**1794
for sties, **4:**1926
for stomachaches, **4:**1929
for sunburn, **4:**1953
for tonsillitis, **4:**2023
for toxic shock syndrome, **4:**2031
for trichomoniasis, **4:**2046
for vaginitis, **4:**2085
for wounds, **4:**2168
California buckeye. *See* Horse chestnut
California buckthorn. *See* Buckthorn
Calluses. *See* Corns and calluses
Cambridge University, **3:**1245
Camellia sinensis. See Tea
Cameron, Ewan, **1:**354
Cammiphora opobalsamum. See Balm
of Gilead
cAMP, **1:**509
Campbell, Don, **4:**1901
Camphor
for bronchitis, **1:**304
for fever, **2:**751
for juvenile rheumatoid arthritis,
2:1135
Campion, Kitty, **2:**680–681
Campylobacter jejuni, **2:**776, 820
Canada balsam, for respiratory dis-
eases, **2:**681
Canada tea. *See* Wintergreen
Canadensis. *See* Elder flower
Canadian College of Naturopathic
Medicine (Toronto), **3:**1434
Cananga odorata. See Ylang ylang
Cancer, **1:345–353,** *346, 347*
AIDS-related, **1:**35–36
allopathic *vs.* alternative medicine
views, **1:**347, 355–356
chills from, **1:**446, 447
environmental therapy and, **2:**690
vs. genital warts, **2:**826, 827
low back pain and, **3:**1234
malignant lymphomas, **3:***1283,*
1283–1286
Mediterranean diet and, **3:**1312
pain control for, **1:**198
potassium and, **3:**1621
veganism and, **4:**2095
See also specific types of cancer
Cancer and Vitamin C (Pauling and
Cameron), **1:**354
Cancer prevention, **1:**352
amygdalin and, **1:**117–118
beta carotene for, **1:**204–206

Craniosacral Therapy Educational Trust, **1**:563
Crataegus species. *See* Hawthorn
Craving (Substance abuse), **4**:1944, 1947
Creatine, **1**:72, **565–567**, **3**:1232
Creating Affluence: Wealth Consciousness in the Field of All Possibilities (Chopra), **1**:176
Creative arts therapy. *See* Art therapy
Creeping Charlie/Jenny/John. *See* Lysimachia
Creeping thyme. *See* Thyme
Creighton University, **2**:871
Cretinism, **2**:1041
Criler, George, Jr., **2**:1029
Crinnion, Walter, **3**:1345
Crisis intervention, **3**:1672
Crocus sativa. See Saffron
Crohn's disease, **1**:**567–571**, *568*, **2**:1072
    glucosamine for, **2**:849
    omega-3 fatty acids for, **3**:1484
    Rosen method for, **3**:1762
    vitamin B12 for, **4**:2108
Cross lateralization of the brain, **2**:649
Cross-linking theory of aging, **1**:29
Croton oil, **1**:56, **1**:539
Croup, **1**:90, **1**:**571–573**, *572*, **2**:997
Crown chakra, **1**:408
Crush wounds, **4**:2166, 2167
Crusted scabies. *See* Scabies
Cryosurgery, for cervical dysplasia, **1**:406
Cryotherapy, **2**:1082, **2**:1142
Cryptotympana species. *See* Cicada
Cryptoxanthin, **1**:363
Crystal healing, **1**:**573–575**, *574*
Cs-4. *See* Cordyceps
CSF. *See* Cerebrospinal fluid
CSR. *See* Craniosacral rhythm
CT scans. *See* Computed tomography scans
CTS. *See* Carpal tunnel syndrome
Cucurbita pepo, for worms, **4**:2162
Cue-controlled relaxation, **3**:1724
Culpeper, Nicholas
    barberry, **1**:182
    calendula, **1**:343
    chickweed, **1**:431, 432
    fennel, **2**:743
    feverfew, **2**:753
    herbal medicine, **2**:951
    horsetail, **2**:1001
    milk thistle, **3**:1358
    nettle, **3**:1445
    parsley, **3**:1554
    rosemary, **3**:1760
    sage, **4**:1777
    valerian, **4**:2088
Culturelle (Probiotic), **3**:1647
Cumin, 1:82, **4**:1928, 1929
Cupping, **1**:**575–577**, *576*
    acupuncture and, **1**:19

    for bronchitis, **1**:305
    for chronic fatigue syndrome, **1**:481
    for neck pain, **3**:1440
    for pinched nerve, **3**:1591
    sports massage, **4**:1914
    for stomachaches, **4**:1929
    Swedish massage, **4**:1957
Cupressus sempervirens. See Cypress
Cuprimine. *See* Penicillamine
Cuprum, **4**:1929, 2149
Curanderas, **1**:577
Curanderismo, **1**:**577–578**
Curanderos, **1**:577
Curcuma augustifolia. See Arrowroot
Curcuma longa. See Turmeric
Curcumin, **3**:1528, **4**:2057
The Cure Is in the Cupboard (Ingram), **3**:1491
Curly dock. *See* Yellow dock
Currant seed oil. *See* Black currant seed oil
Current Medical Diagnosis and Treatment 2000, **2**:1090
Cuscuta, **1**:**578–580**, **4**:1832
Cushing's syndrome, **2**:1017, 1018
Cutaneous field stimulation, for itching, **2**:1113
Cuts and scratches, **1**:**580–582**, *581*, **4**:2166, 2167
    garlic for, **2**:811
    hyssop for, **2**:1046
    osha for, **3**:1501
    prickly pear cactus for, **3**:1643
Cuttlefish, sepia from, **4**:1828
Cutweed. *See* Kelp
CVA (Cerebral vascular accident). *See* Stroke
CVS (Cyclic vomiting syndrome), **4**:2126
Cyanides, amygdalin and, **1**:117–118
Cyanocobalamin. *See* Vitamin B12
Cyclamen europaeum, **2**:1101
Cyclic adenosine monophosphate, **1**:509
Cyclic vomiting syndrome, **4**:2126
Cyclosarin, Gulf War syndrome and, **2**:883
Cyclothymia, **1**:229
Cydonia oblonga. See Quince seed
Cymatic therapy, **1**:**582–583**, **4**:1899, 1901, **4**:1957
Cymbopogon citratus. See Lemongrass
Cymbopogon martinii, for worms, **4**:2162
Cyperus, **1**:**583–585**
Cypress
    for bedwetting, **1**:193
    in hydrotherapy, **2**:1014
    for juvenile rheumatoid arthritis, **2**:1135
    for menstruation disorders, **3**:1339
    for varicose veins, **4**:2092
Cypripedium calceolus. See Lady's slipper

Cysteine
    as antioxidant, **1**:102
    for cataracts, **1**:374
    for gastritis, **2**:816
    for heavy metal poisoning, **2**:931
    for juvenile rheumatoid arthritis, **2**:1135
    for lead poisoning, **3**:1193
Cystic fibrosis, **2**:853, **3**:1221
Cystic Fibrosis Foundation, **2**:853
Cystine kidney stones, **2**:1156
Cystinuria, betaine hydrochloride for, **1**:212
Cystitis. *See* Bladder infections
Cystostatic agents, for dandruff, **2**:593
Cysts
    breast, **2**:756–757, **2**:1090
    knee pain and, **2**:1160
    ovarian, **3**:1519–1524
Cytokines, **3**:1666–1667, **4**:2161
Cytotoxic tests, **2**:611, 691

D

D and C. *See* Dilatation and curettage
Da huang. *See* Rhubarb root
Daidzein, **2**:1005, 1094
Daily allowance. *See* Recommended daily allowance
Dairy products
    calcium in, **1**:340, 341
    linoleic acid and, **3**:1220
    medium-chain triglycerides in, **3**:1313
    veganism and, **4**:2095–2096
    See also Diet
Dalmatian pellitory, **1**:484, 485
Dalton, Christine, **2**:1104
Damiana, **2**:**587–588**
    for binge eating disorder, **1**:218
    for bipolar disorder, **1**:230
    for fatigue, **2**:736
    for postpartum depression, **3**:1614
Dan shen. *See* Sage
Dan zhu ye, for prickly heat, **3**:1640
Dana-Farber Cancer Institute, **3**:1248
Dance of the Deer Foundation, **4**:1836
Dance therapy, **2**:**588–591**, *589*
    for anxiety, **1**:105
    as movement therapy, **3**:1379
    for stress, **4**:1936
Dancing mushroom. *See* Maitake
Dandelion, **2**:**591–593**, *592*
    for acne, **1**:6
    for anemia, **1**:82
    for atopic dermatitis, **2**:607
    for constipation, **1**:537
    for edema, **2**:672
    for endometriosis, **2**:685
    for gallstones, **2**:798
    for hangovers, **2**:895
    for insulin resistance, **2**:1088

Index

Green tea, **2:876–878,** *877*
　for aging, **1:**31
　for anxiety, **1:**105
　for atopic dermatitis, **2:**607
　for cancer, **1:**350, 519
　for coronary heart disease, **2:**917
　for dry mouth, **2:**648
　for heart disease, **2:**922
　for nausea, **3:**1437
　for retinopathy, **3:**1734
Green Unicorn Pill, **1:**257
Grieve, Maude, **4:**1880
Griffonia simplicifolia, **2:**603
Grifola frondosa. See Maitake
Grindelia, **1:**572, **2:**607
Grinder, John, **3:**1451
Grinspoon, Lester, **3:**1290
Groats. *See* Wild oat
Ground berry. *See* Wintergreen
Ground raspberry. *See* Goldenseal
Group therapy, **1:**97, **3:**1671, 1672
　See also Psychotherapy
GSE. *See* Grapefruit seed extract
GSR sensors, **1:**221–222
Guan Zhong, for worms, **4:**2162
Guar gum, for insulin resistance, **2:**1088
Guelder rose. *See* Cramp bark
Guggal resin. *See* Myrrh
Guggul, **2:879–880**
　for coronary heart disease, **2:**917
　for Ménière's disease, **3:**1323
　See also Boswellia
Gugulipids. *See* Myrrh
Gui pi tang, **1:**161
Gui Zhi. *See* Ramulus Cinnamomi Cassiae
Guided imagery, **2:880–882,** **3:**1724–1725
　for bladder cancer, **1:**253
　for bone spur pain, **1:**277
　for breast cancer effects, **1:**291
　for canker sores, **1:**357
　for childbirth, **1:**437
　for colorectal cancer, **1:**518
　for Crohn's disease, **1:**569
　for endometriosis, **2:**685
　for fibromyalgia, **2:**759
　for hangovers, **2:**895
　for heel spurs, **2:**933
　for Hodgkin's disease, **2:**971
　for irritable bowel syndrome, **2:**1105
　for kidney stones, **2:**1157
　for lung cancer, **3:**1242
　for malignant lymphomas, **3:**1284
　for mononucleosis, **3:**1369*t*
　for muscle cramps, **3:**1404
　for osteoarthritis, **3:**1504
　for pain management, **1:**324
　with past life therapy, **3:**1559
　during pregnancy, **3:**1632
　for radiation injuries, **3:**1695
　for stress, **4:**1936

　for stress-related hair loss, **2:**892
　for stroke, **4:**1941
　for substance abuse, **4:**1946
　for Tourette syndrome, **4:**2028
　See also Autogenic training; Relaxation therapy
Guided Imagery and Music, **3:**1406
Guild for Structural Integration. *See* Rolf Institute of Structural Integration
Guillain-Barré syndrome, **3:**1573, 1574
Guinea grains. *See* Grains-of-paradise fruit
Guinea rush. *See* Cyperus
Gulf War syndrome, **2:**690, 723, **882–885**
Gulfweed. *See* Sargassum seaweed
Gum
　chewing, for heartburn, **2:**927
　. *See* Myrrh
Gum bush. *See* Yerba santa
Gum diseases, **1:**1, **2:**885, **885–887,** *886*
　calcium for, **1:**340
　coenzyme Q10 for, **1:**502
　goldenseal for, **2:**858
　grapefruit seed extract for, **2:**870
　green tea for, **2:**876
　selenium for, **4:**1814
　usnea for, **4:**2072
　See also Gingivitis
Gum plant. *See* Comfrey
Gum weed. *See* Grindelia
Gummas, from syphilis, **4:**1965
Guo qi zi. *See* Lycium fruit
Gurmabooti. *See* Gymnema
Gurmar. *See* Gymnema
Gut permeability. *See* Leaky gut syndrome
Gutta percha tree, **2:**718
Guttate psoriasis, **3:**1660
GW 8150 (Hair loss gel), **2:**891
Gymnema, **2:**622, **888–889**
Gynecological disorders. *See* Reproductive system disorders
Gypsy weed. *See* Bugle weed

H

H2 blockers. *See* Histamine receptor blockers
HAART. *See* Highly active antiretroviral therapy
Haas, Elson, **2:**922
Hab Al Baraka. *See* Black cumin
Hachimijiogan, for cataracts, **1:**374
Hackett, George, **3:**1651
Hackmatack. *See* Thuja
Haemophilus influenzae, **2:**659, 662, **3:**1327
Hahnemann Medical Clinic (Albany, California), **2:**984, 987, 992

Hahnemann, Samuel, **1:**310, **2:**982, **4:**1828
　constitutional prescribing homeopathy, **1:**338–339
　hepar sulphuris, **2:**939
　homeopathy and, **1:**285, **2:**951, 980–982, 985, 989
　ledum, **3:**1198
　mercurius vivus, **3:**1341, 1342
　natrum muriaticum, **3:**1421–1422
　silica, **4:**1858
　syphilis, **4:**1968
　testing treatments, **1:**388
　trituration, **1:**337
Hai Zao. *See* Sargassum seaweed
Hair analysis
　detoxification and, **2:**611
　environmental therapy and, **2:**691
　for heavy metal poisoning, **2:**930, 931
　holistic dentistry and, **2:**975
Hair care
　for lice infestation, **3:**1212–1213
　linoleic acid for, **3:**1221
　prickly pear cactus for, **3:**1643
Hair loss, **2:891–893,** *892*
　hibiscus for, **2:**961
　kelp for, **2:**1152
　magnolia for, **3:**1274
　replacement methods, **2:**893
　saw palmetto for, **4:**1786
Hairy leukoplakia of the tongue, **1:**35
Halitosis. *See* Bad breath
Hallucinogenic drugs, **4:**1945, 2185
Hallux valgus. *See* Bunions
Halprin, Anna, **3:**1380
Halvorson, Peter, **4:**2043–2044
Hamamelis virginiana. See Witch hazel
Hambrecht, Rainer, **1:**73, 119
Hamburg parsley. *See* Parsley
Han Dynasty, Chinese food cures and, **1:**452
Hand warts, **4:**2131
Hand-foot syndrome, sickle cell anemia and, **4:**1854
Handicapped persons, Feldenkrais method and, **2:**739
Hands, reflexology and, **3:**1713, 1715–1717
Hangnail. *See* Ingrown nails
Hangovers, **2:893–896**
　See also Alcoholism
Hanna somatic education. *See* Somatics
Hanna, Thomas, **3:**1378, **4:**1894
Hao-shu. *See* Mugwort
Hard measles. *See* Measles
Hardening of the arteries. *See* Atherosclerosis
Hare Krishna movement, **1:**215
Hare's ear. *See* Chinese thoroughwax
Harich, Jacob, **2:**869
Haritaki fruit, **4:**2050
Harner, Michael, **4:**1836

Index

damiana for, **2**:587
echinacea for, **2**:665, 666
elder flower for, **2**:673–674
ephedra for, **2**:696
evodia fruit for, **2**:722
eyebright for, **2**:727
gardenia for, **2**:808
gelsemium for, **2**:822
grapefruit seed extract for, **2**:870
homeopathy for, **2**:982
lemongrass for, **3**:1203
lobelia for, **3**:1224
lomatium for, **3**:1227
mercurius vivus for, **3**:1341
osha for, **3**:1501
pau d'arco for, **3**:1561
rhus toxicodendron for, **3**:1748
Siberian ginseng for, **2**:844
sore throat and, **4**:1896
usnea for, **4**:2072
Influenza vaccine
importance of, **2**:1079
otitis media and, **2**:663
pinellia and, **3**:1594
stroke risk and, **4**:1942
Infusion for Promoting Blood Circulation and Improving Eyesight, **2**:1020
Infusions, defined, **1**:286
Ingham, Eunice D., **3**:1714
Ingram, Cass, **3**:1491
Ingrown nails, **2**:1080–1082, *1081*
INH, for tuberculosis, **4**:2053, 2054
Inhalation (Aromatherapy), **1**:125, **2**:717
Inhalation (Steam). *See* Steam inhalation
Inhaled poisons, **1**:424, **3**:1343
Inheritance. *See* Genetic disorders
Initiation, for shamanism, **4**:1836
Injection therapy, for varicose veins, **4**:2093
Injuries, **2**:851, **3**:1496–1497
See also Wounds
Inner ear. *See* Vestibular system
Inner eye. *See* Mind's eye
INNO-LIA test, for syphilis, **4**:1967
Inorganic mercury, **3**:1343, 1344, 1346
Inositol, **1**:159, **2**:685
Inositol hexaniacinate, **3**:1453, **4**:2111
Insect bites. *See* Bites and stings
Insect repellents
lemon balm, **3**:1200
lemongrass, **3**:1203
for malaria, **3**:1281
myrrh, **3**:1414
neem, **3**:1443
thuja, **4**:2011
wormwood, **4**:2165
Insecticides
aucklandia, **1**:161
brewer's yeast, **1**:300, 301
dalmatian pellitory, **1**:484, 485
feverfew, **1**:485

for lice infestation, **3**:1211, 1212, 1213–1214
lysimachia, **3**:1257, 1258
malaria and, **3**:1281
neem, **3**:1441, 1443
poisoning and, **1**:421
Insoluble dietary fiber
for constipation, **1**:536, 537
defined, **2**:963–964, **3**:1464
sources of, **2**:965
Insomnia, **2**:1082–1087, **4**:1876, 1877
5-HTP for, **2**:762
behavioral modification therapy for, **1**:198
biota for, **1**:225–226
Chinese foxglove root for, **1**:448
Chinese yams for, **1**:457
fo ti for, **2**:773
gastrodia for, **2**:818
Ignatia for, **2**:1049
jet lag and, **2**:1120, 1121
kava kava for, **2**:1144
magnesium for, **3**:1269
marijuana for, **3**:1290
massage therapy for, **3**:1299, 1301
meditation for, **3**:1308
melatonin for, **3**:1316–1317
motherwort for, **3**:1374
nux vomica for, **3**:1469
ophiopogon for, **3**:1489
pulsatilla for, **3**:1676, 1678
Rosen method for, **3**:1762
Russian massage for, **3**:1768
sesame oil for, **4**:1830
shiatsu massage for, **4**:1839, 1840
sulfur for, **4**:1949
Institute for ElectroAcupuncture and ElectroDiagnostics, **2**:676
Institute of Medicine, **1**:206, 207
Institute of Orthomolecular Medicine, **3**:1498
Institute of Thai Massage, **4**:2004–2005
Insulin
blood glucose and, **2**:617
chromium and, **1**:477–478
for diabetes, **2**:622
glucosamine and, **2**:849
hypoglycemia and, **2**:1037, 1039
maitake and, **3**:1276
South Beach diet and, **4**:1903
Zone diet and, **4**:2194
Insulin resistance, **2**:1087–1089
Insulin shock, **2**:1037
Insulin-dependent diabetes mellitus. *See* Diabetes mellitus
Integral yoga, **2**:898
Integrated cancer treatment, **1**:350, **3**:1517
Intention tremor, **4**:2040–2041
Interior design, feng shui and, **2**:742
Interleukin-6, juvenile rheumatoid arthritis and, **2**:1136

Intermittent claudication, **1**:360, **2**:836, **3**:1453
Internal derangement, **4**:1992, 1993, 1994
Internal fixation, **2**:785–786
Internal hemorrhoids. *See* Hemorrhoids
Internal radiation, **1**:350
International Academy of Compounding Pharmacists, **2**:1006
International Alliance of Healthcare Educators, **1**:145
International Association of Infant Massage, **2**:1062, 1064
International Association of Professional Natural Hygienists, **2**:734
International College of Applied Kinesiology, **1**:114, 116–117
International Council on Control of Iodine Deficiency Disorders, **2**:1091
International Foundation for Homeopathy (Seattle), **2**:984, 987, 992
International Fragrance Research Association, **1**:288
International Headache Society, **2**:906
International Institute of Reflexology, **3**:1714
International Iridology Research Association, **2**:1099, 1100
International Jojoba Export Council, **2**:1124
International Myomassethics Federation, Inc., **4**:1932
International School of Shiatsu, **4**:1840
International Shintaido Federation, **4**:1848, 1849
International Society for the Study of Subtle Energies and Energy Medicine, **1**:221
International Therapy Examinations Council, **3**:1769
International Trepanation Advocacy Group, **4**:2044
Internet
tinnitus therapy and, **4**:2021
unreliable information, **1**:287, **2**:953
The Interpretation of Dreams (Freud), **3**:1670
Intertrigo, from diaper rash, **2**:626
Interventions, for alcoholism, **1**:42, 45
Intervertebral disk displacement. *See* Herniated disk
Intestinal dysbiosis, **3**:1648
Intestinal flu. *See* Gastroenteritis
Intestinal gas. *See* Gas (Gastrointestinal)
Intestinal inflammation, **1**:567–568, **2**:1073
Intestinal obstructions, **1**:568, 570
Intestinal parasites. *See* Worms
Intestinal perforations, **1**:568, **2**:1073
Intestinal toxemia. *See* Toxic bowel syndrome
Intestinal worms. *See* Worms
Intoxic dilation of the colon, **2**:1073

K

M

Miliaria. *See* Prickly heat

Milieu therapy. *See* Environmental therapy

Military herb. *See* Yarrow

Milk glands, **2:**756

Milk of magnesia. *See* Magnesium hydroxide

Milk thistle, **3:1358–1360,** *1359*
  for acne, **1:**6
  for alcoholism, **1:**45
  for anxiety, **1:**106
  for breast feeding, **1:**295
  for cervical dysplasia, **1:**406
  for chronic poisoning, **1:**424
  for cirrhosis, **1:**496, **3:**1358
  detoxification and, **2:**612
  for endometriosis, **2:**685
  for gallstones, **2:**798
  for hangovers, **2:**895
  for heavy metal poisoning, **2:**931
  for hepatitis, **2:**943, **3:**1358
  for jaundice, **2:**1118
  for lead poisoning, **3:**1193
  for malaria, **3:**1280
  for menstruation disorders, **3:**1339
  for multiple chemical sensitivity, **3:**1394
  for panic disorder, **3:**1541
  for phobias, **3:**1582
  for stress, **4:**1936
  for substance abuse, **4:**1946

Milk vetch root. *See* Astragalus

Millefoil. *See* Yarrow

Miller, Baron Ferdinand von, **2:**715

Miller, Neal, **1:**219

Mills, John, **1:**111

Milne Institute, **1:**564

Milton, John, **2:**727

Milwaukee brace, for scoliosis, **4:**1807–1808

Mimulus flower remedy, **2:**768*t,* 770

Minamata disease (Japan), **3:**1345

The Mind/Body Effect (Benson), **3:**1724

Mind/Body Medical Institute at Harvard, **1:**297, **3:**1724

Mind/body medicine, **3:1360–1365**
  for asthma, **1:**140
  Benson, Herbert and, **3:**1724
  for bursitis, **1:**326
  for cancer, **1:**349–350
  for cerebral palsy, **1:**356
  for cervical dysplasia, **1:**406
  detoxification and, **2:**612
  for mononucleosis, **3:**1369*t*
  for ovarian cancer, **3:**1516
  for ovarian cysts, **3:**1522
  psychoneuroimmunology and, **1:**350, **3:**1362, 1666–1667
  psychophysiology and, **3:**1667–1669
  psychosomatic medicine and, **3:**1663–1665
  for syphilis, **4:**1968
  uterine cancer and, **4:**2074

See also Holistic medicine

Mindell, Earl, **4:**1816, 1818

Mindfulness meditation, **3:**1309, 1310

Mindfulness-based stress reduction, **1:**105, **3:**1309, 1310, 1363

Mind's eye
  dyslexia and, **2:**650, 651
  trepanation and, **4:**2043

Minerals, **3:**1464–1465
  for ADHD, **1:**159
  chelated, **1:**415–418
  importance of, **1:**416
  trace, **1:**159, 416, **3:**1464–1465, **4:**1974

See also specific minerals

Miner's candle. *See* Mullein

Miner's elbow. *See* Bursitis

Miner's lung. *See* Emphysema

Mini-stroke. *See* Transient ischemic attack

Minor Bupleurum pills, **3:**1370

Minor Bupleurum soup, **2:**736

Miotics, for glaucoma, **2:**847

Mirena intrauterine device, **2:**655

Miscarriage, **1:**248–249, **1:**267, 268

See also Pregnancy

Mishmi bitter. *See* Coptis

Missile wounds, **4:**2166, 2167

Missouri snakeroot. *See* Echinacea

Mistletoe, **3:1365–1368,** *1366*
  for bladder cancer, **1:**252–253
  for common cold, **1:**530

Mitchell, H. K., **2:**1050

Mitchella repens. See Squawvine

Mites, scabies and, **4:**1789–1790

Mitral valve prolapse, **3:**1269

Mittelschmerz, **3:**1520

Mixed hemispheric dominance, **2:**649

Mixed sleep apnea, **4:**1871, 1876

MLD. *See* Lymphatic drainage

MMR vaccine. *See* Measles-mumps-rubella vaccine

Mock pennyroyal. *See* Pennyroyal

Modeling, in behavioral modification therapy, **1:**198

Modern Herbal (Grieve and Leyel), **1:**314, **4:**1880

Modified radical mastectomy, **1:**292

Moist warts. *See* Genital warts

Molybdenum
  for leukemia, **3:**1207
  for lung cancer, **3:**1241
  as trace mineral, **1:**416

Momordica charantia. See Bitter melon

Monascus purpureus Went. *See* Red yeast rice extract

Mondeville, Henri de, **2:**1009

Moneywort. *See* Lysimachia

Monilial infection. *See* Vulvovaginal candidiasis

Monk's pepper. *See* Chasteberry

Monkshood. *See* Aconite

Monoamine oxidase inhibitors
  5-HTP and, **2:**762, 763
  for anxiety, **1:**106
  for bipolar disorder, **1:**231
  for depression, **2:**604
  kola nuts and, **2:**1166

Monocytes, leukemia and, **3:**1205

Mononucleosis, **3:1368–1372,** 1369*t*
  lomatium for, **3:**1227
  sore throat and, **4:**1896, 1897, 1898

Monosodium glutamate, **1:**171, 421–422

Monotherapy, epilepsy and, **2:**704

Mood disorders. *See specific disorders*

Mood stabilizing agents, **1:**230, **2:**761

Moore, Michael, **3:**1501

Moose elm. *See* Slippery elm

Moral issues. *See* Ethics

Moraxella catarrhalis, **2:**659, 663

Mori, Shigeaki, **3:**1721

Morinda citrifolia. See Noni

Mormon tea. *See* Ephedra

Morning sickness, **3:1372–1373,** 1630, 1631–1632
  anise for, **1:**91
  ginger for, **2:**834, 835
  ipecac for, **2:**1092
  sepia for, **4:**1828
  shiatsu massage for, **4:**1840

Morrison, F. R., **4:**1983

Mortality rates
  anorexia nervosa, **1:**97
  appendicitis, **1:**112
  blood poisoning, **1:**264, 265
  cervical cancer, **1:**406
  chickenpox, **1:**429
  cirrhosis, **1:**493
  colorectal cancer, **1:**519
  Crohn's disease, **1:**570
  gangrene, **2:**803, 804
  gastritis, **2:**817
  gastroenteritis, **2:**820
  heart attack, **2:**915, 918
  heart disease, **2:**920
  influenza, **2:**1076, 1079
  irritable bowel syndrome, **2:**1075
  juvenile rheumatoid arthritis, **2:**1136
  lead poisoning, **3:**1190
  leukemia, **3:**1208
  lung cancer, **3:**1238, 1243
  malaria, **3:**1278
  malignant lymphomas, **3:**1285
  malnutrition, **1:**443
  measles, **3:**1305
  meningitis, **3:**1329
  obesity, **3:**1473
  ovarian cancer, **3:**1514, 1517
  pancreatic pseudocyst rupture, **3:**1536
  pancreatitis, **3:**1538
  pneumonia, **3:**1605, 1609
  prostate cancer, **3:**1656, 1659
  SARS, **3:**1608
  systemic lupus erythematosus, **4:**1974

O

eucommia bark for, **2:**719
Premature infants
  cerebral palsy and, **1:**396
  massage therapy for, **2:**1062–1063,
    3:1299, 1301
  music therapy and, **3:**1406
Premenstrual dysphoric disorder,
  3:1336, 1340
  See also Premenstrual syndrome
Premenstrual phase of menstruation,
  3:1336
Premenstrual syndrome, **3:**1337–1338,
  3:1636–1639
  buchu for, **1:**311, 312
  calcium for, **1:**340
  chamomile for, **1:**410
  chasteberry for, **1:**414, **2:**757
  chicory for, **1:**433
  facial massage for, **2:**729
  fish oil for, **2:**761
  flaxseed for, **2:**765
  gamma-linolenic acid for,
    2:800–801
  gingko for, **2:**837
  lemon balm for, **3:**1200
  linoleic acid for, **3:**1221
  magnesium for, **3:**1269
  manganese for, **3:**1286, 1287
  pine bark extract for, **3:**1593
  Rosen method for, **3:**1762
  sesame oil for, **4:**1830
Prenatal care, **3:**1631
Prenatal massage. *See* Pregnancy massage
Prenatal testing, **3:**1631
Preparations of herbs, types of,
  1:286–287
Presbycusis, **2:**912
Presbyopia, **1:**373
Prescription for Nutritional Healing
  (Balch and Balch), **1:**242, **2:**1091
Preservatives (Food). *See* Food additives and preservatives
Preserve Harmony Pill, **4:**2127
President's Council on Physical Fitness
  and Sport, **3:**1412
Pressure sores. *See* Bedsores
Pressure treatment. *See* Compression
  treatment
Preuss, Harry, **3:**1276
Priapism, **4:**1854
Price, Weston A., **2:**972, 974
Price-Pottenger Nutrition Foundation,
  2:974
Prickly ash, **2:**1161, **3:**1707
Prickly heat, **3:1639–1640, 4:**2144
Prickly pear cactus, **3:1640–1644,** *1641*
Priessnitz, Vinzenz, **2:**1012–1013, *1013*
Priest's crown. *See* Dandelion
Prilosec, **2:**960
Primal therapy, **3:**1672
Primary amenorrhea, **3:**1336, 1339
Primary dysmenorrhea, **2:**653, **3:**1337,
  1340

Primary headaches, **2:**906
Primary insomnia. *See* Insomnia
Primary lung cancer, **3:**1238
  See also Lung cancer
Primary osteoarthritis. *See* Osteoarthritis
Primary syphilis, **4:**1965
Primary *vs.* recurrent herpes infections,
  1:506
Pritikin diet, **3:1644–1646**
Pritikin Longevity Center, **3:**1645
Pritikin, Nathan, **1:**149, **3:**1644
*The Pritikin Permanent Weight-Loss
  Manual* (Pritikin), **3:**1645
*The Pritikin Program for Diet and
  Exercise* (Pritikin), **3:**1645
Pritikin, Robert, **1:**149, **3:**1645
PRK. *See* Photorefractive keratectomy
Proanthocyanidins, **1:**224
  for aging, **1:**31
  as antioxidant, **1:**101
  in cranberry, **1:**560, 561
  in grape seed extract, **2:**871
  grapes and, **2:**873–875
  in pine bark extract, **3:**1593
Probiotics, **3:1646–1651**
  for chronic fatigue syndrome, **1:**481
  colonic irrigation and, **1:**516
  for diarrhea, **2:**629–630
  food poisoning and, **2:**778, 780
  for fungal infections, **2:**794
  for gastroenteritis, **2:**821
  for hangovers, **2:**895
  for inflammatory bowel disease,
    2:1074
  kombucha as, **2:**1167, 1168
  for Lyme disease, **3:**1254
  for parasitic infections, **3:**1547
  spirulina as, **4:**1912
  for systemic lupus erythematosus,
    4:1974
  for vaginitis, **4:**2085
  wild oat and, **4:**2153
  See also Acidophilus; Prebiotics
Procaine, in neural therapy,
  3:1450–1451
Procyanidins, **2:**871
Prodromes
  genital herpes, **2:**824
  herpes simplex, **1:**506
  hot flashes, **2:**1004
Productive cough, **1:**554
Progenitor cryptocides, **3:**1222–1223
Progesterone
  cellulite and, **1:**392
  dong quai and, **2:**645
  effect on PMS, **3:**1636
  hot flashes treatment and, **2:**1005,
    1007
  menopause and, **3:**1330, 1333
  menstruation and, **3:**1335, 1336
  natural hormone replacement therapy and, **3:**1424, 1425

synthetic, Mexican yam and,
  3:1352–1353
Progestins, **2:**685, 1007
Programmed senescence theory of
  aging, **1:**29
Progressive myonecrosis. *See* Gas gangrene
Progressive relaxation, **1:**199, **3:**1356,
  3:1723–1724
Progressive Relaxation (Jacobson),
  3:1723
Prokinetic drugs, **2:**928, 1061
Prolactin, **1:**25, 26, 414
Prolapsed disk. *See* Herniated disk
Prolapsed hemorrhoids. *See* Hemorrhoids
Proliferative phase of menstruation,
  3:1335
Proliferative retinopathy. *See* Retinopathy
Prolotherapy, **3:1651–1652**
Pronation, **2:**932, 933
Prophetic medicine. *See* Unani-tibbi
Proscar. *See* Finasteride
Prostaglandins
  aloe vera and, **1:**61
  black cumin and, **1:**245
  black currant seed oil and,
    1:247–248
  borage and, **1:**278
  dysmenorrhea and, **2:**653
  essential fatty acids and, **2:**708, 709,
    3:1487–1488
  for glaucoma, **2:**847
Prostasin blood protein, **3:**1515
Prostate biopsy, **3:**1654, 1657
Prostate cancer, **3:1656–1660,** *1657*
  cuscuta for, **1:**579
  DHEA and, **2:**616
  ganoderma for, **2:**805
  green tea for, **2:**876
  high fiber diet for, **2:**964
  immuno-augmentation therapy and,
    2:1051
  linoleic acid for, **3:**1221
  lycopene for, **1:**363, **3:**1248
  maitake for, **3:**1276
  meditation for, **3:**1310
  selenium for, **4:**1814
  soy isoflavones and, **2:**1005
Prostate enlargement, **3:1652–1656,**
  1653
  androstenedione for, **1:**76
  grape seed extract for, **2:**872
  hyperthermia for, **2:**1029
  kava kava for, **2:**1144
  kelp for, **2:**1152
  nettle for, **3:**1445
  pygeum for, **1:**25–26
  saw palmetto for, **1:**26, **3:**1654,
    1655, **4:**1786–1787
  traditional African medicine for,
    4:2032, 2033
  zinc for, **4:**2191–2192

vitamin E for, **4:**2120–2121
wild oat for, **4:**2153
witch hazel for, **4:**2157–2158
Skin care products
  AHAs, **1:**63–64
  aloe vera, **1:**61–62
  Balm of Gilead, **1:**180
  BHAs, **1:**209
  coix, **1:**504
  dandelion, **2:**592
  French green clay, **2:**786–787
  jojoba oil, **2:**1124–1125
  rosacea and, **3:**1755, 1756
Skin conductance level sensors,
  1:221–222
Skin diseases
  aloe vera for, **1:**61–62
  applied kinesiology and, **1:**115
  arsenicum album for, **1:**130
  barberry for, **1:**182–183
  bitter melon for, **1:**237
  black cumin for, **1:**245
  black currant for, **1:**248
  bloodroot for, **1:**266
  borage for, **1:**279
  brewer's yeast for, **1:**300
  calendula for, **1:**343
  castor oil for, **1:**371
  chamomile for, **1:**410
  chickweed for, **1:**432
  cnidium seeds for, **1:**499
  coltsfoot for, **1:**525
  coptis for, **1:**544
  devil's claw for, **2:**613, 614
  essential oils for, **2:**711
  gamma-linolenic acid for, **2:**800,
    801
  garlic for, **2:**811
  glucosamine for, **2:**849
  gotu kola for, **2:**862, 863
  hepar sulphuris for, **2:**939, 940
  hibiscus for, **2:**960, 961
  horsetail for, **2:**1002
  itching and, **2:**1112
  jojoba oil for, **2:**1125
  juniper for, **2:**1131, 1132
  ledum for, **3:**1199
  light therapy for, **3:**1218, 1219
  lomatium for, **3:**1227
  lycopodium for, **3:**1250, 1251
  marsh mallow for, **3:**1293
  mercurius vivus for, **3:**1341
  mullein for, **3:**1391
  neem for, **3:**1442
  ox-eye daisies for, **1:**485
  pau d'arco for, **3:**1561
  pine bark extract for, **3:**1593
  red cedar for, **3:**1708
  red clover for, **3:**1709–1710
  rhus toxicodendron for, **3:**1748
  scallion for, **4:**1791
  selenium for, **4:**1812
  sheep sorrel for, **4:**1837
  silica for, **4:**1858

slippery elm for, **4:**1880
sulfur for, **4:**1948, 1949
treatment of, **1:**250
urine therapy for, **4:**2070
witch hazel for, **4:**2158
yellow dock for, **4:**2176
yerba santa for, **4:**2178
See also specific diseases
Skin inflammation, **2:**1044
Skin patch tests
  for AHAs, **1:**64
  for black cumin, **1:**246
  for contact dermatitis, **1:**539
  for dermatitis, **2:**607
  for essential oils, **1:**125
  for vitamin E, **4:**2121–2122
Skin pinch test for cellulite, **1:**393
Skin rashes. *See* Rashes
Skin respiratory factor, **1:**301
Skin resurfacing
  for acne, **1:**8
  BHAs for, **1:**208–209, 210
Skin scraping, for neck pain, **3:**1440
Skin tests, for tuberculosis, **4:**2053
Skin ulcers, **4:**1965, **4:**2072
Skinner, B. F., **1:**198, **3:**1671
Skullcap, **4:1867–1870**
  for alcoholism, **1:**45
  for anxiety, **1:**106
  for binge eating disorder, **1:**218
  for bipolar disorder, **1:**230
  for fractures, **2:**784, 785
  for hay fever, **2:**903
  for headaches, **2:**909
  for insomnia, **2:**1084
  for Lyme disease, **3:**1254
  for menopause, **3:**1331
  for migraine, **3:**1356
  for pain, **3:**1528
  for panic disorder, **3:**1541
  for phobias, **3:**1582
  for PMS, **3:**1637
  for postpartum depression, **3:**1614
  for rhinitis, **3:**1743
  for shingles, **4:**1845
  for sleep disorders, **4:**1877
  for substance abuse, **4:**1946
  for tremor, **4:**2041
  See also Chinese skullcap
Skunk cabbage, for whooping cough,
  4:2148
SLE. *See* Systemic lupus erythematosus
Sleep apnea, **4:1870–1874,** *1871,* 1876,
  1878
Sleep deprivation, **1:**192, **2:**893, 894
  See also Insomnia
Sleep disorders, **4:1874–1879,** *1875*
  chronic fatigue syndrome and,
    1:480
  dementia and, **2:**598
  gotu kola for, **2:**863
  hops for, **2:**995, 996
  jet lag and, **2:**1120, 1121

magnetic therapy for, **3:**1272
passionflower for, **3:**1557
See also specific disorders
Sleep endoscopy, **4:**1889
Sleep patterns, fatigue and, **2:**736
Sleep pillows. *See* Dream pillows
Sleep positions
  for sleep apnea, **4:**1872
  for snoring, **4:**1890
Sleep stages, **2:**1083, **4:**1875
Sleep terror disorder, **4:**1876
Sleeping pills. *See* Hypnotics; Sedatives
Sleeplessness. *See* Insomnia
Sleep-onset insomnia, **2:**1083
Sleep-restriction therapy, **2:**1084
Sleepwalking disorder, **4:**1876
Slipped disk. *See* Herniated disk
Slippery elm, **4:1879–1881**
  for bedsores, **1:**191
  for canker sores, **1:**357
  for colic, **1:**511
  for colorectal cancer, **1:**518
  for common cold, **1:**530
  for cradle cap, **1:**557
  for Crohn's disease, **1:**569
  for croup, **1:**572
  in essiac tea, **2:**713, 714
  for gastritis, **2:**816
  for gastroenteritis, **2:**821
  for heartburn, **2:**927
  for influenza, **2:**1078
  for irritable bowel disease, **2:**1075
  for irritable bowel syndrome,
    2:1105
  for laryngitis, **3:**1183
  for mononucleosis, **3:**1370
  for peptic ulcers, **4:**2061
  for rashes, **3:**1701
  for sore throat, **4:**1897
  for stomachaches, **4:**1929
  for teething, **4:**1991
  for tonsillitis, **4:**2023
Slippery root. *See* Comfrey
SMA. *See* Sensory-motor amnesia
Small cell lung cancer, **3:**1238–1239
Small parasites, defined, **3:**1545
Small round-structured viruses, **2:**820
Smallpox, gardenia for, **2:**808
Smarana bhakti, **1:**214
Smell and Taste Research Foundation,
  1:492
Smell, essential oils and, **2:**711
Smoking, **4:1881–1887,** 1882*t,* *1883*
  atherosclerosis and, **1:**149
  bladder cancer and, **1:**252
  bronchitis and, **1:**303, 304, 305
  cancer and, **1:**346
  carotenoids and, **1:**364
  cervical dysplasia and, **1:**404
  cluster headaches and, **2:**907
  emphysema from, **2:**679, *680,* 682
  frostbite and, **2:**793, 793=1
  gum diseases and, **2:**885, 887

U

with dance therapy, **2:**590
for dysmenorrhea, **2:**654
for endometriosis, **2:**685
for hangovers, **2:**895
for headaches, **2:**909
for heartburn, **2:**927
for infertility, **2:**1071
for insomnia, **2:**1084
for Lyme disease, **3:**1254
for migraine, **3:**1356
as mind/body medicine, **3:**1364
for mononucleosis, **3:**1371
for prostate cancer, **3:**1658
for prostate enlargement, **3:**1654
for psoriasis, **3:**1661
for sleep disorders, **4:**1878
for uterine cancer, **4:**2074
for warts, **4:**2133
See also Guided imagery
Visuddha, **1:**408
Vital formula, for menopause, **3:**1332
Vitamin A, **4:2105–2107**
for abscess, **1:**2
for adolescents, **4:**1988
for AIDS, **1:**37
for allergies, **1:**56
animal *vs.* plant sources, **1:**206
as antioxidant, **1:**101, 362
for asthma, **1:**139
for atopic dermatitis, **2:**607
for boils, **1:**272
for bronchitis, **1:**305
for cancer, **1:**350
for cataracts, **1:**374
for cervical dysplasia, **1:**405
for chickenpox, **1:**429
for children, **1:**444
for cuts and scratches, **1:**581
for emphysema, **2:**682
enzyme therapy and, **2:**694
for fever, **2:**751
fish oil supplements and, **2:**761
for fungal infections, **2:**794
for gastritis, **2:**816
for genital warts, **2:**827
for gum diseases, **2:**886
for hay fever, **2:**903
for hearing loss, **2:**913
for heavy metal poisoning, **2:**931
for hyperopia, **2:**1020
for hypothyroidism, **2:**1042
for infections, **2:**1066
for jet lag, **2:**1121
for juvenile rheumatoid arthritis, **2:**1135
for leukemia, **3:**1207
for lung cancer, **3:**1241
for measles, **3:**1305
for meningitis, **3:**1328
for menstruation disorders, **3:**1339
for mononucleosis, **3:**1370
for myopia, **3:**1409
for night blindness, **3:**1456
for ovarian cysts, **3:**1521

for Parkinson's disease, **3:**1550
for peptic ulcers, **4:**2061
for radiation injuries, **3:**1695
for retinopathy, **3:**1735
for rhinitis, **3:**1744
for sore throat, **4:**1897
for sties, **4:**1926
for systemic lupus erythematosus, **4:**1974
toxicity of, **1:**102, 207, 444
for tuberculosis, **4:**2053
for UTIs, **1:**257
for whooping cough, **4:**2149
See also Beta carotene
Vitamin A deficiency, **4:2105–2106**
night blindness and, **3:**1455, 1456
vision disorders and, **1:**204
Vitamin B complex, **4:2109–2112**
ademetionine and, **1:**22
for aging, **1:**30
for asthma, **1:**139
for autism, **1:**172
in brewer's yeast, **1:**300
for canker sores, **1:**357
for cervical dysplasia, **1:**405
for cirrhosis, **1:**496
for cold sores, **1:**507
for coronary heart disease, **2:**917
for dandruff, **2:**593
for dementia, **2:**599
for depression, **2:**603
for dizziness, **2:**641
for dysmenorrhea, **2:**654
for endometriosis, **2:**685
for fungal infections, **2:**794
for hay fever, **2:**903
for hearing loss, **2:**913
for heart disease, **2:**922
for hot flashes, **2:**1006
for infertility, **2:**1070
for jaundice, **2:**1118
for juvenile rheumatoid arthritis, **2:**1135
for knee pain, **2:**1162
for lead poisoning, **3:**1193
for leukemia, **3:**1207
for lung cancer, **3:**1241
for Lyme disease, **3:**1254
for meningitis, **3:**1328
for menstruation disorders, **3:**1339
for mononucleosis, **3:**1370
for neuralgia, **3:**1448
for osteoarthritis, **3:**1504
for Parkinson's disease, **3:**1550
for peptic ulcers, **4:**2061
for radiation injuries, **3:**1695
for retinopathy, **3:**1735
for rosacea, **3:**1755
for shingles, **4:**1845
for systemic lupus erythematosus, **4:**1974
for tinnitus, **4:**2021
for tuberculosis, **4:**2053
for wheezing, **4:**2142

See also individual B vitamins
Vitamin B deficiency, **1:**446, 447, **4:**2110–2111
Vitamin B1. *See* Thiamine
Vitamin B2. *See* Riboflavin
Vitamin B3. *See* Niacin
Vitamin B5. *See* Pantothenic acid
Vitamin B6. *See* Pyridoxine
Vitamin B7. *See* Biotin
Vitamin B9. *See* Folic acid
Vitamin B10. *See* Folic acid
Vitamin B12, **4:2107–2109**
for aging, **1:**30
for Alzheimer's disease, **1:**68
for cervical dysplasia, **1:**405
for chronic fatigue syndrome, **1:**481
for cold sores, **1:**507
for dementia, **2:**599
for dizziness, **2:**641
for gastritis, **2:**816
for headaches, **2:**909
for hives, **2:**969
for ischemia, **2:**1109
for memory loss, **3:**1320
memory loss and, **3:**1318
for Ménière's disease, **3:**1324
for multiple sclerosis, **3:**1398
for muscle cramps, **3:**1404
for sleep disorders, **4:**1877
for smoking cessation, **4:**1882*t,* 1885
in spirulina, **4:**1911
for thrombophlebitis, **3:**1580
veganism and, **4:**2096
vegetarianism and, **3:**1180, **4:**2100
Vitamin B12 deficiency, **4:**2107–2108, 2110
Vitamin B12 deficiency anemia, **1:**80–81, 83
Vitamin C, **4:2112–2116,** 2114*t*
for abscess, **1:**2
for aging, **1:**30
for AIDS, **1:**37
for allergies, **1:**56
as antioxidant, **1:**101
for asthma, **1:**139, 140
for autism, **1:**172
bioflavonoids and, **1:**223, 225
for bipolar disorder, **1:**230
for blood clots, **1:**262
for boils, **1:**272
for bronchitis, **1:**305
for bruises, **1:**307
for cancer, **1:**350, 354
for cataracts, **1:**373, 374
for cerebral palsy, **1:**398
for cervical dysplasia, **1:**405
for chickenpox, **1:**429
for chills, **1:**447
chondroitin and, **1:**473
for cold sores, **1:**507
for common cold, **1:**531
for conjunctivitis, **1:**533
for constipation, **1:**537

Z